George H. Muller, D.V.M.
Clinical Professor of Dermatology Emeritus
Department of Dermatology
School of Medicine
Stanford University
Stanford, California

Robert W. Kirk, D.V.M.
Professor of Medicine Emeritus
Department of Clinical Sciences
New York State College of Veterinary Medicine
Cornell University
Ithaca, New York

Danny W. Scott, D.V.M.
Professor of Medicine
Department of Clinical Sciences
New York State College of Veterinary Medicine
Cornell University
Ithaca, New York

SMALL ANIMAL DERMATOLOGY

FOURTH EDITION

1989
W. B. SAUNDERS COMPANY
Harcourt Brace Jovanovich, Inc.
Philadelphia • London • Toronto • Montreal
• Sydney • Tokyo

W. B. SAUNDERS COMPANY
Harcourt Brace Jovanovich, Inc.

The Curtis Center
Independence Square West
Philadelphia, PA 19106

*Listed here are the latest translated editions of this book together
with the language of the translation and the publisher.*
French (*1st Edition*)—Vigot Frères Editors, Paris, France
Japanese (*1st Edition*)—Gakusosha Company Ltd., Japan
Italian (*2nd Edition*)—Marrapese Editore, Rome, Italy
Portuguese (*3rd Edition*)—Editora Manole Ltda, São Paulo, Brazil

Library of Congress Cataloging-in-Publication Data

Muller, George H.

Small animal dermatology.

Includes index.

1. Dogs—Diseases.   2. Cats—Diseases.   3. Veterinary
   dermatology.   4. Pets—Diseases.   I. Kirk, Robert
   Warren, 1922–   .   II. Scott, Danny W.   III. Title.

SF992.S55M85   1989   636.089′65   88–6466

ISBN 0–7216–2416–2

Editor: John Dyson
Developmental Editor: Linda Mills
Designer: Karen O'Keefe
Production Manager: Bob Butler
Manuscript Editor: Leslie Fenton
Illustration Coordinator: Peg Shaw
Cover Designer: Michelle Maloney
Indexer: Mark Coyle

Small Animal Dermatology   ISBN   0–7216–2416–2

Last digit is the print number: 9   8   7   6   5   4   3   2

Preface and Acknowledgments

This fourth edition of Small Animal Dermatology continues the tradition of the previous three. It is a practical, hands-on guide to a field exploding with new information. Practitioners can readily find answers to perplexing clinical problems; but students and others seeking deeper discussion will not be disappointed. The entire text has been thoroughly and extensively revised, and the selected references are current and provide an entrée to pertinent research. Dozens of new disorders are described. Additional color and black and white illustrations document these new diseases but also expand the coverage of many diseases described in previous editions. We have attempted to keep the nomenclature of diseases up to date, correct, and descriptive. For example, eosinophilic granuloma complex, feline endocrine alopecia, and miliary dermatitis have been replaced with more appropriate titles.

To conserve space for new information, the appendix on drugs has been deleted; and, interesting as it was, the chapter on comparative dermatology has made way for a discussion of new disorders. Chapters on neoplastic diseases, immunology, pathology, and therapy have been expanded.

As in previous editions, dozens of our colleagues in veterinary dermatology have contributed slides, case material, and pro and con suggestions regarding factual material in the text. Their illustrations are acknowledged with appreciation where they appear. We are deeply and especially grateful to dermatologists Carol Foil, Peter Ihrke, and William Miller, each of whom made major contributions to a critique of the old text and to suggestions for the new.

Sue Huber and Helen Kirk typed the manuscript, and John Dyson and Linda Mills of The W. B. Saunders Company did their usual superb job to facilitate production.

This will be the last edition with major input from George Muller and Bob Kirk. The book has been a labor of love that we have thoroughly enjoyed. We trust this and future editions will continue to enhance our colleagues' understanding of small animal dermatology.

G. H. MULLER
R. W. KIRK
D. W. SCOTT

Notice

Extraordinary efforts have been made by the authors and the publisher of this book to insure that dosage recommendations are precise and in agreement with standards officially accepted at the time of publication.

It does happen, however, that dosage schedules are changed from time to time in the light of accumulating clinical experience and continuing laboratory studies. This is most likely to occur in the case of recently introduced products.

It is urged, therefore, that you check the manufacturer's recommendations for dosage, especially if the drug to be administered or prescribed is one that you use only infrequently or have not used for some time.

In addition, some drugs mentioned have been used by the authors as experimental drugs. Others have been used after official clearance for use in one species but not in others. In these cases the authors have reported on their own considerable experience, but readers are urged to view the recommendations with discretion and precaution.

THE AUTHORS

Contents

CHAPTER **15**

Psychogenic Dermatoses ——————————————————— *749*

CHAPTER **16**

Environmental Diseases ——————————————————— *762*

CHAPTER **17**

Nutritional Skin Diseases ——————————————————— *796*

1

Structure and Function of the Skin

What a glorious organ it is! The skin is the largest organ of the body, and the anatomic and physiologic barrier between animal and environment. It provides protection from physical, chemical, and microbiologic injury, and its sensory components perceive heat, cold, pain, pruritus, touch, and pressure. In addition, the skin is synergistic with internal organ systems and thus reflects pathologic processes that are either primary elsewhere or are shared with other tissues. Not only is the skin an organ with its own reaction patterns, but it is also a mirror reflecting the *milieu interieur* and, at the same time, the capricious world to which it is exposed. The skin, hair, and subcutis of a newborn puppy represent 24 per cent of its body weight.[88] By the time of maturity, these structures compose only 12 per cent of body weight.

General Functions of the Skin

The general functions of the skin have been modified to apply to animal skin as follows:[42, 57–63, 90, 106, 123, 126a]

1. *Enclosing barrier.* The most important function of skin is to make possible an internal environment for all other organs by maintaining an effective barrier to the loss of water, electrolytes, and macromolecules.

2. *Environmental protection.* A corollary function is the exclusion of external injurious agents—chemical, physical, and microbiologic—from entrance into the internal environment.

3. *Motion and shape.* The flexibility, elasticity, and toughness of the skin allow motion and provide shape and form.

4. *Adnexa production.* Skin produces keratinized structures such as hair, nails, and the horny layer of the epidermis.

5. *Temperature regulation.* Skin plays a role in the regulation of body temperature through its support of the hair coat, regulation of cutaneous blood supply, and sweat gland function.

6. *Storage.* The skin is a reservoir of electrolytes, water, vitamins, fat, carbohydrates, proteins, and other materials.

7. *Indicator.* The skin may be an important indicator of general health, internal disease, and the effects of substances applied topically or taken internally.

8. *Immunoregulation.* Keratinocytes, Langerhans' cells, and lymphocytes together provide the skin with an immunosurveillance capability that effectively prejudices against the development of cutaneous neoplasms and persistent infections.

9. *Pigmentation.* Processes in the skin (melanin formation, vascularity, and keratinization) help determine the color of the coat and skin. Pigmentation of the skin helps prevent damage from solar radiation.

10. *Antimicrobial action.* The skin surface has antibacterial and antifungal properties.

11. *Sensory perception.* Skin is a primary sense organ for touch, pressure, pain, itch, heat, and cold.

12. *Secretion.* Skin is a secretory organ by virture of its apocrine, eccrine, and sebaceous glands.

13. *Excretion.* The skin functions in a limited way as an excretory organ.

14. *Blood pressure control.* Changes in the peripheral vascular bed affect blood pressure.

15. *Vitamin D production.* Vitamin D is produced in the skin through stimulation with solar radiation. In the epidermis, vitamin D_3 (cholecalciferol) is formed from provitamin D_3 (7-dehydrocholesterol), via previtamin D_3, on exposure to sunlight.[73] The vitamin D–binding protein in plasma translocates vitamin D_3 from the skin to the circlation. Vitamin D_3 is then hydroxylated in the liver to 25-hydroxyvitamin D_3 and again hydroxylated in the kidney to form 12, 25-dihydroxyvitamin D_3, which may be important in the regulation of epidermal proliferation and differentiation. The importance of the skin in vitamin D metabolism, and vice versa, is unknown in dogs and cats.

Ontogeny

Initially, the embryonic skin consists of a single layer of ectodermal cells and a dermis containing loosely arranged mesenchymal cells embedded in an interstitial ground substance. The ectodermal covering progressively develops into two layers (the basal cell layer, or *stratum germinativum*, and the outer *periderm*), three layers (the *stratum intermedium* forms between the other two layers), and then into an adult-like structure.[14, 77, 90, 123] Melanocytes (neural crest origin) and Langerhans' cells (bone marrow origin) become identifiable during this period of ectodermal maturation.

Dermal development is characterized by the increase in thickness and numbers of fibers, the decrease in ground substance, and the transition of mesenchymal cells into fibroblasts. Elastin fibers appear later than do collagen fibers. Histiocytes, Schwann cells, and dermal melanocytes also become recognizable. In humans, fetal skin contains a large percentage of Type III collagen, in contrast to the skin of the adult, which contains a large proportion of Type I collagen.[42, 77, 89] Fat cells (adipocytes, lipocytes) begin to develop into the subcutis from spindle-shaped mesenchymal precursor cells ("prelipoblasts") in the second half of gestation.

The embryonal stratum germinativum differentiates into hair germs (primary epithelial germs), which give rise to hair follicles, sebaceous glands, and apocrine sweat glands. Hair germs initially consist of an area of crowding of deeply basophilic cells in the basal layer of the epidermis. Subsequently, the areas of crowding become buds that protrude into the dermis. Beneath each bud lies a group of mesenchymal cells, from which the dermal hair papilla is later formed.

As the hair germ lengthens and develops into a hair follicle and hair, three bulges appear. The lowest (deepest) of the bulges develops into the attachment for the arrector pili muscle; the middle bulge differentiates into the sebaceous gland; and the uppermost bulge evolves into the apocrine sweat gland. These appendages develop on the ental side of primary hair follicles, while secondary hair follicles develop on the extal side. In general, the first hairs to appear on the fetus are vibrissae and tactile or sinus hairs that develop on the chin, eyebrows, and upper lip. The general body hair appears first on the head and gradually progresses caudally.

Eccrine gland germs also begin as areas of crowding of deeply basophilic cells in the basal layer of the epidermis. They initially differ from hair germs only slightly, by being narrower and by showing fewer mesenchymal cells at their base.

Gross Anatomy and Physiology

At each body orifice, the skin is continuous with the mucous membrane located there (digestive, respiratory, ocular, urogenital). The skin and hair coat vary in quantity and quality among species, breeds within a species, and individuals within a breed; they also vary from one area to another on the body, and according to age and sex.

In general, skin thickness decreases dorsally to ventrally on the trunk and proximally to distally on the limbs.[34, 82, 114, 124, 131] The skin is thickest on the forehead, dorsal neck, dorsal thorax, rump, and base of the tail. It is thinnest on the pinnae and on the axillary, inguinal, and perianal areas. The reported average thickness of the general body skin of cats is 0.4 to 2.0 mm[114] and for the dog, 0.5 to 5.0 mm.[34, 70] The hair coat is usually thickest over the dorsolateral aspects of the body and thinnest ventrally on the lateral surface of the pinnae and on the undersurface of the tail.

The skin surfaces of haired mammals are, in general, acidic. The pH of normal feline and canine skin has been reported to range from about 5.5 to 7.5.[32, 70, 107, 114]

HAIR

Hair, which is characteristic of mammals, is important in thermal insulation and sensory perception and as a barrier against chemical and physical injury to the skin.[83, 90, 106, 122] The ability of hair coat to regulate body temperature correlates closely with length, thickness, and medullation of individual hair fibers. In general, hair coats composed of long, fine, poorly medullated fibers, with coat depth increased by piloerection, are the most efficient for thermal insulation at low environmental temperatures. In addition, coat color is of some importance in thermal regulation, with light-colored coats being more efficient in hot, sunny weather.

Both primary (outercoat, guard) and secondary (undercoat) hairs are medullated in dogs and cats. Thus, the term "lanugo" (nonmedullated) is incorrect when applied to nonfetal dogs and cats. In cats, secondary hairs are far more numerous than primary hairs (10:1 dorsally, 24:1 ventrally).[114] The hairs of the cat have been divided into three types based on gross appearance: (1) guard hairs (thickest, straight, evenly tapered to a fine tip), (2) awn hairs (thinner, possessing subapical swelling below the hair tip), and (3) down hairs (thinnest, evenly crimped or undulating).[105]

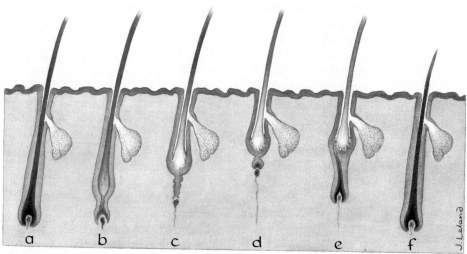

Figure 1:1. The hair cycle. *A*, Anagen: During this growing stage, hair is produced by mitosis in cells of the dermal papilla. *B*, Early catagen: In this transitional stage, a constriction occurs at the hair bulb. The hair above this will become a "club." *C*, Catagen: The distal follicle becomes thick and corrugated and pushes the hair outward. *D*, Telogen: This is the resting stage. The dermal papilla separates and an epithelial strand shortens to form a secondary germ. *E*, Early anagen: The secondary germ grows down to enclose the dermal papilla and a new hair bulb forms. The old "club" is lost. *F*, Anagen: The hair elongates as growth continues.

Hair Cycle

Hairs do not grow continuously, but rather in cycles (Fig. 1:1). Each cycle consists of a growing period *(anagen)* during which the follicle is actively producing hair, and a resting period *(telogen)* when the hair is retained in the follicle as a dead, or "club," hair that is subsequently lost. There is also a transitional period *(catagen)* between these two stages. It is often stated that certain breeds of dogs—poodles, Old English sheepdogs, schnauzers—have continuously growing hair coats.[27] Apparently, there is no scientific investigation that would substantiate such a statement.

The hair cycle, and thus the hair coat, is controlled by photoperiod, ambient temperature, nutrition, hormones, general state of health, genetics, and poorly understood "intrinsic factors."[2, 3, 14, 19, 45, 46, 83, 106, 109, 126a] Hair replacement in dogs and cats is mosaic in pattern (neighboring hair follicles being in different stages of the hair cycle at any one time), is unaffected by castration, and responds predominantly to photoperiod and, possibly, to ambient temperature. Dogs and cats in temperate latitudes such as the northern United States and Canada may shed noticeably in spring and fall. Hair follicle activity, and thus hair growth rate, is maximal in summer and minimal in winter. For example, up to 50 per cent of hair follicles may be in telogen in the summer and may increase to 90 per cent in winter. Catagen hairs always constitute a minor proportion of the total number of hairs, usually accounting for 4 to 7 per cent of the total.[3, 118] Many dogs and cats exposed to several hours of artificial light (e.g., animals housed indoors) will shed, sometimes profusely, throughout the year.[92, 114]

Hair grows until it attains its preordained length, which varies according to body region and is genetically determined, and then it enters the resting phase, which may last for a considerable time. Each region of the body has its own ultimate length of hair beyond which no further growth occurs. This phenomenon is responsible for the distinctive coat lengths of various breeds and is genetically determined. In mongrel dogs, it has been shown that hair growth rates vary at different sites, and the speed of growth was related to the ultimate length of the hair in each particular site.[45] For example, in the shoulder region, where ultimate hair length was about 30 mm, the average rate of hair growth was 6.7 mm/wk, whereas in the forehead region, which has ultimate hair length of about 16 mm, the growth rate was 2.8 mm/wk. Other investigators report daily hair growth rates in dogs of 0.04 to 0.18 mm (greyhound)[19, 23] and 0.34 to 0.40 mm (beagle).[2] In the cat, daily hair growth rate was reported to be 0.25 to 0.30 mm.[14]

Because hair is predominantly protein, nutrition has a profound effect on its quantity and quality (see Chap. 17). Poor nutrition may produce a dull, dry, brittle, or thin hair coat, with or without pigmentary disturbances.

Under conditions of ill health or generalized disease, anagen may be considerably shortened. Accordingly, a large percentage of body hairs may be in telogen at one time. Telogen hairs tend to be more easily lost, so the animal may shed excessively. Disease states may also lead to faulty formation of hair cuticle, resulting in a dull, lusterless hair coat. Severe illnesses or systemic stress may cause many hair follicles to enter synchronously and precipitously into telogen. Thus, shedding of these hairs (telogen defluxion, see p. 699) occurs simultaneously, often resulting in visible thinning of the coat or actual alopecia.

The hair cycle and hair coat are also affected by hormonal changes.[19, 42, 46, 83, 106] In general, anagen is initiated and advanced, and hair growth rate is accelerated, by thyroid hormones (see Hypothyroidism, Chap. 10). Conversely, excessive amounts of glucocorticoids or estrogens inhibit anagen and suppress hair growth rate (see pp. 622 and 584).

Hair growth is a confusing subject that needs much research. It should be remembered that the hair coat of pet animals is a cosmetic or ornamental feature. Every effort should be made to minimize procedures (clipping and shaving) that may affect the animal's appearance for many weeks. Although generalizations can be misleading, normal or short coats usually take about 3 to 4 months to regrow after shaving, while long coats may take as long as 18 months.[92] Occasionally, an unexplained and extremely frustrating failure to regrow hair in an area of skin (usually following clipping and surgical scrubbing) is seen.[118] The skin in affected areas appears grossly normal. Biopsy reveals telogenization of the hair follicles. This frustrating "follicular arrest" disappears spontaneously in 3 to 6 months after clipping.

Recently, attention has focused on the usefulness of *hair analysis* as a diagnostic tool.[123, 143] It is well recognized by most dermatologists and nutritionists in human medicine that mineral and trace element analysis of hair samples is *not* a clinically useful tool to assess nutritional status. The reasons for variability and unreliability include environmental effects (topical agents, geographic location, occupational exposures), differing hair growth rates (health, drugs, age, sex), and lack of standardization in analysis techniques. Until and unless adequate scientific documentation of the validity of such multi-element analysis is forthcoming, it is necessary for both health professionals and the public to be aware of the very limited value of hair analysis and of the potential to be confused and misled.

Scientifically oriented nutritionists do not use hair analyses as a primary method of detecting nutritional problems. Cautious consumers and health professionals should regard practitioners who rely solely on this test with suspicion.[143]

Small (0.16 to 0.42 mm diameter), hairless, knoblike structures are present in the haired skin of cats and dogs (Fig. 1:2).[34, 111, 114] These *tylotrich pads* serve as slow-adapting mechanoreceptors.

Hair Colors and Types

DOG

Although hair types in dogs are extremely diverse, various authors have attempted to classify them on the basis of color, length, type of bristle, and characteristics of the medulla and cortex.[34, 92] Hair types among dogs can be divided into normal (intermediate length), short, and long coats.

Normal Coat. The normal coat is typified by that seen in the German shepherd, the corgi, and wild dogs such as wolves and coyotes. It is composed of primary hairs (coarse guard hairs or bristles) and secondary hairs (fine hairs or undercoat). A high proportion of the hairs, by number but not by weight, are secondary hairs.

The next two classes of hair coats also are made up basically of primary and secondary hairs, but the relative sizes of hairs and their numbers vary markedly from the normal coat.

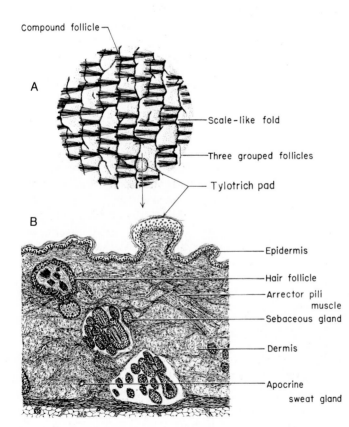

Compound follicle

A

Scale-like fold

Three grouped follicles

Tylotrich pad

B

Epidermis

Hair follicle

Arrector pili muscle

Sebaceous gland

Dermis

Apocrine sweat gland

Figure 1:2. Surface contour, hair arrangement, and histology of the hairy skin. *A,* View of scalelike folds and arrangement of hair follicles. *B,* Histologic section of hair skin. (Modified from Evans, H. E., and Christensen, G. C.: Miller's Anatomy of the Dog. 2nd ed. W. B. Saunders Company, Philadelphia, 1979.)

Short Coat. The short coat can be classified as coarse or fine. The coarse short hair is typified by the rottweiler and many of the terriers. This type of coat has a strong growth of primary hairs and a much lesser growth of secondary hairs. The total weight of hair is less, and the secondary hairs, especially, are less in weight and number than in the normal coat. The fine short coat is exemplified by boxers, dachshunds, and miniature pinschers. This type of coat has the largest number of hairs per unit area. The secondary hairs are numerous and well developed, and the primary hairs are reduced in size, as compared with the normal coat.

Long Coat. The long coat also can be arranged into two subdivisions: the fine long coat and the woolly or coarse long coat. The fine long coat is found in the cocker spaniel, the Pomeranian, and the chow chow. This coat has greater weight of hair per unit area than does the normal coat, except in the toy breeds, in which the weight may be less because the hair is finer. The woolly or coarse long coat is found in the poodle and also in the Bedlington terrier and the Kerry blue terrier. Secondary hairs make up 70 per cent of the total weight of these coats and 80 per cent of the number of hairs. Compared with other secondary-type hairs these are relatively coarse, and the three breeds mentioned have less tendency to shed hair than do many breeds.

The genetic aspects of coat color in dogs is a complex subject.[80, 92] Pigmentation in individual hairs may be uniform throughout the length of the shaft, or it may vary. In the agouti-type hair (German shepherd, Norwegian elkhound) the tip is white or light, the heavy body is pigmented brown or black, and the base is a light yellow or red-brown. Pigment cells in the bulb of the hair deposit pigment in or between the cortical and medullary hair cells. The amount of pigment deposited in the hair and its location there produce different optical effects. However, there are only two types of pigment. The black-brown pigment is designated as eumelanin; the yellow-red pigment is called pheomelanin. In addition, the melanocytes of the follicle may or may not produce pigment throughout the period of growth. In black hair, pigment production obviously remains active throughout the period.

CAT

The colors and types of hair coat in cats have been studied in some detail.[104, 105, 140] A self (solid) cat is a single color throughout. No patterning, shading, ticking, or other variation of color is observed, although it is common for kittens to have slightly tabby markings and scattered white hairs that disappear with maturity. Whatever their coloring, all cats are genetically tabbies, possessing either the Abyssinian, mackerel, or blotched tabby genes or a combination of two of these types. Solid white is dominant over all colors but may be associated with various abnormalities, such as the white cat with blue eyes that has cochlear degeneration and deafness.

The tabby is the basic type of cat, the "wild" type from which all others evolved. The tabby is actually a complex color arising from two component patterns governed by two separate sets of genes. The underlying pattern is agouti, which is characterized by hairs with a bluish base and black tip separated by yellow banding. The tabby genes determine whether the cat has narrow vertical gently curving stripes (mackerel), larger patches (blotch), or an Abyssinian pattern.

"Tipped" hair coats are characterized by hairs that have colored tips (blue, red, black, and so forth) overlying a paler color. Differences in the degree of tipping are great, with the greatest in the smokes and least in the chinchillas (silvers). "Pointed" hair coats are characterized by pale-colored hair on the body with darker hairs on the extremities or "points" (nose, ears, feet, tail). Points arise through a temperature-dependent mechanism and are seen in breeds such as Siamese, Himalayan, Balinese, and Birman. In these breeds, the dark hair color (acromelanism) is due to a temperature-dependent enzyme that converts melanin precursors into melanin by a process of oxidation.[114] With high temperatures the hair is light colored, with low temperatures it is darker; thus, kittens are light at birth, and cats kept indoors or in tropical climates are lighter than those kept outdoors or in cold climates. Inflammation and hyperemia result in light-colored new hair growth. Senility, with poor peripheral circulation, or shaving to remove hair results in dark-colored new hair growth.

Multicolored coats include the tortoiseshell and piebald spotting patterns. The archetypic tortoiseshell is a patchwork of black and orange, but there is a range of color variation among "torties," including chocolate (chestnut), cinnamon, blue, and lilac (lavender), these colors referring to the nonorange areas. The tortoiseshell pattern occurs in females or in males with two X chromosomes. White "spotting" in piebald cats varies in degree from white gloves on the feet, a nose smudge, or a white bib, to extensive white over most of the body.

The *Maltese dilution*, which dilutes black to blue, orange to cream, and seal point (Siamese) to blue, is inherited as an autosomal recessive trait.[101, 102] In normal black-haired cats, numerous small round melanin granules are scattered uniformly throughout the cortex and medulla of the hair and the skin. In the skin from Maltese dilution cats, a nonuniform distribution of very large, irregularly sized melanin granules results from the clumping of small granules.

In a typical short-haired cat, the longest primary hairs average about 4.5 cm in length, in contrast to the silky coat of a good show cat whose primary hairs may exceed 12.5 cm in length. The short-hair is the fundamental "wild" type and is dominant to the others. Various mutant hair coat types have occurred that have been perpetuated as a breed characteristic. The rex mutant is characterized by curly hairs and occurs in two major breeds: the Devon rex and the Cornish (German) rex. The Cornish rex lacks primary hairs, while the Devon rex has primary hairs that resemble secondary hairs. Cornish rex whiskers are often short and curly, while Devon rex whiskers are often absent or stubbled. In some Devon rexes, the coat is completely absent on the chest, belly, and shoulders, a fault many breeders try to eliminate. Cornish and Devon rexes may partially or completely molt, especially during estrus or pregnancy, resulting in a symmetric alopecia, which may be mistaken for an endocrine dermatosis.[35] These breeds are also recommended occasionally as "hypoallergenic" cats to humans with animal dander hypersensitivities, but there appears to be no scientific documentation for this claim.

The wire-hair mutation, seen in the American wirehair, is characterized by a coat that looks and feels wiry, being coarse, crimped, and springy. All hairs are curled in an irregular fashion, the awn hairs resembling a shepherd's crook.

Microscopic Anatomy and Physiology

EPIDERMIS

The outer layer of the skin, or epidermis, is composed of multiple layers of cells ranging from columnar to flat in shape (Fig. 1:3). These are of four distinct

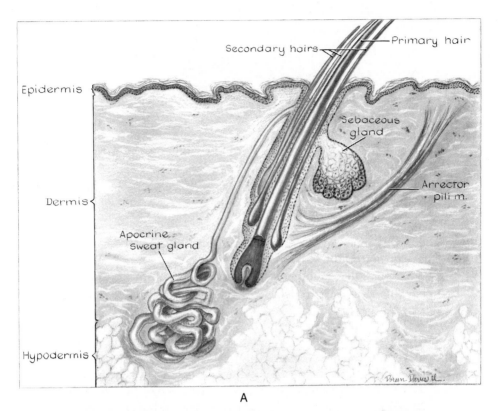

A

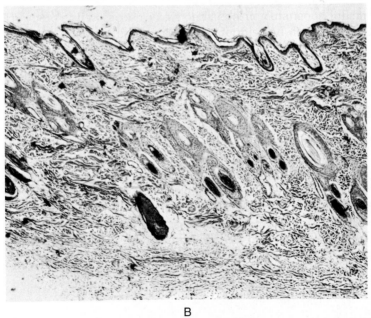

B

Figure 1:3. *A*, Normal canine skin (diagrammatic). *B*, Normal canine skin (low power).

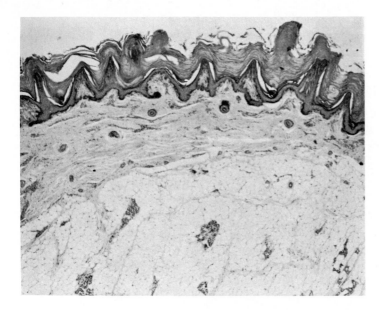

Figure 1:4. Histologic section of canine footpad (low power).

types: keratinocytes (about 85 per cent of the epidermal cells), melanocytes (about 5 per cent), Langerhans' cells (3 to 8 per cent), and Merkel cells (associated with tylotrich pads). For purposes of identification, certain areas of the epidermis are classified as layers and are named, from inner to outer, as follows: basal layer (stratum basale), spinous layer (stratum spinosum), granular layer (stratum granulosum), clear layer (stratum lucidum), and horny layer (stratum corneum). In general, the epidermis of cats and dogs is quite thin (one to three cell layers, not counting the horny layer) in haired skin, ranging from 0.1 to 0.5 mm.[34, 81, 114, 124, 131] The thickest epidermis is found in the footpads (Fig. 1:4) and planum nasale (Fig. 1:5), where it may measure 1.5 mm. The surface of the footpad epidermis is smooth in cats, but quite papillated and irregular in dogs. Rete ridges (projections of the epidermis into the underlying dermis) are not found in normal-haired skin of cats and dogs. However, rete ridges may be found in normal footpad and planum nasale epidermis and in the lightly haired scrotum (Fig. 1:6).

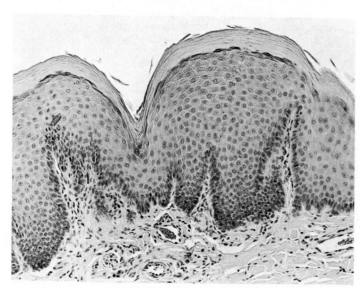

Figure 1:5. Histologic section of the planum nasale.

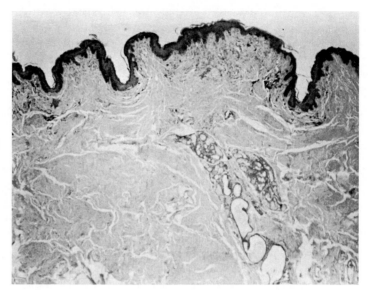

Figure 1:6. Histologic section of scrotal skin showing rete ridges.

Basal Layer

The stratum basale is a single row of columnar to cuboidal cells resting on the basement membrane zone that separates the epidermis from the dermis (Fig. 1:7). Most of these cells are keratinocytes, which are constantly reproducing and pushing upward to replenish the epidermal cells above. The daughter cells move into the outer layers of the epidermis and are ultimately shed as dead horny cells. Mitotic figures and apoptotic (dyskeratotic, necrotic) keratinocytes are occasionally seen, especially in areas of skin with thicker epidermis (e.g., planum nasale, footpad, mucocutaneous junction). Evidence has been pre-

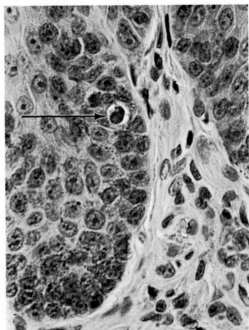

Figure 1:7. Melanocyte or "clear cell" in the basal layer of the planum nasale (high power, H & E stain).

sented that suggests that there is morphologic and functional heterogenicity in basal keratinocytes,[76] some populations serving primarily an anchorage function and others serving a proliferative and reparative function.

MELANOCYTES AND MELANOGENESIS

Melanocytes, the second type of cell found in the basal layer of the epidermis, are also found in the outer root sheath and the hair matrix of hair follicles and in the ducts of sebaceous and sweat glands.[92, 114] Traditionally, melanocytes are divided structurally and functionally into two compartments: epidermal and follicular.[44] Since melanocytes do not stain readily with hematoxylin and eosin (H & E) and because they undergo artifactual cytoplasmic shrinkage during tissue processing, they appear as "clear cells" (Fig. 1:7). In general, there is one melanocyte per every 10 or 20 keratinocytes in the basal cell layer. They are derived from the neural crest and migrate into the epidermis in early fetal life. Although melanocytes are of nondescript appearance, with special stains (dopa reaction, Fontana's ammoniacal silver nitrate) they can be shown to have long cytoplasmic extensions (dendrites) that weave among the keratinocytes. There is an intimate relationship between melanocytes and keratinocytes in which both cells interact and exist as epidermal symbionts—a functional and structural unit called the "epidermal melanin unit."[42, 126a] Ultrastructurally, melanocytes are characterized by typical intracytoplasmic melanosomes and premelanosomes and a cell membrane–associated basal layer lamina. Most of the melanin pigment in skin is located in the basal layer of the epidermis, but in dark-skinned animals melanin may be found throughout the entire epidermis as well as within superficial dermal melanocytes.

Melanin pigments are chiefly responsible for the coloration of skin and hair. Melanins embrace a wide range of pigments, including the brown-black eumelanins, yellow or red-brown pheomelanins, and other pigments whose physiochemical natures are intermediate between the two. Despite the different properties of the various melanins, they all arise from a common metabolic pathway in which dopaquinone is the key intermediate.[37, 42, 44] Tyrosine is converted to dopa, which is then oxidized to dopaquinone. Both reactions are catalyzed by the same copper-containing enzyme, tyrosinase.

Classically, melanin production has been thought to be under the control of genetics and melanocyte-stimulating hormone (MSH) from the pituitary gland.[37, 42, 44, 69, 126a] However, data are accumulating to indicate that β–MSH is not a physiologic hormone, has no role in regulation of pigmentation, and is probably an artifact produced during isolation of β-lipotropin (β-lipotropin is derived from the primordial peptide, pro-opiomelanocortin, produced in the pars intermedia of the pituitary gland).[20, 42, 103] Alpha–MSH is also a fragment of β-lipotropin, and is two to four times *less* potent a pigmenting agent than β-lipotropin. Beta-lipotropin may be the physiologic hormone. Recent interest has focused on the theory that melanogenesis and melanocyte proliferation are, in fact, regulated locally by the keratinocyte and Langerhans' cell more than by distant factors in the pituitary gland. Arachidonic acid and its metabolites (leukotrienes, prostaglandins) are known to affect melanogenesis and melanocyte proliferation. In addition, ultraviolet light and inflammation increase the production of melanin locally in affected skin.[42, 44] Hormones (especially androgens, estrogens, glucocorticoids, and thyroid hormones) are also able to modulate melanogenesis through mechanisms that are poorly understood at present.[42, 44]

Melanogenesis takes place in membrane-bound organelles called melanosomes,[37, 42, 77, 126a] designated Types I through IV according to maturation. Melanosomes originate from the Golgi apparatus, where the tyrosinase enzyme is formed. Type I melanosomes contain no melanin and are electronlucent. As melanin is progressively laid down on protein matrices, melanosomes become increasingly electron-dense. At the same time, they migrate to the periphery of the dendrites, where transfer of melanin to adjacent epidermal cells takes place. Transfer involves the endocytosis of the dendrite tips and of the incorporated Type IV melanosomes, by the adjacent keratinocytes. Melanocytes eject melanosomes into keratinocytes by a unique biologic transfer process called cytocrinia.[42] Dermal melanocytes are often referred to as "continent" melanocytes, because they do not transfer melanosomes as do the epidermal, or "secretory," melanocytes. Skin color is determined mainly by the number, size, type, and distribution of melanosomes. Melanins not only are responsible for coloration but also play important roles in photoprotection and free-radical scavenging.[37, 42, 44]

MERKEL'S CELLS

Merkel's cells are epidermal clear cells confined to the basal cell layer, or just below, and occur only in tylotrich pads.[77, 111, 112, 114, 115] These specialized cells (slow-adapting mechanoreceptors) contain a large cytoplasmic vacuole that displaces the cell nucleus dorsally. They possess desmosomes and characteristic dense-core cytoplasmic granules and paranuclear whorls on electron microscopic examination. Merkel's cells also contain cytokeratin, neurofilament, and neuron-specific enolase, suggesting a dual epithelial and neural differentiation (see Chap. 20).

Spinous Layer

The stratum spinosum ("prickle cell layer") is composed of the daughter cells of the stratum basale.[112, 114, 124, 131] In haired skin, this layer is one to two cells thick. The stratum spinosum becomes much thicker at the footpads, planum nasale, and mucocutaneous junctions, where it may occasionally approach 20 cell layers. The cells are lightly basophilic to eosinophilic, nucleated, and polyhedral to flattened cuboidal in shape. The keratinocytes of the stratum spinosum appear to be connected by intercellular bridges ("prickles"), which are more prominent in nonhaired skin (Fig. 1:8). Ultrastructurally, keratinocytes are characterized by tonofilaments and desmosomes.[42, 47] Immunohistochemically, they are characterized by the presence of cytokeratins.[42] The keratinocytes of the stratum spinosum synthesize *keratinosomes* (lamellar granules, membrane-coating granules, Odland bodies), which are important in the barrier function of the epidermis (see Epidermopoiesis and Keratogenesis in this chapter).[42, 77]

Because of the research efforts directed at defining the pathomechanism of pemphigus, much has been learned concerning the structure and chemical composition of epidermal desmosomes (see Chap. 9).[42] Desmosomes are presently known to consist of keratinocyte tonofilaments and their attachment plaques, the keratinocyte plasma membrane, and the desmosomal core (desmoglea), which is interposed between two adjacent keratinocyte plasma membranes. Numerous desmosomal plaque proteins (tentatively grouped as desmoplakins) and desmosomal core glycoproteins (tentatively grouped as

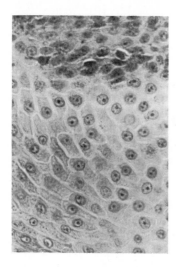

Figure 1:8. Prickle cells from footpad showing intercellular bridges (high power).

desmogleins) have been characterized. Initial studies have suggested that the immunohistochemical staining pattern seen with human pemphigus foliaceus antibody is identical to that seen with an antibody directed at desmoglein I (desmosomal core glycoprotein).

LANGERHANS' CELLS

Langerhans' cells are mononuclear dendritic cells located suprabasally.[42, 77] They are epidermal "clear cells" that do not stain for melanin with dopa. Langerhans' cells in many species have characteristic intracytoplasmic organelles (Birbeck's or Langerhans' granules), which are observed by means of electron microscopy.[42, 77] However, the Langerhans'-like cell studied in dogs does *not* contain these granules.[43, 118, 142] Langerhans' cells are aureophilic (i.e., they stain with gold chloride), and they contain membrane-associated adenosine triphosphatase as well as vimentin and S-100 protein (immunohistochemical markers). They also have Fc-IgG and C3 receptors, and synthesize and express immune response gene-associated antigens. These cells are of bone marrow origin, of monocyte-histiocyte lineage, and serve antigen-processing and alloantigen-stimulating functions. Studies in humans have shown that the number of Langerhans' cells per unit of skin varies from one area of skin to another in the same individual, emphasizing the need to use adjacent normal skin as a control when counting Langerhans' cells in skin lesions.[51]

The Skin as an Immunologic Organ

Advances in the past decade have demonstrated that normal mammalian epidermis functions as the most peripheral outpost of the immune system. Langerhans' cells, keratinocytes, epidermotropic T lymphocytes, and draining peripheral lymph nodes are thought to form collectively an integrated system of "skin-associated lymphoid tissues" ("SALT") that mediates cutaneous immunosurveillance.[17, 18, 21, 66, 126a] *Langerhans' cells* (see previous discussion) stimulate the proliferation of relevant helper T lymphocytes by the presentation of antigen; they also induce cytotoxic T lymphocytes directed to allogeneic and modified self-determinants, produce interleukin 1 and other cytokines, contain numerous enzymes and are phagocytic.[17, 18, 21, 66]

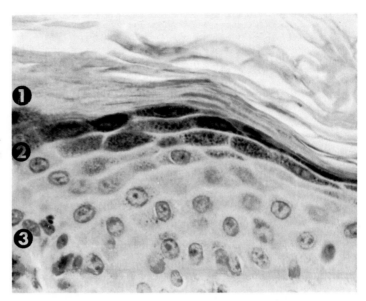

Figure 1:9. *1*, Horny layer; *2*, granular layer; and 3, prickle cell layer from the planum nasale (high power).

The *keratinocyte* also plays an active role in epidermal immunity.[21, 66] Keratinocytes (1) produce "epidermal cell–derived thymocyte-activating factor (ETAF)" that is probably identical to interleukin 1, (2) produce various cytokines (interleukin 3, prostaglandins, leukotrienes, interferon, etc.), (3) are phagocytic, and (4) can express immune response gene-associated antigen in a variety of lymphocyte-mediated skin diseases (presumably as a result of gamma interferon secretion by activated lymphocytes).[17, 18, 21, 66]

Ultraviolet light and topical or systemic glucocorticoids are known to depress Langerhans' cell numbers and function as well as other cutaneous and systemic immune responses.[17, 18, 66, 71] The areas of photoimmunology and photocarcinogenesis are receiving much attention, especially as concerns the pathogenesis of skin cancer.

Granular Layer

The stratum granulosum is variably present in haired skin, ranging from one to two cells thick in areas where it occurs.[112, 114, 124, 131] In nonhaired skin or at the infundibulum of hair follicles, the stratum granulosum may be four to eight cells thick (Fig. 1:9). Cells in this layer are flattened, basophilic, and contain shrunken nuclei and large, deeply basophilic keratohyaline granules in their cytoplasm. Keratohyaline granules are the morphologic equivalents of the structural protein profilaggrin, which is the precursor of filaggrin (see Horny Layer).[39] Profilaggrin is synthesized in the stratum granulosum. The function of keratohyaline granules is incompletely understood but is thought to be concerned with keratinization and barrier function.[42]

Clear Layer

The stratum lucidum is a fully keratinized, compact thin layer of dead cells.[112, 114, 124, 134] This layer is anuclear, homogeneous, and hyaline-like and contains refractile droplets (eleidin). The stratum lucidum is best developed in the footpads, less so in the planum nasale, and is absent from all other areas of skin.

Horny Layer

The stratum corneum is the outer layer of completely keratinized tissue that is contantly being shed.[112, 114, 124, 131] This layer, consisting of flattened, nuclear, eosinophilic cells, is thicker in lightly haired or glabrous skin (Fig. 1:9). Its gradual desquamation normally is balanced by proliferation of the basal cells, which maintains a constant epidermal thickness.

In routinely processed sections, the stratum corneum varies from 3 to 35 μm in thickness in cats and from 5 to 1500 μm in dogs. However, clipping and histologic preparation involving fixation, dehydration, and paraffin embedding result in the loss of about one-half of the stratum corneum.[18] The stratum corneum of canine truncal skin, when measured in cryostat sections, was found to have a mean thickness of 47 cell layers that measured 13.3 μm.[81] The loose, "basket weave" appearance of the stratum corneum is an artifact of fixation and processing.[14, 77, 81]

The keratin proteins (cytokeratins) belong to acidic and basic keratin families.[78, 126a] In any given epidermal cell layer, an acidic keratin is paired with a basic keratin of similar molecular weight. The keratin pairs are characteristic for the state of differentiation of the particular layer of keratinocytes.[42, 78] In the stratum corneum, keratins become highly cross-linked through disulfide bonding. The structural protein *filaggrin* appears to be important in the alignment of cytokeratin filaments.[39] In addition, a cornified cell envelope, consisting of the plasma membrane and a thickened submembranous layer that includes the protein involucrin, bounds the cells of the stratum corneum. *Involucrin* is a structural protein synthesized in the stratum spinosum, cross-linked in the stratum granulosum by a calcium-requiring epidermal transglutaminase enzyme.[121, 126] The cornified cell envelope provides structural support to the cell and resists invasion by microorganisms and deleterious environmental agents, but does not appear to have a significant role in regulating permeability.

Topographic studies have shown that the epidermal surface varies from gently undulating on the densely haired skin of the back to heavily folded on the skin of the abdomen (Fig. 1:10).[81, 112] The hairs arise from the follicle infundibula, which are seen as "pits" in the skin (Figs. 1:11 and 1:12). At their bases the hairs tend to be joined by amorphous material that can also be seen

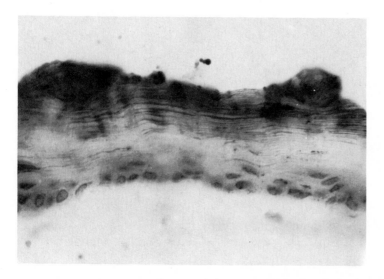

Figure 1:10. Frozen section of skin treated with an alkaline buffer to swell the cornified cells. Sudanophilic material (dark layers) is present in intercellular spaces of the distal stratum corneum (× 900). (From Lloyd, D. H., and Garthwaite, G.: Epidermal structure and surface topography of canine skin. Res. Vet. Sci. *33*:99, 1982.)

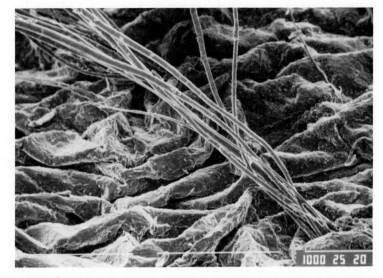

Figure 1:11. Scanning electron micrograph of freeze-dried skin from the posterior abdomen. The skin is heavily folded. White bar marker indicates 1000 μm. (From Lloyd, D. H., and Garthwaite, G.: Epidermal structure and surface topography of canine skin. Res. Vet. Sci. *33*:99, 1982.)

around the squamae adhering to hairs. The surface of the stratum corneum is uneven, especially in the hairy areas (Fig. 1:11). It is covered with a homogeneous film that tends to conceal the structure of the squames and their intercellular junctions. Globular masses that are partially concealed by this film can be seen (Fig. 1:13). Upon closer examination, the surface can be seen to be composed of hexagonal cells and an amorphous substance that appears to be oozing to the surface at the margins of the cells (Fig. 1:14). The bases of the hair follicle infundibula are sealed by an amorphous substance (sebaceous and cutaneous lipids) and squamae. There is no evidence that sebum flows from the hair pore to the interfollicular region, which suggests that rubbing and grooming are important in spreading this emulsion over the skin.

Skin surface lipids of the cat and dog were studied by thin layer chromatography and found to contain *more* sterol esters, free cholesterol, cholesterol esters, and diester waxes, but fewer triglycerides, monoglycerides, free fatty acids, monoester waxes, and squalene than those of humans.[79, 93, 95, 120, 134, 135] It was suggested that the surface lipids of cats and dogs are mainly of epidermal origin, while those of humans are mainly of sebaceous gland origin.

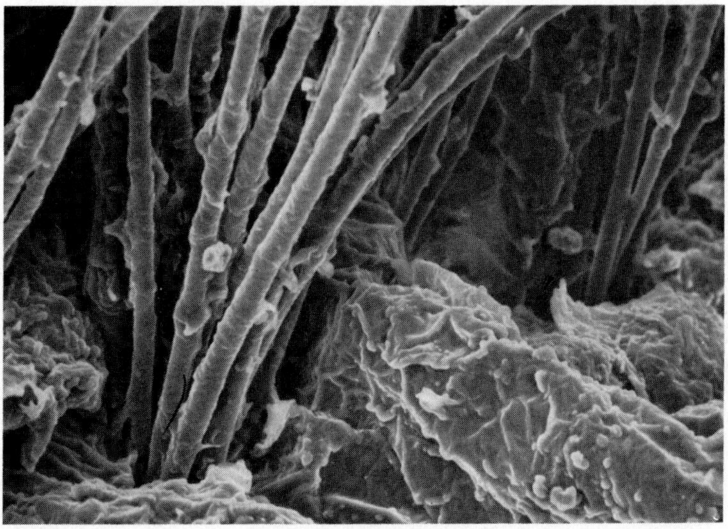

Figure 1:12. Scanning electron micrograph of freeze-dried skin from the anterior abdomen. (From Lloyd, D. H., and Garthwaite, G.: Epidermal structure and surface topography of canine skin. Res. Vet. Sci. *33*:99, 1982.)

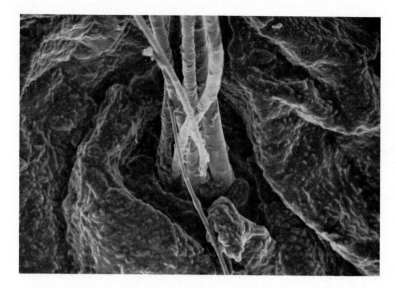

Figure 1:13. High-power view of hair follicle shown in Figure 1:11. ($\times$ 170). Note globular masses on surface. (From Lloyd, D. H., and Garthwaite, G.: Epidermal structure and surface topography of canine skin. Res. Vet. Sci. *33*:99, 1982.)

EPIDERMOPOIESIS AND KERATOGENESIS

The most important product of the epidermis is the highly stable, disulfide bond–containing fibrous protein, keratin. This substance is the major barrier between animal and environment, the "Miracle Wrap" of the body. Prekeratin, the fibrous protein synthesized in the keratinocytes of the stratum basale and stratum spinosum, appears to be the precursor of the fully differentiated stratum corneum proteins.[42, 126a]

The epidermis is ectodermal in origin and normally undergoes an orderly pattern of proliferation, differentiation, and keratinization.[48, 98, 129] The factors controlling epidermal proliferation, differentiation, and keratinization are incompletely understood. Among the intrinsic factors known to play a modulating role in these processes are the dermis,[42] epidermal growth factor,[42, 67] epidermal chalone,[42, 84] epibolin,[48] calmodulin,[42, 128] interferons,[141] acid hydrolases,[40] cyclic AMP,[42, 113] arachidonic acid metabolites,[42, 129] and various hormones (particularly epinephrine and cortisol).[42, 106] In addition, there appears to be a host of hormones and enzymes that can either or both induce and increase the activity

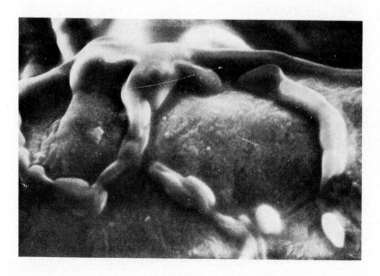

Figure 1:14. Surface of the stratum corneum in the interfollicular region. Amorphous material appears to be oozing onto the surface at the margins of the squames ($\times$ 2300). (From Lloyd, D. H., and Garthwaite, G.: Epidermal structure and surface topography of canine skin. Res. Vet. Sci. *33*:99, 1982.)

of the enzyme ornithine decarboxylase.[42] This enzyme is essential for the biosynthesis of polyamines (putrescine, spermidine, and spermine), which encourage epidermal proliferation. Numerous nutritional factors are also known to be important for normal keratinization, including protein, fatty acids, zinc, copper, vitamin A, and B vitamins (see Chap. 17).[42]

Modern research in epidermal cellular and molecular biology recognizes four distinct cellular events in the process of cornification: (1) keratinization (synthesis of the principal fibrous proteins of the keratinocyte), (2) keratohyaline synthesis (including the histidine-rich protein, filaggrin), (3) formation of the highly cross-linked, insoluble stratum corneum peripheral envelope (including the structural protein involucrin), and (4) generation of neutral lipid-enriched intercellular domains, resulting from the secretion of distinctive keratinosomes. The keratinosomes are synthesized primarily within the keratinocytes of the stratum spinosum and are then displaced to the apex and periphery of the cell as it reaches the stratum granulosum. They fuse with the plasma membrane and secrete their contents (neutral sugars linked to either or both lipids and proteins; hydrolytic enzymes; sterols). Intercellular lipids then undergo substantial alterations and assume an integral role in the regulation of stratum corneum barrier function and desquamation.

Tritiated thymidine labeling techniques have shown that the turnover (cell renewal) time for the viable epidermis (stratum basale to stratum granulosum) of dogs is approximately 22 days.[10] Clipping the hair shortened the epidermal turnover time to approximately 15 days.[11] Surgically induced wounds in the skin of normal dogs greatly increased epidermal mitotic activity.[139] Epidermal turnover time in seborrheic Cocker Spaniels and Irish Setters approximated 7 days.[12]

Recently, the growth characteristics and morphology of canine keratinocytes grown in vitro have been reported.[137] The use of cultured canine keratinocytes should provide a useful model for in vitro studies of epidermal kinetics, the pathogenesis of various dermatologic diseases, and the cutaneous effects of various pharmacologic agents.

CUTANEOUS ECOLOGY

The skin forms a protective barrier without which life would be impossible. This defense has three components: physical, chemical, and microbial.[42, 96,97] Hair forms the first physical line of defense to prevent contact of pathogens with the skin and to minimize external physical or chemical insult to the skin. Hair may also harbor microorganisms.

The stratum corneum forms the basic physical defense barrier. Its thick, tightly packed keratinized cells are permeated by an emulsion of sebum and sweat. This emulsion, concentrated in the outer layers of keratin, also functions as a physical barrier. In addition to its physical properties, the emulsion provides a chemical barrier to potential pathogens. Water-soluble substances in the emulsion include inorganic salts and proteins that inhibit microorganisms. Sodium chloride and the antiviral glycoprotein interferon, albumin, transferrin, complement, glucocorticoid, and immunoglobulins are in the emulsion.[48, 81, 96, 97] In the normal skin of dogs, (1) IgG and IgM are found in the interstitial spaces in the dermis, in dermal blood vessels, and in hair papillae; (2) IgM is found at the basement membrane zone of the epidermis, hair follicles, and sebaceous glands; (3) IgA is found in the apocrine sweat glands (suggesting that it functions as a cutaneous secretory immunoglobulin); and (4) C3 is found in the stratum corneum and in the dermal interstitial spaces.[81]

The single factor with the greatest influence on the flora is the degree of hydration of the stratum corneum.[42, 96, 97] Increasing the quantity of water at the skin surface (increased ambient temperature, increased relative humidity, or occlusion) enormously increases the number of microorganisms. In general, the moist or greasy areas of the skin support the greatest populations of microorganisms.

The normal skin microflora also contributes to skin defense. Bacterial and, occasionally, yeasts and filamentous fungi are located in the superficial epidermis (especially in the intercellular spaces) and the infundibulum of hair follicles. The normal flora is a mixture of bacteria that live in symbiosis. The flora may change with different cutaneous environments, which include such factors as pH, salinity, moisture, albumin level, and fatty acid level. The close relationship between the host and the microorganisms enables bacteria to occupy microbial niches and inhibit colonization by invading organisms.

Some organisms are believed to live and multiply on the skin, forming a permanent population; these are known as residents, and they may be reduced in number but not eliminated by degerming methods.[96, 97] The resident skin flora is not spread out evenly over the surface but is aggregated in microcolonies of various sizes. Other microorganisms are merely contaminants acquired from the environment, can be removed by simple hygienic measures, and are called transients.[96, 97]

Most studies on the normal microbial flora of the skin of cats and dogs have been strictly qualitative. The skin is an exceedingly effective environmental sampler, providing a temporary haven and way station for all sorts of organisms. Thus, only repeated quantitative studies allow the researcher to make a reliable distinction between resident and transient bacteria.

In cats, most studies indicate that *Micrococcus* sp., coagulase-negative staphylococci, α-hemolytic streptococci, and *Acinetobacter* sp. are normal residents of the skin (see Chap. 5).[75, 92, 114] Recent studies have shown that coagulase-negative and coagulase-positive staphylococci are frequently isolated from the skin of normal cats.[26, 31] Of the coagulase-negative staphylococci, *S. simulans* was isolated most frequently and is probably a normal resident. *S. capitis, S. epidermidis, S. haemolyticus, S. hominis, S. sciuri,* and *S. warneri* were isolated primarily from household cats as opposed to cattery cats, suggesting that cats acquire these species of staphylococci through human contact. Of the coagulase-positive staphylococci, *S. aureus* and *S. intermedius* were isolated more commonly from household cats, as opposed to cattery cats. Cats may frequently be asymptomatic carriers of the dermatophyte, *Microsporum canis*, as well (see Chap. 7).[114]

In dogs, most studies indicate that *Micrococcus* sp., coagulase-negative staphylococci, α-hemolytic streptococci, and *Acinetobacter* sp. are normal residents of the skin (see Chap. 5).[92] Recent studies have shown that coagulase-negative and coagulase-positive staphylococci (especially *S. epidermidis* and *S. intermedius*) are regularly isolated from the skin and hair coat of normal dogs and that there are no significant quantitative or qualitative differences in the staphylococci of skin and hair or between species of staphylococci and body site.[74, 136] In addition, it is well known that many saprophytic fungi—including

Malassezia pachydermatis, Alternaria spp., *Aspergillus* spp., and *Penicillium* spp.—can be cultured from the skin and hair of normal dogs and cats (see Chap. 7).[92, 114–116]

Epidermal Histochemistry

Histochemical studies of normal cat and dog epidermis have demonstrated distinct oxidative enzyme activity in all layers except the stratum corneum.[50, 64, 86, 87] In addition, strong reactions for nonspecific esterases were demonstrated, especially in the stratum granulosum. Oxidative enzymes demonstrated included cytochrome oxidase, succinate dehydrogenase, malate dehydrogenase, isocitrate dehydrogenase, lactate dehydrogenase, glucose-6-phosphate dehydrogenase, nicotinamide-adenine dinucleotide phosphate (NADPH), NADH, and and monoamine oxidase. Hydrolytic enzymes demonstrated included acid phosphatase, arylsulfatase, β-glucuronidase, and leucine aminopeptidase. Positive reactions for cholinesterases were not observed. Thus, the enzyme pattern of normal cat and dog epidermis shows only limited similarities to that of humans, especially as concerns esterase distribution.

BASEMENT MEMBRANE ZONE

The basement membrane zone is the physicochemical interface between the epidermis and the dermis.[1, 42, 65, 126a] This zone is important in (1) anchoring the epidermis to the dermis, (2) maintaining a functional and proliferative epidermis, (3) maintaining tissue architecture, (4) wound healing, and (5) functioning as a barrier. The basement membrane zone is often poorly differentiated in H & E preparations, but stains nicely with PAS.[112, 114, 124, 131] It is most prominent in nonhaired areas of the skin and at mucocutaneous junctions. As observed by light microscopy, the basement membrane zone comprises only the fibrous zone of the sublamina densa area and is about 20 times thicker than the actual basal lamina.

Ultrastructurally, the basement membrane zone can be divided into the following four components, proceeding from epidermis to dermis (Fig. 1:15):

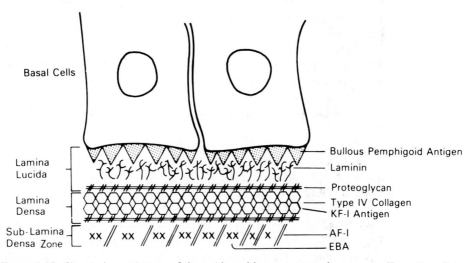

Basal Cells

Lamina Lucida — Bullous Pemphigoid Antigen / Laminin

Lamina Densa — Proteoglycan / Type IV Collagen / KF-I Antigen

Sub-Lamina Densa Zone — AF-I / EBA

Figure 1:15. Chemical constituents of the epidermal basement membrane zone. (From Katz, S. I.: The epidermal basement membrane zone—structure, ontogeny, and role in disease. J. Am. Acad. Dermatol. *11*:1025–1037, 1984.)

Table 1:1. CHARACTERISTICS OF BASEMENT MEMBRANE ZONE COMPONENTS

Component	Localization	Function
Type IV collagen	Lamina densa (± lamina lucida)	Adherence, networking
Type V collagen	Lamina lucida	?
Type VII collagen	Anchoring fibrils	Anchorage
Laminin	Lamina lucida (± lamina densa)	Adherence
Nidogen	Lamina lucida (± lamina densa)	Adherence
Enactin	Lamina lucida (± lamina densa)	Adherence
Heparan sulfate	Lamina densa	Electrical charge barrier, networking
Bullous pemphigoid antigen	Basal cell hemidesmosone and lamina lucida	Adherence
Cicatricial pemphigoid antigen	Lamina lucida	—
Epidermolysis bullosa acquisita antigen	Sublamina densa area (± lamina densa)	Adherence
Fibronectin	Sublamina densa area (± lamina lucida)	Networking
KF-1 antigen	Lamina densa	Adherence
AF-1 and AF-2 antigen	Anchoring fibrils	Adherence

(1) the basal cell plasma membrane, (2) the lamina lucida (lamina rara), (3) the lamina densa (basal lamina), and (4) the sublamina densa area (lamina fibro-reticularis), which includes the anchoring fibrils and the dermal microfibril bundles. The first three components appear to be primarily of epidermal origin. The precise biochemical and functional aspects of the basement membrane zone and its various components are still being unraveled. Presently recognized basement membrane zone components, their localization, and their presumed functions are listed in Table 1:1. The involvement of the basement membrane zone in many important dermatologic disorders has prompted most of the current research interest (Fig. 1:16). The KF-1, AF-1, and AF-2 antigens have been shown to be absent in hereditary dystrophic forms of epidermolysis bullosa in humans.

DERMIS

The dermis (corium) is an integral part of the body's connective tissue system and is of mesodermal origin.[42, 112, 114, 124, 126a, 131] In areas of thick-haired skin, the dermis accounts for most of the depth, whereas the epidermis is thin. In very thin skin, the decreased thickness results from the thinness of the dermis. The dermis is composed of fibers, ground substance, and cells. It also contains the epidermal appendages, arrector pili muscles, blood and lymph vessels, and nerves. Because the normal-haired skin of cats and dogs does not have epidermal rete ridges, dermal papillae are not usually seen. Thus, a true papillary and reticular dermis, as described for humans, is not present in cats and dogs. The terms "superficial" and "deep" dermis are preferred. The dermis accounts for most of the tensile strength and elasticity of the skin, is involved in the remodeling, maintenance, and repair of the skin, and also modulates the structure and function of the epidermis. The dermis of scrotal skin is unique in that it contains numerous large smooth muscle bundles.

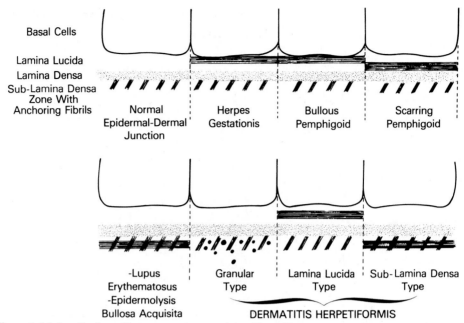

Basal Cells

Lamina Lucida
Lamina Densa
Sub-Lamina Densa
Zone With
Anchoring Fibrils

Normal	Herpes	Bullous	Scarring
Epidermal-Dermal	Gestationis	Pemphigoid	Pemphigoid
Junction			

-Lupus
Erythematosus
-Epidermolysis
Bullosa Acquisita

| | Granular | Lamina Lucida | Sub-Lamina Densa |
| | Type | Type | Type |

DERMATITIS HERPETIFORMIS

Figure 1:16. Localization of immunoreactants at the epidermal basement membrane zone in various skin diseases. (From Katz, S. I.: The epidermal basement membrane zone—structure, ontogeny, and role in disease. J. Am. Acad. Dermatol. *11*:1025–1037, 1984.)

Dermal Fibers

The dermal fibers are formed by fibroblasts and are collagenous, reticular, and elastic. *Collagenous fibers* (collagen) have great tensile strength and are the largest and most numerous (accounting for approximately 90 per cent of all dermal fibers and 80 per cent of the dermal extracellular matrix). They are thick bands composed of multiple protein fibrils and are differentially stained by Masson's trichrome. Collagen contains two unusual amino acids—hydroxyly-sine and 4-hydroxyproline—whose levels in urine have been used as indices of collagen turnover.[42] *Reticular fibers* (reticulin) are fine branching structures that, with age, closely approximate collagen. They can be detected best with special silver stains. Elastic fibers are composed of single fine branches that possess great elasticity and account for about 4 per cent of the dermal extracellular matrix. They are well visualized by Verhoeff's and van Gieson's elastin stains (Fig. 1:17). The major component of elastic fibers is elastin, which contains two unique cross-linked amino acids desmosine and isodesmosine, that are not found in other mammalian proteins.[42, 110]

There are numerous genetically and structurally different types of collagen molecules.[42, 65, 89, 132] Type I, Type III, and Type V collagen predominate in the dermis and account for approximately 80 per cent, 15 per cent, and 5 per cent, respectively, of the dermal collagen. Type IV and Type V collagens are found in basement membrane zone, and Type VII collagen is found in the anchoring fibrils of the basement membrane zone. The biosynthesis of collagen is a complex process of gene transposition and translation, intracellular modifica-tions, packaging and secretion, extracellular modifications, and fibril assembly and cross-linking. Collagen abnormalities may result from genetic defects, deficiencies of vitamin C, iron, and copper, and β-aminopropionitrile poisoning (lathyrism).

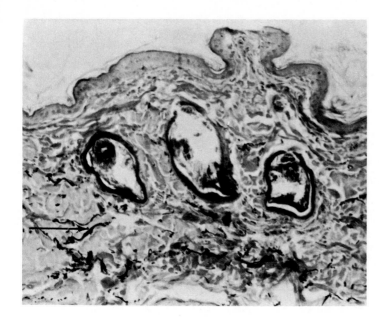

Figure 1:17. Elastic fibers from section of skin stained with elastic van Gieson. Note tylotrich pad (epidermal papilla) at surface of skin (low power.)

In general, the superficial dermis contains fine, loosely arranged collagen fibers that are irregularly distributed and a network of fine elastin fibers. The deep dermis contains thick, densely arranged collagen fibers that tend to parallel the skin surface and elastin fibers that are thicker and less numerous than those in the superficial dermis.

Dermal Ground Substance

The ground (interstitial) substance is a mucoid gel-sol of fibroblast origin composed of proteoglycans, principally hyaluronic acid, dermatan sulfate (chondroitin sulfate B), chondroitin-4-sulfate (chondroitin sulfate A), and chondroitin-6-sulfate (chondroitin sulfate C).[42, 126a] It fills the spaces and surrounds other structures of the dermis but allows electrolytes, nutrients, and cells to traverse it in passing from the dermal vessels to the avascular epidermis. The proteoglycans function in water storage and homeostasis; selective screening of substances; supporting dermal structure; lubrication; and collagen fibrillogenesis, orientation, growth, and differentiation.

Cell surface *fibronectin* is an adhesive glycoprotein produced by keratinocytes, fibroblasts, endothelial cells, and histiocytes.[22, 100] It mediates cell-to-cell interaction and cell adhesion to the substrate and modulates microvascular integrity, vascular permeability, and wound healing. Fibronectin has been implicated in a variety of cell functions, including cell adhesion and morphology, opsonization, cytoskeletal organization, oncogenic transformation, cell migration, phagocytosis, hemostasis, and embryonic differentiation.

Small amounts of *mucin* (a blue-staining, granular-to-stringy appearing substance with H&E stain) are often seen in normal feline and canine skin, especially around appendages and blood vessels. In the Chinese Shar Pei, however, large amounts of mucin are normally found throughout the dermis, which could be confused with pathologic myxedema (mucinosis) in other species.

Dermal Cellular Elements

The dermis is usually sparsely populated with cells (Fig. 1:18).[112, 114, 124, 131] *Fibroblasts* are present throughout. *Melanocytes* may be seen near superficial dermal blood vessels, especially in dark-skinned dogs. Melanocytes may also be seen around the hair bulbs of darkly colored dogs, especially Doberman pinschers.

Mast cells are most abundant around superficial dermal blood vessels and appendages. In dogs, as in cats, many mast cells are easily recognized with routine H&E stain. In cats, the cells have a "fried-egg" appearance with the lightly stained intracytoplasmic granules giving the cytoplasm a stippled appearance. In both species, the mast cells are more easily recognized with special stains such as toluidine blue and acid orcein-Giemsa. In general, normal cat skin contains about 4 to 20 mast cells per high-power microscopic field (HPMF) around superficial dermal blood vessels, with normal dog skin containing about 4 to 12 cells per HPMF.[92, 114]

Other cells that are occasionally seen in very small numbers in normal feline and canine skin include *neutrophils, eosinophils, lymphocytes, histiocytes,* and *plasma cells* (Fig. 1:18).

HAIR FOLLICLES

The hair shaft is divided into medulla, cortex, and cuticle.[42, 77, 112, 114, 131] The *medulla,* the innermost region of the hair, is composed of longitudinal rows of cuboidal cells, or cells flattened from top to bottom. The cells are solid near the hair root, but the rest of the hair shaft contains air and glycogen vacuoles. The *cortex,* the middle layer, consists of completely cornified, spindle-shaped cells, whose long axis is parallel to the hair shaft. These cells contain the pigment that gives the hair its color. Pigment may also be present in the medulla, but there it has little influence on the color of the hair shaft. In general, the cortex accounts for about one-sixth to one-fourth of the width of the hair shaft. The *cuticle,* the outermost layer of the hair, is formed by flat, cornified, anuclear cells arranged like slate on a roof, the free edge of each cell facing the tip of the hair (Fig. 1:19). Secondary hairs have a narrower medulla and a more prominent cuticle than do primary hairs. Lanugo hairs have no medulla. In the cat, the profile of the hair shaft is distinctly serrated.

Hair follicles are usually positioned at a 30- to 60-degree angle to the skin surface. Cats and dogs have a compound hair follicle arrangement (Fig. 1:20). In general, a cluster consists of two to five large primary hairs surrounded by groups of smaller secondary hairs. One of the primary hairs is the largest (central primary hair), while the remaining primary hairs are smaller (lateral primary hairs). Each primary hair has sebaceous and sweat glands and an arrector pili muscle. Secondary hairs may be accompanied by sebaceous glands, but by nothing else. The primary hairs generally emerge independently through separate pores, while the secondary hairs emerge through a common pore. From 5 to 20 secondary hairs may accompany each primary hair. Hairs are present in groups of 100 to 600/cm² in the dog, with 2 to 15 hairs per group. In cats, there are 800 to 1600 groups/cm², with about 10 to 20 hairs per group.[92, 114]

The hair follicle has five major components: the dermal hair papilla, the hair matrix, the hair, the inner root sheath, and other outer root sheath. The

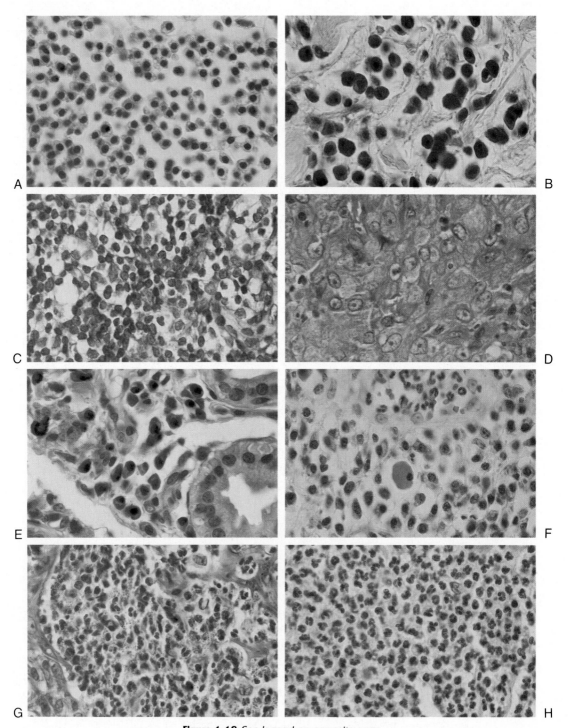

Figure 1:18 *See legend on opposite page*

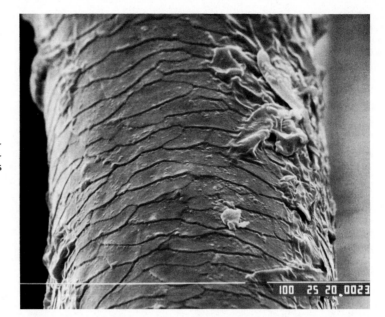

Figure 1:19. Scanning electron-micrograph of canine hair showing shingle-like hair cuticle with globs of amorphous material on its surface.

pluripotential cells of the hair matrix give rise to the hair and the inner root sheath. The outer root sheath represents a downward extension of the epidermis. Large hair follicles produce large hairs. For descriptive purposes, the hair follicle is divided into these three anatomic segments: (1) the *infundibulum*, or pilosebaceous region (the upper portion, which consists of the segment from the entrance of the sebaceous duct to the skin surface), (2) the *isthmus* (the middle portion, which consists of the segment between the entrance of the sebaceous duct and the attachment of the arrector pili muscle), and (3) the *inferior segment* (the lower portion, which extends from the attachment of the arrector pili muscle to the dermal hair papilla).

The inner root sheath is composed of three concentric layers, which from inside to outside include (1) the *inner root sheath cuticle* (a flattened, single layer of overlapping cells that point toward the hair bulb and interlock with the cells of the hair cuticle), (2) the *Huxley layer* (one to three nucleated cells thick), and (3) the *Henle layer* (a single layer of non-nucleated cells). These layers contain eosinophilic cytoplasmic granules called trichohyaline granules. Although it has traditionally been thought that trichohyaline granules are produced in the inner root sheath, recent findings of trichohyaline granules in the hair cortex of humans and guinea pigs have suggested that traditional concepts may require future modification.[53] The inner root sheath keratinizes and disintegrates when it reaches the level of the isthmus of the hair follicle. The amino acid citrulline occurs in high concentrations in hair and trichohyaline granules, and has been used as a marker for hair follicle differentiation.

Figure 1:18. *A*, Feline mast cells. Round-to-oval cells with a central nucleus arnd faintly eosinophilic, poorly visualized cytoplasmic granules (× 400, H & E stain). *B*, Canine mast cells. Round-to-oval cells with a central nucleus that is often obscured by the numerous, deeply basophilic cytoplasmic granules (× 400, H & E stain). *C*, Canine lymphocytes. Round cells with small amounts of basophilic cytoplasm (× 400, H & E stain). *D*, Feline macrophages. Pleomorphic cells with round, oval, or folded nuclei and a large amount of faintly eosinophilic cytoplasm (× 400, H & E stain). *E*, Canine plasma cells. Oval cells with a round, eccentric nucleus, basophilic cytoplasm, and a perinuclear "halo" (clear zone) (× 400, H & E stain). *F*, Feline Russell's body. A large oval cell (center) with an eccentric, round nucleus and a brightly eosinophilic, refractile cytoplasm (× 400, H & E stain). *G*, Canine eosinophils. Round-to-oval cells with segmented (usually bilobed) nuclei and brightly eosinophilic cytoplasmic granules (× 400, H & E stain). *H*, Canine neutrophils. Round-to-oval cells with segmented nuclei and faintly eosinophilic, often indistinct cytoplasm (× 400, H & E stain).

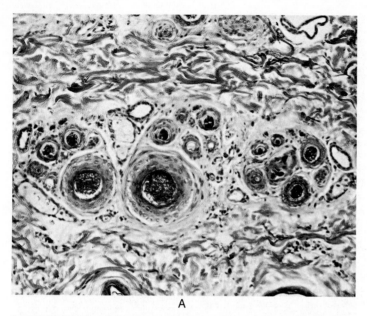

A

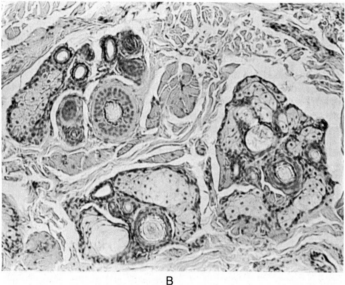

B

Figure 1:20. *A,* Three multiple hair follicle units (high power). *B,* Three apopiloseba-ceous complexes, each showing primary and secondary hairs, sebaceous and apo-crine glands, and arrector pili muscles (high power).

The outer root sheath is thickest near the epidermis and gradually decreases in thickness toward the hair bulb. In its lower portion (from the isthmus of the hair follicle downward), the outer root sheath is covered by the inner root sheath and does not undergo keratinization, and its cells have a clear, vacuo-lated cytoplasm (glycogen). In the middle portion of the hair follicle (isthmus), the outer root sheath is no longer covered by the inner root sheath and undergoes trichilemmal keratinization (keratohyaline granules are not formed). In the upper portion of the hair follicle (infundibulum), the outer root sheath undergoes keratinization in the same fashion as the surface epidermis. The outer root sheath is surrounded by two other prominent structures: a basement membrane zone, or "glassy" membrane (a downward reflection of the epider-mal basement membrane zone), and a fibrous root sheath (a layer of dense connective tissue). Perifollicular mineralization of the basement membrane zone has been described in healthy toy poodle bitches.[119] This may also occur as a senile change in other breeds of dogs[118] and must be differentiated from the perifollicular mineralization seen in dogs with naturally occurring or iatrogenic Cushing's syndrome (see Chap. 10).

The dermal hair papilla is continuous with the dermal connective tissue and is covered by a thin continuation of the basement membrane zone. The inner root sheath and hair grow from a layer of plump, nucleated epithelial cells that cover the papilla. These cells regularly show mitosis and are called the hair matrix.

The hair follicles of animals with straight hair are straight, while those of animals with curly hair tend to be spiral in configuration. Follicular folds have been described in the hair follicles of animals. These structures represent multiple (1 to 23) corrugations of the inner root sheath, which project into the pilary canal immediately below the sebaceous duct opening. These folds are believed to be artifacts of fixation and processing, as they are not seen in unprocessed sections cut by hand.[114]

Two specialized types of tactile hairs are found in mammalian skin: sinus hairs and tylotrich hairs.[92, 114] *Sinus hairs* (vibrissae) are found on the muzzle, lip, eyelid, face, throat, and on the palmar aspect of the carpus of cats (pili carpalis, carpal gland). These hairs are thick, stiff, and tapered distally. Sinus hairs are characterized by an endothelium-lined blood sinus interposed between the external root sheath of the follicle and an outer connective tissue capsule (Fig. 1:21). The sinus is divided into a superior nontrabecular ring or annular sinus, and an inferior cavernous, or trabecular, sinus. A cushion-like thickening of mesenchyme ("sinus pad") projects into the annular sinus. The cavernous sinuses are traversed by trabeculae containing many nerve fibers. Skeletal muscle fibers attach to the outer layer of the follicle. Pacinian corpuscles are

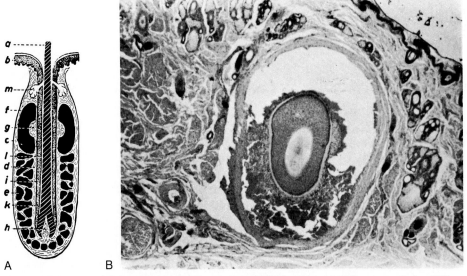

A   B

Figure 1:21. *A*, Hair follicle of sinus hair of cat in longitudinal section, semidiagrammatic ($\times$ 150): *a*, hair; *b*, epidermis; *c*, outer, *d*, inner, layer of the dermal follicle; *e*, the blood sinus (this sinus has been differentiated into a nontrabecular annular sinus *f*, into which projects the sinus pad *g*); *h*, hair papilla; *i*, glassy membrane of the follicle; *k*, outer root sheath; *l*, inner root sheath; *m*, sebaceous glands. *B*, Tactile hair from upper lip of dog showing blood sinus (high power). (*A*, reprinted from Trautmann, A., and Fiebiger, J.: Fundamentals of the Histology of Domestic Animals. Copyright 1952 by Cornell University. Used by permission of Cornell University Press.)

situated close to the sinus hair follicles. Sinus hairs are thought to function as slow-adapting mechanoreceptors.

Tylotrich hairs are scattered among ordinary body hairs. Tylotrich hair follicles are larger than surrounding follicles and contain a single stout hair and an annular complex of neurovascular tissue that surrounds the follicle at the level of the sebaceous glands. Tylotrich hairs are thought to function as rapid-adapting mechanoreceptors. Each tylotrich follicle is associated with a tylotrich pad (Haarscheibe, touch spot, or touch corpuscle) (Fig. 1:2). Tylotrich pads are composed of a thickened and distinctive epidermis underlaid by a convex area of fine connective tissue that is highly vascularized and well innervated. Unmyelinated nerve fibers end as flat plaques in association with Merkel's cells, which serve as slow-adapting touch receptors.

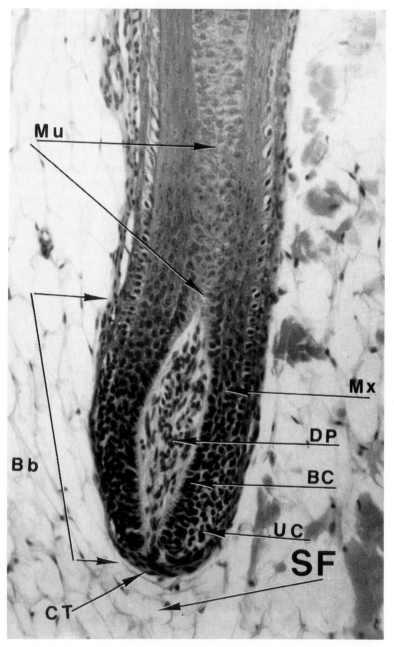

Figure 1:22. Anagen hair follicle. Longitudinal section of a secondary hair follicle at anagen stage, from the saddle region of a 28-month-old beagle. The bulb (Bb) extends into the subcutaneous fat (SF). The spindle-shaped dermal papilla (DP) extends toward the medulla of the hair (Mu), the base of the dermal papilla is continuous with the connective tissue (CT) of the hair follicle. The dermal papilla is surrounded by the matrix cells (Mx) of the bulb (Bb). The basal cells of the matrix are columnar (BC). The lower part of the bulb contains undifferentiated matrix cells (UC). (× 350, H & E.) (From Al-Bagdadi, F. K., Titkemeyer, C. W., and Lovell, J. E.: Histology of the hair cycle in male beagle dogs. Am. J. Vet. Res. 40:1734, 1979.)

The histologic appearance of hair follicles varies with the stage of the hair follicle cycle.[3, 42, 77] The *anagen* hair follicle is characterized by a well-developed, spindle-shaped dermal papilla, which is capped by the hair matrix (the "ball-and-claw" appearance) to form the hair follicle bulb (Fig. 1:22). Hair matrix cells are often heavily melanized and show mitotic activity. The anagen hair follicle extends into the deep dermis and often into the subcutis.

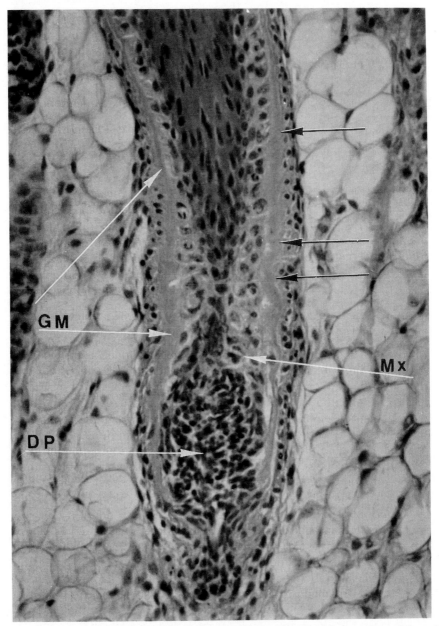

Figure 1:23. Catagen. Longitudinal section of a hair follicle at catagen stage from the saddle region of a 2-week-old beagle. The dermal papilla (DP) is oval in shape. The nuclei are crowded and the matrix cells (Mx) that border the dermal papilla have lost their orientation. The glassy membrane (GM) is thick and straight at the upper part of the hair follicle (single black unlabeled arrow in the upper part of the picture) while above the bulb, the glassy membrane is undulating (two black unlabeled arrows in the lower part of the picture). (× 395, H & E.) (From Al-Bagdadi, F. K., Titkemeyer, C. W., and Lovell, J. E.: Histology of the hair cycle in male beagle dogs. Am. J. Vet. Res. *40*:1734, 1979.)

The *catagen* hair follicle is characterized by a thickened, irregular, undulating basement membrane zone, a thickened middle third of the outer root sheath, a smaller bulb, and an ovoid or round dermal papilla (Fig. 1:23). The *telogen* hair follicle is characterized by the small dermal papilla that is separated from the bulb, a lack of melanin and mitotic activity, an absence of the inner

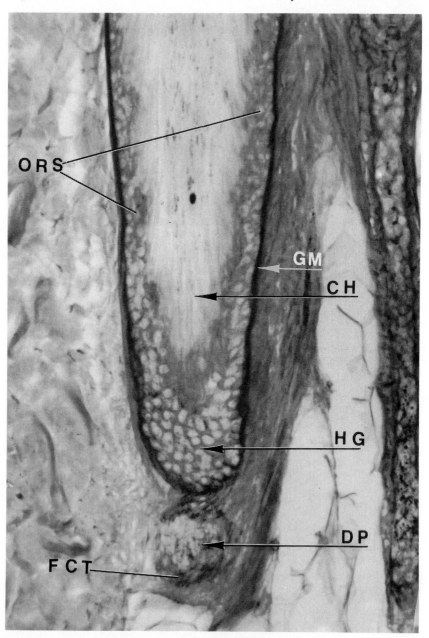

Figure 1:24. Telogen. Longitudinal section of a main hair follicle at telogen stage from the saddle region of a 3-month-old beagle. The dermal papilla (DP) is separated from the matrix cells of hair follicle. It is surrounded by fibrous connective tissue (FCT) and appears to contact the base of the follicle at one point. The hair germ cells (HG) are located at the base of the club hair (CH). The cells of the outer root sheath (ORS) lack glycogen granules. The glassy membrane (GM) is thick and PAS positive. The hair follicle at this stage is surrounded by connective tissue that separates the follicle from the adipose tissue (× 400). (From Al-Bagdadi, F. K., Titkemeyer, C. W., and Lovell, J. E.: Histology of the hair cycle in male beagle dogs. Am. J. Vet. Res. *40*:1734, 1979.)

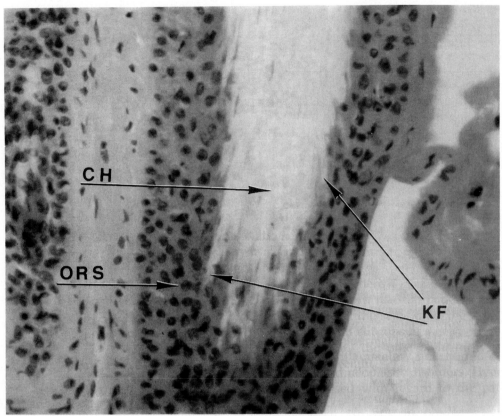

Figure 1:25. Club hair of telogen. Longitudinal section of a main hair follicle at telogen stage from the saddle region of a 24-month-old beagle. The club hair (CH) has many keratinized fibers (KF) that extend between the cells of the outer root sheath (ORS). These keratinized fibers give the club hair a brushlike appearance. (× 465, H & E.) (From Al-Bagdadi, F. K., Titkemeyer, C. W., and Lovell, J. E.: Histology of the hair cycle in male beagle dogs. Am. J. Vet. Res. *40*:1734, 1979.)

root sheath, a club (brushlike) hair, and prominent apoptosis ("dyskeratosis" or "necrosis" of individual keratinocytes) of the external root sheath (Figs. 1:24 and 1:25).

A hair plucked in anagen shows a larger expanded root, which is moist and glistening, often pigmented and square at the end, and surrounded by a root sheath (Fig. 1:26). A hair plucked in telogen shows both a club root with no root sheath or pigment and a keratinized sac (Fig. 1:26).

SEBACEOUS GLANDS

Sebaceous (holocrine) glands are simple or branched alveolar glands distributed throughout all haired skin.[42, 90, 112, 114, 124, 131] The glands usually open through a duct into the pilary canal in the infundibulum (pilosebaceous follicle). Sebaceous glands tend to be largest in areas where hair follicle density is lowest. They are largest and most numerous near mucocutaneous junctions, in the interdigital spaces, on the dorsal neck and rump, on the chin (submental organ), and on the dorsal tail (tail gland, supracaudal organ, preen gland). Sebaceous glands are not found in the footpads and planum nasale.

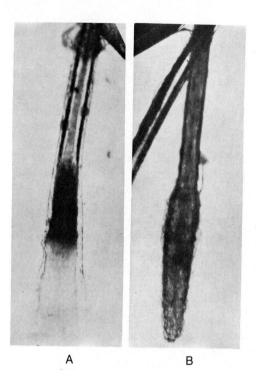

A   B

Figure 1:26. *A,* Anagen hair plucked from hair follicle (low power). *B,* Telogen hair plucked from hair follicle (low power). (Courtesy Drs. E. J. Van Scott and P. Frost, National Institutes of Health, Bethesda, Maryland.)

Sebaceous lobules are bordered by a basement membrane zone, upon which sits a single layer of deeply basophilic basal cells ("reserve" cells) (Fig. 1:27). The cells become progressively more lipidized and eventually disintegrate to form sebum toward the center of the lobule. Sebaceous ducts are lined with squamous epithelium.

The oily secretion (sebum) produced by the sebaceous glands tends to keep the skin soft and pliable by forming a surface emulsion that spreads over the surface of the stratum corneum to retain moisture and thus maintain proper hydration. The oil film also spreads over the hair shafts and gives them a glossy sheen. During periods of illness or malnutrition, the hair coat may

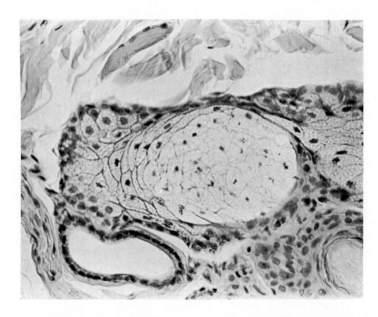

Figure 1:27. Canine sebaceous gland (apocrine duct in lower left corner, hair follicle and hair in lower right corner) (high power).

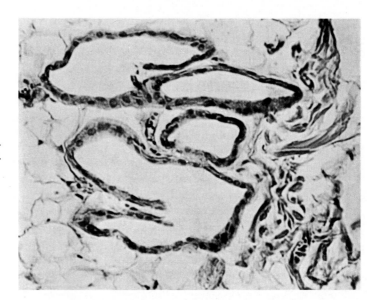

Figure 1:28. Section through coiled portion of apocrine sweat gland (high power).

become dull and dry as a result of inadequate sebaceous gland function. In addition to its action as a physical barrier, the sebum-sweat emulsion forms a chemical barrier against potential pathogens (see Cutaneous Ecology in this chapter). Many of sebum's fatty acid constituents (linoleic, myristic, oleic, and palmitic acids) are known to have antimicrobial actions.

Sebaceous glands have an abundant blood supply and appear to be innervated. Their secretion is thought to be under hormonal control, with androgens causing hypertrophy and hyperplasia, and estrogens and glucocorticoids causing involution. The skin surface lipids of cats and dogs have been studied in some detail and are different from those of humans (see Horny Layer in this chapter). Enzyme histochemical studies have indicated that all mammalian sebaceous glands contain succinic dehydrogenase, cytochrome oxidase, and a few esterases.[91]

SWEAT GLANDS

Apocrine Sweat Glands

Apocrine sweat glands are generally coiled and saccular or tubular and are distributed throughout all haired skin.[34, 42, 94, 112, 114, 124, 131] They are not present in footpads or planum nasale. These glands are localized below the sebaceous glands, and they usually open through a duct into the pilary canal in the infundibulum, above the sebaceous duct opening. Apocrine sweat glands tend to be larger in areas where hair follicle density is lower. They are largest and most numerous near mucocutaneous junctions, in interdigital spaces, and over the dorsal neck and rump.

The secretory portions of apocrine sweat glands consist of a single row of flattened to columnar epithelial (secretory) cells and a single layer of fusiform myoepithelial cells (Figs. 1:28 and 1:29). The apocrine sweat gland excretory duct is lined by two cuboidal to flattened epithelial cell layers and a luminal cuticle, but no myoepithelial cells.[56] In general, apocrine sweat glands do not appear to be innervated.

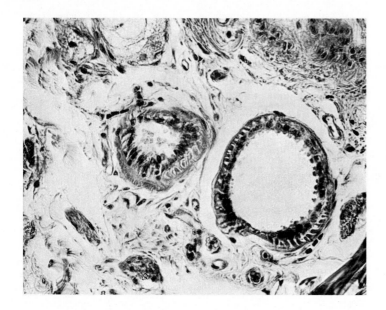

Figure 1:29. Apocrine gland showing secretory epithelium (high power).

Enzyme histochemical studies have demonstrated alkaline phosphatase and acid phosphatase in apocrine sweat gland secretory epithelium.[55, 91]

Eccrine Sweat Glands

Eccrine (merocrine) sweat glands are found only in the footpads.[34, 114, 124, 131] They are small, tightly coiled, and located in the deep dermis and subcutis of the footpads. Secretory coils consist of a single layer of cuboidal to columnar epithelial cells and a single layer of fusiform myoepithelial cells (Fig. 1:30). The intradermal portion of the excretory duct consists of a double row of cuboidal epithelial cells. The excretory duct opens directly to the footpad surface.

Enzyme histochemical studies have demonstrated cytochrome oxidase, succinic and other dehydrogenases, phosphorylases, and alkaline phosphatase

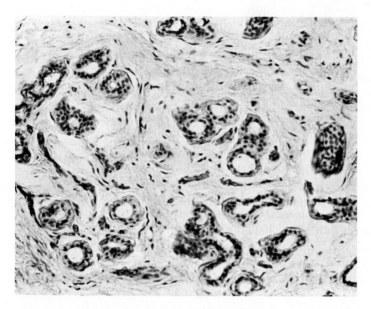

Figure 1:30. Eccrine sweat glands from canine footpad (high power).

in eccrine sweat glands.[91] These glands are richly supplied with cholinesterase-positive nerves.[6, 8, 50, 91, 114, 138]

Sweating and Thermoregulation

Cat and dog skins do not possess the extensive superficial arteriovenous shunts of humans and swine that are designed to disseminate heat in hot weather.[126a] In addition, carnivores lack eccrine sweat glands in the hairy skin.

The frequency of sweating and the circumstances under which sweating occurs in cats and dogs is unclear. Some authors state that the dog shows great variation in the degree of apocrine sweating that takes place and that some breeds (especially German shepherd, Labrador retriever, and other large breeds) may show visible sweating in the axillae, groin, and ventral abdomen.[127] Others state that apocrine sweating is occasionally seen in certain febrile and excited dogs.[94] Still others report that apocrine sweating was not seen in dogs subjected to severe generalized temperature stress or in dogs that were struggling violently.[25] Eccrine sweating has been seen on the footpads of excited or agitated cats and dogs.[92, 127]

In dogs, localized apocrine sweating can be produced by local heat applications and the intradermal injection of various sympathomimetic (epinephrine, norepinephrine) and parasympathomimetic (acetylcholine, pilocarpine) drugs.[4, 5, 24, 54, 94] Because responses to all these can be blocked by atropine, the final physiologic stimulus appears to be cholinergic. It has also been reported that asphyxiation or the intravenous injection of epinephrine or norepinephrine produced generalized apocrine sweating in dogs.[54] Because these responses could not be blocked by adrenal medullectomy but were blocked by sympathetic denervation of skin, it was concluded that canine apocrine sweating was primarily regulated by neural mechanisms, with humoral mechanisms playing a subsidiary role. One group of researchers has concluded—on the basis of available local and systemic pharmacologic data, local and generalized thermal responses, hypothalamic stimulation, and electron microscopic examinations—that canine apocrine sweat glands are not directly innervated and have little, if any, thermoregulatory importance.[15, 25] It has also been suggested that, because the only physiologic stimulus noted to consistently produce apocrine sweating in dogs was copulation, apocrine sweating in dogs served a predominantly pheromonal function.[25]

Eccrine sweating from the footpads of cats and dogs can be provoked by cholinergic stimuli and less so by adrenergic stimuli.[6–8, 114, 125] Atropine blocks glandular responses to these agents. Feline eccrine sweat contains lactate, glucose, sodium, potassium, chloride, and bicarbonate and differs from that of humans by being hypertonic and alkaline, and containing much higher concentrations of sodium, potassium, and chloride.[114]

Mechanisms to Conserve Heat. When the environmental temperature falls, the body attempts to reduce heat loss by vasoconstriction in the skin and erection of the hairs to improve the insulating qualities of the skin and coat. The external temperature at which the heat-retaining mechanisms are no longer able to maintain a constant body temperature and at which heat production has to be increased is known as the *critical temperature*. Normal dogs with intact pelage had a critical temperature of 57°F, but when their coats were shaved off they had a critical temperature of 77°F.[92] Thick subcutaneous fat also acts as efficient insulating material. Nonfasting animals have a lower critical temperature than fasting individuals, and thus the former are better able to stand a low environmental temperature. When the aforementioned mechanisms of heat conservation are no longer effective in preventing a fall in body temperature, an increase in heat production begins. A rapid increase in heat production is accomplished mainly by shivering. In normal dogs shivering begins when the rectal temperature falls by about 2°F.

Mechanisms to Dissipate Heat. Heat is regularly lost from the body by radiation, conduction, and convection; vaporization of water from the skin and respiratory passages; and excretion of urine and feces. The excretory losses are relatively unimportant in heat dissipation. Ordinarily, 75 per cent of the heat loss is attributable to radiation, conduction, and convection. The efficiency of these mechanisms varies with the external temperature and humidity, and is modified further by the animal's vasomotor and pilomotor responses. These become quite ineffective at higher temperatures, and heat loss by vaporization of water from the skin and lungs becomes more influential. Since they do not produce an abundance of eccrine sweat, dogs and cats have developed the ability to vaporize large volumes of water from their respiratory passages. In dogs, as the environmental temperature rises above 80 to 85°F, the rate of breathing also rises, but the depth of breathing (tidal volume) is markedly reduced. This helps to prevent excess carbon dioxide blowoff and severe blood gas changes. At a rectal temperature of 105°F the dog is in danger of thermal imbalance, and at 109°F collapse is imminent.

The rectal temperature of the cat begins to rise at an environmental temperature of 90°F, but as the respiratory rate increases the tidal volume is only slightly reduced, so the cat is more susceptible to a lowering of its blood carbon dioxide level (i.e., to respiratory alkalosis). However, the cat possesses an additional compensatory mechanism. A hot environment, or sympathetic stimulation, produces a copious flow of watery saliva from the submaxillary gland. The cat spreads this on its coat for additional water vaporization, and cooling results. Similar stimulation in dogs produces only a scanty secretion of thick saliva that cannot help the cooling process.[92]

The problem of temperature regulation in dogs and cats is often complicated by the physical condition of the coat and by the environmental temperature. Breeds with heavy coats intended for cold climates are often moved to regions of high temperatures, where they may suffer. The problem is greatly accentuated by a matted, unkempt coat that stifles air circulation through the hair. Proper grooming will greatly increase the comfort of these animals. (See Chap. 4, Care of the Skin and Hair Coat.)

SPECIALIZED GLANDS

Specialized glands include the perianal (circumanal) glands, the glands of the external auditory canal, and the anal sacs (see Chap. 18), as well as the tail gland.

The *tail gland* (supracaudal gland, preen gland) of the *dog* is an oval-shaped area located on the dorsal surface of the tail over the fifth to seventh coccygeal vertebrae, about 5 cm distal to the anus (Fig. 1:31).[34, 92] This gland is consistently present in wild canidae but is regarded as an atavism in dogs, because it is somewhat different in structure, is lacking in function, and is clearly visible in only about 5 per cent of all normal male dogs. However, the gland is present

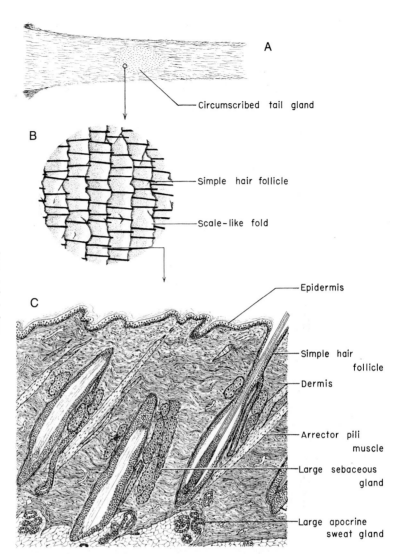

A

Circumscribed tail gland

B

Simple hair follicle

Scale-like fold

Figure 1:31. Surface contour, hair arrangement, and histology of the tail gland area. (Modified from Evans, H. E., and Christensen, G. C.: Miller's Anatomy of the Dog. 2nd ed. W. B. Saunders Company, Philadelphia, 1979. After Lovell and Getty, 1957.)

C

Epidermis

Simple hair follicle

Dermis

Arrector pili muscle

Large sebaceous gland

Large apocrine sweat gland

histologically in most dogs. The hair coat of the region is characterized by stiff coarse hairs, each emerging singly from its follicle. The surface of the skin may be yellow and waxy from the abundant secretion of the numerous large glands in the area. This secretion may aid in olfactory species recognition. This area of the tail may be severely affected in seborrheic skin diseases and may also develop hyperplasia, cystic degeneration, infection, adenoma, and adenocarcinoma.

Histologically, the canine tail gland is composed predominantly of "hepatoid" (perianal) cells, identical to those in the circumanal glands. The glandular ducts empty into hair follicles. The tail gland and the circumanal gland are testosterone-dependent and form a topographic-ethnologic unit.

The tail gland (supracaudal organ) of the *cat* consists of numerous large sebaceous glands that run the entire length of the dorsal surface of the tail.[114, 124] Excess accumulation of glandular secretion in this area is called "stud tail" (see Chap. 14).

ARRECTOR PILI MUSCLES

Arrector pili muscles are of mesenchymal origin and consist of smooth muscle with intracellular and extracellular vacuoles.[34, 42, 106, 114, 124, 131] They are present in all haired skin and are largest in the dorsal neck and rump. Arrector pili muscles originate in the superficial dermis and insert approximately perpendicularly on a bulge of the primary hair follicles (see Fig. 1:33). Branching of these muscles is often seen in the superficial dermis. Arrector pili muscles are about one-fourth to one-half the diameter of central primary hair follicles in most haired skin areas but of equal diameter in the dorsal lumbar, dorsal sacral, and dorsal tail areas.

These muscles receive cholinergic innervation and contract in response to epinephrine and norepinephrine, producing pilorection. Arrector pili muscles probably function in thermoregulation and the emptying of sebaceous glands.

BLOOD VESSELS

Cutaneous blood vessels are generally arranged in three intercommunicating plexuses of arteries and veins (Fig. 1:32).[34, 42, 92, 114] The deep plexus is found at the interface of the dermis and subcutis. Branches from this plexus descend into the subcutis and ascend to supply the lower portions of the hair follicles and the apocrine sweat glands. These ascending vessels continue upward to feed the middle plexus, which lies at the level of the sebaceous glands. The middle plexus gives off branches to the arrector pili muscles, ascending and descending branches that supply the middle portions of the hair follicles and the sebaceous glands, and ascending branches to feed the superficial plexus. Capillary loops that are immediately below the epidermis emanate from the superficial plexus and supply the epidermis and upper portion of the hair follicles. Blood vessel endothelial cells are characterized ultrastructurally by a peripheral basement membrane and intracytoplasmic Weibel-Palade bodies (rod-shaped tubular structures enveloped in a continuous single membrane), as well as by possessing factor VIII antigen, plasminogen activators, prostaglandins, and by being phagocytic.[42, 77]

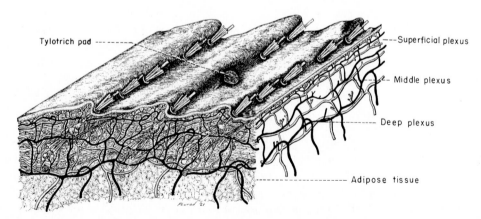

Figure 1:32. Schematic section of skin of the dog, showing tylotrich pad (epidermal papilla, haarscheiben) and blood vessels (veins in black). (Modified from Evans, H. E., and Christensen, G. C.: Miller's Anatomy of the Dog. 2nd ed. W. B. Saunders Company, Philadelphia, 1979.)

Arteriovenous anastomoses are normal connections between arteries and veins that allow arterial blood to enter the venous circulation without passing through capillary beds.[42, 77, 92, 106] Because of the size and position of these anastomoses, they can alter circulation dynamics and the blood supply to tissues. They occur in all areas of the skin but are most common over the extremities (especially the legs and ears). They occur at all levels of the dermis but especially in the deep dermis.

Arteriovenous anastomoses show considerable variation in structure, ranging from simple slightly coiled vessels to such complex structures as the glomus. The glomus is a special arteriovenous shunt located within the deep dermis. Each glomus consists of an arterial and a venous segment. The arterial segment (Sucquet-Hoyer canal) branches from an arteriole. The wall shows a single layer of endothelium, surrounded by a basement membrane zone, and a media that is densely packed with four to six layers of glomus cells. These cells are large and plump, have a clear cytoplasm, and resemble epithelioid cells. Glomus cells are generally regarded as being modifed smooth muscle cells. The venous segment of the glomus is thin walled and has a wide lumen.

Arteriovenous anastomoses are associated with thermoregulation. Constriction or dilatation of the shunt restricts or enhances, respectively, the blood flow to an area. Acetylcholine and histamine cause dilatation, while epinephrine and norepinephrine cause constriction.

Pericytes, varying from fusiform to clublike in appearance, are aligned parallel to blood vessels on the dermal side of the vessels.[42, 52, 77] They are contractile cells, containing actin-like and myosin-like filaments, and are important in regulating capillary flow. The origin of pericytes is uncertain.

Veil cells are flat fibroblast-like cells that surround all dermal microvessels.[16, 42] Unlike pericytes, which are an integral component of the vascular wall and are enmeshed in the mural basement membrane material, veil cells are entirely external to the wall. The veil cell demarcates the vessel from the surrounding dermis and can be considered to be adventitial.

LYMPH VESSELS

Lymphatics arise from capillary networks that lie in the superficial dermis and surround the adnexa.[28, 77, 108] The vessels arising from these networks drain into a subcutaneous lymphatic plexus. Lymph vessels are not usually seen above the middle dermis in routine histologic preparations of normal skin.

The lymphatics are essential for nutrition because they control the true microcirculation of the skin, which is the movement of interstitial tissue fluid. The supply, permeation, and removal of tissue fluid are important for proper function. The lymphatics are the drains that take away the debris and excess matter resulting from daily wear and tear in the skin. They are essential channels for the return of protein and cells from the tissues into the blood stream and for linking the skin and regional lymph nodes in an immunoregulatory capacity.

In general, lymph vessels are distinguished from blood capillaries by (1) possessing wider and more angular lumina, (2) having flatter and more attenuated endothelial cells, (3) having no pericytes, and (4) containing no blood. However, even the slightest injury disrupts the wall of a lymphatic or blood vessel or the intervening connective tissue. Consequently, traumatic fistulae are commonplace. These account for the frequent observation of "blood flow" in the lymphatics in inflamed skin.

NERVES

In general, cutaneous nerve fibers are associated with blood vessels (dual autonomic innervation of arteries), various cutaneous endorgans (tylotrich pad, Pacini's corpuscle, Meissner's corpuscle, and mammalian endorgan), sebaceous glands, hair follicles, and arrector pili muscles and occur as a subepidermal plexus.[42, 92, 114] Some free nerve endings even penetrate the epidermis. Under the light microscope, small cutaneous nerves and free nerve endings can be demonstrated satisfactorily only by methylene blue, metallic impregnation, or histochemical techniques.

In addition to the all-important function of sensory perception (touch, heat, cold, pressure, pain, and itch), the dermal nerves promote the survival and proper functioning of the epidermis (i.e., the so-called trophic influences).

The area of skin supplied by the branches of one spinal nerve is known as its dermatome. Dermatomes have been mapped out for the cat[49, 72] and dog.[9, 68, 133]

Pruritus

Pruritus or itching is an unpleasant sensation that provokes the desire to scratch.[29, 47, 85, 126a] It is the most common symptom in dermatology and may be due to specific dermatologic diseases or may be generalized without clinically evident skin disease. Pruritus may be sharp or well localized (epicritic), or it may be poorly localized with a burning quality (protopathic).

The skin is richly endowed by a network of sensory nerves and receptors (Fig. 1:33). The sensory nerves subserve hair follicles as well as encapsulated structures such as Pacini's corpuscles, Meissner's corpuscles, Ruffini's corpuscles, and Krause's end bulbs.[42, 87, 114] In addition, sensory nerves may end as free nerve endings, referred to as penicillate nerve endings. The penicillate endings arise from the terminal Schwann's cell in the dermis as tuftlike origins and give rise to an arborizing network of fine nerves, and they terminate either subepidermally or intraepidermally. These unmyelinated penicillate nerve endings are limited to the skin, mucous membranes, and cornea.

Although several morphologically distinct end organs have been described, a specific end organ for pruritus has not been found. It is still controversial whether functional specificity of the afferent fibers or temporal coding of stimuli determines the sensation.

On the basis of the properties of afferent units, somatosensory activity can be subdivided into mechanoreceptors, thermoreceptors, and nociceptors. The nociceptors are involved in itch and pain. Nociceptors are supplied by A delta and C fibers. The A delta fibers (myelinated) conduct at about 10 to 20 m/sec and carry fibers for spontaneous (physiologic), well localized, pricking type of itch (epicritic itch). The type C fibers (nonmyelinated) conduct more slowly (2 m/sec) and subserve unpleasant, diffuse burning (pathologic) itch (protopathic itch). Both fibers enter the dorsal root of the spinal cord, ascend in the dorsal column, and cross to the lateral spinothalamic tract (Fig. 1:34). From there the fibers ascend to the thalamus and via the internal capsule to the sensory cortex,

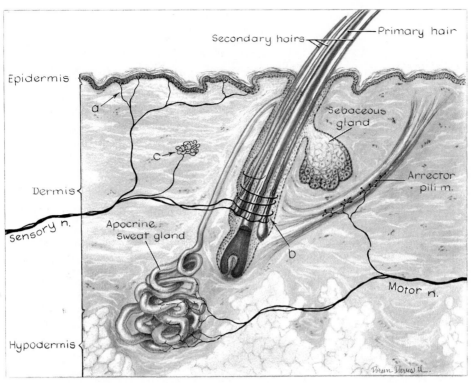

Figure 1:33. Nerve supply of the canine skin. *A*, Dermal nerve network. *B*, Hair follicle network. *C*, Specialized end-organs.

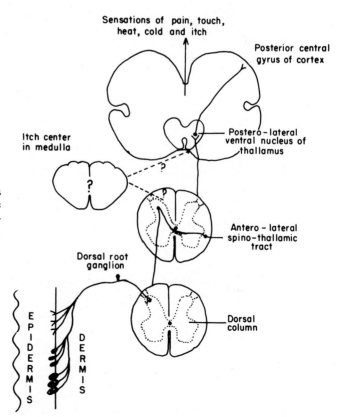

Figure 1:34. Afferent pathways of cutaneous sensations in man. (From Halliwell, R. E. W.: Pathogenesis and treatment of pruritus. J.A.V.M.A. *164*:793, 1974.)

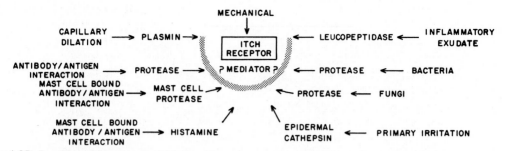

Figure 1:35. Possible pathways in the initiation of pruritus. (From Halliwell, R. E. W.: Pathogenesis and treatment of pruritus. J.A.V.M.A. *164*:793, 1974.)

where the itch sensation may be modified by emotional factors and competing cutaneous sensations.

At present, it has not been possible to isolate a universal mediator to explain pruritus. A host of chemical mediators have been implicated in pruritus, including histamine, proteolytic enzymes or proteases (e.g., kallikrein, cathepsins, leukopeptidases, proteases of microbial origin, plasmin), peptides (e.g., bradykinin, vasoactive intestinal peptide, substance P), prostaglandins, and leukotrienes (Fig. 1:35).[29, 42, 47, 85, 115, 130] It is clear that histamine and prostaglandins are not the most important mediators of itch in dogs, cats, and humans. Presently, proteolytic enzymes are thought to be the major mediators of itch in these species.

Recent clinical investigations have indicated that leukotrienes may be important modulators of pruritus in dogs.[116] In addition, central factors such as anxiety, boredom, or competing cutaneous sensations (e.g., pain, touch, heat, cold) can magnify or reduce the sensation of pruritus by selectively acting on the "gate-control" system. For instance, pruritus is often worse at night because other sensory input is low. Although the mechanisms involved here are not clear, it has been suggested that stressful conditions may potentiate pruritus through the release of various opioid peptides.[38] Various neuropeptides—such as enkephalins, endorphins, and substance P—have been demonstrated to participate in the regulation of such cutaneous reactions as pruritus, pain, flushing, pigmentary changes, and inflammation.[42]

SUBCUTIS

The subcutis (hypodermis) is the deepest and usually thickest layer of the skin.[34, 42, 112, 114, 124, 131] It is a fibrofatty structure, consisting of lobules of fat cells (lipocytes, adipocytes) interwoven with connective tissue. The subcutis functions (1) as an energy reserve, (2) in heat insulation, (3) as a protective padding, and (4) in maintaining surface contours. Recent studies have demonstrated that the subcutis is also an important steroid reservoir, site of steroid metabolism, and site of estrogen production.[30]

Senility

Senile changes have been reported in the skin of aged dogs[13] and cats.[114] The hair of some dogs was dull and lusterless, with areas of alopecia and callus formation over pressure points. An increase in the number of white hairs on the muzzle and body were frequently seen. The footpads and noses of some dogs were hyperkeratotic, and claws tended to become malformed and brittle.

Histologically, one may see orthokeratotic hyperkeratosis of the epidermis and hair follicles, the latter often being atrophic and containing no hairs. Atrophy of the epidermis may be manifested as a single layer of flattened keratinocytes with pyknotic nuclei. Dermal changes may include decreased cellularity, fragmentation and granular degeneration of collagen bundles, and occasional diminution and fragmentation of elastic fibers. The solar elastosis (basophilic degeneration of elastic) that characterizes aging human skin is not usually seen in aged dogs and cats. It is probable that the dense hair coat of dogs and cats protects them from the damaging effects of ultraviolet light.

Variable changes may be seen in the glands of the skin, including cystic dilatation of apocrine sweat glands and the presence of large, yellow, refractile granules in the secretory cells of the apocrine sweat glands. Arrector pili muscles became more eosinophilic, fragmented, and vacuolated.

Extensive studies in humans have demonstrated the following changes in senile skin: epidermal atrophy, decreased adherence of corneocytes, flattening of the dermoepidermal junction; decreased numbers of melanocytes and Langerhans' cells; dermal atrophy (relatively acellular and avascular), altered dermal collagen, elastin, and glycosaminoglycans; atrophy of the subcutis; attenuation of eccrine and apocrine glands; decreased sebaceous gland secretion; reduction of hair follicle density; thinning, ridging, lack of luster of nail plates; decreased growth rate of the epidermis, hair and nails; delayed wound healing; reduced dermal clearance of fluids and foreign materials; compromised vascular responsiveness; diminished eccrine and apocrine secretions; reduced sensory perception; reduced vitamin D production; and impairment of the cutaneous immune and inflammatory responses.[36] Clinical correlates in humans of these intrinsic aging changes of the skin include alopecia, pallor, xerosis (dry skin), increased number of benign and malignant neoplasms, increased susceptibility to blister formation, predispostion to injury of the dermis and underlying tissues, increased risk of wound infections, and thermoregulatory disturbances.[36] Wounds in aged beagles and boxers heal less rapidly than in young dogs.[99]

References

1. Abrahamson, D. R.: Recent studies on the structure and pathology of basement membranes. J. Pathol. 149:257, 1986.
2. Al-Bagdadi, F. A., et al.: Hair follicle cycle and shedding in male beagle dogs. Am. J. Vet. Res. 38:611, 1977.
3. Al-Bagdadi, F. A. et al.: Histology of the hair cycle in male beagle dogs. Am. J. Vet. Res. 40:1734, 1979.
4. Aoki, T., and Wada, M.: Functional activity of the sweat glands in the hair skin of the dog. Science 114:123, 1951.
5. Aoki, T.: Stimulation of the sweat glands in the hairy skin of dogs by adrenaline, noradrenaline, acetylcholine, mecholyl and pilocarpine. J. Invest. Dermatol. 24:545, 1955.
6. Aoki, T.: Cholinesterase activities associated with the sweat glands in the toe pads of the dog. Nature (Lond.) 202:1124, 1964.
7. Aoki, T.: Evidence for the discharge of cholinesterase into canine eccrine sweat. Nature (Lond.) 211:886, 1966.
8. Aoki, T.: Postnatal development of secretory function of sweat glands in the dog foot pads and cholinesterase activities associated with these glands. Tohoku J. Exp. Med. 110:173, 1973.
9. Bailey, C. S., et al.: Cutaneous innervation of the thorax and abdomen of the dog. Am. J. Vet. Res. 45:1689, 1984.
10. Baker, B. B., et al.: Epidermal cell renewal in the dog. Am. J. Vet. Res. 34:93, 1973.
11. Baker, B. B., et al.: Epidermal cell renewal in dogs after clipping of the hair. Am. J. Vet. Res. 35:445, 1974.
12. Baker, B. B., and Maibach, H. I.: Epidermal cell renewal in seborrheic skin of dogs. Am. J. Vet. Res. 48:726, 1987.
13. Baker K. P.: Senile changes of dog skin. J. Small Anim. Pract. 8:49, 1967.
14. Baker, K. P.: Hair growth and replacement in the cat. Brit. Vet. J. 130:327, 1974.
15. Bell, M., and Montagna, W.: Innervation of sweat glands in horses and dogs. Brit. J. Dermatol. 86:160, 1972.

16. Braverman, I. M., et al.: A study of the veil cells around normal, diabetic, and aged cutaneous microvessels. J. Invest. Dermatol. 86:57, 1986.

17. Breathnach, S. M.: Do epidermotropic T cells exist in normal human skin? A re-evaluation of the SALT hypothesis. Brit. J. Dermatol. 115:389, 1986.

18. Breathnach, S. M., and Katz, S. I.: Cell-mediated immunity in cutaneous disease. Human Pathol. 17:161, 1986.

19. Butler W. F., and Wright, A. I.: Hair growth in the greyhound. J. Small Anim. Pract. 22:655, 1981.

20. Chastain, C. B., and Ganjam, V. K.: Clinical Endocrinology of Companion Animals. Lea & Febiger, Philadelphia, 1986.

21. Choi, K. L., and Saunder, D. N.: The role of Langerhans cells and keratinocytes in epidermal immunity. J. Leuk. Biol. 39:343, 1986.

22. Clark R. A. F.: Fibronectin and the skin. J. Invest. Dermatol. 81:475, 1983.

23. Comben, N.: Observations on the mode of growth of the hair of the dog. Brit. Vet. J. 107:231, 1951.

24. Cotton, D. W. K., and van Hasselt, P.: Sweating on the hairy surface of the beagle. J. Invest. Dermatol. 59:313, 1972.

25. Cotton, D. W. K., et al.: Nature of the sweat glands in the hairy skin of the Beagle. Dermatologica 150:75, 1975.

26. Cox, H. U., et al.: Distribution of staphylococcal species on clinically healthy cats. Am. J. Vet. Res. 46:1824, 1985.

27. Craig, J. A., et al.: A practical guide to clinical oncology—4: chemotherapy and immunotherapy. Vet. Med. 81:226, 1986.

28. Daroczy, J.: The structure and dynamic function of the dermal lymphatic capillaries. Brit. J. Dermatol. 109:99, 1983.

29. Denman, S. T.: A review of pruritus. J. Am. Acad. Dermatol. 14:473, 1986.

30. Deslypere, J. P., et al.: Fat tissue: a steroid reservoir and site of steroid metabolism. J. Clin. Endocrinol. Metab. 61:564, 1985.

31. Devriese, L. A., et al.: Identification and characterization of staphylococci isolated from cats. Vet. Microbiol. 9:279, 1984.

32. Draize, H. H.: The determination of the pH of the skin of man and common laboratory animals. J. Invest. Dermatol. 5:77, 1942.

33. El Baze, P., et al.: Distribution of polyamines in human epidermis. Brit. J. Dermatol. 22:393, 1985.

34. Evans, H. E., and Christensen, G. C.: Miller's Anatomy of the Dog. 2nd ed. W. B. Saunders Company, Philadelphia, 1979.

35. Feinman, J. M.: The Rex cat: a mutation for the masses. VM/SAC 78:1717, 1983.

36. Fenske, N. A., and Lober, C. W.: Structural and functional changes of normal aging skin. J. Am. Acad. Dermatol. 15:571, 1986.

37. Fitzpatrick, T. B., et al.: Biology and Diseases of Dermal Pigmentation. University of Tokyo Press, Tokyo, 1981.

38. Fjellner, B., et al.: Pruritus during standardized mental stress. Acta Derm. Venereol. (Stockh) 65:199, 1985.

39. Ford, M. J.: Filaggrin. Int. J. Dermatol. 25:547, 1986.

40. Freinkel, R. K., and Traczyk, T. N.: Acid hydrolases of the epidermis: Subcellular localization and relationship to cornification. J. Invest. Dermatol. 80:441, 1983.

41. Garthwaite, G., et al.: Location of immunoglobulins and complement (C3) at the surface and within the skin of dogs. J. Comp. Pathol. 93:185, 1983.

42. Goldsmith, L. A. (ed.): Biochemistry and Physiology of Skin. Oxford Press, New York, 1983.

43. Goodell, E. M., et al.: Canine dendritic cells from peripheral blood and lymph nodes. Vet. Immunol. Immunopathol. 8:301, 1985.

44. Guaguere, E., et al.: Troubles de la pigmentation melanique en dermatologie des carnivores Iʳᵉ partie: elements de physiopathologie. Point Vet. 17:549, 1985.

45. Gunaratnam, P., and Wilkinson, G. T.: A study of normal hair growth in the dog. J. Small Anim. Pract. 24:445, 1983.

46. Hale, P. A.: Periodic hair shedding by a normal bitch. J. Small Anim. Pract. 23:345, 1982.

47. Halliwell, R. E. W.: Pathogenesis and treatment of pruritus. J. Am. Vet. Med. Assoc. 164:793, 1974.

48. Haloprin, K. M., et al.: Control of epidermal cell proliferation in vitro. Brit. J. Dermatol. 3:13, 1984.

49. Hekmatpanah, J.: Organization of tactile dermatomes, C_1 through L_4, in cat. J. Neurophysiol. 24:129, 1961.

50. Hellman, K.: Cholinesterase and amine oxidase in the skin: a histochemical investigation. J. Physiol. (London) 129:454, 1955.

51. Horton, J. J., et al.: An assessment of Langerhans cell quantification in tissue sections. J. Am. Acad. Dermatol. 11:591, 1984.

52. Imayama, S., and Urabe, H.: Pericytes on the dermal microvasculature of the rat skin. Anat. Embryol. 169:271, 1984.

53. Ito, M., and Hashimoto, K.: Trichohyaline granules in hair cortex. J. Invest. Dermatol. 79:392, 1982.

54. Iwabuchi, T.: General sweating on the hairy skin of the dog and its mechanisms. J. Invest. Dermatol. 49:61, 1967.

55. Iwasaki T.: An electron microscopic study on secretory process in canine apocrine sweat gland. Jap. J. Vet. Sci. 43:733, 1981.

56. Iwasaki, T.: Electron microscopy of the canine apocrine sweat duct. Jap. J. Vet. Sci. 45:739, 1983.

57. Jarrett, A.: The Physiology and Pathophysiology of the Skin I. Academic Press, New York, 1973.

58. Jarrett, A.: The Physiology and Pathophysiology of the Skin II. Academic Press, New York, 1973.

59. Jarrett, A.: The Physiology and Pathophysiology of the Skin III. Academic Press, New York, 1977.

60. Jarrett, A.: The Physiology and Pathophysiology of the Skin IV. Academic Press, New York, 1977.

61. Jarrett, A.: The Physiology and Pathology of the Skin V. Academic Press, New York, 1978.

62. Jarrett, A.: The Physiology and Pathophysiology of the Skin VI. Academic Press, New York, 1978.

63. Jarrett, A.: The Physiology and Pathophysiology of the Skin VII. Academic Press, New York, 1982.

64. Jenkinson, D. M., and Blackburn, P. A.: The distribution of nerves, monoamine oxidase and cholinesterase in the skin of the dog and cat. Res. Vet. Sci. 9:521, 1968.

65. Katz, S. I.: The epidermal basement membrane zone—structure, ontogeny, and role in disease. J. Am. Acad. Dermatol. 11:1025, 1984.

66. Katz, S. I.: The skin as an immunologic organ. A tribute to Marion B. Sulzberger. J. Am. Acad. Dermatol. 13:530, 1985.

67. King, L. E.: What does epidermal growth factor do and how does it do it? J. Invest. Dermatol. 84:165, 1985.

68. Kitchell, R. L., et al.: Electrophysiologic studies of cutaneous nerves of the thoracic limb of the dog. Am. J. Vet. Res. 41:61, 1980.

69. Klein, L. E., and Norlund, J. J.: Genetic basis of pigmentation and its disorders. Int. J. Dermatol. 10:621, 1981.

70. Kral, F., and Schwartzman, R. M.: Veterinary and Comparative Dermatology. J. B. Lippincott Company, Philadelphia, 1964.

71. Kripke, M. L.: Immunology and Photocarcinogenesis. New light on an old problem. J. Am. Acad. Dermatol. *14*:149, 1986.
72. Kuhn, R. A.: Organization of tactile dermatomes in cat and monkey. J. Neurophysiol. *16*:169, 1953.
73. Kuroki, T.: Possible functions of 12, 25-dihydroxy vitamin D_3, an active form of vitamin D_3, in the differentiation and development of skin. J. Invest. Dermatol. *84*:459, 1985.
74. Kwochka, K. W.: Qualitative and quantitative incidence of staphylococci on normal canine skin and haircoat: an investigation into the possibility of two different microbial populations. Proc. Annu. Meet. Am. Acad. Vet. Dermatol. and Am. Coll. Vet. Dermatol., 1986.
75. Kwochka, K. W.: Differential diagnosis of feline miliary dermatitis. Current Veterinary Therapy IX. W. B. Saunders Company, Philadelphia, 1986, p. 538.
76. Lavker, R. M., and Sun, T. T.: Heterogeneity in epidermal basal keratinocytes: Morphological and functional correlations. Science *215*:1239, 1982.
77. Lever, W. F., and Schaumburg-Lever, G.: Histopathology of the Skin VI. J. B. Lippincott Company, Philadelphia, 1983.
78. Levine, A., et al.: Cancer Cell. Vol. I. The Transformed Phenotype. Cold Spring Harbor Laboratory, New York, 1984.
79. Lindholm, J. S., et al.: Variation of skin surface lipid composition among mammals. Comp. Biochem. Physiol. *69B*:75, 1981.
80. Little, C. C.: The Inheritance of Coat Color in Dogs. Comstock Publishing Associates, Ithaca, 1957.
81. Lloyd, D. H., and Garthwaite, G.: Epidermal structure and surface topography of canine skin. Res. Vet. Sci. *33*:99, 1982.
82. Lovell, J. E., and Getty, R.: The hair follicle, epidermis, dermis, and skin glands of the dog. Am. J. Vet. Res. *18*:873, 1957.
83. Lyne, A. G., and Short, B. F.: Biology of the Skin and Hair Growth. American Elsevier Publishing Company, New York, 1965.
84. Marks, F., and Richter, K. H.: A request for a more serious approach to the chalone concept. Br. J. Dermatol. *3*:58, 1984.
85. Martin, J.: Pruritus. Int. J. Dermatol. *24*:634, 1985.
86. Meyer, W., and Neurand, K.: The distribution of enzymes in the epidermis of the domestic cat. Arch. Dermatol. Res. *260*:29, 1977.
87. Meyer, W., and Neurand, K.: Zur leuzinaminopeptidase-aktivitat in normaler und geschadigter katzenhaut. Zbl. Vet. Med. *24*:601, 1977.
88. Miller, M. E., et al.: Anatomy of the Dog. W. B. Saunders Company, Philadelphia, 1964.
89. Minor, R. R.: Collagen metabolism. Am. J. Pathol. *98*:227, 1980.
90. Montagna, W., and Parakkal, P. F.: The Structure and Function of the Skin III. Academic Press, New York, 1974.
91. Montagna, W.: Comparative anatomy and physiology of the skin. Arch. Dermatol. *96*:357, 1967.
92. Muller, G. H., et al.: Small Animal Dermatology III. W. B. Saunders Company, Philadelphia, 1983.
93. Nicolaides, N., et al.: The skin surface lipids of man compared with those of eighteen species of animals. J. Invest. Dermatol. *51*:83, 1968.
94. Neilsen, S. W.: Glands of the canine skin—morphology and distribution. Am. J. Vet. Res. *14*:448, 1953.
95. Nikkari, T.: Comparative chemistry of sebum. J. Invest. Dermatol. *62*:257, 1974.
96. Noble, W. C.: Microbiology of Human Skin II. Lloyd-Luke, London, 1981.
97. Noble, W. C.: Microbial Skin Disease: Its Epidemiology. Butler and Tanner, Ltd., London, 1983.
98. Ogawa, H., and Yoshike, T.: Keratin, keratinization, and biochemical aspects of dyskeratosis. Int. J. Dermatol. *23*:507, 1984.
99. Orentreich, N., and Selmanowitz, V. J.: Levels of biological functions with aging. Trans. N. Y. Acad. Sci. *31*:992, 1969.
100. Quaissi, M. A., and Capron, A.: Fibronectines: structures et fonctions. Ann. Inst. Pasteur Immunol. *136*:12, 1985.
101. Prieur, D. J., and Collier, L. L.: The Maltese dilution of cats. Feline Pract. *14*:23, 1984.
102. Prieur, D. J., and Collier, L. L.: Maltese dilution of domestic cat: a generalized cutaneous albinism lacking ocular involvement. J. Hered. *75*:41, 1984.
103. Prunieras, M.: Melanocytes, melanogenesis, and inflammation. Int. J. Dermatol. *25*:624, 1986.
104. Queinnec, B.: Nomenclatures des robes du chat. Rev. Med. Vet. *134*:349, 1983.
105. Robinson, R.: Genetics for Cat Breeders. Pergamon Press, Oxford, 1977.
106. Rook, A. J., and Walton, G. S.: Comparative Physiology and Pathology of the Skin. Blackwell Scientific Publications, Oxford, 1965.
107. Roy, W. E.: Role of the sweat gland in eczema in dogs. J. Am. Vet. Med. Assoc. *124*:51, 1954.
108. Ryan, T. J., et al.: Lymphatics of the skin. Neglected but important. Int. J. Dermatol. *25*:411, 1986.
109. Ryder, M. L.: Seasonal changes in the coat of the cat. Res. Vet. Sci. *21*:280, 1976.
110. Sandberg, L. B., et al.: Elastin structure, biosynthesis and its relationship to disease states. N. Engl. J. Med. *304*:566, 1981.
111. Schwarz, R., et al.: Die gesunde Haut von Hund und Katze. Kleintierpraxis *26*:395, 1981.
112. Schwarz, R., et al.: Micromorphology of the skin (epidermis, dermis, subcutis) of the dog. Onderstepoort J. Vet. Res. *46*:105, 1979.
113. Schwarz, W., et al.: Cyclic nucleotides in human epidermis—diurnal variations. J. Invest. Dermatol. *82*:119, 1984.
114. Scott, D. W.: Feline dermatology 1900—1978: a monograph. J. Am. Anim. Hosp. Assoc. *16*:331, 1980.
115. Scott, D. W.: Feline dermatology 1979—1982: introspective retrospections. J. Am. Anim. Hosp. Assoc. *20*:537, 1984.
116. Scott, D. W., and Buerger, R. G.: Nonsteroidal anti-inflammatory agents in the management of canine pruritus. J. Am. Anim. Hosp. Assoc. (In press.)
117. Scott, D. W.: Feline dermatology 1983—1985: "The Secret Sits." J. Am. Anim. Hosp. Assoc. *23*:255, 1987.
118. Scott, D. W.: Unpublished observations.
119. Seaman, W. J., and Chang, S. H.: Dermal perifollicular mineralization of toy poodle bitches. Vet. Pathol. *21*:122, 1984.
120. Sharaf, D. M., et al.: Skin surface lipids of the dog. Lipids *12*:786, 1977.
121. Sherertz, E. C.: Misuse of hair analysis as a diagnostic tool. Arch. Dermatol. *121*:1504, 1985.
122. Simon, M., and Green, H.: Enzymatic cross-linking of involucrin and other proteins by keratinocyte particulates in vitro. Cell *40*:677, 1985.
123. Spearman, R. I. C.: The Integument. Cambridge University Press, London, 1973.
124. Strickland, J. H., and Calhoun, M. L.: The integumentary system of the cat. Am. J. Vet. Res. *24*:1018, 1963.
125. Takahashi, Y.: Functional activity of the eccrine sweat glands in the toe-pads of the dog. Tohoku J. Exp. Med. *83*:205, 1964.

126. Thacher, S. M., and Rice, R. H.: Keratinocyte-specific transglutaminase of cultured human epidermal cells. Relation to cross-linked envelope formation and terminal differentiation. Cell 40: 685, 1985.

126a. Thoday, A. J., and Friedmann, P. S.: Scientific Basis of Dermatology. A Physiological Aproach. Churchill Livingstone, New York, 1986.

127. Thomsett, L. R.: Structure of canine skin. Brit. Vet. J. 142:116, 1986.

128. Van De Kerhof, P. C. M., and Van Erp, P. E. J.: Epidermal calmodulin and skin disease. Int. J. Dermatol. 24:507, 1985.

129. Van Scott, E. J., and Yu, R. J.: Hyperkeratinization, corneocyte cohesion, and alpha hydroxy acids. J. Am. Acad. Dermatol. 11:867, 1984.

130. Wallengren, J., et al.: Substance P and vasoactive intestinal peptide in bullous and inflammatory skin disease. Acta Derm. Venereol. (Stockh) 66:23, 1986.

131. Webb, A. J., and Calhoun, M. L.: The microscopic anatomy of the skin of mongrel dogs. Am. J. Vet. Res. 15:274, 1954.

132. Weber, L., et al.: Collagen-type distribution and macromolecular organization of connective tissue in different layers of human skin. J. Invest. Dermatol. 82:156, 1984.

133. Whalen, L. R., and Kitchell, R. L.: Electrophysiologic studies of the cutaneous nerves of the head of the dog. Am. J. Vet. Res. 44:615, 1983.

134. Wheatley, V. R., and Sher, D. W.: Studies of the lipids of dog skin. I. The chemical composition of dog skin lipids. J. Invest. Dermatol. 36:169, 1961.

135. Wheatley, V. R., et al.: Studies of the lipids of dog skin. II. Observations of the lipid metabolism of perfused surviving dog skin. J. Invest. Dermatol. 36:237, 1961.

136. White, S. D., et al.: Occurrence of Staphylococcus aureus on the clinically normal canine haircoat. Am. J. Vet. Res. 44:332, 1983.

137. Wilkinson, J. E., et al.: Long-term cultivation of canine keratinocytes. J. Invest. Dermatol. 88:202, 1987.

138. Winkelmann, R. K., and Schmit, R. W.: Cholinesterase in the skin of the rat, dog, cat, guinea pig and rabbit. J. Invest. Dermatol. 33:185, 1959.

139. Winstanley, E. W.: The rate of mitotic division in regenerating epithelium in the dog. Res. Vet. Sci. 18:144, 1975.

140. Wright, M., and Walter, S.: The Book of the Cat. Summit Books, New York, 1980.

141. Yaar, M., et al.: Effects of alpha and beta interferons on cultured human keratinocytes. J. Invest. Dermatol. 85:70, 1985.

142. Yager, J. A., and Scott, D. W.: The skin and appendages. Pathology of Domestic Animals III. Vol. I. Academic Press, New York, 1985, p. 407.

143. Zlotkin, S. H.: Hair analysis. A useful tool or a waste of money? Int. J. Dermatol. 24:161, 1985.

2

Dermatohistopathology

Dermatohistopathology is a highly developed, vibrant, rapidly progressing, and invaluable science in human medicine. In fact, in 1974 the American Boards of Dermatology and Pathology began examining candidates and awarding Certificates of Special Competence in Dermatopathology. Most of the sophistication in human dermatohistopathology has come about through the efforts of dermatologists who have a special interest in pathology. Such pioneers of the field include Gustav Simon, Paul G. Unna, Jean Darier, Hamilton Montgomery, Walter F. Lever, Herman Pinkus, James H. Graham, J. A. Milne, A. Bernard Ackerman, and Robert W. Goltz.

Dermatohistopathology has only recently received significant attention in veterinary dermatology. This has largely been due to the interest of clinical veterinary dermatologists in studying all aspects of animal skin disease. As a result of this increasing interest in dermatohistopathology, we have witnessed an explosion in the number of "new" skin diseases described in dogs and cats since 1975, e.g., pemphigus vulgaris, pemphigus vegetans, pemphigus foliaceus, pemphigus erythematosus, bullous pemphigoid, systemic lupus erythematosus, discoid lupus erythematosus, toxic epidermal necrolysis, subcorneal pustular dermatosis, sterile eosinophilic pustulosis, erythema multiforme, epidermolysis bullosa, dermatomyositis, morphea, granulomatous sebaceous adenitis, vitamin A–responsive dermatosis, hepatocutaneous syndrome, xanthomatosis, staphylococcal hypersensitivity, leukocytoclastic vasculitis, hyposomatotropism in the mature dog, canine eosinophilic granuloma, organoid nevus, fibrous histiocytoma, malignant histiocytosis, clear cell hidradenoma, tricholemmoma, collagenous nevus, cutaneous phlebectasia, zinc-responsive dermatosis, and inverted follicular keratosis.

The clinical veterinary dermatologist is in a unique and perfect position to examine the historical, physical, laboratory, therapeutic, and prognostic features of animal skin diseases and to establish meaningful histopathologic correlates. As more veterinary dermatologists are trained and certified, we can expect an increasing recognition of "new" skin diseases and a more thorough appreciation of the therapeutic and prognostic value, as well as diagnostic value, of dermatohistopathology in veterinary medicine.

Artifacts in Dermatohistopathology

Even the best dermatohistopathologist cannot read an inadequate, poorly preserved, poorly fixed, or poorly produced specimen. Numerous artifacts can be produced by the improper selection, preparation, taking, handling, fixation, and processing of skin biopsies. It is very important that the clinician and pathologist be cognizant of these potentially disastrous distortions of the truth.

1. Artifacts due to *improper selection* include excoriations and other physicochemical effects (e.g., maceration, inflammation, necrosis, and staining abnormalities caused by topical medicaments).

2. Artifacts due to *improper preparation* include inflammation, staining abnormalities, and removal of surface pathology (surgical scrubbing and use of antiseptics), as well as collagen separation (pseudoedema) and pseudosinus formation (intradermal injection of local anesthetic).

3. Artifacts due to *improper taking and handling* include pseudovesicles, pseudoclefts and shearing (dull punch or poor technique); pseudopapillomas or pseudonodules, pseudosclerosis, pseudosinuses, pseudocysts, and lobules of sebaceous glands within hair follicles or on the skin surface or both (squeeze artifacts due to intervention with forceps); marked dehydration, elongation, and polarization of cells and cell nuclei (electrodesiccation); and intercellular edema, clefts, and vesicles (friction).

4. Artifacts due to *improper fixation and processing* include dermoepidermal separation, intracellular edema, and fractures (autolysis); curling and folding (failure to use wooden or cardboard "splints"); intracellular edema, vacuolar alteration, and multinucleated epidermal giant cells (freezing); "formalin pigment" in blood vessels and extravascular phagocytes (use of nonbuffered formalin); hardening, shrinkage, and loss of cellular detail (alcohol in fixative); poor staining and "soft," easily displaced and distorted tissue (Bouin's solution); thick, fragmented sections (inadequate dehydration during tissue processing); pseudoacanthosis (tangential sections associated with poor orientation of specimen); and dermoepidermal separation and displacement of dermal tissues into epidermis (cutting sections *from* dermis *to* epidermis).

The Vocabulary of Dermatohistopathology

Dermatohistopathology has a specialized vocabulary, because many of the histopathologic changes that occur are unique to the skin. Unfortunately, as is true of most sciences, the dermatologic and general medical literatures abound with confusing and sometimes inappropriate dermatohistopathologic terms. The following is a definition of terms, based on an amalgamation of such considerations as precision of definition, descriptive value, popular usage, and historical precedent, and a discussion of their diagnostic significance in dermatohistopathology.

EPIDERMAL CHANGES

Hyperkeratosis

Hyperkeratosis is an increased thickness of the stratum corneum and may be *absolute* (an actual increase in thickness—the most common situation) or *relative* (an apparent increase due to thinning of the underlying epidermis—a rare situation). The types of hyperkeratosis are further specified by the adjectives *orthokeratotic* (anuclear, Fig. 2:1) and *parakeratotic* (nucleated, Fig. 2:2). Orthokeratotic and parakeratotic hyperkeratoses are commonly, but less precisely,

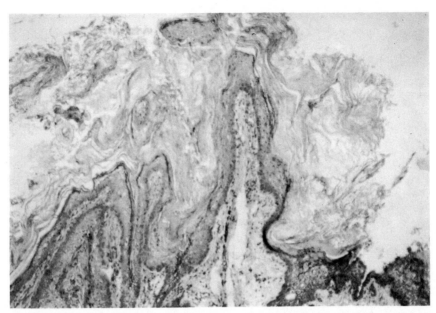

Figure 2:1. Orthokeratotic hyperkeratosis represents an anuclear increase in the horny layer. It may be caused by excessive production of keratin (callus) or by excessive retention of keratin (ichthyosis). The illustration shows extreme orthokeratotic hyperkeratosis (with papillomatosis) from a case of canine ichthyosis.

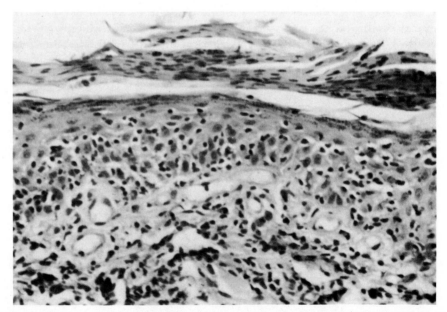

Figure 2:2. Parakeratotic hyperkeratosis is a state of imperfect or abnormal keratinization and is characterized by retention of nuclei in the stratum corneum or the outer root sheath. It is often associated with rapid cell turnover and is seen in a case of seborrhea (above). This figure also demonstrates prominent intercellular edema or "spongiosis."

referred to as hyperkeratosis and parakeratosis, respectively. Other adjectives commonly used to describe further the nature of hyperkeratosis include *basket-weave* (e.g., dermatophytosis and endocrinopathic conditions), *compact* (e.g., lichenoid dermatoses and cutaneous horns), and *laminated* (e.g., ichthyosis).

Orthokeratotic and parakeratotic hyperkeratosis may be seen as alternating layers in the stratum corneum. This observation implies episodic changes in epidermopoiesis. If the changes are generalized, the lesions appear as horizontal layers. If the changes are focal, the lesion is a vertical defect in the stratum corneum. Orthokeratotic and parakeratotic hyperkeratosis are common, non-diagnostic findings in virtually any chronic dermatosis. They simply imply altered epidermopoiesis, whether inflammatory, hormonal, neoplastic, or developmental in nature. However, *diffuse* parakeratotic hyperkeratosis is suggestive of zinc-responsive dermatosis, some vitamin A–responsive dermatoses, thallotoxicosis, generic dog food dermatosis, and the hepatocutaneous syndrome.

Hypokeratosis

The decreased thickness of the stratum corneum, called hypokeratosis, is much less common than hyperkeratosis and reflects an exceptionally rapid epidermal turnover time or decreased cohesion, or both, between cells of the stratum corneum. Hypokeratosis may be found in seborrheic and other exfoliative skin disorders. It may also be produced by excessive surgical preparation of the biopsy site or by friction and maceration in intertriginous areas.

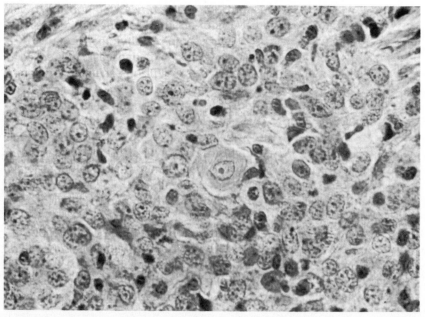

Figure 2:3. Dyskeratosis is abnormal or imperfect keratinization of epidermal cells or adnexal keratinocytes. The change may be seen in benign or malignant conditions. A large dyskeratotic cell in the center of anaplastic carcinoma cells (malignant dyskeratosis) is illustrated. (Photomicrograph courtesy J. D. Conroy.)

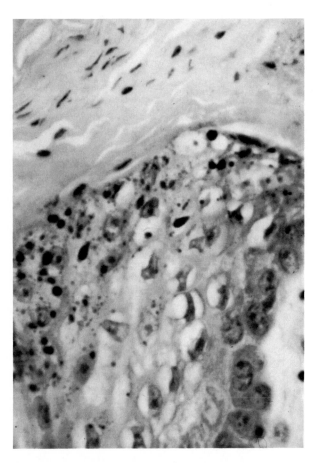

Figure 2:4. Hypergranulosis (keratohyaline granules) is shown as a prominent and thickened granular layer. This is seen in disorders characterized by orthokeratotic hyperkeratosis, such as canine ichthyosis. This figure also shows intracellular edema.

Dyskeratosis

Dyskeratosis is a premature and faulty keratinization of individual cells (Fig. 2:3). The term is also used, although less commonly, to indicate a general fault in the keratinization process and thus in the state of the epidermis as a whole. Dyskeratotic cells are characterized by eosinophilic, swollen cytoplasm and condensed, dark-staining nuclei. Such cells are often difficult to distinguish from *necrotic* keratinocytes on light microscopic examination. The judgment usually depends on whether the rest of the epithelium is thought to be keratinizing or necrosing.

This defect in keratinization may be seen in a number of inflammatory dermatoses (especially the lichenoid dermatoses, the pemphigus complex, zinc-responsive dermatosis, some vitamin A–responsive dermatoses, and generic dog food dermatosis) and neoplastic dermatoses (especially papilloma, squamous cell carcinoma, and keratoacanthoma).

Hypergranulosis and Hypogranulosis

The terms hypergranulosis and hypogranulosis indicate, respectively, an increase and a decrease in the thickness of the stratum granulosum. Both entities are common and nondiagnostic. *Hyper*granulosis may be seen in any dermatosis in which there is epidermal hyperplasia and orthokeratotic hyperkeratosis (Fig. 2:4). *Hypo*granulosis is often seen in dermatoses in which there is parakeratotic hyperkeratosis.

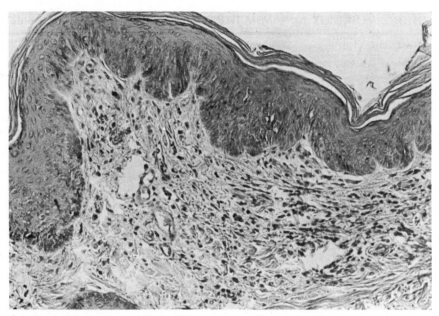

Figure 2:5. Hyperplasia is a thickening of the noncornified epidermis. The thickening is due to increased layers of keratinocytes and may be seen in the surface epidermis or in adnexal keratinocytes. It is present in chronic dermatoses (acanthosis nigricans) or inflammatory processes (chronic flea bite hypersensitivity). The latter is illustrated. Note hyperplasia, rete ridges, a superficial inflammatory infiltrate, and capillary dilatation.

Hyperplasia

An increased thickness of the noncornified epidermis due to an increased number of epidermal cells (Fig. 2:5) is called hyperplasia. The term *acanthosis* is often used interchangeably with hyperplasia. However, acanthosis specifically indicates an increased thickness of the stratum spinosum and may be due to hyperplasia (*true* acanthosis, which is the most common, or hypertrophy or

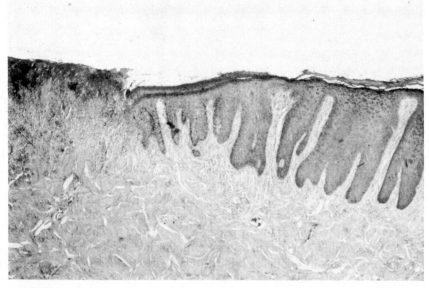

Figure 2:6. Elongated rete ridges are a reaction to chronic irritation and a form of hyperplasia. In this case of acral lick dermatitis, the ulcerated area is to the left. There is fibroplasia, a chronic inflammatory infiltrate, and downward proliferation of the epidermis resulting in rete ridge formation. (Photomicrograph courtesy J. D. Conroy.)

*pseudo*acanthosis, which is uncommon). Epidermal hyperplasia is often accompanied by *rete ridge formation* (irregular hyperplasia resulting in "pegs" of epidermis that appear to project downward into the underlying dermis) (Fig. 2:6). Rete ridges are *not* found in normal *haired* skin of dogs and cats.

The following adjectives further specify the types of epidermal hyperplasia (Fig. 2:7): (1) *irregular*—uneven, elongated, pointed rete ridges with an obliterated or preserved rete-papilla configuration, (2) *regular (psoriasiform)*—more or less evenly elongated rete ridges with preservation of the rete-papillae config-

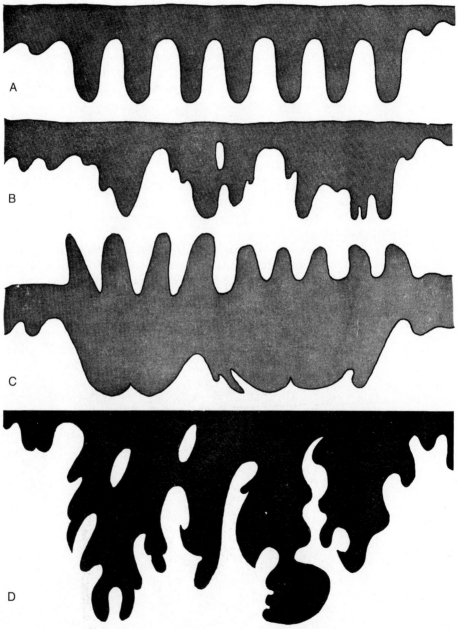

Figure 2:7. Patterns of epidermal hyperplasia: *A*, regular; *B*, irregular; *C*, papillated; *D*, pseudocarcinomatous. (From Ackerman, A. B.: Histologic Diagnosis of Inflammatory Diseases. Lea & Febiger, Philadelphia, 1978.)

uration; (3) *papillated*—digitate projections of the epidermis above the skin surface; and (4) *pseudocarcinomatous (pseudoepitheliomatous)*—extreme, irregular hyperplasia, which may include increased mitoses, squamous eddies, and horn pearls, thus resembling squamous cell carcinoma; although cellular atypia is absent, and the basement membrane zone is not breached (Fig. 2:8). These four forms of epidermal hyperplasia may be seen in various combinations in the same specimen.

Epidermal hyperplasia is a common, nondiagnostic feature of virtually any chronic inflammatory process, and the four types of the condition, for the most part, are useful descriptive terms that have little specific diagnostic significance. Pseudocarcinomatous hyperplasia is most commonly associated with underlying dermal suppurative, granulomatous, or neoplastic processes and with chronic ulcers. Papillated hyperplasia is most commonly seen with neoplasia, callosities, epidermal nevi, seborrheic dermatitis, and zinc-responsive dermatosis. Psoriasiform hyperplasia is most commonly seen with mycosis fungoides and psoriasiform lichenoid dermatosis of springer spaniels.

Hypoplasia and Atrophy

Hypoplasia is a decreased thickness of the noncornified epidermis due to a decrease in the number of cells. *Atrophy* is a decreased thickness of the noncornified epidermis due to a decrease in the size of cells (Fig. 2:9). An early sign of epidermal hypoplasia or atrophy is the loss of the rete ridges in areas of skin where they are normally present (i.e., in the nonhaired skin of dogs and cats).

Epidermal hypoplasia and atrophy are uncommon in skin diseases of dogs and cats but are occasionally seen with hormonal (hyperadrenocorticism, hypothyroidism), developmental (cutaneous asthenia), and inflammatory (discoid lupus erythematosus) dermatoses.

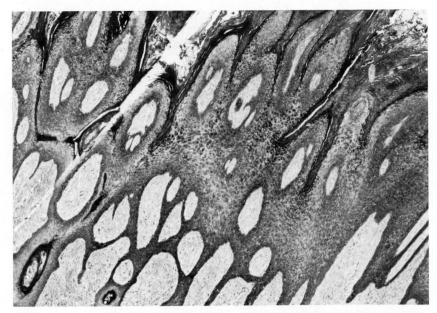

Figure 2:8. Pseudocarcinomatous epidermal hyperplasia in a dog with acral lick dermatitis.

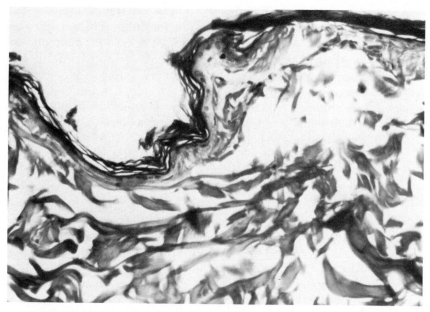

Figure 2:9. Epidermal atrophy in a dog with testosterone-responsive dermatosis.

Necrosis

The term *necrosis* refers to the death of cells or tissues in a living organism and is judged to be present primarily on the basis of nuclear morphology. *Necrolysis* is often used synonymously with necrosis but actually implies a *separation* of tissue due to death of cells (e.g., epidermal necrolysis). Nuclear changes indicative of necrosis include *karyorrhexis* (nuclear fragmentation), *pyknosis* (nuclear shrinkage and consequent hyperchromasia), and *karyolysis* (nuclear "ghosts"). With all three necrotic nuclear changes, individual keratinocytes are characterized by loss of intercellular bridges, with resultant rounding of the cell, and a normal-sized or swollen eosinophilic cytoplasm. Necrosis is further specified by the adjectives *coagulation* (cell outlines preserved but cell detail lost) or *caseation* (complete loss of all structural details, the tissue being replaced by a granular material containing nuclear debris).

Epidermal necrosis may be focal as a result of drug eruptions, microbial infections, or lichenoid dermatoses or may be generalized as a result of physicochemical trauma (primary irritant contact dermatitis, burns, thallotoxicosis), interference with blood supply (vasculitis, thromboembolism, subepidermal bullae, dense subepidermal cellular infiltrates), or an immunologic mechanism (toxic epidermal necrolysis, erythema multiforme). A unique type of epidermal necrosis has been described in graft-versus-host disease in humans and dogs. This *satellite cell necrosis* (satellitosis) is characterized by individual keratinocyte necrosis in association with contiguous ("satellite") lymphoid cells. Satellitosis is also seen in erythema multiforme, lupus erythematosus, and other lichenoid dermatoses.

Intercellular Edema

Intercellular edema *(spongiosis)* of the epidermis is characterized by a widening of the intercellular spaces with accentuation of the intercellular bridges, giving the involved epidermis a "spongy" appearance (Fig. 2:10). Severe intercellular edema may lead to rupture of the intercellular bridges and the formation of *spongiotic vesicles* within the epidermis. Severe spongiotic vesicle formation may, in turn, "blow out" the basement membrane zone in some areas, giving the appearance of *sub*epidermal vesicles. Intercellular edema is a common, nondiagnostic feature of any acute or subacute inflammatory dermatosis. Diffuse spongiosis, which also involves the hair follicle outer root sheath, may be seen with feline eosinophilic plaque and zinc-responsive dermatoses. Spongiosis of the upper one-half of the epidermis, which is overlayed by marked diffuse parakeratosis, is seen in the hepatocutaneous syndrome.

Intracellular Edema

Intracellular edema (hydropic degeneration, vacuolar degeneration, ballooning degeneration) of the epidermis is characterized by increased size, cytoplasmic pallor, and displacement of the nucleus to the periphery of affected cells (see Fig. 2:4). Severe intracellular edema may result in *reticular degeneration* and intraepidermal vesicles.

Intracellular edema is a common, nondiagnostic feature of any acute or subacute inflammatory dermatosis. Caution must be exercised not to confuse intracellular edema with freezing artifact, delayed fixation artifact, or the intracellular accumulation of glycogen seen in the outer root sheath of normal hair follicles and secondary to epidermal injury.

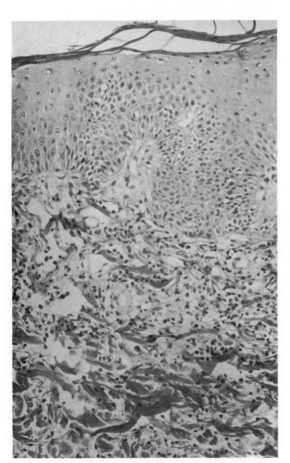

Figure 2:10. Intercellular edema (spongiosis) is edema between keratinocytes. This causes increased distance between individual cells. The illustration is from a case of seborrhea with prominent spongiosis. Also evident are hyperplasia, parakeratotic hyperkeratosis, and a superficial inflammatory infiltrate in the dermis. (Photomicrograph courtesy J. D. Conroy.)

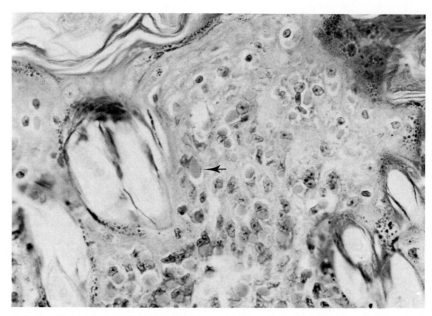

Figure 2:11. Hyperplasia and ballooning degeneration of the epidermis and intracytoplasmic inclusions (arrow) in a cat with feline poxvirus infection.

Ballooning Degeneration

Ballooning (koilocytosis) degeneration is a specific type of degenerative change seen in epidermal cells and characterized by swollen eosinophilic cytoplasm without vacuolization, by enlarged or condensed and occasionally multiple nuclei, and by a loss of cohesion resulting in acantholysis (Fig. 2:11). Ballooning degeneration is a specific feature of viral infections.

Reticular Degeneration

This type of degeneration is caused by severe intracellular edema of epidermal cells in which the cells burst, resulting in multilocular intraepidermal vesicles in which septae are formed by resistant cell walls. It may be seen with any acute or subacute inflammatory dermatosis.

Hydropic Degeneration of Basal Cells

Hydropic degeneration (liquefaction degeneration, vacuolar alteration) of the basal epidermal cells is a term used to describe intracellular edema restricted to cells of the stratum basale (Fig. 2:12). This process may also affect the basal cells of the outer root sheath of hair follicles. Hydropic degeneration of basal cells is usually focal but, if severe and extensive, may result in intrabasal or subepidermal clefts or vesicles owing to dermoepidermal separation. Hydropic degeneration of basal cells is an uncommon finding and is usually associated with lichenoid dermatoses, drug eruptions, lupus erythematosus, toxic epidermal necrolysis, erythema multiforme, dermatomyositis, and epidermolysis bullosa simplex.

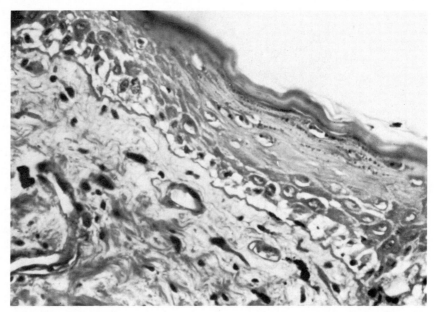

Figure 2:12. Hydropic degeneration of epidermal basal cells in a dog with epidermolysis bullosa simplex. (From Scott, D. W., and Schultz, R. D.: Epidermolysis bullosa simplex in the collie dog. J.A.V.M.A., *171*:721, 1977.)

Acantholysis

A loss of cohesion between epidermal cells, resulting in intraepidermal clefts, vesicles, and bullae (Fig. 2:13), is known as acantholysis (dyshesion, desmolysis, desmorrhexis). Free epidermal cells in the vesicles are called acanthocytes (Fig. 2:14). This process may also involve the outer root sheath of hair follicles and

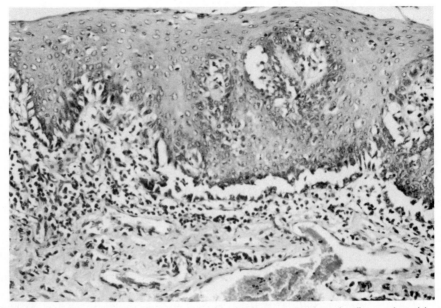

Figure 2:13. Acantholysis indicates a loss of cohesion between epidermal cells or adnexal keratinocytes or both that is due to degeneration or faulty formation of intercellular bridges (desmosomes). This leads to intraepidermal clefts, lacunae, vesicles, and bullae. It is seen above in a case of canine pemphigus vulgaris. This illustrates a suprabasilar cleft and intraepidermal vesicles containing acantholytic cells. (Photomicrograph courtesy A. A. Stannard.)

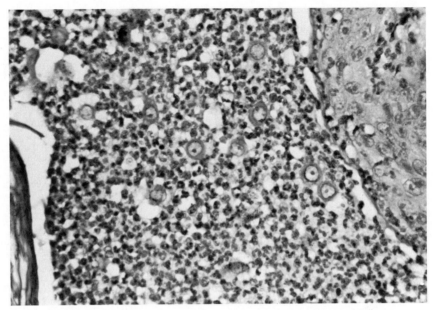

Figure 2:14. Acantholytic cells from a case of canine pemphigus foliaceus.

glandular ductal epithelium. Acantholysis is further specified by reference to the level at which it occurs, i.e., *subcorneal, intragranular, intraepidermal,* or *suprabasilar*.

Acantholysis may be caused by severe spongiosis (any acute or subacute inflammatory dermatosis), ballooning degeneration (viral infection), proteolytic enzymes released by neutrophils (bacterial and fungal dermatoses, subcorneal pustular dermatosis), autoantibodies against intercellular cement substance (pemphigus complex), developmental defects, and neoplastic transformation (squamous cell carcinoma, actinic keratosis).

Exocytosis

The term exocytosis refers to the migration of inflammatory cells or erythrocytes, or both, through the intercellular spaces of the epidermis (Fig. 2:15). Exocytosis of inflammatory cells is a common, nondiagnostic feature of any inflammatory dermatosis. Exocytosis of erythrocytes implies purpura (e.g., vasculitis, coagulation defect). When the condition involves eosinophils in combination with spongiosis, it is often referred to as "eosinophilic spongiosis" and may be seen in ectoparasitism, pemphigus, pemphigoid, sterile eosinophilic pustulosis, eosinophilic plaque, eosinophilic granuloma, and hypereosinophilic syndrome.

Clefts

The slitlike spaces known as clefts (lacunae), which do not contain fluid, occur within the epidermis or at the dermoepidermal junction. Clefts may be caused by acantholysis or hydropic degeneration of basal cells (Max Joseph spaces). However, they may also be caused by mechanical trauma and tissue retraction associated with the taking, fixation, and processing of biopsy specimens.

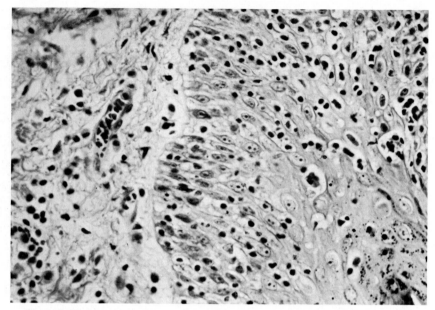

Figure 2:15. Exocytosis of leukocytes through the epidermis in a dog with scabies.

Microvesicles, Vesicles, and Bullae

Microvesicles (Fig. 2:16), vesicles, and bullae are microscopic and macroscopic, fluid-filled, relatively acellular spaces within or below the epidermis. Such lesions are often loosely referred to as *blisters*. These lesions may be caused by severe intercellular or intracellular edema, ballooning degeneration, acantholysis, hydropic degeneration of basal cells, subepidermal edema, or other factors resulting in dermoepidermal separation (e.g., the autoantibodies in bullous pemphigoid). Microvesicles, vesicles, and bullae may thus be further

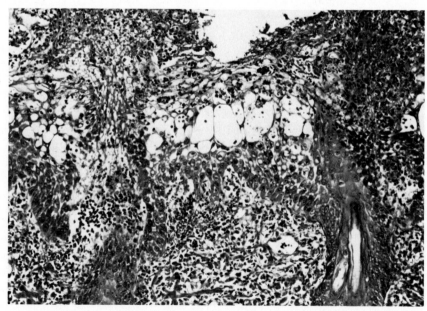

Figure 2:16. Epidermal microvesicles in a cat with eosinophilic plaque.

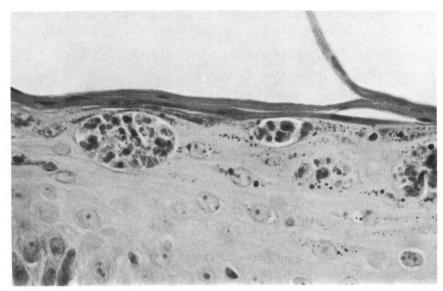

Figure 2:17. Microabscesses are observed in many dermatoses. This illustrates microabscesses containing many eosinophils located within the epidermis. (Photomicrograph courtesy J. D. Conroy.)

described by their location as subcorneal, intragranular, intraepidermal, suprabasilar, intrabasal, or subepidermal. When these lesions contain larger numbers of inflammatory cells, they may be referred to as *vesicopustules*.

Microabscesses and Pustules

Microabscesses and pustules are microscopic or macroscopic intraepidermal and subepidermal cavities filled with inflammatory cells (Fig. 2:17), which can be further described as follows, on the basis of location and cell type: (1) *Spongiform pustule of Kogoj* (Fig. 2:18)—a multilocular accumulation of neutrophils within and between keratinocytes, especially those of the stratum granulosum and stratum spinosum, in which cell boundaries form a spongelike network. It is seen in microbial infections. (2) *Munro's microabscess* (Fig. 2:19)—a small, desiccated accumulation of neutrophils within or below the stratum corneum, which is seen in microbial infections and seborrheic disorders. (3) *Pautrier's microabscess* (Fig. 2:20)—a small, focal accumulation of abnormal lymphoid cells, which is seen in epitheliotropic lymphomas. (4) *Eosinophilic microabscess*—a lesion seen in ectoparasitism, eosinophilic granuloma, eosinophilic folliculitis, sterile eosinophilic pustulosis, bullous pemphigoid, and the pemphigus complex. (5) *Subcorneal microabscesses and pustules*—subcorneal accumulations, predominantly composed of neurophils, that are seen in microbial infections, subcorneal pustular dermatosis, linear IgA dermatosis, pemphigus foliaceus and erythematosus, and systemic lupus erythematosus.

Hyperpigmentation

Hyperpigmentation (hypermelanosis) refers to excessive amounts of melanin deposited within the epidermis and, often, concurrently in dermal melanophages. Hyperpigmentation may be focal or diffuse and may be confined to

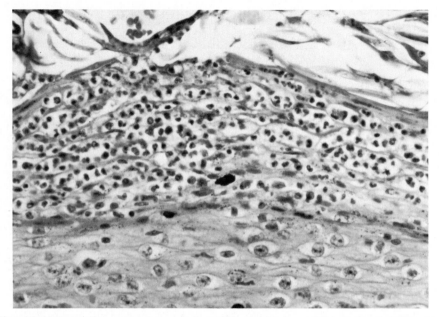

Figure 2:18. Spongiform microabscess in the epidermis of a dog with staphylococcal folliculitis.

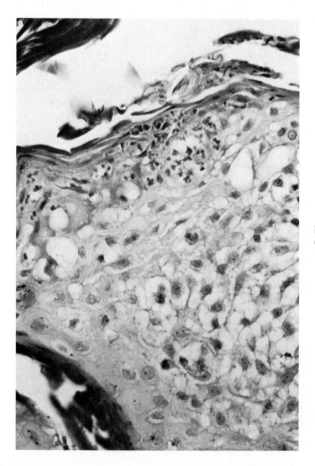

Figure 2:19. Munro's microabscess in the superficial epidermis of a dog with seborrheic dermatitis.

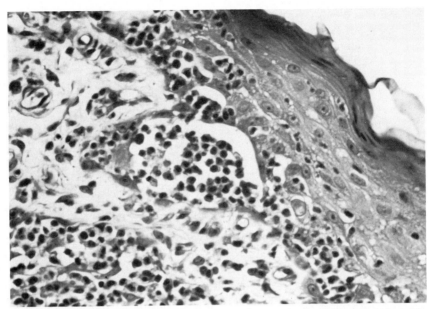

Figure 2:20. Pautrier's microabscess in the lower epidermis of a dog with mycosis fungoides.

the stratum basale or present throughout all epidermal layers (Fig. 2:21). It is a common, nondiagnostic finding in chronic inflammatory and hormonal dermatoses as well as in some developmental and neoplastic disorders. Hyperpigmentation must always be cautiously assessed with regard to the patient's *normal* pigmentation.

Hypopigmentation

Hypopigmentation (hypomelanosis) refers to decreased amounts of melanin in the epidermis. The condition may be associated with congenital or acquired idiopathic defects in melanization (e.g., leukoderma, vitiligo), toxic effects of

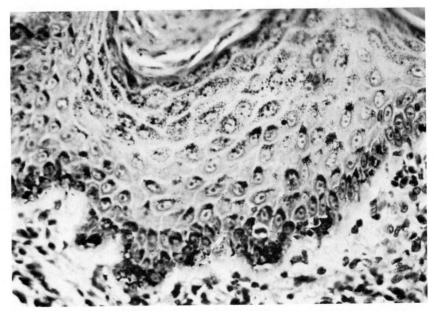

Figure 2:21. Epidermal melanosis (hyperpigmentation) in a dog with acanthosis nigricans.

certain chemicals on melanocytes (e.g., monobenzyl ether of dihydroquinone in rubbers and plastics), inflammatory disorders that affect melanization or destroy melanocytes, hormonal disorders, and dermatoses featuring hydropic degeneration of basal cells (e.g., lupus erythematosus). In the hypopigmented dermatoses associated with hydropic degeneration of basal cells, the underlying superficial dermis usually reveals *pigmentary incontinence*.

Crust

The consolidated, desiccated surface mass called crust is composed of varying combinations of keratin, serum, cellular debris, and often microorganisms. Crusts are further described on the basis of their composition: (1) *serous*—mostly serum (Fig. 2:22), (2) *hemorrhagic*—mostly blood, (3) *cellular*—mostly inflammatory cells, (4) *serocellular* (exudative)—a mixture of serum and inflammatory cells, and (5) *palisading*—alternating horizontal rows of orthokeratotic-to-parakeratotic hyperkeratosis and pus (e.g., dermatophilosis, dermatophytosis).

Crusts merely indicate a prior exudative process and are rarely of diagnostic significance. However, crusts should always be closely scrutinized, because they may contain the following important diagnostic clues: (1) dermatophyte spores and hyphae, (2) the filaments and coccoid elements of *Dermatophilus congolensis*, and (3) large numbers of acantholytic keratinocytes (pemphigus complex). Bacteria, and bacterial colonies, are common inhabitants of surface debris and are of no diagnostic significance.

Dells

These small depressions or hollows in the surface of the epidermis are usually associated with focal epidermal atrophy and orthokeratotic hyperkeratosis. Dells may be seen in lichenoid dermatoses, especially in lupus erythematosus.

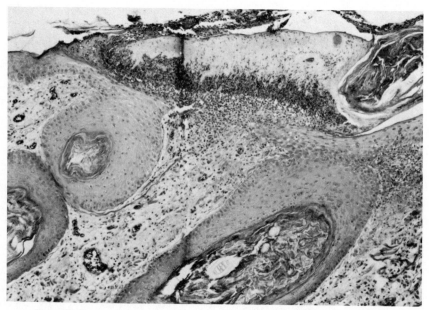

Figure 2:22. Serocellular crust in a cat with primary irritant contact dermatitis.

Epidermal Collarette

The term epidermal collarette refers to the formation of elongated, hyperplastic rete ridges at the lateral margins of a pathologic process that appear to curve inward toward the center of the lesion. Epidermal collarettes may be seen with neoplastic, granulomatous, and suppurative dermatoses.

Horn Cysts, Pseudohorn Cysts, Horn Pearls, and Squamous Eddies

Horn cysts (keratin cysts) are circular cystic structures that are surrounded by flattened epidermal cells and that contain concentrically arranged lamellar keratin. Horn cysts are features of trichoepitheliomas and basal cell tumors. *Pseudohorn cysts* are illusory cystic structures formed by the irregular invagination of a hyperplastic, hyperkeratotic epidermis. They are seen in numerous hyperplastic or neoplastic epidermal dermatoses. *Horn pearls* (squamous pearls) are focal, circular, concentric layers of squamous cells showing gradual keratinization toward the center, often accompanied by cellular atypia and dyskeratosis. Horn pearls are features of squamous cell carcinoma and pseudocarcinomatous hyperplasia. *Squamous eddies* are whorl-like patterns of squamoid cells with no atypia, dyskeratosis, or central keratinization. Squamous eddies are features of numerous neoplastic and hyperplastic epidermal disorders.

Epidermolytic Hyperkeratosis

Epidermolytic hyperkeratosis (granular degeneration) is characterized by (1) perinuclear clear spaces in the upper epidermis, (2) indistinct cell boundaries formed either by lightly staining material or by keratohyaline granules peripheral to the perinuclear clear spaces, (3) a markedly thickened stratum granulosum, and (4) orthokeratotic hyperkeratosis. It is seen in certain types of ichthyosis, linear epidermal nevi, actinic keratoses, seborrheic keratoses, papillomas, keratinous cysts, and squamous cell carcinoma (Fig. 2:23).

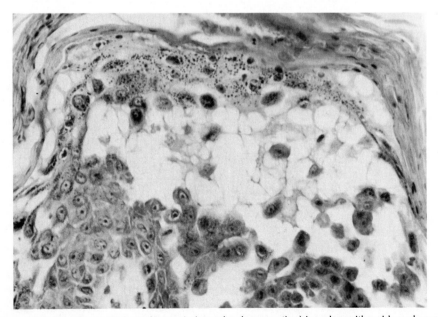

Figure 2:23. Epidermolytic hyperkeratosis (granular degeneration) in a dog with epidermal nevus.

DERMAL CHANGES

Collagen Changes

Dermal collagen is subject to a number of pathologic changes and may undergo the following: (1) *hyalinization*—a confluence and an increased eosinophilic, glassy, refractile appearance, as seen in chronic inflammation and connective tissue diseases; (2) *fibrinoid degeneration*—deposition on or replacement with a brightly eosinophilic fibrillar or granular substance resembling fibrin, as seen in connective tissue diseases; (3) *lysis*—a homogeneous, eosinophilic, complete loss of structural detail, as seen in microbial infections, and ischemia; (4) *degeneration*— a structural and tinctorial change characterized by slight basophilia, granular appearance, and frayed edges of collagen fibers, as seen in canine and feline eosinophilic granuloma; (5) *dystrophic mineralization*—deposition of calcium salts as basophilic, amorphous, granular material along collagen fibers, as seen in hyperadrenocorticism; (6) *atrophy*—thin collagen fibrils and decreased fibroblasts, with a resultant decrease in dermal thickness, as seen in hormonal dermatoses; (7) *disorganization and fragmentation*—cutaneous asthenia; and (8) *alignment in vertical streaks*—elongated, thickened parallel strands of collagen in the superficial dermis, perpendicular to the epidermal surface, as seen in chronically rubbed, licked, or scratched skin, such as that with acral lick dermatitis and hypersensitivity reactions.

Fibroplasia, Desmoplasia, Fibrosis, and Sclerosis

Fibroplasia refers to the formation and development of fibrous tissue in increased amounts and is often used synonymously with *granulation tissue*. The condition is characterized by a fibrovascular proliferation in which the blood vessels with prominent endothelial cells are oriented roughly perpendicular to the surface of the skin. The new collagen fibers, with prominent fibroblasts, are oriented roughly parallel to the surface of the skin. Edema and inflammatory cells are constant features of fibroplasia. *Desmoplasia* is the term usually used when referring to the fibroplasia induced by neoplastic processes.

Fibrosis is a later stage of fibroplasia in which increased numbers of fibroblasts and collagen fibers are the characteristic findings. Little or no inflammation is present. *Sclerosis* (scar formation) may be the endpoint of fibrosis, wherein the increased numbers of collagen fibers have a thick, eosinophilic, hyalinized appearance, and the number of fibroblasts is greatly reduced.

Papillomatosis, Villi, and Festoons

Papillomatosis refers to the projection of dermal papillae above the surface of the skin, resulting in an irregular undulating configuration of the epidermis. Often associated with epidermal hyperplasia, papillomatosis is also seen with chronic inflammatory and neoplastic dermatoses. *Villi* are dermal papillae, covered by one to two layers of epidermal cells, that project into a vesicle or bulla. Villi are seen in pemphigus vulgaris and warty dyskeratoma and occasionally in actinic keratoses and squamous cell carcinoma. *Festoons* are dermal papillae, devoid of attached epidermal cells, that project into the base of a vesicle or bulla. They are seen in bullous pemphigoid, epidermolysis bullosa simplex, and drug eruption.

Pigmentary Incontinence

Pigmentary incontinence refers to the presence of melanin granules that are free within the subepidermal dermis and within dermal macrophages (melanophages). Pigmentary incontinence may be seen with any process that damages the stratum basale and the basement membrane zone, especially with hydropic degeneration of basal cells (lichenoid dermatoses, lupus erythematosus, dermatomyositis, erythema multiforme, epidermolysis bullosa simplex). In addition melanophages may be seen in noninflammatory conditions where melanin production is greatly increased.

Edema

Dermal edema is recognized by dilated lymphatics (not visible in normal skin), widened spaces between blood vessels and perivascular collagen (*perivascular edema*), or widened spaces between large areas of dermal collagen (*interstitial edema*). The dilated lymphatics and widened perivascular and interstitial spaces may or may not contain a lightly eosinophilic, homogeneous, frothy-appearing substance (serum).

Dermal edema is a common, nondiagnostic feature of any inflammatory dermatosis. Severe edema of the superficial dermis may result in subepidermal vesicles and bullae, necrosis of the overlying epidermis, and predisposition to artifactual dermoepidermal separation during handling and processing of biopsy specimens. Severe edema of the superficial dermis may result in a vertical orientation and stretching of collagen fibers, producing the "gossamer" (web-like) collagen effect seen with erythema multiforme and severe urticaria.

Mucinous Degeneration

Mucinous degeneration (myxedema, mucoid degeneration, myxoid degeneration, mucinosis) is characterized by increased amounts of an amorphous, stringy, granular, basophilic material that separates, thins, or replaces dermal collagen fibrils and surrounds blood vessels and appendages in H & E–stained sections. Only small amounts of mucin are ever visible in normal skin, mostly around appendages and blood vessels. Mucin is more easily demonstrated with stains for acid mucopolysaccharides, such as Hale's iron and Alcian blue. Mucinous degeneration may be seen as a focal (usually perivascular) change in numerous inflammatory, neoplastic, and developmental dermatoses. Diffuse mucinous degeneration may be seen with hypothyroidism, acromegaly, lupus erythematosus, mucinoses, and the *normal* Chinese Shar Pei skin.

Grenz Zone

This marginal zone of relatively normal collagen separates the epidermis from an underlying dermal alteration. A grenz zone may be seen in neoplastic and granulomatous disorders.

Follicular Changes

Follicular epithelium is affected by most of the histopathologic changes described for the epidermis. Follicular (poral) keratosis, plugging, and dilatation are common features of such diverse conditions as inflammatory, hormonal, and developmental dermatoses. *Perifolliculitis, folliculitis,* and *furunculosis* (penetrating or perforating folliculitis) refer to varying degrees of follicular inflammation. *Follicular atrophy* refers to the gradual involution and disappearance that are characteristic of hormonal dermatoses. Hair follicles should be closely examined to determine which phase of the growth cycle they are in. *Telogenization,* a predominance of telogen hair follicles, is characteristic of hormonal dermatoses and states of telogen defluxion as associated with stress, disease, and drugs. *Follicular dystrophy* refers to the presence of incompletely and/or abnormally formed hair follicles and is seen in developmental abnormalities such as hypotrichosis and color mutant alopecia. Perifollicular fibrosis is seen in chronic folliculitides and in canine dermatomyositis.

Glandular Changes

Sebaceous and apocrine sweat glands may be involved in various dermatoses. *Sebaceous glands* may be involved in many suppurative and granulomatous inflammations *(sebaceous adenitis).* In dogs and cats an idiopathic granulomatous sebaceous adenitis is seen, which, in the late stages, is characterized by complete absence of sebaceous glands. They may become *atrophic* (reduced in number and size, with pyknotic nuclei predominating) and *cystic* in hormonal and developmental dermatoses, in occasional chronic inflammatory processes, and as a senile change. Sebaceous glands may also become *hyperplastic* in chronic inflammatory dermatoses and in senile nodular sebaceous hyperplasia. Sebaceous gland atrophy and hyperplasia must always be cautiously assessed with regard to the area of the body from which the skin specimen was taken.

Apocrine sweat glands are commonly involved in suppurative and granulomatous dermatoses *(hidradinitis).* Periapocrine accumulation of plasma cells is commonly seen in acral lick dermatitis and chronic pyodermas. The apocrine sweat glands may become *dilated* or *cystic* in many inflammatory, developmental, and hormonal dermatoses; in apocrine cystomatosis; and as a senile change. The light microscopic recognition of apocrine gland *atrophy* is a moot point, since dilated apocrine secretory coils containing flattened epithelial cells are a feature of the normal postsecretory state.

Vascular Changes

Cutaneous blood vessels exhibit a number of histologic changes, including *dilatation* (ectasia), *endothelial swelling, hyalinization, fibrinoid degeneration, vasculitis, thromboembolism,* and *extravasation* (diapedesis) *of erythrocytes* (purpura).

SUBCUTANEOUS FAT CHANGES

The subcutaneous fat (panniculus adiposus, hypodermis) is subject to the connective tissue and vascular changes described above. It is frequently involved in suppurative and granulomatous dermatoses. In addition, subcutaneous fat may exhibit its own inflammatory changes *(panniculitis, steatitis)* without any significant involvement of the overlying dermis and epidermis (sterile nodular panniculitis, feline nutritional steatitis, coccidioidomycosis, bacterial endocarditis, botryomycosis, atypical mycobacteriosis, subcutaneous fat sclerosis, erythema nodosum) and may atrophy in various hormonal, inflammatory (wucher atrophy), and idiopathic dermatoses. Fat micropseudo-cyst formation and lipocytes containing radially arranged needle-shaped clefts are seen with *subcutaneous fat sclerosis*.

MISCELLANEOUS CHANGES

Civatte Bodies. Civatte bodies (colloid bodies, apoptotic bodies, hyaline bodies, ovoid bodies, filamentous bodies) are degenerate basal epidermal cells that appear as round, homogeneous, eosinophilic bodies in the stratum basale or just below. Civatte bodies are features of lichenoid dermatoses (see Fig. 9:68).

Thickened Basement Membrane Zone. Thickening of the light microscopic basement membrane zone appears as focal, linear, homogeneous, eosinophilic bands below the stratum basale. The basement membrane zone is better demonstrated with periodic acid-Schiff (PAS) stain. Thickening of the basement membrane zone is a feature of lichenoid dermatoses, especially lupus erythematosus (see Fig. 9:64).

Papillary Squirting. Papillary squirting is present when superficial dermal papillae are edematous and contain dilated vessels, and when the overlying epidermis is also edematous and often contains exocytosing leukocytes and parakeratotic scale. "Squirting" papillae are a feature of seborrheic dermatitis and zinc-responsive dermatoses.

Dysplasia. This term refers to a faulty or abnormal development of individual cells, and it is also commonly used to describe abnormal development of the epidermis as a whole. Dysplasia may be a feature of neoplastic, hyperplastic, and developmental dermatoses.

Anaplasia. Anaplasia (atypia) is a feature of neoplastic cells, in which there is a loss of normal differentiation and organization (Fig. 2:24).

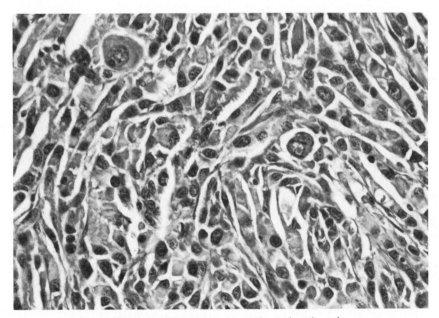

Figure 2:24. Anaplastic cells in a dog with amelanotic melanoma.

Metaplasia. This term is used in reference to a change in the type of mature cells in a tissue into a form that is not normal for that tissue (e.g., osseous metaplasia in skin of a patient with hyperadrenocorticism). Through metaplasia, a given cell may exhibit epithelial, mesothelial, or mesenchymal characteristics, regardless of the tissue of origin.

Nests. Nests (theques) are well-circumscribed clusters or groups of cells within the epidermis or the dermis. Nests are seen in some neoplastic and hamartomatous dermatoses, such as melanomas and melanocytic nevi.

Lymphoid Nodules. These nodules are rounded, discrete masses of primarily mature lymphocytes. They are often found perivascularly in the deep dermis or subcutis, or both. Apparently uncommon in dogs and cats, they are most commonly recognized in the eosinophilic granuloma complex, lupus erythematosus, pseudolymphoma, panniculitis, and feline mast cell tumors.

Multinucleated Epidermal Giant Cells. Multinucleated epidermal giant cells are found in viral infections and in a number of nonviral and nonneoplastic dermatoses characterized by epidermal hyperplasia, dyskeratosis, chronicity, or pruritus.

Squamatization. This refers to the replacement of the normally cuboidal or columnar, slightly basophilic basal epidermal cells by polygonal or flattened, eosinophilic keratinocytes. It may be seen in lichenoid tissue reactions.

Flame Figure. A flame figure is an area of altered collagen surrounded by eosinophils and eosinophilic granules. In chronic lesions the eosinophil content decreases, histiocytes decrease in number, and palisading granulomas may be formed. Flame figures may be seen in canine and feline eosinophilic granuloma, sterile eosinophilic pustulosis, and insect/arthropod bite reactions.

CONFUSING TERMS

Necrobiosis

Necrobiosis is the degeneration and death of cells or tissue followed by replacement. Examples of necrobiosis would be the constant degeneration and replacement of epidermal and hematopoietic cells.

The term necrobiosis has been used in dermatohistopathology to describe various degenerative changes in collagen found in canine and feline eosinophilic granuloma, and human granuloma annulare, necrobiosis lipoidica, and rheumatoid and pseudorheumatoid nodules. The use of the term necrobiosis to describe a *pathologic* change is inappropriate and confusing, both histologically and etymologically, and should be discouraged. It is better to use the more specific terms described previously under Collagen Changes.

Nevus and Hamartoma

A *nevus* is a circumscribed developmental defect in the skin. Nevi may arise from any skin component or combination thereof. Nevi are hyperplastic in nature. The term nevus should never be used alone but always with a modifier such as melanocytic, epidermal, vascular, sebaceous, collagenous, and so on.

Hamartoma literally means a tumor-like proliferation of normal or embryonal cells. In other words, a hamartoma is a macroscopic hyperplasia of normal tissue elements and is often used synonymously with nevus. However, the term hamartoma may be applied to hyperplastic disorders in any tissue or organ system, whereas the term nevus is restricted to the skin.

CELLULAR INFILTRATES

Dermal cellular infiltrates are described in terms of (1) the *types* of cells present and (2) the *pattern* of cellular infiltration. In general, cellular infiltrates are either *monomorphous* (one cell type) or *polymorphous* (more than one cell type). Further clarification of the predominant cells is accomplished by modifiers such as *lymphocytic, histiocytic, neutrophilic, eosinophilic,* and *plasmacytic* (see Fig. 1:11).

Patterns of cellular infiltration are usualy made up of one or more of the following basic patterns: (1) *perivascular* (angiocentric—located around blood vessels), (2) *perifollicular and periglandular* (appendagocentric, periappendageal, periadnexal—located around follicles and glands), (3) *lichenoid* (assuming a "bandlike" configuration that parallels and "hugs" the overlying epidermis), (4) *nodular* (occurring in basically well-defined groups or clusters at any site), and (5) *diffuse* (interstitial—scattered lightly or solidly throughout the dermis).

The types of cells and patterns of infiltration present are important diagnostic clues to the diagnosis of many dermatoses.

Histopathologic Distribution Patterns in the Skin

THE DERMATITIS REACTION

The dermatitis reaction is a nondiagnostic cutaneous inflammatory response with concomitant changes in the epidermis and dermis.

Acute dermatitis is characterized *grossly* by vesicles, papules, erythema, edema, and exudation and *histologically* by spongiotic vesicles, spongiosis, intracellular edema, and leukocytic exocytosis as well as superficial dermal edema, vascular dilatation, and perivascular inflammatory cells.

Subacute dermatitis is characterized *grossly* by erythema, edema, and exudation, with or without crusts, and mild-to-moderate vesiculation. *Histologically*, it is characterized by epidermal and dermal changes similar to those described for acute dermatitis. In addition, there are varying degrees of epidermal hyperplasia and orthokeratotic or parakeratotic hyperkeratosis.

Chronic dermatitis is characterized *grossly* by mild erythema, scaling, crusts, lichenification, and pigmentary disturbances. *Histologically*, it is characterized by variable epidermal hyperplasia and orthokeratotic or parakeratotic hyperkeratosis, and mild-to-moderate degrees of dermal edema, vascular dilatation, and perivascular inflammatory cells.

The dermatitis reaction is not a particularly useful concept from the standpoint of diagnostic or therapeutic specificity. However, it is a useful and frequently employed concept for histopathologic description and morphologic diagnosis. Although the tissue may show no other condition, it is most frustrating to clinicians to receive a histopathologic diagnosis of "chronic dermatitis," "chronic nonsuppurative dermatitis," or "chronic nonspecific dermatitis." Such histopathologic diagnoses should always be amended with the phrase "consistent or compatible with," and a differential diagnosis should be listed.

> **Histopathologic diagnoses should always be amended with the phrase "consistent or compatible with," and a differential diagnosis should be listed.**

DERMATOLOGIC DIAGNOSIS BY HISTOPATHOLOGIC PATTERNS

In 1978, A. B. Ackerman published a textbook on the histopathologic aspects of inflammatory dermatoses in humans.[1] The essence of this book was histopathologic diagnosis by pattern analysis, that is, first categorizing inflammatory dermatoses by their appearance on the scanning objective of the light microscope and then homing in on a specific diagnosis, whenever possible, by the assimilation of fine details gathered on low- and high-power scrutiny. Pattern analysis was introduced to veterinary dermatology in 1983[20] and to veterinary pathology in 1985.[29] This methodology has revolutionized veterinary dermatohistopathology and made the reading of skin biopsies much simpler and much more rewarding (to pathologist, clinician, and patient!). However, as with any histologic method, pattern analysis works only when clinicians supply pathologists with the biopsies most representative of the dermatoses being sampled.

PERIVASCULAR DERMATITIS

In perivascular dermatitis, the predominant inflammatory reaction is centered around the superficial and/or the deep dermal blood vessels. Perivascular dermatitis is subdivided on the basis of accompanying epidermal changes into four types: (1) *pure perivascular dermatitis* (perivascular dermatitis without significant epidermal changes), (2) *interface dermatitis* (perivascular dermatitis with obscuring of the dermoepidermal interface), (3) *spongiotic perivascular dermatitis* (perivascular dermatitis with spongiosis), and (4) *hyperplastic perivascular dermatitis* (perivascular dermatitis with epidermal hyperplasia).

Superficial perivascular dermatitis is by far the most common form of perivascular dermatitis (Fig. 2:25A, B). The usual causes are hypersensitivity reactions (inhalant, dietary, drug, and so forth), ectoparasitisms, seborrheic disorders, and contact dermatitis. *Deep* perivascular dermatitis (Fig. 2:25C) is uncommon and may be seen with systemic disorders (systemic lupus erythematosus, septicemia, hypereosinophilic syndrome, canine histiocytosis), vasculitis, discoid lupus erythematosus, cellulitis, eosinophilic plaque, and tick bite reactions.

Disproportionate orthokeratotic hyperkeratosis, in which the keratin layer is much thicker than the living epidermis, suggests endocrinopathy, vitamin A–responsive dermatosis, ichthyosis, and seborrheic disorders. Disproportionate *follicular* orthokeratotic hyperkeratosis suggests vitamin A–responsive dermatosis. *Diffuse parakeratotic hyperkeratosis* suggests zinc-responsive dermatosis,

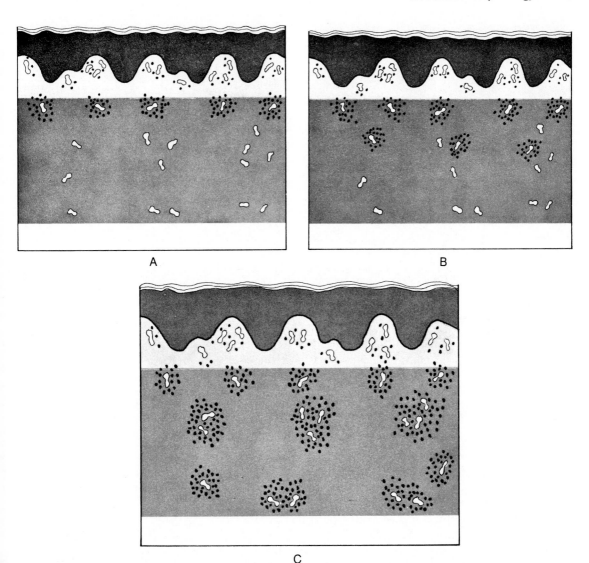

Figure 2:25. *A*, Superficial perivascular dermatitis. Infiltrate is around blood vessels of the superficial plexus. *B*, Superficial perivascular dermatitis. Infiltrate is around blood vessels in upper half of dermis. *C*, Superficial and deep perivascular dermatitis. (From Ackerman, A. B.: Histologic Diagnosis of Inflammatory Diseases. Lea & Febiger, Philadelphia, 1978.)

generic dog food dermatosis, some vitamin A–responsive dermatoses, thallo-toxicosis, and canine hepatocutaneous syndrome.

Focal parakeratotic hyperkeratosis (parakeratotic "caps") may be seen with ectoparasitism, seborrheic disorders, dermatophytosis, and dermatophilosis. When parakeratotic "caps" are combined wtih "papillary squirting," seborrheic dermatitis is likely. Focal areas of "eosinophilic spongiosis" and epidermal necrosis (epidermal "nibbles") are suggestive of ectoparasitism.

Perivascular dermatoses accompanied by numerous *eosinophils* are most likely to represent ectoparasitism or endoparasitism in the dog, and parasitism, hypersensitivity reactions (inhalant, dietary), eosinophilic plaque, and hyper-eosinophilic syndrome in the cat. Perivascular dermatoses accompanied by *vertical streaking of collagen* and/or *sebaceous gland hyperplasia* suggest chronic pruritus (rubbing, licking, chewing), such as that seen with hypersensitivity reactions and acral lick dermatitis.

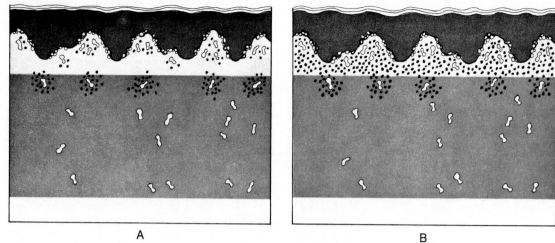

Figure 2:26. *A*, Interface dermatitis with hydropic degeneration. *B*, Interface dermatitis with lichenoid infiltrate. (From Ackerman, A. B.: Histologic Diagnosis of Inflammatory Diseases. Lea & Febiger, Philadelphia, 1978.)

Pure Perivascular Dermatitis (Fig. 2:25)

The cellular infiltrate in perivascular dermatitis may be *monomorphous* or *polymorphous*. The most likely diagnoses include hypersensitivity reactions (inhalant, dietary, drug), urticaria, dermatophytosis, and urticaria pigmentosa.

Interface Dermatitis (Fig. 2:26)

In interface dermatitis, the dermoepidermal junction is obscured by *hydropic degeneration,* (2) *lichenoid cellular infiltrate,* or both. The *hydropic* type of interface dermatitis is seen with drug eruptions, lupus erythematosus, toxic epidermal necrolysis, erythema multiforme, dermatomyositis, epidermolysis bullosa simplex, and graft-versus-host reactions. The *lichenoid* type is seen with drug eruptions, lupus erythematosus, pemphigus, pemphigoid, erythema multiforme, Vogt-Koyanagi-Harada–like syndrome, idiopathic lichenoid dermatoses, and mycosis fungoides. The bandlike cellular infiltration of lichenoid tissue reactions consist predominantly of lymphocytes and plasma cells. If nearby ulceration or secondary infection exits, numerous neutrophils may be present. Uniquely, the lichenoid infiltrate of Vogt-Koyanagi-Harada–like syndrome contains numerous large histiocytes. A lichenoid tissue reaction accompanied by psoriaform epidermal hyperplasia is seen in psoriaform lichenoid dermatosis of springer spaniels. A lichenoid tissue reaction containing many eosinophils suggests an insect/arthropod bite reaction.

Spongiotic Perivascular Dermatitis (Fig. 2:27)

Spongiotic perivascular dermatitis is characterized by varying degrees of spongiosis and spongiotic vesicle formation. Severe spongiotic vesiculation may "blow out" the basement membrane zone, resulting in subepidermal vesicles. The epidermis frequently shows varying degrees of hyperplasia and hyperkeratosis. Spongiotic dermatitis may be *monomorphous* or *polymorphous*. The most likely diagnoses include hypersensitivity reactions, contact dermatitis, ectoparasitisms, seborrheic disorders, and eosinophilic plaque. *Diffuse* spongiosis (involving hair follicle outer root sheaths) suggests eosinophilic plaque and

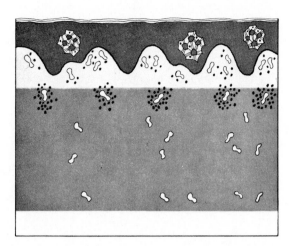

Figure 2:27. Spongiotic dermatitis. (From Ackerman, A. B.: Histologic Diagnosis of Inflammatory Diseases. Lea & Febiger, Philadelphia, 1978.)

zinc-responsive dermatosis. Marked spongiosis and intracellular edema of the upper one-half of the epidermis with overlying diffuse keratosis is seen with the hepatocutaneous syndrome.

Hyperplastic Perivascular Dermatitis (Fig. 2:28)

Hyperplastic perivascular dermatitis is characterized by varying degrees of epidermal hyperplasia and hyperkeratosis, with little or no spongiosis. This is a common, nondiagnostic, chronic dermatitis reaction and is commonly seen with hypersensitivity reactions, contact dermatitis, seborrheic disorders, ectoparasitisms, indolent ulcer, and acral lick dermatitis. *Psoriasiform* perivascular dermatoses (regular, marked epidermal hyperplasia, often with clubbing or fusion of the tips of the rete ridges) are unusual and may represent chronic contact dermatitis, chronic hypersensitivity reactions, acral lick dermatitis, seborrheic disorders, psoriasiform lichenoid dermatosis of springer spaniels, hepatocutaneous syndrome, and dermatophytosis. The most common cause of psoriasiform perivascular "dermatitis" in dogs is mycosis fungoides.

VASCULITIS

Vasculitis is an inflammatory process in which inflammatory cells are present within and around blood vessel walls and there are concomitant signs of

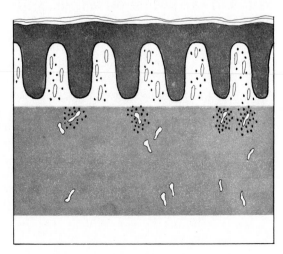

Figure 2:28. Hyperplastic dermatitis. (From Ackerman, A. B.: Histologic Diagnosis of Inflammatory Diseases. Lea & Febiger, Philadelphia, 1978.)

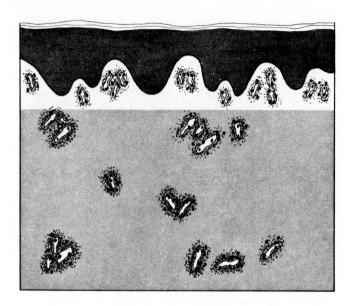

Figure 2:29. Vasculitis. (From Ackerman, A. B.: Histologic Diagnosis of Inflammatory Diseases. Lea & Febiger, Philadelphia, 1978.)

damage to the blood vessels (e.g., degeneration and lysis of vascular and perivascular collagen, degeneration and swelling of endothelial cells, extravasation of erythrocytes, thrombosis, effacement of vascular architecture, and fibrinoid degeneration). Vasculitides are usually classified on the basis of the dominant inflammatory cell within vessel walls, the types being neutrophilic, eosinophilic, and lymphocytic. Fibrinoid degeneration is rare in canine and feline cutaneous vasculitides.

Neutrophilic vasculitis (Fig. 2:29) may be *leukocytoclastic* (associated with karyorrhexis of neutrophils, resulting in "nuclear dust") or *nonleukocytoclastic*, and it is seen in connective tissue disorders (lupus erythematosus, rheumatoid arthritis), "allergic" reactions (drug eruptions, infections, toxins), polyarteritis nodosa, canine staphylococcal hypersenstivity, Rocky Mountain spotted fever, septicemia, and thrombophlebitis from intravenous catheters causing thromboembolism and as an idiopathic disorder.

Lymphocytic vasculitis may be seen in drug eruptions, in ectoparasitism, and as an idiopathic disorder.

NODULAR AND DIFFUSE DERMATITIS, AND GRANULOMATOUS INFLAMMATION

Nodular dermatitis denotes discrete clusters of cells. Such dermal nodules are usually multiple but may occasionally be large and solitary (Fig. 2:30). In contrast, *diffuse dermatitis* denotes a cellular infiltrate so dense that discrete cellular aggregates are no longer easily recognized (Fig. 2:31).

Granulomatous inflammation represents a heterogeneous pattern of tissue reactions in response to various stimuli. There is no simple, precise, universally accepted way to define granulomatous inflammation. A commonly proposed definition of granulomatous inflammation is as follows: a circumscribed tissue reaction that is subacute to chronic in nature and is located about one or more foci, wherein the histiocyte or macrophage is a predominant cell type.[1, 7–12] Thus, granulomatous dermatitis may be nodular or diffuse, but not all nodular

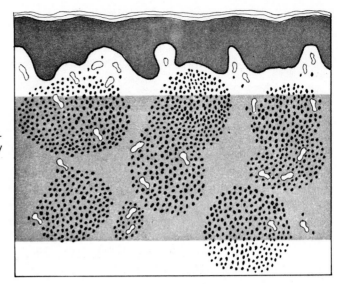

Figure 2:30. Nodular dermatitis. (From Ackerman, A. B.: Histologic Diagnosis of Inflammatory Diseases. Lea & Febiger, Philadelphia, 1978.)

and diffuse dermatoses are granulomatous. Nongranulomatous diffuse dermatoses include eosinophilic plaque, plasma cell pododermatitis, and cellulitis. Pseudolymphoma is an example of a nongranulomatous nodular dermatitis. Granulomatous infiltrates that contain large mumbers of neutrophils are frequently called *pyogranulomatous*. The most common causes of nodular pyogranulomatous dermatitis in dogs are furunculosis and ruptured keratinous cysts.

Cell Types

Nodular dermatitis and diffuse dermatitis are often associated with certain unusual inflammatory cell types.

Foam cells are histiocytes with vacuolated cytoplasm resulting from their contents (lipids, debris, microorganisms).

Epithelioid cells are histiocytes with elongated or oval vesicular nuclei and abundant, finely granular, eosinophilic cytoplasm with ill-defined cell borders.

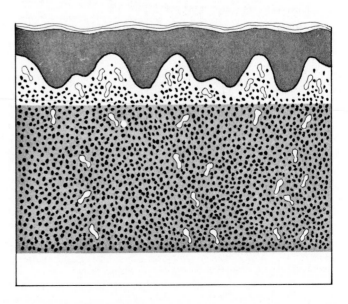

Figure 2:31. Diffuse dermatitis. (From Ackerman, A. B.: Histologic Diagnosis of Inflammatory Diseases. Lea & Febiger, Philadelphia, 1978.)

They are called "epithelioid" because they appear to cluster and adjoin like epithelial cells.

Multinucleated histiocytic giant cells (Fig. 2:32) are histiocytic variants that assume three morphologic forms: (1) *Langhans'* cell (nuclei form a circle or semicircle at the periphery of the cell), (2) *foreign body* (nuclei are scattered throughout the cytoplasm), and (3) *Touton* cell (nuclei form a wreath that surrounds a central, homogeneous, amphophilic core of cytoplasm, which is in turn surrounded by abundant foamy cytoplasm). In general, these three forms of giant cells have no diagnostic specificity, although the Touton variety is fairly specific for xanthomas.

Certain general principles apply to the examination of all nodular and diffuse dermatitides. The processes that should be used are (1) polarizing foreign material, (2) staining for bacteria and fungi, and (3) culturing. In general, microorganisms are most likely to be found near areas of suppuration and necrosis.

Nodular and diffuse dermatitis may be characterized by predominantly neutrophilic, histiocytic, eosinophilic, or mixed cellular infiltrates.

Neutrophils (dermal abscess) often predominate in dermatoses associated with bacteria, mycobacteria, actinomycetes, fungi, prototheca, and foreign bodies.

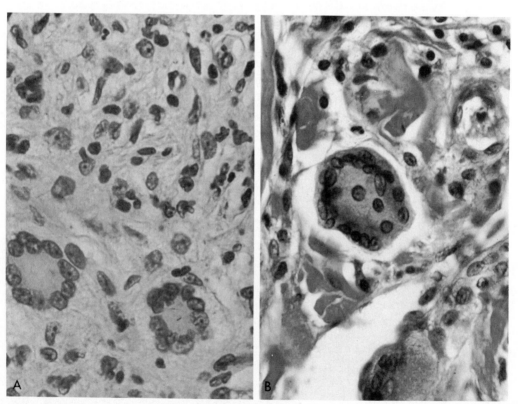

Figure 2:32. Multinucleated histiocytic giant cells are often present in cutaneous granulomas or chronic inflammations localized around foci of irritation. However, one should understand that identification of any one type of giant cell is not diagnostic alone. Several types may be found in a single section, and all are "foreign body" in character. Their different structure is probably related to the physiochemical nature of the foreign material. *A*, Touton-type giant cell. There is a complete ring of nuclei around a "ground glass" center, and all are enclosed within a vacuolated cytoplasm. The illustration is from a human xanthoma. (Photomicrograph courtesy J. D. Conroy.) *B*, Langhans-type giant cell. The peripheral rim of nuclei is arranged in a horseshoe fashion.

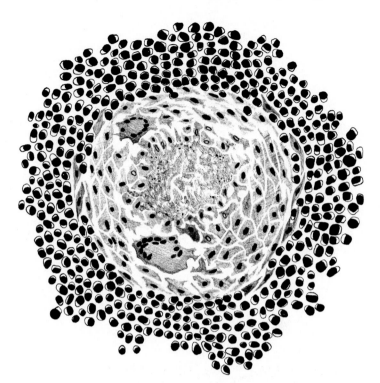

Figure 2:33. Tuberculoid granuloma. (From Ackerman, A. B.: Histologic Diagnosis of Inflammatory Diseases. Lea & Febiger, Philadelphia, 1978.)

Histiocytes may predominate in the chronic stage of any of the entities just listed, in xanthomas, canine histiocytosis (cutaneous and systemic), and in the sterile pyogranuloma/granuloma syndrome. Granulomas that are chiefly composed of histiocytic elements are often referred to as "tuberculoid" (histiocytes and epithelioid cells surrounded by giant cells, followed by a layer of lymphocytes, and finally an outer layer of fibroblasts, as seen in tuberculosis and feline leprosy) (Fig. 2:33) or "sarcoidal" ("naked" epithelioid cells, as seen in canine sarcoidosis) (Fig. 2:34). "Palisading" granulomas are characterized by the alignment of histiocytes like staves around a central focus of collagen degeneration (canine and feline eosinophilic granuloma) (Fig. 2:35), fibrin (rheumatoid nodule), lipids, (xanthoma), or other foreign material (e.g., calcium, as in dystrophic calcinosis cutis and calcinosis circumscripta) (Fig. 2:36).

Eosinophils may predominate in feline and canine eosinophilic granuloma, in certain parasitic dermatoses (dirofilariasis, dracunculosis), and where hair follicles have ruptured. *Mixed* cellular infiltrates are most commonly neutrophils and histiocytes (pyogranuloma), eosinophils and histiocytes (eosinophilic granuloma complex), or some combination thereof.

Plasma cells are common components of nodular and diffuse dermatitis of dogs and cats and are of no particular diagnostic significance. They are commonly seen around glands and follicles in chronic infections. Periapocrine accumulations of plasma cells are commonly seen in acral lick dermatitis. Hyperactive plasma cells may contain eosinophilic intracytoplasmic inclusions (Russell bodies). These accumulations of glycoprotein are largely globulin and may be large enough to push the cell nucleus eccentrically.

Reactions to *ruptured hair follicles* are a common cause of nodular and diffuse pyogranulomatous dermatitis, and any such dermal process should be carefully scrutinized for keratinous and epithelial debris and should be serially sectioned to rule out this possibility.

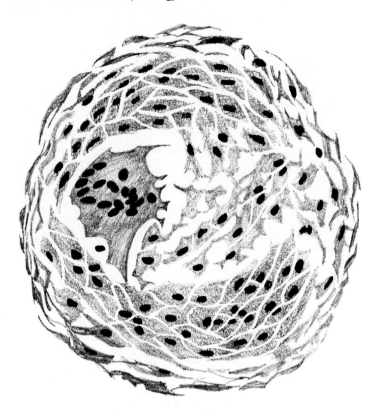

Figure 2:34. Sarcoid granuloma. (From Ackerman, A. B.: Histologic Diagnosis of Inflammatory Diseases. Lea & Febiger, Philadelphia, 1978.)

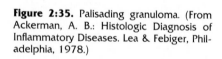

Figure 2:35. Palisading granuloma. (From Ackerman, A. B.: Histologic Diagnosis of Inflammatory Diseases. Lea & Febiger, Philadelphia, 1978.)

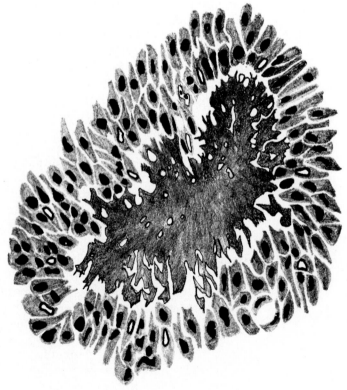

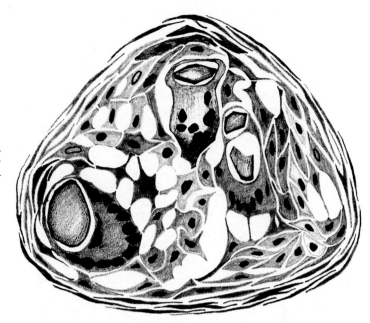

Figure 2:36. Foreign body granuloma. (From Ackerman, A. B.: Histologic Diagnosis of Inflammatory Diseases. Lea & Febiger, Philadelphia, 1978.)

INTRAEPIDERMAL VESICULAR AND PUSTULAR DERMATITIS (Fig. 2:37)

Vesicular and pustular dermatitides show considerable microscopic and macroscopic overlap, because vesicles tend to accumulate leukocytes very early and rapidly. Thus, vesicular dermatitides in dogs and cats frequently appear pustular or vesiculopustular, both macroscopically and microscopically.

Intraepidermal vesicles and pustules may be produced by intercellular or intracellular edema (*any* acute-to-subacute dermatitis reaction), ballooning degeneration (viral infections), acantholysis (the autoantibodies of pemphigus, the proteolytic enzymes from neutrophils in microbial infections and subcorneal pustular dermatosis), and hydropic degeneration of basal cells (lupus erythe-

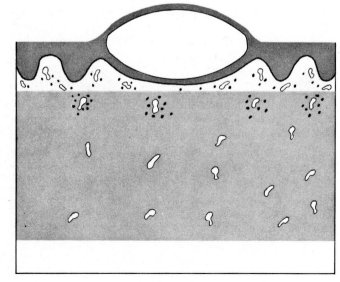

Figure 2:37. Intraepidermal vesicular and pustular dermatitis. (From Ackerman, A. B.: Histologic Diagnosis of Inflammatory Diseases. Lea & Febiger, Philadelphia, 1978.)

matosus, epidermolysis bullosa simplex, erythema multiforme, toxic epidermal necrolysis, dermatomyositis, drug eruptions). It is very useful to classify intraepidermal vesicular and pustular dermatitides as to their anatomic level of occurrence within the epidermis (Table 2:1).

SUBEPIDERMAL VESICULAR AND PUSTULAR DERMATITIS (Fig. 2:38)

Subepidermal vesicles and pustules may be formed through hydropic degeneration of basal cells (lupus erythematosus, epidermolysis bullosa simplex,

Table 2:1. HISTOPATHOLOGIC CLASSIFICATION OF INTRAEPIDERMAL AND SUBEPIDERMAL VESICULAR AND PUSTULAR DERMATOSES

Anatomic Location	Other Helpful Findings
Intraepidermal	
Subcorneal	
Microbial infection	Microorganisms (bacteria, fungi), acantholysis ±
Subcorneal pustular dermatosis	Acantholysis ±
Systemic lupus erythematosus	Acantholysis (mild)
Pemphigus foliaceus and erythematosus	Acantholysis (marked), granular "cling-ons," follicular involvement ±
Sterile eosinophilic pustulosis	Eosinophils, acantholysis (mild), follicular involvement ±
Linear IgA dermatosis	Neutrophils, no microorganisms
Intragranular	
Pemphigus foliaceus and erythematosus	Acantholysis (marked), granular "cling-ons," follicular involvement ±
Intraepidermal	
Spongiotic dermatitis	Eosinophilic exocytosis suggests ectoparasitism, pemphigus, and pemphigoid
Pemphigus vegetans	Acantholysis, eosinophils, papillomatosis
Mycosis fungoides	Atypical mononuclear cells, Pautrier's microabscesses
Hepatocutaneous syndrome	Diffuse parakeratosis, marked edema of upper epidermis
Suprabasilar	
Pemphigus vulgaris	Acantholysis, follicular and glandular duct involvement ±
Intrabasal	
Lupus erythematosus	Hydropic degeneration of basal cells
Epidermolysis bullosa simplex	Hydropic degeneration of basal cells
Drug eruption	Hydropic degeneration of basal cells; necrotic keratinocytes ±
Toxic epidermal necrolysis	Hydropic degeneration of basal cells, epidermal coagulation necrosis
Erythema multiforme	Hydropic degeneration of basal cells, single cell necrosis of keratinocytes
Dermatomyositis	Hydropic degeneration of basal cells, perifolliculitis
Subepidermal	
Bullous pemphigoid	Subepidermal vacuolar alteration, inflammation ±
Epidermolysis bullosa simplex	Hydropic degeneration of basal cells, little or no inflammation
Lupus erythematosus	Hydropic degeneration of basal cells
Drug eruption	Hydropic degeneration of basal cells ±
Toxic epidermal necrosis	Epidermal coagulation necrosis, little or no inflammation
Erythema multiforme	Hydropic degeneration of basal cells, single cell necrosis of keratinocytes, "gossamer" collagen
Dermatomyositis	Hydropic degeneration of basal cells, perifolliculitis
Severe subepidermal edema or cellular infiltration	
Severe intercellular edema	Spongiotic vesicles

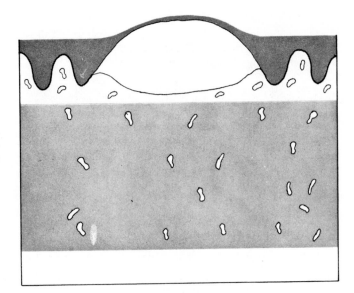

Figure 2:38. Subepidermal vesicular and pustular dermatitis. (From Ackerman, A. B.: Histologic Diagnosis of Inflammatory Diseases. Lea & Febiger, Philadelphia, 1978.)

erythema multiforme, dermatomyositis, drug eruption, toxic epidermal necrolysis), dermoepidermal separation (bullous pemphigoid, drug eruption), severe subepidermal edema or cellular infiltration (especially urticaria, cellulitis, vasculitis, and ectoparasitism), and severe intercellular edema, with "blow out" of the basement membrane zone (spongiotic perivascular dermatitis (Fig. 2:27). Concurrent epidermal and dermal inflammatory changes are important diagnostic clues (see Table 2:1). Caution is warranted when examining older lesions, as re-epithelialization may result in subepidermal vesicles and pustules assuming an intraepidermal location. Such re-epithelialization is usually recognized as a single layer of flattened, elongated basal epidermal cells at the base of the vesicle or pustule.

PERIFOLLICULITIS, FOLLICULITIS, AND FURUNCULOSIS

Perifolliculitis denotes the accumulation of inflammatory cells around a hair follicle and the exocytosis of these cells through the follicular epithelium (Fig. 2:39). *Folliculitis* implies the accumulation of inflammatory cells within follicular

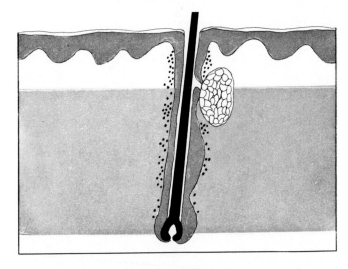

Figure 2:39. Perifolliculitis. (From Ackerman, A. B.: Histologic Diagnosis of Diseases. Lea & Febiger, Philadelphia, 1978.)

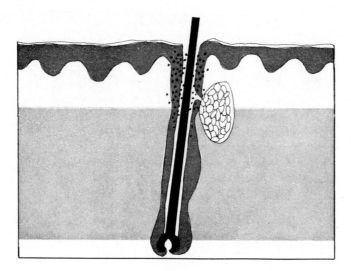

Figure 2:40. Folliculitis. (From Ackerman, A. B.: Histologic Diagnosis of Inflammatory Diseases. Lea & Febiger, Philadelphia, 1978.)

lumina (Fig. 2:40). *Furunculosis* (penetrating or perforating folliculitis) signifies hair follicle rupture (Fig. 2:41). Obviously, perifolliculitis, folliculitis, and furunculosis usually represent a pathologic continuum and may all be present in the same specimen. Follicular inflammation is a common gross and microscopic finding, and one must always be cautious in assessing its importance. It is a common secondary complication in pruritic dermatoses (e.g., hypersensitivities and ectoparasitism), seborrheic dermatoses, and hormonal dermatoses. Thus, a thorough search for underlying causes is mandatory.

Follicular inflammation may be caused by bacteria, fungi, and parasites (*Demodex* spp., *Pelodera strongyloides*) and rarely by atopy, food allergy, and seborrheic dermatitis. The folliculitides associated with bacteria, fungi, and parasites are usually suppurative initially, whereas those occasionally associated with atopy, food allergy, and seborrheic dermatitis are predominantly spongiotic (small numbers of exocytosing mononuclear cells or neutrophils, or both) perifolliculitides. Any chronic folliculitis, particularly where there is furunculosis, can become pyogranulomatous or granulomatous.

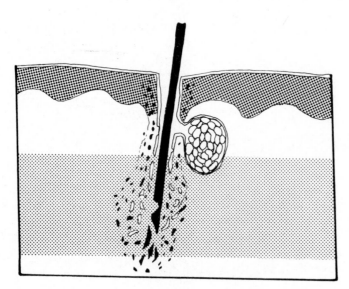

Figure 2:41. Furunculosis.

Furunculosis, regardless of the initiating cause, is frequently associated with moderate to marked tissue eosinophilia. The significance of this finding is unknown but may represent a foreign body reaction (to keratin and so forth). In addition, dogs may rarely develop a sterile, *eosinophilic folliculitis* with sterile eosinophilic pustulosis and sterile eosinophilic pinnal folliculitis.

It must be remembered that involvement of the hair follicle outer root sheath is a feature of pemphigus and that any significant degree of acantholysis mandates a consideration of this disorder. Likewise, the hair follicle outer root sheath may be involved in the hydropic degeneration and lichenoid cellular infiltrates of lupus erythematosus.

Alopecia areata is characterized initially by a perifolliculitis, wherein lymphocytes surround (like a "swarm of bees") the inferior segment of the hair follicle. *Granulomatous sebaceous adenitis* produces an apparent perifolliculitis, until closer inspection reveals no exocytosis of the outer root sheath, and an inflammatory process centered on sebaceous glands.

Dermatomyositis is often associated with marked perifollicular fibrosis.

PANNICULITIS

The panniculus is commonly involved as an extension of dermal inflammatory processes, especially of suppurative and granulomatous dermatoses. Likewise, there is usually *some* deep dermal involvement in virtually all panniculitides.

Panniculitis is conveniently divided on an anatomic basis into the *lobular* type (primarily involving fat lobules), the *septal* type (primarily involving interlobular connective tissue septae) and the diffuse type (Fig. 2:42). In dogs, diffuse panniculitis is the most common pattern, and septal panniculitis is the one most often found in cats. Patterns of panniculitis appear to have little diagnostic or prognostic significance in dogs and cats. Neither does the cytologic appearance (pyogranulomatous, granulomatous, suppurative, eosinophilic, lymphoplasmacytic, fibrosing) appear to have much diagnostic or prognostic significance. In fact, most panniculitides, regardless of the cause, look histologically similar. As with nodular and diffuse dermatitis, polarization, special stains, and cultures are usually indicated. *Septal* panniculitis is seen with vasculitides and erythema nodosum. A rare form of canine panniculitis, one associated with lupus erythematosus (lupus profundus, lupus erythematosus panniculitis), is characterized by lymphoplasmacytic septal to lobular panniculitis, with septal vasculitis, numerous lymphoid nodules, and often an overlying interface dermatitis. *Feline subcutaneous fat sclerosis* is characterized by marked septal fibrosis, fat micropseudocyst formation, and lipocytes that contain radially arranged, needle-shaped clefts.

FIBROSING DERMATITIS

Fibrosis presages the resolving stage of an intense or insidious inflammatory process, and it occurs mainly as a consequence of collagen destruction. Fibrosis that is histologically recognizable does not necessarily produce a visible clinical scar. Ulcers that cause damage to collagen in the superficial dermis only do not usually result in scarring, whereas virtually all ulcers that extend into the deep dermis inexorably proceed to fibrosis and clinical scars.

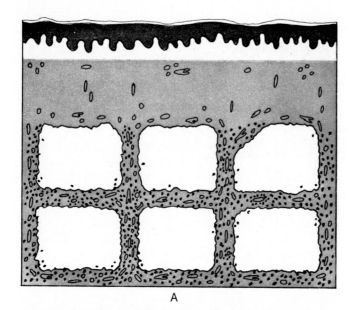

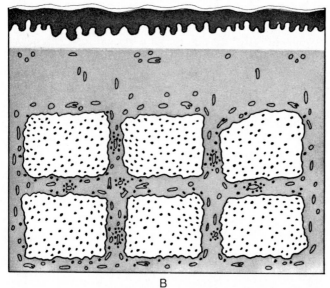

Figure 2:42. *A*, Septal panniculitis. *B*, Lobular panniculitis. (From Ackerman, A. B.: Histologic Diagnosis of Inflammatory Diseases. Lea & Febiger, Philadelphia, 1978.)

Fibrosing dermatitis (Fig. 2:43) follows severe insults to many types to dermal collagen. Thus, fibrosing dermatitis alone is of minimal diagnostic value, other than for its testimony to severe antecedent injury. The pathologist will have to look carefully for telltale signs of the antecedent process, such as furunculosis, vascular disease, foreign material, lymphedema, lupus erythematosus, dermatomyositis, and morphea.

ENDOCRINOPATHY

Endocrine dermatoses are those associated with various documented or presumed hormonal disturbances. These dermatoses have in common many histopathologic findings.[28] The existence of an endocrinopathy is suggested by the following dermatohistopathologic lesions: orthokeratotic hyperkeratosis,

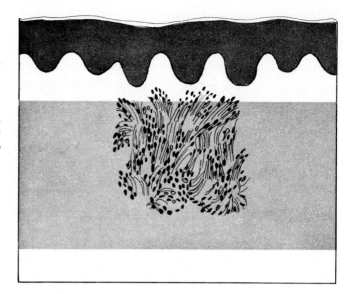

Figure 2:43. Fibrosing dermatitis. (From Ackerman, A. B.: Histologic Diagnosis of Inflammatory Diseases. Lea & Febiger, Philadelphia, 1978.)

follicular keratosis, telogenization of hair follicles, follicular atrophy, follicular dilatation and plugging, hair follicles devoid of hair, and sebaceous gland atrophy (Fig. 2:44). Although these findings are indicative of an endocrinopathy, they are nondiagnostic. Findings indicative of a *specific* endocrinopathy may or may not be present in any given specimen (see Chap. 10).

Inflammatory changes are a frequent and potentially misleading finding in the endocrine dermatoses, and they reflect the common occurrence of secondary seborrhea or pyoderma with these disorders (see Chap. 10). In such cases, it is essential that the clinician supply detailed histoclinical data and that the pathologist "read between the lines" and look beyond the distracting inflammatory changes.

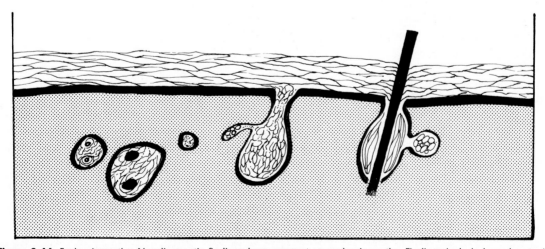

Figure 2:44. Endocrinopathy. Nondiagnostic findings here suggest an endocrinopathy. Findings include hyperkeratosis, follicular keratosis, follicular atrophy, follicular dilatation and plugging, mostly telogen hair follicles, epidermal hyperpigmentation, and sebaceous gland atrophy.

ENDOCRINE IMPERSONATORS

Certain dermatoses are characterized by clinical and pathologic findings that may be suggestive of an endocrinopathic condition. Various *genetic hypotrichoses* (hypotrichosis, black hair follicle dysplasia, color mutant alopecia) are characterized by follicular keratosis and atrophy and by telogenization. However, dystrophic hair follicles (poorly developed, anomalous shapes, abortive attempts to form hairs) are usually observed, and other signs of dermal atrophy are usually not present. *Nutritional deficiencies* may be characterized by varying degrees of cutaneous atrophy as well as by anomalous and curled ("corkscrew") hair shafts. *Telogen defluxion* is characterized by telogenization but by no other signs of cutaneous atrophy. In the chronic stage, *alopecia areata* is characterized by follicular atrophy as well as by "orphaned" cutaneous glands and arrector pili muscles. In the chronic stage, granulomatous sebaceous adenitis is characterized by complete absence of sebaceous glands and variable degrees of hyperkeratosis.

INVISIBLE DERMATOSES

Generations of dermatohistopathologists have struggled with biopsy specimens from diseased skin that appear to be normal under the microscope. Since normal skin is rarely biopsied in clinical practice, one must assume that some evidence of disease is present. From the perspective of the dermatohistopathologist, the *invisible dermatoses* are clinically evident skin diseases that show a histologic picture resembling normal skin.[2] Technical problems must be eliminated, such as sampling errors that occur when normal skin on an edge of the biopsy specimen has been sectioned and the diseased tissue has been left in paraffin.

When confronted with an invisible dermatosis, the dermatohistopathologist should consider the following possible disorders and techniques for detecting them: dermatophytosis (special stain for fungi in keratin), ichthyosis (surface keratin removed?), pigmentary disturbances (hypermelanoses and hypomelanoses, such as lentigo and vitiligo), amorphous deposits in the superficial dermis (Congo red stain for amyloid depositis), urticaria, urticaria pigmentosa (toluidine blue stain for mast cells), connective tissue disorder (cutaneous asthenia), and connective tissue nevi.

Conclusion

A skin biopsy can be diagnostic, confirmatory, and helpful, or it can be inconclusive, depending on the dermatosis, the selection, handling, and processing of the specimen and the skill of the histopathologist.

The dermatologist has no right to make a diagnosis of nonspecific dermatitis or inflammation. Every biopsy specimen is a sample of some specific process, but the visible changes may be "noncharacteristic" and may not permit a diagnosis.[12]

The clinician should always accept the terms "nonspecific changes" and "nonspecific dermatitis" only with great reserve. Many pathologic entities that are now well recognized were once regarded as nonspecific! *Recourse to serial sections (the key pathologic changes may be very focal), special stains, second opinions, and further biopsies may be required.*

References

1. Ackerman, A. B.: Histopathologic Diagnosis of Inflammatory Skin Diseases. Lea & Febiger, Philadelphia, 1978.
2. Brownstein, M. H., and Rabinowitz, A. D.: The invisible dermatoses. J. Am. Acad. Dermatol. 8:579, 1983.
3. Burgdorf, W. H. C., Nasemann, T., Janner, M., and Schutte, B.: Dermatopathology. Springer-Verlag, New York, 1984.
4. Dorland's Illustrated Medical Dictionary. 26th ed. W. B. Saunders Company, Philadelphia, 1981.
5. Fitzpatrick, T. B., et al.: Dermatology in General Medicine. 2nd ed. McGraw-Hill Book Company, New York, 1979.
6. Graham, J. H., et al.: Dermal Pathology. Harper & Row, New York, 1972.
7. Hirsh, B. C., and Johnson, W. C.: Concepts of granulomatous inflammation. Int. J. Dermatol. 23:90, 1984.
8. Hirsh, B. C., and Johnson, W. C.: Pathology of granulomatous diseases. Epithelioid granulomas, Part I. Int. J. Dermatol. 23:237, 1984.
9. Hirsh, B. C., and Johnson, W. C.: Pathology of granulomatous diseases. Epithelioid granulomas, Part II. Int. J. Dermatol. 23:306, 1984.
10. Hirsh, B. C., and Johnson, W. C.: Pathology of granulomatous diseases. Histiocytic granulomas. Int. J. Dermatol. 23:383, 1984.
11. Hirsh, B. C., and Johnson, W. C.: Pathology of granulomatous diseases. Foreign body granulomas. Int. J. Dermatol. 23:531, 1984.
12. Hirsh, B. C., and Johnson, W. C.: Pathology of granulomatous diseases. Mixed inflammatory granulomas. Int. J. Dermatol. 23:585, 1984.
12a. Hood, A. F., et al.: Primer of Dermatopathology. Little, Brown & Company, Boston, 1984.
13. Leider, M., and Rosenblum, M.: A Dictionary of Dermatological Words, Terms, and Phrases. McGraw-Hill Book Company, New York, 1968.
14. Lever, W. F., and Schaumburg-Lever, G.: Histopathology of the Skin. 6th ed. J. B. Lippincott Company, Philadelphia, 1983.
15. Lugo, M., and Putong, P. B.: Metaplasia. An overview. Arch. Pathol. Lab. Med. 108:185, 1984.
16. McMillan, E. M.: Monoclonal antibodies and cutaneous T cell lymphoma. J. Am. Acad. Dermatol. 12:102, 1985.
17. Milne, J. A.: An Introduction to the Diagnostic Histopathology of the Skin. Williams & Wilkins, Baltimore, 1972.
18. Montgomery, H.: Dermatopathology. Harper & Row, New York, 1967.
19. Moschella, S. L., et al.: Dermatology. 2nd ed. W. B. Saunders Company, Philadelphia, 1983.
20. Muller, G. H., et al: Small Animal Dermatology. 3rd ed. W. B. Saunders Company, Philadelphia, 1983.
21. Nishioka, K., et al.: Eosinophilic spongiosis in bullous pemphigoid. Arch. Dermatol. 120:1166, 1984.
21a. Okun, M. R., and Edelstein, L. M.: Gross and Microscopic Pathology of the Skin. Dermatopathology Foundation Press, Boston, 1976.
22. Mehregan, A. H.: Pinkus' Guide to Dermatohistopathology. 4th ed. Appleton-Century-Crofts, New York, 1986.
24. Penney, N. S.: Immunoperoxidase methods and advances in skin biology. J. Am. Acad. Dermatol. 11:284, 1984.
25. Robinson, J. K.: Fundamentals of Skin Biopsy. Year Book Medical Publishers, Inc., Chicago, 1986.
26. Rook, A., et al.: Textbook of Dermatology. 3rd ed. Blackwell Scientific Publications, Oxford, 1979.
27. Scott, D. W.: Lichenoid reaction in the skin of dogs: Clinicopathologic correlations. J.A.A.H.A. 20:305, 1984.
28. Scott, D. W.: Histopathologic findings in the endocrine skin disorders of the dog. J.A.A.H.A. 18:173, 1982.
29. Yager, J. A., and Scott, D. W.: The skin and appendages. *In* Pathology of Domestic Animals. 3rd ed. Academic Press, Inc., New York, 1985, p. 407.
30. Turner, R. R., et al.: Histiocytic malignancies. Morphologic, immunologic, and enzymatic heterogeneity. Am. J. Surg. Pathol. 8:485, 1984.

3

Diagnostic Methods

The Systematic Approach

If the veterinarian examines patients with skin disease in a cursory manner and attempts to make snap judgments, confusion and incorrect diagnoses will often result. In no other system of the body is a careful plan of examination and evaluation more important than in skin. Ideally, a thorough examination and appropriate diagnostic procedures should be accomplished the first time the patient is seen and before any masking treatments have been initiated. The following points should be systematically considered and correlated for a rational, accurate dermatologic diagnosis.

Steps to a Dermatologic Diagnosis

1. *Clinical Examination: Record age, sex, breed, and general medical and dermatologic history. The inquiry should determine the chief complaint and data about the original lesion's location, appearance, onset, and rate of progression. Also determine the presence and degree of pruritus, contagion to other animals or people, and possible seasonal incidence. Relationship to diet and environmental factors and the response to previous medications are also important.*
2. *Physical Examination:*
   a. *Determine the distribution pattern and the regional location of affected areas.*
   b. *Closely examine the skin to identify primary and secondary lesions. Evaluate alopecias or hair abnormalities.*
   c. *Observe the configurations of specific skin lesions and their relationship to each other; certain patterns are diagnostically significant.*
3. *Diagnostic and Laboratory Aids: Diagnostic aids such as skin scrapings, Wood's light examination, impression smears, and fungal or bacterial cultures should be done routinely. Biopsies, hormonal assays, chemistry panels, and other special tests are also performed when indicated by clinical findings.*
4. *Correlation of the Data: Make a list of differential diagnoses.*
5. *Narrowing the List of Differential Diagnoses: Plan additional tests, observations of therapeutic trials, and so on to narrow the list and provide a definitive diagnosis.*

Clinical Examination

RECORDS

Recording historical facts, physical findings, and laboratory data in a systematic way is particularly important in patients with skin disease. Many dermatoses are chronic, and skin lesions are slow to change. For this reason, outline sketches of the patient enable the clinician to draw in the location and extent of lesions. One sketch is worth many words, and comparison of sketches made at different intervals graphically portrays changes in the lesions over time.

Figure 3:1 illustrates a satisfactory record form for noting physical and laboratory findings for dermatology cases. The special form enables one to circle pertinent descriptive terms, saves time, and ensures that no important information is omitted. This form details only dermatologic data and should be used as a supplement to the general history and physical examination record. A special dermatologic history form is also useful, especially for allergic and chronic cases (Fig. 3:2).

HISTORY

The clinician should obtain a complete medical history in all cases. Some dermatologists prefer to examine the skin quickly at first, so that pertinent questions can be emphasized in taking the history, while inappropriate items can be omitted. However, it is vital to use a systematic, detailed method of examination and history taking so that important information is not overlooked.

AGE

Some dermatologic disorders are age related, so age is important in the dermatology history. For example, demodicosis usually begins in young dogs before sexual maturity. Allergies tend to appear in more mature individuals, probably because repeated exposure to the antigen must occur before clinical signs develop. Hormonal disorders tend to occur in animals between 6 and 10 years of age, and most neoplasms develop in mature-to-older patients. Most of the ages listed in Table 3:1 refer to the usual age at the beginning of the disease.

SEX

The sex of the patient obviously limits the incidence of certain problems, but it is especially important in sex hormone imbalances. Perianal adenomas are seen almost exclusively in male dogs. One should determine whether the patient is sexually intact and, if so, whether the skin problem bears any relationship to the estrual cycle.

BREED

Breed predilection determines the incidence of some skin disorders. For example, seborrhea is common in cocker spaniels; acanthosis nigricans usually occurs in dachshunds; adult-onset hyposomatotropism occurs in Pomeranians, keeshonds, and chow chows; dermatomyositis is found in Shetland sheepdogs and collies; zinc-responsive dermatosis occurs in Siberian huskies and Alaskan malamutes; and many of the wire-coated terrier breeds (Scotties, Cairns,

NEW YORK STATE COLLEGE OF VETERINARY MEDICINE—VETERINARY TEACHING HOSPITAL

DERMATOLOGY

DATE: _____

REF. DVM _____

CLINICIAN _____

SECONDARY # _____

PRIMARY LESIONS (Circle)

Macule	Patch	Papule	Plaque
Vesicle	Bulla	Pustule	Wheal
Nodule	Tumor		

SECONDARY LESIONS (Circle)

Scale   Epidermal collarette   Scar
Ulcer   Erosion   Crust   Excoriation
Fissure   Comedone   Cyst   Abscess
Hypopigmentation   Hyperpigmentation   Erythema
Hyperkeratosis   Callus   Alopecia

Pruritus:

Parasites:

SKIN CHANGES

Elasticity + −   Extensibility + −
Thickness + −

QUALITY OF HAIR COAT   OTHER FACTORS

Epilation: + −   Footpads
Pelage is: Dry,   Nails
  Brittle, Dull, Oily   Hyperhidrosis

CONFIGURATION OF LESIONS

Linear   Annular (Target)   Grouped

DIFFERENTIAL DIAGNOSIS

DISTRIBUTION OF LESIONS

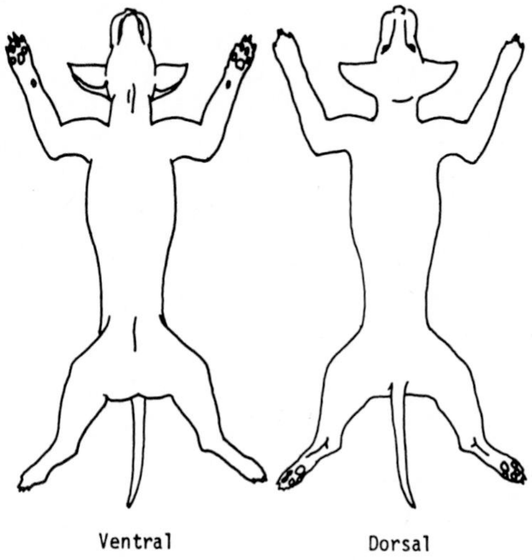

Ventral   Dorsal

LABORATORY TESTS

Scotch Tape: _____Wood's Light + −
Skin Scraping: _____
KOH Digestion: _____
Direct Smear: _____
Fungal Culture: _____
Bacterial Culture: _____
Sensitivity: _____
Allergy: _____
_____
Endocrine: _____
Immune:
  D.I.T.: _____
  I.I.T.: _____
ANA: _____
Other: _____
Biopsy:

Figure 3:1. Dermatology examination sheet.

NEW YORK STATE COLLEGE OF VETERINARY MEDICINE—VETERINARY TEACHING HOSPITAL

DATE: _____   DERMATOLOGY HISTORY SHEET

CHIEF COMPLAINT(S) _____

_____

_____

_____

AGE PURCHASED _____

REF. DVM _____   KENNEL ____PET SHOP ____PRIVATE ____WHERE ___

CLINICIAN _____   HAS ANIMAL BEEN OUT OF AREA? YES ____NO _____

SECONDARY #_____   IF YES—WHERE _____

_____

Date Problem First Noticed _____ Age _____Is It Year Round? Yes _____No _____

If Seasonal, Is It Worse: Spring _____Summer _____Fall _____Winter _____

Where Did Problem Begin? _____

What Did It Look Like Then? _____

How Has It Changed or Spread? _____

Are Other Animals or People Affected? Yes _____No _____If So Describe _____

When Did You Last See Fleas? _____

Describe Animal's Indoor Environment _____

Time Indoors _____% _____

Describe Animal's Outdoor Environment _____

Time Outdoors _____%_____

Does Animal Itch? Yes _____   No _____   When? Constantly _____Sporadically _____Night _____

Animal's Diet _____

What Medications Have Been Used? List Effects and Dates Used _____

_____

_____

_____

Other Illnesses of Animal _____

What Other Facts Do You Think Would Be Helpful? _____

_____

_____

_____

(Use Reverse Side If Needed)

Figure 3:2. Dermatology history sheet.

Table 3:1. SKIN DISEASE WITH FREQUENT AGE-RELATED ONSET (STRONG CLINICAL IMPRESSION)

Age	Disease
Less than 6 months	Acanthosis nigricans
	Acne, canine
	Alopecia universalis
	Black hair follicle dysplasia
	Color mutant alopecia
	Cutaneous asthenia
	Demodicosis, generalized
	Demodicosis, localized
	Dermatomyositis
	Dermatophytosis
	Epidermolysis bullosa
	Ectodermal defect
	Hypotrichosis
	Ichthyosis
	Impetigo
	Infantile pustular dermatosis
	Juvenile cellulitis
	Lymphedema
	Mucopolysaccharidosis
	Other congenital hereditary defects
	Pituitary dwarfism
	Tyrosinemia
	Viral papillomatosis (oral)
	Zinc-responsive dermatosis
1 to 3 years	Atopy
	Food allergy, skin fold dermatitis
	Hyposomatotropism in the mature dog
	Seborrhea
Over 6 years	Endocrine imbalances
	Hepatocutaneous syndrome
	Lip fold dermatitis
	Neoplasms
Senile dogs	Alopecia
	Decubital ulcer
	Nasodigital hyperkeratosis
	Thin, fragile skin

Sealyhams, West Highland whites, Irish terriers, and Welsh terriers) seem to be particularly predisposed to allergic skin disease (see Table 3:2).

In a study of dogs in northern California conducted at the University of California at Davis, thirty-one breeds were found to be at elevated risk for the development of skin diseases, including Doberman pinscher, Irish setter, Dalmatian, dachshund, golden retriever, various terrier breeds, Shar Pei, chow chow, and akita.[1] In the same study, decreased risk for skin disease was found for dogs of mixed breeding and for twelve purebred breeds, including St. Bernard, standard poodle, beagle, basset hound, German short-haired pointer, Afghan hound, and Australian shepherd.

OWNER'S COMPLAINT

The owner's complaint or chief cause of concern is often the major sign used in compiling a differential diagnosis. The clinician who can "draw out" a complete history in an unbiased form has, indeed, a valuable skill. It is

Table 3:2. BREED PREDILECTION FOR SKIN DISEASES (STRONG CLINICAL IMPRESSION)

Breed	Disease	Breed	Disease
Abyssinian cat	Idiopathic ceruminous otitis externa Psychogenic dermatitis/alopecia	Collie	Bullous pemphigoid Dermatomyositis Discoid lupus erythematosus
Afghan hound	Hypothyroidism		Fibrous histiocytoma
Airedale	Hyposomatotropism Melanoma		Keratoacanthoma Nasal pyoderma Pemphigus erythematosus
Akita	Granulomatous sebaceous adenitis Pemphigus foliaceus Vogt-Koyanagi-Harada–like syndrome		Sertoli's cell tumor Systemic lupus erythematosus
		Dachshund	Acanthosis nigricans Demodicosis
Basenji	Immunoproliferative enteropathy		Folliculitis and pododermatitis
Beagle	Demodicosis Lymphosarcoma, perianal gland tumor, sebaceous gland tumor		Histiocytoma Hyperadrenocorticism Hypothyroidism Juvenile cellulitis
Bernese Mountain dog	Hemangiosarcoma Malignant histiocytosis Systemic histiocytosis		Linear IgA dermatosis Lipoma, liposarcoma Mastocytoma Nodular panniculitis
Boston terrier	Atopy, calcinosis circumscripta, fibroma, melanoma Demodicosis Hyperadrenocorticism Mastocytoma Sebaceous gland tumor Tail fold dermatitis		Pattern alopecia (ears) Pattern alopecia (ventral) Pemphigus foliaceus Sebaceous gland tumor Sterile pyogranuloma syndrome Sternal callus Vasculitis
Boxer	Acne, canine Atopy, calcinosis circumscripta Demodicosis Dermoid cyst Fibroma, hemangioma Hemangiopericytoma Histiocytoma Hyperadrenocorticism Hypothyroidism, lymphosarcoma Mastocytoma Pododermatitis Sertoli's cell tumor Squamous cell carcinoma Sterile pyogranuloma syndrome Sternal callus	Dalmatian	Atopy Demodicosis Folliculitis and furunculosis Squamous cell carcinoma
		Doberman pinscher	Acne, canine Acral lick dermatitis Color mutant alopecia (blue) Demodicosis Flank sucking Folliculitis and pododermatitis Hypopigmentation (lip, nose) Hypothyroidism Sterile pyogranuloma syndrome
Bull Terrier	Furunculosis, bacterial Mastocytoma Squamous cell carcinoma Zinc deficiency	English bulldog	Acne Demodicosis Facial fold dermatitis Folliculitis and pododermatitis Hypothyroidism
Cats (general)	Abscess Acne Dermatophytosis Eosinophilic plaque, eosinophilic granuloma, indolent ulcer Feline symmetric alopecia Flea bite hypersensitivity Otodectic otitis Plasma cell pododermatitis Psychogenic dermatitis/alopecia Solar dermatitis Stud tail		Mastocytoma Perianal gland tumor Sterile pyogranuloma syndrome Tail fold dermatitis
		German shepherd	Calcinosis circumscripta Cellulitis (folliculitis and furunculosis) Collagenous nevi Collagen disorder of footpads Discoid lupus erythematosus Fly dermatitis of ear tips Hemangioma—hemangiosarcoma Hemangiopericytoma Keratoacanthoma Lymphosarcoma Multiple perianal fistulas Nasal pyoderma
Chihuahua	Demodicosis		
Chow chow	Hyposomatotropism Hypothyroidism Pemphigus foliaceus		*Table continued on following page*

Table 3:2. BREED PREDILECTION FOR SKIN DISEASES
(STRONG CLINICAL IMPRESSION) *Continued*

Breed	Disease	Breed	Disease
German shepherd (Continued)	Otitis externa Pemphigus erythematosus Pituitary dwarfism Seborrhea Systemic lupus erythematosus	Pointers	Acral mutilation Demodicosis Juvenile cellulitis
		Pomeranian	Hyposomatotropism
Golden retriever	Acral lick dermatitis Acute moist dermatitis Atopy Folliculitis and furunculosis Hypothyroidism Juvenile cellulitis Lymphosarcoma	Poodle	Basal cell tumor Ectodermal defect Epiphora Granulomatous sebaceous adenitis Hyperadrenocorticism Hyposomatotropism Hypothyroidism Otitis externa Pilomatrixoma Sebaceous gland tumor Squamous cell carcinoma
Great Dane	Acne Acral lick dermatitis Callus formation, hygroma Demodicosis Dermoid cyst Histiocytoma Hygroma Hypothyroidism Pododermatitis—folliculitis		
		Pug	Atopy Facial fold and tail fold dermatitis
		Rhodesian ridgeback	Dermoid sinus in midline of back
Great Pyrenees	Acute moist dermatitis Demodicosis	Rottweiler	Folliculitis Vasculitis Vitiligo
Irish setter	Atopy Acral lick dermatitis Color mutant alopecia Folliculitis and furunculosis Hypothyroidism Seborrhea	Samoyed	Perianal gland tumor
		Schipperke	Pemphigus foliaceus
		Shar Pei	Atopy Demodicosis Fold dermatitis Folliculitis Hypothyroidism Seborrhea
Irish wolfhound	Hygroma Hypothyroidism		
Keeshond	Castration responsive dermatosis Keratoacanthoma Hyposomatotropism Hypothyroidism	Siamese cat	Hypotrichosis Periocular leukotrichia Psychogenic dermatitis/alopecia
Labrador retriever	Acral lick dermatitis Acute moist dermatitis Atopy Folliculitis and furunculosis Lipoma Mastocytoma Seborrhea	Schnauzer	Atopy Hypothyroidism Schnauzer comedo syndrome Subcorneal pustular dermatosis
		Shetland sheepdog	Dermatomyositis Discoid lupus erythematosus Epidermolysis bullosa (?) Folliculitis Histiocytoma Systemic lupus erythematosus
Lhasa apso	Atopy		
Malamute	Zinc-responsive dermatosis Castration-responsive dermatosis		
		Siberian husky	Castration responsive dermatosis Discoid lupus erythematosus Eosinophilic granuloma Zinc-responsive dermatosis
Norwegian elkhound	Keratoacanthoma Sebaceous gland tumor		
Old English sheepdog	Demodicosis Folliculitis—pododermatitis	Spaniels (cocker and springer)	Apocrine gland tumor Basal cell tumor Cutaneous asthenia Epidermoid cyst Fibrosarcoma Hypothyroidism Lichenoid psoriasiform dermatosis Lip fold dermatitis
Pekingese	Facial fold dermatitis Sertoli's cell tumor Squamous cell carcinoma		
Persian cat	Facial fold dermatitis Dermatophytosis Hair mats		

Table 3:2. BREED PREDILECTION FOR SKIN DISEASES
(STRONG CLINICAL IMPRESSION) *Continued*

Breed	Disease	Breed	Disease
Spaniels (cocker and springer) *(Continued)*	Lipoma Lymphosarcoma Melanoma Otitis externa Papilloma Perianal gland tumor Sebaceous gland tumor Seborrhea Trichoepithelioma	Scottish	Atopy Folliculitis Lymphosarcoma Melanoma Squamous cell carcinoma
		West Highland white	Atopy Epidermal dysplasia Seborrhea
Terriers		Wire-haired fox	Atopy Neurofibroma
Cairn	Atopy		Sebaceous gland tumor
Kerry blue	Dermoid cyst Footpad keratoses (corns) Otitis externa Papilloma Pilomatrixoma	Viszla	Granulomatous sebaceous adenitis
		Weimaraner	Lipoma Mastocytoma Sertoli's cell tumor Sterile pyogranuloma syndrome

important that the questions presented to the client do not suggest answers or tend to shut off discussion. A friendly "Let's help this patient together" attitude often stimulates the client to reveal more information. Some owners purposely or unconsciously withhold pertinent facts, especially about neglect, diet, previous medication, or other procedures they feel may not be well received by the examining veterinarian. The skillful clinician is ever tuned to listen for side comments by the client or by the children. These may be veritable "pearls" of information in a mass of trivia.

Next, the following information should be obtained from the owner: date of onset, original locations of the lesions, description of the initial lesions, tendency to progression or regression, factors affecting the course, and previous treatment (home, proprietary, or pet shop remedies used, as well as veterinary treatment).

Almost all animals with skin disorders have been bathed, dipped, sprayed, or larded with one or more medications, and the owner may be reluctant to disclose a complete and honest list of previous treatment. It is important that the types of medication and dates of application be completely divulged, since a modification of pertinent signs may have resulted.

Although the patient cannot relate subjective findings (symptoms), it is possible to determine the degree of hyperesthesia, pruritus, and pain reasonably well.

Pruritus is one of the most common presenting complaints and in many cases is a hallmark of cutaneous allergy. The presence and degree of itching is a most important criterion in the differential diagnosis of many skin diseases.

> **The presence or absence of pruritus is one of the most important clinical facts in the differential diagnosis of dermatoses.**

The owner's idea of the intensity of itching, however, may vary considerably from that of the veterinarian. Consequently, it is helpful to ask the questions, "How many times daily do you see your dog scratch?" "Does he itch in many sites, or just a few?" "Does he shake his head?" "Does he lick his paws?"

The same type of specific question is helpful when discussing diets, as the owner often remembers the atypical feedings. A more representative answer is often secured if one asks, "What did your pet eat yesterday (or over the past 48 hours)?"

Since contact irritants or allergens are important, it is necessary to inquire about the dog's environment. Does he live in an apartment or is he outdoors in the fields and forests? Does he sleep in a dog house or in the owner's bed? Does the bedding consist of straw, shavings, or wool blankets?

In determining contagion, one should inquire about the skin health of other animals on the premises. The presence of skin disease in the people associated with the patient also may be highly significant in some disorders (scabies and dermatophytosis).

At this point, the clinician usually has a general idea of the problem and is ready to proceed with a careful physical examination. In some cases the clinician may want to come back to the general medical history, if further developments indicate a more serious or underlying systemic disease. Table 3:3 lists some systemic diseases with cutaneous lesions.

Physical Examination

In dermatology the clinician can observe the pathologic lesions directly and need not rely on radiologic shadows or referred sounds to determine abnor-

Table 3:3. SYSTEMIC DISEASES WITH CUTANEOUS LESIONS

Disease	Skin Lesions or Symptoms
Atopy	Pruritus
Castration responsive dermatosis	Alopecia
Cold agglutinin disease	Erythema, purpura, necrosis, ulceration
Diabetes mellitus	Atrophy, ulceration, pyoderma, seborrhea
Dirofilariasis	Erythema, alopecia, pruritus, nodules
Erythema multiforme	Macules, papules, vesicles, wheals
Feline leukemia virus infection	Pyoderma, seborrhea, poor healing, cutaneous horns on footpads
Hepatocutaneous syndrome	Mucocutaneous crusts and ulcers, footpad hyperkeratosis and ulcers
Hyperadrenocorticism	Alopecia, hyperpigmentation, calcinosis cutis, pyoderma, seborrhea, phlebectasias, thin and hypotonic skin
Hypothyroidism	Alopecia, hypothermia, seborrhea, pyoderma, hyperpigmentation, myxedema, galactorrhea
Leishmaniasis	Erythema, nodules, ulceration, exfoliative dermatitis
Male feminizing syndrome	Alopecia, seborrhea, hyperpigmentation, gynecomastia, galactorrhea
Mycoses, deep	Nodules, ulceration, fistulas
Mycosis fungoides	Erythroderma, plaques, nodules, ulceration
Ovarian imbalances	Alopecia, hyperpigmentation, seborrhea
Pemphigus	Purulent exudate, crusting, vesiculation, ulceration/erosion
Pituitary dwarfism	Alopecia, cutaneous degeneration, hyperpigmentation
Sertoli's cell tumor	Alopecia, gynecomastia, hyperpigmentation
Systemic lupus erythematosus	Pyoderma, seborrhea, ulceration, pruritus, erythema
Thallium toxicosis	Alopecia, erythema, ulceration
Toxic epidermal necrolysis	Ulceration, blisters, pain
Tuberculosis	Nodules, ulceration, fistulas

mality, as skin lesions are clearly visible. By careful, systematic inspection alone, the diagnosis of many dermatoses becomes apparent.

> **Good lighting is of paramount importance.**

Normal daylight without glare is best, but any artificial light of adequate candle power is sufficient if it produces bright, uniform lighting. The lamp should be adjustable to illuminate all body areas. A combination loupe and light provides magnification of the field as well as good illumination.

Before concentration on the individual lesions begins, the entire animal should always be observed from a distance of several feet for a general impression of abnormalities and to observe distribution patterns.

Does he appear to be in good health? Is he fat or thin, unkempt or well groomed? Is the problem generalized or localized? What is the distribution of the lesions? Are they bilaterally symmetric or unilaterally irregular?

In order that some of these questions can be answered, the patient must be examined more closely. The dorsal aspect of the body should be inspected by viewing it from the rear, as elevated hairs are more obvious from that angle. Then, carefully, the lateral surfaces should be observed. Next, the clinician should turn the patient over for a careful examination of the ventral region.

CLOSE EXAMINATION OF THE SKIN

After an impression is obtained from a distance, the skin should be examined more closely. Palpation now becomes important too. What is the texture of the hair? Is it coarse or fine, dry or oily, and does it epilate easily? A change in the amount of hair present is often a dramatic finding. Alopecia is a complete lack of hair in areas where it is normally present. Hypotrichosis implies a partial alopecia that may be developmental, hormonal, neoplastic, inflammatory, or idiopathic. Hypertrichosis is excess hair and, although very rare in animals, is usually hormonal or developmental in nature.

The texture, elasticity, and thickness of the skin should be determined and impressions of heat or coolness recorded. It is important to examine every inch of skin and mucous membranes. It is easier to find important skin lesions in some breeds than in others, depending on the thickness of the coat. There is a variation in density of an individual's coat in different body areas. Lesions can be discerned more easily in sparsely haired regions. However, the clinician must part or clip the hair in many areas to observe and palpate lesions that are partially covered. It is useful to clip hair over an area of abnormal skin with a surgical blade (such as No. 40 Oster) to expose the area for identification of lesions. The clipped area is then cleansed with alcohol. Lesions previously hidden by hair and debris can now be clearly seen and interpreted. It is as if a "window" appears giving a new view of the skin disease. When abnormalities are discovered it is important to establish their general distribution as well as their configuration within an area (Fig. 3:3). Are they single, multiple, discrete, diffuse, grouped, or confluent? With sharp observation, linear or annular configuration of the lesions may be noted (Table 3:4).

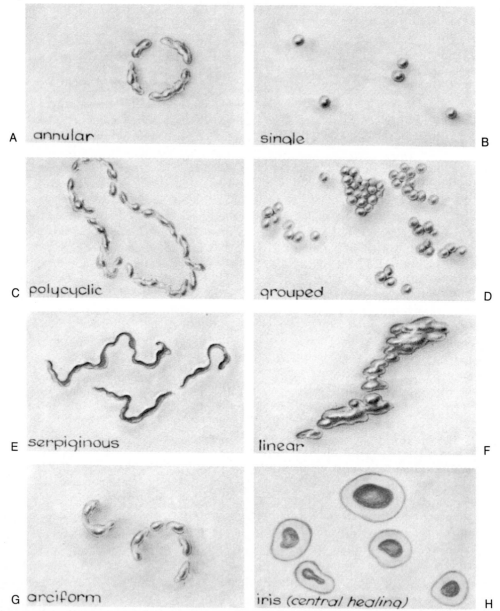

Figure 3:3. Configuration of skin lesions. *A,* Annular configuration has a clear or less involved center and is found in local seborrhea and certain dermatomycoses. *B,* Single lesions are typified by canine acne, acral lick dermatitis, cysts, and many tumors. *C,* Polycyclic configurations often result from the confluence of lesions or a spreading process. Examples are demodicosis or acute moist dermatitis. *D,* Grouped lesions are clusters, often the result of new foci developing around an old lesion. They are seen in folliculitis, nasal pyoderma, contact dermatitis, and calcinosis cutis. *E,* Serpiginous lesions develop as a result of spreading, such as in canine scabies or demodicosis. *F,* Linear configurations are best typified by linear granuloma of cats or by contact with irritant materials streaked along the skin. *G,* Arciform lesions may result from spreading, as in canine scabies and demodicosis. *H,* Central-healing (target) configurations are produced when the skin heals behind an advancing front of a disease process. It is typical of certain dermatophytoses, demodicosis, and folliculitis.

Table 3:4. DERMATOLOGIC DESCRIPTION
(OTHER THAN PRIMARY AND SECONDARY LESIONS)

Distribution	***Consistency***
Generalized	Indurated
Localized	Soft
Bilateral symmetric	Rolled border
Asymmetric	Fluctuant
Patchy	Atrophied
Scattered	
Multifocal	***Quality***
	Dry
Arrangement	Moist
Discrete	Greasy
Confluent	Oozing
Well defined	Bleeding
Poorly defined	Secondarily infected
	Purulent
Configuration	
Annular	***Color***
Arciform	Erythematous
Grouped	Violaceous
Polycyclic	Yellow
Linear	Brown
Serpiginous	White
Central healing	Gray
	Black
Depth	
Elevated	
Surface	
Deep	

Two special techniques of close examination of the skin are noteworthy:

1. *Diascopy* is a technique that involves pressing a clear piece of plastic or glass over an erythematous lesion. If the lesion blanches on pressure, the reddish color is due to vascular engorgement. If it does not, there is hemorrhage into the skin (petechia or ecchymosis).

2. *Nikolsky's sign* is elicited by applying pressure on a vesicle or at the edge of an ulcer or erosion or even on normal skin. It is positive when the outer layer of the skin is easily rubbed off or pushed away. It indicates poor cellular cohesion, as found in the pemphigus complex.

At this point one should focus upon individual lesions and examine them minutely with good light and a hand lens or a head loupe with 4- to 6-power magnification.

Examine individual lesions minutely with a magnifying head loupe or other magnifying device.

Lesional Changes

The evolution of lesions should be determined either by history or by finding different stages of lesions on the same patient. Papules often develop into vesicles and pustules, which may rupture to leave erosions or ulcers and finally crusts. An understanding of these processes helps in the diagnostic process. As lesions develop in special patterns, they also involute in characteristic ways.

Acute lesions often appear suddenly and disappear quickly and completely. Chronic lesions may leave diagnostically important pigmentation or scars that persist for months or permanently (i.e., chronic generalized demodicosis and juvenile cellulitis, respectively).

MORPHOLOGY OF SKIN LESIONS

> **Search for individual lesions: scrutinize and identify.**

Morphology of skin lesions is the essential feature of dermatologic diagnosis and sometimes is the *only* guide if laboratory procedures yield no useful information. The clinician must learn to recognize primary and secondary lesions! A primary lesion is one that develops spontaneously as a direct reflection of underlying disease. Secondary lesions evolve from primary lesions or are artifacts induced by the patient or by external factors such as trauma or medications. Careful inspection of the diseased skin will frequently reveal a primary lesion suggestive of a specific dermatosis. In many cases, however, the significant lesion must be differentiated from the mass of secondary debris. The ability to discover a characteristic lesion and understand its significance is the first step toward mastering dermatologic diagnosis. Variations are common, since early as well as advanced stages exist in most skin diseases. In addition, the appearance of skin lesions may change with medication, self-inflicted trauma, and secondary infection.

Most skin diseases, however, are characterized by a single type of lesion. This primary lesion varies slightly from its initial appearance to its full development. Later, through regression, degeneration, or traumatization, it changes in appearance and in its new, altered form becomes a secondary lesion.

The diagrams and photographs of this chapter help, in a graphic way, to identify the primary and secondary lesions. The definitions and examples explain the importance and relationship of skin lesions to canine and feline dermatoses.

The skin lesions depicted in the diagrams that follow graphically demonstrate how the pathologic morphology varies from normal (Figs. 3:4 to 3:21).

Primary Lesions (Lesions of first diagnostic importance)

Macule—patch	Pustule	Tumor—neoplasm	Wheal
Papule—plaque	Nodule	Vesicle—bulla	

Secondary Lesions (Evolutionary or complicating lesions of secondary diagnostic importance)

Scale—epidermal collarette	Comedo	Pigmentary abnormalities
Crust	Fissure	(hyperpigmentation or
Scar	Excoriation	hypopigmentation)
Erosion—ulcer	Lichenification	Hyperkeratosis-callus

NORMAL CANINE SKIN

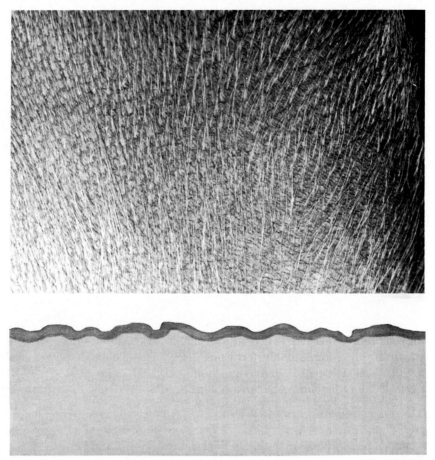

Figure 3:4. Normal canine skin. In the diagram, the dark (upper) zone represents the epidermis, which in canine skin is thin and without prominent epidermal pegs. The light (lower) zone represents the dermis.

DISTRIBUTION PATTERNS OF SKIN LESIONS

A dramatic change becomes apparent when a skin disorder affects an animal whose body is covered with a dense hair coat. Even the most casual observer is aware of the loss of hair in certain areas. The alopecic pattern, which is often sharply demarcated, assumes a new meaning when it is accurately interpreted. When alopecia and other hair changes are evaluated according to their distribution pattern over the entire body, significant diagnostic clues can be recognized. Comparatively speaking, only on the human scalp is alopecia as striking and meaningful.

Text continued on page 122

> *Recognizing the distribution pattern of skin lesions and hair changes is a valuable diagnostic aid.*

PRIMARY LESION—MACULE

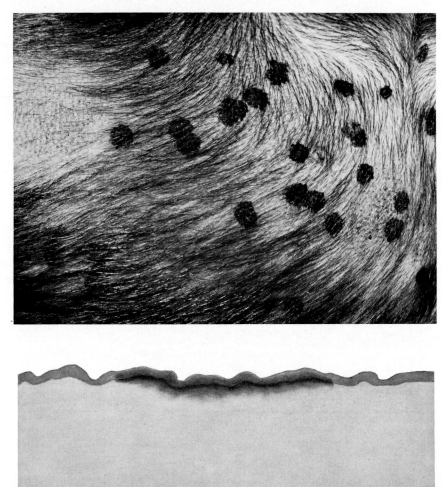

Figure 3:5. *Macule*—a circumscribed, flat spot up to 1 cm in size characterized by change in color of the skin. The discoloration can result from several processes: increase in melanin pigmentation, depigmentation, and erythema or local hemorrhage. Examples are the hyperpigmented patches in the axillae of dogs with acanthosis nigricans, erythematous macules in many types of acute dermatitis, lentigo, and pigmented nevi. (Photograph illustrates lentigo). Types of macules are as follows: *patch*—a macule over 2 cm in size; *purpura*—a type of macule caused by bleeding into the skin. It is usually dark red but changes to purple as absorption proceeds; *petechia*—pinpoint macules that are much less than 1 cm in diameter and that are due to hemorrhage; *ecchymoses*—patches greater than 1 cm in diameter that are due to hemorrhage.

PRIMARY LESION—PAPULE

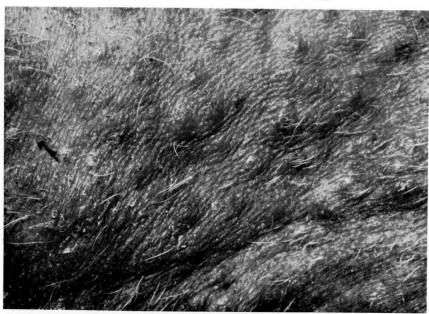

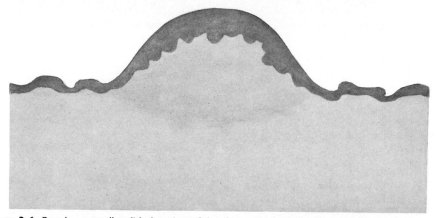

Figure 3:6. *Papule*—a small, solid elevation of the skin up to 1 cm in diameter. A papule can always be palpated as a solid mass. Many papules are pink or red swellings produced by tissue infiltration of inflammatory cells, by intraepidermal and subepidermal edema, or by epidermal hypertrophy. Papules may or may not involve hair follicles. Examples are the erythematous papules seen in chronic allergic contact dermatitis of dogs after exposure to plants. (Photograph illustrates allergic contact dermatitis.) *Plaque*—a larger flat-topped elevation formed by the extension or coalition of papules. A plaque that is made up of closely packed projecting elevations often covered by crusts is called a vegetation.

PRIMARY LESION—NODULE

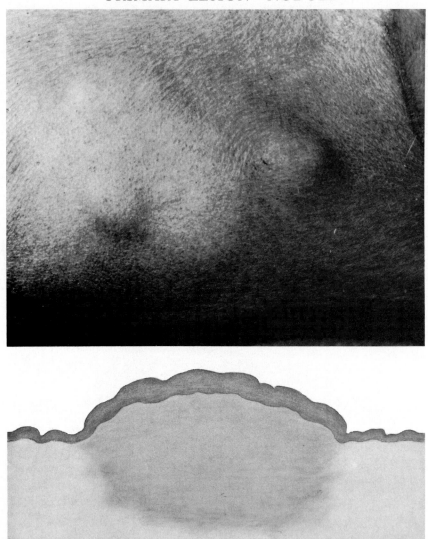

Figure 3:7. *Nodule*—a small circumscribed, solid elevation greater than 1 cm in diameter that usually extends into the deeper layers of the skin. Nodules usually result from massive infiltration of inflammation or neoplastic cells into the dermis or subcutis. Deposition of fibrin or crystalline material also produces nodules. (Photograph illustrates nodular panniculitis.)

PRIMARY LESION—TUMOR

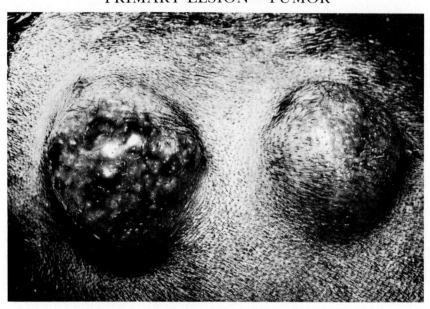

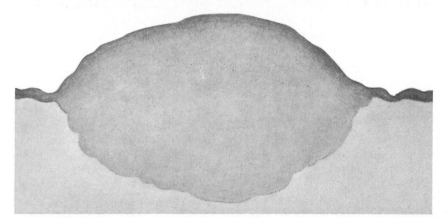

Figure 3:8. *Tumor*—a neoplastic enlargement that may involve any structure of the skin or subcutaneous tissue. Examples are fibromas, mastocytomas, melanoma, and carcinomas. (Photograph illustrates calcifying epitheliomas.) *Cyst*—an epithelium-lined cavity containing fluid or a solid material. It is a smooth, well-circumscribed fluctuant-to-solid mass. Skin cysts are usually lined by adnexal epithelium (hair follicle, sebaceous, or apocrine) and filled with cornified cellular debris or sebaceous or apocrine secretions.

PRIMARY LESION—PUSTULE

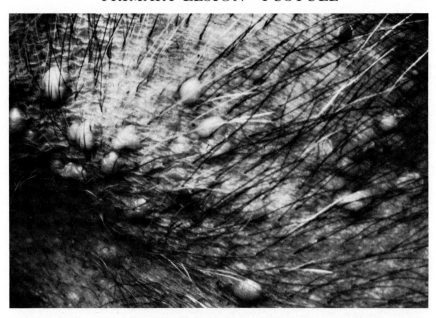

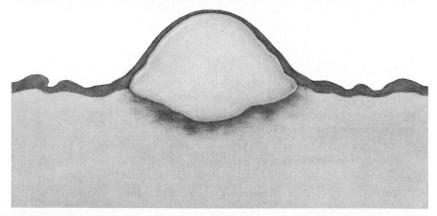

Figure 3:9. *Pustule*—a small, circumscribed elevation of the epidermis filled with pus. It is technically a small abscess (occasionally sterile) that may be intraepidermal or follicular in location. The color is usually yellow but may be pink or red. Examples are acne, folliculitis, and the pustules seen on the abdomen of puppies with impetigo. (Photograph illustrates nonfollicular pustules from subcorneal pustular dermatosis.) *Abscess*—a demarcated fluctuant lesion resulting from a dermal or subcutaneous accumulation of pus. The pus is not visible on the surface of the skin until it drains to the surface. Abscesses are usually larger and deeper than pustules.

PRIMARY LESION—WHEAL

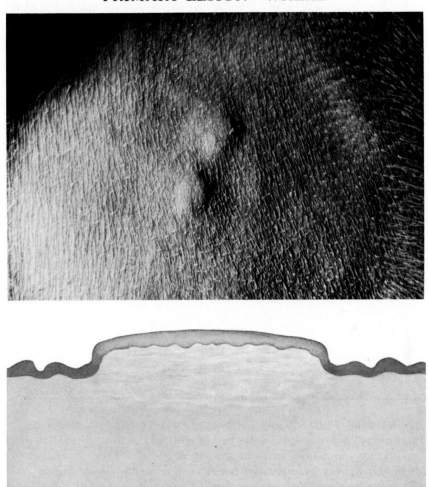

Figure 3:10. *Wheal*—a sharply circumscribed, raised lesion consisting of edema that appears and disappears within minutes or hours. Wheals are characteristically white-to-pink elevated ridges or round edematous swelling that only rarely have pseudopods at their periphery. They blanch upon diascopy (viewing the skin through a glass slide that is pressed firmly against the lesion). A huge hive of a distensible region such as the lips or eyelids is called angioedema. Urticarial lesions persist for days and consist of mixed cell infiltrate as well as edema. In dogs they produce characteristic raised areas of the hair coat that are especially prominent on the back. Examples of wheals are hives, insect bites, and positive reactions to allergy skin tests. (Photograph illustrates hives.)

PRIMARY LESION—VESICLE

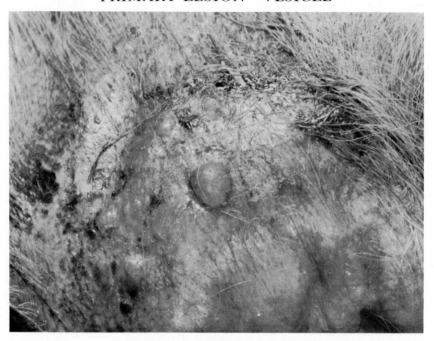

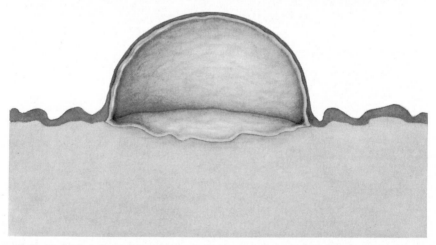

Figure 3:11. *Vesicle*—a sharply circumscribed elevation of the epidermis filled with clear fluid. They are rarely seen in dogs and cats, since they are fragile and transient. Lesions up to 1 cm in diameter are called vesicles and are seen in viral or autoimmune dermatoses, or dermatitis caused by irritants. They may be intraepidermal or subepidermal in location. *Bulla*—vesicle greater than 1 cm in diameter. (Photograph illustrates several vesicles on the medial surface of a canine pinna caused by a chemical irritant.

SECONDARY LESION—SCALE

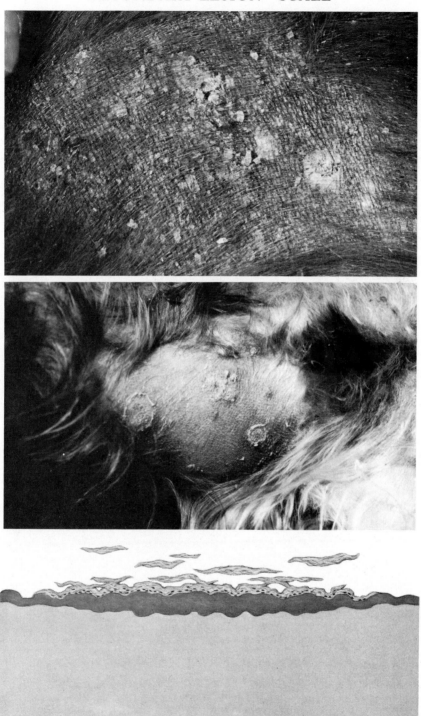

Figure 3:12. *Scale*—an accumulation of loose fragments of the horny layer of the skin (cornified cells). The scale is the final product of epidermal keratinization. The consistency of flakes varies greatly, and they can appear branny, fine, powdery, flaky, platelike, greasy, dry, loose, adhering, or "nitlike." The color varies from white, silver, yellow, or brown to gray. Scales are seen in seborrhea, generalized demodicosis, and chronic allergic dermatitis. (Top photograph illustrates seborrhea). *Epidermal collarette*—a special type of scale arranged in a circular rim of loose keratin flakes. It represents the remnants of the epidermal tissue layers that once formed the "roof" of a vesicle, bulla, or pustule. (Bottom photograph illustrates a healing pustule of staphylococcal folliculitis.)

SECONDARY LESION—CRUST

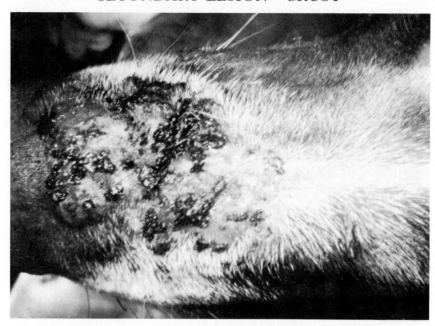

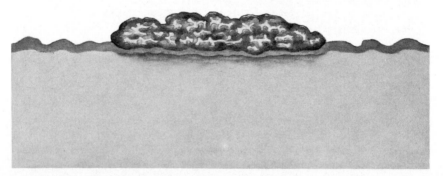

Figure 3:13. *Crust*—formed when dried exudate, serum, pus, blood, cells, scales, or medications adhere to the surface and often mingle with hair. Unusually thick crusts are found in hairy areas because the dried material tends to adhere more tightly than in glabrous skin. Hemorrhagic crusts in pyoderma are brown or dark red; yellowish-green crusts appear in some cases of pyoderma; tan, lightly adhering crusts are found in impetigo. *Vegetations*—heaped-up crusts seen in pemphigus vegetans. (Photograph illustrates nasal pyoderma.)

SECONDARY LESION—SCAR

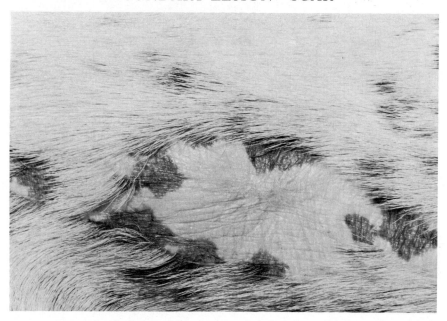

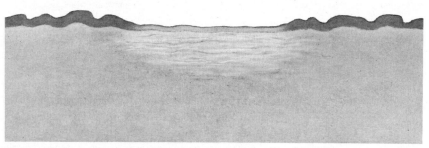

Figure 3:14. *Scar*—an area of fibrous tissue that has replaced the damaged dermis or subcutaneous tissue. Scars are the remnants of trauma or dermatologic lesions. Most scars in dogs and cats are alopecic, atrophic, and depigmented. Proliferative scars do occur and in dark-skinned dogs scars can be alopecic and hyperpigmented. Scars are observed following severe burns and in deep pyoderma. (Photograph illustrates burn scarring.)

SECONDARY LESION—ULCER

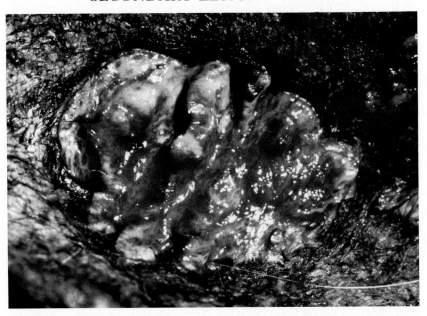

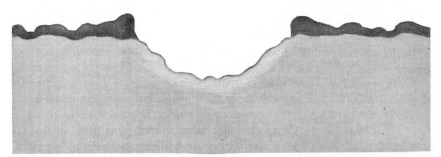

Figure 3:15. *Ulcer*—a break in the continuity of the epidermis, with exposure of the underlying dermis. A severe pathologic process is required to form an ulcer; therefore, a search for the cause is always indicated. It is important to note the structure of the edge, the firmness of the ulcer, and the type of exudate in the crater. A scar is often left after healing of ulcers. Examples are feline eosinophilic ulcer syndrome and chronic solar dermatitis. (Photograph illustrates an ulcer on the abdomen of a dog with staphylococcal furunculosis.) *Erosion*—a shallow ulcer that does not penetrate the basal laminar zone and consequently heals without scarring.

SECONDARY LESION—EXCORIATION

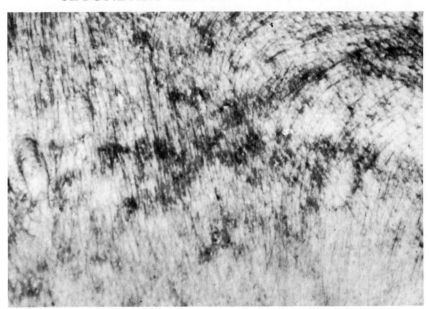

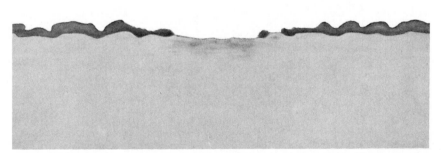

Figure 3:16. *Excoriation*—a superficial removal of epidermis caused by scratching, biting, or rubbing. Excoriations are self-produced and caused by pruritus; they invite secondary bacterial infection. Acute moist dermatitis caused by self-inflicted trauma is such an example. (Photograph illustrates linear excoriations on the side of a dog with scabies.)

SECONDARY LESION—LICHENIFICATION

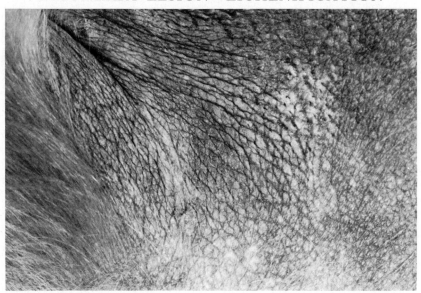

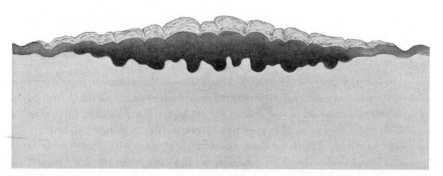

Figure 3:17. *Lichenification*—a thickening and hardening of the skin characterized by an exaggeration of the superficial skin markings. Lichenified areas frequently result from friction. They may be normally colored but more often are hyperpigmented. Examples are the hyperpigmented, lichenified flanks in the male feminizing syndrome and the axillae in acanthosis nigricans. (Photograph illustrates the axilla of a dog with chronic atopic dermatitis; lichenification here is a result of rubbing.)

SECONDARY LESION—HYPERPIGMENTATION

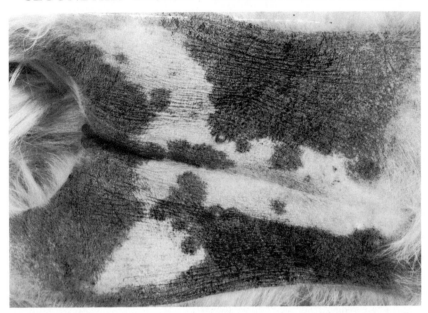

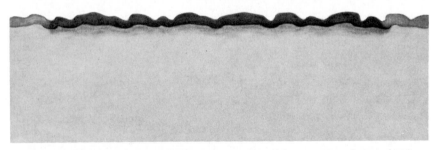

Figure 3:18. *Abnormal pigmentation*—skin coloration caused by a variety of pigments, but most commonly melanin, which is responsible for a variety of skin colors: black—melanin present throughout the epidermis (lentigo); blue—melanin within melanocytes and melanophages in the middle and deep dermis (blue nevus); gray—diffuse dermal melanosis (metastatic melanoma); tan, brown, black—various shades of normal skin color in breeds are due to melanin; brown—hemochromatosis is due primarily to melanin, not hemosiderin. Other pigments are as follows: Red-Purple—hemorrhage in the skin is red at first, becoming dark purple with time (bruises). Yellow-Green—accumulations of bile pigments (icterus). Other terms are the following: *hypopigmentation (hypomelanosis)*—loss of epidermal melanin (postinflammatory lesions). Leukoderma is a general term for white skin, whereas vitiligo refers to a specific disease. Lack of pigment in hair is called leukotrichia or achromotrichia; *hyperpigmentation (hypermelanosis, melanoderma)*—increased epidermal and occasionally dermal melanin. Melanophages may be found in the superficial dermis. (Postinflammatory, chronic, traumatic, and endocrine skin lesions.) Excess pigment in hair is called melanotrichia. (Photograph illustrates postinflammatory hyperpigmentation.)

SECONDARY LESION—COMEDO

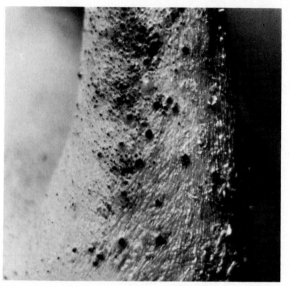

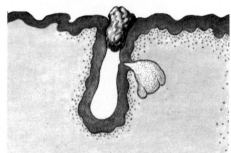

Figure 3:19. *Comedo*—a dilated hair follicle filled with cornified cells and sebaceous material. It is the initial lesion of acne and may predispose the skin to bacterial folliculitis. A comedo is produced secondary to seborrheic skin disease and seborrhea, or to occlusion with greasy medications, or by systemic or topical corticosteroids. A *sinus* is an epithelium-lined channel from a cavity to the skin surface. (Photograph, illustrating comedones of skin on the tail of a dog, courtesy of W. H. Miller, Jr.)

SECONDARY LESION—HYPERKERATOSIS

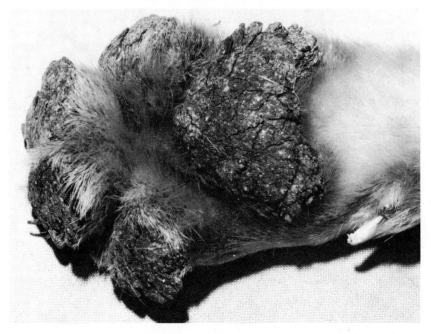

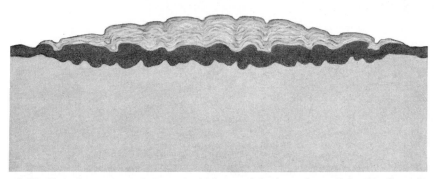

Figure 3:20. *Hyperkeratosis*—an increase in thickness of the horny layer of the skin. Examples are callus formation and nasodigital hyperkeratosis (hardpad). The keratogenic hyperplasia can occur in plaques, ridges, circular areas, or even "feathered" projections of digital pads. In the planum nasale and digital pads, increased thickness of the horny layer of the epidermis is normal. (Photograph illustrates digital hyperkeratosis.)

SECONDARY LESION—FISSURE

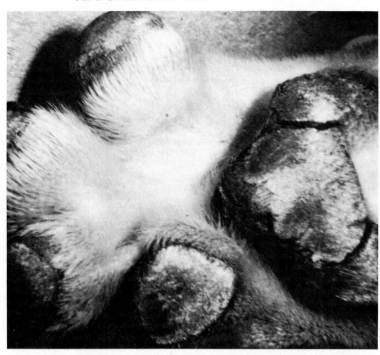

Figure 3:21. *Fissure*—a linear cleavage into the epidermis, or through the epidermis into the dermis caused by disease or injury. Fissures may be single or multiple tiny cracks or large clefts several centimeters long. They have sharply defined margins and may be dry or moist and straight, curved, or branching. They occur when the skin is thick and inelastic and then subjected to sudden swelling from inflammation or trauma, especially in regions of frequent movement. Examples are found at ear margins, and at ocular, nasal, oral, and anal mucocutaneous borders. (Photograph illustrates two fissures in footpad.) *A,* The dermogram shows a tiny split through the normal epidermis covered with a small crust. *B,* The split enlarges and becomes a fissure as it penetrates into the dermis causing inflammatory infiltration and capillary dilatation. It is still covered with a hemorrhagic crust. *C,* The well-established deep fissure extends deeply into the upper half of the dermis, causing more extensive vascular dilatation and inflammatory infiltration. The epidermal margins on each side of the fissure become acanthotic.

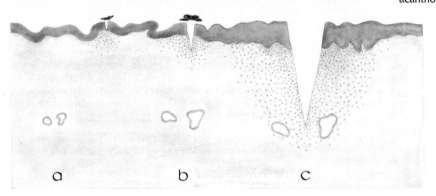

a   b   c

In animals, the primary or secondary skin lesions are often hidden under the hair coat; in fact, it requires painstaking observation to see them. In short-coated animals, if you stand behind the patient and use both hands to roll the skin into a horizontal fold, it is possible to see between the erected hair shafts to the skin surface. By rolling the fold forward away from you, you can see progressively new areas of skin surface and get "an impression" of the distribution of lesions. Only when the animal is clipped can the distribution pattern of such lesions be seen with ease and accuracy. Consequently, in animals there are two distinctly different patterns that aid diagnosis: (1) the changes in external hair coat and (2) the definition and distribution of primary and secondary skin lesions. These two factors do not necessarily have a reciprocal relationship. In addition, it is important to recognize whether the

Bilaterally Symmetric Lesions

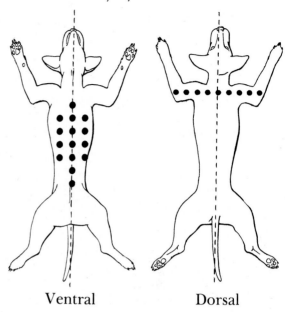

Ventral   Dorsal

Figure 3:22. When a line is drawn from the tip of the nose to the end of the tail and the distribution of the lesions is the same on the right side as on the left side, the pattern is called bilaterally symmetric. Most such skin disorders have an internal cause; frequently the skin becomes a reflection of internal disease. Examples are hypothyroidism, hyperadrenocorticism, and Sertoli's cell tumor.

lesions present a symmetric distribution on either side of the midline or an asymmetric distribution (Figs. 3:22 and 3:23).

Different Stages

As a skin disease progresses from its earliest appearance to its final, fully developed state, the pattern must necessarily change. A small patch of alopecia can enlarge into almost total hair loss in some cases. Obviously, if all interme-

Asymmetric Distribution Pattern

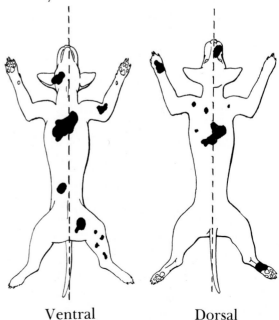

Ventral   Dorsal

Figure 3:23. When a line is drawn from the tip of the nose to the end of the tail and the lesions on one side are not identical with those on the other side, the distribution pattern is asymmetric. External environmental causes, such as ectoparasites, fungi, or contact allergens, are examples of disorders which cause such skin patterns.

diate stages of such a disease were drawn diagrammatically, the result would be more confusing than helpful. Therefore, it is necessary to select for each skin disorder the single distribution pattern that is of greatest diagnostic value. Different stages of each disease exist, and the total impact of the diagram should be interpreted with that fact constantly in mind. In addition, note whether the distribution pattern represents alopecia or changes of the skin surface or both. Diagrams representing typical distribution patterns are presented with the discussion of each dermatosis.

REGIONAL DIAGNOSIS

When a dermatosis is confined to a specific region, several diagnoses are often possible. Table 3:5 lists areas or parts of the body along with the skin diseases that are commonly localized or especially severe in those areas. The chart should be useful in suggesting a number of differential diagnoses.

Table 3:5. REGIONAL DIAGNOSIS

Area	Disease	Area	Disease
Head	Atopy	Eyelid	Hordeolum
	Demodicosis	(Continued)	Seborrheic blepharitis
	Dermatophytosis		Trichiasis
	Facial fold dermatitis	Nasal Area	Contact dermatitis (plastic, rubber)
	Feline food allergy		Demodicosis
	Feline leprosy		Dermatophytosis
	Juvenile cellulitis		Discoid lupus erythematosus
	Otic vascular necrosis		Facial fold dermatitis
	Pemphigus erythematosus		Folliculitis, bacterial
	Pemphigus foliaceus		Nasodigital hyperkeratosis
	Scabies, feline		Pemphigus erythematosus
	Sporotrichosis		Pemphigus foliaceus
	Sterile pyogranuloma syndrome		Sporotrichosis
	Systemic lupus erythematosus		Squamous cell carcinoma
	Vasculitis		Sterile pyogranuloma syndrome
	Zinc-responsive dermatosis		Vitiligo-like lesions
Ear	Alopecia, pattern		Vogt-Koyanagi-Harada–like syndrome
	Atopy		
	Ceruminal gland tumor	Lip	Acne, canine and feline
	Cold agglutinin disease		Candidiasis
	Demodicosis		Contact dermatitis (plastic, rubber)
	Fly dermatitis		Demodicosis
	Frostbite		Indolent ulcer, feline
	Melanoderma and alopecia of		Juvenile cellulitis
	Yorkshire terriers		Lip fold dermatitis
	Otitis externa		Oral papillomatosis, canine
	Bacterial		Vitiligo-like lesions
	Candidiasis		Vogt-Koyanagi-Harada–like syndrome
	Ceruminous		
	Demodicosis	Oral Cavity	Bullous pemphigoid
	Malassezia (yeast)	(Mucosal Lesions)	Candidiasis
	Otodectes cynotis		Discoid lupus erythematosus
	Trombiculidiasis		Eosinophilic granuloma, canine and feline
	Scabies, canine and feline		Eosinophilic plaque, feline
	Seborrhea, marginal (pinna)		Erosions, chemical
	Solar dermatitis, feline		Erosions, viral, feline
	Sterile eosinophilic pinnal folliculitis		Fibrosarcoma
Eyelid	Chalazion		Fusospirochetal stomatitis
	Demodicosis		Gingival hypertrophy
	Dermatophytosis		Indolent ulcer, feline
	Distichiasis		Malignant melanoma
	Entropion		
	Folliculitis, bacterial		

Table 3:5. REGIONAL DIAGNOSIS *Continued*

Area	Disease	Area	Disease
Oral Cavity (Mucosal Lesions) *(Continued)*	Marginal gingivitis, ulcerative, dental Mycosis fungoides Oral papillomatosis Pemphigus vulgaris Plasma cell stomatitis, feline Squamous cell carcinoma Systemic lupus erythematosus Thallium toxicosis Vegetative glossitis (foreign body)	Abdomen	Bullous pemphigoid Calcinosis cutis Contact dermatitis (ventral abdomen) Eosinophilic plaque, feline Feline symmetric alopecia Folliculitis, bacterial Hookworm dermatitis Hyperadrenocorticism Impetigo Mycobacteriosis, atypical, feline Panniculitis, sterile, feline *Pelodera* dermatitis Psychogenic dermatitis/alopecia, feline Subcorneal pustular dermatitis Trombiculidiasis
Mucocutaneous Margins	Bullous pemphigoid Candidiasis Erythema multiforme Hepatocutaneous syndrome Mycosis fungoides Pemphigus vulgaris Systemic lupus erythematosus Thallium toxicosis Toxic epidermal necrolysis	Flanks	Bullous pemphigoid Folliculitis, bacterial Hyposomatotropism Mechanical irritation (flank suckers) Ovarian imbalance
Chin	Acne, canine and feline Demodicosis Juvenile cellulitis Eosinophilic granuloma, feline Furunculosis, bacterial	Tail	Acute moist dermatitis Cold agglutinin disease Cryoglobulinemia Feline symmetric alopecia Flea bite hypersensitivity Frostbite Hyperplasia of tail gland, stud tail Mechanical irritation (tail suckers) Psychogenic dermatitis/alopecia, feline Tip of tail trauma
Neck	Contact dermatitis (collars) Dermoid sinus Flea bite hypersensitivity, feline Flea collar dermatitis		
Lower chest	Contact dermatitis Fibrovascular papilloma Sternal callus		
Axilla	Acanthosis nigricans Atopy Bullous pemphigoid Contact dermatitis Pemphigus vulgaris	Anus	Anal sac dermatitis Anal sac disease Bullous pemphigoid Perianal adenoma Perianal fistulas Perianal gland hyperplasia
Back	Atopy Calcinosis cutis Cheyletiellosis Comedo syndrome, schnauzers Flea bite hypersensitivity Folliculitis, bacterial Food hypersensitivity Hypothyroidism Pediculosis Psychogenic dermatitis/alopecia, feline	Legs	Acral lick dermatitis Calcinosis circumscripta Contact dermatitis Decubital ulcers Demodicosis Elbow callus Elbow callus pyoderma Hygroma Eosinophilic granuloma, feline Feline leprosy Lymphangitis, bacterial, fungal Lymphedema *Pelodera* dermatitis Scabies, canine
Trunk	Demodicosis, generalized Eosinophilic plaque, feline Folliculitis, bacterial Hyperadrenocorticism Hyposomatotropism Hypothyroidism Male feminizing syndrome Ovarian imbalance Panniculitis, sterile Sebaceous adenitis Sertoli's cell tumor Sterile eosinophilic pustulosis Subcorneal pustular dermatosis Vitamin A–responsive dermatosis	Feet	Acral mutilation Atopy Collagen disease of German shepherd footpads Contact dermatitis Demodicosis Dermatophytosis Digital hyperkeratosis of Irish terriers

Table continued on following page

Table 3:5. REGIONAL DIAGNOSIS *Continued*

Area	Disease	Area	Disease
Feet *(Continued)*	Digital pad hyperkeratosis	Nails	Hyperthroidism, feline
	Food hypersensitivity		Leishmaniasis
	Hepatocutaneous syndrome		Nail deformities
	Hookworm dermatitis		Onychogryphosis
	Interdigital foreign bodies (foxtails, thorns)		Onychomadesis
			Bullous pemphigoid
	Leishmaniasis		Pemphigus vulgaris
	Pelodera dermatitis		Systemic lupus erythematosus
	Pemphigus foliaceus		Onychomycosis
	Pododermatitis		Onychorrhexis
	Plasma cell, feline		Paronychia
	Traumatic		Arteriovenous shunt
	Sterile pyogranuloma syndrome		Bacterial
	Trombiculidiasis		Feline leukemia
	Tyrosinemia		Trauma
	Zinc-responsive dermatosis		Traumatic injury

Dermatologic Laboratory Procedures

Diagnostic tests and laboratory procedures are useful whenever a definitive diagnosis cannot be made from the case history and clinical examination alone. Some tests should be done routinely since (1) the skin has a number of clinical reaction patterns, and many dermatoses of vastly different etiology look the same, and (2) many dermatoses are complex problems with more than one cause. It would be embarrassing to miss the diagnosis of demodicosis, scabies, or dermatomycosis because a simple test was not performed. Laboratory procedures can confirm many clinical diagnoses and provide a logical basis for successful therapeutic management.

> **A routine laboratory procedure will frequently solve an undiagnosed dermatosis.**

EXAMINATION FOR PARASITES

Skin Scraping

This is one of the most frequently used tests in veterinary dermatology and always should be performed. Its purpose is to enable the clinician to find and identify small and microscopic ectoparasites. The equipment needed to perform a skin scraping is mineral oil, a scalpel blade with or without a handle, microscopic slides, coverslips, and a microscope.

Not all skin scrapings are made in the same way. Success in finding parasites is enhanced if the technique of scraping is adapted to the specific parasite that the clinician expects to find. The method of scraping for demodectic mites is different from scrapings for sarcoptic mites. *Cheyletiella, Dermanyssus,* cat fur mites, and ear mites each require a slightly different scraping technique.

The following discussions elaborate the special techniques needed to enhance the effectiveness of scraping for specific parasites.

Demodectic Mites. The affected skin should be squeezed between the thumb and forefinger to help extrude the mites from the hair follicles. This same technique can be used to express demodectic mites from the skin of the proximal external ear canal of occasional dogs and cats with demodectic mange. The extruded material is scraped up and placed on a microscope slide. It is helpful to apply a drop of mineral oil to the skin site being scraped, or to the scalpel blade, to facilitate the adherence of material to the blade. Then, additional material is obtained by scraping the skin more deeply, until capillary bleeding is produced. Not more than two drops of mineral oil are added to the usual amount of scraped material on the microscopic slide. Too much or too little oil used in the preparation will make it difficult to examine only one layer microscopically. The oil is mixed with the scraped material using a wooden applicator stick to obtain an even mixture. Always place a coverslip on the material to be examined to ensure a uniform layer.

> *Examining material from a skin scraping without a coverslip can cause false-negative results.*

Diagnosis is made either by the demonstration of many adult mites or by finding an increased ratio of immature forms (ova, larvae, and nymphs) to adults. Observing whether the mites are alive or dead is of prognostic value while the animal is being treated. Finding only an occasional adult mite is consistent with a diagnosis of normal skin, *not* demodicosis. It would seem that skin scraping is a straightforward, easy laboratory procedure; however, every year the authors continue to receive referred demodicosis cases that were misdiagnosed owing to false-negative skin scrapings. Skin scrapings are mandatory in all cases of canine pyoderma and seborrhea, because generalized demodicosis may be the primary cause of the conditions. Dogs harbor only one species of mite, *Demodex canis*, while cats have two species, *Demodex cati* (which resembles the canine mite) and a second, as yet unnamed species that is short and squat.

Canine Scabies Mites. Canine sarcoptic mites, *Sarcoptes scabiei (var. canis)*, are hard to find, so multiple deep scrapings are indicated. Fifteen or 20 extensive scrapings should be made, with emphasis on the ears and elbows. For scraping, select skin sites that have not been excoriated, and look for red raised papules with yellowish crusts on top (see Fig. 8:40A,B).

Extensive amounts of material should be accumulated in the scrapings and spread on microscope slides. It is sometimes very useful to use a second microscope glass slide instead of a coverslip to compress the thick crusts. Examine each and every field until a mite is found; one mite is diagnostic. However, dark brown, round or oval fecal pellets or ova from adult mites may also be found and are diagnostic (see Fig. 8:40C,D). In difficult cases it may be useful to accumulate an even larger amount of hair and keratin debris from scrapings. Place the material in a warm solution of 10 per cent KOH for 20 minutes to digest keratin, and then stir the mixture and centrifuge. Mites are thus concentrated and can often be picked off the surface film and identified with a microscope.

Feline Scabies Mites. The feline scabies mite, *Notoedres cati*, is much easier to find than the canine mite; otherwise, the techniques described for canine scabies are appropriate here. The best place to scrape is the face or ears, under crusts and scales.

Cheyletiella Mites. *Cheyletiella* mites are very large and can even be seen with a magnifying glass. They look like small white scales that move, and they are jokingly called "walking dandruff." To examine for them microscopically, clip a swath of scaly, scurfy skin, and obtain scales by superficially scraping the skin surface, using a scalpel blade covered with mineral oil. At no time is a deep scraping needed, since the mites are surface dwellers and do not burrow as do sarcoptic mites or live in hair follicles as do demodectic mites. *Cheyletiella* mites move about rapidly in pseudotunnels in the epidermal debris. The scraped material and mineral oil are placed on a slide for examination as described above. These mites are usually easy to find in dogs but may be very difficult to demonstrate in cats. The acetate tape method and the flea comb can be very useful for demonstrating this infestation.

Chigger Mites. The most common chigger mite is *Eutrombicula alfreddugesi*. These mites can be seen with the naked eye, especially easily on the medial pinna of the ear. They appear as bright orange objects adhering tightly to the skin. They are easily distinguished from ear mites by their larger size and intense color. They should be covered with mineral oil and picked up with a scalpel blade. A true skin scraping is not needed. However, when removed from the host for microscopic examination they should immediately be placed in mineral oil, or they will jump away.

Poultry Mites. *Dermanyssus gallinae* is a mite that attacks poultry, wild and cage birds, and dogs and cats, as well as humans. It is red when engorged with blood; otherwise it is white, gray, or black. When the animal shows evidence of itching and the history indicates there is exposure to bird or poultry housing, a skin scraping for *Dermanyssus* mites is indicated. One or two mites on the dog or cat can cause much itching and localized, self-inflicted trauma. The best place to find the mites is directly at the excoriated site. Remove the debris, scales, and crusts that harbor the mites. Place the material on a microscopic slide, and add several drops of mineral oil. Cover it with another glass slide instead of a coverslip. Squeeze the two slides firmly together to crush any crusted material. *Dermanyssus* mites are very active, and the motion of their wildly moving legs will often be noticed even before the mites are seen. Make more than one scraping, have patience, and hope for good luck. The acetate tape method of collection can often be used successfully.

Cat Fur Mites. *Lynxacarus radovsky* can be demonstrated microscopically by searching for "salt and pepper" hairs. The mites are usually located along the topline, attached to the terminal parts of the hairs. A true superficial skin scraping can be made if the mites are suspected to be on the skin, but plucking affected hairs and examining them in a mineral oil preparation may be diagnostic. The acetate tape impression can also be used.

Ear Mites. *Otodectes cyanotis* mites usually are most at home in the external ear canal of dogs and cats. However, they may also be found on the surface skin, the head, and the body, especially around the rump and tail. They can be found by superficial scraping or acetate tape method, such as described for *Cheyletiella* mites, and identified by microscopic examination.

Smears of the External Ear Canal

Waxy, mucoid, or purulent exudates of the external ear canal can be collected carefully, using a metal loop or cotton swab, and smeared gently on a microscopic slide. The material may be mixed with mineral oil for better visualization of otodectic and demodectic mange mites. The smear can also be air-dried and stained with Diff Quik or new methylene blue for better visualization of yeasts, bacteria, and cells (see p. 139). When infection is present, other stains should be used to determine the types of bacteria and inflammatory cells present and whether or not the organisms are being phagocytized.

Acetate Tape Impression

Acetate tape (only the *clear* transparent form) can be used to collect small parasites and other epidermal debris for identification. If one wraps the clear, transparent tape around one's fingers "sticky side out" and presses the tape firmly against areas containing loose debris or suspected parasites, the material is trapped on the sticky tape. The tape is then pressed onto a microscope slide for further examination under magnification. Collected objects are immobilized between the tape and the microscope slide. The method is especially useful for small rapidly moving parasites, such as biting lice or fleas, and for round objects that are hard to find and hold, such as flea eggs. It is a useful technique for identification of fleas, flea feces, flea eggs, lice, nits, *Cheyletiella* mites and eggs, *Otodectes* mites and eggs, miscellaneous mites such as *Dermanyssus*, *Walchia*, *Lynxacarus*, and *Eutrombicula*, and small ticks. The method is also useful for examining skin scales, crusts, and keratin debris. If one wishes to examine the proximal or distal ends of hairs to determine the stage of hair cycle or whether hairs are bitten-off or frayed, a group of hair shafts can be plucked from the skin, aligned, and pressed into the acetate tape for secure orientation while the observations are made (trichogram).

EXAMINATION FOR DERMATOPHYTES

Culture and Examination of Fungi

Fungal culture is mandatory for proper identification of fungi.

To ascertain the cause of a dermatophytosis, proper specimen collection, isolation, and correct identification are necessary.

WOOD'S LIGHT

One aid used to assist in specimen collection is Wood's light. This is an ultraviolet light with a light wave of 253.7 nm filtered through a cobalt or nickel filter.

A useful unit has two light tubes, one on either side of a central magnifying glass, and the entire complex is contained in a plastic rim with a comfortable handle (Fig. 3:24). When an animal is to be examined, the Wood's light should be allowed to warm up for 5 to 10 minutes, since the stability of the light's wave length and intensity is temperature dependent. The animal should be placed in a dark room. When exposed to the Wood's light, hairs invaded by *Microsporum canis* may result in a yellow-green fluorescence in about one-half of the isolates (see Fig. 7:8F). The fluorescence is due to tryptophan metabolites

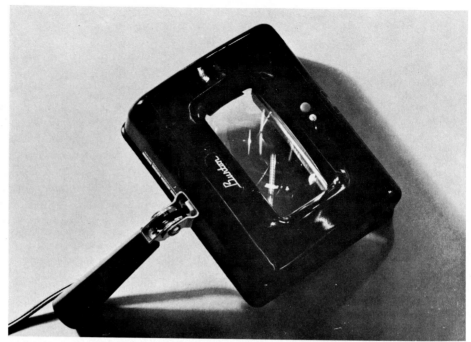

Figure 3:24. Wood's light with magnifying glass for examination of fungal materials for fluorescence.

produced by the fungus. These metabolites are produced only by fungi that have invaded actively growing hair and cannot be elicited from an in vitro infection of hair. Fluorescence is not present in scales or crusts or in cultures of dermatophytes. Other less common dermatophytes that may fluoresce include *M. distortum, M. audouinii,* and *Trichophyton schoenleinii.*

Many factors influence fluorescence. Medication such as iodine will destroy it. Bacteria such as *Pseudomonas aeruginosa* and *Corynebacterium minutissimum* may fluoresce, but with a different color. Keratin, soap, petroleum, and other medication may fluoresce and give false-positive reactions. If the short stubs of hair are producing fluorescence, the proximal end of hairs extracted from the follicles should fluoresce. These fluorescing hairs should be picked with forceps and used for inoculating fungal medium or for microscopic examination.

Summary of Wood's light diagnosis:
1. *Positive fluorescence suggests fungal infection.*
2. *Lack of fluorescence is inconclusive (patient may be free of fungal infection or affected by the presence of a nonfluorescent dermatophyte).*

SPECIMEN COLLECTION

Accurate specimen collection is necessary to isolate dermatophytes.

Hair. Hair is the specimen most commonly collected for the isolation of fungi. With forceps, select hairs that fluoresce with the Wood's light. Another means of collecting infected hair is the toothbrush method. A sterile toothbrush is gently brushed through the animal's coat to accumulate hair and keratin debris. The toothbrush is then shaken or gently pressed onto the isolation medium. The technique has proved to be especially valuable in cats that may be carriers of *M. canis*.

Hair may be collected from large dogs using a sterile hairbrush. Some clinicians achieve good results using sterile carpet squares gently rubbed over the animal's coat. These carpet squares are pressed into the medium and removed. The hairs obtained by these methods can be used for culture or microscopic examination.

Skin. Suspected skin lesions should be cleaned of extraneous debris before keratin scales are collected. If the lesion is grossly contaminated, it can be wiped gently with gauze (not cotton) that has been soaked in 70 per cent alcohol. If the lesion is reasonably clean, the scraping can be made without wetting the area. The specimens for examination or inoculation should be obtained from both the periphery of the growing lesion and an area adjacent to the lesion.

Dermatophytes can often be cultured from the normal skin near the periphery of the lesion but also from the active lesion. In contrast, the *Candida* species may best be cultured from the lesion itself.

Nail. To examine and culture nail infections, part of the nail should be removed. The nail should be ground or clipped into tiny pieces for inoculation or for digestion by KOH. Material under the nail and near the edge of the nail should be collected.

Hair and nail collected from suspected lesions can be placed in a clean, labeled envelope or Petri dish. Scrapings of skin should never be placed in closed containers such as screw-capped tubes, which will increase moisture and encourage growth of contaminating bacteria and thus make it more difficult to isolate the dermatophytes.

CLEARING KERATIN

This procedure requires practice and expertise. It uses either 20 per cent KOH or a chloral hydrate solution, both of which are very irritating to the skin or eyes of the operator. Be careful! Because most animal fungal infections are ectothrix, clearing is not as necessary as it is for infections involving humans. In fact, one of the authors (D. W. S.) uses only mineral oil in which to suspend suspected hairs. The procedure may also be useful in clearing excess keratin debris from scrapings being examined for ectoparasites. The equipment necessary is 20 per cent KOH, microscope slides and coverslips, an alcohol or Bunsen burner, forceps, and a scalpel handle and blade.

Material is collected as for a skin scraping, together with plucked hairs or nails, and deposited on a slide. Several drops of 20 per cent KOH are applied to the slide, a coverslip is added, and the slide is gently heated (avoid boiling) for 15 to 20 seconds. Alternately, the preparation may be allowed to stand for 30 minutes at room temperature. An excellent result is obtained if the mount is placed on the microscope lamp for gentle heating. The preparation will be ready for examination in 15 to 20 minutes, and the structures will be better preserved.

Another procedure is to add one part of a 1.2 per cent dye solution of Permanent Black Super Quink or India ink to two parts of 20 per cent KOH.

The addition of this dye may aid in interpretation of the KOH preparation by staining the hyphae and conidia.

Two clinicians, Schwartzman and Foil, use the following formula as a replacement for the KOH solution in the digestion process to clear keratin: 50 gm of chloral hydrate are added to 25 ml liquid phenol and 25 ml of liquid lactic acid. Several days may pass before the crystals go into solution, but when they do, no precipitate forms. The slide can be read almost immediately after hair and keratin are added to this chloral hydrate solution.

MICROSCOPIC EXAMINATION

Examination of cleared or stained scrapings from mycotic lesions may reveal yeasts, conidia, hyphae, or pseudohyphae. The hyphae of the common dermatophytes are usually uniform in diameter (2 to 3 μm), septate, and variable in length and degree of branching. Older hyphae are usually wider and may be divided into beadlike chains of rounded cells (arthroconidia).

> *Hyphae may be confused with artifacts such as threads, wisps of cotton, fiber glass or elastic fibers, and early KOH crystal formations from overheated or dried-out slide preparations (Fig. 3:25).*

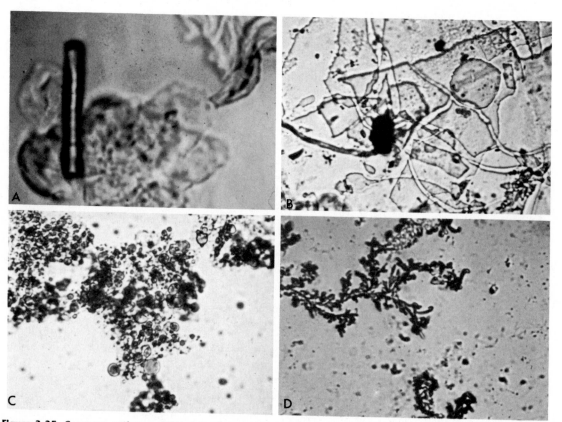

Figure 3:25. Common artifacts in KOH-cleared specimens. *A,* Plastic, resin, or fiber glass "hair." *B,* Cracked keratinized cells and cholesterol crystals. Note cotton wisp at left side of illustration. *C,* Oil drops from topical medication may look like budding yeast culture. *D,* Crystals from dried-out KOH preparations. (Courtesy Paul Jacobs.)

The artifacts described above may cause false positive identifications. In addition, keratinized cell wall "skeletons" and cholesterol crystals that make up the so-called mosaic fungus may be most difficult to differentiate from fungal hyphae.

In skin scales, the branched septate hyphae of different dermatophytes are identical to one another and require isolation and culture for identification. However, the arrangement of conidia in or on the hair is of interest. In hair, the downward growth of the fungus keeps pace with the growth of the hair and never advances to the edge of the mitotically active area in the bulb (Fig. 7:1). The hyphae in the older portions of the hair may break up into a large number of conidia. The way in which these arthroconidia affect the hair is typical of certain fungi. This is less important in veterinary than in human medicine, since most animal dermatophytes have ectothrix distribution.

In an *ectothrix invasion* of hair, hyphae may be seen within the hair shaft, but they grow outward and show a great propensity to form arthroconidia in a mosaic pattern on the surface of the hair (Fig. 3:26A). The hairs may fluoresce, which is typical of *M. canis*, *M. audouinii*, and *M. distortum*. Hairs infected by the following fungi do not fluoresce. Large conidia (5 to 8 μm) in sparse chains outside the hairs are seen in *M. gypseum* and *M. vanbreuseghemii* infections. Intermediate-sized conidia (3 to 7 μm) in dense chains are seen with *Trichophyton mentagrophytes*, *T. verrucosum*, and *T. equinum* infections.

An *endothrix infection* is characterized by conidia formation within the hair shaft (Fig. 3:26B). The hair cuticle is not broken, but the hair may break off or curl. Endothrix invasion is rarely seen in animals but is typical of *T. tonsurans* infections in humans.

FUNGAL CULTURE

Sabouraud's dextrose agar has traditionally been used in veterinary mycology for isolation of fungi; however, other media are available with bacterial and fungal inhibitors, such as Dermatophyte Test Medium (DTM), potato dextrose agar, and rice grain medium. Mycosel and Mycobiotic agar are formulations of Sabouraud's dextrose agar with cycloheximide and chloramphenicol added to inhibit fungal and bacterial contaminants. If a medium with cycloheximide is used, fungi sensitive to it will not be isolated. Some organisms sensitive to cycloheximide include *Cryptococcus neoformans*, many members of the Zygomycota, some *Candida* species, *Aspergillus* species, *Pseudoallescheria boydii*, and many agents of phaeohyphomycosis. DTM is essentially a Sabouraud's dextrose agar containing cycloheximide, gentamicin, and chlortetracycline as antifungal and antibacterial agents. The pH indicator phenol red has been added. Dermatophytes first utilize protein in the medium, with alkaline metabolites turning the medium to red (Fig. 3:27A). When the protein is exhausted the dermatophytes utilize carbohydrates, giving off acid metabolites. The medium changes from red to yellow. Most other fungi utilize carbohydrates first and proteins only later; they, too, may produce a change to red in DTM— but only after a prolonged incubation (10 to 14 days or more). Consequently, DTM cultures should be examined daily for the first 10 days. Fungi such as *Blastomyces dermatitidis*, *Sporothrix schenckii*, *Histoplasma capsulatum*, *Coccidioides immitis*, *Pseudoallescheria boydii*, some *Aspergillus* species, and others may cause a change to red in DTM, so microscopic examination is essential to avoid an erroneous presumptive diagnosis. Since DTM may depress development of

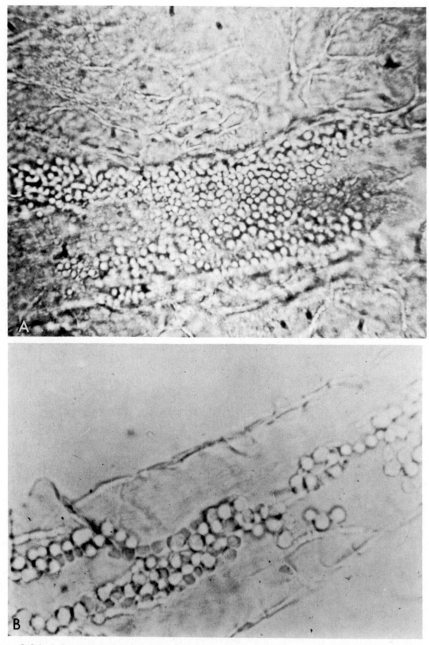

Figure 3:26. *A,* Ectothrix invasion of hair. Masses of conidia form a mosaic pattern on the surface of the hair, and hyphae may penetrate the shaft. *B,* Endothrix invasion. Conidia are within the hair shaft. (Courtesy C. Pinello.)

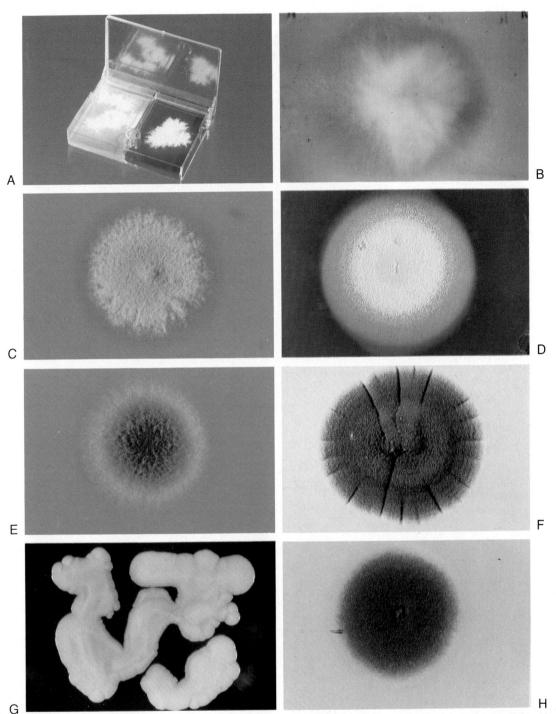

Figure 3:27. Fungal colonies. *A*, Seven-day culture of *M. canis.* Left side, plain Sabouraud's dextrose agar; right side, DTM medium. *B*, Gross colony of *M. canis. C*, Gross colony of *M. gypseum. D*, Gross colony of *T. mentagrophytes. E*, Gross colony of *Aspergillus. F*, Gross colony of *Penicillium. G*, Gross colony of *Candida albicans. H*, Gross colony of *Alternaria. (A, C, E, H,* courtesy C. Pinello. *B, D, F, G,* courtesy Paul Jacobs.)

conidia, mask colony pigmentation, and inhibit some pathogens, fungi re-covered on DTM should be transferred to plain Sabouraud's dextrose agar for identification.

Fungal growth on DTM must be evaluated daily for 10 days. After that, nondermatophytes can turn the medium to red.

Potato dextrose agar is useful for promoting sporulation and observing pigmentation. On potato dextrose agar, *M. canis* has a lemon-yellow pigment, whereas *M. audouinii* has a salmon- or peach-colored pigment. Rice agar medium promotes conidia formation in some dermatophytes, especially *M. canis* strains, which produce no conidia on Sabouraud's dextrose agar.

Skin scrapings, nails, and hair should be inoculated onto Sabouraud's dextrose agar and DTM, Mycosel, or Mycobiotic agar. Cultures should be incubated at 30°C with 30 per cent humidity. A pan of water in the incubator usually provides enough humidity. Cultures should be checked daily for fungal growth. DTM may be incubated for 10 to 14 days, but cultures on Sabouraud's dextrose agar should be allowed to develop for 30 days. Figure 3:27 illustrates the gross colony morphologic patterns of some common fungi.

IDENTIFICATION OF FUNGI

Identification of fungi that have been isolated requires careful microscopic examination. Slide preparations and slide cultures are two techniques that have been used for microscopic examination (Fig. 3:28).

Slide preparations can be used to identify fungal structures. Hyphae and conidia from mature colonies may be teased apart and spread on a microscope slide. The slide is flooded with saline or lactophenol cotton blue stain, protected with a coverslip, and examined.

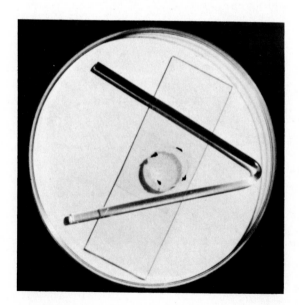

Figure 3:28. Fungal slide culture made in Petri dish. (Courtesy C. Pinello.)

An alternate method is the "acetate tape" method. Preparations by this method are easily made with pressure-sensitive tape from stationery stores. To make the preparation, a "flag" of tape that measures 1 cm by 1 cm is fastened to the end of a wooden applicator stick or wire needle, or is grasped in forceps, and the sticky surface of the flag is touched to the surface of the culture colony just proximal to the advancing periphery. The tape is then pressed, sticky side down, on a slide with a drop of water or lactophenol cotton blue stain and examined under the microscope (Fig. 3:29).

Fungal slide cultures can also be used to grow fungal specimens for identification (Figs. 3:30 to 3:32).*

Salient facts useful in identifying the three major dermatophytes are briefly described below.

Microsporum Canis. These lesions may fluoresce as yellow-green. Hairs that fluoresce should be plucked for culture or microscopic examination. Examination of a KOH preparation may reveal conidia present in masses on the hair shaft.

Colony Morphology. On Sabouraud's dextrose agar, *M. canis* produces a white cottony-to-woolly colony (see Fig. 3:27A,B). With age the colony becomes more powdery, has a central depressed area, and may show radial folds. The pigment on the reverse surface is yellow-orange, becoming dull orange-brown. On potato dextrose agar, the pigment is lemon yellow. *M. canis*, unlike *M. audouinii*, grows well on rice medium.

Microscopic Morphology. *M. canis* usually forms abundant spindle-shaped macroconidia with thick echinulate walls. The echinulations (spines) are more pronounced at the terminal end, which often forms a knob. The macroconidia are composed of six or more cells (Figs. 3:30A and 3:31A). One-celled microconidia may be seen. Conidia develop best on rice agar medium and poorly or not at all on Sabouraud's dextrose agar.

Diagnostic Criteria. The distinctive macroconidia and the lemon-yellow reverse pigment are characteristic of *M. canis*.

Microsporum Gypseum. Fluorescence is rare and if present is very dull. The conidia (ectothrix) on hair shafts are larger than those of *M. canis*.

Colony Morphology. Colonies are rapid growing with a flat-to-granular texture and a buff-to-cinnamon brown color (Fig. 3:27C). Sterile white mycelia may develop in time. The reverse pigmentation is pale yellow to tan.

Microscopic Morphology. Echinulate macroconidia contain up to six cells with relatively thin walls (Figs. 3:30B and 3:31B). The abundant ellipsoid macroconidia lack the terminal knob present in *M. canis*. One-celled microconidia may be present.

Diagnostic Criteria. The abundant ellipsoid macroconidia and flat-to-granular texture of the colony are definitive features.

Trichophyton Mentagrophytes. No fluorescence is seen with Wood's light. Ectothrix chains of arthroconidia may be observed on hair.

Colony Morphology. Colony morphology is variable. Most zoophilic forms produce a flat colony with a white to cream-colored powdery surface (Fig. 3:27D). The color of the reverse pigment is usually brown to tan but may be dark red. The anthropophilic form produces a colony with a white cottony surface.

---

*Detailed descriptions of these and other fungal colonies can be found in Muller, G. H., Kirk, R. W., and Scott, D. W.: Small Animal Dermatology, 3rd ed. W. B. Saunders, Philadelphia, 1983.

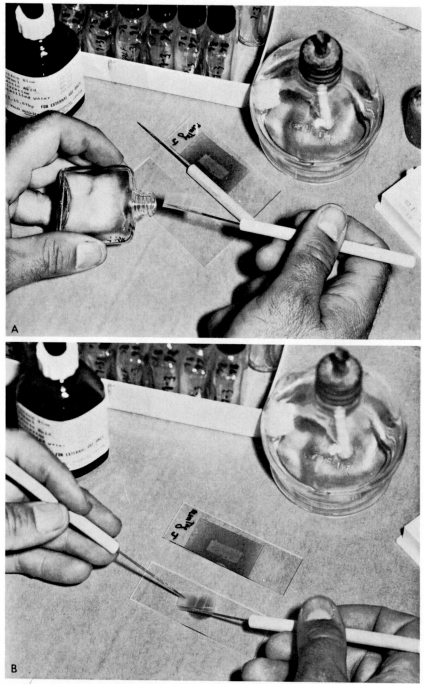

Figure 3:29. *A,* Inserting acetate tape "flag" into fungus culture bottle to pick up conidia. *B,* Tape is pressed down on a drop of water or lactophenol cotton blue stain. A coverslip is added, and the preparation is ready for microscopic examination. Note completed slide preparation in the background.

Microscopic Morphology. The zoophilic form of *T. mentagrophytes* produces globose microconidia that may be arranged singly along the hyphae or in grapelike clusters. Macroconidia, if present, are cigar shaped with thin smooth walls (Figs. 3:30C and 3:31C). Some strains produce spiral hyphae, which may also be seen in other dermatophytes.

Diagnostic Criteria. The colony morphology, spiral hyphae, macroconidia, and microconidia are useful characteristics for identifying *T. mentagrophytes.* When grown on potato dextrose agar, *T. mentagrophytes* does not produce a dark red pigment like that formed by *T. rubrum.* Strains of *T. mentagrophytes* are more apt to be urease positive than is *T. rubrum.* Because *T. rubrum* may be incorrectly identified as *T. mentagrophytes,* the above differential features are important.

EXAMINATION FOR BACTERIA

Veterinarians frequently take specimens for bacterial culture, but they rarely grow and identify the cultures in their own practice. Specimens should be collected for culture and rapidly sent to a skilled microbiologist in a laboratory equipped to provide prompt, accurate identification and antibacterial sensitivities.

Selection of appropriate lesions for culturing is critical. Ideally, an intact pustule should be opened with a sterile needle and swabbed. Alternatively, one can perform a gentle surgical scrub of papules, plaques, or nodules and then perform a punch biopsy and submit the tissue specimen in a sterile vial for culture. Cultures taken from draining tracts and ulcers and beneath crusted, exudative material are rarely meaningful and usually misleading.

Although a definitive identification of bacteria by making direct smears of exudates and impression smears of denuded surfaces is not possible, clinicians can gain much helpful information in a few minutes by this method. The type and relative number of organisms, their Gram-stain characteristics, and the effectiveness and type of inflammatory response can be rapidly documented in the office laboratory. More details can be found in the following section, Cutaneous Cytology.

Cutaneous Cytology

An enormous amount of vital diagnostic data can be obtained by microscopically examining stained material, such as impression smears of tissue or fluids, during a clinical examination. It is possible to accomplish this with minimal equipment and in less than 5 minutes. The equipment includes a clean microscope slide, a coverslip, and a stain. The stain of choice in clinical practice is Diff Quik or new methylene blue. In laboratories or for special projects, the longer, more complicated Wright's stain or Giemsa stain is of course very nice, but the longer time and additional skill may not be justified during an office call.

Materials for cytologic examination can be gathered by *needle aspiration* of fluid-filled lesions (pustule, vesicle, abscess, cyst) or solid lesions (nodule, tumor); or by *impression smears* of ulcers, the cut surfaces of nodules and tumors, or the surface of "pricked" papules, pustules, and vesicles. The material

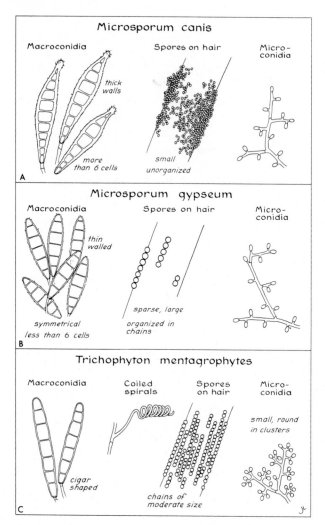

Figure 3:30. A, Characteristic microscopic morphology of *M. canis*; B, characteristic microscopic morphology of *M. gypseum*; C, characteristic microscopic morphology of *T. mentagrophytes*. The conidia and spirals are microscopic structures. The hair shafts are much larger.

obtained is spread thinly on the glass slide and allowed to dry. It is then stained for microscopic examination. By use of these methods it is often possible to distinguish between bacterial skin infection and bacterial colonization of some other dermatosis, determine whether the pustule contains bacteria or is sterile, discover yeasts and fungi, identify various cutaneous neoplasms, or find the acantholytic cells of the pemphigus diseases.

Bacteria are a frequent finding in impression smears from skin and can be seen as basophilic-staining organisms in specimens stained with new methylene blue or Diff Quik. Although identification of the exact species of bacteria is not possible with a stain (as it is in a culture), it is possible to distinguish cocci

Figure 3:31. Microscopic detail of typical fungal organisms. A, Macroconidia, *M. canis*. B, Macroconidia, *M. gypseum*. C, Macroconidia, microconidia, and mycelia, *T. mentagrophytes*. D, Microscopic detail of *Aspergillus*. E, Microscopic detail of *Penicillium*. F, Microscopic detail of *Scopulariopsis*. G, Microscopic detail of *Alternaria*. H, Microscopic detail of *Cladosporium*. (A, D–H, courtesy M. R. McGinnis. B, from McGinnis, M. R., D'Amato, R. F., and Land, G. A.: Pictorial Handbook of Medically Important Fungi and Aerobic Actinomycetes. Praeger Press, New York, 1982. C, from McGinnis, M. R.: Laboratory Handbook of Medical Mycology. Academic Press, Inc., New York, 1980.)

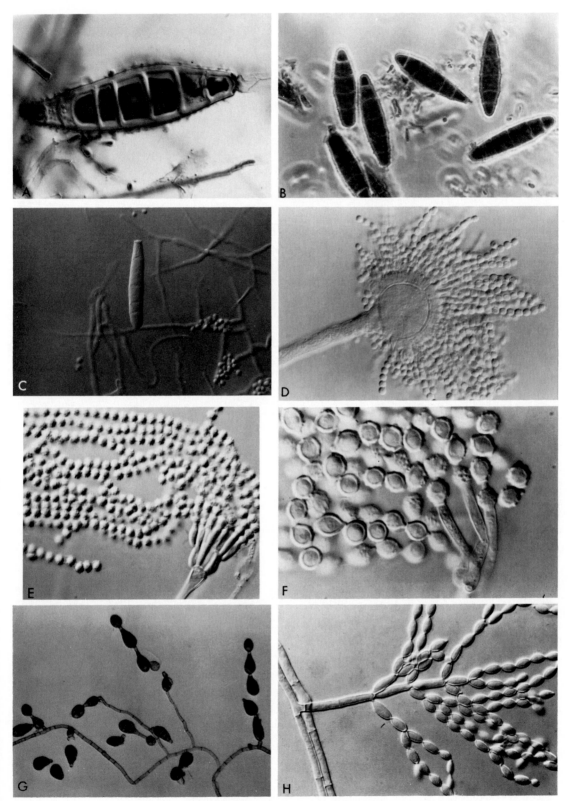

Figure 3:31 *See legend on opposite page*

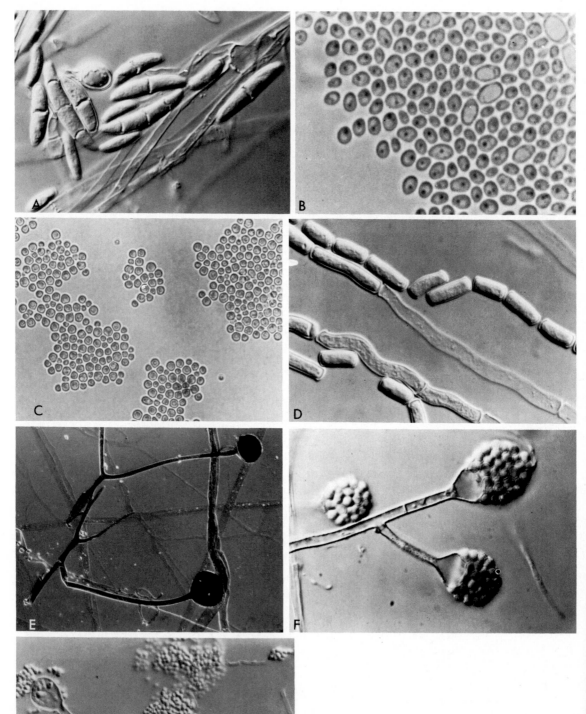

Figure 3:32. Microscopic detail of typical fungal organisms. A, Fusarium. B, Candida. C, Rhodotorula. D, Geotrichum. E, Rhizopus. F, Absidia. G, Mucor.

from rods (see Fig. 3:33A,B), determine whether they are Gram-positive or Gram-negative (with a Gram stain), and often institute very appropriate and effective antibiotic therapy without performing a culture and antibiotic sensitivity (see p. 175). If no bacteria are found in the stained fluid, the clinical condition is probably not a pyoderma.

Next, one looks for the cytologic response of the skin. Are there inflammatory cells? (Fig. 3:33A–E.) Are they eosinophils, neutrophils, or mononuclear cells? If neutrophils are present, do they exhibit degenerative or "toxic" cytologic changes, which would suggest infection? If bacteria and inflammatory cells are found on the same preparation, is there phagocytosis? (Fig. 3:33A,B.) Are the bacteria ingested by individual neutrophils, or are they engulfed by macrophages and multinucleated histocytic giant cells? Are there many bacteria, but few or no inflammatory cells, none of which exhibit degenerative cytologic changes or phagocytes?

Cytologic examination may allow the rapid recognition of: (1) unusual infectious agents (actinomycetes, mycobacteria, subcutaneous and deep mycoses, leishmania) (Fig. 3:33C), (2) sterile pustular dermatoses (pemphigus, sterile eosinophilic pustulosis, subcorneal pustular dermatosis) (Fig. 3:33D), (3) autoimmune dermatoses (pemphigus) (Fig. 3:33F), and neoplastic conditions (Fig. 3:33G,H).

A synopsis of cytologic findings and their interpretation is presented in Table 3:6. Cytomorphologic characteristics of neoplastic cells are presented in Table 20:4, p. 175.

The Biopsy

Skin biopsy is *not* performed as often as it should be, and when it is carried out it is often too late, with poor specimen selection or poor technique or both. Skin biopsy should *not* be regarded as merely a diagnostic aid for the difficult case. It provides a permanent record of the pathology present at a particular moment in time, and knowledge of this pathology acts as a stimulus for the clinician to think more deeply about the basic cellular changes underlying the disease.

WHEN TO BIOPSY

Hard and fast rules on when to perform a skin biopsy cannot be made. The following suggestions are offered as general guidelines. Biopsy should be performed on (1) all obviously neoplastic or suspected neoplastic lesions, (2) all persistent ulcerations, (3) a dermatosis that is not responding to apparently rational therapy, (4) any dermatosis that, in the experience of the clinician, is unusual or appears serious, and (5) any suspected condition for which the therapy is expensive, dangerous, or time-consuming enough to necessitate a definitive diagnosis before beginning treatment. In general, skin biopsy should be performed within 3 *weeks* in any dermatosis that is not responding to what appears to be appropriate therapy. This early intervention: (1) helps obviate the nonspecific, masking, and misleading changes of chronicity, topical and systemic medicaments, excoriation, and secondary infection, and (2) allows more rapid institution of specific therapy, thus reducing permanent disease

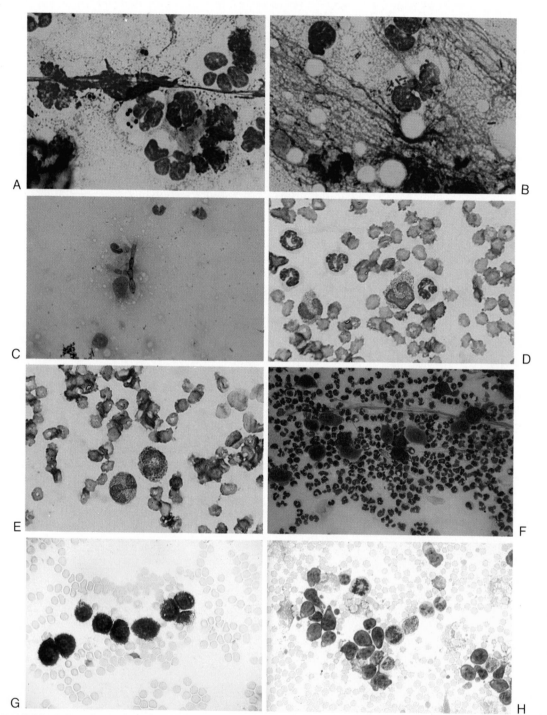

Figure 3:33. *A,* Degenerate neutrophils with phagocytized cocci *(Staphylococcus sp)* from a dog with pyoderma. *B,* Degenerate neutrophils with phagocytized rods *(Pseudomonas sp)* from a dog with otitis externa. *C,* Macrophage containing fungal hypha from a cat with phaeohyphomycosis. *D,* Canine eosinophil from sterile eosinophilic pustulosis. *E,* Basophil and eosinophil from feline flea allergy dermatitis. *F,* Acantholytic cells and neutrophils from a dog with pemphigus foliaceus. *G,* Mast cells from a dog with a cutaneous mast cell tumor. *H,* Malignant lymphocytes from a dog with cutaneous lymphosarcoma.

Table 3:6. CYTOLOGIC DIAGNOSIS FROM STAINED* SMEARS

Finding	Diagnostic Considerations
Neutrophils	
Degenerate	Bacterial infection
Nondegenerate	Sterile inflammation (e.g., canine allergy, subcorneal pustular dermatosis, linear IgA dermatosis)
Eosinophils	Ectoparasitism, endoparasitism, feline allergy, furunculosis, eosinophilic granuloma, feline eosinophilic plaque, pemphigus, sterile eosinophilic pustulosis, mast cell tumor, sterile eosinophilic pinnal folliculitis
Basophils	Ectoparasitism, endoparasitism, feline allergy
Mast cells	Ectoparasitism, feline allergy, mast cell tumor
Lymphocytes, macrophages, and plasma cells	
Granulomatous	Infections (especially furunculosis) vs. sterile (e.g., foreign body, sterile granuloma syndrome, sterile panniculitis)
Pyogranulomatous (many neutrophils, too)	(same as for granulomatous)
Eosinophilic granulomatous	Furunculosis, ruptured keratinous cyst, eosinophilic granuloma
Plasma cells	Plasma cell pododermatitis, plasmacytoma
Acanthocytes	
Few	*Any* suppurative dermatosis
Many	Pemphigus
Bacteria	
Intracellular	Infection
Extracellular *only*	Colonization
Yeast†	
Peanut-shaped	*Malassezia* or *Candida*
Fungi	
Spores, hyphae	Fungal infection (see Chap. 7)
Atypical/monomorphous cell populations‡	
Clumped and rounded	Epithelial neoplasm
Individual, rounded, and numerous	Lymphoreticular or mast cell neoplasm
Individual, rounded, or elongated, and sparse	Mesenchymal neoplasm

*Diff Quik or New Methylene Blue
†Commonly seen, *rarely* pathogenic (must see phagocytosis)
‡See Chapter 20.

sequelae (scarring, alopecia), patient suffering, and needless financial involvement of the owner. Anti-inflammatory agents can dramatically affect the histologic appearance of many dermatoses. Such agents, especially glucocorticoids, should be stopped for 2 to 3 weeks prior to biopsy.

WHAT TO BIOPSY

In most instances, the histologic examination of a fully developed primary lesion will give more information than the examination of early or late lesions. Exceptions to this rule are vesicular, bullous, and pustular lesions, of which very early lesions are selected in order to eliminate secondary changes that can obscure the diagnosis (degeneration, regeneration, or secondary infection). As these fluid-filled lesions are often quite fragile and transient in canine and feline skin (lasting only 2 to 6 hours), it may be necessary to examine patients every 2 to 4 hours in order to find early intact lesions for biopsy. Vesicles, bullae, and pustules that have been present for over 12 hours should not be biopsied.

Often, the histologic diagnosis is facilitated by taking multiple biopsies. By using this technique, lesions in different stages of development are sampled, and it is probable that one sample will establish the diagnosis. Together, the samples document a pathologic continuum. Whenever possible, perform the biopsy with spontaneous, primary lesions (macules, papules, pustules, vesicles, bullae, nodules, and tumors), and avoid lesions that are marred by excoriation, chronicity, or medication.

HOW TO BIOPSY

In general, a 4- to 6-mm biopsy *punch* provides an adequate specimen. It is imperative *not* to include any significant amount of normal skin margin with punch biopsies. Unless the person taking the biopsy personally supervises the processing of the specimen in the tissue block, rotation in the wrong direction may result in failure to section the lesional portion of the specimen.

Excisional biopsy with a scalpel is often indicated (1) for larger lesions, (2) for vesicles, bullae, and pustules (the rotary and shearing action of a punch may damage the lesion), and (3) when disease of the subcutaneous fat is suspected (punches often fail to deliver diseased fat).

Skin biopsy is usually easily and rapidly accomplished using physical restraint and local anesthesia. Desired lesion sites are gently clipped (if needed), and the surface is *gently* cleansed by daubing or soaking with a solution of 70 per cent alcohol. *Under no circumstances* should biopsy sites be scrubbed or prepared with other antiseptics (e.g., iodophors). Such endeavors remove important surface pathology and create iatrogenic lesions, all of which render the specimen useless or misleading. After the surface has air dried, the desired lesion is undermined with an appropriate amount, usually 1 to 2 ml, of local anesthetic (2 per cent lidocaine) injected subcutaneously. An exception to this procedure would be made when disease of the fat is suspected, in which case regional or ring blocks or general anesthesia should be used, because injection into the fat will distort the tissues. The local injection of lidocaine stings, and some animals object strenuously. The desired lesion is then punched or excised, including the underlying fat. Great care should be exercised when manipulating the biopsy specimen, avoiding the use of large forceps and instead using tiny mosquito hemostats, Adson thumb forceps, or the syringe needle through which the local anesthetic was injected. The biopsy site is then sutured closed. The use of chromic gut eliminates the need for suture removal.

COMPLICATIONS OF SKIN BIOPSY

Complications following skin biopsy are very rare. Caution should be exercised when biopsying patients with *bleeding disorders*, including patients taking aspirin and anticoagulants. Such medications should be stopped, if possible, for 1 to 2 weeks prior to biopsy. *Wound healing problems* should be anticipated in patients with hyperadrenocorticism and hypothyroidism, in patients with various collagen defects (such as cutaneous asthenia), and in patients taking glucocorticoids or antimitotic drugs. Such drugs should be stopped 2 to 3 weeks before biopsy, if possible. *Wound infections* are very rare. Caution should be exercised when injecting lidocaine, which contains *epinephrine*, near extremities (ear tips, digits, and so forth) and into patients with impaired circulation, cardiovascular disease, or hypertension, or patients receiving phenothiazines, beta-adrenergic receptor blockers, monoamine oxidase inhibitors (e.g., amitraz), or tricyclic depressants. Finally, be careful of the total amount of lidocaine injected into very small kittens and puppies, since it could produce myocardial depression, muscle twitching, or neurotoxicity. Do not exceed 0.5 ml per kitten or puppy.

WHAT TO DO WITH THE BIOPSY

Skin biopsy specimens should be gently blotted to remove artifactual blood and placed with the subcutaneous side down on pieces of wooden tongue depressor or cardboard. They should be gently pressed flat for 30 to 60 seconds to facilitate adherence. Placing the specimens on a flat surface allows proper anatomic orientation and obviates potentially drastic anatomic artifacts associated with curling and folding. The specimen and its adherent splint are then immersed in fixative within 1 to 2 minutes, since artifactual changes develop rapidly in room air.

In most instances, the fixative of choice is 10 per cent neutral phosphate-buffered formalin (100 ml 40 per cent formaldehyde, 900 ml tap water, 4 gm acid sodium phosphate monohydrate, and 6.5 gm anhydrous disodium phosphate). The volume of the fixative should be 10 to 20 times that of the specimen, and the specimen should be fixed for at least 24 hours. This formalin fixative freezes at about $-11°C$, and specimens exposed to cold prior to fixation will develop freezing artifacts. This situation can be avoided by keeping fixed specimens at room temperature for at least 6 hours prior to exposure to cold or by using an *alcoholic* formalin solution (formol). This is composed of 100 ml 40 per cent formaldehyde and 900 ml 95 per cent ethyl alcohol. Alternatively, a 70 per cent ethyl or isopropyl alcohol can be used. The latter two alternatives are less desirable, as alcohol solutions produce tissue hardening and shrinkage, resulting in significant artifacts.

The last critical consideration regarding what to do with a skin biopsy is deciding *whom* to send it to. Obviously, the clinician wants to send it to someone who can provide the most information. The choices should be prioritized as follows: (1) a veterinary dermatologist or pathologist with a special interest and expertise in dermatohistopathology, (2) a general veterinary pathologist, or (3) a physician pathologist. A word of caution is in order here: Physician pathologists are often singularly unhelpful or misleading in the interpretation of animal skin pathology.

A frequent and unfortunate omission concerning skin biopsies submitted by clinicians is that of adequate clinical information. The clinician and pathologist are a diagnostic team, and the diagnosis (and the patient!) is best served when each member of the team does his/her part. A concise description of the history, physical findings, results of laboratory examinations and therapeutic trials, and the clinician's differential diagnosis should always accompany the biopsy specimen. Remember that old (but ever so appropriate!) cliché, "garbage in, garbage out."

Table 3:7. STAINING CHARACTERISTICS OF VARIOUS CUTANEOUS COMPONENTS WITH ACID ORCEIN-GIEMSA (AOG)

Test Component	Color
Nuclei	Dark blue
Cytoplasm of keratinocytes	Blue-purple
Cytoplasm of smooth muscle cells	Light blue
Keratin	Blue
Collagen	Pink
Elastin	Dark brown to black
Mast cell granules	Purple
Some acid mucopolysaccharides	Purple
Melanin	Dark green to black
Hemosiderin	Yellow-brown to green
Erythrocytes	Green-organge
Eosinophil granules	Red
Cytoplasm of histiocytes, lymphocytes, and fibrocytes	Light blue
Cytoplasm of neutrophils	Clear to light blue
Cytoplasm of plasma cells	Dark blue to gray-blue
Amyloid	Sky blue to gray-blue
Hyaline	Pink
Fibrin and fibrinoid	Green-blue
Keratohyalin	Dark blue
Trichohyalin	Red
Bacteria, fungal spores, and hyphae	Dark blue
Serum	Light blue

TISSUE STAINS

Hematoxylin and eosin (H & E) is the most widely used routine stain for skin biopsies. In the laboratory of one of the authors (D.W.S), *acid orcein-Giemsa (AOG)* is also used as a routine stain for skin biopsies. The routine use of AOG markedly reduces the need for ordering special stains (Table 3:7). Table 3:8 contains guidelines for the use of various special stains.

SPECIAL PROCEDURES

In the last decade, a number of techniques have been developed for studying biopsy specimens. These techniques were usually developed to allow the identification of special cell types. Examples of such procedures include immunofluorescence testing, electron microscopy, enzyme histochemistry, and immunocytochemistry. The latter two procedures have not yet been extensively investigated in small animal dermatology, but should become increasingly used and invaluable diagnostic tools in the future.

Immunofluorescence testing is routinely done in veterinary medicine (see p. 441). Biopsies for immunofluorescence testing must be carefully selected and either snap-frozen or placed in Michel's fixative. *Electron microscopy* is best performed on small specimens (1 to 2 mm in diameter) fixed in 3 per cent glutaraldehyde. *Enzyme histochemistry* is performed on frozen sections or on tissues fixed in 2 per cent paraformaldehyde, dehydrated in acetone, and embedded in glycol methacrylate (see Chap. 20). *Immunocytochemistry* may be

Table 3:8. STAINING CHARACTERISTICS OF VARIOUS SUBSTANCES WITH SPECIAL STAINS

Stain	Tissue and Color
van Gieson's	Mature collagen, *red;* immature collagen, keratin, muscle, and nerves, *yellow*
Masson's trichrome	Mature collagen, *blue;* immature collagen, keratin, muscle, and nerves, *red*
Verhoeff's	Elastin and nuclei, *black*
Gomori's aldehyde fuchsin	Elastin, sulfated acid mucopolysaccharides, and certain epithelial mucins, *purple*
Oil red O*	Lipids, *dark red*
Sudan black B*	Lipids, *green-black*
Scarlet red*	Lipids, *red*
Gomori's or Wilder's reticulin stain	Reticulin, melanin, and nerves, *dark brown to black*
Periodic acid–Schiff	Glycogen, neutral mucopolysaccharides, fungi, and tissue debris, *red*
Alcian blue	Acid mucopolysaccharides, *blue*
Hale's colloidal iron	Acid mucopolysaccharides, *blue*
Toluidine blue	Acid mucopolysaccharides and mast cell granules, *purple*
Gomori's methenamine silver	Fungi, *black*
Gram's or Brown and Brenn	Gram-positive bacteria, *blue* Gram-negative bacteria, *red*
Fite's modified acid-fast	Acid-fast bacteria, *red*
Fontana's ammoniacal silver nitrate	Premelanin and melanin, *black* (hemosiderin usually positive too, but less intense)
Prussian blue	Ferrous and ferric iron, *dark blue*
von Kossa's	Calcium salts, *dark brown to black*
Alizarin red	Calcium salts, *red*
Congo red (can be performed on routine sections but best on frozen sections)	Amyloid, *orange to red* with green birefringence on polarized light
Thioflavin T	Amyloid, *blue to green* with fluorescence microscopy
Foot's or Snook's silver nitrate	Nerves and reticulum, *black*
Giemsa's	Mast cell granules, *purple;* eosinophil granules, *red;* Leishman-Donovan bodies, *red*
Dopa reaction—fresh frozen tissues	Peroxidase-containing cells—melanocytes, granulocytes, and mast cells—positive
Feulgen's reaction	Deoxyribonucleic acid (DNA), *magenta*
Methyl green—pyronine	Ribonucleic acid (RNA), *pink;* DNA, *green*
Warthin-Starry	Spirochetes, *black*

*Require frozen sections of formalin-fixed tissue.

performed on formalin-fixed, routinely processed tissues (e.g., immunoperoxidase methods), or on frozen sections (e.g., lymphocyte markers), depending on the substance being studied (see Chap. 20).

Reference

1. Ihrke, P. J., Franti, C. E.: Breed as a risk factor associated with skin diseases in dogs seen in northern California. Calif. Vet. *39*:13, 1985.

Dermatologic Therapy

Topical Treatment

CLEANING THE SKIN

The skin surface constantly accumulates debris. The normal skin surface film contains excretory products of skin glands, exfoliated flakes of the horny layer, and extraneous dirt. Excessive amounts of these together with exudates, blood, and crusts are found in the surface film of abnormal skin. For health, the skin and coat should be groomed to minimize these accumulations (see p. 230). If proper skin and coat care is neglected, skin irritation may result, or accumulations of debris may have adverse effects on a skin disease that is already present.

Most cases of skin disease that need topical medication require clipping, cleansing, and application of therapeutic agents as logical steps to effective treatment. Clipping is most desirable to enable close scrutiny of the lesions. It also permits thorough cleaning, adequate skin contact, and economical application of the desired medicament. In many cases, complete removal of the coat may be necessary, but usually clipping the local area suffices. This should be done neatly to avoid disfigurement. If the hair over the involved area is clipped closely (against the grain with a No. 40 clipper), while a border around this is clipped less closely (with the grain), the regrowth of hair more quickly "blends" the area into the normal coat pattern. When the cosmetic effects of clipping may be severe, they should always first be discussed with the owner to obtain approval. This contact is especially important when treating show animals or those with long coats, such as Yorkshire terriers, Old English sheepdogs or Afghan hounds. All needless clipping should be avoided. During clipping, a vacuum cleaner can be used advantageously to remove all loose, dry hair and debris. The lesions are inspected carefully before further procedures are determined.

Clipping and cleaning the lesion works wonders! Then add topical medication.

Acute and subacute dermatoses, especially when vesiculation and oozing are present, are damaged by vigorous washing with soap and water. Topical cleansing should be avoided in these cases. In other instances wet dressings, warm oil baths, and cosmetic cleansing creams can be used safely. For certain problems, judicious use of alcohol or ether may be effective. Agents such as gasoline, paint remover, and cleaning fluids should *never* be used on dog or cat skin. They are extremely irritating and highly toxic. Road tar on the feet or legs of dogs or cats can be treated satisfactorily by using scissors to cut off the large masses of tar and hair. The remaining tar can be soaked in an emollient oil with a surface active agent for 24 hours to soften the mass. A simple shampoo then usually removes any residuum. Paint on the coat is best removed by clipping the affected hair after the paint has hardened.

HYDROTHERAPY

> *Plain tap water is one of the most effective agents in the treatment of skin diseases. It is often forgotten—or misused.*

Water is a component of many lotions. Water may also be applied as a wet dressing or in baths. Frequent periodic renewal of wet dressings (15 minutes on, several hours off) prolongs the effect; but if more continuous therapy or occlusive coverings are used, the skin temperature rises and an undesirable maceration occurs. This is less likely to happen if the wet dressing is left open. Hydrotherapy can be used to hydrate or to dehydrate the skin, depending on how it is managed. Loose, damp gauze compresses applied for 15 minutes on and for 1 hour off promote evaporation of water from the gauze and from the skin surface and are drying to the underlying tissues too. If lots of water is maintained on the skin surface by wet towels, soaks, or baths, the skin hydrates as water is taken up by keratin and hair. If a film of oil is applied immediately after soaking, evaporation of water (transpiration) is hindered and the skin retains moisture.

> *Oils soften the skin by blocking transpiration and thus increasing the moisture content of the stratum corneum (Fig. 4:2D).*

The water temperature may be cool or above body temperature, and the effect can thus be modified as needed. Whirlpool baths, with or without detergents and antiseptics added, make gentle, effective cleaning possible (Fig. 4:1). These treatments may be used to remove crusts and scales, to cleanse wounds and fistulas, to rehydrate skin (Fig. 4:2C), and to prophylactically manage patients prone to decubital problems, urine scalds, and other ills. Ten to 15 minutes of therapy once or twice daily is adequate. The patient should be toweled and placed in an air-stream drier to dry. Other topical medications can be applied later, if needed.

In hydrotherapy, moisture is the specific agent, and various additives change its effects only slightly. In general, water treatment removes crusts, bacteria, and other debris and greatly reduces the possibility of secondary infection. It promotes epithelialization and allays the symptoms of pain, pruritus, and burning. It also softens keratin. Studies have demonstrated that

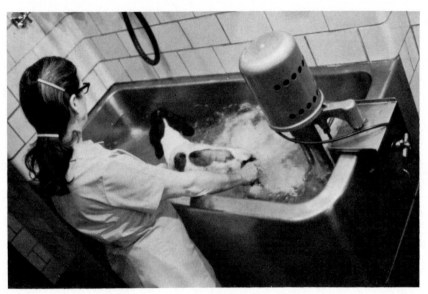

Figure 4:1. Patient enjoys a warm, antiseptic whirlpool bath that gently cleanses and hydrates the skin.

the suppleness and softness of the skin are due to its water content, not to the oils on the surface (Fig. 4:2).

MEDICATIONS USED WITH WATER

Astringents, antiseptics, or antibiotics added to water create other effects, in addition to the cooling and cleansing of compresses and baths. Astringents precipitate proteins and prevent exudation. Aqueous medications are the topical treatments of choice in acute exudative dermatoses.

Aluminum acetate (Burow's solution USP) is available commercially as Domeboro. It is drying, astringent, and mildly antiseptic. The usual solution is 1:40 in cool water, and soaks are repeated three times daily for 30 minutes. (One packet of powder, or one tablet, is added to 0.5 L [1 pt] or 1 L [1 qt] of water.)

Magnesium sulfate 1:65 solution (1 tbsp per L [qt] of warm water) is a mildly hypertonic solution for wet dressings. It tends to dehydrate or "draw" water from the tissues. *Isotonic sodium chloride* solution for wet dressings can be made by adding 5 ml (1 tsp) of table salt to 0.5 L (1 pt) of water.

Silver nitrate 0.25 per cent solution may be applied to moist, weeping, denuded areas as an antiseptic, coagulant, and stimulating agent. It should be used infrequently and sparingly.

Potassium permanganate 1:1000 to 1:30,000 solution (1 grain $KMnO_4$ tablet or 5 ml [1 tsp] to 15 ml [1 tbsp] of crystals per 1 L [1 qt] of water) may be applied in fresh preparations for soaks or irrigations. It is astringent, antiseptic, and antimicrobial and toughens and stains the skin.

Boric acid is ineffective and dangerous and should *not* be used.

Antibiotic wet dressings may be made from many antibiotics. Neomycin sulfate has excellent stability, is bactericidal, and is effective against many gram-positive and gram-negative bacteria. However, it has been known to

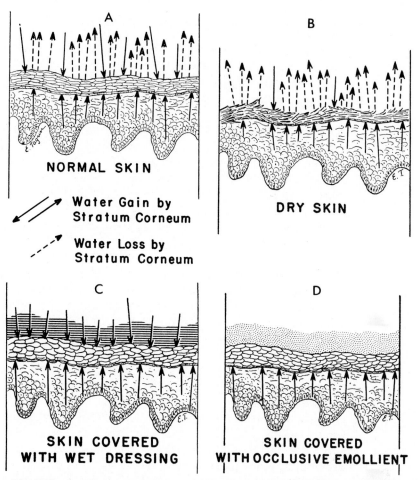

Figure 4:2. *A*, Water exchange through the stratum corneum of normal skin in equilibrium with the environment. Water is being received from the underlying tissues and from the environment. In addition, water is being lost to the environment, and there is a net transfer from the underlying tissues to the environment. *B*, Water exchange through the stratum corneum of skin that has been transferred from a high to a low environmental humidity. The water loss to the environment is temporarily increased and that received from the environment is decreased. The stratum corneum becomes dehydrated, since the amount of water it can receive from the underlying tissues is limited. *C*, Water exchange through the stratum corneum when the skin is covered with a wet dressing. The stratum corneum hydrates, since water is being received both from the underlying tissues and the external water. *D*, Water exchange through the stratum corneum when the skin is covered with an occlusive emollient. The stratum corneum hydrates, since water is being received from the underlying tissues and water loss to the environment is prevented. (From Frazier, E. N., and Blank, I. H.: A Formulary for External Therapy of the Skin. Charles C Thomas, Springfield, Ill., 1954.)

cause sensitization. Ordinarily, 500 mg is added to 25 ml of saline for wet dressings and irrigating solutions.

Bath oils, which are commonly used in human medicine (Nutraspa, Domol, Lubath), have limited use for animals. They are most commonly used in the management of dry skin (seborrhea sicca). Products such as Alpha-Keri, HY-LYT efa, Humilac, and other skin and coat conditioners are available in sprays, which can be applied to the dry coat and massaged to produce improved sheen. Solutions are also available to add to a small volume of water and to use after a bath as a rinse. They contain dewaxed, oil-soluble fraction of lanolin, mineral oil, and a nonionic emulsifier and produce a nice gloss after the coat dries. Used in excess, they make the coat greasy and cause it to rapidly collect dirt.

Lactic acid and urea have hygroscopic and keratolytic actions that aid in normalizing the epidermis and especially the quality of the stratum corneum. The application of urea in a cream or ointment base has a softening and moisturizing effect on the stratum corneum and makes the vehicle feel less greasy. While it acts as a humectant in concentrations of 2 to 20 per cent, above that level it is keratolytic. That action is a result of the solubilization of prekeratin and keratin and the fact that it may break hydrogen bonds that keep the stratum corneum intact.[124] Humilac contains both urea and lactic acid, and it can be used as a spray or rinse. To make a rinse, 5 capfuls of Humilac are added to 1 L (1 qt) of water. The mixture is rinsed over the dog's coat and allowed to dry.

Soaps and shampoos are cleansing agents for the skin and hair. Soluble soaps are sodium (hard soap) or potassium (soft soap) salts of high molecular weight (i.e., monobasic aliphatic acids). They usually contain preservatives, essential oils, and coloring matter. The osmotic effect and detergent action of soaps may irritate the skin. Irritation is caused by the mechanical effect of the foam, emulsification of the skin oils and grease, and softening of the epidermis. The most bland soaps and shampoos are made from coconut or other vegetable oils. No matter how bland the soap, it should always be thoroughly rinsed from the skin. Coconut oil shampoo, hexachlorophene liquid soap USP (hexachlorophene 10 per cent in potassium soap), and Alpha-Keri soap are examples of simple cleansing agents commonly used.

Medicated soaps and shampoos contain additional ingredients that supposedly enhance or add other actions to that of the shampoo. It is incongruous, in some cases, to add medications to a drug whose primary purpose is to remove substances from the skin. However, some medicaments may have enough opportunity for effect or for limited absorption during a prolonged shampoo, and their addition may be justified (e.g., insecticides, salicylic acid, sulfur, tar, selenium, antiseptics).

Pharmaceutical companies provide a multitude of "medicated shampoos." They often have specific indications and contraindications. It is important to become familiar with a few (perhaps one of each type) and to understand thoroughly the ingredients and their concentration and action. Always choose the mildest shampoo that will produce the desired actions. Strong shampoos can be harmful as well as helpful. Shampoos can be classified as follows:

1. Nonmedicated or "hypoallergenic" shampoos are primarily meant for cleansing. An inexpensive human hair shampoo or dishwashing liquid (e.g., Joy, Ivory) removes dirt and debris from the skin nicely. Among the veterinary mild detergent shampoos are Mycodex Pearlescent, HY-LYT efa, and Allergroom Emollient Shampoo.

2. Antiseborrheic shampoos usually contain salicylic acid, sulfur, and tar in various combinations and strengths. *Sulfur* is keratolytic, keratoplastic, antibacterial, antifungal, antiparasitic, antipruritic, and mildly "follicular flushing"; *salicylic acid* is mildly antipruritic, bacteriostatic, and keratolytic: and *tar* is keratolytic, keratoplastic, antipruritic, and vasoconstrictive. Sebbafon, Seba-Lyt, and Sebulex contain sulfur and salicylic acid. LyTar, Mycodex Tar and Sulfur, and Allerseb T contain tar, sulfur, and salicylic acid. Adams Sulfur Shampoo contains only sulfur in a shampoo vehicle.

3. Benzoyl peroxide (OxyDex, Pyoben)-containing shampoos have been

used for "follicular flushing" in dermatology for acne. They are keratolytic, antibacterial, antipruritic, and degreasing.

4. Selenium shampoos (Selsun Blue) are keratolytic and degreasing. They contain selenium sulfide, prolong epidermal turnover time, and are antifungal.

Soap substitutes can be obtained in the form of detergents or cleaning creams. Because these products do not foam vigorously, they are not especially effective unless the hair has been removed. They cause little irritation to sensitive skin and are particularly effective in removing greasy films or glandular exudates such as sebum. pHisoDerm, a hypoallergenic emulsion containing entsulfon, wool fat cholesterols, lactic acid, and petroleum, is an example of an aqueous detergent cleanser; on the other hand, Nivea Creme or oil, an emulsion of neutral aliphatic hydrocarbons in water with wool fat cholesterol, is an example of a nonaqueous cleansing cream. Allergroom and HY-LYT efa are gentle nonmedicated shampoos whose detergent and soap-free formulas produce a rich lather that thoroughly cleans normal and dry hair. They may be used on an animal whose skin is intolerant of soap and are often useful in dogs and cats with dry skin.

Although many types of solid debris can be removed from the skin by various soaps and detergents, removal of excess keratin (hyperkeratosis) is dependent on maceration of the scales. Here *alkaline* soaps or detergents are more effective. The removal of bacteria is affected by the electric charge of the skin and the organisms. Since soap or markedly alkaline detergents make both skin and organisms more negative electrically, they are more efficient in removing bacteria than are less alkaline detergents.

HAIR CARE PRODUCTS

Many products of the human cosmetic line have been used on dogs' coats, and some have been modified especially for use in grooming dogs. This discussion will cover the effects some of these products have on the hair itself. Hair is an inert keratinous substance, and "life," bounce, glossiness, body, "flyaway," and manageability are terms used in describing the condition of inert hair. Different effects are needed on different hair coat types, e.g., collie, Yorkshire terrier, Scottish terrier, and beagle.

Shampoos should remove external dirt, grime, and sebum and leave the hair soft, shiny, and easy to comb. To accomplish this, they should lather well, rinse freely, leave no residue, cause no eye damage, and remove soil rather than natural oils. Some shampoos still have a soap base, but most are surfactants or detergents with a variety of additives that function as thickeners, conditioners, lime-soap dispersants, protein hydrolysates, and perfumes. There are dozens of products on the market.

Soap shampoos work well in soft water, but in hard water they leave a dulling film of calcium-magnesium soap on the hair unless special lime-dispersing agents are added to bind calcium-magnesium and heavy metal ions and overcome the problem.

Detergent shampoos are synthetic surfactants, usually salts of lauryl sulfate. They do not react with hard water, but they tend to be harsher cleansing agents than soap. This disadvantage is partially overcome by various additives. Glycol, glyceryl esters, lanolin derivatives, oils, and fatty alcohols are considered to be superfatting or emollient additives that prevent the complete removal of natural oils or tend to replace them. They also give the hair more luster and, as "lubricants," make it easier to comb.

Baby shampoos are expensive detergents that are milder and less effective cleansing agents. They do not irritate the eyes and are adequate shampoos, if heavy oils and excessive grime are not the problem.

Dry shampoos are mixtures of absorbent powders and mild alkali. They are dusted into the hair and removed by brushing. They are not good cleansers, and the brushing greatly increases static electricity in the hair. They are *not* recommended.

Hair conditioners have two main purposes: to reduce static electricity so that coarse hair does not snarl or become "flyaway," and give "body" to limp hair or thin hair. Normal hair maintains electric neutrality. However, clean, dry hair in a low-humidity environment or when brushed excessively picks up increased negative electric charges. Adjacent hairs that are similarly charged repel one another and produce the condition known as "flyaway." Conditioners or "cream rinses" are cationic (positively charged) surfactants or amphoteric materials that neutralize the charge and eliminate "flyaway." They are slightly acidic, which hardens keratin and removes hard water residues. They also contain a fatty or oily component that adds a film that provides luster. Thus, these products make hair lie flat and comb easily, but they do not provide the "body" or fluff that some coats require. Protein conditioners or "body builders" contain oil and protein hydrolysates. Oils add luster, while protein hydrolysates coat the hair and make it "thicker." This may be a slight advantage in hair with a dried, cracked, outer-cuticle layer, but the effect is actually minimal. Only a thin film is added, so hair is not strengthened. If the protein is added to a shampoo rather than used separately, most of it will be washed away during rinsing, further reducing the effect.

FACTORS THAT INFLUENCE DRUG EFFECTS ON THE SKIN

Topical medications consist of active ingredients incorporated in a vehicle that facilitates application to the skin. In selecting a vehicle, one must consider the solubility of the drug in the vehicle, the rate of release from the vehicle, the ability of the vehicle to hydrate the stratum corneum, the stability of the active agent in the vehicle, and the interactions (chemical and physical) of the vehicle, the active agent, and the stratum corneum. The vehicle is not always inert, and in fact many have important therapeutic effects.[124] The pharmaceutic characteristics of a medication may be important but the pharmacologic actions are paramount.

With topical medications, one basic question is whether or not the drug penetrates the skin and if so, how much. Absorption is highly variable, and most drugs penetrate only 1 to 2 per cent after 16 to 24 hours.[41] Clinical efficacy and absorption are not synonymous; absorption is only one factor in efficacy. Some drugs in insoluble form in the vehicle have only a surface effect.

Absorption of drugs through the skin involves three major variables.

1. *Concentration* of the drug and its solubility in the vehicle. The package label gives the percentage of drug concentration, not the percentage of solubility. Newer propylene glycol vehicles for topical corticosteroids increase solubility and drug delivery, so systemic effects following topical use are common— and dangerous.

2. *Movement* of the drug from the vehicle to the skin barrier. The solubility of the drug in the horny layer relative to its solubility in the vehicle is described by the partition coefficient. The concentration of the drug *in the barrier*, not in the vehicle, is what determines the diffusion force. Increased lipid solubility favors drug penetration, because the stratum corneum is lipophilic.

3. *Diffusion coefficient* is a measure of the extent to which the barrier interferes with drug mobility. The stratum corneum is unsurpassed as an unfavorable environment for drug penetration. Physical disruption of the epidermal barrier by the use of lipid solvents, keratolytic agents, or cellulose tape "stripping" of the top layers of cells increases absorption potentials. DMSO facilitates cutaneous penetration of some substances. Moisture and occlusive dressings enhance percutaneous absorption as well. Conversely, large molecular size means poor mobility and poor absorption.

Iontophoresis is a process that applies direct electric current through a charged drug solution and the patient to increase drug absorption.[148] It may be useful to produce high drug concentrations in superficial local lesions such as ulcers.

TOPICAL FORMULATIONS

Powders

Powders are pulverized organic or inorganic solids that are applied to the skin in a thin film. They may be added to liquids to form "shake lotions," or to ointments to form pastes. Some powders (talc, starch, zinc oxide) are inert and have a physical effect; others (sulfur) contain active ingredients that have a chemical or antibacterial effect. Powders are used as drying agents and to cool and lubricate intertriginous areas. The affected skin should be cleaned and dried before the powder is applied. Powder build-up or caking should be avoided, but if it occurs, wet compresses or soaks will gently remove the excess. On long-coated animals, a fine powder is an acceptable retention vehicle for insecticides and fungicides.

Lotions

Lotions are liquids for topical use, in which medicinal agents are dissolved or suspended. Some are essentially "liquid powders," because when the liquid evaporates, a thin powder film is left on the skin. Lotions tend to be more drying (because of their water or alcohol base) than liniments, which have an oily base. These medications tend to be cooling, antipruritic, and drying (depending on the base). They are vehicles for active ingredients such as sulfur (Adams Sulfur Lotion). The liquid preparations can be applied repeatedly, but when they tend to "cake" or build up, they should be removed gently by wet dressings. In general, lotions are indicated for acute oozing dermatoses and are contraindicated in dry, chronic conditions.

An example of a soothing, antipruritic lotion is calamine lotion (USP), which contains calamine, zinc oxide, glycerin, bentonite magma, and calcium hydroxide solution. Astringent lotions contain tannic acid, alum, and acetic acid.

Emulsions

Emulsions are oily or fatty substances that have been dispersed in water. As a group, they are classified by composition between lotions and ointments. Emulsions are thicker than lotions but thinner than ointments. Emulsions are of two types: oil dispersed in water and water dispersed in oil. Although both types are used as vehicles, the former dilutes with water, loses water rapidly, and therefore is cooling. The latter type dilutes with oil and loses its water slowly. In both cases, once the water evaporates, the action of the vehicle on the skin is no different from that of the oil and emulsifying agent alone. Thus, the characteristics of the residual film are those of the oily phase of the vehicle. This can be illustrated by comparing cold cream and vanishing cream. Cold cream is mostly oil with a little water. The oils have a low melting point, so when the water evaporates a thick, greasy film is left on the skin. A vanishing cream, on the other hand, is mostly water with oils that have a high melting point. When the water evaporates, a thin film of fat is left on the skin. This waxlike film does not feel greasy. Urea added to creams also decreases the greasy feel.

Emulsions are commonly used as vehicles for other agents. They have the advantage of easy application, give mechanical protection, and are soothing, antipruritic, softening, and fairly penetrating. The disadvantage in the hairy skin of animals is that they can be occlusive, greasy, heat-retaining, and messy.

Creams and Ointments

Creams, ointments, salves, and pastes are mentioned here in the order of increasing viscosity. All spread fairly easily and maintain contact between the drug and the skin. They act merely as vehicles in most cases, but may disrupt the horny layer so that penetration is enhanced or may interfere with water loss and glandular secretion. These effects may serve to hydrate the skin somewhat, but also may produce a folliculitis because of occlusion of pilosebaceous orifices.

Creams and ointments are mixtures of grease or oil and water that are emulsified with high-speed blenders. Emulsifiers, coloring agents, and perfumes are often added to improve the physical characteristics of the product. Pastes are highly viscous ointments into which large amounts of powder are incorporated. While pastes may be tolerated on slightly exudative skin (the powder takes up water), in general, creams and ointments are contraindicated in oozing areas.

Creams and ointments function to lubricate and smooth skin that is roughened. They form a protective covering that reduces contact with the environment, and certain occlusive types may reduce water loss. They also serve to transport medicinal agents into follicular orifices and keep drugs in intimate contact with the horny layer. This type of medication should be applied with gentle massage several times daily to maintain a *thin* film on the skin. Thick films are wasteful, occlusive, and messy to surroundings. An obvious film of ointment left on the skin surface means too much has been applied. Usually ointments disappear spontaneously, but thick films can be softened and removed by water or oil soaks and gentle massage.

Water-washable ointment bases such as Carbowax 1500 can be readily removed with water. Oily bases are not freely water washable. It is important for the clinician to understand the uses and advantages of these types of bases, because the total effect on the skin is caused by the vehicle as well as its "active" ingredient.

Simple petroleum jelly soothes and protects inflamed skin.

Hydrophobic oils mix poorly with water. They contain few polar groups (-OH, -COOH, and so on). These oils get in close contact with the skin and spread easily. Since they are hydrophobic, it is difficult for water to pass through a film of these oils, and they are occlusive for the skin. They retain heat and water, and thick films of the more viscid forms (petroleum) produce an uncomfortable sensation to the patient. The oily forms (mineral oil) are often incorporated into emulsion-type vehicles.

Hydrophilic oils are miscible with water. They contain many polar groups, and those with the greatest number are most soluble in water. Although they are ointments only in regard to their physical characteristics, the polyethylene glycols are alcohols that are readily miscible with water. Polymers with a molecular weight greater than 1000 are solid at room temperature, but a slight rise to body temperature causes melting to form an oily film. Carbowax 1500 is such a product. It mixes with skin exudates well, is easily washed off with water, and is less occlusive than other bases.

Gels

Gels are topical formulations composed of combinations of propylene glycol, propylene gallate, disodium EDTA, and carboxypolymethylene, with HCl added to adjust the pH. They act as a clear, colorless, thixotrophic base and are greaseless and water miscible. The active ingredients incorporated in commercially used bases of this type are completely in solution. Gels are being more widely used, since, despite their oily appearance, they can be rubbed into the skin to disappear completely and do not leave the skin with a sticky feeling.[103] Gels are especially useful for animals, because they pass through the hair coat to the skin and are not messy. Examples of gels used in veterinary medicine are OxyDex and Pyoben, which are antimicrobial, keratolytic, and degreasing. KeraSolv is a keratolytic, humectant gel for hyperkeratotic conditions.

Dimethyl Sulfoxide (DMSO)

DMSO is a simple, hygroscopic, organic solvent. Because it is freely miscible with lipids, organic solvents, and water, it is an excellent vehicle. When exposed to the air, concentrated solutions will take in water to become hydrated at 67 per cent. However, stronger concentrations tend to cross the skin barrier better. DMSO penetrates skin (within 5 minutes) but also mucous membranes and the blood barrier, as well as cell, organelle, and microbial membranes. Unlike most solvents, penetration is achieved without membrane damage.[16] It facilitates absorption of many other substances across membranes, especially corticosteroids. On a cellular level, DMSO and steroids exert a synergistic effect.

DMSO has properties of its own as a cryoprotectant, radioprotectant and anti-ischemic, anti-inflammatory, and analgesic agent. It also has variable antibacterial, antifungal, and antiviral properties, depending on the concentration (usually 5 to 50 per cent) and the organism involved. Although its mechanism of action is incompletely understood, the systemic toxicity and teratogenicity of this solvent in its pure form are considered low. Toxicity may be of concern, depending on dose, route, species, and individual reaction. Impurities or combinations with other agents may make DMSO dangerous as a result of its ability to enhance transepidermal absorption. Industrial forms of DMSO should never be used for medical purposes, since the impurities it contains will be absorbed and may be toxic.

At present, DMSO is only FDA approved in the United States for musculoskeletal problems in horses and as a vehicle for a topical otic product (Synotic).

When approved, potential uses might include topical application to cutaneous ulcers, burns, open wounds, skin grafts, reduction of exuberant granulation tissue, and acral lick dermatitis. One formula shown to be safe and useful contains Burow's solution, hydrocortisone, and 90 per cent DMSO. Equal parts of 90 per cent DMSO and H/B 101 [1 per cent hydrocortisone and 2 per cent Burow's solution in a water and propylene glycol base] are mixed. The formulation is applied daily to benefit patients with acute moist dermatitis and acral lick dermatitis.

EMOLLIENTS, KERATOLYTICS, AND DRY SKIN

Emollients are agents that soften or soothe the skin; keratolytics are agents that promote separation or peeling of the horny layer of the epidermis. Both types of drugs are useful in hydration and softening of the skin.

"Dryness of the skin" is recognized when any one of the following is present: roughness of the surface, inflexibility of the horny layer, or fissuring with possible inflammation.

Normal skin is not a waterproof covering but is constantly losing water to the environment by transpiration (Fig. 4:2A). This loss is dependent on body temperature, environmental temperature, and relative humidity (Fig. 4:2B). The barrier layer of the epidermis is the major deterrent to water loss, although the normal lipid film on the surface plays a minor role too. This film is derived from sebum and from degenerated epidermal cells. Dry keratin is highly insoluble and can be soaked in oil for months without any effect. If it is immersed in water for a short period, however, it quickly softens.

The hydration of keratin is a basic principle of softening the skin.

If all cells at the surface of the skin were to desquamate completely and evenly, the surface of the skin should remain smooth. However, because they are lost in flakes and patches, the skin surface is rough. This is accentuated when excessive use of soap and defatting agents removes lipids and causes the alternation of excess hydration and drying. This allows clumps of cells to be loosened prematurely and fissures to form, accentuating the roughness (i.e., chapped skin). Sebum on the skin or externally applied lipid films have a tendency to make the surface feel smoother. The flexibility of keratin is directly related to its moisture content. Because the barrier in the epidermis limits the amount of water that the horny layer can receive from below, the moisture content of that layer is dependent on the environment. Water content of the horny layer can be increased by occlusive dressings to prevent loss (Fig. 4:2D), by adding water with baths or wet dressings (Fig. 4:2C), or by using hygroscopic medications to attract water (glycerin). For maximum softening, the skin should be hydrated in wet dressings, dried, and covered with an occlusive hydrophobic oil (petrolatum). The barrier to water loss can be further strengthened by covering the local lesion with plastic wrap under a bandage. Nonocclusive emollients are relatively ineffective in retaining moisture.

Keratolytic agents do not dissolve keratin but soften excessively keratinized tissue so that it can be removed mechanically. Excessive hydration causes maceration of tissue, which then can be easily removed. Salicylic acid 6 per cent, propylene glycol 50 per cent, and urea 20 per cent are keratolytic agents that are present in many ointments. Ointment under an occlusive dressing causes water to accumulate in the horny layer. Some of the moisture leaches salicylic acid out of the ointment, and the resulting reduction of the skin pH allows the keratin to absorb more water than at its normal pH. Thus, the cornified epidermis is macerated and can be removed. Sulfur and tar are also good keratolytic agents. Benzoyl peroxide (OxyDex or Pyoben) is keratolytic, degreasing, and a "follicular-flushing" agent.

TOPICAL ANTIPRURITICS

Antipruritic agents attempt to provide temporary relief of itching, but no really satisfactory medication exists. Most of the antipruritic agents listed here have other actions and are discussed in detail in other sections of this chapter. Corticosteroids, administered systemically and topically, offer much help, but they are not without risk. Hydrocortisone 1 per cent is necessary for good topical effect; however, the fluorinated corticosteroids are more potent and penetrate better. Antihistamines that are administered systemically are occasionally useful, but applied topically they are useless. Topical anesthetics may be partially effective, but they may be toxic (methemoglobinemia) or have sensitizing potentials (phenol 0.5 per cent, tetracaine and lidocaine 0.5 per cent).[177]

Cool wet dressings are often helpful, and in general any volatile agent provides a cooling sensation that might be palliative. This is the basis for using menthol (1 per cent), thymol (1 per cent), and alcohol (70 per cent) in antipruritic medications. In addition, menthol has a specific action on local sensory nerve endings. Cool water baths alone or accompanied by Burow's solution soaks (Domboro) or colloidal oatmeal (Aveeno) may be helpful for a period lasting from hours to days.

In general, antipruritics give relief from itching by means of four methods:

1. Substituting some other sensation, such as heat or cold, for the itch. Examples of such agents are menthol 0.12 to 1 per cent, camphor 0.12 to 5 per cent, thymol 0.5 to 1 per cent, heat (warm water soaks or baths), or cold (ice packs).

2. Protecting the skin from external influences such as scratching, biting, trauma, temperature changes, humidity changes, pressure, and irritants. This can be done with bandages or any impermeable protective agents.

3. Anesthetizing the peripheral nerves by using local anesthetics such as benzocaine, tetracaine, lidocaine, benzoyl peroxide, or tars.

4. Using specific biochemical agents, such as topical glucocorticoids.

TOPICAL ANTIMICROBIAL AGENTS

No group of drugs is employed more widely than antimicrobial agents. The terminology used to describe the actions of drugs on microbes is somewhat confusing because of discrepancies between strict definitions of terms and their general usage. *Antiseptics* are substances that kill or prevent growth of microbes (the term is used especially for preparations applied to living tissue). *Disinfectants* are agents that prevent infection by destruction of microbes (the term is used especially for substances applied to inanimate objects). Antiseptics and disinfectants are types of *germicides*, which are agents that destroy microbes. Germicides may be further defined by the appropriate use of terms such as *bactericide, fungicide,* and *virucide.*

In a discussion of such heterogeneous compounds as antimicrobials, some method of classification is desirable. So varied are the compounds, with respect to chemical structure, mechanism of action, and use, that too strict a classification may be more confusing than elucidating. The following classification is a compromise.

The antiseptic agents are listed with brief comments so that their purposes can be appreciated when they are recognized as ingredients in proprietary formulations. The usage of some of these agents is described in other sections of the text.

Alcohols. These act by precipitating proteins and dehydrating protoplasm. They are bactericidal (not sporicidal), astringent, cooling, and rubefacient. However, they are irritating to denuded surfaces and are generally contraindicated in acute inflammatory disorders. Seventy per cent ethyl alcohol and 70 to 90 per cent isopropyl alcohol are the most effective concentrations and are bactericidal within 1 to 2 minutes at 30° C.

Glycols. *Propylene glycol* is a fairly active antibacterial and antifungal agent. A 40 to 50 per cent concentration is best. It is primarily used as a vehicle for other powerful antimicrobial agents. In dilute solution, it is an effective humectant because it is hygroscopic. In a 60 to 75 per cent solution it denatures and solubilizes protein and therefore is keratolytic.

Phenols. Phenols, cresols, resorcinol, hexylresorcinol, thymol, and picric acid act by denaturing microbial proteins. They are also antipruritic and somewhat antifungal. However, they are quite irritating and currently have few legitimate uses on the skin. One exception is the chlorinated phenol *hexachlorophene,* which is a good antibacterial agent (*not* to be used for *Pseudomonas* spp.). However, organic material and tissue extracts hinder its activity, and alarming toxicities (especially in young animals) have greatly curtailed its use. Phenols are contraindicated in cats.

Chlorhexidine. Chlorhexidine is a phenol-related biguanide antiseptic that has many stellar properties: it is *highly effective* against many fungi, viruses, and most bacteria, except perhaps some *Pseudomonas* and *Serratia* strains; it is nonirritating, rarely sensitizing, not inactivated by organic matter, and persistent in action; and it is effective in shampoo, ointment, surgical scrub, and solution formulations containing 0.5 to 2.0 per cent concentrations of chlorhexidine diacetate. A 0.05 per cent dilution in water is an effective, nonirritating solution for wound irrigation. This agent is safe for cats.

Formaldehyde. A 1:200 solution of formaldehyde kills bacteria, fungi, mycobacteria, viruses, and spores in 1 to 6 hours, but it is too irritating for the skin.

Balsams. Balsams are naturally occurring mixtures of resins, volatile oils, and organic acids. They are weak antimicrobials and antiparasitics and are mild counterirritants (e.g., Peruvian balsam).

Acids. In general, acids are weak antibacterials and antifungals. Benzoic and salicylic acids are moderate keratolytics. One per cent *acetic acid* has been found to be beneficial in superficial *Pseudomonas* infections of skin and the external ear.

Halogenated Agents

Iodine. This is one of the oldest antimicrobials. Elemental I is the active agent (mechanism unknown). It is rapidly bactericidal, fungicidal, virucidal, and sporicidal and is used in the following forms: (1) *Tincture of iodine*—2 per cent iodine and 2 per cent NaI in alcohol is a most effective skin antiseptic. It is irritating and sensitizing, especially in cats. (2) *Lugol's iodine*—5 to 7 per cent iodine and 10 per cent potassium iodide (KI) in water. It also is irritating and sensitizing in cats. (3) *Povidone-iodine* (Betadine)—iodine with polyvinyl pyrrolidone, which slowly releases iodine to tissues. It is less irritating than other halogenated agents to skin and mucous membranes, and can be used under tapes and bandages. Povidone-iodine has a prolonged action (4 to 6 hours), is nonstinging and non-staining, and is not impaired by blood, serum, necrotic debris, or pus. However, even these "tamed" iodines can be irritating, especially in cats and in inflammatory conditions of the scrotum and external ear in dogs.

Sodium Hypochlorite and Chloramines. These are effective bactericidal, fungicidal, sporicidal, and virucidal agents. Their action is thought to be due to liberation of hypochlorous acid. Fresh preparations are needed. Sodium hypochlorite 5.25 per cent (Clorox) diluted with water 1:10 (modified Dakin's solution) is usually well tolerated. Organic material greatly reduces its antimicrobial activity.

Oxidizing Agents. *Hydrogen peroxide* is a *weak* germicide that acts through the liberation of nascent oxygen (e.g., 3 per cent H_2O_2 used in dilute water solution). It has limited usefulness.

Potassium permanganate ($KMnO_4$) acts as a bactericidal, astringent, and fungicidal agent (especially against *Candida* spp.). Its action is thought to involve liberation of nascent O_2. This agent stings and stains and is inhibited by organic material. $KMnO_4$ 1:10,000 to 1:30,000 solution can be used to irrigate weeping skin lesions.

Benzoyl peroxide is a potent, broad-spectrum antibacterial agent that is also keratolytic, antipruritic, and degreasing. It has a "follicular-flushing" action but can be irritating. Available as a 5 per cent gel and a 2.5 per cent shampoo (OxyDex, Pyoben), benzoyl peroxide is an excellent adjunct to the antibiotic therapy of superficial and deep pyodermas and for seborrheic disorders. *Do not use proprietary or more concentrated formulations on animals, as they are irritating.*

Synthetic Organic Dyes. These are a variety of *weak* antimicrobial agents are available that have few indications, including the following: (1) *azo dyes*—phenazopyridine, scarlet red, (2) *acridine dyes (flavines),* and (3) *rosaniline dyes*—gentian violet, crystal violet, fuchsine (rosaniline).

Surface-acting Agents. These agents in the form of emulsifiers, wetting agents, or detergents act by altering "energy relationships" at interfaces, thus disrupting or damaging cell membranes. They also denature proteins and inactivate enzymes. The most commonly used examples are the *cationic detergents* (quaternary ammonium compounds), especially *benzalkonium chloride* (Zephiran). Benzalkonium chloride is a broad-spectrum antibacterial agent (not effective against *Pseudomonas* spp.). However, anionic soaps inactivate it, and it is toxic to cats, producing skin and muscle necrosis.

Heavy Metals. *Mercury derivatives* precipitate proteins and block sulfhydryl bonds of enzymes; they are antibacterial and astringent but quite sensitizing, staining, and inferior to other current agents.

Silver salts precipitate proteins and interfere with bacterial metabolic activities; they are antibacterial and astringent but irritating (escharotic), staining, and stinging (e.g., silver nitrate 0.5 per cent). Silver sulfadiazine is effective for superficial burns.

Zinc salts precipitate proteins; they are antibacterial, antifungal, and astringent, but can be irritating (e.g., zinc sulfate 0.2 to 1 per cent, zinc oxide 20 per cent, and zinc undecylenate 1 to 10 per cent).

Sulfur. The bacteriostatic factor in sulfur is thought to be pentathionic acid. Sulfur is used in a 1 to 10 per cent concentration. It is an effective fungicide and parasiticide.

Oxyquinolines. These agents are weakly antibacterial and antifungal: their mechanism of action is unknown. The most commonly used is iodochlorhydroxyquin (Vioform).

Antibiotics. Many potent antibacterial agents are available in topical form (ointments are most common). The most commonly used are neomycin, bacitracin, polymyxin B, gramicidin, nitrofurazone, and thiostrepton (e.g., Neo-Polycin, Furacin). Important considerations for some of them are as follows: (1) *neomycin* (great potential for allergic sensitization), (2) *nitrofurans* (sensitizing, plasma and blood inhibit their action), and (3) *sulfonamides* (sensitizing, of questionable benefit topically, so they should not be used). In general, the same agent should not be used topically and systemically.

There is very little indication for the topical use of these antimicrobial agents by themselves in veterinary dermatology. Antibiotic-steroid combinations (Neo-Aristovet, Neo-Synalar, Neo-Polycin-HC, Tresaderm, Panalog) are occasionally indicated in chronic, dry, lichenified, secondarily infected dermatoses (seborrhea complex, allergic dermatoses) and are commonly indicated in otitis externa. Several clinical and bacteriologic trials in humans have shown these antibiotic-steroid combinations to be superior to either agent alone.[124]

Antibiotic medications are used topically for many types of skin infections. Wet dressings are not popular because of the difficulty of maintaining the effect; therefore most medications are incorporated in ointment bases. Neomycin (5 mg/gm), bacitracin (500 units/gm), polymyxin B (5000 units/gm), and tyrothricin (0.5 mg/gm) are antibiotics commonly used topically. Nitrofurazone (0.2 per cent) is an antibacterial agent that is effective in liquid or dressing form.

TOPICAL ANTIFUNGAL AGENTS

Local therapy of dermatophytoses in dogs and cats may not be highly effective. Because of the heavy hair coat and the organisms' habitat deep in the hair follicle, contact with topical agents is incomplete. Clipping the hair and using liquid, low-surface-tension vehicles are helpful in obtaining more penetration.

Some patients have thick keratin scales, and keratolytic agents may promote good contact. Powder vehicles are of little value, and creams are useful only on glabrous areas. Iodine solutions are fungicidal, but may be highly irritating if used repeatedly. Iodochlorhydroxyquin in a cream form (Vioform), however, is a nonirritating form of iodine. Sodium hypochlorite solution (0.5 per cent stock solution), can be diluted to 1:20 and used safely on all animals; and commercial lime-sulfur solutions diluted to 2.5 per cent are also effective. Chlorhexidine (Nolvasan) is an excellent antifungal agent and is available as a solution, ointment, and shampoo. Tolnaftate, which is effective on the glabrous skin of man, is not effective on the hairy skin of dogs and cats. Four antifungal agents that are chemically related to ketoconazole have a broader spectrum of activity, are extremely effective in localized infections, and are nonirritating and consequently are topical drugs of choice. The products are haloprogin (Halotex), econazole (Spectrazole), miconazole (Micatin, Conofite), and clotrimazole (Lotrimin, Veltrim), and each is described in the following discussion. Nystatin suspension, amphotericin B suspension, clotrimazole, econazole, and miconazole are useful for *Candida* infections. Topical enilconazole has been highly successful in the treatment of canine nasal aspergillosis.[147]

Many dermatophytic infections are self-limiting and heal spontaneously. Numerous therapeutic fallacies have resulted, giving useless drugs undeserved credit. To clarify this confusion, a number of common antifungal and anticandidal drugs are listed and described as follows:

1. *Amphotericin B* (Fungizone) is effective against *Candida* infections and other intermediate and deep mycoses of the skin. It is used in 3 per cent cream, lotion, or ointment.

2. *Chlorines* can be used for localized or generalized dermatophytoses (see p. 163).

3. *Captan* is effective against dermatophytes; it is also antibacterial. Captan may be used for localized or generalized dermatoses. Although it is safe, nontoxic, and nonirritating, it is a contact sensitizer in humans (e.g., Orthocide, 30 ml [1 oz] to 4 L [1 gal] of water).

4. *Chlorhexidine* is a broad-spectrum antibacterial and antifungal agent. It is described with antimicrobials on p. 162.

5. *Clotrimazole* (Lotrimin) in a 1 per cent concentration is effective against dermatophytes and *Candida* spp. It is safe and nontoxic, with little irritation.

6. *Econazole* (Spectrazole) is available as a 1 per cent topical cream.

7. *Haloprogin* (Halotex) in a 1 per cent cream or solution is effective against dermatophytes and yeasts. It is nontoxic and nonirritating.

8. *Iodines* are most effective as povidone-iodine compounds and may be used for localized lesions (Betadine ointment and solution) or for generalized lesions and to reduce contagion (Betadine shampoo and whirlpool concentrate). Caution is necessary for use in cats!

9. *Miconazole* (Conofite) in a 2 per cent cream or lotion is effective against yeasts and dermatophytes; it is safe, nontoxic, and usually nonirritating.

10. *Nystatin* is effective against yeasts only (e.g., Panolog ointment and Nystatin cream).

11. *Sulfur* is effective for dermatophytes. It may be used for localized lesions (Adams Lotion of Sulfur) or for generalized lesions and to reduce contagion (Lym Dyp, Adams Sulfur Shampoo).

12. *Thiabendazole* is effective for dermatophytes. It is safe, nontoxic, and nonirritating and is best used for local lesions, especially acute, exudative, or kerion-like reactions (e.g., Tresaderm). A 13 per cent aqueous solution has

been used successfully as a dip applied three times a week for 4 weeks in cases of generalized dermatophytosis.[58]

13. *Enilconazole* (0.2 per cent solution) has been reported to be very effective in dermatophytosis when applied as a total body dip twice weekly for four weeks.[178]

TOPICAL ANTIPARASITIC AGENTS

Numerous products are available for use on dogs and cats.[88] The active ingredients are incorporated into dips, shampoos, sprays, powders, and lotions. Many of them would be highly toxic if applied in a vehicle that promoted absorption, or in a form that enabled the animal to ingest quantities by licking the medication. Cats are especially prone to licking habits and are particularly susceptible to toxic reactions with chlorinated hydrocarbons and organophosphate products.

With the emphasis on new, more effective drugs we sometimes forget that sulfur and its derivatives are excellent parasiticides. The commercial lime-sulfur solution mentioned on p. 404 is safe for dogs and cats and is a cheap, effective treatment for several mite infestations, as well as being fungicidal, bactericidal, keratolytic, and antipruritic. Adams Sulfur Shampoo or Adams Lotion of Sulfur and 10 per cent sulfur ointment USP are other forms of sulfur medications. One to five per cent sulfur is effective against many mites, chiggers, lice, and some fleas. In concentrations above 3 per cent, it is keratolytic and may be irritating. Sulfur is *not* an effective flea repellent.

Pyrethrin. This agent is a volatile oil extract of the chrysanthemum flower. It contains six active pyrethrins that as contact poisons have a fast knock-down action and "flushing" action on insects, but no residual activity. There is no cholinesterase suppression. Pyrethrin demonstrates a rapid kill but low toxicity, and the low concentration of 0.06 to 0.4 per cent is effective *if* synergized with 0.1 to 2.0 per cent piperonyl butoxide (PBO). Cats may develop CNS signs in response to PBO, but otherwise toxicity is very low. Pyrethrins are effective against fleas, flies, lice, and mosquitoes.

Pyrethroids (D-transallethrin, resmethrin, tetramethrin and D-phenothin). These are synthesized chemicals that are modeled after pyrethrin. In action and toxicity they are comparable to pyrethrin, but are less expensive. They produce a quick kill that is improved by the addition of a synergist and, also, of pyrethrin. Many degrade on exposure to ultraviolet light, and there is little or no residual activity. Microencapsulation of pyrethroids (and other insecticides) has prolonged their effective action from 1 day to 5 or more weeks. This process suspends the insecticide in microcapsules that are inactive while suspended in liquid. When sprayed onto a surface they become active, and as they dry or are exposed to light, small amounts of insecticide keep moving up to the surface of the capsules. This reservoir effect prolongs the action and reduces the toxicity to the host. An insect touches a capsule and sticks to it. The insecticide is then absorbed through its chitin with toxic effect. Some products provide a mix of microencapsulated pyrethrins and natural pyrethrins for quick knock-down and prolonged effect (Sectrol).

Chlorinated Hydrocarbons. These dangerous insecticides persist in the environment and animal tissue for very long times (for years, in some cases). Representatives of this group are DDT, lindane, chlordane, dieldrin, and methoxychlor. The last drug, the only one now used, is administered occasionally as a flea powder. It is safe, even for cats, but better choices are available. The other compounds are tightly restricted or their use is prohibited.

Cholinesterase Inhibitors. Two kinds of cholinesterase inhibitors are available, carbamates and organophosphates.

Carbamates. Those are typified by *carbaryl* (Sevin) and are safe for dogs and cats in 3.0 to 5.0 per cent concentration in powders (Diryl), and 0.5 to 2.0 per cent sprays (Mycodex), and in dips (Mycodex). Although lower concentration products may be used on kittens and puppies older than 6 weeks, it is probably safer to use only pyrethrin until they are several months old. Fleas tend to develop resistance to Sevin. *Bendiocarb* (Ficam) is a carbamate used by exterminators for premises flea control. It is safe, odorless, and nonstaining and has good residual activity. *Propoxur* (Sendran) is relatively insoluble in water, but it is used in collars and powders because of its rapid knock-down and reasonable residual effect. As other carbamates, it may be used in combination with other insecticides, such as pyrethrins.

Organophosphates. The most toxic insecticides in use are organophosphates. They are potent cholinesterase inhibitors, and a cumulative effect may be seen if animals are exposed to similar insecticides in another preparation or in lawn and garden applications. None of this group should be used on kittens, and most are also dangerous to adult cats. Malathion is different in some respects from the rest of the group. It provides a quick insect knock-down, and it can be used carefully on adult cats. Some of the commonly used organophosphates are the following:

1. *Chlorfenvinphos* (Supona, Dermaton) is used for fleas and ticks or premises sprays. It is not a good scabicide.

2. *Chlorpyrifos* (Dursban) is popular for sprays and dips for fleas in the southeastern United States. It is used by commercial exterminators and has been microencapsulated for a truly long residual effect (Duratrol).

3. *Cythioate* (Proban) is a systemic insecticide (see p. 181).

4. *Diazinon* is popular for premises use for fleas and ticks. It has a long residual effect and insects do not easily become resistant. Available as powder, liquid, or in microencapsulation.

5. *Dichlorvos* (Vapona) has been used in fly strips and flea collars. It has fast knock-down but little residual action.

6. *Fenthion* (Pro-Spot, Spotton) is a topical medication that is absorbed through the skin for systemic effect (see p. 181).

7. *Malathion* is a commonly used organophosphate with good effect on fleas and relatively low toxicity. It is often combined with other insecticides (not other cholinesterase inhibitors) for use on dogs and cats and can be used on the premises.

8. *Phosmet* (Paramite dip) is used for flea control on mature dogs and cats. It is not a reliable scabicide.

Insect Growth Regulators (IGRs). These are natural chemicals in insects that control early stages of their metabolism, morphogenesis, and reproduction. Final maturation and pupation of flea larvae proceed only in the absence of the IGR that was essential for early larval growth. Methoprene (Precor) is a chemical with structure and biochemical activities that mimic those of the natural IGR. Application of methoprene to the premises by spray or fogger will prevent maturation of pupal fleas if they are exposed to it. There are several problems in ensuring contact, one being that the chemical is light-sensitive so that it has little value outdoors. Another is the difficulty in driving the product deep into rugs, cracks, and recessed places where the larvae are developing. A further problem is the fact that methoprene affects the flea late in its growth cycle, so that results will be delayed for several weeks. This is corrected by simultaneous spraying or mixing with insecticides that kill adult fleas (Siphotrol Plus II).

Formamidines. These newly formulated acaricidal agents act by inhibition of monoamine oxidase. Amitraz (Mitaban), the veterinary form, is effective against demodectic cheyletiella, otodectes, and sarcoptic mites but not against fleas. The drug is unstable and rapidly oxidizes on exposure to air or sunlight, so it is important to not use expired products or to divide contents of a bottle for use on different days. Its other actions include α-adrenergic agonism and prostaglandin inhibition. Side-effects of treatment often include transient sedation and pruritus, hypothermia, bradycardia, hypotension, and hyperglycemia. The vehicle, xylene, is thought to participate in toxicity problems.[168, 181]

Use of amitraz in demodicosis is discussed on p. 391. In the United States, official approval for treatment dictates dipping every 14 days with 250 ppm solution. Better results are obtained with weekly dips.[78]

Repellents. Although these chemicals are capable of keeping insects away, they require frequent application—often every few hours, depending on temperature, humidity, density of insects, movement of animal, and drying effect of the wind. Many are oily and irritating, stain clothes, and dissolve plastic. New spray repellents may avoid some of these drawbacks but they are too new to evaluate. There is some concern about systemic toxicity. Compounds with repellent action include pyrethrum and diethyltoluamide ("DEET," DMT-50, Deep Woods OFF); ethohexadiol; and dimethyl phtholate and butopyronoxyl (Indolone), neither of which repels ticks. Two products used in insecticidal mixtures are MGK-11 and MGK-326.[88] Avon's bath oil (Skin So Soft) has been shown to be an effective repellent.

In summary, literally thousands of commercial products are marketed as insecticides. The preceding comments, it is hoped, provide some insight into ingredient actions. In using the products, following the manufacturers' directions is paramount. General directions for treatment of specific problems such as fleas, lice, and ticks can be found in appropriate chapters in this text.

Most insecticides come in the following pharmaceutical forms: (1) Dips, which are the most effective residual form. A dip is applied after a bath and allowed to dry on the skin. It may be repeated in 7 to 10 days. (2) Powders, which are the next most effective residual form. Apply these twice weekly or as needed, deep into the coat. Powders may be messy, drying to the skin and hair coat, and irritating to mucous membranes. (3) Sprays, which have less residual effect. The hissing noise of pressurized aerosols may alarm the pet, and the use of hand pump aerosols overcomes this "startle" effect. Ruffle up the coat and spray down at the skin (not messy). Sprays may be applied as needed. (4) Shampoos, which have no residual benefit. (5) Solutions, which are used for local or spot treatment. They may be messy.

TOPICAL ANTI-INFLAMMATORY AGENTS

Wet dressings, previously discussed, are among the simplest and safest agents that reduce inflammation. In recent years, topical corticosteroid preparations have been used effectively and safely to reduce inflammation. There is little evidence to suggest that they have caused dissemination of cutaneous infections, but if they are used in the presence of known infections, specific antibacterial or antifungal agents should be added to the preparation.

In high concentration, in abraded skin, or under occlusive dressings, small amounts of these corticosteroids are absorbed, but they rarely produce serious untoward clinical effects. However, Moriello and colleagues[102] found that short-term application (7 days) of topical otic products (Panalog, Tresaderm) can adversely affect the adrenocortical response to exogenous adrenocorticotropic hormone (ACTH). Marked adrenocortical suppression was still present 14 days after therapy was discontinued. These products also produced elevations in routinely monitored liver enzyme tests (e.g., serum alkaline phosphatase, leucine aminotransferase). Similarly, Zenoble and Kemppainen reported that the daily application of triamcinolone, fluocinonide, or betamethasone to the skin of normal dogs for 5 days produced suppression of adrenocortical responses to ACTH, which persisted for 3 to 4 weeks after the last application.[179] Finally, Glaze and coworkers reported that daily application of ophthalmic preparations containing glucocorticoids also suppressed adrenocortical responses to ACTH and produced elevations in hepatic enzymes in normal dogs.[180] It may be concluded that topical glucocorticoids should not be considered innocuous drugs. They maintain a "pool" in the skin, enough that once-daily application may suffice to continue topical effect. *People handling these medications should wear gloves to prevent exposure and toxic effects.* The most commonly used topical corticosteroids are methylprednisolone (Medrol 0.25 to 1 per cent), hydrocortisone (1 per cent), prednisolone (0.5 per cent), dexamethasone (Decadron 0.25 per cent), triamcinolone acetonide (Kenalog 0.1 to 0.25 per cent), betamethasone-17-valerate (Valisone 0.1 per cent), and fluocinolone acetonide (Synalar 0.025 per cent). The fluorinated steroids are more potent, penetrate better, and thus are more effective. Table 4:1 lists therapeutic concentrations of several topical glucocorticoids and provides brand-name examples.

TOPICAL ANTISEBORRHEICS

Antiseborrheic drugs include keratolytics and keratoplastics.[146, 182] The seborrheic complex comprises important and common skin diseases, such as primary seborrhea (in cocker and springer spaniels), secondary seborrhea (accompanying atopy, scabies, and demodicosis), schnauzer comedo syndrome, tail gland hyperplasia, and stud tail. Antiseborrheics can be applied as ointments, creams, gels, and lotions, but the most popular form for hairy skin is the antiseborrheic shampoo. Antiseborrheics are commercially available in various different combinations. The clinician must make the decision as to which combination of drugs to use and needs to know the drugs' actions and concentrations. Ideal therapeutic response depends on the correct choice. For dry and scaly seborrhea (sicca) a different preparation is needed than for oily and greasy seborrhea (oleosa). Sulfur, for instance, is very useful in seborrhea but is *not* a good degreaser. Benzoyl peroxide, on the other hand, degreases very well but can be too keratolytic for dry, brittle skin. The following discussion may help the clinician to understand and distinguish the correct medication from among the myriad of commercially available pharmaceuticals.

Sulfur has an action on the skin that is mainly twofold, keratoplastic and keratolytic. The best keratolytic action occurs when sulfur is incorporated in petrolatum. (This is in sharp contrast to the findings with salicylic acid, which produces its effect faster when employed in an emulsion base.) The keratolytic effect of sulfur results from its superficial effect on the horny layer and the

Table 4:1. RELATIVE EFFICACY OF TOPICAL CORTICOSTEROIDS
IN VARIOUS FORMULATIONS

Lowest efficacy

0.25–2.5%	Hydrocortisone
0.25%	Methylprednisolone acetate (Medrol)
0.04%	Dexamethasone* (Hexadrol)
0.1%	Dexamethasone* (Decaderm)
1.0%	Methylprednisolone acetate (Medrol)
0.5%	Prednisolone (Meti-Derm)
0.2%	Betamethasone* (Celestone)

Low efficacy

0.01%	Fluocinolone acetonide* (Fluonid, Synalar)
0.01%	Betamethasone valerate* (Valisone)
0.025%	Fluorometholone* (Oxylone)
0.025%	Triamcinolone acetonide* (Aristocort, Kenalog, Triacet)
0.1%	Clocortolone pivalate* (Cloderm)
0.03%	Flumethasone pivalate* (Locorten)

Intermediate efficacy

0.2%	Hydrocortisone valerate (Westcort)
0.1%	Hydrocortisone butyrate (Locoid)
0.025%	Betamethasone benzoate* (Benisone, Flurobate, Uticort)
0.025%	Flurandrenolide* (Cordran)
0.1%	Betamethasone valerate* (Valisone)
0.05%	Desonide (Tridesilon)
0.025%	Halcinonide* (Halog)
0.05%	Desoximetasone* (Topicort L.P.)
0.05%	Flurandrenolide* (Cordran)
0.1%	Triamcinolone acetonide*
0.025%	Fluocinolone acetonide*

High efficacy

0.05%	Betamethasone dipropionate* (Diprosone)
0.1%	Amcinonide* (Cyclocort)
0.25%	Desoximetasone* (Topicort)
0.5%	Triamcinolone acetonide*
0.2%	Fluocinolone acetonide* (Synalar-HP)
0.05%	Diflorasone diacetate* (Florone)
0.1%	Halcinonide* (Halog)
0.05%	Fluocinonide* (Lidex, Topsyn)

*Fluorinated steroids.
Reproduced, with permission, from Katzung, B. G., (ed.): Basic and Clinical Pharmacology. 3rd ed. Copyright Appleton & Lange, Los Altos, 1987, p. 775.

formation of hydrogen sulfide. The keratoplastic effect is caused by the deeper action of the sulfur on the basal layer of the epidermis. This effect also is produced by giving sulfur orally or by injection, but the best keratoplastic changes occur when sulfur in an emulsion base is applied topically. Ten per cent precipitated sulfur in lotions or ointments may intensify epidermal peeling and is useful for seborrheic and intertriginous dermatoses. Weaker concentrations in other vehicles may be used effectively for bacterial, fungal, and parasitic infections.

In summary, sulfur is keratolytic, keratoplastic, antibacterial, antifungal, antiparasitic, a mild "follicular flusher," but *not* a good degreaser. It is available in ointments in concentrations from 2 to 10 per cent. Its most popular form is in shampoos, such as Sebbafon, LyTar, Mycodex Tar and Sulfur, Adams Sulfur Shampoo, Sebalyt, and Allerseb T.

Salicylic acid (0.1 to 2 per cent) is keratoplastic and exerts a favorable influence on the new formation of the keratinous layer. It is also mildly antipruritic and bacteriostatic. It is a common ingredient in most of the antiseborrheic shampoos previously listed. In stronger concentrations (3 to 6 per cent) it acts as a keratolytic (Keralyt 6 per cent), causing shedding and softening of the stratum corneum. When salicylic acid is *combined with sulfur* it is believed that a synergistic effect occurs. A common combination is a 2 to 6 per cent concentration of each drug. In human dermatologic practice a 40 per cent salicylic acid plaster is used for the treatment of calluses and warts.

Tar preparations are derived from destructive distillation of bituminous coal or wood. Birch tar, juniper tar, and coal tar are crude products listed in order of increasing capacity to irritate. Coal tar solution (5 to 10 to 20 per cent) produces a milder, more readily managed effect. Most pharmaceutical preparations for dermatology have been highly refined to decrease the staining effect and the strong odor. In this refining process some of the beneficial effects of tar are lost, but its potential carcinogenic danger is also decreased. Straight tar lotions have no place in small animal practice because of their toxicity and tendency to cause local irritation. Cats are especially sensitive to coal tar. All tars are odiferous, potentially irritating and photosensitizing, and carcinogenic. Some may stain light-colored hair coats.

Popular veterinary ointments that make use of some of the principles just listed include those containing cetyl alcohol, coal tar, and sulfur as well as salicylic acid in an emulsion base (Pragmatar), sulfur ointment (USP), ichthammol ointment (USP), zinc oxide, and thuja.

Tar shampoos are widely used, however, and seem to be helpful in managing seborrhea. They are keratolytic, keratoplastic, and mildly degreasing. They include LyTar, Pragmatar, Mycodex Tar and Sulfur, and Allerseb T.

Propylene glycol is an agent that is primarily used as a solvent and vehicle. In concentrations above 50 per cent it is usually a primary irritant and will produce erythema and superficial desquamation of the horny layer. Below concentrations of 20 per cent its effects are not irritating. It is an excellent lipid solvent and defats the skin; however, its chief value is probably the ability to enhance percutaneous penetration of drugs. Propylene glycol is also a potent and reliable antibacterial agent. For most dermatologic cases it can be used in concentrations of 30 to 40 per cent.

Benzoyl peroxide (5 per cent) is keratolytic, antibacterial, degreasing, antipruritic, and "follicular flushing." It is available as a gel (OxyDex, Pyoben) and as a shampoo (OxyDex and Pyoben Shampoos).

Miscellaneous Antiseborrheic Topical Preparations

Vitamin A Acid 0.05 Per Cent (Retinoic Acid, Tretinoin). This is a popular item in human dermatology (used for acne and ichthyosis). It increases the epidermal turnover time and reduces cohesiveness of keratinocytes. Local irritation is a significant problem for many people (e.g., Retin-A). (See also p. 197.)

Alpha-Hydroxyacids 5 to 10 Per Cent. These include lactic, citric, pyruvic, glutamic, glycolic, and tartaric acids. Recently, outstanding success has been shown in modulating keratinization, especially in human ichthyosis (related to biosynthesis of mucopolysaccharides). *Fatty acids* are keratolytic and fungistatic; examples are caprylic, propionic, and undecylenic acids. The best of these (although it is weak) is undecylenic acid (e.g., Desenex).

Selenium Sulfide 1 to 2.5 Per Cent. This acts as a keratolytic and cytostatic agent on cells of the epidermis and follicular epithelium to reduce desquamation. The veterinary products, especially, can be irritating and staining. If the use of selenium sulfide is desired, Selsun Blue, Selsun, or Exsel is recommended.

Bath Oils. These are highly dispersible or spreading oils that have surfactant activity and are indicated in seborrhea sicca as an adjunct to keratolytic shampoos. Shampoo first, rinse well, then apply bath oil rinse and let dry (e.g., Alpha-Keri oil or spray, HY-LYT efa oil or spray).

Humectants. These preparations use components of the natural moisturizing factor, such as carboxylic acid, urea, and lactic acid, to rehydrate the skin without oil (e.g., Humilac).

Astringents. These agents precipitate proteins and in general do not penetrate deeply. They are indicated in acute, subacute, and some chronic exudative dermatoses.

Vegetable Astringents. Tannins from oak trees, sumac, or blackberries are especially recommended for more potent action. *Tan Sal* (5 per cent tannic acid and 5 per cent salicylic acid, in 70 per cent alcohol QS) is a potent astringent and should not be used more than once on the same lesion (may cause irritation and/or sloughing).

Emollients. These agents soften the stratum corneum, and they protect and soothe the skin. They are occasionally used alone but are most commonly used as vehicles for other drugs. They include the following:
1. *Vegetable oils*—olive, cotton seed, corn, peanut.
2. *Animal oils*—lard, whale oil, anhydrous lanolin (wool fat), lanolin with 25 to 30 per cent water (hydrous wool fat).
3. *Hydrocarbons*— paraffin, petrolatum (mineral oil).
4. *Waxes*—whitewax (bleached beeswax), yellow wax (beeswax), spermaceti.

SUNSCREENS

A dense hair coat protects most small animals from excessive exposure to sunlight. However, dogs with discoid lupus erythematosus, systemic lupus erythematosus, and pemphigus erythematosus may react to exposure to the sun of the eyelids and hairless portions of the planum nasale. In white cats, the tips of the ears are prone to sunburn, and in white-coated dogs that like to sunbathe (especially Dalmatians and bull terriers), the glabrous skin of the abdomen may burn. (See p. 762.)

The greater the wavelength of light that reaches the skin, the deeper its penetration.[132a] Thus, ultraviolet B with wavelengths between 280 and 320 nm produces erythema and acute and chronic carcinogenic light reactions. Its energy is almost all expended in the epidermis. Ultraviolet A (UVA) has wavelengths of 320 to 400 nm. It induces direct pigmentation but may also contribute to photodamage. Visible light has the greatest wavelengths, 400 to 800 nm, and penetrates to the subcutis.

The skin reacts to protect itself by producing melanin, which scatters and absorbs ultraviolet (UV) and visible light, and by quenching free radicals. It also reacts with acanthosis and hyperkeratosis and produces indirect pigmentation, which is longer lasting than the direct melanin produced by UVA. Much of the high-energy short-wave radiation is absorbed by various protein complexes in the superficial tissue. DNA repair mechanisms also help cope with light damage.

Protection from the sun can be attained by staying indoors from 10:00 AM to 3:00 PM, by hardening the skin (a process of building up pigmentation and light acanthosis and hyperkeratosis), and by the use of topical or oral sunscreens. Topical sunscreens may act physically or chemically. In chemical screens, para-aminobenzoic acid (PABA) or benzophenone derivatives act to absorb UV. They are clear, cosmetically acceptable lotions or gels. Physical sunscreens are agents that include chemicals like zinc oxide or titanium dioxide, which reflect and scatter light by forming an opaque barrier. These agents are messy—especially in long hair coats. Topical sunscreens are rated for efficiency by a sun protective factor (SPF) number. Numbers 2 to 4 are mild blockers, 8 to 10 give good protection, and 15 gives maximum blockage. These numbers are only guides, since frequency and thickness of application, temperature, humidity, potency of light exposure, patient's sensitivity, and many other factors modify results. Usually, sunscreen needs to be applied three to four times a day for greatest effectiveness.

Oral sunscreens are chemicals such as β-carotene and chloroquine that act to quench free radicals and to stabilize membranes. They have not been proved to prevent sunburn in people but have been useful in cases of light-induced dermatosis.[83a] A β-carotene derivative has been used in cats and dogs to reduce phototoxicity (see pp. 769, 770). Canthaxanthin (β-carotene-4,4'-dione) is a red-orange pigment found in plants and other sources. The "safety" of this product has been challenged. Side-effects include orange-brown skin, brick-red stools, crystalline gold deposits on the retinae, orange plasma, and lowered amplitudes on electroretinograms (ERGs). The usual maximum dose for humans is 25 mg/kg daily, but some companies recommend four 30-mg capsules once daily: Golden Tan, Orobronze. In toxicity studies of dogs, the long-term and short-term LD_{50} is greater than 10,000 mg/kg.

PHYSICAL THERAPY

The use of heat, cold, light, and radiation therapy for treatment of skin disorders is not new, but recent advances have made the therapies more specific and more effective. In addition to this discussion, freezing, heat, electricity, and laser light are presented as surgical techniques on p. 213.

Photochemotherapy

Photochemotherapy is a technique that uses lightwaves to excite or increase the energy of a photosensitive drug that causes a selective cytotoxic effect on tumors. The drug is a hematoporphyrin derivative (Photofrin-V).[164] The drug also has a much greater affinity for tumor tissue than for surrounding normal cells. Light is only effective on a few layers of surface cells, except red-range lights, which can penetrate as much as 1 to 2 cm. The light source is a laser system that produces a red laser beam that passes through low-attenuation fiberoptic tracts. These are directed through 19-gauge needles into the appropriate areas of tumor. Treatment takes about 20 minutes, and repeated exposures are no problem, although patients should be kept out of sunlight for 3 to 4 weeks. Roughly 50 per cent of tumors respond completely, and an additional 30 per cent show partial responses.[163] The most favorable results were obtained with malignant melanoma, fibrosarcoma, mast cell tumor, adamantinoma, and synovial cell sarcoma. Mixed responses were seen in squamous cell carcinoma, adenocarcinoma, leiomyosarcoma, and hemangio-pericytoma. In treatment of human cancer, when photochemotherapy is followed by hyperthermia the results are better than with either treatment alone.[46]

Hyperthermia

Local current-field radiofrequency is used to produce enough heat in a local superficial area to cause tissue necrosis. Two groups have used a temperature of 50°C for 30 to 60 seconds to treat feline tumors.[54, 71] The heat was controlled to affect only the tumor and 2 to 3 mm of surrounding normal tissue. Results were much better with lesions less than 5 mm in diameter by 2 mm deep. In these cases approximately 70 per cent of tumors completely regressed, and an additional 20 per cent partially regressed. With larger tumors, the results were much poorer. Favorable responses were obtained with squamous cell carcinomas, fibrosarcomas of cats, and perianal tumors of dogs. There were no serious side-effects. This therapy should not be used on the pinna of the ear, as it may cause necrosis and sloughing.

Hyperthermia has also been used for topical treatment of localized dermatophytosis.[86] By using the same system and producing heat of 50°C for 30 seconds in an area 4 mm deep by 1 cm in diameter, successful results were achieved with proven dermatophyte infections after only one treatment.[86] For large lesions, the heat probe was moved sequentially to new areas of 1 cm in diameter until the whole lesion was treated. Fluorescence disappeared within 48 hours, and healing was complete in 2 to 6 weeks. Hyperthermia was considered to be the treatment of choice for localized dermatophytosis.

Heat is also used in electrosurgical procedures, such as fulguration, to destroy tissue. (See Electrosurgery, p. 217.)

X-ray Therapy

X-ray therapy has important benefits to contribute to treatment of skin tumors, feline indolent ulcer, and acral lick dermatitis. Because not all cells are equally sensitive to radiation, these rays act selectively. Cells that divide rapidly, such as carcinoma cells and the basal cells of the hair papilla and vascular endothelium, are damaged more easily than those of the remaining skin. X-ray beams that are "filtered" through aluminum or copper sheets to remove soft rays penetrate deeply into the tissues because of their short wavelengths. Radiation delivered at about 80 KV with little or no filtration (0.5 mm Al) has longer wavelengths, and its energy is dissipated very superficially.

Before considering x-ray therapy for a patient, the clinician must be certain of the following:
1. The treatment has good potential for benefit and little potential for harm.
2. No safer form of therapy will suffice.
3. Proper, safe equipment and facilities are available in order that (a) the exact dose can be administered, (b) the patient can be anesthetized or restrained for therapy without exposure to personnel, (c) proper shielding of unaffected parts is provided.
4. Adequate records will be kept for future references.
If these points can be accomplished, x-ray therapy may be considered.

In superficial skin diseases, such as indolent ulcer in cats or acral lick dermatitis, or in slightly deeper inflammations, such as cellulitis or elbow pyoderma, soft-to-medium rays are helpful. The usual dosage is 300 to 500 R (half value layer [HVL] = 1 mm Al) repeated within 3 days (total 600 to 1000 R). In deeper, more chronic inflammations, the individual dosage may be 300 R, but with filtration up to 0.5 mm copper and repeated at 3- to 4-day intervals for a total dose of 1000 to 1500 R.

In deeper conditions, where it is necessary to deliver tumoricidal doses of radiation, a much larger total dosage is needed. Malignant lesions may require 2000 to 4000 R for effect, but the various types have specific sensitivities. With these higher doses, shielding of unaffected tissue is vitally important, and treatment of the lesion from different angles by using different portals of entry for the x-ray beam is desirable to spare the tissues that cannot be shielded. Only a qualified radiologist should deliver these treatments.

Perianal gland tumors are highly sensitive to radiation. Benign lesions (hyperplasia, adenoma) receive 1000 to 2000 R; malignant lesions (adenocarcinoma) should receive 2000 to 4000 R.

Transmissible venereal tumors also are exquisitely radiosensitive, so this method is an excellent treatment. A dose of 1000 to 2000 R produces complete remission.

Mast cell tumors are usually radiosensitive, but multiple sites and rapid extension complicate the treatment problems. Usual dose is 2000 to 4000 R.

Squamous cell carcinoma may be sensitive, but some tumors are highly resistant. If surgical excision is not possible, 3000 to 4000 R may be beneficial.

Malignant melanoma should be removed surgically by wide excision. Since it metastasizes very early, secondary palliative radiation may be temporarily useful. Dosage is 3000 to 4000 R.

Fibrosarcoma should be treated surgically if possible, but palliative radiation therapy, 3000 to 4000 R, may be used adjunctively.

Neurofibrosarcomas are highly resistant to radiation therapy.

Systemic Therapy

SYSTEMIC ANTIBIOTICS

Antibiotic agents for systemic use in skin disorders have rather special and specific indications. The only use of antibiotics is to kill bacteria or to so inhibit organisms that the host can dispose of them. Since the overwhelming majority of canine skin infections are caused by coagulase-positive *Staphylococcus intermedius*, antibiotics that affect these bacteria and concentrate in the skin are of primary interest here. Occasionally *Proteus* spp., *Pseudomonas* spp., and *Escherichia coli* are involved as secondary invaders in deeper soft-tissue infections. In cats, the primary bacteria are *Pasteurella multocida* and β-hemolytic streptococci.[139] Thus, the penicillins and ampicillins are the antibiotics of choice for cats.

The principles of proper antibiotic usage should first require that the antibiotic inhibit the specific bacteria, preferably in a bactericidal manner. The drug should have a narrow spectrum, so that it produces little effect on organisms of the natural flora of the skin or intestinal tract (for oral medications). Bacteriostatic drugs also are completely effective as long as the host is not compromised or immunosuppressed. The antibiotic should be inexpensive, should be easily given and absorbed (orally, if it is to be prescribed for home use), and should have no adverse effects.

The most important factors influencing the effectiveness of antibiotics are the distribution to the skin in effective levels and the level of activity in that tissue milieu. It has been shown that only about 4 per cent of the cardiac output of blood reaches the skin, compared with 33 per cent that reaches muscle.[9] This variation will be reflected in the relative distribution of antibiotics among organs. In studies of the different regions of skin, penicillin-type antibiotic levels in the hypodermis reached about 60 per cent, and dermoepidermal junction levels reached about 40 per cent, of the peak serum levels in dogs.[93] Although the epidermis is relatively avascular, studies on skin infections showed that the systemic route of therapy is better than the topical route for all but the most superficial infections.[93] The stratum corneum is a major permeability barrier to effective topical drug penetration. These facts lead to the inescapable conclusion that the skin is one of the most difficult tissues in which to obtain high antibiotic levels.

Four factors that may reduce the effectiveness of a therapeutic plan are the following:

1. The organism is resistant to the antibiotic.
2. The dosage is inadequate to attain inhibitory concentrations in the skin and maintain them adequately.
3. The organism may be protected by enzymes such as β-lactamase or by surviving inside macrophages where they are not exposed to the antibiotic effect.
4. The duration of therapy is inadequate to eradicate the infection.

Reedy[122] reported on antibiotic sensitivity tests on 100 isolates of coagulase-positive *Staphylococcus* spp. from canine pyoderma (see Table 4:2). When antibiotics have been given previously, the incidence of susceptibility decreases.[75] There may also be other interesting variables. In the United States about 60 per cent of coagulase-positive *Staphylococcus* spp. isolates are resistant to amoxicillin and ampicillin, while in the United Kingdom only about 5 per cent are resistant.[93] This and other factors suggest that culture and sensitivity tests should be performed on chronic, refractory cases of pyoderma to better guide selection of the most effective drug. However, for superficial, initial infections direct smears and evaluation of Gram's stain or other quick stains of exudates may provide adequate information to start rational therapy immediately.[63, 64] This approach may presuppose a "feel" for the most effective drugs being reported in other laboratory cultures in your practice.

Table 4:2. RESULTS OF ANTIBIOTIC SENSITIVITY TESTS*

Drug	Number of Sensitive Patients	Number of Resistant Patients	Number of Patients Previously on the Drug
Ampicillin	59	41 (12)†	20
Cephalosporin	99	1 (1)	21
Chloramphenicol	89	11 (2)	16
Oxacillin	87	13 (2)	4
Erythromycin	74	26 (9)	33
Tetracycline	51	49 (11)	16
Lincomycin	59	41 (15)	33
Tribrissen	57	43 (21)	46

*On 100 isolates of coagulase-positive *Staphylococcus* spp. from canine pyoderma.
†Number of resistant patients previously on the drug.

Knowledge of antibiotic susceptibility to β-lactamase I (penicillinase) should guide selection of therapy to avoid that problem, and long-term therapy will help avoid the resistance gained by intracellular protection.

Dosage is a critical question. Although some clinicians believe that intermittent dosage and fluctuating blood levels are satisfactory therapy[93] (especially for penicillin-type drugs), the authors believe that constant, high blood levels are imperative. Antibiotic combinations are unnecessary and usually contraindicated. Antibiotics that are well absorbed and that distribute well to tissues are desirable. Chloramphenicol, a trimethoprim-sulfonamide combination, and amoxicillin distribute well to superficial tissues, while lincomycin, erythromycin, and the synthetic penicillins do not. These characteristics must be matched against the spectrum of activity, route and ease of dosage, cost, and resistance factors when decisions are made on the drug of choice. The drugs that are used commonly for skin infections include cefadroxil, cephalexin, chloramphenicol, erythromycin, amoxicillin with clavulanate potassium, lincomycin, oxacillin or cloxacillin, and trimethoprim-sulfadiazine. Any of these must be given in maximum dose for at least 14 to 21 days, once treatment for an infection has begun, and for 30 to 60 days in more complex infections. Many of these drugs can be used sequentially with good effect. They should not be used in combination simultaneously. Those that distribute well to many tissues are chloramphenicol and trimethoprim-sulfadiazine.

Table 4:3 contains the dosage of antibiotics that are more commonly used for skin infections. Patients should be weighed, and medications should be administered in full dose at specified intervals for the optimum length of time. In general, treatment should be continued until 7 days *after* clinical "cure." Remember how hard it is to reach effective antibiotic levels in the skin! For instance, a common mistake is to administer chloramphenicol at a dosage of less than the recommended 50 mg/kg TID, the lower dosage being much less effective.

Recently there has been much interest in the use of rifampin in canine pyoderma.[183] Rifampin is a broad-spectrum antibiotic effective against many gram-positive and gram-negative bacteria including coagulase-positive staphylococci. This antibiotic also has the unique capacity to kill intracellular microorganisms. A major disadvantage of rifampin is that resistance develops rapidly so the drug must be given with other antibiotics. It is also potentially hepatotoxic. Specific indications and dosages of rifampin in canine pyoderma are currently being studied.

Table 4:3. DOSAGES OF SYSTEMIC ANTIBIOTICS COMMONLY USED FOR SKIN INFECTION

Drug	Route	Dose/kg	Frequency (Interval)
Amoxicillin with clavulanate*	oral	15 mg	12 hours
Cefadroxil*	oral	22 mg	12 hours
Cephalexin	oral	30 mg	12 hours
Chloramphenicol	oral	50 mg	8 hours
Erythromycin	oral	15 mg	8 hours
Lincomycin	oral	15 mg	8 hours
Oxacillin	oral	20 mg	8 hours
Trimethoprim-sulfadiazine	oral	30 mg	12 hours

*Anecdotal reports suggest that this drug was ineffective at the recommended frequency, but successful when given every 8 hours.

No drug is without potential hazard, but most of the above are quite safe. Comments about several possible problems deserve attention. Chloramphenicol commonly causes a mild reversible anemia in dogs when given beyond 2 to 3 weeks. This effect is especially serious, however, in cats and chloramphenicol should be used with care in that species. In cats, the dosage is repeated once every 12 hours for only 1 week. Erythromycin, lincomycin, and oxacillin may produce vomiting. Administer them with food, and switch to another drug if vomiting persists. Gentamicin is inactivated by pus, is potentially ototoxic and nephrotoxic, is expensive, and must be given every 8 hours by injection for best effect. A high dosage of trimethoprim-sulfadiazine is needed to reach optimum levels in skin. It should never be given to Doberman pinschers, as they seem to have a genetic predisposition to a sulfadiazine-caused type-III hypersensitivity reaction and nonseptic polyarthritis.[44]

In summary, the initial antibiotic for uncomplicated pyodermas probably should be erythromycin or lincomycin. Chloramphenicol or high doses of trimethoprim-sulfadiazine are worthy alternatives. Oxacillin and cloxacillin can be used interchangeably but only when sensitivities indicate they are needed. Amoxicillin with clavulanate has impressive laboratory data, but some clinicians have been disappointed by case results. Gentamicin and cephalosporins should be reserved for specific isolates of known sensitivities or for severe infections in which other therapy is not adequate. In the United States penicillin, ampicillin/amoxicillin, tetracyclines, and sulfonamides are usually ineffective for canine bacterial skin infections.

SYSTEMIC ANTIFUNGAL AGENTS

The ideal antifungal agent should have a wide therapeutic index and tissue distribution, a broad spectrum of antifungal activity, high efficacy, and an oral dosage form.[39] Ketoconazole comes close to this, but other agents fall short, especially because they have a low therapeutic index. Guidelines for indications and dosages of these agents are given in Table 4:4.[39]

Table 4:4. GUIDELINES FOR SYSTEMIC CHEMOTHERAPY OF SELECTED MYCOSES

Mycosis	Drug(s) of Choice	Dosage and Administration
Microsporum canis infection	Griseofulvin (microsize)	20–50 mg/kg divided BID, 4–6 wk
	Griesofulvin in PEG	5–10 mg/kg daily, 4–6 wk
Trichophyton infection	Griseofulvin (microsize)	20–50 mg/kg divided BID until culture neg.
	Griseofulvin in PEG	5–10 mg/kg daily until culture neg.
Sporotrichosis	Na or K iodide (20%)	Dogs: 1 ml/5 kg daily, 6 wk Cats: 0.5 ml/5 kg daily, 6 wk
Blastomycosis	Amphotericin B and ketoconazole	0.5 mg/kg 3 times weekly to total dose 6 mg/kg 10–20 mg/kg divided, 3–6 months 30 mg/kg for CNS, bone, eye
Cryptococcosis	Amphotericin B and ketoconazole	0.25–0.5 mg/kg 3 times weekly to 4 mg/kg total dose 5–10 mg/kg divided, 3–6 months
CNS cryptococcosis	Amphotericin B and 5-flucytosine	0.5 mg/kg 3 times weekly to total dose 4 mg/kg 100–200 mg/kg/day divided TID

From Foil, C.: Antifungal agents in dermatology. *In* Kirk, R. W. (ed.): Current Veterinary Therapy. 10th ed. W. B. Saunders, Philadelphia, 1986, p. 563.

Iodides of sodium and potassium are given orally in daily doses of saturated solutions. They have a disagreeable taste and may cause nausea and iodism, especially in cats. Although widely distributed in the body, their mechanism of action is unknown since they have no efficacy against fungal organisms in vitro. They are highly effective in the treatment of sporotrichosis. In dogs, use a 20% solution of sodium and give 40 mg/kg/day SID or BID (1 ml per 5 kg body weight). Give cats 20 mg/kg or 0.5 ml/5 kg/day SID.

Griseofulvin is a fungistatic antibiotic obtained by fermentation from several species of *Penicillium*.[39] Its antifungal activity results from the inhibition of cell wall synthesis, nucleic acid synthesis, and mitosis. This agent is only active against growing cells, which are killed, while older, more dormant cells may only be inhibited from reproducing.[57] Following oral administration in humans, the drug reaches peak serum levels in 4 to 8 hours and at that time can also be detected in the stratum corneum.[32] The highest concentrations are in the outermost layers and the lowest are in the basal layers.[124] The drug is secreted in sweat and is deposited in keratin precursor cells and remains tightly bound during the differentiation process. Consequently, new growth of hair or claws is the first to be free of disease. Holzworth has suggested that animals (cats) be placed on griseofulvin for several days prior to clipping, so that unaffected hair would grow out and most of the affected hair would be clipped away.[61]

Griseofulvin is in a state of flux in the skin, and, consequently, a dosage administered once or twice daily is needed to maintain constant blood levels. This drug is only indicated for dermatophyte infections (*Microsporum, Trichophyton,* and in humans *Epidermophyton*). It is not generally effective topically or against yeasts (*Candida, Malassezia*).

The dosage and concern for the toxicity of griseofulvin have been controversial. It should be given with a fatty meal to enhance absorption. Griseofulvin has a disagreeable taste and nausea is common. Dividing daily doses increases absorption and reduces nausea. Particle size of the drug also affects absorption and this influences the dosage. There are two common forms, a microsize crystal (dose 20 to 50 mg/kg BID) and ultramicrosize in polyethylene glycol (PEG) for which the dose is only 5 to 10 mg/kg once daily. This difference is important to recognize or toxicities may result. Griseofulvin PEG should not be given to kittens less than 6 weeks of age. In problem cases, the daily dose of *microsize* griseofulvin can be increased to at least 100 mg/kg/day with reasonable safety. Kunkle and Meyer gave cats 110 to 145 mg/kg daily for 11 weeks without any signs of clinical, hematologic, or hepatic toxicity. They concluded that abnormalities developing with the use of high-dose griseofulvin therapy may be an idiosyncratic reaction found only in a few cats.[77]

Major toxicities are teratogenicity (it is absolutely contraindicated in pregnant animals, especially in very early stages) and gastrointestinal upsets. Anemia, leukopenia, depression, ataxia, and pruritus have also been reported.[57] They supposedly regress when the drug is withdrawn, but hemograms every 2 weeks and careful observation are advisable during therapy to monitor those blood parameters and the early onset of toxicity.

Ketoconazole (Nizoral) is a synthetic fungal imidazole derivative that is active against many fungi and yeasts, including dermatophytes, *Candida, Malassezia,* and numerous dimorphic fungi responsible for systemic mycoses.[123a] It acts by inhibiting the synthesis of ergosterol, the main membrane lipid of fungal cells. With decreased ergosterol the cell is unable to maintain membrane integrity, and the results are increased permeability, cell degeneration, and death. This effect is delayed, and the onset of action of ketoconazole takes 5 to 10 days.

Consequently, in serious cases amphotericin B, which acts rapidly, is often used in combination with ketoconazole to compensate for this initial delay. Because *Leishmania* are rich in ergosterol, ketoconazole may be effective for leishmaniasis.[101]

Ketoconazole is insoluble in water but soluble in dilute acid solutions with low pH. When it is given with food, especially tomato juice, absorption will be enhanced. It should not be given with gastric antacids or drugs like cimetidine, or anticholinergics. There are many reports of its use without FDA approval in dogs and cats with a suggested dosage of 10 to 20 mg/kg/day for as long as 6 to 8 weeks.[4] For systemic mycoses such as blastomycosis, 30 mg/kg/day has been used.[26] However, because ketoconazole does not enter the CNS well, a dose of 40 mg/kg/day may be necessary for life-threatening CNS and nasal mycoses.

Although this agent is relatively well tolerated, canine side-effects occur, including inappetence, pruritus, alopecia, and a reversible lightening of the hair coat.[101] At dosages higher that 40 mg/kg/day there were anorexia, nausea, and increased liver enzyme levels. Cats are more sensitive and have anorexia, fever, depression, vomition, diarrhea, and neurologic abnormalities; therefore, lower doses or even alternate-day therapy may be necessary. Ketoconazole may be teratogenic. In normal doses (10 to 30 mg/kg/day) it has been shown to suppress basal cortisol concentration and response to ACTH, suppress serum testosterone concentrations, and increase serum progesterone concentrations.[105] When the drug is halted, a sharp testosterone rebound occurs. In therapeutic use, one should be aware of the possible effect on libido and breeding effectiveness in males and the possibility of inducing or exacerbating prostatic disease, as well as the potential for managing prostate disease, mammary carcinoma, and spontaneous hyperadrenocorticism.[18] It has been recently reported that ketoconazole has various immunomodulating effects, including suppression of granulocyte chemotaxis and lymphocyte blastogenic responses.[79a]

In veterinary medicine ketoconazole is effective in the treatment of dermatophytosis (some strains of microsporum are resistant), candidiasis, blastomycosis,[26] coccidioidomycosis,[176] histoplasmosis,[107] and cryptococcosis.[8, 109] In humans and experimental animals it produced good results in candidiasis, dermatophytosis, histoplasmosis, and paracoccidioidomycosis; moderate results with coccidioidomycosis, chromoblastomycosis, and aspergillosis; but poor results with mycetomas, aspergillomas, and phaeohyphomycoses.[157] Ketoconazole is often prescribed in combination with amphotericin B for systemic infections, as the antifungal activity of both seems to be enhanced.[22] Protocols for the drug are complex, and the reader is referred to Moriello[101] or Greene[51] for details.

Itraconazole is a new imidazole derivative for the systemic treatment of mycoses.[185] In humans it is highly effective in dermatophytoses, candidiasis, and intermediate and deep mycoses. The drug is given orally and produces higher tissue levels than the corresponding peak plasma levels. Itraconazole is bound to keratinocytes and is secreted in sweat and sebum. This new imidazole has attractive possibilities in veterinary medicine.

Amphotericin B (Fungizone) is a fungicidal antibiotic that disrupts fungal (and bacterial) cell membranes by binding with ergosterol. It also binds to mammalian cell membranes and therefore is relatively toxic. Amphotericin B is most effective for blastomycosis, histoplasmosis, coccidioidomycosis, cryptococcosis, and candidiasis—in the first two cases when combined with ketoconazole and in the last two when combined with flucytosine. These combination protocols are used to take advantage of the prompt action of amphotericin B and to reduce its toxicity. Problems of therapy include nephrotoxicity (especially in dehydrated and hyponatremic animals), anemia, phlebitis, and hypokalemia.[131] Organisms tend to develop resistance to the drug.

Amphotericin given systemically must be given intravenously dissolved *only* in 5 per cent dextrose and water. A reasonable dose for dogs is 0.5 mg/kg on alternate days and for cats, which are more sensitive, 0.15 mg/kg. Treatment with this drug is dangerous and complicated, and clinicians are advised to consult other references for specific guidelines.[51, 101, 131]

Flucytosine (Ancobon) is an orally administered fluorinated pyramidine that has been useful against *Candida*, *Cryptococcus* and *Aspergillus*. Fungal cells are susceptible if they convert flucytosine to fluorouracil, which interferes with DNA synthesis. Resistant, mutant organisms emerge regularly and rapidly in the presence of the drug, one reason for its being used in combination with amphotericin B. The oral dose is 60 mg/kg TID, but it is used as a second-line treatment. With drugs such as ketoconazole available, the future of flucytosine is not bright.

SYSTEMIC ANTIPARASITIC AGENTS

Systemic parasiticidal agents are given orally, by injection, or by placement on the skin for transepidermal absorption to produce effective blood levels of insecticide. When the parasite bites the host and ingests blood, it gets a toxic dose of medication and dies. Unfortunately for allergic hosts, the antigenic saliva has been injected and the allergic reaction continues. Although these systemics may reduce the insect (flea) population, they are only part of a complete flea control program (see p. 416). Owners may become complacent and rely too much on these medications. Systemics also have great potential for toxicity, especially if the owners apply another topical insecticide that uses a drug of the same type.

Cythioate (Proban) is a popular, orally dosed organophosphate that has been heavily promoted to dog owners. It is marketed in a 1.6 per cent solution or in 30-mg tablets for oral use. The dose of 3 mg/kg twice weekly for weeks apparently has a wide margin of safety. However, severe overdosing sharply decreases serum cholinesterase levels without clinical signs. The levels return to normal 42 days after medication is halted.[133] Although this agent has not been approved for cats, Battistella[13] used it in a series of cats at a dosage of 1.5 mg/kg twice weekly. If no toxicity was observed and fleas were not controlled, the dose was increased to 3 mg/kg twice weekly. It was concluded that cythioate was reasonably safe and provided good control.

Several problems may cause concern. Effective blood levels are only maintained for 6 to 12 hours after medication and an increase in dose frequency may produce toxicity. Administration to dogs with heartworms or liver disorders may be dangerous. The use of cythioate in animals with flea bite hypersensitivity will not stop the cause of the hypersensitivity reaction.

Fenthion (Pro-Spot, Spotton) is a highly toxic, very stable organophosphate used primarily as a large animal pour-on for hypoderma larvae. It is an oily liquid with a disagreeable odor. It has been used for fleas in dogs for many years in the southeastern United States in an unapproved form (Spotton).[85]

The suggested dose was 20 to 30 mg/kg (0.75 ml per 5 kg) applied to the skin of the back of dogs and repeated every 10 days. A maximum of 0.3 ml per cat is applied to the *skin* at the base of the skull or between the shoulders and repeated every 10 days.[85] The dose should be tapered to once-a-month treatment if flea control is maintained. Recently, a liquid dosage form of fenthion (Pro-Spot) has been approved for dogs with a recommended dose of 8 mg/kg repeated every 14 days and applied as described above.[7, 12] Mason and colleagues[94] showed in a field study that an optimum canine dose of 20 mg/kg every 14 to 21 days was safe and highly effective. Although it decreased serum cholinesterase levels significantly, they were essentially reactivated after 14 days.[134] Significant toxicity is seen after a dosage of 90 mg/kg every 14 days for three doses; death occurs after a single dose of 270 mg/kg.[88]

Use of this drug has been controversial, as unintentional toxicity is common and it has unpredictable effects. It is dangerous to patients and owners! If used at all, it should be applied at the minimum effective dose and with proper supervision.

Ivermectin is a derivative of avermectin B, a macrocyclic lactone from fermentation products of *Streptomyces avermitilis*. It acts as a broad-spectrum parasiticidal agent in a variety of host species. This drug is noted for activity against nematodes, microfilaria, and sarcoptic, cheyletiella, notoedric, and otodectic mites; however, it is not effective against demodex mites.

Ivermectin probably paralyzes nematodes and arthropods by stimulating the presynaptic release of gamma-aminobutyric acid (GABA) and by potentiating its binding to its receptors. The result is a blockade of the postsynaptic transmission of nerve impulses, and thus parasites become paralyzed and slowly die.[14] GABA is a peripheral neurotransmitter of affected parasites, while in mammals it is a CNS neurotransmitter; ivermectin does not readily cross the blood–brain barrier, except possibly in some collies.

Ivermectin does not affect trematodes and cestodes, because GABA is not involved in neurotransmission in those species. Parasite paralysis is the main action of ivermectin but it also suppresses reproduction. Ticks are not killed, but their egg production and molting are suppressed.

Ivermectin can be given parenterally or orally with good absorption. However, the polysorbate 80 in the injectable form of ivermectin for horses is highly toxic to small animals. Ivermectin is rapidly absorbed orally but persists in the tissues for prolonged periods. This is important because it does not have a rapid killing effect on affected parasites. Ivermectin is only approved in the United States for small animals at a very low dosage for heartworm prophylaxis (Heartgard 30). Experimental reports indicate that single oral doses of 200 μg/kg are effective for canine and feline scabies, and feline and canine otodectes infestations.[14, 15, 40, 88] Recently, the bovine injectable ivermectin (Ivomec) has been administered subcutaneously to dogs and cats (300 μg/kg, repeated in 3 weeks) for the successful treatment of cheyletiellosis.[186] *The use of ivermectin in a collie, Shetland sheepdog, or any dog resembling a collie is contraindicated.* In addition, ivermectin should not be administered to puppies less than 3 months of age, as toxicity may be seen in *any* breed. Ivermectin should *not* be used concurrently with other GABA–potentiating drugs (e.g., diazepam). The vehicle has no effect on toxicity of the oral dosage form,[111] and injectable doses of 1/200 of the lethal dose for beagles killed collies having a wide range of sensitivity. Collies that died had high levels of ivermectin in the CNS. Signs of toxicity advanced from ataxia, depression, mydriasis, tremors, recumbency, and vomiting to death.[121] Some animals respond to supportive care but IV picrotoxin is the only drug with the potential to reverse the toxicity.[14] No adverse effects on spermatogenesis, fertility, or reproductive performance were seen when ivermectin was given to male beagles at 600 μg/kg orally per month for eight treatments.[187] When officially released, this drug may have interesting potential uses in small animal dermatology. At the time of this writing, many clinicians in the United States are using the injectable cattle medication Ivomec for oral dosage of dogs and cats even though it has not been officially approved.

HYPOSENSITIZATION

Hyposensitization is a biologic therapy for atopic patients that involves giving multiple increasing doses of reactive agents (allergens) parenterally.[76] The patient responds by forming IgG antibodies against each specific antigen. These circulating antibodies are protective because they bind with invading allergens before those allergens reach tissue-fixed IgE. This blocking antibody theory may be only a partial explanation of hyposensitization, since other mechanisms are proposed, such as a decrease in cellular sensitivity or a long-term diminution of the reaginic antibody available to sensitize mediator-releasing cells (tolerization). (See Chap. 9, p. 461, for a more detailed discussion.)

IMMUNOMODULATING AGENTS

The remarkable gains in basic immunologic knowledge have outpaced improvements in available agents or techniques that can be used to clinically modify the immune response.[11] Many biologic and synthetic immunomodifiers, adjuvants, and drugs with both specific and nonspecific effects on immunity have been investigated.[150] Many of the therapies currently available are still in the developmental stage. However, it appears likely that important gains of the next decade will come from the sphere of immunomodulation. When the mechanism of actions of the many immunomodulating agents are more completely understood, specific sequential combinations will be used to achieve desired clinical results. Therapy for immunomodulation can be divided into three broad categories: (1) agents that facilitate a normal immune response (i.e., immunorestoration), (2) agents that stimulate the immune response (i.e., immunostimulation), and (3) noncytotoxic agents that suppress the immune response (i.e., immunosuppression). These will be discussed briefly, with more attention being given to those agents that have some present clinical use.

Immunorestoration

The concept of restoring a dysfunctional or failing immune system has many parallels to other organ systems in the body. The most obvious in immunology relate to immunoglobulin replacement, interferon therapy, administration of thymic hormones, and bone marrow and fetal liver transplantation. In addition, T-cell–produced soluble mediators such as lymphokines and the recently identified interleukins transmit growth and differentiation signals among immunocytes.

Immunoglobulins have long been used to passively immunize patients with primary and secondary humoral immunodeficiency disorders with exogenous antibody. Immune and hyperimmune serum globulins have been used in a variety of primary B-cell deficiencies (agammaglobulinemia) and secondary immunodeficiencies (burns, exfoliative dermatitis, chronic lymphocytic leukemia) of humans, but the expense and high incidence of adverse reactions are major concerns.

Interferon is a natural, broad-spectrum antiviral glycoprotein that is species-specific and produced by virtually all nucleated animal cells.[149] Three types are known: alpha, produced by monocytes; beta, produced by fibroblasts; and gamma, produced by T cells. When a cell is invaded by a virus, it responds by synthesizing and releasing interferon. The interferon binds to the surface of uninfected neighboring cells and stimulates them to produce a group of protective proteins that inhibit viral reproduction in a manner that is not fully understood. Interferon also activates macrophages and increases the destructive capacity of cytotoxic T cells and natural killer cells. It inhibits the division of cells, including some tumor cells. Although the therapeutic potential of interferon is promising, all types are pyrogenic, and there are many serious side-effects.

Thymic hormones are peptides that circulate in peripheral blood and are important in the development and maintenance of the immune system. Thymosin and its thymic fractions control the maturation and differentiation of T cells leading to normal function. With aging, there are decreased production and a rise in frequency of autoantibodies. These changes lead to increased susceptibility to infections, decreased resistance to tumor growth, and increased incidence of autoimmune diseases.[159] It is anticipated that thymic hormones may have future therapeutic relevance in problems of the aged and in management of some of the disease states common to that group of patients.[159]

Immunostimulation

Immunomodulating agents that act as potentiators of the immune response may act at several points in the immunologic scheme without a specific target cell. Some, such as transfer factor, are antigen specific, and others, such as levamisole, are entirely nonspecific in their action on a disordered immune system. Other agents require a functional immune system to function (bacille Calmette-Guérin, BCG). Bacterial antigens may act as immunostimulants to patients with poor immune responses or as hyposensitizing agents to those with staphylococcal hypersensitivities.

Levamisole is a synthetic chemical derivative of tetramisole, first introduced as a broad-spectrum anthelmintic. It acts directly on lymphocytes, macrophages, and granulocytes to modify their mobility, secretion, and proliferation. Its exact mechanism of action is unknown, but its effects are most pronounced in increasing the number and function of T lymphocytes in aged, diseased, or immunocompromised hosts.[17] There is no effect on B cells or antibody production and the drug does not increase immune responses above normal levels. Although levamisole is a potent anthelmintic it is not toxic to bacteria, viruses, protozoa, fungi, or normal or tumor cells. It may increase the protective effect of some vaccines and stabilize tumor remission. Its potentiating effects are enhanced by the parallel administration of a primary stimulus such as an antigen. In humans no effect is observed in young people, but in older people the drug restores to normal a variety of immunologic functions. Levamisole has been used in humans with rheumatic, hypersensitivity, and neoplastic diseases, but the adverse effects of granulocytopenia, skin hypersensitivity, gastrointestinal disturbances, and immune suppression have made it a less desirable agent. Canine toxicity was reported following its use in a case of dirofilariasis at a dose of 12 mg/kg SID.[100] The dog developed ataxia, diarrhea, dyspnea, salivation, bradycardia, and stupor but responded within 4 days to treatment with atropine, isoproterenol, glycopyrrolate, and supportive care.[62] Levamisole is also a potential cause of cutaneous drug eruptions, erythema multiforme, and toxic epidermolysis in dogs. In veterinary immunology it may be useful for chronic or recurrent infections involving skin or soft tissues and in primary and secondary immunodeficiency states.[191] The dosage is critical, since levamisole has a so-called window effect: doses that are higher or lower than optimum may produce immunosuppression rather than stimulation.[127] Clinicians presently use 2.2 mg/kg orally repeated three times weekly.

Thiabendazole (Mintezol) may be used as an immunostimulant in a manner somewhat similar to levamisole in doses of 5 to 10 mg/kg orally three times weekly.

Bacterial antigens may be useful in recurrent staphylococcal skin infections.[10, 188, 191] There is much debate about their effectiveness and method of action.[20, 87] Cell-wall-containing antigens may stimulate T cells, and they may also act as hyposensitizing agents. Autogenous bacterins are expensive and have not been highly effective. Staphoid A-B is a *Staphylococcus aureus* cell-wall antigen and toxoid mixture of both alpha and beta toxins from whole cultures of *S. aureus* (phage types I, III, and V), which are inactivated in formalin. This antigen is used in cases of so-called bacterial hypersensitivity, according to the dosage schedule in Table 4:5 with 67 to 88 per cent success.[120] In the patients that respond, many need to be on monthly boosters indefinitely to prevent relapse.

Staphylococcal phage lysate (Staphage Lysate) also is effective for recurrent pyodermas.[3, 20, 120, 128] The antigens are prepared by lysing parent cultures of *S. aureus*, serologic types I and III, with a polyvalent staphylococcal bacteriophage. After ultrafiltration, the lysates contain antigenic fractions of *S. aureus* and active bacteriophage. The phage is polyvalent and has lysed in vitro a significant proportion of field strains of staphylococci. Its ability to lyse staphylococci in vivo has been shown in experimental animals. Clinical benefits following vaccination have been attributed to stimulation of antibacterial antibodies; however, benefits may also result from a favorable effect of the antigen on the state of cellular sensitivity to staphylococci.

A positive effect on T-cell depression (measured by lymphocyte blastogenesis) has been shown in canine staphylococcal dermatitis patients treated with Staphage Lysate. For the injection schedule see Table 4:6.

Table 4:5. STAPHOID A-B DOSAGE SCHEDULE

Day	Intradermal (ml)	Subcutaneous (ml)	Total Dosage (ml)
1	0.1	0.15	0.25
2	0.1	0.40	0.50
3	0.1	0.65	0.75
4	0.1	0.90	1.00
5	0.1	1.15	1.25
12	0.1	1.40	1.50
19	0.1	1.65	1.75
26	0.1	1.90	2.00
Monthly	0.1	1.90	2.00

Table 4:6. STAPHAGE LYSATE INJECTION SCHEDULE

Week	ml of Staphage Lysate*
1	0.25
2	0.50
3	0.75
4	1.00
Can be increased to 2.0 ml every 3–21 days, if necessary, for maintenance.	

*Injected subcutaneously

The use of bacterial antigens should be reserved for patients with a history of bacterial dermatoses that respond to long-term antibiotic therapy that is followed by relapse when therapy is discontinued. Antibiotic therapy is used in addition to the antigen injections for the first month; then phage lysate is used alone. Staphage Lysate and Staphoid A-B are not licensed for use in dogs and cats.

Protein A is a constituent of the cell wall of *S. aureus* Cowan 1 (SAC) and many other staphylococci. When plasma is perfused over protein A, it reacts with the Fc region of immunoglobulins and combines with immune complexes. In the laboratory it will bind, and thus it can remove almost all canine IgG and IgM and substantial amounts of IgA from canine serum.[97] This phenomenon has been used in extracorporeal immunoabsorption and has been shown to have antiviral and antitumor activity in humans, dogs, and cats.[89, 189] It may also have great future potential in immune complex diseases. The mechanism may include the following: removal of circulating immune complexes by Fc binding of IgG complexes, activation of plasma factors after contact with protein A, enhanced cytotoxic T-lymphocyte induction, induction of gamma interferon production, enhanced natural killer cell activity, enhanced antibody dependent cell-mediated cytotoxicity, or release into the plasma of bacterial products that may have immunomodulatory activity.[89, 189]

Bacterial products (bacterial antigens, protein A, BCG, and propionibacteria) exert the following major effects on the immune system of the host: activate B and T lymphocytes, natural killer cells, and macrophages; abrogate suppressor cell inductions; intensify antibody-dependent cell-mediated toxicity; induce immune interferon; and elaborate tumor cell necrosis factor.

Propionibacterium acnes (ImmunoRegulin) has been introduced recently as an immunostimulant for recurrent canine pyoderma. Initial reports suggested giving IV injections twice weekly for 2 weeks, then once weekly until improvement is seen, with once-monthly injections for maintenance. Over 50 per cent of the cases were said to be in complete remission (Immuno Vet, company report). Tinsley and Taylor reported its use in the successful management of a multicentric malignant mast cell tumor in a dog.[166] Other field reports have been equivocal or disappointing;[191] therefore, much additional work is needed to properly evaluate this product in small animal dermatology.

Immunosuppression

Since 1940 the corticosteroids have been used in many treatment protocols to control excessive immune responses (see p. 198). Azathioprine and (in humans) heterologous antilymphocyte serum have been used as well. Cytotoxic drugs also have been used to induce immune tolerance by destroying replicating cells. The cytotoxic drugs are divided into (1) cell-cycle drugs that destroy rapidly multiplying cells (antimetabolites and folic acid antagonists) and (2) noncycle drugs that are injurious to all cells and usually result in a depletion of small lymphocytes (alkylating agents) (see below).[11]

More recently, cyclosporine has appeared as an agent unlike any other immunosuppressant agent in that it allows selective alteration of the immune system. Ordinarily, it does not block primary antibody response but acts to inhibit lymphokine production by impairing interleukin-2 production by quiescent and activated helper T cells. It does not have specific toxic effects on lymphocytes and myelocytes but does have significant nephrotoxicity and other less serious, reversible, dose-related side-effects. It is primarily used in organ transplantation; however, rapid taper protocols, lower doses, and use in combination with corticosteroids (which block interleukin-1 production) offer promise of its future application in autoimmune disease.[11]

CYTOTOXIC AGENTS

Cyclophosphamide

Cyclophosphamide (Cytoxan) is an alkylating agent that is used alone or in combination chemotherapy for tumors, as well as for its immunosuppressive activity in nonmalignant diseases and organ transplants.[151] It acts to revert mitoses by interference with DNA replication and RNA translation. Able to kill cells in all phases of the cell cycle, this type of cytotoxic drug is more effective in slow-growing tumors than are phase-specific drugs that act only during a specific time of the cell cycle. It is most effective against rapidly dividing cells.[125] Lymphocytes are especially sensitive to cyclophosphamide.

Major toxicities include sterile hemorrhagic cystitis, bladder fibrosis, teratogenesis, infertility, alopecia, nausea, inflammation of the gastrointestinal tract, increased susceptibility to infections, and depression of the bone marrow and hematopoietic systems. Its effects should be monitored with periodic hemograms.

Cyclophosphamide is immunosuppressive to both the humoral and cell-mediated immune systems but is more effective against B cells than against T cells. Cyclophosphamide suppresses antibody production. Maximum effect is seen if the drug is given shortly after the antigenic stimulus, when it suppresses primary and secondary humoral responses.

Clinical indications include lymphoreticular tumors for which the drug is best if combined with corticosteroids or vincristine. It can be given after high doses of corticosteroids to maintain improvement (with fewer side-effects) with immune-mediated diseases such as systemic lupus erythematosus, vasculitis, pemphigus vulgaris, bullous pemphigoid, idiopathic thrombocytopenia, hemolytic anemia, gammopathies, and rheumatoid arthritis.[191] Tumor dosage is 50 mg/M^2 body surface area (BSA) for 4 days, then off 3 days; repeat each week. For immunosuppression, the oral dose is 1.5 to 2.5 mg/kg every other day.

Azathioprine

Azathioprine (Imuran) is a synthetic modification of 6-mercaptopurine (6-MP) that can be given orally or by injection. It slowly releases 6-MP at various sites in the body, where it interferes with DNA and RNA metabolism and primarily affects rapidly proliferating cells.[125] It affects cell-mediated immunity and T-lymphocyte–dependent antibody synthesis. Primary antibody synthesis is affected more than secondary antibody synthesis. Azathioprine is preferred to 6-MP because it has a more favorable therapeutic index. Even so, it is a potent drug with serious potential toxicities, which include leukopenia, thrombocytopenia, vomiting, hypersensitivity, pancreatitis, elevated serum alkaline phosphatase levels, skin rashes, and alopecia. Patients should be monitored by at least monthly complete blood counts and platelet counts.

Azathioprine has been used for prevention of human transplant rejections and for rheumatoid arthritis that is not responsive to other treatment. In small animals it may be useful for pemphigus complex, bullous pemphigoid, and systemic lupus erythrematosus as well as other autoimmune and immune-mediated disorders.[191] The oral dose for dogs is 2.2 mg/kg once daily until clinical response is achieved and then is continued every other day.[125] Corticosteroids can be given on the alternate days when azathioprine is not given.

Cats are very susceptible to azathioprine toxicity (including fatal leukopenia, thrombocytopenia), and this drug should be used *very* cautiously, if at all, in this species.

Chlorambucil

Chlorambucil (Leukeran) is an orally administered alkylating agent that is one of the slowest acting and least toxic of that group of drugs.[125] Although serious toxicity is rare at regular doses, myelosuppression is possible; consequently, hemograms should be monitored every 2 to 4 weeks.

Chlorambucil may be useful in the pemphigus complex, bullous pemphigoid, systemic lupus erythematosus, immune-mediated vasculitis, and cold agglutinin disease as well as in lymphocyte and plasma-cell malignancies.[191] Chlorambucil may be used to replace cyclophosphamide if hemorrhagic cystitis develops during the use of that drug. The oral dose in dogs and cats is 2.2 mg/M^2 once daily for 4 consecutive days, then off 3 days; repeat each week. Larger doses have been given safely, and doses from 0.2 mg/kg to 1.4 mg/kg have been used for convenience.

CYCLOSPORINE

Cyclosporine (Sandimmune Cyclosporine A) is a fat-soluble peptide antibiotic that is a highly effective immunosuppressive agent in human organ transplantation and in the treatment of graft-versus-host (GVH) syndrome in bone marrow transplantation. In animal models it has been used with similar excellent results.[170] Immunosuppressants such as corticosteroids, azathioprine, and cyclophosphamide are nonspecifically cytotoxic; high doses kill normal cells.[170] Cyclosporine, however, has low cytotoxicity relative to its immunosuppressive potency. It has a selective effect on T lymphocytes, especially T helper cells, to produce immunosuppression without inhibiting T suppressor cells or depressing bone marrow.[110] While the exact mechanism of action of cyclosporine is unknown, its immunosuppressive effects are dose dependent, reversible with drug withdrawal, and most marked when the drug is administered before the antigenic stimulation. Thus, it is useful in tissue transplantation.

A high incidence of nephrotoxicity and hepatic toxicity is seen in people. Dogs may develop gingival hyperplasia and papillomatosis, vomiting, diarrhea, bacteriuria, bacterial skin infection, anorexia, nephropathy, bone marrow suppression, and a lymphoplasmacytoid dermatosis.[203, 204] Cats are reported to have only minor side-effects.[53]

The clinical indications of cyclosporine are organ transplantation and inhibition of delayed-hypersensitivity reactions of many immune-mediated diseases. It is used in pemphigus foliaceus and immune-mediated myasthenia gravis, thyroiditis, neuritis, uveitis, and arthritis. In addition, it is used in humans who have pemphigus vulgaris, bullous pemphigoid, collagen vascular disorders, and graft-versus-host syndrome. Initial studies in dogs and cats with immunologic dermatoses such as pemphigus foliaceus, pemphigus erythematosus, and discoid lupus erythematosus have shown cyclosporine by itself to be rarely effective.[191] Cyclosporine has been ineffective in the treatment of canine and feline epitheliotropic lymphoma (mycosis fungoides). The oral dosage for dogs and cats is 20 mg/kg daily, the dosage for cats being divided and given twice daily.[79, 170] In dogs, this dosage resulted in serum concentrations of 200 to 1000 ng/ml; levels above 200 ng/ml produce continuous immunosuppression. Variable absorptions may occur among individuals and with day-to-day administration, so it is possible that doses of 10 mg/kg/day may be effective.

NONSTEROIDAL ANTI-INFLAMMATORY AGENTS

Although corticosteroids are highly effective in managing many hypersensitivity disorders, the serious side-effects stimulate constant investigations for alternative drugs or methods that will allow a reduction in dose. Eicosapentaenoic acid (EPA) is available in a fatty acid formulation that appears promising (see p. 191). Scott and Buerger[142] used that agent and five others in a nonblinded study of nonsteroidal anti-inflammatory agents in the management of 45 cases of canine pruritus. Thirty-two dogs had atopy and/or flea bite hypersensitivity, and thirteen had idiopathic nonseasonal pruritus. As a group, the six drugs controlled itching in 40 per cent of the cases with improvement in another 15 per cent. However, side-effects were seen in 46 per cent of the cases, being severe enough in 33 per cent to cause treatment with one or more of the drugs to be halted.

The six drugs included three antihistamines (H_1 blockers, each from a different chemical class), an antibiotic, aspirin, and the EPA formulation (Derm Caps). Good-to-moderate improvement of pruritus was obtained for each medication, as seen in Table 4:7.

Although these results show promise, further studies are needed to evaluate the merits of nonsteroidal anti-inflammatory agents in the management of pruritus in dogs that is due to hypersensitivity reactions.

Histamine in humans is an important mediator of immediate allergic and inflammatory reactions.[23] In small animals it probably plays a smaller, though perhaps a contributory, part in allergy and pruritus. The effects of histamine can be blocked in three ways: by physiologic antagonists (epinephrine), by release inhibitors that reduce the degranulation of mast cells (cromolyn), and by histamine-receptor antagonists. One group of the latter are antihistamines,

Table 4:7. RESULTS OF STUDY OF NONSTEROIDAL ANTI-INFLAMMATORY AGENTS IN 45 CASES OF CANINE PRURITUS

Drug	Dosage	Number Controlled	Number Improved	Number Side-Effects
Chlorpheniramine	4 mg TID	4	4	12
Diphenhydramine	25–50 mg TID	3	7	7
Hydroxyzine	2.2 mg/kg TID	3	8	7
Erythromycin	11 mg/kg TID	2	4	4
EPA formula	1 cap/9 kg SID	5	5	4
Aspirin	25 mg/kg TID	1	4	2

a term that refers to H_1 receptor blockers such as chlorpheniramine and diphenhydramine. In addition to their histamine-blocking action, they have therapeutic value because of the sedation, antinausea, anticholinergic, antiserotonin, and local anesthesia effects they produce.

Antihistamines are chemicals that block the action of histamines at receptor sites. However, not all the effects of histamine are blocked by H_1 receptor-site antihistamines. There are six drug classes of antihistamines with variable sedation as a side-effect. All the drugs are well absorbed and are 70 to 80 per cent effective in humans against allergic rhinitis and conjunctivitis, although they may potentially be followed by a rebound of clinical signs.[38] They are more effective if given in addition to an alpha receptor agonist (pseudoephedrine). Hydroxyzine gave the best antipruritic effect with human atopy patients.

H_2 receptor blockers may have a role in modifying the cutaneous inflammatory response. Cimetidine (Tagamet) and ranitidine, which is more powerful and longer acting, are available for clinical use but are not FDA approved for small animals. H_2 antihistamines (cimetidine) should not be given alone since they inhibit the negative feedback histamine exerts on mediators released by mast cells, thus potentially exacerbating an inflammatory dermatosis.[5] The combination of H_1 and H_2 blockers counteracts the action of any circulating histamine by blocking all of the available histamine receptors. H_1 and H_2 antagonists have no effect on the receptor sites of each other.

Cimetidine is not a first-line drug in human dermatology, but is used in combination with H_1 antihistamine for urticarial, allergic, and immunologic dermatoses when other therapy fails. It has also been used as an antipruritic in dermatoses related to systemic disorders and as an immunorestorative in cases of T-cell lymphoma, mycosis fungoides, and candidiasis.[5] In a study of 15 dogs with allergic skin disease cimetidine alone was helpful in only one dog, and no dog responded better to the combination of H_2 (cimetidine) and H_1 (diphenhydramine) blockers than to the H_1 blocker alone.[193]

Cimetidine appears safe for dogs and cats at a dosage of 5 to 10 mg/kg orally every 6 to 8 hours.[25] It may be useful in some cases of chronic recurrent pyoderma with pruritus.[20, 191] Much more evaluation remains to be done in small animal dermatology, however.

In human dermatology the nonsteroidal anti-inflammatory drugs are under intense study, since they may prove beneficial in many inflammatory dermatoses where more conventional therapy has failed. Elevated levels of inflammatory mediators of the prostaglandin and leukotriene series have been found in psoriasis, ultraviolet B inflammation, leukocytoclastic vasculitis, contact dermatitis, bullous pemphigoid, and many other disorders. Drugs in this category include salicylate, indomethacin, ibuprofen, and naproxen.

FATTY ACID SUPPLEMENTS

Some nutritional supplements (such as Efa-Z Plus) are formulations of high-potency essential fatty acids, vitamins A and E, pyridoxine, biotin, inositol, and zinc. They are said to be useful for seborrhea, dry skin, and excessive shedding of dry, dull hair, which are often thought to be caused by dietary or environmental abnormalities. When effective, response may take 8 to 12 weeks to be evident. (See Chap. 17, Nutritional Skin Diseases.)

Recent interest has centered on the use of increased ingestion of fatty acids to modify the arachidonic acid inflammatory cascade and thus to reduce pruritus associated with hypersensitivity reactions such as atopy (Fig. 4:3).[99] In atopy, sensitized mast cells exposed to an allergen degranulate and release a variety of mediators of inflammation into the tissues. In dogs and cats these include histamine, heparin, proteolytic enzymes, leukotrienes, prostaglandins, and other chemotactic factors. Prostaglandins and leukotrienes are products of fatty acid metabolism.

Fatty acids are metabolized by shared enzyme systems. If their metabolism could be directed to pathways that produced fewer inflammatory end products, reduced pruritus might ensue. Arachidonic acid has been most widely studied, and its metabolism leads to the production of the 2-series prostaglandins and the 4-series leukotrienes, agents that are highly inflammatory.[49, 82, 167] Arachidonic acid is stored in cells in an unavailable form until it is released by the action of phospholipase A_2 in order that its metabolism can proceed. Phospholipase A_2 is blocked by cortisol. Arachidonic acid metabolites have been identified in many cell types, besides mast cells, that participate in hypersensitivity reactions (neutrophils, eosinophils, lymphocytes, monocytes, macrophages, keratinocytes, and vascular endothelial cells).

The effects of prostaglandins on the skin include alteration of vascular permeability, potentiation of vasoactive substances such as histamine, modu-

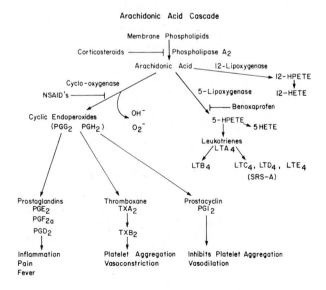

Figure 4:3. Arachidonic acid cascade. PG = prostaglandin. HPETE = hydroperoxyeicosatetraenoic acid. HETE = hydroxyeicosatetraenoic acid. LT = leukotriene. Tx = thromboxane. SRS-A = slow-reacting substance of anaphylaxis. (From Lichtenstein, J., Flowers, F., and Sherertz, E.F.: NSAID in dermatology. Int. J. Dermatol. 26:80, 1987.)

lation of lymphocyte function, and potentiation of pain and itch. Prostaglandins and leukotrienes potentiate each other. The effects of leukotrienes on the skin are to alter vascular permeability, to activate neutrophils, to modify lymphocyte function and to cause potent neutrophil and eosinophil chemotaxis. Manipulation of fatty acid metabolism by using the shared enzyme system to competitively inhibit formation of some of the above substances seems possible.

The omega-3 fatty acids are not essential, but as pharmacologic agents they play an important part in manipulation of fatty acid metabolism, and in humans in the reduction of serum cholesterol. These agents include eicosapentenoic acid (EPA), docosapentenoic acid (DPA), and docosahexanoic acid (DHA). They are derivatives of linolenate and originate in algae and phytoplankton, which are consumed by krill and later by larger marine fish. The muscles of krill, herring, mackerel, and salmon and the liver of cod are high in omega-3 fatty acids.

Miller and colleagues[99] used 93 pruritic dogs in a study using a special formulation of fatty acids (Derm Caps). Each capsule contains EPA 15.0 mg, gamma-linolenic acid 10.2 mg, linoleic acid 269.0 mg, and linolenic acid 0.4 mg, and those amounts were considered to be a daily dose for a 9.1-kg dog. Dogs with flea or food allergies were excluded. No other treatment was allowed. Within 2 weeks 35 per cent of the dogs showed a good to excellent response and about half of those were completely controlled. If medication was stopped, itching returned; if medication was resumed, improvement was observed. Other dogs that were being controlled with corticosteroids had their dose requirements decreased by 50 per cent when they were given the fatty acid capsules.

The pharmacologic mechanism responsible for the decrease in pruritus is unknown, but it probably involves modulations of the arachidonic acid cascade away from the highly inflammatory 2-series prostaglandins and the 4-series leukotrienes and toward the 1- and 3-series prostaglandins and the 5-series leukotrienes, which have much less inflammatory potential.[99] EPA inhibits the formation of 4-series leukotrienes by serving as a competitive inhibitor of 5-lipoxygenase activity.[48, 167]

Since the fatty acid supplementation would have no effect on histamine or proteolytic enzymes, which are pruritogenic agents in many dogs, H_1 antihistamines and cortisol may be useful in reduced dose or, if necessary, in full dose in nonresponsive cases. This fatty acid formulation appears to be a safe and somewhat effective nonsteroidal anti-inflammatory agent for management of atopy in some dogs. Further work with this fascinating concept is eagerly awaited.

Recently EPA (Derm Caps) has been reported to be effective in a small number of cocker spaniels with idiopathic seborrhea, but was of no benefit in West Highland white terriers with epidermal dysplasia or in springer spaniels with psoriasiform lichenoid dermatosis.[192]

CHRYSOTHERAPY

Chrysotherapy is the use of *gold* as a therapeutic agent in disease. Gold compounds are capable of modulating many phases of immune and inflammatory responses, but the exact mechanisms of this effect are unknown.[136] Gold is available in two dosage forms, which have dissimilar pharmacokinetics:

oral compounds (Ridaura or Auranofin) and the parenteral compound auro-thioglucose (Solganol). Neither form is approved for use in dogs and cats, but the distribution, metabolism, and actions have been established in humans and laboratory animals. Studies in humans show that the oral forms are 25 per cent absorbed and attain blood levels with a 21-day half-life, but only small amounts can be detected in tissues and skin.[165] In a very few trials in dogs the results were equivocal, but no adverse side-effects were observed.[171] The parenteral form is 100 per cent absorbed but has only a 6-day half-life in blood. It is 95 per cent protein bound and is well distributed to cells of the mononuclear phagocytic system, liver, spleen, bone marrow, kidneys, and adrenals. Much lesser amounts are detected in skin.

In humans, gold may act at several levels of inflammation and immune response. Auranofin appears to have an additional immunomodulating action, but both oral and parenteral golds inhibit bacteria, the first component of complement, and the epidermal enzymes that may be responsible for blister formation in pemphigus. Both also reduce the release of inflammatory mediators such as lysosomal enzymes, histamine, and prostaglandins and interfere with immunoglobulin-synthesizing cells.

Toxic effects are worrisome in humans, among whom 33 per cent of patients have some problem, although 80 per cent of them are minor. Most common are skin eruptions, oral reactions, proteinuria, and bone marrow depression. During the induction phase a hemogram and urinalysis should be checked weekly, and monthly thereafter.[36] Kummel reported three cases of fatal toxic epidermal necrolysis in dogs that had been treated with Solganol for 3 to 9 months.[73] This may be enhanced by previous or concurrent administration of azathioprine.[191]

Parenteral gold (Solganol) has been reported to be effective in treatment of all three types of canine and feline pemphigus that were unresponsive to glucocorticoids.[172] It has been useful for the treatment of canine bullous pemphigoid and feline plasma cell pododermatitis.[191] It has also been suggested as a treatment for unresponsive rheumatoid arthritis. Although most adverse reactions develop late in therapy, it is suggested that a small IM test dose of 1 mg be given to patients under 10 kg body weight and that 5 mg be given to larger patients in the first week. Dosage is increased to 1 mg/kg IM weekly until remission occurs. If no response is seen after twelve weeks of therapy the dose can be increased to 1.5 to 2.0 mg/kg.[191] After remission one dose is given every 2 weeks, and then once monthly for several months. It is advisable to eventually halt medication for observation, since some patients go into complete remission, while others can be maintained on a reduced dosage. Two points of caution: (1) The treatment takes 6 to 12 weeks for full effect to occur, so that other medication (if needed) should be maintained at full dosage until this lag period is passed. (2) Gold compounds should not be administered simultaneously with other cytotoxic drugs (such as azathioprine, cyclophosphamide), as toxicity is thereby enhanced.

The oral form of gold (auranofin) has been used in only a few dogs with pemphigus (3 to 6 mg/day) with little success. In addition, this oral form is very expensive.

Gold is seldom the first-choice drug for pemphigus. Patients are usually started on glucocorticoids, with cyclophosphamide or azathioprine added to reduce the steroid dosage. In cases with excessive side-effects, gold is a logical second choice. It may be especially useful in cats.[95, 191]

Gold has given equivocal results in treatment of human cases of systemic lupus erythematosus and epidermolysis bullosa.[165]

SULFONES AND SULFONAMIDES

Dapsone. This is an anti-inflammatory, antibacterial chemical (4,4'-diaminodiphenyl sulfone); its precise mechanism of action is unknown.[84] It has anti-inflammatory effects and inhibits lysosomal enzymes, degranulation of mast cells, synthesis of IgG, IgA and prostaglandins, and neutrophil chemotaxis.[42] Dapsone is an antioxidant scavenger and also inhibits proteases. Its metabolism has not been studied in dogs, but in humans it is rapidly absorbed orally and reaches peak concentrations in 4 to 8 hours, although the serum half-life varies from 10 to 50 hours. Dapsone is useful in various diseases characterized by accumulations of neutrophils. It is often effective for vasculitis with lupus erythematosus or systemic lupus erythematosus–like disorders in humans. In these cases the human dosage regimen starts low and rapidly builds to 150 mg/day. This dosage is held until response occurs and then is gradually decreased and stopped after 4 to 10 months. In many cases there is no relapse—the patients remain disease free. Treatment with dapsone is also effective in human leprosy, dermatitis herpetiformis, subcorneal pustular dermatosis, and some cases of pemphigus, pemphigoid, and rheumatoid arthritis. In dogs, dapsone has been used with benefit in cases of subcorneal pustular dermatosis, leukocytoclastic vasculitis, linear IgA dermatosis, and pemphigus foliaceus and erythematosus.[144] Dapsone is most useful in the first two diseases, although not all cases were controlled. In the last three diseases only about half the cases showed benefit. However, in some cases of pemphigus that were successfully treated with immunosuppressive combinations (such as azathioprine with corticosteroids) the addition of dapsone permitted lowering the dose of the corticosteroid.

Dapsone is not approved for use in dogs and cats in the United States, but journal reports suggest a dosage of 1 mg/kg TID orally for 2 to 3 weeks until lesions clear and then a reduction of the dose to BID or SID. The maintenance dose should be further reduced to once or twice weekly, or even stopped, since toxicity is somewhat dose related.

Potential toxicity can be serious. During induction, mild anemia, leukopenia, and moderate elevations of serum alanine aminotransferase (ALT) may be expected but do not necessitate stopping treatment if the animal remains clinically normal. Blood dyscrasias, skin reactions, and hepatic toxicity can be serious. Patients should be monitored every 2 weeks during induction with hemograms, blood urea nitrogen (BUN) urinalysis, and serum ALT determination. Cats are especially susceptible to dapsone toxicity, with hemolytic anemia and various neurotoxicities reported.

Sulfasalazine (Azulfidine). This chemical is converted in the colon to sulfapyridine 5-aminosalicylate, which has anti-inflammatory action.[124, 144] The dosage is 20 mg/kg TID orally. Dosage may be reduced or even changed to every other day and still maintain clinical remission. A serious side-effect is the production of a high incidence of keratitis sicca, and therefore tear production should be checked regularly. Scott has reported that two dogs with subcorneal pustular dermatosis were managed satisfactorily with sulfasalazine after becoming refractory to dapsone.[144]

COLCHICINE

Colchicine is a toxic alkaloid of plants, primarily used for human gout, which has application in dermatology as a second-line drug for inflammatory diseases characterized by connective tissue abnormalities with leukocyte chemotaxis.[6] It interferes with leukocyte functions and inhibits histamine release, formation of leukotriene B_4, collagen synthesis, and movement of melanin granules to melanophages, while increasing collagenolytic activity. In humans it is used for dermatitis herpetiformis, dermatomyositis, necrotizing vasculitis, and systemic sclerosis. Although it has severe gastrointestinal side-effects, in combination with topical agents it may have future application in veterinary medicine.

ANTIMALARIALS

Several antimalarials have been useful in treatment of humans with discoid lupus erythematosus, polymorphous light eruption, solar urticaria, and scleroderma.[66] There are also anecdotal reports of response with cutaneous leishmaniasis, cutaneous cryptococcosis, epidermolysis bullosa, and lymphocytic skin infiltrations.[160] Antimalarials may have future use in problem cases involving animals with such diseases. Their specific mode of action is unknown, but the drugs stabilize lysosomal membranes and thus are anti-inflammatory. They inhibit protein synthesis, viral replication, and cell-mediated immunity. They do not affect the development of primary or secondary antibody response but do inhibit complement; consequently, they may inhibit the formation of immune complexes, which explains their effectiveness in systemic lupus erythematosus (SLE) and related autoimmune disorders. The drugs are seldom used alone for first-line therapy and in humans are usually given with salicylates or small doses of corticosteroids. Side-effects are numerous, the most serious affecting the eyes.

The four drugs most commonly used in humans are quinacrine (Atabrine), chloroquine (Aralen), amodiaquin (Camoquin), and hydroxychloroquine (Plaquenil). Their place in veterinary dermatology has yet to be determined although quinacrine has been used as a treatment for canine giardiasis, and anecdotal reports have suggested that the antimalarials may be beneficial in canine lupus erythematosus. (See p. 525.)

MEDICATIONS RELATED TO NUTRITION

Nutritional factors that influence the skin are exceedingly complex. It is obvious, however, that for proper skin health and function, the diet must be complete in all essential nutritional factors. When deficiencies in nutrition are produced experimentally, they often result in cutaneous disorders, but these are seldom characteristic enough to allow specific diagnosis. Furthermore, because of the interaction of nutrients, a deficiency of one item may upset delicate balances; therefore, the skin manifestation may be the result of the imbalance rather than the initial deficiency. For these reasons it is felt that a complex diet of well-balanced, wholesome, and fresh ingredients is the proper approach to providing adequate nutrition for skin health. It is necessary in some cases to modify the diet or to use nutritional supplements to improve skin health, but the cliché "Add more fat to the diet" is an overworked suggestion that seldom is helpful.

General overeating leads to obesity, which may cause intertriginous dermatitis and bacterial infections or, by increasing the fat layer, may make heat dissipation more difficult. It has been reported that the incidence of skin problems was 40 per cent higher in overweight dogs than in dogs at optimum body weight.[28]

General malnutrition, on the other hand, causes the skin to become dry, inelastic, and scaly. The skin may become more susceptible to infection and may show hemorrhagic tendencies and pigment disturbances. Undernourishment can develop through interference with intake, absorption, or utilization, through increased requirements or excretion, or through inhibition.

Specific nutritional factors are most difficult to evaluate; a great number of nutrients have been determined to have an influence on skin health. These include essential fatty acids, amino acids and protein, vitamins, and minerals. (See Chap. 17, Nutritional Skin Diseases.) A survey of 20 Canadian commercial nutritional supplements revealed that none of them met all the requirements of dogs for vitamins A and E, zinc, and linoleic acid if given at the manufacturers' recommended dose.[1] Only two products provided adequate amounts of three of the four nutrients. If doses of some products were increased to meet adequate levels of the most deficient nutrient, severe imbalances and toxicity were possible, and the cost of medication also increased.

Individual vitamins, minerals, and fatty acids are being used to treat specific dermatoses. The conditions may not reflect dietary deficiencies, and the nutrients may be acting to produce pharmacologic effects.[35] Vitamins A and E, zinc, and essential fatty acids are of most concern as specific medical supplements for skin health.

Vitamin A (retinol) must be available to cats, as they cannot convert β-carotene. In addition to its use for normal growth and differentiation of keratinocytes, vitamin A has important roles in the biosynthesis of mucopolysaccharides, labilization of lysosomal enzymes, inhibition of abnormal keratinization proliferation, suppression of size and function of sebaceous glands, modulation of neutrophil and macrophage function, and synthesis of prostaglandins. It has been useful in large doses for treating a specific follicular keratosis called vitamin-A–responsive dermatosis (see pp. 726, 799). An oral daily dosage of 1000 IU/kg is suggested, although larger doses can be given initially, with lower doses later in the course. Normal nutritional maintenance dose approximates 100 IU/kg/day, and the toxic dose is approximately 20,000 IU/kg daily.

A discussion of the retinoids (analogs of vitamin A) is found on p. 197.

Vitamin E is a fat-soluble natural antioxidant that is a mild antagonist to leukotriene formation. Excessive supplementation with fatty acids (especially unsaturated) may make vitamin E less available and may produce pansteatitis. Vitamin E has been used in the treatment of discoid lupus erythematosus, pemphigus erythematosus, epidermolysis bullosa, and acanthosis nigricans with variable results.[191] Recommended dosage of dl-α tocopherol acetate is 100-400 mg per animal twice daily for at least 30 to 60 days before its effect may be seen. Recently oral vitamin E was found to be of little if any value in treating dogs with allergic skin disease.[193]

Zinc is an important factor in many enzyme systems, and it also stabilizes cell and lysosomal membranes, depresses neutrophil and macrophage function, interferes with complement, is a lymphocyte mitogen, and generates specific cells involved in immunologic recognition.[1] Anecdotal comments have suggested it for treating burns, seborrhea, and recurrent pyoderma and to stimulate wound healing.[35]

Zinc has been shown to be effective in treating two specific dermatoses. One results from a probable genetic defect that is characterized by decreased intestinal absorption of zinc. This condition is seen primarily in Siberian huskies and Alaskan malamutes, but also in other large breeds such as Doberman pinschers and Great Danes. The other is a zinc-responsive dermatosis in dogs (often puppies) that are fed diets with excess ingredients that interfere with zinc absorption. These excess ingredients include calcium phytate (vegetable fiber and soybean meal), iron, tin, and copper. This interference provides a classic example of how excess use of nutritional supplements with a multitude of ingredients may do more harm than good. Recently oral administration of zinc was found to be of no value in treating dogs with allergic skin disease.[193]

Oral administration of zinc usually causes rapid resolution of the skin lesions.[135] However, others have reported that in zinc-related dermatosis of Siberian huskies (genetic problem) zinc sulfate is only effective if given intravenously.[173] Ten to 15 mg/kg IV is given every week for 4 to 6 weeks (without adverse effects) and then used as needed for maintenance. In the first type of disorder supplementation may be needed for life, while in the second, once the patient responds, zinc supplements can be halted if the dietary imbalances are corrected. Several zinc salts are effective. Zinc methionine (Zinpro) is said to be better absorbed, and therefore a dosage of 2 mg/kg/day elemental zinc is adequate. Zinc sulfate at a dosage of either 10 mg/kg/day (of the salt) or 4 mg/kg/day (of the elemental zinc) is appropriate. Zinc gluconate also is a satisfactory dosage form. More research is needed to determine the efficacy of different methods of zinc administration.

Fatty acids can be supplemented for their effect on the arachidonic acid cascade (p. 191) or as nutritional additions of essential (unsaturated) fatty acids. Of the three essential fatty acids—linoleic, linolenic, and arachidonic—dogs can synthesize the remaining two from linoleic acid. Cats, however, cannot synthesize arachidonic acid (found in fish oil and animal fats), and it must be supplied. This is one reason clinicians often suggest that home fat supplements be 50:50 animal fat and vegetable oil. Fatty acids are a source of calories, are vehicles for absorption of the fat-soluble vitamins, and are necessary for the synthesis of steroids and phospholipids. About 2 per cent of the caloric intake, or 0.22 gm/kg/day, of linoleic acid is needed for maintenance. Excessively high intakes will interfere with utilization of vitamin E and high fat intake may cause diarrhea, pansteatitis, or pancreatitis.

Retinoids

Naturally occurring vitamin A is an alcohol, all-trans retinol. It is oxidized in the body to retinal and retinoic acid. Each of these compounds has variable metabolic and biologic activities, although both are important in the induction and maintenance of normal growth and differentiation of keratinocytes. Depending on the amount present, retinoids can have either stimulatory or inhibitory effects on epidermal growth.[24] In normal skin, retinoids stimulate epidermal proliferation, but if skin lesions are already present, they reduce such proliferation. They are immunodulators with anti-inflammatory, antikeratinizing effects. They also reduce the size and output of sebaceous glands.

There are hundreds of synthetic agents related to vitamin A, and many of these are being evaluated for their ability to inhibit the formation of chemical-induced papillomas in mice, while producing no symptoms of vitamin A toxicity. Two compounds have been used clinically: isotretinoin (13-cis-retinoic acid), a natural metabolite of retinol marketed as Accutane; and etretinate, a synthetic retinoid only approved for use in Europe. Etretinate is more effective in psoriasis, but it is stored in the liver and therefore is potentially toxic.[30] Isotretinoin is used for people who have cystic acne and keratinization disorders (ichthyosis, pityriasis, multiple warts, keratoacanthoma, actinic keratosis, papillomatosis as well as basal cell tumors, and precancerous epithelial lesions). Although the side-effects are numerous and mimic hypervitaminosis A, the patients have normal vitamin A serum levels.

To date, these agents have not been highly effective in small animal dermatology. Topical forms are irritating and not easily adaptable to the hair-covered animal skin. Systemic use of isotretinoin in 10 cats with squamous cell carcinoma and preneoplastic lesions of the head was without benefit.[33] Fadok reported discouraging results of her own study and those of several other investigators who used isotretinoin for idiopathic (primary) seborrhea.[35] Isotretinoin has been used successfully in some cases of canine ichthyosis (see p. 747), feline acne (see p. 740), schnauzer comedo syndrome, granulomatous sebaceous adenitis, and epitheliotropic lymphoma (mycosis fungoides).[194] It was ineffective for epidermal dysplasia in West Highland white terriers.[194] A dosage of 0.25 to 1.0 mg/kg twice daily can be tried for 1 to 2 months, as long as patients are monitored periodically with physical examination, CBC, and serum chemistry findings, including triglycerides and cholesterol levels. Toxicities in small animals include conjunctivitis, periorbital erythema and edema, anorexia and lethargy, and xerostomia. Teratogenicity, skeletal exostoses, cheilitis, conjunctivitis, erythema, and pruritus have commonly been seen in humans.

HORMONAL AGENTS

Hormonal agents are an enigma. Dosage levels are critical, and maintenance of constant, uniform levels or planned fluctuating levels by replacement therapy may be crucial to a proper response. Many doses are determined empirically. Only a few preparations are prescribed effectively for specific skin effects.

Glucocorticoid Hormones

Glucocorticoid hormones have potent effects on the skin and are the most frequently prescribed drugs for dermatologic therapy. They profoundly affect immunologic and inflammatory activity. They block movement of neutrophils, eosinophils, and lymphocytes to the site of inflammation. T lymphocytes seem to be more affected than other lymphocyte populations. A wide range of lymphocyte functions important in inflammatory and immunologic responses is suppressed, including the following: cell activation, proliferation, and differentiation; mediator production and release; response to mediators; antigen recognition; and cytotoxic effector function.[126] Glucocorticoids also stabilize lysosomal membranes of neutrophil granules to inhibit release of enzymes important in the inflammatory response. Fibroblastic activity is reduced, synthesis of histamine is delayed, and complement is inhibited. Antibody production is not suppressed, but there is a decreased antibody response and effect. Prostaglandin and leukotriene production and release may also be affected, as cortisol blocks phospholipase A_2, which helps release arachidonic acid to start its inflammatory cascade. Glucocorticoid response to inflammatory stimuli is nonspecific. (It is the same whether it is a response to infection, trauma, toxin, or immune complex deposition.) The drug must reach the local site of inflammation to be effective, and the degree of response and cellular protection from injury is proportionate to the concentration of glucocorticoid in the inflamed tissue.[126] Thus, doses and dose intervals should vary depending on the patient's specific needs.

Several other factors influence the tissue glucocorticoid effect. One is the relative potency of the drug. Synthetic compounds made by adding methyl or fluoride groups to the basic steroid molecule increase the potency and the duration of action. Another factor is the effect of protein binding. Only free glucocorticoid is metabolically active.

Corticosteroid-binding globulin is a specific glycoprotein that binds glucocorticoids but it has a relatively low binding capacity. When large doses of glucocorticoids are administered, its capacity is exceeded, and albumin becomes the protein used for binding. Animals with low serum albumin have a lower binding capacity, and the excess unbound glucocorticoid becomes freely available, possibly producing toxicity.[55] In addition, the route of administration and water solubility affect the duration of action. Oral glucocorticoids, given as the free base or as esters, are rapidly absorbed. Parenteral glucocorticoids are usually esters of acetate, diacetate, phosphate, or succinate. The latter two are very water soluble and produce rapid serum levels of active drug, even when given intramuscularly. The acetate and diacetate esters, on the other hand, are not very water soluble and are slowly absorbed. As a result, they produce continuous low levels of glucocorticoid for days or weeks. The long effect produces significant adrenal suppression, a problem that can be avoided by giving short-acting glucocorticoids orally every other day.

Many of the desirable effects of glucocorticoids can be responsible for adverse effects if present in excess or at the wrong time. It is imperative to make an accurate diagnosis in order that the needed type, duration, and level of glucocorticoid can be provided. Except in the case of hypoadrenocorticism, glucocorticoids do not correct a primary cause, but act symptomatically or palliatively. The anti-inflammatory and immunosuppressive actions desired for one therapeutic need may facilitate the establishment or spread of concomitant infections or parasitic diseases. Animals treated with glucocorticoids have a tendency to develop bacterial infections of the skin, urinary, and respiratory systems.[55]

Indications for Use. The major indications for glucocorticoid therapy are hypersensitivity dermatoses (flea bite hypersensitivity, atopy, food hypersensitivity), pyotraumatic dermatitis ("hot spot"), contact dermatitis (irritant or hypersensitivity), autoimmune dermatoses (pemphigus, pemphigoid, lupus erythematosus), and acral lick dermatitis (see Table 4:8). Glucocorticoids are usually only *part* of the management employed for most dermatoses, and the clinician must control or minimize other predisposing, precipitating, and complicating factors to keep the glucocorticoids in their proper perspective, that is, to use them (1) as infrequently as possible, (2) at as low a dose as possible, (3) in alternate-day regimens whenever possible, and (4) only when other less hazardous forms of therapy have failed or could not be employed.[70]

Table 4:8. CANINE AND FELINE DERMATOSES AMENABLE TO ANTI-INFLAMMATORY AND IMMUNOSUPPRESSIVE DOSES OF GLUCOCORTICOIDS

Anti-inflammatory	Immunosuppressive
Pyotraumatic dermatitis	Pemphigus
Allergic dermatitis (parasitic, inhalant, food, drug)	Pemphigoid
Contact dermatitis (irritant, hypersensitive)	Lupus erythematosus (systemic, discoid)
Urticaria/angioedema	Cold hemagglutinin disease
Seborrheic dermatitis	Vasculitis
Acral lick dermatitis	Epidermolysis bullosa simplex
Solar dermatitis	Sterile panniculitis
Acanthosis nigricans	Vogt-Koyanagi-Harada–like syndrome
	Canine sterile eosinophilic pustulosis
	Sterile pyogranuloma syndrome
	Feline indolent ulcer
	Feline eosinophilic plaque
	Feline and canine eosinophilic granuloma

Administration. For dermatoses, glucocorticoids are usually administered orally, by injection (intramuscularly, subcutaneously, intralesionally), topically, or in some combination thereof. In any one patient, the decision as to which route or routes to employ depends on various factors.

Of the systemic routes, oral administration is preferred because (1) it can be more closely regulated (a daily dose is more precise than with a repository injection; the drug can be rapidly withdrawn if undesirable side-effects occur), and (2) it is the *only* safe, therapeutic, physiologic way to administer glucocorticoids for more long-term therapy.[27, 130, 138, 141]

Injectable glucocorticoids are usually administered intramuscularly or subcutaneously. Although most injectable glucocorticoids are licensed for intramuscular use, many clinicians administer them subcutaneously. The reasons for choosing the subcutaneous route are (1) there are fewer patient objections (and fewer pet owner crises!), and (2) it is clinically as effective as intramuscular administration. There is a theoretic preference for using the intramuscular route in the obese patient, since subcutaneous deliveries could be sequestered in fat tissue.

Intralesional injections of glucocorticoids are often thought of as local, intracutaneous therapy, devoid of any systemic effect. Intralesional therapy is employed for solitary or multiple cutaneous lesions, but it has systemic effects, some of which can be serious.

Choosing a Glucocorticoid. The choice of a glucocorticoid may be difficult. One cannot establish a single rule or set of rules that will apply to all patients with any given glucocorticoid-responsive dermatosis. Factors that must be considered include the duration of therapy, the personality of the patient, the personality and reliability of the owner, the response of the patient to the drug, the response of the patient's *disease* to the drug, and other patient–disease considerations.

The personality of the patient can significantly influence the choice of glucocorticoid; witness the attempts to pill the obstreperous cat that is a blur of fur, fangs, and claws. Likewise, the reliability of the owner can be the deciding factor—remember that there are owners who cannot, or will not, give oral medicaments to their pets.

The clinician will learn, by history or personal experience, that some glucocorticoids do not seem to work as well as others in certain patients. The problem probably reflects dosage, absorption, and metabolic differences. As a corollary, the clinician should note that in some patients a glucocorticoid that once was satisfactory apparently loses its effectiveness. For example, in an atopic dog that initially did well on prednisolone, the prednisolone seemed to lose its effect. Subsequently, the dog responded well to equipotent doses of orally administered triamcinolone. In most cases, after a variable length of time, the clinician would be able to return to successfully managing the dog with prednisolone. This well-recognized but poorly understood phenomenon is called steroid tachyphylaxis.[27]

Finally, the clinician may discover, by history or personal experience, that a patient can receive certain glucocorticoids without significant adverse effects, but not others. Hence, a dog may develop colitis or behavioral changes on prednisolone but not on triamcinolone.

Therapeutic Dosage. Optimal therapeutic doses have not been scientifically determined for *any* glucocorticoid in *any* canine or feline dermatosis. Presently espoused "anti-inflammatory," "antipruritic," "antiallergic," or "immunosuppressive" glucocorticoid doses have been determined through years of clinical experience. Moreover, it is imperative to remember that every patient is an individual and that *glucocorticoid therapy must be individualized.* Recommended glucocorticoid doses are guidelines and nothing more.

Use the smallest possible dose for the shortest possible time.

The two most commonly used oral glucocorticoids are prednisolone and prednisone. For all practical purposes, these two drugs are identical (the choice of one or the other usually is made on the basis of cost). Remember, however, that prednisone must be converted in the liver to prednisolone, the active form. Dosage recommendations in this text will be based on prednisolone (prednisone) equivalents. Table 4:9 contains information on approximately equipotent dosages of other oral glucocorticoids.

Table 4:9. CHARACTERISTICS OF VARIOUS GLUCOCORTICOIDS FOR ADMINISTRATION*

Drug	Glucocorticoid Potency†	HPA‡ Axis-Suppressive Activity	Suitable for Alternate-Day Steroid Therapy	Equivalent Dose (mg)
Short-Acting				
Hydrocortisone	1.0	+	No	20
Prednisolone	4.0	+	Yes	5
Prednisone	4.0	+	Yes	5
Methylprednisolone	5.0	+	Yes	4
Intermediate-Acting				
Triamcinolone	5.0	+ +	No	4
Long-Acting				
Flumethasone	15.0	+ + +	No	1.5
Dexamethasone	30.0	+ + +	No	0.75
Betamethasone	30.0	+ + +	No	0.60

*From Scott, D. W.: Dermatologic use of glucocorticoids. Vet. Clin. North Am. (Small Anim. Pract.) *12*:19, 1982.
†Compared with hydrocortisone on a mg-for-mg basis.
‡HPA = hypothalamic-pituitary-adrenal.

"Physiologic" doses of glucocorticoids are those that approximate the daily cortisol (hydrocortisone) production by normal individuals. In dogs, daily cortisol production has been reported to be 0.2 to 1 mg/kg per day.[104, 138, 141, 145] No such information is available for cats. "Pharmacologic" doses of glucocorticoids are those that exceed physiologic requirements. Significantly, *any* pharmacologic dose of glucocorticoid, no matter how large or small, suppresses the hypothalamic-pituitary-adrenal axis.[27, 126, 141, 152]

Dermatologically speaking, clinicians usually talk in terms of anti-inflammatory versus immunosuppressive doses of glucocorticoids. A commonly used *anti-inflammatory* (as in allergic dermatoses) *induction* dose of oral glucocorticoid in dogs is 1.1 mg prednisolone/kg/day SID. A commonly used *anti-inflammatory maintenance* dose for dogs is 0.55 to 1.1 mg prednisolone/kg every other morning. For autoimmune dermatoses, a commonly used *immunosuppressive induction* dose for dogs is 2.2 to 4.4 mg prednisolone/kg/day SID. A commonly used *immunosuppressive maintenance* dose for dogs is 1.1 to 2.2 mg prednisolone/kg every other morning.

In general, compared with dogs, cats require about twice the dose of glucocorticoid orally for induction and maintenance therapy.[23] In addition, maintenance doses of glucocorticoid in cats are administered every other evening.[138, 139, 145] It is probable that the diurnal rhythm of dogs and cats is not dramatic, and timing dosages to morning or evening hours is less important than was previously thought. It is important, however, to maintain the 24-hour alternate-day freedom from medication in order that adrenal suppression is avoided.

An excellent injectable anti-inflammatory glucocorticoid is methylprednisolone aetate (Depo-Medrol). Clinically, dogs are given doses of 1.1 mg/kg, subcutaneously or intramuscularly, and the effect usually lasts for 1 to 3 weeks. In cats, this product is administered at a dose of 5.5 mg/kg (20 mg per cat), subcutaneously or intramuscularly, and the effect may last for 1 week to 6 months. Other commonly used injectable glucocorticoids (and their clinical duration of effect) include prednisolone (1 to 2 days), dexamethasone (1 to 7 days), and betamethasone (7 to 60 days).

Methylprednisolone acetate can be used for intralesional therapy (as in acral lick dermatitis or feline indolent ulcers, eosinophilic granuloma, and eosinophilic plaques). In practice, " intralesional" is a misnomer. Owing to the nature of these dermatoses, most injections are in fact sublesional. In general, a volume of methylprednisolone acetate (20 mg/ml) should be used that is sufficient to undermine the lesion (10 to 40 mg total dose). The usual recommendation for intralesional glucocorticoid therapy in humans is 0.1 ml of triamcinolone acetonide (10 mg/ml) per site.[90] Remember these injections are in fact systemic and will produce systemic effects. Use care in establishing dosage.

Recently glucocorticoid "pulse" therapy has been used in humans and dogs with various immunologic dermatoses which were refractory to standard glucocorticoid regimens.[194] Dogs were hospitalized and given 11 mg/kg methylprednisolone sodium succinate intravenously in 250 ml of 5 per cent dextrose and water during a 1-hour period for 3 consecutive days. The reported advantages of glucocorticoid pulse therapy include immediate symptomatic relief, avoidance of side-effects seen with high-dose oral dosage of glucocorticoids, and the ability to lower the dosage or discontinue the use of oral glucocorticoids after the pulse therapy. In humans, potential side-effects (uncommon) of pulse therapy include duodenal ulcers, sudden electrolyte shifts, cardiac arrest, anaphylaxis, and sudden death. This treatment modality requires further evaluation in veterinary medicine.

Regimen. Glucocorticoid regimens will vary with the nature of the dermatosis, the specific glucocorticoid being used, and the use of induction versus maintenance therapy.

In general, dermatoses requiring anti-inflammatory doses of oral glucocorticoid require smaller doses and shorter periods of daily induction therapy to bring about remission, as compared with dermatoses requiring immunosuppressive doses. Anti-inflammatory induction doses are usually given for 5 to 10 days, whereas immunosuppressive induction doses are often administered for 10 to 21 days.

The key, in therapy, is to continue daily induction doses until disease activity is completely suppressed.

Maintenance therapy with oral glucocorticoid is best accomplished with prednisolone, prednisone, or methylprednisolone (see Table 4:9) on an alternate-day basis.[23, 37a, 104, 141, 145, 152] With alternate-day therapy, the daily dose of glucocorticoid used for successful induction therapy is given as a single massive dose, every other morning for dogs and every other evening for cats. This alternate-day dose is reduced by 50 per cent, 1 week at a time, until the lowest satisfactory maintenance dose is achieved. This regimen does not eliminate adrenal atrophy, but it is less severe and its onset is delayed. *It is the only dosage system that should be used for long-term therapy of steroid-responsive diseases in small animals.* In some animals, alternate-day glucocorticoid therapy can be extended to every third or fourth day. Rarely, anti-inflammatory alternate-day glucocorticoid therapy with the preferred prednisolone, prednisone, or methylprednisolone will not be successful. In these cases, the clinician has three therapeutic options (assuming that glucocorticoid therapy is all that can be done): (1) administer prednisolone, prednisone, or methylprednisolone on a *daily* basis, informing the owner of the inevitability of iatrogenic hyperglucocorticoidism; (2) switch to a more potent oral glucocorticoid on an alternate-day basis; or (3) switch to injectable glucocorticoids. Although the more potent oral glucocorticoids are usually not satisfactory for alternate-day therapy (because of potency and duration of effect, they do not spare the hypothalamic-pituitary-adrenal axis [see Table 4-9]), they can occasionally be employed with few or no significant side-effects, especially in cats. Clinically, the most satisfactory agents in this respect appear to be triamcinolone, dexamethasone, and flumethasone. Some animals can be satisfactorily managed only with injectable glucocorticoids.

In the long-term management of animals on glucocorticoid therapy, periodic urinalysis and urine cultures should be obtained to recognize urinary tract infections that are not clinically apparent.

In contrast to anti-inflammatory glucocorticoid therapy, dermatoses requiring immunosuppressive induction doses are often unmanageable with alternate-day glucocorticoid maintenance therapy. For example, with pemphigus and pemphigoid, glucocorticoids were unsatisfactory as the sole form of therapy in over 50 per cent of the cases.[143]

While intramuscular or subcutaneous glucocorticoid therapy is usually fine for induction therapy, it is often unsatisfactory for dermatoses that require chronic maintenance therapy. Although definitive studies are needed for dogs and cats, clinical experience suggests that (as is usually the case in humans) if repository glucocorticoids (methylprednisolone acetate, triamcinolone acetonide) are given no more often than every 2 months, side-effects will usually be negligible. It has been shown that a single intramuscular injection of methylprednisolone acetate (Depo-Medrol) is capable of altering adrenocortical function in dogs for at least 5 weeks.[68, 69] In another study,[141] it was shown that a single intramuscular injection of triamcinolone acetonide (Vetalog) was capable of altering adrenocortical function in dogs for up to 4 weeks.

Intralesional injections of glucocorticoids are usually repeated every 7 to 10 days until the dermatosis is in remission (usually two to four treatments) and then given as needed.

Side-Effects. The side-effects associated with systemic glucocorticoid therapy are best discussed under two separate categories: those seen with anti-inflammatory doses and those seen with immunosuppressive doses.[37a, 45, 104, 140, 145, 152]

Expected side-effects with anti-inflammatory induction therapy include polydipsia, polyuria, and polyphagia. These are usually unavoidable, of little health significance, tolerated by most owners, and eliminated or greatly minimized when alternate-day maintenance therapy is achieved. Far less common, but much more alarming, are behavioral changes (depression, somnolence, viciousness), panting, and diarrhea (may be bloody). These usually necessitate stopping therapy (herein lies a major advantage of *oral* therapy!) and can often be minimized or eliminated by switching to a different glucocorticoid.

Side-effects with alternate-day anti-inflammatory maintenance regimens are usually minimal, the most common being polydipsia and polyuria on the day of glucocorticoid administration and a tendency toward minor weight gain and a dull, dry hair coat. Occult urinary tract infections can be troublesome, and patients on long-term alternate-day steroid therapy should receive occasional urinalyses. Again, switching to a different glucocorticoid may reduce or eliminate some of these side-effects. Methylprednisolone has less tendency to produce polydipsia and polyuria than prednisone or prednisolone.

Immunosuppressive induction and maintenance regimens produce side-effects that are much more common and much more severe. Obviously, this effect is related to the dose of glucocorticoid required to control the dermatoses in question. The traditional immunosuppressive dose of prednisolone (2.2 mg/kg/day) may be ineffective. The clinically superior immunosuppressive dose of prednisolone (4.4 to 6.6 mg/kg/day) may be satisfactory in less than 50 per cent of cases and may result in death due to acute pancreatitis after 7 to 10 days of therapy. It may produce unacceptable side-effects (extreme polydipsia, polyuria, and polyphagia; muscle weakness and wasting; hepatopathy; severe depression; and diarrhea) or lack of efficacy.[143]

In summary, significant side-effects with appropriate anti-inflammatory systemic glucocorticoid regimens are uncommon in dogs, occurring in less than 10 per cent of the animals treated. However, with immunosuppressive regimens, the incidence and severity of glucocorticoid side-effects escalate alarmingly, and less than 50 per cent of the dogs so treated can be satisfactorily managed.

It must be emphasized that alternate-day therapy with prednisolone is not a panacea. Occasionally, some dogs (and people) cannot be successfully managed with such therapy without developing iatrogenic hyperglucocorticoid-ism.[37a, 143] This probably reflects differences in serum protein levels or in absorption, metabolism, or clearance of glucocorticoid in those individuals. Additionally, occasional dramatic individual variation is observed in suscepti-bility to acute or chronic glucocorticoid side-effects[145]; therefore, (1) one can see various degrees of iatrogenic hyperglucocorticoidism after as little as 3 weeks to as long as 7 years of therapy, and (2) one may see only calcinosis cutis or full-blown Cushing's syndrome as an individual dog's manifestation of hyper-glucocorticoidism.[140, 141, 145] Although clinically effective doses of systemic glu-cocorticoids in cats are usually twice those needed in dogs, significant side-effects are rare.[139, 141, 145] Polydipsia, polyuria, polyphagia, a tendency for weight gain, depression, and diarrhea are occasionally seen. Significant iatrogenic hyperglucocorticoidism has been produced in cats only after the *weekly* subcu-taneous administration of methylprednisolone acetate for 10 weeks. Obviously, such therapy would never be either employed or indicated in clinical situa-tions.

Significant side-effects following intralesional glucocorticoid therapy have not been reported in dogs and cats. Local cutaneous atrophy and local inflammatory reactions (presumably due to crystalline material left at the injection site) are rarely seen. These side-effects, as well as panniculitis, sterile abscesses, necrosis, and pigmentary disturbances, are well recognized in humans.[45, 90, 152]

A potentially much more significant side-effect of intralesional therapy is systemic hyperglucocorticoidism.[11, 18, 34] Normal dogs given subconjunctival injections of methylprednisolone acetate had suppressed adrenocortical re-sponses to exogenous adrenocorticotropic hormone (ACTH) for 9 to 20 days.[123] Additionally, dogs that received intracutaneous or subconjunctival injections of methylprednisolone or betamethasone were unresponsive to intradermal histamine and skin test allergens for up to 4 weeks.[138] Even short-term topical glucocorticoid medications have been shown to depress adrenal function for at least 2 weeks.[102] The health significance of such findings in dogs and humans is unknown. Certainly such medications could influence interpretation of results of hematologic, adrenal function, and intradermal allergy skin tests.

Evaluation. Evaluation of results during corticosteroid therapy is very important. When appropriate systemic anti-inflammatory glucocorticoid ther-apy is given to an otherwise healthy dog or cat, the risks are minimal. The risks associated with immunosuppressive doses are of greater concern, espe-cially since the medication is usually prescribed for serious or life-threatening diseases. Significant concurrent dysfunction of major organ systems will also drastically increase the risks. Some owners balk at the expense, risk, and unpleasant side-effects or at the complex therapy protocol, and they refuse treatment. Occasionally, the clinician may be forced to choose between using drugs that may not be in the animal's best long-term interest or performing euthanasia at the owner's request.

When long-term systemic therapy is started, owners should be instructed to observe their animals closely and report immediately any significant side-effects. A physical check-up and urinalysis are advised every 3 to 4 months before more medication is dispensed. The ACTH response test is useful in such cases. Animals (except cats) on such regimens often have depressed ACTH responses and elevated serum alkaline phosphatase levels, but otherwise they usually are clinically normal.

Thyroid Hormones

Thyroid hormones can be replaced successfully by oral medication and are indicated as replacement therapy for primary, secondary, and tertiary hypothyroidism, for adjunctive management of some canine pyodermas and of idiopathic seborrhea syndromes, and for feline symmetric alopecia (feline endocrine alopecia).[129] The administration of thyroid hormones can force varying degrees of hair growth in normal dogs as well as in dogs and cats with various nonthyroidal dermatoses.

The metabolically active thyroid hormones are L-thyroxine (T_4), which is the main secretory product of the thyroid gland, and L-triiodothyronine (T_3), which is 3 to 5 times more potent than T_4 and secreted in small amounts by the thyroid gland. L-thyroxine acts as a prohormone, being deiodinated by peripheral tissues to the more potent T_3, as needed. In dogs, 40 to 60 per cent of T_3 is derived this way.[37] This control mechanism serves to safeguard against T_3 deficiency in critical tissues. In addition, the liver and kidneys can concentrate thyroid hormone and may exchange hormone rapidly with the plasma, if necessary. As is true of many other hormones, only thyroid hormones that are unbound (to protein) are metabolically active. In dogs, only about 0.1 per cent of total serum T_4 and 1.0 per cent of serum T_3 are free. The plasma half-life of T_4 is 10 to 16 hours, while that of T_3 is 5 to 6 hours. These figures reflect plasma disappearance and do not indicate the extent of biologic half-life. Although T_4 and T_3 are measured in thyroid hormone serum levels, approximately 50 to 60 per cent of the body's T_4 and 90 to 95 per cent of the T_3 are intracellular. Thus, laboratory data, especially of T_3, do not provide a highly accurate estimate of the total body pool.

The *bioavailability* and efficacy of administered thyroid hormones depend on the route of administration, absorption, peripheral metabolism, quantity of pooled hormone in cellular stores, and persistence of biologic effects.[37]

Dogs are thought to absorb only 10 to 50 per cent of an oral dose of T_4, while absorption of T_3 may be much higher.[34] In peripheral tissues, conversion of T_4 to T_3 may be impaired by starvation, surgery, diabetes mellitus, and other chronic illnesses such as liver and renal disease. These nonthyroid illnesses produce a syndrome called the "euthyroid sick syndrome," characterized by low tissue levels of T_3 and T_4 (see p. 578). It may be an adaptive mechanism to limit the catabolic state of illness or malnutrition. Low laboratory-derived hormone levels in this syndrome or in drug-induced T_3 reductions do not constitute an indication for thyroid hormone supplementation.

There are four types of thyroid hormone medications. (1) Crude preparations from desiccated thyroid tissue (Thyroid USP) have a variable hormone content and an uncertain shelf life. They should not be used. (2) Synthetic thyroid hormone combinations are intended to mimic the T_4:T_3 ratio in humans (4:1). However, since the ratio in dogs is 6:1, these products are expensive, they introduce complex dosage problems, and they have an increased potential for causing thyrotoxicosis. These, also, should not be used.

(3) Synthetic L-thyroxine is the medication of choice for hypothyroidism. It is the main natural secretory product and, by virtue of being the prohormone, provides the hormone replacement in a physiologic manner. It also aids in the proper feedback for thyroid-stimulating hormone (TSH) release and is inexpensive. It has been recommended that only Synthroid or Soloxine be used, *not* the generic products. However, many clinicians use the generic products with

few or no problems. Recommended oral dosages vary from 0.02 to 0.04 mg/kg daily with a total daily maximum of 0.9 mg per patient, to 20 µg/kg BID (Table 4:10). For maximum absorption, this should be given when the patient is in a fasted state. Since the dosage is proportional to the metabolic rate, a better schedule might be 0.5 mg/M_2 BSA.[22] Dividing the dose and giving it every 12 hours may produce a more physiologic effect and is recommended at least for the 4 to 6 week induction period as tissue storage levels are replenished.

The dosage in cats (for hypothyroidism following treatment to ablate thyroid glands in hyperthyroidism) is 0.05 to 0.20 mg per cat daily.[37]

(4) Synthetic L-triiodothyronine (Cytobin, Cytomel) is the active intracellular hormone, but usually it should not be used for routine treatment of hypothyroidism, as it by-passes the normal physiologic and cellular regulatory pathway. Because it has a short half-life, even administration at short intervals tends to produce frequent high peaks of the drug, which favors toxicity. It may be indicated in so-called poor converters—those very rare individuals who cannot convert T_4 to T_3. It may also be indicated when thyroid replacement is needed with simultaneous administration of drugs that inhibit conversion of T_4 to T_3 (i.e., pharmacologic doses of glucocorticoids). Oral dosage, if needed, would be 4 to 6 µg/kg TID or perhaps BID. Dosage in cats has been reported as starting at 20 µg per cat twice daily, but increasing gradually to 50 µg twice daily by 2 weeks.[162]

Response to therapy with either of the above medications will be seen with increased activity and mental alertness in 10 to 14 days; hair regrowth will be observed at 4 to 6 weeks, but 4 to 5 months are necessary for complete regrowth; reduction in hyperpigmentation will be seen in 3 to 6 months; and reduction of recurrent pyoderma will occur in 3 to 4 months. In treatment for feline symmetric alopecia, total hair regrowth has occurred by 12 weeks.[162]

Table 4:10. DOSE RECOMMENDATIONS FOR INITIATION OF THYROID HORMONE REPLACEMENT THERAPY*

Preparation†	Generic Name	Dog	Cat
L-thyroxine (T_4)	Levothyroxine	20–40 µg/kg‡ given once daily (use higher dose per kg for smaller animals) or 20 µg/kg§ given every 12 hours	20 µg/kg§ given every 12 or 24 hours
L-triiodothyronine (T_3)	Liothyronine	4.4–6.6 µg/kg‖ given every 8 hours	
L-thyroxine and L-triiodothyronine combined (T_4:T_3)		20 µg/kg T_4: 5 µg/kg T_3 given every 12 hours (dosage actually computed on basis of T_4 content of product)¶	

*Modified from Rosychuk, R. A. W.: Thyroid hormones and antithyroid drugs. Vet. Clin. North Am. (Small Anim. Pract.) *12*:111, 1982.
†Approximate biologic dose equivalents: 0.1 mg T_4 = 25 µg T_3 = 1 grain (65 mg) desiccated thyroid/thyroglobulin.
‡20–32 µg/kg = 0.02–0.032 mg/kg or 0.1 mg per 7–11 lbs.
§20 µg/kg = 0.1 mg/11 lbs. See text for rationale.
‖4.4 µg/kg = 2 µg/lb.
¶Computed on the basis of T_4 content of product: 1 grain equivalent of these products equals 50–60 µg T_4 and 12.5–15 µg T_3 and is equivalent in biologic potency to 1 grain desiccated thyroid.

While these clinical evaluations are the best measure of successful replacement, there may be equivocal responses that should be studied by measuring serum hormone levels. T_3 is primarily intracellular and difficult to measure, and a protocol is not well delineated. T_4, however, can be measured by the post pill test. This should only be done when the animal is in a "steady state," having been on regular medication for at least 1 month. For dogs on adequate, once-daily medication, testing just before medication should show normal or low normal serum thyroxine (T_4) levels. Animals on once- or twice-daily medication should be checked 4 to 8 hours after receiving a dose, when the serum levels should be high normal, or slightly higher. If levels are not normal, the dosage should be increased and testing should be repeated 1 month later.

Complications with therapy involve medication for patients with concurrent cardiac or adrenal insufficiencies or thyrotoxicosis. Initiating T_4 medication may rapidly increase tissue metabolism and exhaust the cardiac reserve of a marginally coping heart or may exacerbate an adrenal crisis. With cardiac patients, start T_4 at one-fourth the recommended dosage and increase slowly to full dose by 4 weeks (see p. 651). Patients with hypoadrenocorticism should have glucocorticoid therapy instituted prior to T_4 replacement. Thyrotoxicosis is rare in dogs but may be evidenced by polyuria and polydipsia, nervousness, panting, weight loss, tachycardia, hypertension, and pruritus. Stop medication, perform a serum thyroxine determination, and reinstitute medication at a lower dose after clinical status improves.

Growth Hormone

Growth hormone (GH) deficiency can be divided into two groups: primary GH deficiency, and GH deficiency secondary to causes such as hypothyroidism, hyperadrenocorticism, or zinc deficiency. In the secondary forms, treatment of the primary cause produces a satisfactory response, since secretory capacity of GH returns to normal.[29] There are two canine syndromes that respond to GH therapy: pituitary dwarfism and hyposomatotropism in the mature dog (see pp. 611, 615.)

Growth hormone is expensive and difficult to obtain. Human GH is active in phylogenetically lower animals such as dogs. Nonprimate GH preparations (feline, canine, bovine, porcine, ovine) are immunologically interrelated, and all except ovine appear to be effective for small animal therapy.

Treatment must be given by subcutaneous injections. For pituitary dwarfism, 10.0 IU of bovine GH, or 2.0 IU of porcine GH, can be given three times a week for 4 to 6 weeks. For hyposomatotropism in mature dogs (pseudo-Cushing's disease), either of the above products can be given every other day for 10 injections. For dogs less than 14 kg body weight, the dose is 2.5 IU per injection, and for those over 14 kg body weight it is 5.0 IU per injection.

With successful therapy, hair growth should be evident in 4 to 6 weeks. If alopecia develops again, GH treatment can be repeated. Some dogs may become unresponsive, perhaps because antibodies develop against GH, which decrease its biologic activity.

Limited supplies of synthetic human GH manufactured by recombinant DNA techniques have become available and seem to hold promise for human use. Their effect in animals is unknown at this date. The future use of GH-releasing factor for dogs that have hypothalamic disease resulting in GH deficiency may hold promise.[29]

Therapy with GH involves some risks. Diabetes mellitus may develop, although it may resolve when treatment is halted. Acromegaly may be produced, or patients may develop anaphylaxis during retreatment.

Sex Hormones

When it comes to replacement therapy, sex hormones are an enigma. Most hormones are present in both sexes and their levels in blood fluctuate markedly during the day. The available assays are expensive and often unsatisfactory, in part because there are many compounds related to one hormone and the assay system only measures one compound.

In addition, androgens and estrogens are produced by the adrenal glands and gonads, or by peripheral conversion. Abnormalities of sex hormone tissue receptors and sex hormone binding protein may markedly affect the biologic availability of hormones. (Over 90 per cent of sex steroids are protein bound and inactive.)[98] All the doses of sex hormones given in this section are empirical. Please refer to Chap. 10, Cutaneous Endocrinology, and to the references for more detailed information.

Estrogens are indicated in estrogen-responsive dermatosis of female dogs (ovarian imbalance type II) and have been used in a repositol injectable form at a 1:20 ratio with testosterone for the treatment of feline symmetric alopecia of cats. In dogs, diethylstilbestrol 0.02 mg/kg up to 1 mg total can be given orally once daily for 14 days, then every other day for 14 days, and then twice weekly (see p. 627). Long-term maintenance can be continued with that dose once or twice weekly.[129] Initial hair regrowth should be evident in 2 to 4 weeks, with complete response in 2 to 3 months. Do not continue the treatment for more than 3 months if there is no response.

Complications of estrogen therapy include: induction of estrus, bone marrow suppression in dogs (anemia, leukopenia, thrombocytopenia),[161] and hepatotoxicity. Cats are highly sensitive to estrogens, and lethal effects are common with a total dose of 10 mg, even when the hormones are administered over several weeks. With intact females, the possibility of abortion or pyometra should be considered, while in males, prostatic hyperplasia may result.

Androgens are indicated in testosterone-responsive dermatosis of male dogs, idiopathic male feminizing syndrome, and feline symmetric alopecia, which also is probably not an endocrine disorder. Methyltestosterone (Metandren) and fluoxymesterone (Halotestin) can be given every other day in oral doses of 0.5 mg/kg, up to a total maximum of 30 mg. Testosterone propionate aqueous suspension in propylene glycol/alcohol or in oil can be given once weekly IM at doses of 0.5 to 1.0 mg/kg.[129] The latter drug can be given once IM to cats with feline symmetric alopecia in a total dose of 12 mg. It is often combined with 0.6 mg of repositol stilbestrol or 0.5 mg of repositol estradiol. Successful treatment should produce significant regrowth of hair within 2 to 3 months.

Complications include aggressive behavior and hepatotoxicity. It is advisable to have baseline liver profiles prior to initiating therapy. In addition, cats on testosterone may spray urine the first few days.

PROGESTAGENS

Progestational compounds have been used rather indiscriminately in recent years in the management of behavioral disorders and the treatment of a variety of nonspecific inflammatory dermatoses. They suppress release of gonadotropin and ACTH and have variable effects on androgens and estrogens in different species, depending on the dose and the target organ.[74] They also induce GH release and act on the hypothalamus and the limbic system.

Two synthetic progestagens are used in small animal dermatology and have rather similar effects. They can often be used interchangeably, although in some cases one product is better than the other.[108]

Megestrol acetate (MA) (Ovaban, Megace) is an oral drug originally marketed to suppress canine estrus and still not approved in the United States for feline dermatoses. It has potent anti-inflammatory effects, especially in cats; but in the usual dose has been shown to produce more and longer lasting adrenal suppression than anti-inflammatory doses of prednisolone.[96] It has also been blamed for development of diabetes mellitus, but one study showed no change in glucose tolerance curves after 3 weeks of therapy with MA.[92] Dosage of MA in dogs with behavioral dermatoses is 2 to 4 mg/kg daily. For induction with cats, the dosage is 2.5 to 5.0 mg per cat every other day, declining to 2.5 to 5.0 mg every 7 to 14 days for maintenance. This is a potent drug with serious toxic potential, and it should not be used if alternative therapy is available (see following discussion).

Medroxyprogesterone acetate (MPA) (Depo-Provera) is an injectable repository progestagen. Repository progesterone in oil is also available. Because progestagens can have serious side-effects, injectable long-lasting dosage forms should only be used if the short-acting (and thus, safer) oral products present problems of administration. Dosages are 50 to 100 mg per cat and 20 mg/kg for dogs. Repeat only if needed in 3 to 6 months.

Clinical usage of the above progestagens has been rather empirical, and much of the rationale revolves around behavioral modification to prevent self-trauma.

In dogs, boredom dermatoses may be ameliorated with this treatment, and so flank sucking, acral lick dermatitis, tail biting, and foot sucking are some of its typical uses. Canine hormonal alopecias that do not respond to other hormone therapy may benefit from a short course and low dosage of MA.[74]

In cats, progestagen therapy may benefit indolent ulcers, eosinophilic plaques, and eosinophilic granulomas, but especially alopecias that are due to licking and itching. It has been helpful in feline symmetric alopecia (so-called feline endocrine alopecia) and feline hyperesthesia syndrome.[74] Because it has antiandrogen effects, it has been advocated for stud tail in male cats.

Several major side-effects must be considered when progestagen therapy is contemplated. Truly hormonal problems are decreased spermatogenesis, development of pyometra, and postponement of estrus. GH levels increase and acromegaly may develop. Mammary gland fibroadenomatous hyperplasia is seen in both intact and neutered male and female cats and has little correlation with dose or frequency of medication. Some cases regress when treatment is halted, but in others the mammary tissue ulcerates and neoplasms may develop, necessitating surgical removal.

Diabetes mellitus has been reported in cats being treated with MA.[113] Some cases require insulin, but usually the disorder is transient and spontaneously regresses.

Behavioral abnormalities are common. Often the animals are more affectionate and slightly lethargic and have polydipsia and polyphagia. Consequently, they gain weight.

The most serious side-effect is adrenocortical suppression, which occurs with even low doses and persists for many weeks, probably because of the long half-life of the progestagens.[96] *This suppression is a major reason to avoid these drugs.*

The *gonadotropins and prolactin* are adenohypophyseal hormones that are stimulated by hypothalamic releasing factors and that regulate endogenous sex hormones. They are involved in complex interhormonal reactions, and specifically targeted effects are not possible. Until small animal hormone relationships are better understood and more easily measured, these compounds will not be useful in routine dermatology practice.

Skin Surgery

Skin surgery can be an important part of small animal dermatology. From skin biopsies for diagnosis to cryosurgery for specialized procedures, many new developments have been seen in recent years. It is essential to know what equipment is needed and to have appropriate knowledge to use the equipment properly. Cold steel surgery, cryosurgery, laser surgery, and electrosurgery will be discussed in this chapter. Biopsy techniques are covered in Chapter 3, Diagnostic Methods.

Dermatologists recommend plastic surgery for correction of anatomic defects causing dermatoses of facial, tail, vulva, and lip folds.[153] Skin grafting (pinch,[60] strip,[154] mesh,[156] and pedicle[67] grafts) is useful to repair defects of skin of the extremities where tumors or lesions such as acral lick dermatitis have been removed surgically. Plastic repair of ear flaps and the external ear canal[91, 116] may be helpful in correcting associated dermatologic or cosmetic problems. Plastic surgery techniques will not be discussed in this chapter, but information on them can be found in the references.[31, 153]

COLD STEEL SURGERY

Excision of small tumors and other lesions is a minor procedure that often can be done on an outpatient basis but usually is better performed if the animal is held in the hospital for several hours. This enables the practitioner to use tranquilization, sedation, or general anesthesia as needed to promote control and relaxation of the patient. Patients requiring extensive surgery with plastic repair procedures and grafts need an operating room with complete aseptic routine. Even minor cases, however, must be handled with proper preparation, sterile instruments, and other measures to accomplish a scrupulously clean operation.

The dermatologist who employs surgical treatment for human diseases usually performs minor techniques on skin that is relatively hairless; therefore the cosmetic effects are crucial. Most procedures appear complex because avoidance of scarring is a primary consideration. In veterinary dermatology the clinician should, of course, avoid disfigurement; but because of the dense pelage, small scars are relatively unimportant.

With any surgical procedure it is necessary to clip the hair closely, wash the unbroken skin surface carefully until it is clean using a surgical scrub solution such as 1 per cent chlorhexidine diacetate (Nolvasan) or 0.75 per cent povidone-iodine (Betadine), and rinse thoroughly. Defat the skin by wiping the surface in a circular fashion from the center outward, using sterile swabs soaked in 70 per cent alcohol. The skin can then be sprayed or swabbed with 0.5 per cent solution of chlorhexidine diacetate or, as a second choice, 1 per cent solution of povidone-iodine. The surgical site is then ready to drape.

Basic instruments needed for skin surgery are in the average emergency or spay pack. The following additional instruments are useful for the delicate work in many skin surgical procedures:

1. Bard-Parker handles and blades, Nos. 10, 11, and 15
2. Small curved mosquito hemostats
3. Allis's tissue forceps
4. Skin hooks (sharp single prong)
5. Iris forceps (mouse-toothed)
6. Olsen-Hegar needle holder with suture scissors
7. Skin punches sizes 1 to 9 mm
8. Small automatic skin retractor

The lesions should be outlined by elliptic scalpel incisions that extend through the skin. The specimen or lesion is dissected free from the underlying tissue with scissors or hemostats or both. Healing and final results will be better if the long axis incisions are oriented parallel to the tension lines shown in Figure 4:4. For closure, nylon sutures such as Vetafil will produce good approximation with minimal scarring. Many quality suture materials are available, and the exact selection is a matter of personal preference. Swaged-on needles can further reduce the chance of infection and result in smaller scars. In routine cases with small incisions, the sutures can be removed in 10 to 14 days.

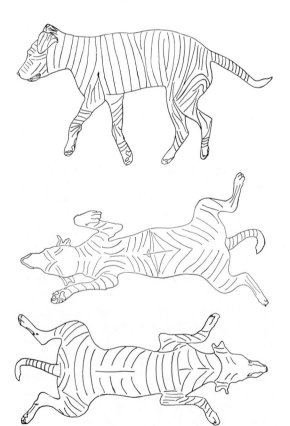

Figure 4:4. Composite drawing of the lateral, ventral, and dorsal aspects of a dog to show skin tension lines (based on six cases). (From Irwin D.H.G.: Tension lines in the skin of the dog. J. Small Anim. Pract. 7:593, 1966.)

CRYOSURGERY

Cryosurgery is the controlled use of freezing temperatures to destroy undesirable tissue, while doing minimal damage to surrounding healthy tissue. Cryosurgery was used clinically in human medicine in the early 1960s, and its use has become more widespread in dermatology since that time. In veterinary medicine, reports of its clinical use for malignant neoplasms began appearing from about 1970 to 1972. Further reports on the use of cryosurgery in small animal practice appeared for neoplastic and dermatologic conditions.[47, 59, 72] By 1982 it became clear that cryosurgery was especially useful in many conditions in which cold steel surgery was less effective. The anal and oral areas are preferred sites for cryosurgery, and there is indication for its use in selected acral lick dermatitis cases (lick granulomas). Specific conditions in which cryosurgery may be indicated include perianal fistulas, oral tumors, rectal tumors, nasal mucosal tumors, tail gland hyperplasia, feline indolent ulcers, and acral lick dermatitis. In the nasal, oral, and rectal areas where surgical access and hemostasis would be difficult, cryosurgery has real advantages. In large lesions of acral lick dermatitis that cannot be removed by cold steel surgery, cryosurgery offers a favorable alternative to skin grafting. For readers who are seriously considering using cryosurgery, an excellent reference is the book *Symposium on Cryosurgery*,[174] which covers all phases of small animal cryosurgery.

Discussion of cryosurgery will be divided into four sections: Basic Principles, Freezing Agents, Cryosurgical Units, and Dermatologic Indications for Cryosurgery.

Basic Principles of Cryosurgery

The lethal effect of subzero temperatures on cells depends on five factors:
1. Type of cell being frozen
2. Rate of freezing
3. Final temperature (must be at least $-20°C$)
4. Rate of thawing
5. Repetition of the freeze–thaw cycle

Cell damage is more severe with rapid freezing, slow thawing, and three freeze–thaw cycles. A final temperature of $-70°C$ is reached at the surface of the probe with nitrous oxide equipment, so that it can cool only a limited mass of tissue below the required $-20°C$, thereby restricting its application to small, superficial lesions. A final temperature of $-185°C$ can be reached at the tissue junction using liquid nitrogen. This enables the forming of a larger "ice ball" of tissue and allows larger areas to be effectively frozen.

A spray of liquid nitrogen offers the most effective way to freeze large tumor masses but also offers the greatest potential hazard if used carelessly. One advantage is that the base or periphery of a mass can be frozen first, by careful spraying around a delineated area extending 3 to 5 mm beyond the visible edge. The remaining tissues within this frozen "stockade" can be treated by spraying in ever-decreasing circles.[50] Used with care, the spray may prevent "escape" of malignant cells in the circulation, and it enables the operator to form superficial, solid frozen plaques on the surface without damaging deeper structures. In contrast, a probe must freeze a hemisphere as deep as the visible radius. It is important to use needle thermocouples at the deep margins of the tissues to be frozen in order to monitor the effect and to prevent excess damage to normal tissue.

In human dermatology practice, it is common to apply liquid nitrogen with an ordinary cotton applicator stick, which is dipped into the thermos of liquid and touched to the lesion, frequently a small tumor or wart. The applicator stick is touched intermittently to the lesion until the desired area and depth are frozen. Dermatologists with experience in using this method get very good results. The pain is minimal and well tolerated by most patients without local anesthesia.

Many soft tissues, especially glandular tissues, are particularly susceptible to freezing. On the other hand, bone, fascia, tendon sheath, perineurium, and walls of large blood vessels are fairly resistant. A knowledge of relative tissue susceptibility is of great practical importance.

To ensure that no cells escape destruction, the freeze–thaw cycle should be repeated two or more times. Thawing usually takes one and one-half to two times as long as freezing. Freezing is accomplished much more rapidly during the second and third freeze, since circulation to the target area has been compromised.

It has been speculated that useful immunologic effects are possible with cryosurgery. When a cell mass is frozen and left to die in situ, membrane lipoprotein complexes, and hence antigen-antibody complexing and receptor sites, are inevitably disrupted or altered. They are probably not totally destroyed. The nucleus may remain relatively intact. Thus, for a short time antigenicity may be enhanced. Enough antigen is released systemically to produce a strong specific humoral response that may kill escaped cells of the same tumor species. One investigator found that the same immune response occurs in both humans and animals.[50]

Following cryosurgery of canine skin tissue, histopathologic changes occur in an orderly progression of edema, erythema, infiltration of inflammatory cells, tissue necrosis, sloughing, repair by granulation, and re-epithelialization.[21]

ADVANTAGES OF CRYOSURGERY

This method of skin surgery has the following advantages:

1. Lesions can be removed in areas where the skin is so tight or the lesion so large that closure with sutures is impossible. Large lesions of acral lick dermatitis or tumors on lower portions of the leg are examples.

2. Where conventional excision surgery would produce shock or excessive blood loss, cryosurgery results in minimal hemorrhage. This is particularly effective in old or debilitated patients. Scarring is slight and the cosmetic effect is good.

3. Selective destruction of diseased or neoplastic skin is possible with little damage to normal tissue. With premalignant lesions, chances for spread of tumor cells are reduced.[111]

4. Cryosurgery has a possible immunotherapeutic effect on malignant neoplasms.[106]

DISADVANTAGES OF CRYOSURGERY

Cryosurgery has the following disadvantages:

1. The surgeon performing cryosurgery must be experienced and has to

acquire the skill in postgraduate training. Without specialized knowledge and skill, undesirable sequelae can result.

2. The necrosis and sloughing of frozen tissue are an effect that is unpleasant and malodorous for 2 to 3 weeks following cryosurgery.

3. Regrowth of depigmented, white hair on the surgery site sometimes leaves a cosmetic defect.

4. Vital structures surrounding the frozen lesion may be damaged. This applies especially to blood vessels, nerves, tendons, ligaments, and joint capsules. In cryosurgery for multiple perianal fistulas, for instance, fecal incontinence can result if the anal sphincter is damaged. Freezing of bone can result in pathologic fractures.

5. Large blood vessels frozen during cryosurgery for tumor removal may start bleeding 30 to 60 minutes later, when postoperative attention has been relaxed. Air embolism is possible if sprays are used on open vessels.[114]

Freezing Agents

Liquid nitrogen and nitrous oxide are the agents of choice in veterinary medicine. Carbon dioxide and Freon have also been used, but not commonly by veterinarians.

Liquid nitrogen is the most popular freezing agent in cryosurgery.[174] It is a clear, colorless, odorless liquid. It is not flammable and produces a temperature of $-195.8°C$ ($-320.5°F$).[19] It usually can be obtained from the medical supply companies that sell oxygen or from welding gas suppliers. Liquid nitrogen is delivered in various-sized vacuum-insulated Dewar's flasks. It can easily be poured from the flask into the cryosurgical unit. When small quantities are sufficient, physicians keep liquid nitrogen in ordinary quart thermos bottles that are refilled as needed by the supplier. If not agitated, it will remain active in the thermos for about 2 days. Liquid nitrogen can be kept active for a limited time period. Usually, 1 month is the maximum, if the original container is opened several times.

Nitrous oxide is the second most popular cryosurgery agent and is most effective for removing small tumors (under 3 cm) or for treating superficial skin lesions. It requires cryosurgical units specifically designed for its use. Applied with probes, it produces a temperature of $-89°C$.[19] Although it is more expensive on a unit basis than liquid nitrogen, there is no waste, and nitrous oxide is readily available in veterinary hospitals that use gas anesthesia (halothane, nitrous oxide, and oxygen). One large tank can be used for many months, since it is usually connected directly to the unit and is not poured, as is liquid nitrogen.

Cryosurgery differs in many ways from cold steel and electrosurgery. Although it has specific uses, it is never a total replacement for conventional surgery. Proponents of cryosurgery feel it has an excellent place in small animal practice, but knowledge, skill, and experience are necessary for best results. Detractors may have used the technique for the wrong conditions or without proper training, consequently experiencing poor results or complications. Some clinicians were once enthusiastic about cryosurgery but now use it less frequently. As improved units are manufactured, some designed especially for veterinary surgery, the practitioner will find it easier to select the proper cryosurgical apparatus and use it effectively.

Cryosurgical Units

Cryosurgical units deliver the freezing action by spray or probe. Some units (smaller, hand-held bottles) are designed only to spray the gas. Other units have both spray and probe attachments.

Some cryosurgery units deliver gas to a probe that is held against the tissue or inserted into crevices, fistulas, or other tracts to be destroyed. Cryoprobes use the Joule-Thompson effect: Rapid expansion of the gas under pressure provides low freezing temperatures. This is the method used with nitrous oxide. A great variety of probes are available, each for a different purpose. They can be round, flat, curved, pointed, or needle-sharp. A special probe has even been devised for anal sac destruction.

There is a recent trend toward the use of the spray units.[83] Some look like modified thermos bottles with a spraying tip at the top. A mixture of liquid and vaporized liquid nitrogen is sprayed directly on the area to be treated. Different spray devices deliver different mixtures of liquid nitrogen, vapor, and liquid. This can vary from 15 per cent vapor and 85 per cent liquid to 55 per cent vapor and 45 per cent liquid.[19] The higher the percentage of liquid in the spray, the lower the temperature and the more potent the freeze.

Dermatologic Indications for Cryosurgery

Podkonjak reported a series of dermatologic problems treated with cryosurgery. Success rate after one treatment was 86 per cent, and after one or more treatments, 93 per cent. Cases included melanoma, squamous cell carcinoma, fibrosarcoma, papilloma, mast cell tumor, basal cell tumor, hemangioma, histiocytoma, and trichoepithelioma. Also treated were epidermoid cyst, non-healing ulcers, granulation tissue, proliferative tissue in the external ear canal, tail gland hyperplasia, perianal fistula, rectal polyps, and anal adenoma.[115]

Tumors. Cryosurgery does not and should not replace conventional surgery. However, scalpel surgery is difficult or impossible to use in some situations.

Oral Cavity. By means of conventional surgical instruments, access to the oral cavity may be difficult and hemorrhage may be hard to control. Cryosurgery is a simple and more effective method of therapy. It is an alternative in treating recurrent tumors, for cases in which other surgical procedures have failed, especially for malignant neoplasms. Oral cavity squamous cell carcinomas may respond well to cryosurgery. Gingival epulis can be frozen and sloughing will occur without need for hemostasis.

Anal Area. The main advantage of cryosurgery in managing anal tumors, especially perianal adenomas, is that it involves less risk of damaging the anal sphincter or the vital anal nerve supply. In general, though, careful cold steel surgery is still the preferred method of removing perianal adenomas. The rarer perianal adenocarcinoma, on the other hand, may be an appropriate indication for cryosurgery combined with chemotherapy.

Acral Lick Dermatitis (Lick Granulomas). Cryosurgery is indicated in acral lick dermatitis when the lesion is so large that the skin cannot be stretched for suturing after surgical excision. Skin grafting has been used successfully but only by those highly skilled in plastic surgery. It is difficult to keep dogs from damaging the grafted area, since it is their favorite place to lick. Freezing the large lick lesion will destroy the thickened skin, which is then replaced by granulation tissue that is covered by normal epithelium from the wound margins. Since cryosurgery temporarily deadens the sensory nerves, there is less licking and less chance for recurrence at the same site for up to 6 months. Care must be taken not to freeze the underlying bone. In order to have complete control of the depth of freezing, it is essential to insert thermocouples under the lesion. After the lesion heals, the resulting scar and white hair are seldom objectionable in these difficult cases.

Multiple Perianal Fistulas. Perianal fistulas (see p. 383) are difficult to treat by any method, but favorable results have been described using cryosurgery.[59, 72, 83, 175] This method of therapy for perianal fistulas reached a high level of popularity in the late 1970s, but some veterinary surgeons are now returning to the use of surgical excision. The number of lengthy cryosurgical procedures (two or more times) and frequent recurrences of fistulas are two reasons that it has lost favor. Anal sac removal is always recommended before cryosurgery. However, the anal sac area is usually difficult to see because of scar and granulation tissue surrounding the perianal area. Every attempt must be made to avoid the complication of fecal incontinence, which can be a greater problem than the original fistulas. This can be done by carefully controlling the depth of freezing. Freeze only the fistula—not the sphincter or its nerve supply.

LASER SURGERY

Laser surgery is highly successful in some branches of medicine, but its place in dermatology is still unclear. It is not a first-line choice in human disorders except in the treatment of angiomas. Otherwise, laser surgery is reserved for instances when other treatments are not helpful. The technique has been useful in treating warts, vascular lesions, and extensive superficial skin tumors, but questions need to be considered about when to treat the condition, the age of the patient, and the potential for scarring. Standardization of treatments is necessary for humans, and, as this modality becomes more available for animals, the issue must also be resolved for them.[169] In veterinary medicine laser therapy has been reported to be useful in certain cases of feline indolent ulcer and eosinophilic granuloma, acral lick dermatitis, excessive granulation tissue, and skin tumors of the eyelid, pinna, and tail.[190]

ELECTROSURGERY

Just as heat cautery was replaced by electrocautery, the latter has been improved by modern electrosurgery. However, electrocautery equipment is still used to destroy tissue and to control hemorrhage by means of specialized tips that are heated to a bright cherry red, producing incandescent heat. The healing of tissue following the use of electrocautery is like that following a third-degree burn. This will not be discussed further, since the newest electrosurgical units are more efficient. High-frequency electrosurgical units are capable of cutting, cutting and coagulation, desiccation, fulguration, and coagulation (Figs. 4:5 to 4:7). An electrosurgical unit can be extremely useful in small animal dermatology.[52] It has a special niche in the surgical dermatologic armamentarium. The main *advantages* of electrosurgery are (1) reduction of surgery time, (2) reduction of total blood loss, (3) ease of coagulation when ligature application is difficult,

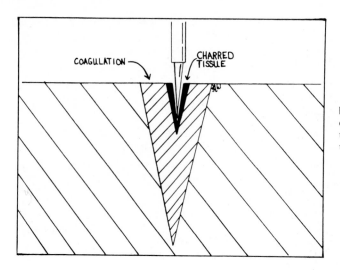

Figure 4:5. Desiccation. This technique is used for dehydration and where deliberate destruction of tissue is desired. (From Greene and Knecht: Electrosurgery. Vet. Surg., *9*:29, 1980.)

Figure 4:6. Fulguration. This technique is used for superficial dehydration or coagulation of the tissue. (From Greene and Knecht: Electrosurgery. Vet. Surg. *9*:29, 1980.)

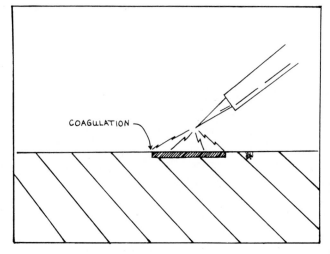

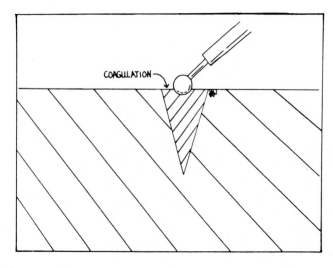

Figure 4:7. Coagulation. This is the sealing of small blood vessels. The electrode is left in contact with the tissue for a period of time until a deep white coagulum is formed. (From Greene and Knecht: Electrosurgery. Vet. Surg. *9*:29, 1980.)

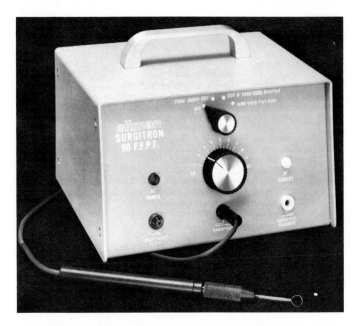

Figure 4:8. Modern electrosurgical unit that generates currents that perform cutting and coagulation simultaneously. (Surgitron, Ellman International Mfg., Hewlett, N.Y., 11557.)

and (4) reduction of foreign material left in the wound.[9] The *disadvantages* are (1) improper use leading to greater tissue damage, (2) presence of necrotic tissue within a wound, (3) delay in wound healing, (4) reduced early tensile strength of wound, up to 40 days after surgery, (5) decreased resistance to infection, (6) greater scar width on the skin, and (7) inability to suture most electrosurgical wounds.

The greatest practical use of electrosurgery is for the removal of small skin tumors. Next in value is hemostasis during both conventional surgery and electrosurgery. The newest electrosurgical units generate currents that perform cutting and coagulation functions simultaneously (Fig. 4:8).

Mechanism and Instrumentation

Electrosurgery uses electric currents to selectively destroy tissues. Electrosurgery is possible because electric current of greater than 10,000 Hz passes through the body without causing pain or muscle contractions, while the tissues and fluid of the body have electric impedance. Low frequencies (3000 Hz) result in pain and muscle contractions. At moderate frequencies (3000 to 5000 Hz) heat is produced, which causes tissue damage. Heat production is directly related to the power and concentration of the current delivered, the duration of time of application to the tissue, and the resistance of the tissue.

With a biterminal electrosurgical unit (Fig. 4:9), current passes from the unit to the active electrode in the handpiece and through the body. The current is conducted over a large surface area, which reduces resistance and current density, and it leaves the patient through the (indifferent) electrode or patient ground plate and returns to the unit. This plate should be as large as possible and covered with electrode paste or alcohol-soaked sponges to prevent secondary heating and burns.

The wave form of the current produced by the electrosurgical unit determines the tissue effect. Continuous, undamped sine waves are used for cutting

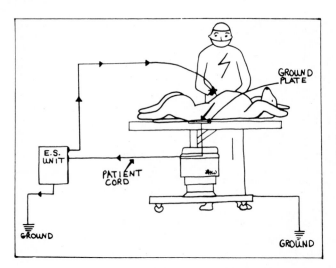

Figure 4:9. Current flow of high-frequency current from the electrosurgery (E.S.) unit through the patient to the electrode plate and patient cord and back to the unit. (From Greene and Knecht: Electrosurgery. Vet. Surg., 9:29, 1980.)

but have poor hemostatic qualities. Interrupted or damped sine waves have poor cutting properties but achieve excellent hemostasis. Modulated, pulsed sine waves produce simultaneous cutting and coagulation.

Recently, a new electric unit that produces a square wave was developed. When the waves are continuous, cutting without coagulation is possible; when the pulses of square waves are interrupted, coagulation without cutting results; and when a combined wave form is produced, both cutting and coagulation are possible.

The currents are generated by a spark gap, by radio tubes, or by battery-operated electrolysis machines. The machines range from inexpensive office units to high-priced hospital models. A unit in the medium price range is practical and versatile enough for use in most veterinary hospitals. Two main types of current are used: spark gap and electronic currents. These are converted from ordinary 110V house current by a high-frequency generator in the electrosurgical unit. In all cases it is mandatory for the patient to be grounded to the machine.

Cutting (Electroincision). Bipolar cutting current is produced in a spark gap machine by increasing the frequency of successive wave trains.

Cutting without Coagulation. Of any electrosurgical method, cutting without coagulation makes an incision with the least damage to surrounding tissue. It can be done in relatively nonvascular tissues. When simultaneous hemostasis is needed, however, a combination of cutting and coagulation gives the most satisfactory results.

Desiccation. Electrodesiccation is the application of a *monopolar* electric current (short spark) of high frequency and high tension to diseased or neoplastic tissue. It is "dried up" by the current.

In dermatology, electrodesiccation can be combined with curettage. If a biopsy is required, the lesions can be first removed surgically by "shaving" the dome-shaped portion above the skin level (shave biopsy). This can be done with a scalpel blade held parallel to the skin or with small curved scissors with the convex surface toward the skin. The tissue remaining below the surface is then destroyed by desiccation and removed by curettage. Such electrodesiccation and curettage are especially useful for removing many sebaceous adenomas, perianal adenomas, fibrovascular papillomas, nevi, actinic keratoses, seborrheic keratoses, and small basal cell tumors.

Coagulation. Electrocoagulation is used to seal small blood vessels by "boiling" the vessels' endothelial cells with the current from the ball-like probe.

There are two methods of applying coagulation. One is to touch the electrode (ball) directly to the small blood vessel until the vessel wall shrinks and the hemorrhage is stopped by the tissue coagulation. The other method is to grasp the small blood vessel with a hemostat, which is then touched with the electrode (a flat probe is best), and the current is turned on with the foot switch. It is important to be sure that a good seal of the vessel is produced by either method, since new hemorrhage will result from insufficient coagulation of the vessel walls.

Fulguration. Electric fulguration is the destruction of tissue by electric sparks generated by a high-frequency current. Direct fulguration occurs when the metal point of the probe is connected to the uniterminal of the high-frequency unit and a spark of electricity is directed to the tissue to be treated. Electrosurgery units capable of fulguration usually have a special probe into which the handpiece is inserted. Some units use the same handpiece, while others have special fulguration handpieces that cannot be plugged into cutting or coagulation plugs. Fulguration is used for destruction of superficial warts and tumors. Without need to touch the lesion, the current dehydrates and coagulates the tissue at the same time. This tissue does not have to be curetted but is allowed to slough. Most fulguration probes have a sharp point.

Electrolysis. Electric epilation of hair can be done by battery operated units or electrosurgical units that can be used at very low power. The probe must be a special tiny wire of such small diameter that it can be introduced into the hair follicle. With skill and experience, and under magnification, epilation can be accomplished. A too-low current will allow epilated hair to grow back, while a current that is too high or an application that is too long can cause scarring. This method has been used for the removal of cilia in trichiasis and distichiasis (see Eyelid Diseases, p. 818).

WOUND HEALING

Veterinary dermatologists are involved in minor surgical procedures and in the management of ulcers and other skin defects. Therefore, a basic understanding of wound healing is essential.[119] In addition to the discussion that follows, more in-depth information can be found in references such as that by Swaim,[153] which is excellent and served as the source for this section.

Wound healing is divided into four stages: (1) inflammation, (2) débridement, (3) repair, and (4) maturation. These stages progress along a continuum, and they may overlap considerably. An incised wound begins to heal by 5 to 8 days with re-establishment of epidermal continuity and a proliferation of fibroblasts from the subcutaneous tissue. There also is minor growth of connective tissue from the papillary layer of the dermis. Thus, healing occurs from the bottom of the wound upward, and the incision site may appear "dished" or inverted until production of underlying connective tissue pushes the epithelium up into an everted position (Fig. 4:10).

In the *inflammatory stage* the immediate reaction to a full-thickness skin loss is for the normal elasticity of skin and muscle tension to enlarge and distort the defect. Vessels contract and constrict for 5 to 10 minutes to limit hemorrhage.

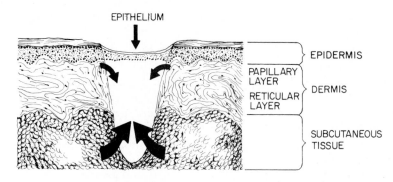

EPITHELIUM

EPIDERMIS

PAPILLARY LAYER

RETICULAR LAYER

DERMIS

SUBCUTANEOUS TISSUE

Figure 4:10. General pattern of wound healing. The wound epithelializes, with most of the connective tissue proliferating from the subcuticular areas upward into the wound (large arrows). A smaller amount of connective tissue proliferates from the papillary layer of the dermis into the wound (small arrows). The reticular layer of the dermis takes part in producing connective tissue to fill the intradermal area. (From Swaim, S. F.: Surgery of Traumatized Skin. W. B. Saunders, Philadelphia, 1980, p. 71.)

Vasodilation then occurs, which together with leakage from venules provides fibrinogen and other clotting elements. Bleeding and lymphatic drainage are controlled by these mechanisms. If lymphatic obstruction is prevented or if the clot is dissolved, such as occurs when fibrinolysin is produced during streptococcal infection, inflammation and infection can spread rapidly.

Later in the inflammatory stage, vascular and cellular responses serve to dispose of microorganisms, foreign material, and devitalized tissue. These mechanisms also set the stage for wound repair. Blood flow increases to the area, and plasma escapes into the tissue to dilute toxins and bring in enzymes, proteins, antibodies, and complement. Leukocytes stick to the capillary endothelium, escape through the vessel wall by diapedesis, and travel through the tissues to the site of injury.

The *débridement stage* begins about 6 hours after injury when neutrophils and monocytes migrate to the wound (Fig. 4:11). Neutrophils phagocytize organisms and then degenerate and die, releasing enzymes that facilitate further breakdown of necrotic debris by the monocytes. Wound healing could proceed without neutrophils, but monocytes are essential. They become macrophages when they enter the wound and phagocytize necrotic tissue. Some coalesce to form multinucleate giant cells, while others evolve into epithelioid cells and histiocytes. Macrophages also attract fibroblasts to the wound and influence them to undergo maturation and maximal collagen synthesis. As leukocytes die and lyse, the exudate takes on the character of pus (even without bacteria) and the protease and collagenase it contains impair wound healing by solubilizing connective tissue. Thus, adequate drainage of an infected wound is important in order to remove exudate and allow healing to progress.

The *repair stage* proceeds quickly when clots, necrotic tissue, and other barriers to healing are removed from the wound. During this stage the following processes occur: proliferation of fibroblasts, capillary infiltration, epithelial proliferation and migration, and, eventually, wound contraction (Fig. 4:12). In simple wounds, fibroblast proliferation and capillary infiltration start by the third to the fifth day. In open wounds, evidence of these processes is recognized as granulation tissue. Fibroblasts are most active in a wound for 14 to 21 days, and they advance along lines of fibrin within a clot and along capillaries that are growing into a wound. At first the fibrin, fibroblasts, and new collagen fibers are vertically oriented in a wound, but after about 6 days they are horizontally aligned, parallel to the wound surface.

The fibroblasts secrete various glycoproteins that constitute the ground substance of the wound. Collagen synthesis by the fibroblasts begins on the fourth or fifth day, and the tiny fibrils bond together into larger fibers that

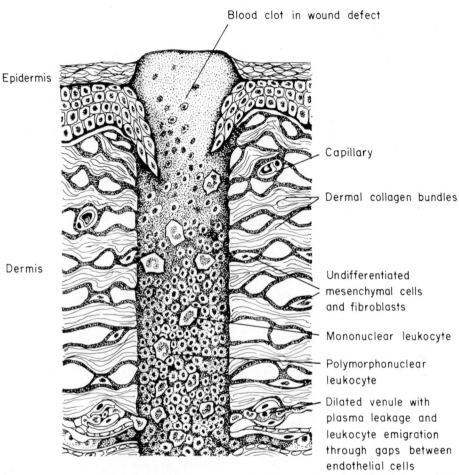

Figure 4:11. The débridement stage of wound healing. It has also been considered part of the inflammatory phase. (From Swaim, S. F.: Surgery of Traumatized Skin. W. B. Saunders, Philadelphia, 1980, p. 75.)

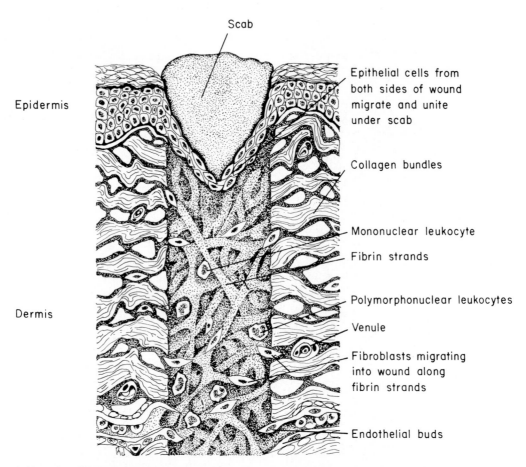

Scab

Epithelial cells from
both sides of wound
migrate and unite
under scab

Epidermis

Collagen bundles

Mononuclear leukocyte

Fibrin strands

Polymorphonuclear leukocytes

Venule

Dermis

Fibroblasts migrating
into wound along
fibrin strands

Endothelial buds

Figure 4:12. Early repair stage of wound healing. It has also been classified as the migratory phase. (From Swaim, S. F.: Surgery of Traumatized Skin. W. B. Saunders, Philadelphia, 1980, p. 78.)

become ever stronger and less soluble. As sufficient collagen is formed, the number of fibroblasts in the wound decreases, marking the end of the repair stage. Elastic fibers play little part in wound repair—a fact that explains the lack of scar elasticity.

Capillary infiltration of the healing wound is important to ensure optimum oxygen supply for the fibroblasts. Without optimum oxygen tension, fibroblasts cannot synthesize collagen adequately. The capillaries are a major part of the bright red granulation tissue that appears in open wounds from 3 to 6 days after injury. In small wounds, this occurs beneath a scab and is not visible. The proliferating capillaries form loops or "knuckles" that give the wound a granular surface. The new vessels anastomose freely and differentiate progressively into arterioles and venules (Fig. 4:13). Lymphatic vessels develop in a similar manner, but a little later in the healing process.

Epithelial proliferation and migration are the first obvious signs of rebuilding and repair. An intense epidermal reaction occurs up to 5 mm back from the wound edge, and the number of epidermal cell layers dramatically increases. The cells lose their firm attachment to the underlying dermis, and they flatten and extend outward and downward over the incised dermis. In simple wounds with clean, close approximation of edges, the defect may be covered by epithelium in 24 hours. In larger wounds, granulation tissue must form *before*

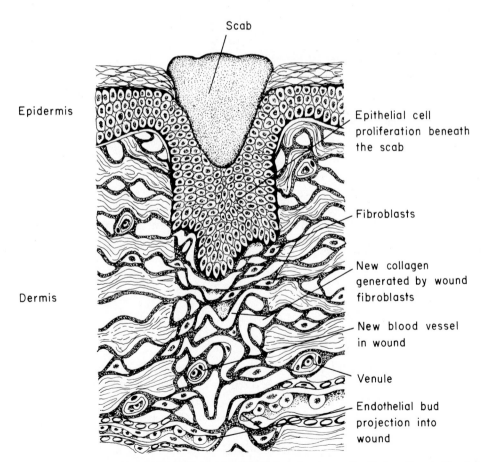

Figure 4:13. Later repair stage of wound healing. It has also been classified as the proliferative phase. (From Swaim, S. F.: Surgery of Traumatized Skin. W. B. Saunders, Philadelphia, 1980, p. 80.)

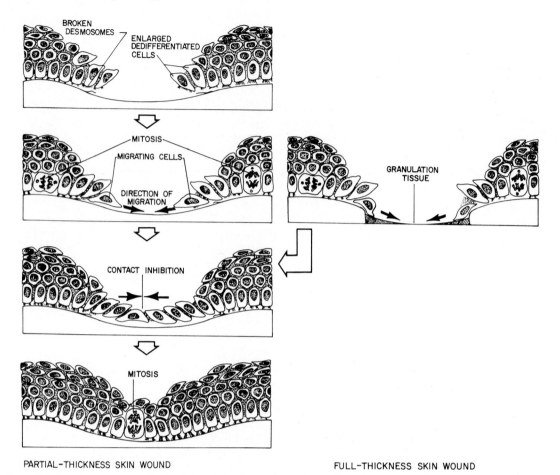

BROKEN DESMOSOMES

ENLARGED DEDIFFERENTIATED CELLS

MITOSIS

MIGRATING CELLS

DIRECTION OF MIGRATION

GRANULATION TISSUE

CONTACT INHIBITION

MITOSIS

PARTIAL-THICKNESS SKIN WOUND   FULL-THICKNESS SKIN WOUND

Figure 4:14. Basic processes of epithelial proliferation and migration. (From Swaim, S. F.: Surgery of Traumatized Skin. W. B. Saunders, Philadelphia, 1980, p. 84.)

wound epithelialization can start, and the process may take days or even weeks to complete (Fig. 4:14). If hair follicles are damaged, they participate in healing because the ends of the cut follicles are deep in the dermis and closer to the depth of the wound (Fig. 4:15). The new epithelium has a smooth undersurface with weak attachment to the connective tissue so it is easily traumatized and may be knocked from a healing wound. With the passage of time, new sebaceous glands and hair follicles may regenerate by differentiation of migrating epidermal cells.

Wound contraction is the reduction in size of an open wound as a result of centripetal movement of the whole-thickness skin that surrounds the lesion. Contraction can serve a useful purpose in loose skin, as it decreases the size of the wound that must be covered with epithelium. Over joints, and in areas of "tight skin," contractures can cause deformities. Contracture takes place between 5 and 45 days after injury. It is thought to result from a pulling action by modified fibroblasts in granulation tissue that take on some of the characteristics of smooth muscle cells. These cells are called myofibroblasts, and they are also capable of producing collagen.

The *maturation stage* is a period of consolidation, strengthening, and remodeling of the wound (Fig. 4:16). In a fresh wound, a lag phase occurs (4

Figure 4:15. Hair follicle contribution to wound epithelialization. The edge of the wound that is situated in the direction of hair flow becomes oblique (forms an obtuse angle) with the wound. The cut lower parts of the hair follicles lie 1 to 2 mm closer to the wound center than does the epidermal edge. Epithelialization occurs from the ends of the cut follicles and from the epidermal edge. (From Swaim, S. F.: Surgery of Traumatized Skin. W. B. Saunders, Philadelphia, 1980, p. 85.)

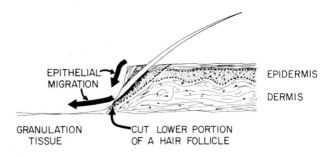

EPITHELIAL MIGRATION

EPIDERMIS

DERMIS

GRANULATION TISSUE

CUT LOWER PORTION OF A HAIR FOLLICLE

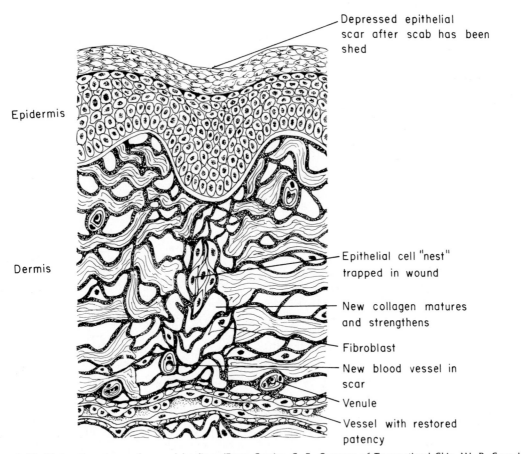

Depressed epithelial scar after scab has been shed

Epidermis

Dermis

Epithelial cell "nest" trapped in wound

New collagen matures and strengthens

Fibroblast

New blood vessel in scar

Venule

Vessel with restored patency

Figure 4:16. Maturation stage of wound healing. (From Swaim, S. F.: Surgery of Traumatized Skin. W. B. Saunders, Philadelphia, 1980, p. 88.)

to 5 days), during which there is little gain in wound strength. The initial strength is due to the fibrin clot, adhesive forces of epithelialization, coagulation of protein in the wound, and ingrowth of capillaries, fibroblasts, and collagen fibrils. Collagen increases rapidly during the first 3 weeks of healing, and then reaches a state of equilibrium. Over a long period of time, maturation and remodeling takes place by cross-linkage and changes in the physical weave of the collagen fibers. The strength of skin and fascia increases but always remains 15 to 20 per cent weaker than surrounding normal tissue. All repair activity is confined to an area within approximately 15 mm of the wound.

Initially, scar tissue is vascular and cellular and appears pink and raised. As maturation occurs, the scar becomes white, hard, and flattened in appearance.

The following general factors are often considered to enhance or hasten wound healing: young age, anabolic steroids, topical and systemic vitamin A, bandaging with nonadherent dressing, rest, lack of movement of the part but ambulation of the patient, warm environment, and general good health. The latter would preclude such disorders as dehydration, anemia, endocrine imbalances, and cardiac, renal, and liver disease.

Ultrasound therapy has been found to benefit wound healing when connective tissue is needed.[2] Although it increases inflammation and delays epithelialization, it stimulates fibroblasts and collagen production and enhances vascularization of granulation tissue.

Factors that generally delay or are detrimental to wound healing, in addition to the poor health factors mentioned above, include obesity and old age, steroids and steroid-related factors, denervation, foreign bodies, infection, insulin deficiency, hypoproteinemia, movement, neoplasia, tissue anoxia, radiation and cytotoxic drugs, seromas and hematomas, cold temperatures, excessive trauma, and exposure during surgery. Nutritional deficiencies, especially of vitamins A, K, E, and C, the B complex, and zinc, are also detrimental to wound healing.

Management of Special Skin Trauma

EPIDERMAL ABRASIONS

Margins of an abraded area are shallow and usually involve only the epidermis. Centrally, the defect may extend into the dermis. Initially, the injury fills with a blood clot and necrotic debris that dehydrate to form a scab. The epidermal adnexa may be injured, but they remain and regenerate. The only care needed is initial gentle cleansing, allowing the scab to form, and protection from infection while the epidermal cells slide under the scab to re-epithelialize the exposed dermis.

CONTAMINATED WOUNDS

The early time following a wound is called the golden period—an interval of about 6 hours during which prophylactic antibiotics are effective. The initial first aid for wounds should only involve covering the wound with dry, clean, nonadhering material to control bleeding and minimize contamination until definitive care can be provided.

For proper care, it may be necessary to use sedation or anesthesia, if allowed by the status of the patient. Otherwise, flushing the wound with 1 per cent lidocaine or using regional anesthesia may be sufficient for proper wound manipulation. *Prophylactic* antibiotics are completely effective for only up to 3 hours post-trauma, and therefore systemic agents should be given *first*. One of the cephalosporins and gentamicin provide broad, effective coverage. The wound can be filled with a water-soluble gel (like K-Y jelly) to protect it from further contamination while the area is prepared for surgery. Mineral oil or petroleum jelly can be applied to clippers to cause the hair to adhere to the blades while the area is being clipped. A vacuum is used to collect and direct debris away from the wound. The skin is prepared with chlorhexidine *surgical scrub* and gently cleansed with alcohol wipes. The clinician should then *thoroughly* irrigate the wound with large volumes of chlorhexidine *solution* (0.05 per cent) to remove the gel and all foreign particles such as hair, dirt, and clotted blood.

Chlorhexidine is preferred to povidone-iodine solution, since it has a wide spectrum of antibacterial effectiveness, immediately reduces the bacterial flora, and has a residual effect as a result of binding to the stratum corneum so tightly that it cannot be removed with alcohol.[155] In the above dilution, it is nonirritating and does not delay healing. Systemic absorption, toxicity, and inactivation by organic matter are not a problem. However, if the tympanic membrane is ruptured, chlorhexidine solution should not be used in the external ear canal, as it may cause ototoxicity.

Clay is by far the most deleterious of the soil contaminants. Pressure lavage (10 psi applied with an 18-gauge needle and 30-ml syringe or 70 psi pulsating, as provided with a dental water pick as in Fig. 18:2) may be used to decontaminate the wound. These pressures have not been found to spread infection.

The wound can then be draped and explored for special problems. Layered débridement with sharp dissection is used to remove devitalized or severely traumatized tissue. Wound closure is made with properly placed sutures to approximate skin and to obliterate dead spaces. Proper placement of drains, if needed, and bandaging as appropriate complete the initial treatment.

DECUBITAL ULCERS

Debilitated, paralyzed patients have poor circulation, and their immobility allows pressure between bony prominences and their bedding to further restrict circulation to a local tissue area. The area becomes red, and a punched-out ulcer develops later. The ulcer may have a gray fibrous coating with surrounding necrotic tissue.

Prevention by frequent turning, gentle massage and flexion of muscles and joints, and placing the patient on a water bed are most important. Once it has developed, treatment of the ulcer should entail cleaning with 0.05 per cent chlorhexidine solution to remove necrotic tissue, pus, and debris. The ulcer should be covered with wet to dry bandages or a nonadherent film, and protected from pressure by "doughnut" rings or bandage rolls. While mild antibacterial dressings are often useful initially, the use of a live yeast cell derivative in shark liver oil ointment (Preparation H) increases oxygen utilization and collagen formation in tissues, and it increases wound healing. It also lubricates and protects the ulcer. When the patient becomes mobile, the ulcers **heal** spontaneously.

Care of the Skin and Hair Coat

Although it is true that the skin is a reflection of general health, many vigorous, normal pets have unkempt hair coats—mainly because of neglect. The veterinarian is vitally concerned with the health of the patient's skin but should leave the styling, grooming, and cosmetic aspects of its hair coat to others. We do not visit a physician for a haircut; neither should we take our dog to the veterinarian for a trim. (However, some veterinarians do employ others to operate separate grooming facilities.) Styles change, and variations in clipping can enhance or mask aspects of conformation that complement the animal's appearance. These nuances of style are the province of owners, breeders, handlers, and commercial grooming establishments. Much of the following discussion is presented as background for students, or for transmittal to clients.

Grooming Procedures in Veterinary Practice

In everyday practice, clinicians are often faced with the need to clip, shave, or otherwise alter a patient's coat for medical reasons. The cosmetic effects may be drastic and if not carefully explained may provoke intense client resentment. Shaving prior to surgical procedures, of course, is understandably important, but needlessly clipping the hair over a vein for a simple intravenous injection may produce a hairless defect that will be unsightly for several months. Hair removed from Yorkshire terriers, Old English sheepdogs, and Afghan hounds may take as long as 18 months to replace. Poodles and beagles tend to grow hair rapidly; schnauzers grow hair slowly.

> **Remember the cosmetic effects of clipping hair, and try to avoid drastic disfigurement.**

Even necessary clipping can be made less obvious if the area is blended into the normal coat by beveling the edges of the lesion. Then, as hair regrows the line of demarcation is not so abrupt and is not obtrusive.

Proper use of the groomer's tools to remove hair mats and snarls will often obviate extensive clipping. Most clients sincerely appreciate attempts to remove crusts, debris, and mats by grooming procedures rather than by hasty clipping. However, when vigorous methods are indicated, they must be used. Remember, a year of neglect cannot be corrected by a 2-hour grooming session—even by a professional groomer.

Routine Grooming Care

Dog and cat breeds have many different coat types, so generalization of grooming details is difficult. A few important principles can be emphasized—the most critical being frequency of care. When a schedule of grooming is found to suffice for keeping the pet "looking sharp," it should be followed religiously; it is better to spend a few minutes grooming regularly than many hours sporadically. Since the impetus to do the job depends partly on motivation, making it easy is important. If proper facilities, effective tools, and a cooperative patient are combined, the task of grooming can be fun. A solid, convenient table with a nonskid surface and a grooming post with a neck or body sling are helpful. A grooming stand with a chair is also satisfactory. It should be located in a quiet area free of distractions. The proper grooming tools should be clean and in good repair. Comb, brush, nail clipper and file, towels, cotton, and swab sticks are the vital implements needed for most breeds. Shampoo, ear cleaning solution, hair lotion, and flea dips are also necessary. Specialized tools, to be described later, are essential for grooming and conditioning some coats.

The animal and his training can make a world of difference in the ease of grooming. Regular habits of good behavior during grooming, established early in life, result in complete cooperation. Most properly trained pets thoroughly enjoy their grooming care.

Prospective pet owners should contemplate grooming problems before purchasing a pet. If time and expense are likely to be problems, one should not choose a pet from a long-haired, wiry- or woolly-coated breed, but instead select a short-coated, easy-to-groom animal. An owner should perform simple daily or weekly grooming chores, but should periodically take advantage of a professional grooming service. The grooming needs of five typical coat types wil be discussed later.

Grooming Tools

Various grooming implements are needed (Fig. 4:17), the number and type depending on the breed and coat. Books are available in large bookstores covering the fine points of grooming individual breeds.

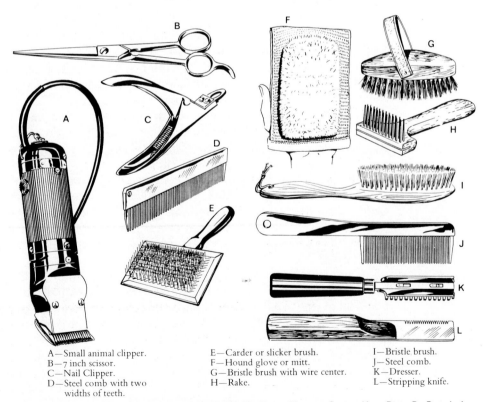

A—Small animal clipper.
B—7 inch scissor.
C—Nail Clipper.
D—Steel comb with two widths of teeth.
E—Carder or slicker brush.
F—Hound glove or mitt.
G—Bristle brush with wire center.
H—Rake.
I—Bristle brush.
J—Steel comb.
K—Dresser.
L—Stripping knife.

Figure 4:17. Grooming implements. (From Miller, D.: Know How to Groom Your Dog. By Permission of Pet Library Ltd., a subsidiary of Sternco Industries, Inc., New York City.)

Electric clippers specially designed for small animals are best. They should have changeable heads or a selection of different-sized blades. Clippers should be held gently on the skin surface and moved slowly. The moving parts should be clean, sharp, and well lubricated. If the blades become hot, are forced, or are pointed down at the skin, severe irritation and "burns" may result. The delicate skin of the genital, eye, and ear regions is most susceptible. Much of the so-called clipper burn is caused by dull blades pulling live hair from the follicle. This may occur in the ear canal by plucking hair, or by strenuous combing and brushing to try and rapidly refurbish a neglected coat. Clipping against the "lay" of the hair produces a shorter cut with any blade than cutting with the hair. Clipping blades are numbered—the larger the number, the closer the cut is made to the skin and the more hair is removed. The No. 40 blade produces a shaven appearance when used against the hair. Only a slight stubble is left when it is used with the hair. No. 15 also cuts closely. No. 10 blades leave enough hair to show the natural color of the coat. Two (Nos. 10 and 15) have general purpose uses, especially around the face, feet, and ears of many breeds. No. 7 blade leaves hair about 0.25 inch long, and No. 5 leaves about 0.5 inch. These latter blades (Nos. 5 and 7) are used for "machine clipping" wiry-coated breeds. Machine clipping cuts all hairs the same length but leaves the dead hair in place—not a desirable practice. Clipper blades (Oster) are now available that will leave 1 inch or 1.5 inch of coat intact.

Dogs should be carefully introduced to the clipper during the first session. The owner can be helpful in this step by training at home. By holding an electric razor near the dog and rubbing it over his coat several times daily he will help the dog to soon become accustomed to its vibration and noise. Gentle firmness and frequent short "breaks" for relaxation are necessary during the clipping sessions.

Shears are often used in conjunction with a comb. Barber scissors about 7 inches long with blunt tips are used to trim long hair and whiskers around the eyes, ear, face, and feet. They are often needed to remove mats and tags. Thinning shears have one solid blade and one serrated blade, so that large bulky coats can be thinned without obvious signs. It is well to insert the shears deeply under the surface of the coat to avoid destroying the external color of coats in which the undercoat and the outer coat are different colors.

Mat and tangle splitter slices mats so they can be removed more easily leaving *some* hair as compared with clipping.

Combs should have rounded teeth to avoid scratching the skin. Combs should always be inserted their full depth into the coat to perform efficiently. Different tooth-spacing is needed for each coat type. Metal, plastic, and bone combs are available. The material is not as important as the design. Forced combing or pulling at tangled mats extracts live and dead hairs and can easily ruin a coat.

The *rake* is an instrument that is especially useful in hacking through the heavy mats in a badly tangled coat. The rake has a single row of long metal teeth set at right angles to the handle. It can inflict serious wounds, especially inside the hock and thigh, and should be used with the utmost care. It can also "pull" live hair needlessly and thus produce irritations.

A *carder* is a square "board" with a short handle. It has bent, fine-wire teeth set close together. The teeth are placed near the skin, and the carder is twisted outward from the skin. This serves to loosen the coat and to remove dead hair and some of the smaller hair mats.

Brushes may be used in the same way on long coats, and if the hair is meant to stand away from the skin, the hair should be brushed (with short strokes) against its natural growth. Smooth-coated dogs should be brushed with the "lay" of the hair. Most groomers feel that nylon or synthetic bristles accumulate static electricity and cause hair breakage. They prefer natural pig bristles or soft wire brushes. Brushes for longer coats have wider-spaced, longer bristles that are firmly set into the rubber-base handle. Excessive brushing breaks hair and pulls it out. Except on short coats, surface brushing does not get the job done. The hair will mat from the skin outward, while the surface looks fine. The hair should be combed or brushed from the skin in small amounts at a time. Place the dog on his side, feet toward you. Hold the coat with the left hand and use the right hand to brush or comb small amounts of hair from under the left hand. Work upwards toward the back, making nice clean parts right down to the skin.

Hound gloves have a palm consisting of boar hair, wire, or fiber bristles. They are used on short-haired dogs to remove the dead undercoat and to give polish to the outer coat.

Stripping combs are also referred to as "dressers." They may be a type with a razor blade encased in serrated teeth, or merely a serrated metal blade attached to a wooden handle. These instruments are used to help "pull out" dull, dead hair. Hair is grasped between the thumb and the comb and removed with a twisting motion. Chalk is sometimes used on the coat to make the hair easier to grip firmly. If the hair is grasped between the thumb and forefinger and extracted, the process is called "plucking." The purpose of stripping and plucking, as applied to terrier-type breeds whose coats are "blown" (loose or ripe), is to remove the dead hair but retain the live. When these animals are "clipped" with a No. 5 or No. 7 blade, both live and dead hairs are shortened. Although the machine clip is fast, it is obviously much less desirable.

Hand rubbing and toweling are used to rub out dead hairs, to stimulate skin circulation, and to give a gloss or glow to the hair. They should be used only on short-coated breeds, or they may increase tangles.

SPECIAL GROOMING NEEDS PRIOR TO BATHING

Prior to bathing dogs, the nails should be clipped or filed to keep them short. Only the Chihuahua breed can be tolerated (in shows) with moderately long nails. For all other breeds the nails should be kept short to keep the feet compact and tight. With frequent filing the quick will recede and the nail can be maintained properly. Also, check between the toes for foreign objects and remove hair under the foot between the pads. Be careful using scissors between pads. Clippers are safer, as they are less apt to produce lacerations.

Teeth should be scaled periodically with a hook-shaped tartar scraper. Occasional scrubbing with cotton dipped in sodium bicarbonate helps keep them white. Periodic ultrasonic cleaning under deep sedation is recommended. The interval between these procedures varies from 3 to 18 months depending on the individual's tartar-building capacity.

The anal sacs should be palpated and expressed, if necessary, prior to bathing so any soilage can be removed during the bath. Place cotton over the anus and with thumb on one side of the anus and fingers on the other press forward and together to express the sacs. A more complete expression of sac contents can be performed by inserting a gloved finger into the rectum to express each sac separately.

The ears, too, should receive attention and care prior to bathing. Some terriers and poodles may have large amounts of hair growing in the ear canals. Excess hair should be plucked from the external ear canal or it may allow cerumen accumulation and irritation. The process of plucking may cause irritation in normal ears and should only be used when it is obviously necessary. Antibacterial and anti-inflammatory medication should be used in the ear canal after the plucking is complete and the canal is clean and dry. A cotton swab dampened with alcohol will usually serve admirably to remove waxy exudates. Pledgets of cotton should be placed firmly in each ear canal prior to bathing to block the entrance of soap and water. After the bath the cotton is removed, and the ears are carefully examined as well as cleaned and dried thoroughly if necessary.

In addition to the foregoing, the dog's eyes should be protected from soap during bathing by applying a small amount of boric acid or cod-liver-oil ointment into the conjunctival sac. If the dog is unkempt and severely matted, the tags and mats should be cut out *before* they are wet; otherwise the mats will be "set" and be almost impossible to remove later without much cutting.

All medium- and long-coated dogs should be combed out completely before bathing. They also should be thoroughly combed after bathing while still damp.

Bathing

The dog is placed in a raised tub and is wet completely with warm water. A shower spray hose is almost essential for easy bathing. Use a bland, liquid flea shampoo for most dogs. *Mild* dishwashing liquids such as Joy or Ivory are satisfactory shampoos for normal coats. Powdered detergents specially designed for dogs are very effective and rinse off easily without leaving a dull film. However, they should be dissolved completely before application and only used in small amounts. The shampoo is applied to the neck and topline of the dog. More water is added and a vigorous lather is worked up. The lather should be rubbed into short-haired dogs but squeezed into long coats, as rubbing may mat the long hair excessively. Work a small brush back and forth through the coat to clean the skin and remove any foreign materials from the hair. The dog's face should be washed carefully and rinsed carefully. A wash cloth is useful to control lather and keep soap from the dog's eyes. Then the entire coat is rinsed thoroughly. A second lather and rinse may be needed to wash the dog until the water runs off clear. Thorough rinsing is essential. If the outer coat is rinsed but soap is left close to the skin, irritation will result. The hair should squeak. Special vinegar, lemon, or bleaching rinses are not recommended except for special problems. However, a small amount of Alpha-Keri or similar oil can be added to a pan of water for the last rinse and will add gloss to the coat. Flea dips also may be necessary in some cases.

The coat should be squeezed to eliminate water and the dog wrapped in a towel and lifted from the tub to a table. Short-coated dogs can be toweled almost dry and then pinned into a large towel to help "set" the coat smoothly.

The towel can be pinned under the abdomen and at the neck. The dogs should be confined to a small cage until dry. Dogs with long coats should be placed in a stream of warm air and the coat combed, brushed, and fluffed as needed to accomplish the desired effect. All animals should be protected from chilling during a bath and for several hours afterward, until thoroughly dry.

All breeds should be bathed before major trimming or stripping sessions, as the bath loosens dead hair. The frequency of a grooming routine depends on the breed and the individual's needs. It is necessary to keep animals clean, but baths tend to soften those coats that should be hard and wiry and may remove natural oils so that the coat becomes dull. Products such as Alpha-Keri, Mr. Groom, or St. Aubrey Coatasheen or Coat Dressing often work wonders in restoring luster and keeping hair manageable.

DRY BATHS

To avoid the drying influence of water baths, dry powder products can be used, especially in long coats. Talc, boric acid powder, or superior special products such as St. Aubrey powder can be dusted into the coat and then thoroughly brushed out. With a *careful* job the coat is left clean and lustrous. However, dry baths are good only for a quick cosmetic clean-up. Shampoo and water baths are still the most effective way to really clean the coat. Powder cleaners are actually very inefficient; they dry the coat and increase its static electricity. Don't use them.

Grooming Needs of Individual Coat Types

For grooming purposes dogs' coats can be divided into five types: the long coat, the silky coat, the nonshedding curly coat, the smooth coat, and the wiry coat. Special grooming greatly enhances the appearance of each dog, but he must have a good natural coat and good conformation for the best effect. The ability to grow a good coat depends largely on inherited factors.

Medications, lotions, and special nutrients, either internal or external, have only limited effects on the coat of a healthy dog. Many owners fail to understand this and expect veterinary miracles to produce a show coat in every dog.

THE LONG COAT WITH UNDERCOAT

Typical breeds include Newfoundlands, German shepherds, collies, Old English sheepdogs, Siberian huskies, Samoyeds, and Welsh corgis.

Necessary implements for grooming them include a rake, natural bristle brush, Hinds 3060 wire brush, and regular and fine Resco combs.

These dogs should be bathed twice yearly—in spring and fall—and the coat saved during the winter. In many cases more frequent bathing may be needed. A rake should be used to remove dead hair. The coat should be combed and brushed forward over the top and sides, backward over the flanks. A fine comb is necessary for the hair under the chin and tail and behind the ears. Dry cleaning with powder brushed through the hair can be used for minor cleaning problems.

THE SILKY COAT

Typical breeds include spaniels, Afghan hounds, Maltese and Yorkshire terriers, setters, Lhasa apso, and Pekingese.

Necessary implements include Hinds or St. Aubrey wire brushes, medium and fine steel combs, natural bristle brushes, Oster clipper with blades Nos. 7, 10, and 15, Duplex stripping knife, and barber scissors.

While all long coats require frequent regular brushing, silky coats in addition require fairly frequent bathing to prevent mats and skin irritation. It may be necessary to use oils or products such as Alpha-Keri to keep the hair soft and lubricated and to prevent snarls and hair breakage. Dry hair tends to respond to static electricity by matting. To brush out these coats the hair can be lifted with the hand and combed or brushed down until it is free of snarls to the skin. Spaniels grow two or three coats per year and should be stripped or clipped about every 3 months.

THE NONSHEDDING CURLY OR WOOLLY COAT

Typical breeds include poodles, Bedlington terriers, and Kerry blue terriers.

Necessary implements include Oster clipper with blades Nos. 7A, 10, and 15, natural bristle brush, fine, medium and coarse steel combs (Twinco or Resco), and scissors.

The three breeds listed above must be clipped every 4 to 6 weeks for best appearance. The puppies should be exposed to grooming from 8 weeks of age so that they will accept the clippers. The first clip should be between 8 and 12 weeks of age, when just the face, feet, and tail are shaved. Only the scissors should be used under the tail, as that skin is very tender and easily irritated.

White, silver, and apricot poodles seem to have especially sensitive skin. A soothing lotion such as Vaseline Intensive Care lotion or Nivea Creme should be applied to areas of possible abrasion.

Since dead and loose hairs from these coats are mostly secondary hairs that become enmeshed in the coat, neglect causes a felt matting. All dead hair must be completely combed out before bathing.

Routine care of this group includes daily combing and wire brushing or carding.

THE SMOOTH COAT

Typical breeds include the hounds, the retrievers, dachshunds, Dalmatians, beagles, whippets, Doberman pinschers, smooth terriers, and boxers.

Necessary implements include only a hound glove or a rubber hound brush and scissors.

Dogs of this group should be bathed only when necessary for cleanliness. The scissors are used to trim off the tactile hairs on the face or to shape the fringes on the tail, ears, and brisket. The coat can be rubbed to shiny sleekness using the hound glove, the hands, or towels. This also removes dead hairs. The natural oils in a person's bare hand provide gloss and the dogs love caressing.

THE WIRY COAT

Typical breeds include the wire-haired fox terrier, Welsh terrier, Airedale terrier, Lakeland terrier, schnauzer, and Sealyham terrier.

Necessary implements include the Oster clipper blades Nos. 7, 10, and 15, a Duplex stripping knife, a Hinds slicker brush, fine and medium steel combs, a hound glove, and barber scissors.

Pups of these breeds should be started on a grooming routine at four months of age by trimming the head, ears, and tail. As adults they require machine clipping every 6 to 8 weeks or hand stripping about every 12 weeks. However, clippers should *never* be used on the body of animals being shown, since that softens the coat by removing the coarse guard hairs. Unfortunately, the change seems to be permanent, and dogs such as miniature schnauzers may be ruined for future showing. Hand stripping should only be done when the coat is *ready*. New hair should not be stripped except to tidy up a bit.

The fingers can best be used to pluck excess hair from the vicinity of the eyes.

THE CORDED COAT

The Komondor and the puli, two Hungarian breeds, are dogs with this type of coat.

Necessary implements are few. Only mild shampoo, *diluted 10:1 with water before application* (so it can be rinsed out easily), a heavy-duty water spray, and a heavy-duty dryer are required.

Dogs with corded coats should *never* be clipped or combed. They are rarely washed or groomed in any way. These dogs have a thick double coat that forms naturally into tassel-like cords described as controlled matting. Sometimes puppies' coats must be teased with a comb to encourage the formation of even cording. The cording is usually complete when the dogs are 1 to 2 years old, and the adult coat does not shed. Pulis may be shown corded *or* with the coat brushed out. Komondors are only shown corded. If the coats become very dirty, bathing can be done carefully. Always use very dilute shampoo. Squeeze it into the coat—do not brush or rub vigorously. Then thoroughly rinse with large volumes of warm water sprayed into the coat with pressure to lift and float out the dirt and shampoo. *Rinse thoroughly!* Do not rub dry with towels or combs, but dry with warm air blowers. It is best to handle them like a good wool sweater. Squeeze water out by hand and allow to drip dry. This takes a long time. Nothing ruins these coats faster than grooming. Always refer dogs with corded coats to knowledgeable professional handlers for proper coat care. This is not a do-it-yourself project!

Special Grooming Problems

Mats can usually be teased apart and combed out if they are small. Very small ones behind the ears and under the legs can be cut off. Larger mats can be slit with a special knife or an Oliver mat and tangle splitter and then teased with one or two teeth of a comb. Some badly neglected long-coated cats or dogs may have an almost complete covering of felt matting. These mats do not form close to skin. The only solution to some of these unfortunate cases is general anesthesia and complete, close clipping. Extreme care is necessary to avoid cutting or irritating the skin. Sometimes the teeth of a comb can be slipped between the mat and the skin to serve as a shield so that the mat can be safely scissored away.

Tar or *paint* embedded in the coat may be difficult to remove. Small deposits should be allowed to harden and then cut off. Tar masses can be soaked in vegetable oil or an emollient oil with a surfactant for 24 hours (bandaged if needed) to soften the tar, and then the entire mass can be washed out with soap and water. *Never* use paint removers or organic solvents such as kerosene, turpentine, or gasoline to remove tar or paint! They produce severe caustic burns. Ether may be used carefully for small areas.

Odors about a coat usually originate from places such as the mouth, ears, feet, or perineum. These should be checked and washed carefully. A rinse with a dilute chlorophyl solution or dilute sodium hypochlorite (in a white animal only) may help remove traces of odors. Highly scented dressings and sprays are objectionable to many people and do not reliably mask odors. The odor of skunks can be greatly ameliorated with a soap and water bath, and a rinse in *dilute ammonia water* (one or two tsp of household ammonia in 1 qt of water). (The tomato juice soak is effective but messy.) Once the dog dries the odor will be gone, but when wet, the hair may have a faint skunk scent for several weeks.

Comments on Grooming Cats

The grooming implements used for dogs in general serve adequately for cats too. However, grooming details have special applications that are outlined here. There is absolutely no substitute for routine daily grooming or for grooming every second or third day. Cats detest bathing and dematting and can be most resentful of rough treatment. Even when you just pet a cat, many of them will slip away afterwards to thoroughly rearrange their haircoat by licking and grooming themselves. From the grooming standpoint, cats have three types of coats—the short hair, single coat; the short hair, double coat; and the long hair.

The short hair, single coat is typified by the Siamese, Burmese, Havana brown, rex, korat, and the domestic shorthair. These cats can be bathed in shampoo and water, quickly dried to avoid chilling, and brushed and combed against the coat to remove dead hair. Final brushing is with the hair. A fine metal comb and natural boar bristle brush are the only implements needed.

The short hair, double coat is typified by the Abyssinian, Manx, Russian blue, and the American shorthair. The double coat is composed of two sets of hair. The long guard hair gives the coat its color, and the dense, short undercoat provides warmth. Both sets of hair are essential in these breeds. The basic coat care of this group is similar to that used for single coats except that caution must be employed as overgrooming can destroy the coat. Loss of the long guard hairs may make the coat look patchy or moth-eaten.

The long hair is typified by Persians and Himalayans. Several sizes of metal combs and a boar bristle brush are necessary for grooming these breeds. The kittens should be started with grooming at 4 weeks of age.

Older kittens and adults can be bathed with mild shampoo and water. Place them on a slanted window screen in a tub. (They feel secure on the wire and stay put, yet water passes through easily.) Rinse well and dry quickly with a towel and warm air blower. This fluffs the coat and gives it body. Do not bathe frequently and not within 2 weeks preceding a show. *Cats almost never require bathing!*

Mats tend to form behind the ears and under the chin, legs, and tail. The skin under the mat becomes irritated. Mats can be prevented by daily combing and brushing.

Some breeders dry clean the coats, with powder or talc sprinkled into the coat and carefully brushed out with a motion up and away from the body. This is rarely a satisfactory grooming method. If powder is left in the hair, it resembles unsightly dandruff and is highly objectionable.

Never clip the ruff or tail of a long-haired cat. The eyes and nasal area should be cleaned to remove exudates that may accumulate.

Special Feline Grooming Problems

A cat's nails should be clipped only if necessary. They soon grow out again and are honed sharply.

Cats' ears are much less prone to infection than dogs' ears, but they should always be checked and cleaned if needed. Young cats are especially predisposed to ear mite infections.

The large supracaudal organ on the dorsal surface of the tail is a mass of hyperactive sebaceous glands that may cause trouble if neglected. Breeders call the problem "stud tail," although it occurs in both sexes. A waxy, unsightly accumulation builds up in the area if proper hygiene is neglected. The exudate can be removed by applying powder to soak it up, by applying a thin oil to soften it, or by sponging the area with alcohol or detergents as solvents. Following this preparation, the oil usually can be brushed or washed off with shampoos satisfactorily. Periodic cleansing should prevent any future problem.

References

1. Ackerman, L.: Nutritional supplements in canine dermatoses. Can. Vet. J. 28:29, 1987.
2. Al-Sadi, H. I.: Effects of ultrasonic therapy on wound healing. Canine Pract. 11:50, 1984.
2a. American Kennel Club: The Complete Dog Book, 17th ed. Howell House, New York, 1985.
3. Anderson, R. K.: Canine pododermatitis. Compend. Cont. Ed. 2:361, 1980.
4. Angarano, D. W., and Scott, D. W.: Use of ketoconazole in treatment of dermatophytosis in a dog. J.A.V.M.A. 190:1433, 1987.
5. Aram, H.: Cimetidine in dermatology. Int. J. Dermatol. 26:161, 1987.
6. Aram, H.: Colchicine in dermatologic therapy. Int. J. Dermatol. 22:566, 1983.
6a. Hubbell, S. J.: Personal communication, 1982.
7. Arther, R. G., and Cox, D. D.: Evaluating the efficacy of fenthion for control of fleas on dogs. Vet. Med. (S.A.C.) 80:28, 1985.
8. Attleberger, M. H.: The systemic mycoses. In Kirk, R. W., (ed.): Current Veterinary Therapy VIII. W. B. Saunders Company, Philadelphia, 1983.
9. Ayliffe, T. R.: Penetration of tissue by antibiotics. Br. Vet. Dermatol. Newsl. 5:233, 1980.
10. Baker, E.: Staphylococcal disease. Vet. Clin. North Am. 4:107, 1974.
11. Bardana, E. J.: Recent developments in immunomodulatory therapy. J. Allergy Clin. Immunol. 75:423, 1985.
12. Barnes, L. E.: Adapting the use of fenthion to special cases. Vet. Med. (S.A.C.) 81:492, 1986.
13. Battistella, M. W.: Evaluating the safety of cythioate for feline flea control. Vet. Med. (S.A.C.) 81:475, 1986.
14. Bennett, D. G.: Clinical pharmacology of ivermectin. J.A.V.M.A. 189:100, 1986.
15. Blogburn, B. L., Hendrix, C. M., et al.: Anthelmintic efficacy of ivermectin in naturally parasitized cats. Am. J. Vet. Res. 48:670, 1987.
16. Brayton, C. F.: Dimethyl sulfoxide (DMSO), a review. Cornell Vet. 76:61, 1986.
17. Brunner, C. J., and Muscoplat, C. C.: Immunomodulatory effects of levamisole. J.A.V.M.A. 176:1159, 1980.
18. Bruyette, D. S., and Feldman, E. C.: Efficacy of ketoconazole in the management of spontaneous canine hyperadrenocorticism. Resident's Forum, University of California, Davis, 1987.
19. Bryne, M. D.: Cryosurgical instrumentation. Vet. Clin. North Am. (Small Anim. Pract.) 10:771, 1980.
20. Breen, P. T.: Bacterial hypersensitivity. Can. Acad. Vet. Dermatol. 4:1, 1987.
21. Bushby, P. A., Hoff, E. S., et al.: Microscopic tissue alterations following cryosurgery of canine skin. J.A.V.M.A. 173:177, 1978.
22. Chastain, C. B., and Ganjam, V. K.: Clinical Endocrinology of Companion Animals. Lea & Febiger, Philadelphia, 1986.
23. Chastain, C. B., and Graham, C. L.: Adrenocortical suppression in dogs on daily and alternate day prednisolone administration. Am. J. Vet. Res. 40:936, 1979.
24. Chytil, E.: Vitamin A and the skin. In Goldsmith, L. A., (ed.): Biochemistry and Physiology of the Skin. Oxford Press, New York, 1983.
25. DeNovo, R. C.: Therapeutics of gastrointestinal diseases. In Kirk, R. W., (ed.): Current Veterinary Therapy IX. W. B. Saunders Company, Philadelphia, 1986.
26. Dunbar, M., et al.: Treatment of canine blastomycosis with ketoconazole. J.A.V.M.A. 182:156, 1983.

27. duVivier, A., and Stoughton, R. B.: Tachyphylaxis to the action of topically applied corticosteroids. Arch. Dermatol. *111*:581, 1975.
28. Edney, A. T. B., and Smith, P. M.: Study of obesity in dogs visiting veterinary practices in the United Kingdom. Vet. Rec. *118*:391, 1986.
29. Eigenmann, J. E.: Growth hormone-deficient disorders associated with alopecia in the dog. *In* Kirk, R. W. (ed.): Current Veterinary Therapy IX. W. B. Saunders Company, Philadelphia, 1986.
30. Ellis, C. N., and Voorhees, J. J.: Etretinate therapy. J. Am. Acad. Dermatol. *16*:267, 1987.
31. Epstein, E., and Epstein, E., Jr.: Skin Surgery. 4th ed. Charles C Thomas, Springfield, Illinois, 1977.
32. Epstein, W. L., Shaw, V. P., et al.: Griseofulvin levels in stratum corneum. Arch. Dermatol. *106*:344, 1972.
33. Evans, A. G., Madewell, B. R., et al.: A trial of 13-cis-retinoic acid for treatment of squamous cell carcinoma and preneoplastic lesions of the head in cats. Am. J. Vet. Res. *46*:2553, 1985.
34. Evinger, J. V., and Nelson, R. W.: The clinical pharmacology of thyroid hormones in the dog. J.A.V.M.A. *185*:314, 1984.
35. Fadok, V. A.: Nutritional therapy in veterinary dermatology. *In* Kirk, R. W. (ed.): Current Veterinary Therapy IX. W. B. Saunders Company, Philadelphia, 1986, p. 591.
36. Fadok, V. A.: Thrombocytopenia and hemorrhage associated with gold salt therapy for bullous pemphigoid in a dog. J.A.V.M.A. *181*:261, 1982.
37. Ferguson, D. C.: Thyroid hormone replacement therapy. *In* Kirk, R. W. (ed.): Current Veterinary Therapy IX. W. B. Saunders Company, Philadelphia, 1986.
37a. Fine, R. M.: Physiologic effects of systemic corticosteroids in dermatology. Cutis *11*:217, 1973.
38. Flowers, F. P., Avaujo, O. E., et al.: Antihistamines. Int. J. Dermatol. *25*:224, 1986.
39. Foil, C. S.: Antifungal agents in dermatology. *In* Kirk, R. W. (ed.): Current Veterinary Therapy IX. W. B. Saunders Company, Philadelphia, 1986.
40. Franc, M., Dorchies, P. H., et al.: Studies on the therapy of otoacariasis of cats with ivermectin. Rev. Med. Vet. *136*:683, 1985.
41. Franz, T. J.: Kinetics of cutaneous drug penetration. Int. J. Dermatol. *22*:499, 1983.
42. Fredenberg, M. F., and Malkinson, F. D.: Sulfone therapy in the treatment of leukocytoclastic vasculitis. J. Am. Acad. Dermatol. *16*:772, 1987.
43. Fridinger, T. L.: Designing the ultimate weapon against fleas. Vet. Med. (S.A.C.) *79*:1151, 1984.
44. Giger, U., Werner, L., et al.: Sulfadiazine-induced allergy in six Doberman pinschers. J.A.V.M.A. *186*:479, 1985.
45. Goette, D. K., Odom, R. B.: Adverse effects of corticosteroids. Cutis *23*:477, 1979.
46. Goldman, L.: Photodynamic therapy and hyperthermia. Derm. Dialog. *5*:2, 1986.
47. Goldstein, R. S., and Hess, P. W.: Cryosurgery of canine and feline tumors. J.A.A.H.A. *12*:340, 1976.
48. Goldyne, M. E.: Leukotrienes: Clinical significance. J. Am. Acad. Dermatol. *10*:659, 1984.
49. Greaves, M. W.: Pharmacology and significance of nonsteroidal anti-inflammatory drugs in the treatment of skin diseases. J. Am. Acad. Dermatol. *16*:751, 1987.
50. Green, C. J.: Cryosurgical treatment of skin tumours. Vet. Dermatol. Newsl. The British Veterinary Dermatology Study Group *4*:16, 1979.
51. Greene, C. E., (ed.): Clinical Microbiology and Infectious Diseases of the Dog and Cat. W. B. Saunders Company, Philadelphia, 1984.
52. Greene, J. A., Knecht, C. D.: Electrosurgery: a review. Vet. Surg. *9*:27, 1980.
53. Gregory, C. R., Taylor, N. J., et al.: Response to isoantigens and mitogens in the cat: Effects of cyclosporin A. Am. J. Vet. Res. *48*:126, 1987.
54. Grier, R. L., Brewer, W. G., et al.: Hyperthermic treatment of superficial tumors in cats. J.A.V.M.A. *177*:227, 1980.
55. Griffin, C.: Systemic glucocorticoid therapy in veterinary medicine. Presentation, Am. Acad. Vet. Dermatol., New Orleans, March, 1986.
56. Halliwell, R. E. W., and Harman, D. W.: Ineffectiveness of elemental sulfur (Lyfe) as a flea repellent in dogs. J.A.A.H.A. *22*:249, 1986.
57. Helton, K. A., Nesbitt, G. H., et al.: Griseofulvin toxicity in cats: Literature review and report of seven cases. J.A.A.H.A. *22*:453, 1986.
58. Heymann, L. D.: Thiabendazole treatment of ringworm in a cat. Med. Vet. Pract. *67*:545, 1986.
59. Hoffer, R. E.: Cryotherapy. *In* Kirk, R. W., (ed.): Current Veterinary Therapy VII. W. B. Saunders Company, Philadelphia, 1980.
60. Hoffer, R. E., and Alexander, J. W.: Pinch grafting. J.A.A.H.A. *12*:644, 1976.
61. Holzworth, J.: Diseases of the Cat. W. B. Saunders Company, Philadelphia, 1987.
62. Hsu, W. H.: Toxicity and drug interactions on levamisole. J.A.V.M.A. *176*:1166, 1980.
63. Ihrke, P. J.: Antibacterial therapy in dermatology. *In* Kirk, R. W., (ed.): Current Veterinary Therapy IX. W. B. Saunders Company, Philadelphia, 1986.
64. Ihrke, P. J.: Antibiotic therapy in canine skin disease—dermatologic therapy III. Compend. Cont. Ed. *11*:177, 1980.
65. Ihrke, P. J.: Topical therapy—uses, principles and vehicles. Dermatologic therapy (Parts 1 and 2). Compend. Cont. Ed. *2*:28 and *2*:156, 1980.
66. Isaacson, D., Elgart, M. et al.: Antimalarials in dermatology. Int. J. Dermatol. *21*:379, 1982.
67. Johnson, D. E.: The repair of skin loss on the foot by means of a double-pedicle abdominal flap. J.A.A.H.A. *12*:593, 1976.
68. Kemppainen, R. J., et al.: Adrenocortical suppression in the dog after a single dose of methylprednisolone acetate. Am. J. Vet. Res. *42*:822, 1981.
69. Kemppainen, R. J., et al.: Adrenocortical suppression in the dog given a single intramuscular dose of prednisone or triamcinolone acetonide. Am. J. Vet. Res. *42*:204, 1982.
70. Kemppainen, R. J.: Principles of glucocorticoid therapy in nonendocrine disease. *In* Kirk, R. W., (ed.): Current Veterinary Therapy IX. W. B. Saunders Company, Philadelphia, 1986.
71. Kobay, M. J., and Jones, B. R.: Local current field radiofrequency hyperthermia for the treatment of superficial skin tumours in cats. N. Z. Vet. J. *31*:173, 1983.
72. Krahwinkel, D. W., Merkley, D. F., et al.: Cryosurgical treatment of cancerous and non-cancerous diseases of dogs, horses and cats. J.A.V.M.A. *169*:201, 1976.
73. Kummel, B.: Treatment of autoimmune disease. Derm. Dialog. *4*:2, 1985.
74. Kunkle, G. A.: Progestagens in dermatology. *In* Kirk, R. W., (ed.): Current Veterinary Therapy IX. W. B. Saunders Company, Philadelphia, 1986.
75. Kunkle, G. A.: Sensitivity of staphylococcal isolates in canine pyoderma. Proceedings, Am. Acad. Vet. Dermatol. Phoenix, March 19, 1987.
76. Kunkle, G. A.: The treatment of canine atopic disease. *In* Kirk, R. W., (ed.): Current Veterinary Therapy VII. W. B. Saunders Company, Philadelphia, 1980.
77. Kunkle, G. A., and Meyer, D. J.: Toxicity of high doses of griseofulvin in cats. J.A.V.M.A. *191*:322, 1987.
78. Kwochka, K. A.: Canine demodicosis. *In* Kirk, R. W., (ed.): Current Veterinary Therapy IX. W. B. Saunders Company, Philadelphia, 1986.

79. Latimer, K. S., Rakich, P. M., et al.: Effects of cyclosporin A administration in cats. Vet. Immunol. Immunopath. 11:161, 1986.

79a. Lesher, J. L., and Chalker, D. K.: Response of the cutaneous lesions of Reiter's syndrome to ketoconazole. J. Am. Acad. Dermatol. 13:161, 1985.

80. Lewis, L. D.: Cutaneous manifestations of nutritional imbalances. Lecture notes, 1982.

81. Lewis, L. D., Morris, M. L., et al.: Small Animal Clinical Nutrition III. Morris, Topeka, 1987.

82. Lichtenstein, J., Flowers, F., et al.: Nonsteroidal anti-inflammatory drugs. Their use in dermatology. Int. J. Dermatol. 26:80, 1987.

83. Lisca, W. D.: Anorectal and perianal cryosurgery. Vet. Clin. North Am. 10:803, 1980.

83a. Lober, C. W.: Canthaxanthin: The "tanning" pill. J. Am. Acad. Dermatol. 13:660, 1985.

84. Long, P. G.: Sulfones and sulfonamides in dermatology today. J. Am. Acad. Dermatol. 1:479, 1979.

85. Lorenz, M.: Managing flea-allergy dermatitis—2: Should you use systemic therapy to control flea-allergy dermatitis? Vet. Med. (S.A.C.) 79:1148, 1984.

86. Lueker, D. C., and Kainer, R. A.: Hyperthermia for the treatment of dermatomycosis in dogs and cats. Vet. Med. (S.A.C.) 76:658, 1981.

87. MacDonald, K. R., Greenfield, J., et al.: Remission of staphylococcal dermatitis by autogenous bacteria therapy. Can. Vet. J. 13:45, 1972.

88. MacDonald, J. M., and Miller, T. A.: Parasiticide therapy in small animal dermatology. In Kirk, R. W., (ed.): Current Veterinary Therapy IX. W. B. Saunders Company, Philadelphia, 1986.

89. MacEwen, E. G.: Approaches to cancer therapy using biological response modifiers. In Brown, N., (ed.): Vet. Clin. North Am. (Small Anim. Pract.) 15:667, 1985.

90. Maibach, H. I., and Stoughton, R. B.: Topical corticosteroids. Med. Clin. North Am. 57:1253, 1973.

91. Mandelker, L.: Use of an autogenous skin graft to correct a defect in a canine ear. Vet. Med. (S.A.C.) 75:833, 1980.

92. Mansfield, P. D., and Kemppainen, R. J.: Effects of megestrol acetate treatment on glucose concentration and insulin response to glucose administration in cats. J.A.A.H.A. 22:515, 1986.

93. Marshall, A. B.: Antibiotic therapy of small animal dermatitis. Br. Vet. Dermatol. Newsl. 5:2, 45, 1980.

94. Mason, K. V., Ring, J., et al.: Fenthion for flea control on dogs under field conditions: Dose response efficacy studies and effect on cholinesterase activity. J.A.A.H.A. 20:591, 1984.

94a. McLain, N.: Personal communication, 1987.

95. Medleau, L., et al.: Ulcerative pododermatitis in a cat: immunofluorescent findings and response to chrysotherapy. J.A.A.H.A. 18:449, 1982.

96. Middleten, D. J., Watson, A. D. J., et al.: Suppression of cortisol responses in cats during megestrol acetate and prednisolone therapy. Can. J. Vet. Res. 51:60, 1987.

97. Miele, J. A., and Krakowha, S.: Quantitative aspects of binding of canine serum immunoglobulins and Staphylococcus aureus protein A. Am. J. Vet. Res. 42:2065, 1981.

97a. Miller, D.: Know How to Groom Your Dog. The Pet Library Ltd., New York.

98. Miller, W. H.: Sex hormones and the skin. In Kirk, R. W., (ed.): Current Veterinary Therapy X. W. B. Saunders Company, Philadelphia. In preparation, 1989.

99. Miller, W. H., Griffin, C. E., et al.: Clinical trial of DVM Derm Caps in the treatment of allergic disease in dogs: a nonblinded study. J.A.A.H.A., 1987.

100. Montgomery, R. D., and Pidgeon, D. L.: Levamisole toxicity in a dog. J.A.V.M.A. 189:684, 1986.

101. Moriello, K. A.: Ketoconazole: Clinical pharmacology and therapeutic recommendations. J.A.V.M.A. 188:303, 1986.

102. Moriello, K. A., Fehrer, S. L., et al.: Effect of otic glucocorticoids on adrenal and hepatic function. Report to Am. Acad. Vet. Dermatol., Phoenix, March 19, 1987.

103. Moschella, S. L., Pillsbury, D. M., et al.: Dermatology. 2nd ed. W. B. Saunders Company, Philadelphia, 1983.

104. Mulnix, J. A.: Corticosteroid therapy in the dog. Proceedings, A.A.H.A. annual meeting, 1977, p. 173.

105. Nachreiner, W. R., McDonald, R., et al.: Ketoconazole-induced changes in selected canine hormone concentrations. Am. J. Vet. Res. 47:2504, 1986.

106. Neel, H. B., III: Immunotherapeutic effect of cryosurgical tumor necrosis. Vet. Clin. North Am. (Small Anim. Pract.) 10:763, 1980.

107. Noxon, J. O., et al.: Disseminated histoplasmosis in a cat: Successful treatment with ketoconazole. J.A.V.M.A. 181:817, 1982.

108. Noxon, J. O.: Progestational compounds in dermatology. Presentation, Am. Acad. Vet. Dermatol., New Orleans, March, 1986.

109. Noxon, J. O., Monroe, W. E., et al.: Ketoconazole therapy in canine and feline cryptococcosis. J.A.A.H.A. 22:179, 1986.

110. Page, E. H., Wexler, D. M., et al.: Cyclosporin A. J. Am. Acad. Dermatol. 14:785, 1986.

110a. Pathak, M. A.: Sunscreens, topical and systemic approaches for protection of human skin against harmful effects of solar radiation. J. Am. Acad. Dermatol. 7:285, 1982.

111. Paul, A. J., Tranquilli, W. J., et al.: Clinical observations of collies given ivermectin orally. Am. J. Vet. Res. 48:684, 1987.

112. Pentlarge, V. W., and Martin, R. A.: Treatment of cryptococcosis in three cats using ketoconazole. J.A.V.M.A. 188:536, 1986.

113. Peterson, M. E., et al.: Insulin-resistant diabetes mellitus associated with elevated growth hormone concentrations following megestrol acetate treatment in a cat. Proceedings, American College of Veterinary Internal Medicine 63, 1984.

114. Podkonjak, K. R.: Veterinary Cryotherapy—1. Vet. Med. (Small Anim. Clin.) 77:51, 1982.

115. Podkonjak, K. R.: Veterinary Cryotherapy—2. Vet. Med. (Small Anim. Clin.) 77:183, 1982.

116. Pohlman, D. L.: A modified surgical approach to chronic otitis externa. Vet. Med. (S.A.C.) 76:334, 1981.

117. Popkin, G. L.: Electrosurgery. In Epstein, E., and Epstein, E., Jr., (eds.): Techniques in Skin Surgery. Charles C Thomas, Springfield, Illinois, 1979.

118. Powers, D. L.: Preparation of the surgical patient. In Slator, D. H., (ed.): Textbook of Small Animal Surgery. W. B. Saunders Company, Philadelphia, 1985.

119. Probst, C. W., and Bright, R. M.: Wound healing. In Slator, D. H., (ed.): Textbook of Small Animal Surgery. W. B. Saunders Company, Philadelphia, 1985.

120. Pukay, B. P.: Treatment of canine bacterial hypersensitivity by hyposensitization with Staphylococcus aureus bacterin-toxoid. J.A.A.H.A. 21:479, 1985.

121. Pulliam, J. D., Seward, R. L., et al.: Investigating ivermectin toxicity in collies. Vet. Med. Small Anim. Clin. 80:30, 1985.

122. Reedy, L. M.: The role of staphylococcal bacteria in canine dermatology. Proceedings, A.A.H.A. annual meeting, April, 1982, p. 71.

123. Regnier, A., et al.: Adrenocortical function and plasma biochemical values in dogs after subconjunctival treatment with methylprednisolone acetate. Res. Vet. Sci. 32:306, 1982.

123a. Restrepo, A. K., Stevens, D. A., et al.: First international symposium on ketoconazole. Rev. Infect. Dis. 2:519, 1980.

124. Robertson, D. B., and Maibach, H. I.: Dermatologic Pharmacology. In Katzung, B. G., (ed.): Basic and Clinical Pharmacology. 2nd ed. Lange Medical Publications, Los Altos, 1984.

125. Rosenthal, R. C.: Cytotoxic drugs in dermatologic therapy. Presentation, Am. Acad. Vet. Dermatol., New Orleans, March, 1986.

126. Rosenthal, R. C., and Wilcke, J. R.: Glucocorticoid therapy. In Kirk, R. W., (ed.): Current Veterinary Therapy VIII. W. B. Saunders Company, Philadelphia, 1983.

127. Rosser, E.: Presentation, A.A.H.A. annual meeting, Las Vegas, April, 1982.

128. Rosser, E.: Recurrent pyodermas. Am. Acad. Vet. Dermatol. annual meeting, Phoenix, March, 1987.

129. Rosychuk, R. A. W.: Hormone therapy in veterinary dermatology. Presentation, Am. Acad. Vet. Dermatol., New Orleans, March, 1986.

130. Rosychuk, R. A. W.: Management of hypothyroidism. In Kirk, R. W., (ed.): Current Veterinary Therapy VIII, W. B. Saunders Company, Philadelphia, 1983.

131. Rubin, S. I.: Nephrotoxicity of amphotericin B. In Kirk, R. W., (ed.): Current Veterinary Therapy IX, W. B. Saunders Company, Philadelphia, 1986.

132. Rubin, S. I.: Nonsteroidal anti-inflammatory drugs, prostaglandins, and the kidneys. J.A.V.M.A. 188:1065, 1986.

132a. Schauder, S., and Ippen, H.: Photodermatoses and light protection. Int. J. Dermatol. 21:241, 1982.

132b. Saunders, B.: How to Trim, Groom and Show Your Dog. Howell House, New York, 1967.

133. Schmidt, J. A., Kohlenberg, M. L., et al.: Assessing the safety of long-term cythioate therapy. Vet. Med. Small Anim. Clin. 79:1159, 1984.

134. Schmidt, J. A., Kohlenberg, M. L., et al.: Safety studies evaluating the effect of fenthion on cholinesterase concentrations. Vet. Med. Small Anim. Clin. 80:21, 1985.

135. Schwartzman, R. M.: Topical Dermatologic Therapy. In Kirk, R. W., (ed.): Current Veterinary Therapy VI. W. B. Saunders Company, Philadelphia, 1977.

136. Scott, D. W.: Chrysotherapy (gold therapy). In Kirk, R. W., (ed.): Current Veterinary Therapy VIII. W. B. Saunders Company, Philadelphia, 1983.

137. Scott, D. W.: Clinical assessment of topical benzoyl peroxide in treatment of canine skin diseases. Vet. Med. Small Anim. Clin. 74:808, 1979.

138. Scott, D. W.: Dermatologic use of glucocorticoids. Vet. Clin. North Am. 12:19, 1982.

139. Scott, D. W.: Feline dermatology 1900–1978. J.A.A.H.A. 16:331, 1980.

140. Scott, D. W.: Hyperadrenocorticism. Vet. Clin. North Am. 9:3, 1979.

141. Scott, D. W., and Green, C. E.: Iatrogenic secondary adrenocortical insufficiency in dogs. J.A.A.H.A. 10:555, 1974.

142. Scott, D. W., and Buerger, R. G.: Nonsteroidal anti-inflammatory agents in the management of canine pruritus. J.A.A.H.A., accepted 1987.

143. Scott, D. W., et al.: Observations on the immunopathology and therapy of canine pemphigus and pemphigoid. J.A.V.M.A. 180:48, 1982.

144. Scott, D. W.: Sulfones and sulfonamides in canine dermatology. In Kirk, R. W., (ed.): Current Veterinary Therapy IX. W. B. Saunders Company, Philadelphia, 1986.

145. Scott, D. W.: Systemic glucocorticoid therapy. In Kirk, R. W., (ed.): Current Veterinary Therapy VII. W. B. Saunders Company, Philadelphia, 1980.

146. Scott, D. W.: Topical cutaneous medicine, or "Now what should I try?" Proceedings, A.A.H.A. 46:89, 1979.

147. Sharp, N.: Personal communication. 1987.

148. Sloan, J. B., and Lotlani, K.: Iontophoresis in dermatology. J. Am. Acad. Dermatol. 15:671, 1986.

149. Smalley, R. V., and Borden, E. C.: Interferon: Current status and future directions of this prototypic biological. Springer Seminars in Immunopathology. 9:73, 1986.

150. Solomon, S. E.: Drugs and the immune system. In Katzung, B. G., (ed.): Basic and Clinical Pharmacology. 2nd ed. Lange Medical Publishers, Los Altos, 1984.

151. Stanton, M. E., and Legendre, A. M.: Effects of cyclophosphamide in dogs and cats. J.A.V.M.A. 188:1319, 1986.

152. Storrs, F. J.: Use and abuse of systemic corticosteroid therapy. J. Am. Acad. Dermatol. 1:95, 1979.

153. Swaim, S. F.: Surgery of Traumatized Skin: Management and Reconstruction in the Dog and Cat. W. B. Saunders Company, Philadelphia, 1980.

154. Swaim, S. F., Lee, A. H., et al.: Evaluation of strip skin grafts in dogs. J.A.A.H.A. 23:155, 1987.

155. Swaim, S. F., and Lee, A. H.: Topical wound medications: a review. J.A.V.M.A. 190:1588, 1987.

156. Swaim, S. F., Pope, E. R., et al.: Evaluation of a practical skin grafting technique. J.A.A.H.A. 20:637, 1984.

157. Symoens, J., et al.: An evaluation of two years of clinical experience with ketoconazole. Rev. Infect. Dis. 2:674, 1980.

158. Symoens, J., and Rosenthal, M.: Levamisole in the modulation of the immune response: the current experimental and clinical state. J. Reticuloendothel. Soc. 21:176, 1977.

159. Sztein, M. B., and Goldstein, A. L.: Thymic hormones—a clinical update. Springer Seminars in Immunopathology 9:1, 1986.

160. Tannenbaum, L., and Tuffanelli, D. L.: Antimalarial agents. Arch. Dermatol. 116:587, 1976.

161. Teske, E.: Estrogen-induced bone marrow toxicity. In Kirk, R. W., (ed.): Current Veterinary Therapy IX. W. B. Saunders Company, Philadelphia, 1986.

162. Thoday, K.: Differential diagnosis of symmetrical alopecia in the cat. In Kirk, R. W., (ed.): Current Veterinary Therapy IX. W. B. Saunders Company, Philadelphia, 1986.

163. Thoma, R. E.: Phototherapy. In Kirk, R. W., (ed.): Current Veterinary Therapy VIII. W. B. Saunders Company, Philadelphia, 1983.

164. Thoma, R. E., Stein, R. M., et al.: Phototherapy: a promising cancer therapy. Vet. Med. Small Anim. Clin. 78:1693, 1983.

165. Thomas, I.: Gold therapy and its indications in dermatology. J. Am. Acad. Dermatol. 16:845, 1987.

166. Tinsley, P. E., and Taylor, D. O.: Immunotherapy for multicentric malignant mastocytoma in a dog. Mod. Vet. Pract. 68:225, 1987.

167. Tolman, E. L., Mezick, J. A., et al.: The arachidonic acid cascade and skin disease. In Stone, J., (ed.): Dermatologic Immunology and Allergy. Mosby, St. Louis, 1985.

168. Turnbull, G. J.: Animal studies in the treatment of poisoning by amitraz and xylene. Human Toxicol. 2:579, 1983.

169. Wheeland, R. G., Walker, N. P. J.: Lasers—25 years later. Int. J. Dermatol. 25:209, 1986.
170. White, J. V.: Cyclosporine: Prototype of a T-cell selective immunosuppressant. J.A.V.M.A. 189:566, 1986.
171. White, S.: Oral gold therapy. Derm. Dialog. 5:2, 1986.
172. White, S.: Report: Gold therapy. A.A.H.A. annual meeting, Las Vegas, April, 1982.
173. Willemse, T.: Intravenous ZnSO₄ for zinc related dermatoses in Siberian huskies. Derm. Dialog. 5:1, 1986.
174. Withrow, S. J., (ed.): Symposium on Cryosurgery. Vet. Clin. North Am. 10:753, 1980.
175. Withrow, S. J., and Lisca, W. D.: Cryosurgery. Vet. Clin. North Am. (Small Anim. Pract.) 10:4, 1980.
176. Wolfe, A. M., and Poppagianis, D.: Canine coccidioidomycosis: treatment with a new antifungal agent, ketoconazole. Calif. Vet. 5:25, 1981.
177. Wilkie, D. A., Kirby, R.: Methemoglobinemia associated with dermal application of benzocaine cream in a cat. J.A.V.M.A. 192:85, 1988.
178. Bussieras, J. et al: Le troitment des teignes des carnivores domestiques au moyen de derivatives recents de l'imidazole. Prat. Med. Chirurg. Anim. Comp. 19:152, 1984.
179. Zenoble, R. D., Kemppainen, R. J.: Adrenocortical suppression by topically applied corticosteroids in healthy dogs. J.A.V.M.A. 191:685, 1987.
180. Glaze, M. R., et al: Ophthalmic corticosteroid therapy: Systemic effects in the dog. J.A.V.M.A. 192:73, 1988.
181. Hsu, W. H., Schaffer, D. D.: Effects of topical application of amitraz on plasma glucose and insulin concentrations in dogs. Am. J. Vet. Res. 49:130, 1988.
182. Guaguere, E.: Topiques keratomodulateurs en dermatologie des carnivores. Point Vet. 17:475, 1985.
183. Ackerman, L.: Cutaneous bacterial granuloma (botryomycosis) in five dogs: Treatment with rifampin. Mod. Vet. Pract. 68:404, 1987.
184. Harris, R., et al: Orally administered ketoconazole: Route of delivery to the human stratum corneum. Antimicrob. Agents Chemother. 24:876, 1983.
185. Cauwenbergh, G., et al: Pharmacokinetic profile of orally administered intraconazole in human skin. J. Am. Acad. Dermatol. 18:263, 1988.
186. Paradis, M., Scott, D. W.: Personal communication, 1988.
187. Daurio, C. P., et al: Reproductive evaluation of male beagles and the safety of ivermectin. Am. J. Vet. Res. 48:1755, 1987.
188. Chaudieu, G.: Essai d'anatoxines staphylococciques pour le traitement des staphylococcies cutanees du chien. Point Vet. 11:67, 1981.
189. Weiss, R. C.: Immunotherapy for feline leukemia using staphylococcal protein A for heterologous interferons: Immunopharmacologic actions and potential use. J.A.V.M.A. 192:681, 1988.
190. Breen, P. T.: Lasers in dermatology. Current Veterinary Therapy X. W. B. Saunders Company, Philadelphia, 1989 (in press).
191. Rosenkrantz, W.: Immunomodulating drugs in dermatology. Current Veterinary Therapy X. W. B. Saunders, Philadelphia, 1989 (in press).
192. Miller, W. H.: Fatty acid supplements as anti-inflammatory agents. Current Veterinary Therapy X. W. B. Saunders Company, Philadelphia, 1989 (in press).
193. Miller, W. H.: Non-steroidal anti-inflammatory agents in the management of canine and feline pruritus. Current Veterinary Therapy X. W. B. Saunders Company, Philadelphia, 1989 (in press).
194. White, S. D., et al: Corticosteroid (Methylprednisolone sodium succinate) pulse therapy in five dogs with autoimmune skin disease. J.A.V.M.A. 191:1121, 1987.

5

Bacterial Skin Diseases

Cutaneous Bacteriology and Normal Defense Mechanisms

The skin forms a protective barrier, without which life would be impossible. The defense has three components: physical, chemical, and microbial.[52] Hair forms the first physical line of defense to protect the contact of pathogens with the skin. It may also harbor bacteria, especially staphylococci.[17, 82] However, the dense, relatively inert stratum corneum forms the basic physical defense layer. Its thick, tightly packed keratinized cells are permeated by an emulsion of sebum and sweat (see pp. 33–38). The emulsion is concentrated in the outer layers of keratin, where some of the volatile fatty acids vaporize, leaving a fairly impermeable superficial sebaceous crust.[51] Together, the cells and the emulsion function as an effective physical barrier.

In addition to its physical properties, the emulsion provides a chemical barrier to potential pathogens. Fatty acids, especially linoleic acid, have potent antibacterial properties. Water-soluble substances in the emulsion include inorganic salts and proteins that inhibit bacteria. Sodium chloride and the antiviral glycoprotein interferon, transferrin, complement, and immunoglobulins IgA, IgG, IgG_1, IgG_2a, IgG_2b, IgG_2c, IgM, and IgE are present in the emulsion.[70] Immunoglobulin levels in the skin do not parallel those in the serum, and specific immunoglobulins are concentrated in different locations in the skin and its adnexa. This suggests specific roles in a defense mechanism.[51]

The normal skin microflora also contributes to skin immunity. Bacteria are located in the superficial epidermis and in the infundibulum of the hair follicles, where sweat and sebum provide nutrients.[51] The normal flora is a mixture of bacteria that live in symbiosis, probably exchanging growth factors. The flora may change with different cutaneous environments. This includes such factors as pH, salinity, moisture, albumin level, and fatty acid level. The close relationship between the host and the microorganisms enables bacteria to occupy the microbial niches and inhibit colonization by invading organisms. In addition, many bacteria (*Bacillus* spp., *Streptomyces* spp., *Streptococcus* spp., and *Staphylococcus* spp.) are capable of producing antibiotic substances, and some are capable of producing enzymes (i.e., β-lactamase) that inhibits antibiotics.

Bacteria cultured from the skin are called normal inhabitants and are classified as resident or transient, depending on their ability to multiply in that habitat.[45, 46] Bacteria on the skin were collected from seven body locations (top of head, lumbar area, tail gland, chin, toe, groin, and axilla) and reported as follows.

Resident Organisms. Resident organisms are normally harmless and will re-establish themselves if removed.

Dog	Cat
Staphylococcus sp (coagulase positive)	*Micrococcus sp.*
Staphylococcus sp. (coagulase negative)	*α-hemolytic streptococci*
	Acinetobacter sp.
Micrococcus sp.	*Staphylococcus simulans* (coagulase negative)
α-hemolytic streptococci	
Acinetobacter sp.	

Bacteria were least numerous in the lumbar area and most abundant from the chin and interdigital web. Micrococci prefer the top of the head. Cats are well known for their fastidious habits, and in one study 50 per cent of the skin cultures were sterile.[46]

Coagulase-negative novobiocin-resistant staphylococci have been isolated from the skin of animals and man. Many species occur: *S. cohnii, S. saprophyticus, S. xylosus, S. sciuri, S. capitus, S. epidermidis, S. haemolyticus, S. hyicus, S. warneri,* and *S. simulans* have been isolated from the skin of dogs or cats.[17] Organisms of this group are commonly isolated from the surface of meat at slaughterhouses and from the skin of workers whose professions bring them into contact with animals or fresh meat. They have been recognized as causative agents of mastitis in cows and goats, urinary tract infections of dogs and human beings, and exudative epidermitis of pigs. Unpublished data confirm that coagulase-negative staphylococci can cause skin disease in dogs, too. In bacterial cultures they could be misdiagnosed as micrococci, which are considered nonpathogenic and therefore not completely identified and studied.

Transient Organisms. Transient organisms may be routinely cultured from the skin but do not multiply there and are of no significance unless they become involved in a pathologic process as secondary invaders.

Dog	Cat
Escherichia coli	β-hemolytic streptococci
Proteus mirabilis	*Escherichia coli*
Corynebacterium sp.	*Proteus mirabilis*
Bacillus sp.	*Pseudomonas* sp.
Pseudomonas sp.	*Alcaligenes* sp.
	Bacillus sp.
	Staphylococcus sp. (coagulase positive)
	Staphylococcus sp. (coagulase negative)

The primary skin pathogen of dogs is *Staphylococcus intermedius.*[18] Because of incomplete laboratory identification in the past, all coagulase-positive staphylococci were routinely reported as *Staphylococcus aureus*. Recent taxonomic studies have shown that the genus *Staphylococcus* can be divided into at least 10 coagulase-negative species (see above) and three coagulase-positive species (*S. aureus, S. intermedius,* and *S. hyicus*). A recent study classified the biotypes of 72 coagulase-positive staphylococci from the skin of healthy dogs and from various surgical and pyogenic lesions. The results showed 70 of the 72 to be *S. intermedius*, and 2 of the 72 to be *S. aureus*. All the *S. intermedius* isolates were coagulase positive with canine plasma.[7] A recent study found the *S. intermedius* isolates from dogs and cats produced as much extracellular protein A as did *S. aureus* isolates from people.[19] The presence of protein A in these isolates could contribute to the pathogenesis of staphylococcal infections of animals in a way similar to that shown for *S. aureus* infections in people. That remains to be proved, however.

There has been speculation about the means by which only a small number of a vast array of bacteria in the environment are able to colonize or infect the skin. The potent cleansing forces of dilution, wash-out, drying, and desquamation of surface cells prevent many organisms from colonizing on the skin. It is now recognized that bacterial adhesion is a prerequisite to colonization and infection.[28] Bacterial adhesion correlates with bacterial virulence, tissue tropism, and host susceptibility to infecting agents. Many bacteria possess surface adhesin, such as lipoteichoic acid (LTA), which binds to specific receptor molecules on cell walls (fibronectin) to fix the organisms to the host. Protein A, for example, is thought to act as an adhesin for staphylococcal organisms to the skin of atopic people. Certain strains of bacteria seem to adhere better to certain regions of the host, and this may play a great part in the variable virulence often observed. Much more investigation needs to be done to explain the potential of this mechanism of infection.

Other organisms from the transient group may be pathogenic in rare cases. Gram-negative organisms tend to flourish in moist, warm areas and to predominate when medications depress the gram-positive flora. Cats infrequently develop pyoderma, but commonly have subcutaneous abscesses. Since these are often from bite wounds, the mouth flora of the cat is an important factor. It includes *Pasteurella multocida*, β-hemolytic streptococci, *Corynebacterium*, *Actinomyces*, fusiform bacilli, and *Bacteroides* sp.

Anaerobic bacteria are usually abundant in gastrointestinal secretions; therefore, fecal contamination is a cause of soft-tissue infections due to these organisms. Anaerobic bacteria isolated from dog and cat infections include *Actinomyces* sp., *Clostridium perfringens*, *Clostridium* sp., *Peptostreptococcus anaerobius*, *Bacteroides melaninogenicus*, *Bacteroides* sp., and *Fusobacterium necrophorus*, *Fusobacterium* sp., and *Propionibacterium* sp.[5, 49] They are usually found in granulomas, cellulitis, abscesses, fistulas, and other soft-tissue wounds, but they may also be cultured from pyoderma, otitis, or stomatitis cases.[25] The aminoglycosides such as gentamicin are notoriously ineffective in therapy of anaerobic bacteria. Metronidazole is usually highly effective.

Antibacterial sensitivity for obligate anaerobic bacteria has been rated as follows:[5, 6, 37]

≥90 per cent ampicillin, amoxicillin, carbenicillin, chloramphenicol, and clindamycin
75 to 90 per cent cephalosporins, lincomycin, penicillin G (except *Bacteroides* sp., which is resistant to penicillin, ampicillin, and cephalothin)
50 to 75 per cent tetracycline, erythromycin
< 25 per cent gentamicin

Staphylococci are among the most resistant of the non–spore-forming organisms. They resist dehydration, are relatively heat resistant, and tolerate antiseptic medications better than the vegetative forms of most bacteria. Many strains produce one or several toxins. These may cause tissue necrosis at the point of infection. Repeated injections of heat-killed staphylococci will protect rabbits against otherwise fatal doses of *S. aureus*. Bacterins may be valuable in combating chronic infections in dogs and cats.

Staphylococcal skin infections are the major concern in pyodermas, and systemic antibiotics are important in therapy. In two studies of strains of coagulase-positive staphylococci from dog and cat infections, the following resistance data were produced.[36, 53] All strains were susceptible to erythromycin, cloxacillin, gentamicin, kanamycin, and neomycin. Fifty per cent were β-lactamase (penicillinase) producers and were therefore resistant to penicillin (and possibly ampicillin). Other resistance figures include lincomycin 20 per cent, tetracycline 25 per cent, trimethoprim-sulfadiazine (Tribrissen) 50 per cent, bacitracin 50 per cent, streptomycin 17 per cent, and chloramphenicol 7 per cent. Organisms have only become resistant to the last drug very recently.[53] Of the strains evaluated, 40 per cent were resistant to one antibiotic, 30 per cent to two antibiotics, and 70 per cent each to three and to five antibiotics. The last two percentage groups were usually isolated from cases of otitis and presumably had been exposed to several agents in previous therapy. Streptococcal organisms are usually highly susceptible to the penicillin group of antibiotics but more resistant to the aminoglycosides and tetracycline.

Generalizations about data on resistance of bacteria to antimicrobials are imprecise at best. Data vary according to geographic areas, the popularity of certain drugs used, the prevalence of patients who have had prior therapy, and even along with the dosage and length of treatment prescribed. Kunkle[48] studied two groups of dogs treated for pyoderma: one group treated in 1981 to 1982 and the other in 1985 to 1986. There was no emerging pattern of resistance of staphylococcal organisms, but dogs who had not received prior antimicrobial drugs were sensitive to a wider spectrum of drugs than those who had received treatment. Another report[57] stated that *S. intermedius* isolates generally were susceptible to cephalothin, methicillin, and gentamicin but were frequently resistant to ampicillin, tetracycline, and penicillin G. Resistance was not associated with depth of skin infection or previous antibiotic use. However, increased resistance to chloramphenicol, clindamycin, and erythromycin (bacteriostatic agents) was associated with previous antimicrobial therapy.

The numbers of resident bacteria on the skin tend to vary with individuals—some have many organisms, while others have few. The number per individual may remain constant, unless disturbed by antibacterial treatment or changes in climate. More bacteria are found on the skin in warm, wet weather than in cold, dry weather. Moist, intertriginous areas tend to have large numbers, and individuals with oily skin have higher counts. Total aerobic counts for normal skin ranged from 10^0 to 10^3 organisms per square centimeter, while similar counts from seborrheic skin ranged from 10^3 to 10^7 per square centimeter.[38] Disease states have an influence on the species and numbers of bacteria present. In seborrheic skin, coagulase-positive staphylococci predominate.[38] This is also true in most pyodermas and in most other bacterial infections of the skin. In patients with various dermatoses (atopy, seborrheic dermatitis, and allergic and irritant dermatitis in humans), increased numbers of resident bacteria are found in all areas of the skin, not just in the affected areas.[45] Compared with dogs that are normal, those with dermatoses have a more prolific growth of aerobic organisms, a greater number of sites carrying coagulase-positive staphylococci, and a higher number of gram-negative microorganisms. Thus, these animals are heavily colonized with potentially patho- genic bacteria, a fact to consider when providing basic therapy for the primary dermatosis. Microorganisms isolated from an intact lesion such as a pustule are evidence of infection, not colonization. Colonization means that a potential pathogen is living on the skin or in a lesion but that *its presence is causing no reaction in the host*. The problem in evaluating a pyoderma culture is to separate secondary colonization from secondary infection. The presence of many degen- erate neutrophils, and phagocytosed bacteria, is direct evidence of a host reaction and is compatible with infection. This can be determined by direct smears of lesion exudates, a technique that may be more informative than cultures.[55]

Skin Infections. Animals at risk for skin infections include those in whom:[8]

1. The surface integrity of the skin has been breached by trauma, surgical incision, or insertion of medical devices (tubes).

2. The skin has become moistened and macerated by constant contact with body fluids, by occlusive dressings, or by constant exposure to water.

3. The normal bacterial flora has been altered or ablated by antimicrobial therapy or by other mechanisms.

4. The local vascular or lymphatic circulation is impaired.

5. The immunocompetence of host, either localized (e.g., seborrheic skin disease) or generalized (e.g., excessive glucocorticoid therapy), has been im- paired to allow opportunistic pathogens to prevail.

Infected skin may be a source of systemic infection, and, conversely, systemic infections may be expressed by various cutaneous manifestations.

It can be accepted as a general rule that if skin infections are to be established, some predisposition is necessary. The predisposing factors are almost always local, since constitutional influences such as anemia and mal- nutrition are rarely important. The many local factors include friction and trauma, excessive moisture (endogenous or exogenous), accumulated dirt and matted hair, chemical irritants, freezing and burns, irradiation, and seborrhea. Bacterial infections may complicate dermatophytosis and insect and parasite infestations. In some instances, the bacterial infection is of major importance and is the primary problem; in others, it is incidental. Thus, skin infections may be classified as primary or secondary.

Primary infections occur in otherwise healthy skin. One species of organism is isolated, a characteristic disease pattern is evident, and the infection is cured by appropriate chemotherapeutic or antibacterial medication.

Secondary infections occur in diseased skin. More than one microorganism may be isolated, a less characteristic disease pattern is present, therapeutic agents are less effective, and treatment of the primary (or underlying) disease is vital to success.

The normal skin puts up a remarkable defense against pathogenic organisms, but damaged skin provides a much more favorable environment for their growth.

STERILIZATION OF THE SKIN

Total sterilization is a practical impossibility, in spite of the superficial location of most bacteria. A 2-minute scrub with soap and water followed by a 2-minute soaking in a 70 per cent alcohol solution is usually adequate for practical purposes. The resident organisms soon return to their original levels; however, 99.9 per cent of bacteria are removed by repeated application of a hexachloro-phene cream (pHisoHex) followed by a final rinse of 0.5 per cent chlorhexidine in alcohol. Since hexachlorophene-containing products are in disfavor, chlor-hexidine scrubs and solutions are popular and effective skin cleansers. In any method, the most important principle is mechanical removal with vigorous brushing.

The healthy, intact integument is remarkably resistant to bacterial infection, although potentially pathogenic bacteria continually threaten its integrity.

Surface Bacterial Infections

Pyotraumatic dermatitis occurs in two histopathologic patterns. One, clinically referred to as acute moist dermatitis, is a superficial, ulcerative inflammatory process caused by trauma. It is discussed on p. 791. The other pattern, pyotraumatic folliculitis, is a deep suppurative folliculitis. It is discussed on page 261.

Intertrigo or skin fold dermatitis is a surface irritation and inflammation caused by frictional trauma of skin rubbing against skin. It is discussed on page 792.

Superficial Bacterial Infections
(Superficial Pyodermas)

Superficial pyodermas are bacterial infections that involve the skin down to and including intact hair follicles. They include impetigo, superficial bacterial folliculitis, and dermatophilosis.

IMPETIGO
(Puppy Pyoderma)

Impetigo is characterized by subcorneal pustules that affect nonhairy areas of the skin.

CAUSE AND PATHOGENESIS

This is a bacterial disease with coagulase-positive *Staphylococcus* sp. organisms invariably the cause of the disease when it affects young dogs prior to or at the time of puberty. It is not contagious, but is often a secondary infection associated with parasitism, viral infections, a dirty environment, immune-mediated disease, or poor nutrition. In older animals, a bullous impetigo may be associated with hyperadrenocorticism, diabetes mellitus, hypothyroidism, or other debilitating diseases, and in these cases other bacteria such as *Pseudomonas* sp. and *Escherichia coli* may be present.[39]

A superficial pustular dermatitis has been described in kittens in association with overzealous "mouthing" by the queen. Cultures revealed *Pasteurella multocida* and/or β-hemolytic streptococci.[72]

CLINICAL FEATURES

Small superficial pustules that do not involve hair follicles are found primarily, but not exclusively, in the glabrous areas of the inguinal and axillary folds in dogs (Figs. 5:1A and 5:2). They are not painful or pruritic but are easily ruptured, and the dried exudate forms yellowish crusts. This is a relatively benign problem that often heals spontaneously and may be noted only incidentally. In kittens, lesions are found mostly on the back of the neck, head, and withers. In bullous impetigo the nonfollicular pustules are large and flaccid, and large sheets of superficial epidermis may be seen to peel away. Coagulase-positive staphylococci are usually cultured from the lesions. Diagnosis is made by the history and the clinical appearance and by documentation of the bacterial cause by direct smears and stains or by cultures of the pustular exudate. Histopathologic findings show nonfollicular subcorneal pustules (Fig. 5:3). Bacteria may or may not be seen within the pustules.

CLINICAL MANAGEMENT

Impetigo may regress spontaneously, but therapy with daily antibacterial shampoos, such as povidone-iodine, chlorhexidine scrub, or benzoyl peroxide shampoo, and wet soaks with drying, astringent agents such as aluminum acetate solution will hasten recovery. In rare cases, systemic antibiotics for staphylococci may be needed for 10 to 14 days (see p. 175). It is desirable to check health management procedures in order to eliminate debilitating factors that may have influenced the onset of the disorder.

Impetigo-like lesions in mature dogs require more careful consideration and may carry a more guarded prognosis, since immune suppression and other serious disorders mentioned above may be involved in the pathogenesis. Bullous impetigo usually responds rapidly to appropriate bacteriocidal antibiotics and treatment of the underlying disease.

Superficial Bacterial Folliculitis

This is a very common bacterial infection that is confined to the superficial portion of the hair follicle.

CAUSE AND PATHOGENESIS

In most cases, superficial folliculitis in dogs is caused by *Staphylococcus intermedius*, although other staphylococcal species and, in fact, other bacteria may be involved. Organisms may be introduced by local trauma, by bruising or scratching, or as an infection that is secondary to dirty coats, poor grooming, seborrhea, parasites (especially demodicosis), hormonal factors, local irritants or allergies. The three most common etiologic agents in canine folliculitis are staphylococci, dermatophytes, and demodectic mites. Superficial folliculitis may progress to deep folliculitis, furunculosis, and even cellulitis.

Folliculitis may or may not be pruritic. It is not clear why these two types of folliculitis exist, or even if the two syndromes (pruritic and nonpruritic) are separate dermatoses. The clinical lesions and histopathologic findings are identical for both types, the only difference between the two being the pruritus. A few cases may be due to bacterial hypersensitivity (so-called pruritic super-

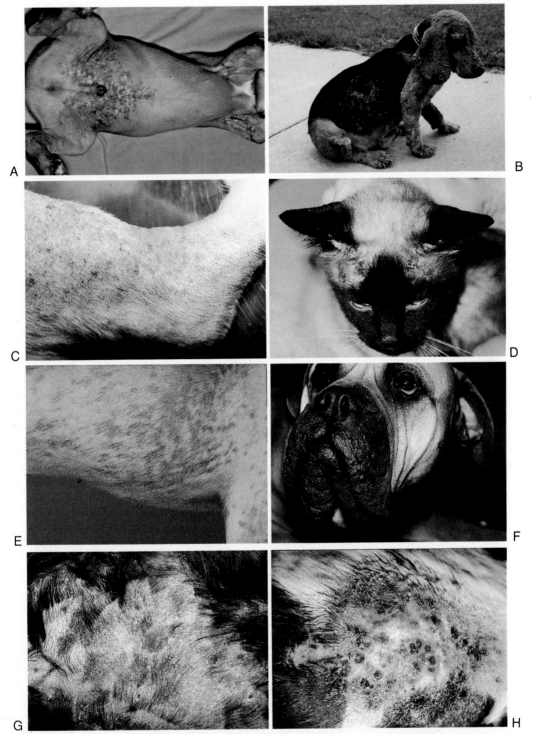

Figure 5:1. Impetigo, dermatophilosis, folliculitis. *A*, Severe impetigo (superficial pustular dermatosis) with clusters of subcorneal pustules on the glabrous skin of the abdomen and axilla. *B*, Dermatophilosis. Beagle has superficial crusts and erosions over ears, body, and legs. (Courtesy M. H. Attelberger.) *C*, Superficial folliculitis, lateral leg. Note follicular pattern. (Courtesy W. H. Miller, Jr.) *D*, Staphylococcal folliculitis on face and ears of Siamese cat. *E*, Lateral thorax of Shar Pei with superficial folliculitis. Note moth-eaten appearance. *F*, Mastiff with muzzle folliculitis. Note multiple papules and nodules on the chin and lips. (Courtesy W. H. Miller, Jr.) *G*, Staphylococcal folliculitis. Target lesions (ringworm-like). Note epidermal collarettes, erythematous ring and hyperpigmentation. (Courtesy W. H. Miller, Jr.) *H*, Rump of a springer spaniel with deep folliculitis and furunculosis. (Courtesy W. H. Miller, Jr.)

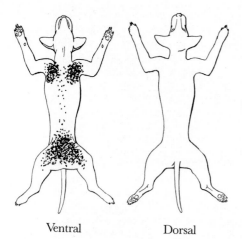

Ventral   Dorsal

Figure 5:2. Impetigo. Distribution pattern.

ficial pyoderma). Because staphylococcal folliculitis can be very pruritic, and because so many pruritic dermatoses (e.g., hypersensitivities and ectoparasitisms) are frequently complicated by "secondary" staphylococcal folliculitis, the old adage "Is it a rash that itches or an itch that rashes?" is a crucial and apt question.

CLINICAL FEATURES

The primary feature of folliculitis, regardless of the cause, is a tiny, inflammatory pustule with a hair shaft protruding from the center.

Look for a pustule with a protruding hair—it is diagnostic of folliculitis.

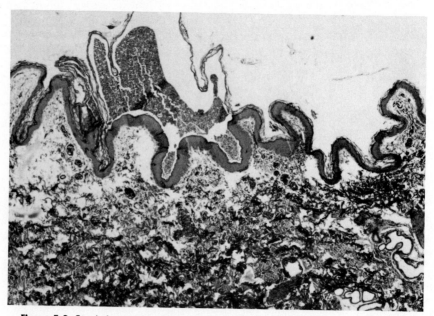

Figure 5:3. Staphylococcal impetigo in a dog. Note nonfollicular subcorneal pustule.

The typical pustule may be difficult to find, since the disease has a long course that is manifested first as papules, then as pustules (often transiently), crusts, epidermal collarettes, hyperpigmentation, excoriation, and alopecia (Fig. 5:1C,D,G). The "bulls-eye" or "target" lesions (Fig. 5:1G) may be highly suggestive, but many vesicular and highly inflammatory processes that begin from a point (such as impetigo and pemphigus) may produce similar circular lesions.

> *"Target" or "bulls-eye" lesions are not specific for folliculitis but suggest a bullous or pustular dermatosis.*

Superficial folliculitis has several distribution patterns. It may appear to be like impetigo in the groin and axilla but usually occurs in older animals and always involves hair follicles. It is much more resistant to treatment than impetigo. More generalized folliculitis may be seen, and although lesions may be concentrated or more easily observed on the ventrum, many lesions are found dorsally (Fig. 5:4). Often, the papular, truncal form of staphylococcal folliculitis in short-coated dogs is misdiagnosed as urticaria. Because of the chronicity, staphylococcal folliculitis may be most apparent as a moth-eaten alopecia (Fig. 5:1E). If these alopecic areas are inflamed (erythema, crusts, hyperpigmentation, scales), folliculitis is commonly misdiagnosed as dermatophytosis. If these alopecic areas are noninflammatory (common in the Shar Pei), folliculitis is often misdiagnosed as an endocrine imbalance. Such lesions in the Shar Pei may be focal cutaneous mucinosis. Distribution patterns previously identified as "short-coated pyoderma" (many breeds), and "Dalmatian bronzing syndrome" are, in most instances, cases of superficial bacterial folliculitis. The hair loss results from follicular inflammation that stops the growth of hair, which subsequently "falls out." When the inflammation subsides, a new hair will grow in the next anagen phase of the follicle. If severe infection destroys the hair bulb, the hair loss will be permanent.

DIAGNOSIS

Since folliculitis is often secondary, every attempt must be made to find the underlying cause. Many factors have been mentioned in the above discus-

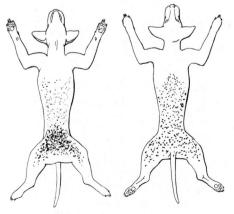

Figure 5:4. Superficial folliculitis. Distribution pattern.

Ventral   Dorsal

sion. The most essential diagnostic techniques are: collection of pus for making stained smears to identify fungal or bacterial organisms, phagocytosis, and the presence or absence of acantholytic cells; culture of pus for organism identification and antibiotic sensitivity; skin scraping for dermatophyte or parasite (demodex, pelodera) identification. Hematology, serum chemistry, hormonal evaluations, and allergy testing may be needed in complex refractory cases. Skin biopsy of individual papules and pustules may be especially helpful.

The histopathologic study of bacterial folliculitis shows a neutrophilic exudate within the hair follicles (Fig. 5:5). Bacteria may or may not be seen within the infected follicles. If a biopsy is done on chronic nonpustular lesions, one often finds perifolliculitis, perifollicular fibrosis, or intraepidermal neutrophilic microabscesses or some combination thereof.

CLINICAL MANAGEMENT

Removal of primary factors predisposing the skin to folliculitis is paramount. Cleansing, antibacterial, antiseborrheic shampoos are indicated after diagnostic specimens have been obtained. Benzoyl peroxide shampoos have a follicular flushing action and are especially effective. If the skin is already too dry, benzoyl peroxide may make matters worse. An emollient chlorhexidine shampoo may be preferable in such cases. Whirlpool baths or soaks with dilute antiseptic solutions such as chlorhexidine may be repeated two to three times daily, if lesions are localized.

Systemic antibiotics are always indicated. If response is evident within the first week, therapy is continued for at least 7 to 10 days after clinical cure. For uncomplicated cases, this time period is usually 3 to 4 weeks. When the response is equivocal, an evaluation of the antibiotics is important. There is much regional variation in antibiotic usage and efficacy. In instances of mixed infections, or if antibiotics are being used empirically, it is important to always use those that will be effective against *Staphylococcus intermedius*.[16] In this regard,

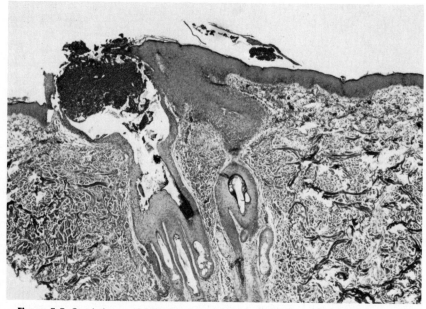

Figure 5:5. Staphylococcal folliculitis in a dog. Note cellular exudate within hair follicle.

some of the best antimicrobials are oxacillin, erythromycin, and chloramphenicol. Somewhat less effective are lincomycin and trimethoprim-sulfonamide. Trimethoprim-sulfonamide should be used with great caution in the Doberman.[41] Cephalexin, cephadroxil, and amoxicillin with clavulanic acid are excellent but should not be used as first-line drugs. The latter has not produced clinical results that were as good as laboratory tests predicted. These three antibiotics are best reserved for infections for which sensitivities indicate that other antibiotics will not be effective. Antibiotics not recommended for empirical use include penicillin, ampicillin, amoxicillin, tetracycline, and *non*trimethoprim potentiated sulfonamides. On sensitivity tests, aminoglycosides are often shown to be effective for these infections; however, they should be reserved for special cases. Coagulase-positive staphylococci have been shown to develop substantial resistance to aminoglycosides over a period of time.[16] These drugs must be given by injection, and toxicity potentials are a concern.

In recurrent, nonpruritic infections, it is necessary to rule out endocrine abnormalities such as hypothyroidism, hyperadrenocorticism, hyperestrogenism in females, and Sertoli's cell tumors in males.[67] Pyodermas involving endocrinopathies often have very large pustules. If the skin remains too dry or too oily after the infection is cleared, consider the various causes of seborrhea as possible underlying causes (see p. 720). Disorders of the immune system causing folliculitis are extremely rare.

In treating folliculitides that are associated with pruritus *do not* use corticosteroids with the antibiotic therapy. If the antibiotics resolve the pyoderma but not the pruritus, rule out atopy, flea bite hypersensitivity, food hypersensitivity, and scabies. If the antibiotic therapy resolves both the folliculitis and the pruritus, the cause was the bacterial infection. If relapse occurs, it must be proved that the pyoderma is in fact, recurrent, and then truly long-term antimicrobial therapy is indicated. Biologic therapy (autogenous and commercial vaccines), immunomodulation (levamisole), or cimetidine may be helpful in some cases (see Chapter Four).

Some cases that relapse repeatedly may be satisfactorily maintained by long-term administration of once-a-day to every-other-day antibiotic therapy (see p. 175) or perhaps even a full day's dose of an antibiotic given once weekly.[48] These methods should be avoided if at all possible. A safer, although less frequently effective, means of prophylaxis is regular bathing (daily, or as needed) with a benzoyl peroxide or chlorhexidine shampoo.[41, 52a]

DERMATOPHILOSIS
(Cutaneous Streptotrichosis)

Dermatophilosis is an actinomycetic disease that produces a superficial, crusted dermatitis caused by *Dermatophilus congolensis*. It is very rare in small animals.

CAUSE AND PATHOGENESIS

The organism is a gram-positive coccus that has not been found in the environment and therefore is thought to come only from carrier animals, usually farm animals.[10, 58] The clinical disease often develops shortly after the rainy season begins and is uncommon in dry climates, because moisture that releases the infectious zoospores is an essential initiating factor. Affected animals usually have minor skin defects from ectoparasites, minor trauma, maceration, inflammation, or infection. Thus, the organism is usually a secondary invader that is easily found by stained smears or cultures.[79] These are motile organisms that eventually form flagellated zoospores. That form is highly resistant and may persist in affected crusts for several years. The motile cocci are chemotropically attracted toward CO_2 diffusing from the surface of the skin. There they germinate to produce a filament that invades the living epidermis and proliferates within it, causing the production of characteristic crusts.[50]

> **The pathogenesis requires the organism, water, and inciting factors to produce the disease.**

Although nutrition and body condition are not thought to be factors in the disease, in large animal species it is associated with sarcoptic and chorioptic mange and sheep scab.[79]

CLINICAL FEATURES

This is a rare disease in small animals, but it may be more common than is realized in moist warm climates such as northern Australia, New Zealand and the southeastern United States. It should be suspected in cases of acute moist dermatitis, chronic folliculitis, seborrheic dermatitis, and other crusted dermatoses in which excessive moisture is present. It has been reported to affect dogs[14, 64, 79] and cats,[10, 58, 72] and one report suggests that the fox is the only natural canine host.[64]

Lesions may involve all parts of the hairy or glabrous skin, and in cats the organism has been isolated from soft-tissue fistulas and granulomatous lesions of the lymph nodes, mouth, and bladder. With skin lesions, the crusts usually are concentrated on the dorsal back and over the scapula and lateral thigh (Fig. 5:1B). The face, ears, and feet may also be affected, and pain is evident, as the animals appear to be unhappy and are disinclined to move around.

Local lesions may start as erythematous papules and pustules with crusts that occasionally thicken and expand to several centimeters in diameter. They may be isolated, circular lesions or may coalesce into larger areas. The classic lesion is an exudative, purulent dermatitis below raised tufts of hair and crusts (Fig. 5:1E). In early lesions, these crusts and the imbedded hairs are easily removed ("paintbrush lesions") to reveal greenish pus on an oval, bleeding, ulcerated surface. The healing lesions are characterized by dry crusts, scaling, hyperpigmentation, and alopecia.

DIAGNOSIS

The purulent exudate or crushed crusts can be made into a direct smear and stained with Giemsa's, Wright's, or Gram's stain or Diff Quik. The organisms appear as two to six parallel rows of gram-positive cocci that look like "railroad tracks" (Fig. 5:6).

For isolation and culture of the organisms, crusts are ground with sterile distilled water and let stand for 30 minutes. The inoculum is taken from the top of the water mixture and placed in antibiotic-enriched (polymyxin B) media.

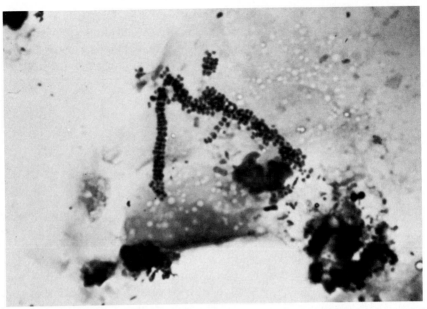

Figure 5:6. Dermatophilosis. Note branching chains of cocci ("railroad tracks") characteristic of *Dermatophilus congolensis* in this direct smear of pus.

Many media, such as blood agar, are satisfactory, but Sabouraud's agar and MacConkey's agar should be avoided. Growth of a rough colony (later becoming smooth) occurs in 3 days, but organisms are small at first and may be missed in the midst of others. With a scanning electron microscope, the colony appears as a mass of fine meshed filaments that become striated and divide into segments (cocci).

Skin biopsy of affected skin is diagnostic and is especially useful in chronic cases. Histopathology shows a hyperplastic superficial perivascular dermatitis or perifolliculitis-folliculitis with a "palisading" crust of orthokeratotic-para-keratotic hyperkeratosis and leukocytes. Organisms are usually easily demonstrated within the keratin on hematoxylin and eosin (H & E), acid orcein-Giemsa (AOG), or Brown and Brenn (B & B) stains.

Differential diagnosis should include seborrheic dermatitis, pustular dermatitis (impetigo, subcorneal pustular dermatosis, pemphigus foliaceus), acute moist dermatitis, staphylococcus folliculitis, dermatophytosis, and zinc-responsive dermatosis.

CLINICAL MANAGEMENT

Eliminate the primary inciting factors, and many cases of dermatophilosis clear up spontaneously. This involves removing the moisture, parasites, or trauma that may be present.

The dermatophilus organism should be eliminated from the skin. Since it does not thrive in an acid pH, topical therapy and good skin hygiene are useful. Crust removal and disposal are essential. Daily soaks with 10 per cent povidone-iodine or 3 per cent lime-sulfur solution given for 1 week and repeated weekly for 3 to 4 weeks are helpful. The systemic use of antibiotics is most effective and should be the primary focus of treatment. The organism is usually sensitive to ampicillin, cephalosporins, cloxacillin, lincomycin, tetracycline, tylosin, and high doses of penicillin. It resists erythromycin, novobiocin, sulfonamides, polymyxin B, and low doses of penicillin.

Therapy with tetracycline or high levels of penicillin for 7 to 10 days is usually adequate. Positive cultures can often be obtained from the skin of healed cases for 7 to 8 months and up to 15 months, an important factor in recurrence of the disease.[79]

Deep Bacterial Infections

(Deep Pyodermas)

Deep pyodermas are serious bacterial infections that often involve tissues deeper than the hair follicle. They invade the dermis and often the subcutaneous tissue as well.

In almost all cases, deep pyodermas are secondary to other contributing conditions; these can be local, such as foreign bodies (foxtails or plant awns, thornapple thorns, and wood slivers), pressure trauma, and nail bed infections, or they may be extremely generalized. With extensive lesions, an immunodeficiency should be considered. Some of the most common general problems contributing to deep pyodermas are demodicosis (probably the foremost), other parasites or dermatophyte infections, hypothyroidism, hyperadrenocorticism, and immunosuppression (naturally occurring or iatrogenic) from infectious diseases, neoplasia, or immunosuppressive chemotherapy. Fortunately, the diagnosis of deep pyodermas is usually clear, but the therapy itself may cause major problems since the patient's response to it is unpredictable. Because of the serious nature of the infection and its difficult treatment, skin scrapings, direct smears, fungal cultures, biopsy, and bacterial culture with antibiotic sensitivity tests are always indicated. Long-term antibiotic therapy and vigorous topical therapy with antibacterial shampoos and whirlpool baths form the cornerstone of therapy; however, the possible underlying factor must be thoroughly investigated and treated. Rare underlying causes of recurrent or severe deep pyoderma include neutrophil defects (diabetes mellitus) (see p. 639); hereditary disorder of Irish setters (see p. 431); cyclic hematopoiesis of gray collies (see p. 710); complement deficiencies (hereditary disorder of Brittany spaniels) (see p. 434); immunoglobulin deficiencies (hereditary IgA deficiency in beagles and Shar Pei) (see p. 429); and miscellaneous defects of humoral and/or cellular immunity (such as hereditary combined immunodeficiency syndrome of basset hounds) (see p. 429); and hereditary zinc deficiency of bull terriers (see p. 674).

Deep skin infections occur as a general syndrome that is usually the continuation of a process that started as a superficial infection or superficial folliculitis. The infection goes deeper into the follicles and breaks through the follicular wall to produce furunculosis or an infection in the dermis and subcutis. The infection follows tissue planes and may extend to the surface, producing multiple fistulas, or move deeper to invade subcutaneous and fatty tissues, producing cellulitis and panniculitis. The terminology for the condition depends on the location of the most obvious lesion and may be called folliculitis and furunculosis, dermal fistulas, or cellulitis and panniculitis. In addition, many infections have distribution patterns that reflect areas of the body most subject to surface trauma (Fig. 5:7). Remembering that the basic pathogenesis is the same, we will discuss these common clinical syndromes in more detail: deep

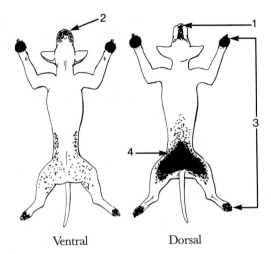

Figure 5:7. Deep folliculitis, furunculosis, cellulitis. Distribution patterns: 1, nasal folliculitis/furunculosis; 2, muzzle folliculitis/furunculosis; 3, pododermatitis; 4, German shepherd folliculitis, furunculosis, cellulitis.

Ventral   Dorsal

folliculitis, furunculosis, and cellulitis; pyotraumatic folliculitis and furunculosis; nasal folliculitis and furunculosis; muzzle folliculitis and furunculosis; pododermatitis; German shepherd folliculitis, furunculosis and cellulitis; anaerobic cellulitis; and subcutaneous abscesses.

DEEP FOLLICULITIS, FURUNCULOSIS, AND CELLULITIS

This is a follicular infection that breaks through the hair follicle to produce furunculosis and cellulitis.

CAUSE AND PATHOGENESIS

Folliculitis and furunculosis (F & F) starts as a surface or follicular infection from a bacterial, fungal, or parasitic cause. With a generalized distribution one should suspect causes such as generalized demodicosis (Figs. 8:28 and 8:31), generalized dermatophyte infection (Figs. 7:7 and 7:8), drug eruptions, endocrine abnormalities, seborrhea, or immunosuppression. Bacteria present usually are *Staphylococcus intermedius*, but deep skin infections are more apt to have secondary infections from *Proteus* sp., *Pseudomonas* sp., and *E. coli* than other pyodermas. Sensitivity to these agents is not predictable, and therefore culture and antibiotic sensitivity tests are imperative. In addition, skin scrapings, direct smears, fungal cultures, and biopsy form a minimum data base for diagnosis.

Histologic examination of biopsy samples may be useful in understanding the mechanism, etiology, and stage of development of the folliculitis and furunculosis syndrome (see p. 85). Folliculitis is an exceedingly common gross and microscopic finding in dogs, and because it is often a secondary development, a thorough search for an underlying cause is mandatory. Folliculitis associated with bacteria, fungi, or parasites is usually suppurative initially, whereas the occasional case associated with atopy, food hypersensitivity, or seborrheic dermatitis is usually spongiotic and mononuclear. Any chronic folliculitis, especially where there is furunculosis, can become granulomatous or pyogranulomatous (Fig. 5:8). Furunculosis, regardless of cause, is usually associated with a tissue eosinophilia, which is assumed to suggest the presence of a foreign body (keratin, hairs). The absence of tissue eosinophilia with furunculosis usually implies immunosuppression, especially due to concurrent glucocorticoid therapy or demodicosis.

CLINICAL FEATURES

Affected areas develop follicular pustules that soon rupture and form dark brown or reddish crusts on the surface (Fig. 5:1*H*). There may be open fistulas from which pus can be expressed by gentle pressure. The irritation of the exudate combined with licking by the patient soon causes a local alopecia and ulceration. Some of the lesions may have a "ringworm-like" appearance (Fig. 5:1*G*). Lesions are most common over the abdomen, trunk, and pressure points and are especially found in short-coated breeds such as the Doberman, Great Dane, Weimaraner, bull terrier, boxer, pointer, and Dalmatian. Of the long-coated breeds, German shepherds (see p. 267), golden retrievers, and Irish setters appear predisposed to the condition.

Pyodermas are rare in cats.

Bacterial folliculitis and furunculosis are rare in the cat. When they appear, follicular papules and pustules are usually located on the face and head (Fig. 5:1*D*) or over the dorsum in a feline–flea bite hypersensitivity pattern. Cultures from these lesions have most commonly grown coagulase-positive staphylococci, and occasionally β-hemolytic streptococci and *Pasteurella multocida*. Feline chin folliculitis and furunculosis may be seen as a secondary infection complicating cases of feline acne (see p. 740).

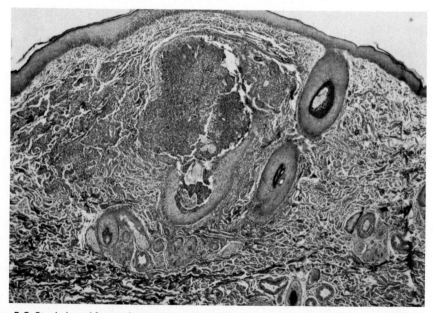

Figure 5:8. Staphyloccal furunculosis in a dog. Note follicular rupture with resultant pyogranulomatous dermal reaction around hair follicle.

CLINICAL MANAGEMENT

Although bacteremia and septicemia usually do not develop, these are serious infections that require careful, thorough, long-term treatment. Since many are secondary infections, treatment or removal of the underlying factor is essential to complete response. Because mixed infections may be found, culture and sensitivity tests are mandatory for proper antibiotic selection (see p. 175). In mixed infections, if all the organisms are not sensitive to a single antibiotic, or if they are only sensitive to an aminoglycoside or cephalosporin, it may be necessary to choose an antimicrobial that is effective against the staphylococcus alone. Antibiotic therapy should be continued for 7 to 10 days beyond clinical cure; in some cases, this may require 8 to 10 weeks or longer.

Treating the **Staphylococcus intermedius** *alone will often put the disease into remission.*

Local whirlpool baths given daily, or wet soaks using dilute chlorhexidine or povidone-iodine solutions given several times a day, promote drainage and healing. They improve circulation and reduce pain.

PYOTRAUMATIC FOLLICULITIS

Clinicians have long recognized that not all cases of pyotraumatic dermatitis (acute moist dermatitis, hot spots) respond to therapy rapidly and completely.

A recent study[63] reported a series of these cases and discovered they could be classified histologically into two groups. In one group, the lesion did not have a large bacterial component. It was a superficial, ulcerative, inflammatory process of undetermined cause and pathogenesis (true pyotraumatic dermatitis or acute moist dermatitis) that responded readily to simple cleansing and corticosteroids (see p. 792) (Fig. 16:14A).

The second group also had superficial ulceration, but in addition had deep suppurative and necrotizing folliculitis and occasional furunculosis (see Fig. 5:9G). Clinically, this type of lesion is thickened, plaquelike, and surrounded by "satellite" papules and pustules. Numerous gram-positive cocci were present in the deep follicles, and it was common to observe panniculitis and hidradenitis with a neutrophilic infiltrate. The authors speculated that the folliculitis was merely a complicating factor in some cases of pyotraumatic dermatitis. There was a strong tendency for young dogs to be affected; this pattern was observed in 70 per cent of the golden retrievers and St. Bernards presumed to have pyotraumatic dermatitis but in only 20 per cent of all other breeds. These cases represent true local pyodermas.

In managing pyotraumatic folliculitis, treatment should include early administration of a systemic antibiotic effective against *S. intermedius*. It should be continued for 7 to 10 days beyond clinical cure. Local clipping, cleaning, and daily application of agents such as Burow's solution (Domeboro) or chlorhexidine soaks, or calamine lotion are often helpful. Elizabethan collars may be indicated, but chemical sedation or analgesia are rarely necessary. Glucocorticoids are contraindicated.

NASAL FOLLICULITIS/FURUNCULOSIS

(Nasal "Pyoderma")

Nasal folliculitis/furunculosis is an uncommon, painful, localized deep infection of the bridge of the nose and the area around the nostrils (Fig. 5:9A,B). It is most common in the German shepherd, collie, pointer, and hunting-type (dolichocephalic) breeds. The cause is unknown but may start from rooting or other local trauma. The onset is rapid, and with proper therapy the course is short (14 to 21 days). Lesions start as papules and pustules, but deep folliculitis and furunculosis soon develop. The deep infection produces scarring, which can be aggravated by overly vigorous cleansing or topical therapy.

Differential diagnosis is extensive and includes the immune-mediated diseases such as discoid or systemic lupus erythematosus, pemphigus foliaceus or erythematosus, demodicosis, dermatophytosis (especially that caused by *Trichophyton mentagrophytes* or *M. gypseum*), drug eruptions, dermatomyositis, subcorneal pustular dermatosis, zinc-responsive dermatosis, trauma, and solar dermatitis.

Clinical management should include a careful consideration of underlying causes, especially if bacterial smears and cultures are negative for bacteria or fungi. The bacterial infections are usually secondary, and they may be caused by a variety of organisms. Appropriate systemic antibiotics should be given in full dosage for 7 to 10 days beyond clinical cure. Gentle topical therapy with wet soaks using Burow's solution or chlorhexidine, three to five times daily for 10 minutes, is excellent. This must be applied gently to prevent further trauma to the tender, inflamed tissues. Elizabethan collars or sedation are rarely needed to alleviate pain and prevent self-induced trauma during the first few days of treatment.

MUZZLE FOLLICULITIS/FURUNCULOSIS

(Canine "Acne")

This is a chronic inflammatory disorder of the chin and lips of young dogs characterized by a deep folliculitis and furunculosis (see Fig. 5:1F).[39] It is most common in short-coated breeds, such as boxers, Doberman pinschers, English bulldogs, Great Danes, Weimaraners, mastiffs, and German short-haired pointers.

Sometimes the disease is discovered by accident, as the lesions are often innocuous and self-limiting. They often disappear with the onset of puberty. Dogs that still have lesions after 1 year of age are unlikely to be cured. Because this is a follicular disease of the face of young dogs, demodicosis and dermatophytosis are the two diseases to be ruled out in a differential diagnosis.

Figure 5:9. Folliculitis—deep pyodermas. *A,* Nasal folliculitis (pyoderma) of pointer's nose. Pustules and crusts are typical of painful lesions. *B,* Nasal folliculitis (pyoderma) showing pustules on dorsum of the nose. *C,* Pododermatitis (interdigital pyoderma) showing pustules and draining fistulas. *D,* Pododermatitis (interdigital pyoderma) with severe edema, cellulitis, and draining sinuses. *E,* Lateral rump and thigh of a German shepherd with furunculosis. *F,* Rump, thigh, and trunk of a German shepherd with furunculosis. Note flea bite hypersensitivity type of distribution pattern. *G,* Pyotraumatic folliculitis (pyotraumatic dermatitis) with severe secondary self-trauma. Note satellite lesions. (Courtesy W. H. Miller, Jr.) *H,* Clostridial cellulitis and necrosis associated with mastitis. (Courtesy W. H. Miller, Jr.)

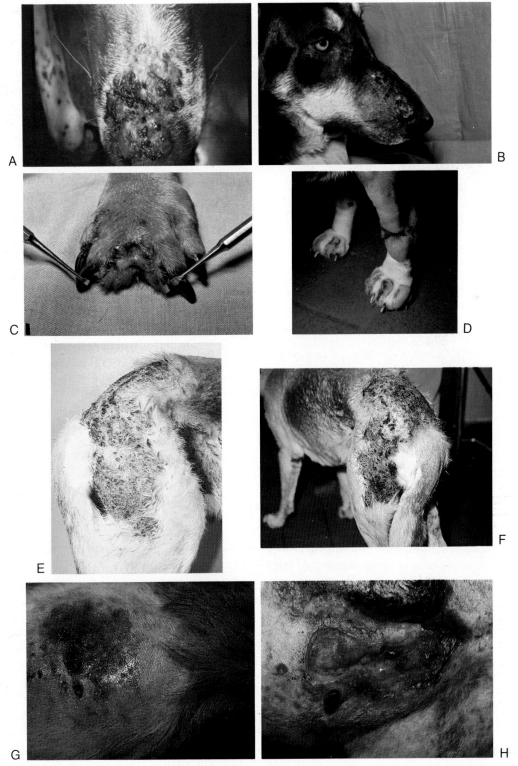

Figure 5:9 *See legend on opposite page*

Treatment may be limited to benign observation or to daily shampoos with benzoyl peroxide, for its follicular flushing action. Benzoyl peroxide gels may also be useful. Only rarely are systemic antibiotics indicated. For chronic cases in adult dogs, an initial course of appropriate antibiotic therapy followed by a penetrating topical glucocorticoid (e.g., Synotic [fluocinolone in DMSO]) applied daily for the first week, then tapered to maintenance (twice a week) is often effective. Presumably hair and keratin can act as cutaneous foreign bodies and cause persistent disease.

PODODERMATITIS
(Interdigital Pyoderma)

Pododermatitis is an inflammatory, multifaceted disease complex that affects the feet of dogs.[2, 71]

CAUSE AND PATHOGENESIS

The cause of this disease is often unknown, but in no cases are the resulting lesions "cysts." The disease is complex and may be frustrating to diagnose and treat.[54] Local factors may be common and relatively easy to find and correct. These include foreign bodies (such as foxtails, awns, thorns, wood slivers, and seeds) and local trauma. When a single foot is affected, a foreign body or local injury should be suspected, especially when there is only one interdigital fistula. The feet are subject to a great variety and intensity of trauma, the front feet more so than the rear. Hunting or field dogs commonly are afflicted with bruises from stones, stubble, and briars; animals walking in sticky substances may accumulate masses of sand, stones, tar, and hair that initiate injury. Contact with irritant chemicals, fertilizers, or weed may cause trouble too. Clipper "burns" from grooming procedures, irritation from housing on wire or rough stones, and inflammation from contact, inhalant, or food hypersensitivities have all initiated pododermatitis. Any of these factors may cause intense licking, which accentuates the irritation.

Fungal infections associated with pododermatitis include dermatophytosis, candidiasis, mycetoma, sporotrichosis, blastomycosis, and cryptococcosis. These are reasonably rare but should be suspected in cases that are refractory to usual antibiotic therapy. Bacterial infections are always secondary and can include a wide variety of organisms. Bacterial hypersensitivity may be a complication (see p. 493).

Parasitic pododermatitis is particularly common, with demodicosis being its most troublesome cause. Every case of chronic interdigital pyoderma must be carefully scraped to look for demodectic mites. Biopsy may be necessary to make the diagnosis of parasitic pododermatitis in chronically inflamed and fibrosed feet. It is often missed! Other parasites involved may include *Pelodera* spp., *Ancylostoma* spp., and *Uncinaria* spp. Ticks and chiggers favor the interdigital webs and may initiate inflammation.

Psychogenic dermatitis may be manifested as excessive licking of the feet by high-strung, nervous individuals—especially poodles, terriers, and German shepherds.

Sterile pyogranulomas may occur on the feet. The cause is unknown, but they are most common in smooth, short-coated breeds such as English bulldogs, dachshunds, Great Danes, and boxers (see p. 552). Osteomyelitis or local neoplasms more characteristically involve a single foot.

Cases of pododermatitis that involve several feet or that are recurrent or refractory to treatment should be evaluated for immunity or neutrophil function that is compromised.[71] Pododermatitis may also be the only clinical sign of hypothyroidism or demodicosis with secondary suppression of cell-mediated immunity. One report suggests that the flat foot and the scoop-shaped web of breeds like the Pekingese and some terriers predispose the area to folliculitis and pedal dermatitis.[83]

Cases of pododermatitis with significant footpad involvement (hyperkeratosis, ulceration) may have an autoimmune basis (pemphigus, pemphigoid, or lupus erythematosus) or may be a manifestation of a drug eruption, zinc-responsive dermatitis, hepatocutaneous syndrome, or canine distemper.

In spite of all these possibilities, a substantial number of cases are idiopathic, recurrent bacterial infections. These can be exceedingly frustrating to manage.

CLINICAL FEATURES

Pododermatitis may affect dogs of any age, sex, or breed, but males of short-coated breeds, such as the English bulldog, Great Dane, basset hound, mastiff, bull terrier, boxer, dachshund, Dalmatian, German shorthaired pointer, and Weimaraner, are more commonly represented. Longer-coated breeds that are commonly affected include German shepherd, Labrador retriever, Golden retriever, Irish setter, and Pekingese. Front feet are more often affected, but one or all four feet may be involved.

Affected tissue may be red and edematous with nodules, ulcers, fistulas, hemorrhagic bullae, and a serosanguinous exudate (Fig. 5:9C). The feet may be grossly swollen (Fig. 5:9D). Pitting edema of the metacarpal and metatarsal areas can be marked. The skin may be alopecic and moist from constant licking, and varying degrees of pain, pruritus, and paronychia may be present. The pain may produce lameness. In some cases the interdigital nodules are nontender and unresponsive to treatment and may be scarred from former lesions. Although the regional lymph nodes are enlarged, other systemic signs seldom occur.

DIAGNOSIS

In some cases, a careful history and physical examination provide the diagnosis of pododermatitis. Because of the complex pathogenesis, all cases for which a cause is not quickly and easily discerned should undergo multiple skin scrapings, a Gram's or Diff Quik stained smear, fungal culture, bacterial culture and antibiotic sensitivity tests, and a representative skin biopsy for H & E stain and direct immunofluorescence testing. The direct smear may provide early clues of the cause by establishing the presence or absence of neutrophils or phagocytized bacteria and their staining property or by showing large numbers of eosinophils, mycetoma or pseudomycetoma "grains," yeast, or largely mononuclear cell exudate. Radiographs for bony changes and opaque foreign bodies may also be needed. In some instances, an evaluation of the immune status might include a hemogram, serum protein electrophoresis, serum immunoglobulin quantification, neutrophil function studies (bactericidal assay, chemotaxis), cell-mediated immunity studies (lymphocyte blastogenesis), serum complement levels, and thyroid-stimulating hormone (TSH) response and dexamethasone suppression tests.

Histopathologic studies are essential to look for foreign bodies (including free hair shafts or keratin in the tissue), bacteria, parasites, fungi, and neoplasia, and to evaluate the cellular response. Special stains may be needed. In general, the histologic response is that of perifolliculitis, folliculitis, or furunculosis; and with the last, a nodular-to-diffuse pyogranulomatous inflammation is common (see p. 78). Direct immunofluorescence testing can be done to pursue the possibility of autoimmune disorders being a cause.

CLINICAL MANAGEMENT

The etiologic factors underlying pododermatitis must be considered. Therapeutic measures depend on the test results and the final diagnosis.

Intensive medical and surgical therapy should be started regardless of the underlying cause. The animal is given a systemic antibiotic suggested by the physical examination and preliminary direct smear or culture (cephalosporin, amoxicillin with clavulanic acid, or chloramphenicol may be useful). General anesthesia is then administered, and the affected feet are prepared for surgery. The surgical objective is to extensively incise and explore all fistulous tracts and to excise all nodules and areas of devitalized tissue. Even when properly performed, this can be a grossly hemorrhagic and unpleasant operation. The feet are cleaned, packed in a topical antibacterial medication, such as nitrofurazone, povidone-iodine, or chlorhexidine dressing, and bandaged firmly enough to stop bleeding for 24 hours. When the dressings are removed, the feet are placed in a whirlpool or in wet soaks for 15 to 20 minutes twice daily. Antibacterial solutions of povidone-iodine or chlorhexidine are beneficial (see p. 162). Systemic antibiotics indicated by sensitivity tests are continued for 7 to 10 days beyond clinical cure (often 8 to 12 weeks), and water soaks are continued until the surgical wounds are healed. Do not give corticosteroids.

Pododermatitis associated with bacterial hypersensitivity or that of idiopathic origin may respond to bacterin or staphylococcal phage lysate therapy (see p. 497).

Cases associated with yeast or dermatophyte infections should be treated locally with 3 per cent lime-sulfur solution or a 1:200 dilution of Captan soaks (p. 165), as well as systemic treatment with griseofulvin or ketoconazole.

Demodicosis is common as a cause of pododermatitis, and therapy for infection without addressing the parasites is futile. This topic is discussed in more detail on page 390. One of the authors (G.H.M.) has obtained excellent results with topical treatment using a mixture of 0.5 ml amitraz (Mitaban) in 30 ml of mineral oil. This is shaken well and gently rubbed into the lesions every third day. The mixture must be made up freshly every week. In cases in which demodectic pododermatitis is associated with generalized demodicosis, the entire animal must be treated as described on page 391. Local therapy alone is not adequate! Never use systemic corticosteroids with demodectic pododermatitis.

The most effective therapy for *sterile pyogranuloma complex* is systemic prednisone or prednisolone, 2.2 mg/kg SID orally until healed, and then alternate morning therapy, which should be reduced or withdrawn as dictated by the animal's response (see p. 555).

If hypothyroidism, natural or iatrogenic hyperadrenocorticism, or demodicosis is corrected, the pododermatitis may show dramatic improvement because of reversal of an immunodeficiency state. Nonspecific therapy for immunosuppression that is occasionally beneficial is a bacterial vaccine series (see p. 185), or an immune modulator such as levamisole can be used (see p. 184). These therapeutic measures may need to be continued indefinitely.

GERMAN SHEPHERD FOLLICULITIS, FURUNCULOSIS, AND CELLULITIS
(Deep Pyoderma of German Shepherds)

This is a deep folliculitis, furunculosis, and in some cases cellulitis, seen almost exclusively in middle-aged German shepherd dogs.

CAUSE AND PATHOGENESIS

A bacterial origin of the disease is suggested, as hemolytic staphylococci, both coagulase positive and coagulase negative, have been commonly isolated.[44] *Staphylococcus intermedius* is probably the major cause, although hemolytic streptococci and *Escherichia coli* have also been isolated.[85] Recent literature suggests that coagulase-negative staphylococci can cause disease in many human organ systems, including skin.[15]

There are certainly predisposing causes affecting the onset of this disorder. Almost all individuals started their disease with pruritus, and since lesions commonly involve the rump, back and thighs, flea bite hypersensitivity would be a prime suspect. Atopy and hypothyroidism have been present in some dogs. Bacterial hypersensitivity, genetic predisposing factors, immune deficiencies, and hypothyroidism have all been considered as precipitating or complicating factors.[44, 59, 85]

CLINICAL FEATURES

The disease almost exclusively affects middle-aged German shepherd dogs, and it is not sex related or influenced by gonadal status. A familial history is occasionally given. Almost all dogs were intensely pruritic and most had fleas. The distribution pattern is typical, with the rump, back, ventral abdomen, and thighs being affected in all cases (Fig. 5:7). Some individuals have more generalized lesions spreading to the chest and neck. The front legs, head, and ears are usually much less involved.

Lesions are usually follicular in origin with clusters of papules, pustules, erosions, and crusts followed by ulcers, fistulas, furunculosis, alopecia, and hyperpigmentation (Figs. 5:9E,F). There may be a great deal of excoriation from the pruritus. Some individuals have seborrhea and hyperkeratosis, and cellulitis is evident in deeper infections. Peripheral lymphadenopathy is common. Animals with the disorder are usually in general good health, although there may be weight loss, poor appetite, and pyrexia. The lesions are usually painful.

The course of the disease is long and stormy with frequent stages of partial healing and exacerbation. This is usually produced by improper selection or inadequate dosage and duration of antibiotics, the concurrent use of corticosteroids, or failure to resolve predisposing factors.

DIAGNOSIS

The physical examination makes the diagnosis highly suggestive. A bacterial culture and antibiotic sensitivity test must be completed, and a hemogram, serum chemistry panel, and thyroid-stimulating hormone (TSH) response test are important to rule out complicating medical problems or to suggest further evaluation of immunocompetence. Fungal culture, skin scraping (demodicosis), and direct smears of exudates are also helpful. The latter usually demonstrates degenerate neutrophils and phagocytized cocci and gives early support to the diagnosis and guidance in initial antibiotic selection.

In one series of cases, histopathologic examination of skin biopsy tissues revealed folliculitis, furunculosis, and cellulitis as the most common findings.[44] Perifollicular pyogranulomatous inflammation was often seen, which supports the follicular origin of the disease. Only a few biopsies showed the large number of eosinophils expected when furunculosis occurs. Another report described the histopathology of 23 cases in the Netherlands, which had hyperkeratosis, acanthosis, and a poorly demarcated, predominantly proliferative dermatitis.[85] Dermal edema was observed, with an exudate predominantly composed of neutrophils and mononuclear cells. In only four cases was the subcutis involved. All of the dogs in this series responded partially and temporarily to 3 to 6 weeks of antibacterial therapy, but relapsed after cessation of the relatively short treatment.

CLINICAL MANAGEMENT

Corticosteroids have no place in the therapy of this disease although one of the authors (GHM) has used them in cases that fail to respond to antibiotic therapy. Aggressive, appropriate antibiotic therapy is the keystone of successful management. Narrow-spectrum antibiotics are indicated; these are selected to be effective against the isolated pathogen. Therapy is re-evaluated after 10 days and continued for at least 7 to 10 days beyond clinical cure.

Topical therapy is essential. It is wise to at least partially clip the animal in the owner's presence so that the shock of its appearance and the magnitude of the problem will be evident. It is essential to sedate the dog, perform a whole body clip, and gently cleanse its entire body with an antibacterial shampoo. After drying, it is amazing how much better the lesions often appear. Whole-body whirlpool baths (see p. 151) and long-term (6 to 10 weeks) systemic antibiotic therapy (see p. 175) are always indicated. Many cases relapse when antibiotics are withdrawn. If this happens, bacterin therapy, immune modulation, or long-term once-a-day or once-a-week antibiotic therapy should be considered (see p. 183). If an immunosuppressed state is confirmed, bactericidal antibiotics should be used. Complicating diseases such as demodicosis, hypothyroidism, atopy, food hypersensitivity, or dermal parasitisms should be handled appropriately.

This is a disease that is easily diagnosed, often initially treated successfully, but that frequently relapses. It may be poorly named. Much more study is needed to explain heritability and the influence of predisposing factors, such as immune defects, in the pathogenesis and management of the disease.

ANAEROBIC CELLULITIS

Cellulitis is a severe, deep, suppurative infection in which the area of infection is poorly defined and tends to dissect through tissue planes. There may be extensive edema, and the skin is often friable, darkly discolored, and devitalized.[27] The weakened tissues may be sloughed or removed easily in the process of treatment so that the affected areas may appear to be more extensive than they really are.

These deep, soft-tissue infections with gangrene and crepitant cellulitis may develop in areas of trauma, surgery (Fig. 5:9H), severe bruising with ischemia, burns, malignancy, and foreign-body introduction. They also may be introduced via poorly managed indwelling catheters; *Serratia marcescens* is a serious nosocomial pathogen that can produce local infection and septicemia in this way.[137] Conditions that create a local decrease in oxygen tension predispose to anaerobe infections. Cellulitis may be seen secondary to cases of diabetes mellitus, demodicosis, or with immunodeficiency. Contamination of predisposed areas with body fluids, but especially with feces, provides the necessary bacterial inoculum for infection. Organisms may include *Clostridia* sp., *Bacteroides* sp., Peptostreptococci, and Enterobacteriaceae such as *Serratia marcescens*.[20] These infections cause mild local pain and skin changes that are minimal at first but later progress rapidly. Systemic toxicity soon develops, and tissue gas accumulation may be extensive. Pure clostridial infections rarely emit foul odors, while mixed anaerobe or nonclostridial crepitant cellulitis frequently is putrid.[25, 27]

Surgery is almost always indicated in treatment of these infections. Necrotic tissue must be removed, since neither host defenses nor antibiotics are effective in necrotic areas. Tissue hypoxia must be remedied too. Proper cleaning, whirlpool therapy, drainage, and high levels of antibiotics are mandatory. For *clostridia*, very high levels of penicillin are suggested; for most other anaerobes, clindamycin, amoxicillin, chloramphenicol, or metronidazole may be useful.[25] Aminoglycosides are usually ineffective.

Serratia marcescens and *Klebsiella pneumoniae* may be especially troublesome, and therefore sensitivity studies are advised. In one report, amikacin (7 mg/kg IM q6h) with piperacillin sodium (40 mg/kg IM q6h) was used for 7 days to cure a dog with *S. marcescens* infection of the leg.[3]

These infections are always serious, and a careful, thorough plan of management is essential.

SUBCUTANEOUS ABSCESSES

Subcutaneous abscesses are most commonly encountered in cats. Bacteria from claw or fang are injected under the skin when it is punctured by a bite or scratch during a cat fight. The wound is small and seals rapidly—and a local infection develops in 2 to 4 days. Some bite wounds are handled well by the cat's normal defense mechanisms. Those that abscess are most commonly found around the tail base and the neck and shoulders. Abscess from bite wounds is one of the most common cat diseases handled in a small animal practice. Untreated, the abscess may rupture, drain, and heal over a period of 2 to 3 weeks. However, the treatment of choice is liberal surgical drainage and thorough flushing of the area with saline, hydrogen peroxide, chlorhexidine solution, or povidone-iodine solution, together with high doses of penicillin or ampicillin systemically for 5 to 7 days. These antibiotics effectively cover the organisms normally found in the cat's mouth and often in the abscess (*Pasteurella multocida*, fusiform bacilli, β-hemolytic streptococci, and *Bacteroides* sp.).

Periodically, a clinician comes up with the suggestion of aspirating the fluid pus from the abscess and injecting an antibiotic solution. This practice should be condemned. The proper treatment for any localized infection is thorough surgical drainage!

Castration of intact male cats has been shown to be a helpful preventive measure, resulting in either rapid or gradual decline in fighting and roaming behavior in 80 to 90 per cent of the cats so treated.[20a, 59]

Recurrent or nonhealing feline abscesses should prompt a consideration of feline leukemia virus infection, immunosuppression, and other infectious agents (*Actinomyces* sp., *Nocardia* sp., *Yersinia pestis*, mycobacteria, mycoses, or sterile panniculitis).[59] *Corynebacterium equi*, resistant to penicillium and tetracycline, was isolated from a feline abscess.[21a] Many anaerobic organisms sometimes are found in feline abscesses.[74] Mycoplasma-like organisms have been isolated from cats with chronic subcutaneous abscesses.[42a] These abscesses were characterized by (1) red-brown nonodorous pus, (2) degenerate neutrophils but no visible microorganisms in direct smears of pus, (3) absence of microbial growth using standard aerobic and anaerobic culture techniques, and (4) failure to respond to routine medical/surgical therapy. All abscesses healed rapidly with tetracycline therapy.

BACTERIAL PSEUDOMYCETOMA
(Cutaneous Bacterial Granuloma, Botryomycosis)

Bacterial pseudomycetoma is a chronic, suppurative, granulomatous disease caused by nonbranching bacteria. They form "grains" of compact colonies in tissues that are surrounded by pyogranulomatous inflammation.[78] Botryomycosis is common in many species but is rarely reported, probably often misdiagnosed or overlooked. The causative bacteria are usually coagulase-positive staphylococci, but in some cases other bacteria, alone or associated with staphylococci, may be responsible. There may be *Pseudomonas* sp., *Proteus* sp., *Streptococcus* sp., and *Actinobacillus* sp. In cases involving dogs and cats, Walton and colleagues reported isolation of multiple organisms.[78]

Most cases involving the skin are initiated by local trauma from bites or other wounds, and some are associated with a foreign body. There may also be muscle or bone involvement. The granuloma develops because a delicate balance exists between the virulence of the organism and the response of the host. The host is able to isolate and contain the infection but unable to eradicate it. This also may be a type of bacterial hypersensitivity, or the grain formation may be associated with the formation of a polysaccharide slime coating produced by the bacteria or a glycoprotein covering resulting from a localized antigen-antibody reaction on the surface of the microorganisms.[10]

Clinically, the skin form of the disease appears as firm solitary or multiple nodules with draining fistulas (Fig. 5:10A). The purulent exudate may have small white granules similar to grains of sand (Fig. 5:11). Special bacterial and fungal stains are necessary to differentiate the granules from those found in actinomycosis, nocardiosis, or mycetomas.

Histopathologically, there is a nodular-to-diffuse dermatitis or nodular-to-diffuse panniculitis, with tissue granules surrounded by a granulomatous-to-pyogranulomatous infiltrate of histiocytes, plasma cells, lymphocytes, neutrophils, and histiocytic giant cells (Fig. 5:10B). The edges of the bacteria masses (granules) may show clubbing and may stain brightly eosinophilic with H & E (Hoeppli-Splendore material). The bacteria are best demonstrated with Gram's tissue stain or Brown and Brenn stain.

Differential diagnosis must include actinomycosis, nocardiosis, eumycotic

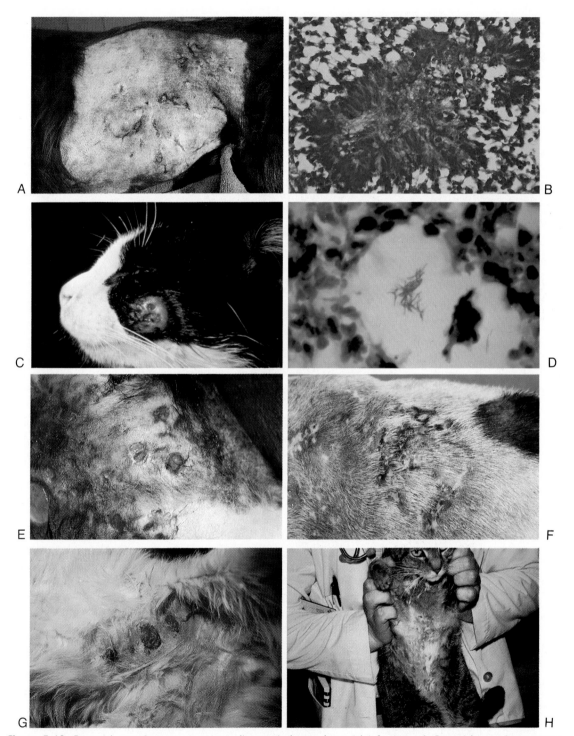

Figure 5:10. Bacterial pseudomycetoma, nocardia, atypical mycobacterial infections. *A*, Bacterial pseudomycetoma (botryomycosis) on dog trunk. Area has been clipped to show nodules and draining tracts. *B*, Bacterial pseudomycetoma (botryomycosis) biopsy section. Note tissue grain. *C*, Ulcerated lesion of feline leprosy on face of a cat. (Courtesy, G. T. Wilkinson.) *D*, Acid-fast organisms in center of clear vacuole in tissue biopsy of atypical mycobacterial granuloma. (Courtesy T. L. Gross and G. A. Kunkle.) *E*, Multiple necrotic granulomatous lesions on the body of a cat associated with *M. fortuitum* infection. (Courtesy W. H. Miller, Jr.) *F*, Soft-tissue infection with draining fistulas on thorax of a dog with atypical mycobacterial granuloma due to *M. chelonei*. (Courtesy G. A. Kunkle.) *G*, Atypical mycobacteriosis (with panniculitis) on the abdomen of a cat. (Courtesy W. H. Miller, Jr.) *H*, Cutaneous nocardiosis (with panniculitis) in a cat. (Courtesy W. H. Miller, Jr.)

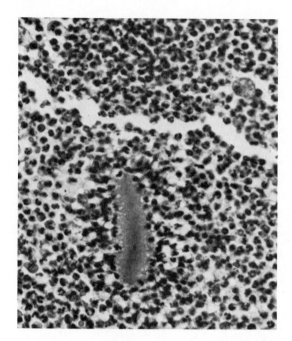

Figure 5:11. Bacterial pseudomycetoma. Pyogranulomatous dermatitis with central tissue grain.

mycetoma, systemic mycoses, subcutaneous dermatophytosis, foreign-body reactions, and chronic bacterial abscesses. Because of the variable prognoses and therapeutic formats, it is imperative that a specific diagnosis be made.

Simple surgical drainage with systemic antibiotic therapy is not usually an adequate treatment, and frequent relapses are the rule. Therapy is essentially limited to complete surgical excision, since the granulomatous mass is relatively impermeable to antibiotics.[78] Appropriate postsurgical antibiotic therapy is essential.

MYCOBACTERIAL GRANULOMAS

Mycobacteria can be divided into three groups: obligate pathogens such as *Mycobacterium tuberculosis* and *M. lepraemurium*, which do not multiply outside vertebrate hosts; facultative pathogens, which normally exist as saprophytes in the environment but sporadically cause disease; and environmental saprophytes, which almost never cause disease.[80] Mycobacteria and the disease syndromes they cause can be further classified as follows:

1. True tuberculosis mycobacteria. *M. tuberculosis*, both bovine and human types. In endemic areas they cause small animal tuberculosis. They are photochromogenic and slow growers, and if injected into guinea pigs they cause death in 6 to 8 weeks—opportunistic mycobacteria do not (see discussion that follows).

2. Leprosy mycobacteria. *M. lepraemurium* causes rat leprosy, which is possibly transmitted to small animals. It is scotochromogenic and does not grow on laboratory media. Many acid-fast organisms are usually found in histologic sections. (See also discussion of Feline Leprosy p. 274).

3. Opportunistic mycobacteria. These can be divided into groups according to their rate of growth and pigment production.

One group of slow-growing organisms (more than 7 days) is nonchromogenic and pathogenic only to cold-blooded animals. Another group of slow-growing mycobacteria of this group include *M. kansasii, M. marinum, M. ulcerans,* and *M. avium* and are facultative pathogens.

The fast-growing (2 to 3 days, or less than 7 days) mycobacteria in the "atypical" or opportunistic group include *M. fortuitum, M. chelonei, M. balnei, M. phlei,* and *M. smegmatis.* Organisms may be scattered through tissues so that a careful search must be made for them. They are often found in small vacuoles in the granulomatous tissue. (See Opportunistic Mycobacterial Granulomas, p. 276).

Natural water may be teeming with saprophytic mycobacteria, including some that are facultative or opportunistic pathogens. These can produce infection by contamination when predisposing factors are present.[80] In trying to isolate and identify individual species, decontamination of saprophytes from cultures, differentiation by biochemical tests, and immunodiffusion analysis are difficult. Recent data suggest that *M. fortuitum* and *M. chelonei* are almost identical culturally. Many cases reported to be caused by the former may actually have been caused by *M. chelonei.*[80] The pathogenicity, prognosis, and epidemiology of the two are not comparable and are more serious with *M. chelonei.*

Cutaneous Tuberculosis

The incidence of cutaneous tuberculosis of dogs and cats has decreased with the decrease of the disease in humans and cattle.[76] It is a rare disease in most parts of the world unless pets experience a high degree of exposure.[60] Animals that live where there are large numbers of people (restaurants or public places), have close contact with an infected owner (i.e., sleeping in the sick person's room), or are fed a variety of unprocessed meat or milk from areas of endemic disease have an increased chance of infection. One per cent of dogs and 3 per cent of cats autopsied at Alfort Veterinary College in 1965 had tuberculosis; of these cases, about 65 per cent were the human type. Others have reported 75 per cent of cases in the dog were due to *M. tuberculosis,* the balance being due to *M. bovis.*[29] Dogs are relatively resistant to *M. avium,* but a few cases have been reported. The predominant lesions in small animals are respiratory and digestive, but there are some skin lesions too.[60] In cats, clinical signs may be insidious, and because diagnostic tests are unreliable, epidemiologic data are of questionable validity.[72, 76]

CLINICAL FEATURES

Cutaneous lesions are single or multiple ulcers, abscesses, plaques, and nodules. Nodules may be in the skin or adherent to subcutaneous tissues (Fig. 5:12). They fail to come to a head and may discharge a thick yellow-to-green pus with an unpleasant odor. The lesions are most common on the head, neck, and limbs. Patients usually appear sick; they have anorexia, weight loss, fever, and lymphadenopathy.[72]

DIAGNOSIS

Diagnosis is by history, physical examination, radiograph, biopsy, culture, bacille Calmette-Guérin (BCG) test (dogs),[60] or lymphocyte blastogenesis test

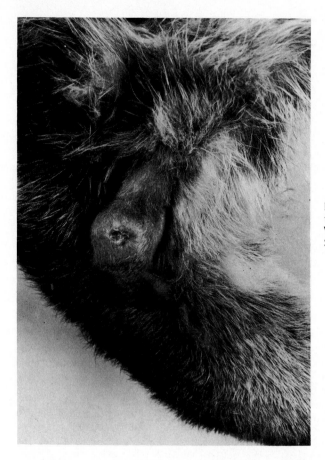

Figure 5:12. An ulcerated skin nodule of cutaneous tuberculosis on the leg of a cat. (Courtesy G. T. Wilkinson and Department of Pathology, Royal [Dick] School of Veterinary Studies, Edinburgh.)

(cats).[43] Biopsy may show a nodular-to-diffuse dermatitis due to pyogranulomatous inflammation (with necrosis and caseation), rare histiocytic giant cells and mineralization, and few-to-many acid-fast organisms. Smears or biopsy will not differentiate between true tuberculosis and opportunistic mycobacterial granulomas. Injection of cultures into guinea pigs causes death in 6 to 8 weeks, but not if the organism is nontuberculous.

BCG prepared for humans can be used to test dogs for tuberculosis. Intradermal injection of 0.1 ml is read at 48 to 72 hours (no sooner). Erythema that resorbs by that time is a negative test. Severe erythema with central necrosis progressing to ulceration *at 10 to 14 days* is significant. Ulceration *after 18 to 21 days* may occur in normal dogs.[60]

CLINICAL MANAGEMENT

With a positive diagnosis, the animal should be euthanized and public health authorities notified. This disease is too dangerous to human beings to justify the risk of treating animals.

Feline Leprosy

Feline leprosy is a granulomatous, nodular, cutaneous infection associated with nonculturable, acid-fast bacteria.

CAUSE AND PATHOGENESIS

It appears that *Mycobacterium lepraemurium* is not the etiologic agent.[56, 68a] Guinea pigs injected with homogenized fresh tissue from spontaneous feline cases are resistant, but rats and cats develop typical local cutaneous and lymph node lesions with demonstrable mycobacteria. In addition, many of the experimental rats develop a generalized granulomatous mycobacterial disease.[68] *M. lepraemurium* injections cause no lesions in cats but produce characteristic lesions of murine leprosy in rats. Local lesions appeared in cats 2 to 6 months after experimental injections of tissue from naturally occurring lesions. The long incubation time is consistent with the higher incidence of diagnosis (50 per cent of the cases) in western Canada during the winter months following exposure in the summer. Live *M. leprae* (leprosy bacillus of humans) has been found in mosquitoes, fleas, and ticks, so it may also be possible for feline leprosy to be transmitted by these vectors too. However, the natural mode of infection is unknown. The disease has been reported in New Zealand, Australia, Great Britain, France, the Netherlands, the United States, and Canada.

Human leprosy is closely associated with immunodeficiency, but the immunologic status of cats with feline leprosy is largely unknown. One experimental cat that was affected naturally, several years previously, failed to develop lesions when inoculated with a homogenate of infectious tissue.[68] McIntosh inoculated five affected cats intradermally with lepromin.[56] Those with tuberculoid leprosy reacted positively, while those with lepromatous leprosy were negative. Lymphocyte stimulation assays were normal in all cats.

In human leprosy, the type of tissue reaction is thought to be a reflection of the immune status of the host. Similar types of reactions are seen in feline leprosy. In refractory individuals that can mount a cell-mediated response, a tuberculoid granulomatous reaction results with few, if any, bacilli present. Susceptible individuals, on the other hand, respond with a lepromatous granuloma and a huge number of bacteria are present.

CLINICAL FEATURES

Lesions are single or multiple cutaneous nodules, which may or may not be ulcerated, from various areas of the body. There may be abscesses or fistulas that show no signs of healing (Fig. 5:10C). However, they do not spread. Lesions also have been found on the nasal, buccal, and lingual mucosae. Regional lymphadenopathy is often seen, but without local pain or systemic illness. There is no sex prevalence, but two-thirds of cases occur in cats 1 to 3 years of age.

DIAGNOSIS

Diagnosis is made on the basis of history, physical examination, and the finding of acid-fast bacilli in direct smears and biopsies (Ziehl-Neelsen stain or Fite-Faraco modification) (Fig. 5:10D). Tissue homogenates should be cultured and also inoculated into guinea pigs to eliminate tuberculosis.

Histopathology may reveal two types of reactions. One is the tuberculoid response with caseous necrosis with relatively few organisms, and those are often only in the areas of necrosis. These epithelioid granulomas are usually surrounded by zones of lymphocytes, which are also commonly aggregated around vessels (Fig. 5:13). The second type reaction (lepromatous leprosy) is a

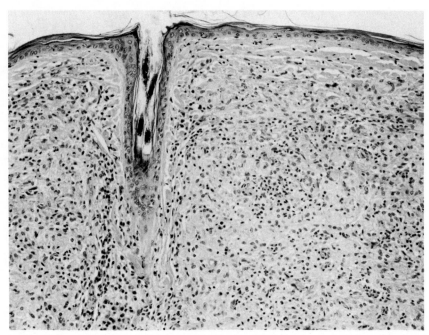

Figure 5:13. Granulomatous inflammation of dermis in a cat. Epidermis intact (H & E stain). (From Schiefer, B., Gee, B. R., and Ward, G. E.: A disease resembling feline leprosy in western Canada. J.A.V.M.A. *165*:1085, 1974.)

granuloma composed of solid sheets of large foamy macrophages containing significant numbers of acid-fast bacilli. The organisms are clustered in globi in a parallel stacking arrangement. Multinucleated histiocytic giant cells often contain bacilli and lymphocytes, and plasma cells may surround vessels (Fig. 5:14). Many polymorphonuclear leukocytes may be present and may cause the lesion to resemble a pyogranuloma.

Differential diagnosis includes: tuberculosis; granulomas due to opportunistic mycobacteria or foreign bodies; deep mycotic infections such as kerion, mycetoma, and phaeohyphomycosis; chronic bacterial infection; eosinophilic granuloma complex and neoplasms such as mast cell tumors, carcinomas, histiocytoma, or lymphoreticular tumors.

CLINICAL MANAGEMENT

Surgical excision is the treatment of choice when there are solitary or circumscribed lesions. Dapsone has been used in doses of 1.0 mg/kg BID to 50 mg BID with variable results. It needs to be used for several weeks and has the potential for producing hemolytic anemia and other toxicities. It is not approved for use in cats. Clofazimine was used to successfully treat one cat at a dosage of 8.0 mg/kg per os once daily for 6 weeks.[90] There were no side-effects. The drug is not approved for cats.

The public health significance of feline leprosy has not been determined.

Opportunistic Mycobacterial Granulomas
(Atypical Mycobacterial Granulomas)

Opportunistic mycobacterial granulomas in dogs and cats can be caused by several "atypical mycobacteria" that are facultative pathogens.

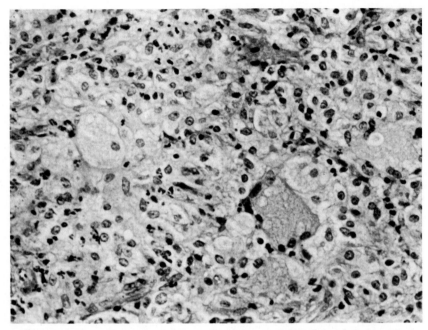

Figure 5:14. Histiocytes with foamy cytoplasm and giant cells (H & E stain). (From Schiefer, B., Gee, B. R., and Ward, G. E.: A disease resembling feline leprosy in western Canada. J.A.V.M.A. *165*:1085, 1974.)

CAUSE AND PATHOGENESIS

Organisms reported to cause cutaneous granulomas in dogs and cats include *Mycobacterium fortuitum*, *M. chelonei*, *M. phlei*, *M. xenopi*, *M. thermoresistible*, and *M. smegmatis*.[13, 24, 30, 47, 81, 84] Because *M. fortuitum* and *M. chelonei* share several metabolic characteristics and are facultative pathogens that result in similar clinical signs, they may be referred to as the M. fortuitum-chelonei complex. The disease has been reported most commonly in cats (perhaps because infection may be introduced through cat bite wounds), but cases in mongrel dogs, a boxer, and a bull mastiff have been recorded.[24, 30]

These mycobacteria are ubiquitous, free-living organisms that are normally harmless and are commonly found in nature. They are found in the soil, but they especially favor water tanks, swimming pools, and sources of natural water.[13] Following injury or injection, they cause chronic subcutaneous abscesses and fistulas. The history of cases of these granulomas occurring in humans commonly cites instances of the disease following a contaminated injection or an infected wound.

These factors appear to cause disease more commonly in animals than in humans. The disease is characterized by chronicity, resistance to antituberculous drugs, and spontaneous resolution.[80]

CLINICAL FEATURES

Following injection, infection of a wound, or other trauma, the lesion develops slowly over a period of several weeks. The course is prolonged and often has been present as a nonhealing wound for several months. Chronic soft-tissue abscessation occurs, with ulcers and draining fistulas (Fig. 5:10*E,F*).

Lesions may localize around the face and head but are commonly on the thorax and abdomen, especially the groin (Fig. 5:10G). The lesions may or may not be painful, and regional lymph nodes are not always enlarged. Systemic illness, such as fever or anorexia, is rarely observed, and the animal feels well.

DIAGNOSIS

Diagnosis is made by finding acid-fast organisms in smears, cultures, or biopsies (Fig. 5:10D). They may be difficult to find on direct smears. Cultures usually grow rapidly and should be made on blood agar and Lowenstein-Jensen (L-J) medium or Stonebrink's medium at 37°C. Because cultural and biochemical tests for positive identification may be complex, the laboratory handling the cultures should be informed that a mycobacterial infection is suspected.

Histopathologic examination may be very helpful. There is a nodular-to-diffuse dermatitis or panniculitis, or both, due to pyogranulomatous inflammation. Stains such as Ziehl-Neelsen or Fite-Faraco modification should be used, and a careful search may be needed to find organisms (Fig. 5:15). They are often clumped in the center of a clear vacuole and surrounded by clusters of neutrophils within the mature granuloma (Fig. 5:16). Alcohol processing in paraffin embedding may cause the acid-fast organism to stain poorly.[81] Rapid Ziehl-Neelsen stain or snap freezing the formalin-fixed tissues with subsequent acid-fast stain enables the bacilli to be seen.[81]

CLINICAL MANAGEMENT

The course is long and the prognosis guarded, but lesions often regress spontaneously after several months, with or without treatment. The most successful therapy is wide surgical excision, débridement, and local treatment. Sutured wounds often break open, and recurrent fistulas are common. It is better to allow wounds to heal by granulation, with appropriate daily local antiseptic lavage. The cases usually do not respond to antitubercular drugs or antibiotics; however, in some cases, laboratory antibiotic sensitivity to kanamycin, gentamicin, and amikacin, has been reasonably reliable, with less dependable sensitivity to erythromycin, chloramphenicol, tetracycline, and polymyxin. It is not clear that these drugs influence the course of the infection.[47]

ACTINOMYCOSIS

This is a rare pyogranulomatous, suppurative disease of many species caused by *Actinomyces* sp. organisms. *A. bovis, A. viscosus, A. baudetii* and *A. hordeovulneris*[9] have been suggested as being causative. They are gram-positive, non–acid fast, catalase-positive, filamentous anaerobic rods that are opportunistic, commensal inhabitants of the oral cavity and bowel.[26a, 72, 73] Infection occurs from trauma and contamination of penetrating wounds, especially those involving foreign bodies such as awns and quills.[33] Hunting or field dogs in southern climates are most commonly affected. Signs take from months to 2 years to develop after the injury; however, organisms can be found in the exudate within 2 weeks.

Clinical lesions may occur as cutaneous granulomas, but subcutaneous abscesses of the face and neck, empyema, or osteomyelitis may develop in

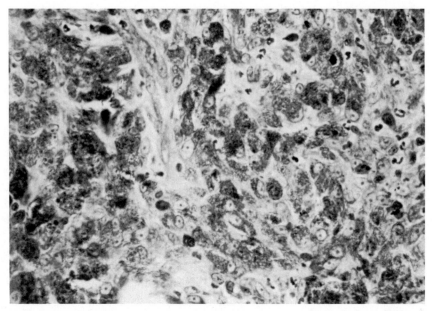

Figure 5:15. Feline atypical mycobacterial granuloma. Note numerous acid-fast organisms within dermal macrophages (Fite-Faraco stain).

Figure 5:16. Histologic section of biopsy from atypical mycobacterial granuloma stained with H & E. Note clear vacuole surrounded by clusters of neutrophils. (Organisms do not stain.) (Courtesy T. Gross and G. Kunkle.)

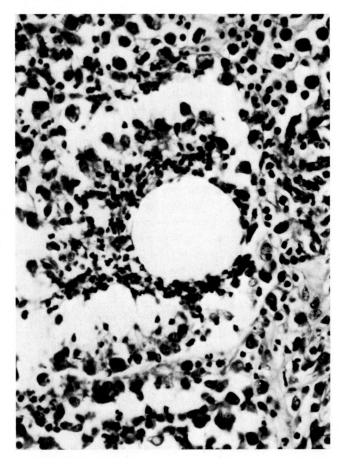

disseminated disease. Draining tracts (mycetoma-like) may discharge a thick yellowish gray or thin hemorrhagic, foul-smelling exudate that contains yellow "sulfur granules."

Diagnosis is by anaerobic culture, direct smears of the granules, and biopsy using special stains (Gram's, Brown and Brenn, or Gomori's methenamine silver). Histopathology reveals a nodular-to-diffuse dermatitis and panniculitis or both due to suppurative or pyogranulomatous inflammation (Figs. 5:17 and 5:18). Tissue grains ("sulfur granules") are usually present. The granules are basophilic and often have a clubbed, eosinophilic periphery (Hoeppli-Splendore material). The gram-positive, non–acid fast, filamentous, occasionally beaded organisms are found within the granules, but they are not easily seen in ordinary H & E preparations. Actinomycosis must be differentiated from nocardiosis, a disease that it closely resembles (p. 282). Since the latter is not highly responsive to penicillin (if treated incorrectly due to misdiagnosis), it may spread rapidly, affecting body cavities and the central nervous system.

Clinical management is based on long-term therapy with antibiotics. High doses of penicillin (100,000 U/kg/day), sulfonamides (10 mg/kg BID), or tri-methoprim-potentiated sulfonamide (5 mg/kg BID) may suffice. Moderately effective drugs are erythromycin, lincomycin, cephalothin, chloramphenicol, tetracycline, and minocycline. The treatment must continue at least 1 month after remission—usually for a total of several months. Local therapy includes surgical débridement and drainage, irrigation of sinuses, and a careful search for foreign bodies. Prognosis is guarded, but one series resulted in over 85 per cent recovery with vigorous therapy.[33] Actinomycosis is not thought to be a contagious disease. (See also therapy for nocardiosis p. 282).

ACTINOBACILLOSIS

Actinobacillosis is a disease of several animal species caused by *Actinobacillus lignieresii*. It resembles actinomycosis in many of its clinical manifestations, but the causative organism is a gram-negative, aerobic coccobacillus that does not survive for a long time outside the host animal. It is a commensal organism found in the mouth of many animals, and clinical lesions often follow bite wounds or injuries around the face and mouth. Infection develops over a period of weeks to months, and its course is long.

Clinical features include single or multiple thick-walled abscesses of the head, neck, mouth, and limbs.[11] They discharge a thick white-to-green odorless pus with soft yellow granules. Diagnosis is made on the basis of aerobic cultures of pus, direct smears, or biopsy of affected tissues.

Histopathology reveals a nodular-to-diffuse dermatitis or panniculitis, or both, due to suppurative or pyogranulomatous inflammation. Tissue grains ("sulfur granules") are usually present. The grains are basophilic and usually surrounded by eosinophilic Hoeppli-Splendore material. Special stains (Gram's or Brown and Brenn) are required to demonstrate the gram-negative organisms.

Clinical management includes surgical extirpation or drainage and curettage. Sodium iodide (0.2 ml/kg of 20 per cent solution, orally BID) and high doses of streptomycin or sulfonamides have been suggested for therapy. The organism also is usually sensitive to tetracycline and chloramphenicol. The course is long, and the prognosis is guarded.[11]

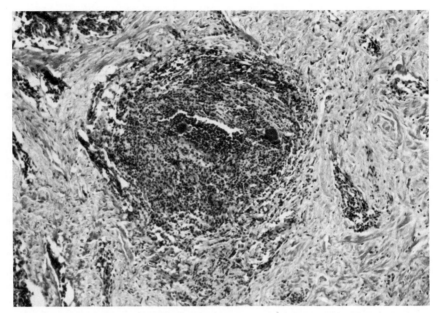

Figure 5:17. Actinomycosis in a dog. Note focal pyogranuloma with two tissue grains.

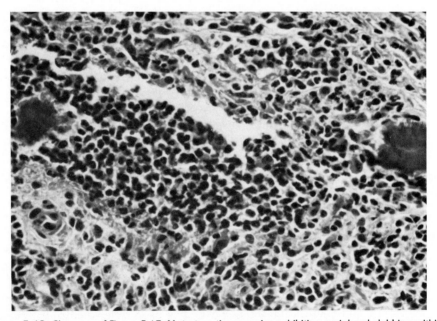

Figure 5:18. Close-up of Figure 5:17. Note two tissue grains exhibiting peripheral clubbing within a pyogranuloma.

NOCARDIOSIS

Nocardiosis is a rare disease characterized by pyogranulomatous and suppurative infection of the skin or lungs, or both, caused by *Nocardia* sp.[26a] The organisms involved, including *N. asteroides, N. braziliensis,* and *N. caviae,* are common soil saprophytes that produce infection by wound contamination, inhalation, and ingestion, particularly in immunocompromised animals. Nocardia are gram-positive, partially acid-fast, branching filamentous aerobes that (except for *N. braziliensis*) have worldwide geographic distribution.

Clinical features are cellulitis, ulcerated nodules, and abscesses that often develop draining sinuses (Fig. 5:10*H*). The exudate has a brownish red, "tomato soup" color and consistency. Sulfur granules are not usually present except with *N. braziliensis* and *N. caviae* infections. Lesions are often found on the limbs, especially the feet, and are often accompanied by lymphadenopathy. Pyothorax may be present, along with other systemic signs, such as weakness, anorexia, fever, depression, and dyspnea, and neurologic signs may be present.[1, 4, 21]

Diagnosis is by direct smear, aerobic culture, and biopsy. Histopathology reveals nodular-to-diffuse dermatitis or panniculitis or both, with or without tissue grains. Special stains (Gram's, Brown and Brenn) are needed to demonstrate organisms. *Nocardia* sp. can be distinguished from *Actinomyces* sp. because they are partially acid fast (modified Fite-Faraco stain) and usually branch at right angles. When branched and beaded, the organisms are similar in appearance to characters of the Chinese alphabet. Differential diagnosis includes actinomycosis and the pyogranulomatous diseases listed on page 276.

Clinical management includes surgical drainage of infected tissues, but antibacterial therapy is the primary need. Large doses of penicillin and a sulfonamide, or sulfadiazine by itself, are helpful. *Equal parts* of sulfadiazine and trimethoprim are probably best.[33] Erythromycin, lincomycin, streptomycin, tetracycline, or minocycline may also be useful. The course of treatment usually continues for several months and should not stop until 4 weeks after clinical remission. Prognosis is guarded. Nocardiosis is not a contagious disease.

Recently, treatment with amikacin, with or without concurrent trimethoprim-sulfamethoxazole, was reported to be very effective for actinomycotic mycetoma (most cases caused by *Nocardia brasiliensis*) in humans.[80a] These patients previously had poor responses to traditional pharmacologic agents, and many had important extracutaneous involvement of organ systems, such as lung, bone, and spinal cord.

Miscellaneous Bacterial Infections

BRUCELLOSIS

Brucellosis may produce a specific secondary scrotal dermatitis resulting from licking the skin over painful epididymitis and orchitis.[69] Some cases may involve necrosis of the testis, with severe inflammation of the entire scrotum, and draining ulcers. *Brucella canis* has been isolated from the exudate.[69]

Brucella canis has also been isolated from a 15-month-old female laboratory beagle with chronic exudative lesions that resembled acral lick dermatitis. Over a period of 16 months, expanding painful lesions developed on both hocks and the dorsum of the right carpus. The lesions were hyperemic, edematous, and granulomatous, with an irregularly pitted surface. A sanguinopurulent exudate was present, and the regional lymph nodes were enlarged. Histologic examination revealed dermal, subcutaneous, and tendinous edema; pronounced lymphoid nodules; a prominent infiltration of macrophages, plasma cells, and lymphocytes; and scattered neutrophils. The enlarged lymph nodes were characterized by sinusoidal histocytosis and medullary cord plasmacytosis. These findings are typical of the tissue response to *Brucella* infection.[22] Diagnosis is made by culture or by tube agglutination tests.

Therapy for canine brucellosis is not recommended because of concerns for public health and concerns for other dogs. In no case should these animals be used for breeding. Castration and long-term therapy with tetracycline or minocycline are suggested in unusual cases in which therapy is undertaken.

PLAGUE

The bubonic plague is an acute, febrile, infectious disease that has a high mortality rate and is caused by the gram-negative organism *Yersinia pestis*, a bipolar ovoid rod of the family Enterobacteriaceae. It is an aerobic, nonmotile, non–spore forming organism that cannot penetrate unbroken skin but can invade mucous membranes. Of the three forms of the disease, the most common is the bubonic, in which localized abscesses form near the site of infection (especially the head and neck). The septicemic and pneumonic forms may be more serious, since they may be undiagnosed until it is too late for effective treatment.

The incubation period is 2 to 6 days, and the course is fulminating and often leads to death. Plague is found in Africa and Asia and in the arid pinion-juniper biomes of the southwestern states of Texas, New Mexico, Arizona, Colorado, California, Utah, and Oregon, where it is an endemic disease. Rodents and cats are highly susceptible, dogs less so, and other domestic animals are resistant. It primarily affects rodents, especially rock and ground squirrels and rats.[66]

Plague is transmitted by fleas or by direct contact with infected animals or exudates. *Diamanus montanus* and four less common rodent-hosted fleas are the primary vectors—the common dog and cat fleas are not normally involved.[68]

An epizootic plague can develop if susceptible rodents come in contact with the *Yersinia* organisms, causing a massive die-off to occur in the rodent colony. The sick rodents become easy prey to cats or other carnivores, and the fleas seek new hosts. Cats can spread the infection to humans by mechanical transmission of infected fleas, by bringing dead or affected rodents home (thus facilitating human contact with the rodent or its fleas), or by direct infection. The latter occurs by bites, contact with pus or by inhalation of droplets from a sneezing or salivating cat. Plague can be a most serious public health problem for people exposed to infected material from clinical cases.[67a]

Animal health personnel handling supposed cat abscesses in endemic plague areas have contracted the disease. In endemic areas, all cats with abscesses should be handled carefully by personnel using disposable gloves and masks, and all animals with plague should be kept in isolation. Oral medications should be avoided, as well as any unnecessary handling, to reduce exposure. Dead animals should be placed in double plastic bags and should be frozen and given to public health authorities for diagnosis and disposal.

Rodents and cats are highly susceptible, dogs less so, and other domestic animals are resistant to plague. Dogs develop mild fevers, whereas cats have severe fevers and subcutaneous abscesses, and 50 per cent may die. Systemic signs are fever, depression, anorexia, and lymphadenopathy. The local signs are single or multiple abscess formations on the limbs, neck, or face—areas that may have been bitten by rodents.

Diagnosis is made by culturing the exudate, by immunofluorescence of impression smears, or by serologic confirmation based on a fourfold increase in antibody titers, from acute to convalescent. The latter is only useful in epidemiologic investigations. It is important to be cautious about the diagnosis, since *Pasteurella multocida* is often cultured from the abscess too. Differential diagnosis should include cat abscesses, wound infections, and other pyogranulomatous diseases listed with feline leprosy (p. 276).

Clinical management includes antibiotic therapy with IM streptomycin (the therapy of choice), tetracycline, or chloramphenicol. The local abscesses must be opened, drained, and irrigated daily with antibacterial solutions (povidone-iodine 1 per cent). Flea control is very important to prevent further spread of infection.

LYME DISEASE
(Borreliosis)

This complex multisystem disorder is caused by a tick-transmitted spirochete *Borrelia burgdorferi*.[53a] Ixodid ticks, especially *Ixodides dammini* are the most common vectors, but other ticks, flies, the cat flea, and mosquitoes have been implicated as possible vectors.

Early stages of the disease in humans show an expanding ring-like rash (erythema chronicum migrans) at the site of the tick bite, which is considered pathognomonic. The macule and/or papule that develops over 1 to 2 weeks has been produced experimentally at an area of shaved rabbit skin. This has not been reported in canine cases, although it may have been present but unobserved due to the heavy coat. Early antibiotic therapy is essential to prevent serious sequelae.[68]

Recently, recurrent pyotraumatic dermatitis (hot spots) has been recognized as a manifestation of canine borreliosis.[86] The lesions are usually solitary, occur over the back and trunk, and exhibit the clinical features of pyotraumatic dermatitis. Histologically, the lesions are characterized by nodular to diffuse pseudolymphoma in the deep dermis. The diagnosis is corroborated by serology (ELISA or IFA).[53a, 86] The lesions have responded rapidly to oral tetracycline therapy.

TRICHOMYCOSIS AXILLARIS

Trichomycosis axillaris is a bacterial infection of the hair shafts of humans. It involves mainly axillary and pubic hair. A similar infection with *Corynebacterium* sp. has been reported in a beagle dog.[62] The animal had a diffuse, irregular, and patchy alopecia that affected the neck and flank regions. There was no dermatitis. In the involved areas, some hairs were broken off and some hair shafts displayed small, hard nodules. Masses of bacteria ensheathed the hair at those locations. Inoculated hair developed nodules that eventually involved the whole hair. Inoculation of normal hair from other dogs produced no alopecia and no bacterial growth. This is not a fungal disease, in spite of its name, and no fungal elements were seen or isolated on culturing.

This is an uncommon and inconsequential disorder that should respond readily to clipping the hair and to frequent use of antibacterial shampoos (OxyDex, Betadine scrub, Nolvasan, Sebbafon).

Pseudopyodermas

There is a group of dermatoses, of variable etiology, which are not pyodermas, although they resemble them. This group includes the following:
1. Callus "pyoderma" (see p. 785)
2. Infantile pustular dermatitis (see p. 841)
3. Juvenile cellulitis (see p. 840)
4. Perianal fistulas (see p. 838)
5. Other pyoderma-like dermatoses
   a. Acne (see p. 739)
   b. Intertrigo (fold dermatitis) (see p. 792)
   c. Linear IgA dermatosis (see p. 541)
   d. Sterile panniculitis (see p. 831)
   e. Pemphigus erythematosus (see p. 505)
   f. Pemphigus foliaceus (see p. 502)
   g. Sterile eosinophilic pustulosis (see p. 549)
   h. Sterile pyogranuloma syndrome (see p. 552)
   i. Subcorneal pustular dermatosis (see p. 828)
   j. Zinc-responsive dermatosis (see p. 801)

References

1. Ackerman, N., Grain, J., et al.: Canine Nocardiosis. J.A.A.H.A. 18:147, 1982.
2. Anderson, R. K.: Canine pododermatitis. Compend. Cont. Ed. 2:361, 1980.
3. Armstrong, J. P.: Systemic Serratia marcescens infections in a dog and a cat. J.A.V.M.A. 184:1154, 1984.
4. Attleberger, M. H.: Actinomycosis, nocardiasis, and dermatophilosis. In Kirk, R. W., (ed.): Current Veterinary Therapy VIII. W. B. Saunders Company Philadelphia, 1983, p. 1184.
5. Berg, J. N., Fales, W. H., et al.: The occurrence of anaerobic bacteria in diseases of the dog and cat. Am. J. Vet. Res. 40:877, 1979.
6. Berg, J. N., Scanlan, C. M., et al.: Clinical models for anaerobic bacterial infection in dogs and their use in testing the efficacy of clindamycin and lincomycin. Am. J. Vet. Res. 45:1299, 1984.
7. Berg, J. M., Wendell, D. E., et al.: Identification of the major coagulase-positive Staphylococcus sp. of dogs as Staphylococcus intermedius. Am. J. Vet. Res. 45:1307, 1984.
8. Bisno, A. L.: Cutaneous infections: Microbiologic and epidemiologic considerations. Am. J. Med. 76:172, May 1984.
9. Buchanan, A. M., and Scott, J. L.: Actinomyces hordeovulneris, a canine pathogen that produces L-phase variants spontaneously with coincident calcium deposition. Am. J. Vet. Res. 54:2552, 1984.
10. Carakostas, M. C., Miller, R. I., et al.: Subcuta-
neous dermatophilosis in a cat. J.A.V.M.A. 185:675, 1984.
11. Carb, A. V., and Liu, S. K.: Actinobacillus lignieresii infection in a dog. J.A.V.M.A. 154:1062, 1969.
12. Chandler, F. W., Kaplan, W., et al.: Histopathology of Mycotic Diseases. Year Book Medical Publishers, Chicago, 1980.
13. Chapman, J. S.: The ecology of the typical mycobacteria. Arch. Environ. Health 22:41, 1971.
14. Chastain, C. B., et al.: Dermatophilosis in two dogs. J.A.V.M.A. 169:1079, 1976.
15. Christensen, G. D.: Coagulase-negative staphylococci—saprophyte or parasite? Int. J. Dermatol. 22:463, 1983.
16. Cox, H. U., Hoskins, J. D., et al.: Antimicrobial susceptibility of coagulase positive staphylococci isolated from Louisiana dogs. Am. J. Vet. Res. 44:2039, 1984.
17. Cox, H. U., Hoskins, J. D.: Distribution of staphylococcal species on clinically healthy cats. Am. J. Vet. Res. 46:1824, 1985.
18. Cox, H. U., Newman, S. S., et al.: Species of staphylococcus isolated from animal infections. Cornell Vet. 74:124, 1984.
19. Cox, H. U., Schmeer, N.: Protein A in Staphylococcus intermedius isolates from dogs and cats. Am. J. Vet. Res. 47:1881, 1986.
20. Crowe, D. T., and Kowalski, J. J.: Clostridial cellulitis with localized gas formation in a dog. J.A.V.M.A. 169:1094, 1976.

21. Davenport, D. J., and Johnson, G. C.: Cutaneous nocardiosis in a cat. J.A.V.M.A. 188:728, 1986.
22. Dawkins, B. G., Machotka, S. V., et al.: Pyogranulomatous dermatitis associated with Brucella canis infection in a dog. J.A.V.M.A. 181:1432, 1982.
23. DeVries, L. A.: Identification and characterization of staphylococci isolated from cats. Vet. Microbiol. 9:279, 1984.
24. Donnelly, T. M., Jones, M. R., et al.: Diffuse cutaneous granulomatous lesions associated with acid-fast bacilli in a cat. J. Small Anim. Pract. 23:99, 1982.
25. Dow, S. W., Jones, R. L., et al.: Anaerobic bacterial infections and response to treatment in dogs and cats: 36 cases (1983–1985) J.A.V.M.A. 189:930, 1986.
26. Emerson, J. K.: Plague. Canine Practice 12:43, 1985.
26a. Fadok, V. A.: Granulomatous dermatitis in dogs and cats. Sem. Vet. Med. Surg. 2:186, 1987.
27. Feingold, D. S.: Gangrenous and crepitant cellulitis. J. Am. Acad. Dermatol. 6:289, 1982.
28. Feingold, D. S.: Bacterial adherence, colonization, and pathogenicity. Arch. Dermatol. 122:161, 1986.
29. Foster, E. S., Seavelli, T. D., et al.: Tuberculosis in a dog. J.A.V.M.A. 188:1188, 1986.
30. Gross, T. L., and Connelly, M. R.: Nontuberculous mycobacterial skin infections in two dogs. Vet. Pathol. 20:117, 1983.
31. Halliwell, R. E. W.: Pyoderma. Proceedings, A.A.H.A. Annual Meeting, 1979, pp. 83–85.
32. Halliwell, R. E. W.: Antibiotic therapy in canine skin disease. Small Anim. Vet. Med. Update Series 12:1, 1978.
33. Hardie, E. M., and Barsanti, J. A.: Treatment of canine actinomycosis. J.A.V.M.A. 180:537, 1982.
34. Hart, B. L., and Barrett, R. E.: Effects of castration on fighting, roaming, and urine spraying in adult male cats. J.A.V.M.A. 163:290, 1973.
35. Higgins, R., Paradis, M.: Abscess caused by Corynebacterium equi in a cat. Can. Vet. J. 21:63, 1980.
36. Hinton, M., Marston, M., et al.: The antibiotic resistance of pathogenic staphylococci and streptococci isolated from dogs. J. Small Anim. Pract. 19:229, 1978.
37. Hirsch, D. C., Indiveri, M. C., et al.: Changes in prevalence and susceptibility of obligate anaerobes in clinical veterinary practice. J.A.V.M.A. 186:1086, 1985.
38. Hurvitz, L., and Ihrke, P. J.: Canine seborrheas. In Kirk, R. W., (ed.): Current Veterinary Therapy VI. W. B. Saunders Company, Philadelphia, 1977.
39. Ihrke, P. J.: The management of canine pyodermas. In Kirk, R. W., (ed.): Current Veterinary Therapy VIII. W. B. Saunders Company, Philadelphia, 1983.
40. Ihrke, P. J.: Therapeutic strategies involving antimicrobial treatment of the skin in small animals. J.A.V.M.A. 185:1165, 1984.
41. Ihrke, P. J.: An overview of bacterial skin disease in the dog. Brit. Vet. J. 143:112, 1987.
42. Ihrke, P. J.: Antibacterial therapy in dermatology. In Kirk, R. W., (ed.): Current Veterinary Therapy IX, W. B. Saunders Company, Philadelphia, 1986.
42a. Keane, D. P.: Chronic abscesses in cats associated with an organism resembling mycoplasma. Can. Vet. J. 24:289, 1983.
43. Kramer, T. T.: Immunity to bacterial infections. Vet. Clin. North Am. 8:683, 1978.
44. Krick, S. A., and Scott, D. W.: Bacterial folliculitis, furunculosis, and cellulitis in the German shepherds: A retrospective analysis of 17 cases. J.A.A.H.A., in press, 1987.
45. Kristensen, S., and Krogh, H. V.: A study of skin diseases in dogs and cats. III. Microflora of the skin of dogs with chronic eczema. Nord. Vet. Med. 30:223, 1978.
46. Krogh, H. V., and Kristensen, S.: A study of skin diseases in dogs and cats. Nord. Vet. Med. 28:459, 1976.
47. Kunkle, G. A., Gulbas, N. K., et al.: Rapidly growing mycobacteria as a cause of cutaneous granulomas: Report of five cases. J.A.A.H.A. 19:513, 1983.
48. Kunkle, G. A.: New considerations for rational antibiotic therapy of cutaneous staphylococcal infection in the dog. Sem. Vet. Med. Surg. 2:212, 1987.
49. Love, D. N., Gailey, M., et al.: Antimicrobial susceptibility patterns of obligately anaerobic bacteria from subcutaneous abscesses and pyothorax in cats. Aust. Vet. Pract. 10:168, 1980.
50. Lloyd, D. H., and Jenkinson, D. M.: The effect of climate on experimental infection of bovine skin with Dermatophilas congolensis. Br. Vet. J. 136:122, 1980.
51. Lloyd, D. H.: Skin surface immunity. Br. Vet. Dermatol. Grp. Newsletter 5:10, 1980.
52. Lloyd, D. H.: The cutaneous defense mechanisms. Br. Vet. Dermatol. Grp. Newsletter 1:9, 1976.
52a. Lloyd, H., and Reyss-Brion, A.: Le peroxide de benzoyle: efficacite clinique et bacteriologique dans le traitement des pyodermites chroniques. Prat. Med. Chirurg. Anim. Comp. 19:445, 1984.
53. Love, D. N., et al.: Characterization of strains of staphylococci from infections in dogs and cats. J. Small Anim. Pract. 22:195, 1981.
53a. Madigan, J. E., and Teitler, J.: Borrelia burgdorferi borreliosis. J.A.V.M.A. 192:892, 1980.
54. Manning, T. O.: Canine pododermatitis. Dermatol. Rep. 2:1, 1983.
55. Marples, R. R.: Fundamental cutaneous microbiology. In Moschella, S. L., Pillsbury, D. M., and Hurley, H. J., Jr., (eds.): Dermatology. W. B. Saunders Company, Philadelphia, 1975, pp. 489–516.
56. McIntosh, D. W.: Feline leprosy: A review of forty-four cases from western Canada. Can. Vet. J. 23:291, 1982.
57. Medleau, L., Long, R. E., et al.: Frequency and antimicrobial susceptibility of Staphylococcus spp. isolated from canine pyodermas. Am. J. Vet. Res. 47:229, 1986.
58. Miller, R. I., and Ladds, P. W.: Probably dermatophilosis in two cats. Aust. Vet. J. 60:155, 1983.
59. Muller, G. H., Kirk, R. W., and Scott, D. W.: Small Animal Dermatology. 3rd ed. W. B. Saunders Company, Philadelphia, 1983.
59a. Mundell, A. C.: Effectiveness of clofazimine in the treatment of feline leprosy. Proceedings, A.A.V.D. and A.C.V.D. Apr. 16, 1988, Washington, D.C., p. 44.
60. Parodi, A., et al.: Mycobacteriosis in the domestic carnivora: present-day epidemiology of tuberculosis in the cat and dog. J. Small Anim. Pract. 6:307, 1965.
61. Phillips, W. E., Kloos, W. E.: Identification of coagulase positive Staphylococcus intermedius and Staphylococcus hyicus subsp. hyicus isolate from veterinary clinical specimens. J. Clin. Microbiol. 14:671, 1981.
62. Phillips, W. E., Williams, B. J.: Antimicrobial susceptibility patterns of canine Staphylococcus intermedius isolates from veterinary clinical specimens. Am. J. Vet. Res. 45:2377, 1984.
63. Reinke, S. I., Stannard, A., et al.: Histopathologic features of pyotraumatic dermatitis. J.A.V.M.A. 190:57, 1987.
64. Richard, J. L., Pier, A. C., et al.: Experimentally induced canine dermatophilosis. Am. J. Vet. Res. 34:797, 1973.
65. Rolfo, N. L.: Bubonic plague in a cat. J.A.V.M.A. 188:534, 1986.

66. Rollag, O. J., et al.: Feline plague in New Mexico: report of five cases. J.A.V.M.A. *179*:1381, 1981.
67. Rosser, E.: Presentation, Annual Meeting, A.A.H.A., Phoenix, March, 1987.
67a. Rosser, W. W.: Bubonic plague. J.A.V.M.A. *191*:406, 1987.
68. Ryan, C. P.: Selected arthropod-borne diseases; plague, lyme disease, babesiosis. *In* August, J. R., Loar, A. S., (eds.): Zoonotic Diseases. Vet. Clin. North Am. *17*:179, 1987.
68a. Schiefer, H. B., and Middleton, D. B.: Experimental transmission of a feline mycobacterial skin disease (feline leprosy). Vet. Pathol. *20*:460, 1983.
69. Schoeb, T. R., and Morton, R.: Scrotal and testicular changes in canine brucellosis. J.A.V.M.A. *172*:598, 1978.
70. Schultz, R. D.: Basic veterinary immunology and a review. *In* Symposium on Practice Immunology. Vet. Clin. North Am. *8*:569, 1978.
71. Scott, D. W.: Canine pododermatitis. *In* Kirk, R. W., (ed.): Current Veterinary Therapy VII. W. B. Saunders Company, Philadelphia, 1980.
72. Scott, D. W.: Feline dermatology 1900–1980: a monograph. J.A.A.H.A. *16*:331, 1980.
73. Scott, D. W.: Nocardiosis and actinomycosis. *In* Kirk, R. W., (ed.): Current Veterinary Therapy VI. W. B. Saunders Company, Philadelphia, 1977.
74. Scott, D. W.: Feline dermatology, 1979–1982, introspective retrospections J.A.A.H.A. *20*:537, 1984.
75. Scott, D. W.: Feline dermatology, 1983–1985, the secret sits. J.A.A.H.A. *23*:255, 1987.
76. Snider, W. R.: Tuberculosis in canine and feline populations. Review of the Literature. Am. Rev. Respir. Dis. *104*:877, 1971.
77. Studdert, V. P., Phillips, W. A., et al.: Recurrent and persistent infections in related Weimaraner dogs. Aust. Vet. J. *61*:261, 1984.
78. Walton, D. K., Scott, D. W., et al.: Cutaneous bacterial granuloma (Botryomycosis) in a dog and cat. J.A.A.H.A. *19*:537, 1983.
79. Walton, G. S.: Dermatophilosis. Presentation, A.A.H.A. Annual Meeting, Las Vegas, April, 1982.
80. Ward, J. M.: *M. fortuitum* and *M. chelonei*: fast growing mycobacteria. Br. J. Dermatol. *92*:453, 1975.
80a. Welsh, O., et al.: Amikacin alone and in combination with trimethoprim-sulfamethoxazole in the treatment of actinomycotic mycetoma. J. Am. Acad. Dermatol. *17*:443, 1987.
81. White, S. D., Ihrke, P. J., et al.: Cutaneous atypical mycobacteriosis in cats. J.A.V.M.A. *182*:1218, 1983.
82. White, S. D., Ihrke, P. J., et al.: Occurrence of *S. aureus* on the clinically normal canine hair coat. Am. J. Vet. Res. *44*:332, 1983.
83. Whitney, J. C.: Some aspects of interdigital cysts in the dog. J. Small Anim. Pract. *11*:83, 1970.
84. Willemse, T., Groothuis, D. G., et al.: *Mycobacterium thermoresistible*: extrapulmonary infection in a cat. J. Clin. Microbiol. *21*:854, 1985.
85. Wisselink, M. A., Willemse, A., et al.: Deep pyoderma in the German shepherd dog. J.A.A.H.A. *21*:773, 1985.
86. Von Tscharner, C.: Personal Communication, Bad Kreuznach, Germany, 1988.

6

Viral, Rickettsial, and Protozoal Skin Diseases

These dermatoses are apparently rare in dogs and cats. Additionally, many of those that have been reported are associative or circumstantial in nature. The following is a brief overview of proven and suspected skin diseases of viral, rickettsial, and protozoal origin in dogs and cats.

Viral Diseases

FELINE LEUKEMIA VIRUS INFECTION

Feline leukemia virus infection has been implicated in a number of feline skin disorders, including chronic or recurrent pyoderma (abscess, cellulitis), chronic paronychia, poor wound healing, seborrhea, and generalized pruritus.[21] Its true relationship to some of these conditions is speculative. Chronic or recurrent pyoderma and paronychia are thought to be caused by the well-known immunosuppressive effects of feline leukemia virus infection. Supportive diagnostic data include laboratory rule-outs and positive tests for the virus.

FELINE T-LYMPHOTROPIC LENTIVIRUS INFECTION

Feline T-lymphotropic lentivirus infection is a recently described retrovirus disease of cats.[10a] The virus attacks T lymphocytes, resulting in severe acquired immunodeficiency. Among the clinical signs of immunodeficiency seen in affected cats are pustular dermatitis, gingivitis, and stomatitis. Positive antibody tests for the virus are diagnostic.

FELINE POXVIRUS INFECTION

Since the middle 1970s, several cases of poxvirus infection have been reported in domestic and exotic felines in Europe.[24] Based on these initial observations, it is thought that the prevalence of clinical disease in cats is low. However, because of the similarity between the viruses isolated from cats and the cowpox virus, and because of the susceptibility of cows and humans to infection with cowpox virus, much interest has been generated in the feline disease.

The precise identity of the poxvirus isolated from cats is currently controversial. Cowpox virus is a member of the *Orthopoxvirus* genus, as are smallpox and vaccinia viruses. All orthopoxviruses have similar morphology and share common antigens, so that differentiation between isolates of these viruses is not always readily achieved or clear. Initial descriptions of the poxvirus isolated from cats led to the conclusion, on the basis of morphologic and cross-neutralization studies, that the isolates were cowpox virus. However, a recent study involving the transmission of the virus isolated from a cat to cattle concluded that the virus was unlikely to be cowpox virus. These investigators suggested that the feline virus be named after the host of origin (e.g., catpox virus or feline poxvirus).

Feline poxvirus infection has been recorded in cats from 2 months to 12 years of age, with no apparent predilections for breed or sex. The most common presenting sign is the development of multiple, circular, 5- to 10-mm diameter skin lesions, which include crusted papules, plaques, nodules, and crateriform ulcers (Figs. 6:1A,B). Pruritus is variable, and the lesions occur most commonly on the face, limbs, paws, and dorsal lumbar area. Initial skin lesions may develop at the site of a reported bite wound. Systemic signs may or may not be present and include some combination of anorexia, lethargy, pyrexia, vomiting, diarrhea, conjunctivitis, dyspnea, and jaundice.

Feline poxvirus infection has also been reported to cause ulcerated, crusted skin lesions in humans who have been exposed to infected cats.[5a, 26]

The differential diagnosis includes bacterial and fungal infections, eosinophilic granuloma, and neoplasia (especially mast cell tumor and lymphosarcoma). Definitive diagnosis is made by skin biopsy, serologic testing, and virus isolation.[1] Dermatohistopathologic findings include hyperplasia, ballooning degeneration, reticular degeneration, microvesicle formation, and necrosis of affected epidermis and the outer root sheath of the hair follicle (Fig. 6:1C). Eosinophilic intracytoplasmic inclusion bodies are found within keratinocytes. Serum samples and fresh biopsy or scab material in viral transport medium are submitted to an appropriate diagnostic laboratory for serologic examination and viral isolation (hemorrhagic pocks are produced on the chorioallantoic membranes of hen eggs), respectively. Histopathology and electron microscopy allow a rapid presumptive diagnosis, but *only* virus isolation allows precise identification.[1]

Therapy is administered based on symptoms. Most cats recover spontaneously within 1 to 2 months. Glucocorticoids are contraindicated.

The epizootiology of feline poxvirus infection is poorly understood. It is hypothesized that cats become infected accidentally and that the virus reservoir is some small wild mammal that is yet unidentified.

CANINE DISTEMPER ✓

Canine distemper is caused by a paramyxovirus.[6] In addition to severe respiratory, gastrointestinal, and neurologic disorders, the virus may produce variable degrees of hyperkeratosis of the footpads (so-called hardpad disease) and nose.

CONTAGIOUS VIRAL PUSTULAR DERMATITIS
(Orf, Contagious Ecthyma)

Contagious viral pustular dermatitis is a disease, primarily found in sheep and goats, that is caused by a paravaccinia virus.[22] Contagious viral pustular

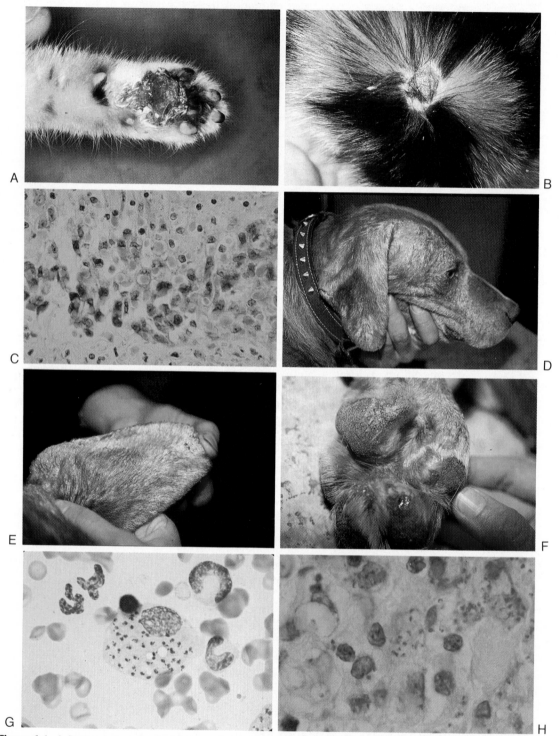

Figure 6:1. *A,* Footpad ulceration in feline poxvirus infection. (Courtesy R. Gaskell.) *B,* Crusted ulcer over dorsal thorax of cat with feline poxvirus infection. (Courtesy R. Gaskell.) *C,* Ballooning degeneration and eosinophilic intracytoplasmic inclusion bodies in feline poxvirus infection. *D,* Exfoliative dermatitis on the head and pinnae of a dog with leishmaniasis. (Courtesy Z. Alhaidari.) *E,* Scaling, crusting, erythema, and alopecia of the pinna in canine leishmaniasis. (Courtesy Z. Alhaidari.) *F,* Purpura, ulceration, and crusting on the paw of a dog with leishmaniasis. (Courtesy Z. Alhaidari.) *G,* Macrophage containing numerous Leishman-Donovan bodies. (Courtesy T. French.) *H,* Skin biopsy in leishmaniasis. Macrophages containing Leishman-Donovan bodies (Giemsa's stain).

dermatitis was reported in a pack of hounds allowed to feed on sheep carcasses.[25] Lesions consisted of circular areas of acute moist dermatitis, ulceration, and crusts. The predilection site was around the head. Skin biopsy revealed epidermal hyperplasia, ballooning degeneration, acantholysis within the stratum spinosum, and marked infiltration of neutrophils. Saline suspensions of skin biopsies were applied to the scarified skin of a normal sheep. Crusts removed from the inoculation sites were processed for electron microscopy, and paravaccinia virus particles were readily seen.

Therapy for contagious viral pustular dermatitis is topical and according to symptoms. The usual course of the disease in animals is 1 to 4 weeks. The disease may be transmitted to humans on exposure of broken skin to lesion material or contaminated objects. Generally, contagious viral pustular dermatitis is a benign disease in humans and results in the formation of a solitary lesion, especially on the hands. Lesions in humans are characterized by macules that progress through a papular, nodular, and papillomatous stage. The lesions are usually centrally umbilicated. Occasionally, lesions will be bullous. Complications of contagious viral pustular dermatitis in humans include regional lymphadenopathy, lymphangitis, secondary bacterial infection, and, rarely, generalized or systemic disease.

FELINE HERPESVIRUS INFECTION

Feline herpesvirus infection has been associated with oral and cutaneous ulceration in cats.[8] Cutaneous ulcers were usually superficial and multiple, and they affected all areas of the skin, including the footpads. In some cases, it was thought that the trauma of shaving the skin or the stress of surgery, or both, precipitated the cutaneous ulcers. Skin biopsies were nondiagnostic, revealing variable degrees of ulceration, chronic inflammation, intraepidermal pustular dermatitis, and folliculitis. Herpesvirus was isolated from skin and oral swabs. Whether or not the cutaneous ulcers and the herpesvirus infection have any cause-and-effect relationship is presently unknown. The course of disease in reported cats varied from rapid-to-prolonged recovery to death.

FELINE CALICIVIRUS INFECTION

"Paw and mouth disease" was reported in a cat in association with calicivirus infection.[4] Clinical signs included swollen, painful feet, with ulceration of the footpads and interdigital webs, and blisters and ulcers on the tongue, palate, and lips. Calicivirus was isolated from skin and oral swabs. Histopathologic examination of affected tissues was not performed. No cause-and-effect relationship between the calicivirus and the "paw and mouth disease" has been established to date.

NEOPLASIA

Papovaviruses cause cutaneous and mucosal papillomas (warts) in the dog (see p. 848). Feline sarcoma virus produces cutaneous fibrosarcomas in young cats (see p. 881). Feline leukemia virus and feline sarcoma virus have been associated with the development of lymphosarcoma, liposarcoma, melanoma, hemangioma, and multiple cutaneous horns in cats (see Chap. 20).

Rickettsial Diseases

CANINE ROCKY MOUNTAIN SPOTTED FEVER

Rocky Mountain spotted fever is caused by the rickettsial agent, *Rickettsia rickettsii*, and is transmitted by ticks.[9, 9a, 18] It is a seasonal disease in the United States, with cases occurring between April and September. Infected dogs develop fever, anorexia, lethargy, peripheral lymphadenopathy, and signs of neurologic dysfunction, which may be accompanied by erythema, petechiation, edema, and occasionally necrosis and ulceration of oral, ocular, and genital mucous membranes and the skin of the ventrum and pinnae. Edema of the extremities is frequently seen. Male dogs may have painful, swollen epididymides. Hematologic changes may include anemia, leukopenia, or leukocytosis and thrombocytopenia. Skin biopsy reveals necrotizing vasculitis.

Dogs with Rocky Mountain spotted fever have a fourfold rise in serum antibody titer to *R. rickettsii*. Direct immunofluorescence testing for *R. rickettsii* antigen in formalin-fixed skin biopsy specimens is frequently positive (antigen seen within vascular endothelium).[9, 9a]

Therapy includes tetracycline, 22 mg/kg TID orally or choramphenicol, 20 mg/kg TID orally for 2 to 3 weeks, and supportive care. The dog presents a potential public health danger when infested with *R. rickettsii*–infected ticks, or when blood or tissues from rickettsemic dogs are handled without suitable protection.

FELINE HEMOBARTONELLOSIS

Feline hemobartonellosis (feline infectious anemia) is an acute or chronic disease of domestic cats characterized by fever, depression, anorexia, and macrocytic hemolytic anemia.[11] It is caused by the rickettsia *Haemobartonella felis*. "Cutaneous hyperesthesia" and "alopecia areata" have been reported to occur in cats with acute and chronic hemobartonellosis.[10] No pictures, photomicrographs, or details of any kind were provided to substantiate these cutaneous diagnoses.

Protozoal Diseases

FELINE TOXOPLASMOSIS

Toxoplasmosis is a multisystemic disease caused by the coccidian *Toxoplasma gondii*.[11] Toxoplasmosis has been rarely reported to cause various cutaneous lesions in humans,[1a] and firm nodules in the skin of the legs in cats.[11] Histopathologic findings in cats were reported to be "necrotizing dermatitis with *Toxoplasma*."[11]

CANINE CUTANEOUS NODULES ASSOCIATED WITH COCCIDIA-LIKE ORGANISMS

Coccidia-like organisms have been seen in granulomatous cutaneous nodules from dogs.[19, 23] The dogs had multiple nodules that were dermal to subcutaneous and up to 2 cm in diameter, over the body. Some nodules were exudative.

Histopathologic findings included diffuse-to-nodular pyogranulomatous dermatitis with numerous eosinophils. Numerous cell types contained one to ten spherical cytoplasmic inclusions, which were composed of coccidia-like elements on light and electron microscopic examination.

LEISHMANIASIS

Leishmaniasis, a disease predominantly of humans and dogs but also occasionally of cats, occurs in the Mediterranean basin, the Middle East and Far East, South America, and in focal endemic areas in Oklahoma and Texas.[6, 7, 11–14, 16, 16a, 17, 20] The disease has various clinical presentations that may be explained by different *Leishmania spp.*[14] Dogs and cats have been infected with *L. donovani* and *L. chagasi.*[12, 13, 15] The disease is transmitted to humans and animals by bloodsucking sandflies of the genus *Lutzomyia* in the New World and *Phlebotomus* in the Old World. Dogs, both domestic and wild, as well as rodents and other wild mammals are the reservoir. Because of the occurrence of open lesions, some investigators have expressed concern regarding the possibility of direct or mechanical transmission from dog to dog or from dog to humans.[16, 16a, 20]

The incubation period varies from weeks to several years. The disease primarily affects dogs less than 5 years old. Classically, dogs are nonpruritic and have an exfoliative dermatitis, which is especially prominent on the face, pinnae, and feet (Figs. 6:1D–F). Periocular alopecia ("lunettes") and marked wasting of temporal muscle are often seen. Silvery white, asbestos-like scales are concentrated in areas of alopecia. Peripheral lymphadenopathy is usually prominent. As the disease advances, pruritic nodules, ulcers, and crusts may develop. Nasal depigmentation, erosion, and ulceration may be seen. The nails may become long and brittle. Intermittent fever, weight loss, lethargy, hepatosplenomegaly, keratoconjunctivitis, lameness, and muscle wasting may be present.

Leishmaniasis is rarely reported in cats,[11, 20] and they are quite resistant to experimental infection with *L. donovani* and *L. chagasi.*[15] Reported cutaneous lesions include crusted ulcers on the lips, nose, eyelids, and pinnae.

The differential diagnosis includes bacterial folliculitis, dermatophytosis, demodicosis, pemphigus foliaceus, systemic lupus erythematosus, zinc-responsive dermatosis, and mycosis fungoides.

Laboratory findings usually include nonregenerative anemia, hyperglobulinemia, hypoalbuminemia, and proteinuria. Indirect immunofluorescence testing for anti-*Leishmania* antibodies is useful, if it is available. The diagnosis is confirmed by finding the organism either in macrophages or free in the tissue in aspirates or biopsies of skin, lymph nodes, or bone marrow (Fig. 6:1G).

Skin biopsy reveals varying degrees of perivascular to nodular or diffuse dermatitis. Orthokeratotic and parakeratotic hyperkeratoses are usually prominent. Foamy macrophages, lymphocytes, and plasma cells predominate. The *Leishmania* organisms are found intracellularly and extracellularly (Fig. 6:1H). They are round to oval, 2 to 4 μm in size, and contain a round, basophilic nucleus and a small rodlike kinetoplast. Although visible in routine stains, *Leishmania* organisms are best seen when Giemsa's stain is utilized.

The classic treatment for canine leishmaniasis is meglumine antimonate (Glucantime).[6, 7, 16, 20] Two test doses of 50 mg/kg daily are followed by 100 mg/kg given subcutaneously daily for 10 days and repeated in 2 weeks. In France, Glucantime is often given intravenously at 200 to 300 mg/kg, every other day, for 15 to 20 treatments.[7] Recently, studies in humans and dogs have suggested that the antileishmanial activity of liposome-encapsulated meglumine antimonate is vastly superior to that of the unencapsulated drug.[2, 3] Clinical signs usually recur at 6- to 18-month intervals, which necessitates retreatment.

Other drugs that have been used in canine leishmaniasis include: (1) sodium stibogluconate (Pentostam) given intravenously or intramuscularly, 20 mg/kg for 8 days and repeated after an 8-day rest, (2) pentamidine (Lomidine) given intramuscularly, 4 mg/kg every other day for at least 15 days, (3) metronidazole (Flagyl) given orally, 10 to 15 mg/kg BID for 15 days, and (4) ketoconazole (Nizoral) given orally, 15 to 30 mg/kg/day for 2 months or longer.[7]

Successful treatment of feline leishmaniasis has not been reported.

In humans, many other drugs have been occasionally advocated for the treatment of leishmaniasis, including rifampicin, 8-aminoquinolines, levamisole, allopurinol, amphotericin B, and dapsone.[3, 5, 24a]

References

1. Bennett, M., et al: The laboratory diagnosis of orthopoxvirus infection in the domestic cat. J. Small Anim. Pract. 26:653, 1985.
1a. Binazzi, M.: Profile of cutaneous toxoplasmosis. Int. J. Dermatol. 25:357, 1986.
2. Chapman, W. L., et al: Antileishmanial activity of liposome-encapsulated meglumine antimonate in the dog. Am. J. Vet. Res. 45:1028, 1984.
3. Chong, H.: Oriental sore. A look at trends in and approaches to the treatment of leishmaniasis. Int. J. Dermatol. 25:615, 1986.
4. Cooper, L. M., and Sabine, M.: Paw and mouth disease in a cat. Aust. Vet. J. 48:644, 1972.
5. Dogra, J., et al: Dapsone in the treatment of cutaneous leishmaniasis. Int. J. Dermatol. 25:398, 1986.
5a. Egberink, H. F., et al: Isolation and identification of a poxvirus from a domestic cat and a human contact case. J. Vet. Med. B 33:237, 1986.
6. Ettinger, S. J.: Textbook of Veterinary Internal Medicine II. W. B. Saunders Company, Philadelphia, 1983.
7. Euzeby, J.: Therapeutique de la leishmaniose generale du chien. Actualite-perspectives. Rev. Med. Vet. 133:383, 1982.
8. Flecknell, P. A., et al: Skin ulceration associated with herpesvirus infection in cats. Vet. Rec. 104:313, 1979.
9. Greene, C. E., et al: Rocky Mountain spotted fever in dogs and its differentiation from canine ehrlichiosis. J.A.V.M.A. 186:465, 1985.
9a. Greene, C. E.: Rocky Mountain spotted fever. J.A.V.M.A. 191:666, 1987.
10. Gretillati, S.: Feline hemobartonellosis. Feline Pract. 14:22, 1984.
10a. Hardy, W. D.: Feline lymphotropic lentivirus: retrovirus-induced immunosuppression in cats. J.A.A.H.A. 24:241, 1988.
11. Holzworth, J.: Diseases of the Cat—Medicine & Surgery. W. B. Saunders Company, Philadelphia, 1987.
12. Keenan, C. M., et al: Visceral leishmaniasis in the German Shepherd dog. I. Infection, clinical disease, and clinical pathology. Vet. Pathol. 21:74, 1984.
13. Keenan, C. M., et al: Visceral leishmaniasis in the German Shepherd dog II. Pathology. Vet. Pathol. 21:80, 1984.
14. Kerdel-Vegas, F.: American leishmaniasis. Int. J. Dermatol. 21:291, 1982.
15. Kirkpatrick, C. E., et al: Leishmania chagasi and L. donovani: experimental infections in domestic cats. Exp. Parasitol. 58:125, 1984.
16. Longstaffe, J. A., et al: Leishmaniasis in imported dogs in the United Kingdom; a potential human health hazard. J. Small Anim. Pract. 24:23, 1983.
16a. Longstaffe, J. A., and Guy, M. W.: Canine Leishmaniasis—United Kingdom update. J. Small Anim. Pract. 27:663, 1986.
17. Nelson, D. A., et al: Clinical aspects of cutaneous leishmaniasis acquired in Texas. J. Am. Acad. Dermatol. 12:985, 1985.
18. Rutgers, C., et al: Severe Rocky Mountain spotted fever in five dogs. J.A.A.H.A. 21:361, 1985.
19. Sangster, L. T., et al: Coccidia associated with cutaneous nodules in a dog. Vet. Pathol. 22:186, 1985.
20. Schawalder, P.: Leishmaniose bei Hund und Katze. Kleintier-Praxis 22:237, 1977.
21. Scott, D. W.: Feline dermatology 1900–1978: a monograph. J.A.A.H.A. 16:331, 1980.
22. Scott, D. W.: Large Animal Dermatology. W. B. Saunders Company, Philadelphia, 1988.
23. Shelton, G. C., et al: A coccidia-like organism associated with subcutaneous granulomata in a dog. J.A.V.M.A. 152:263, 1968.
24. Thomsett, L. R.: Feline poxvirus infection. In Kirk, R. W.: Current Veterinary Therapy IX. W. B. Saunders Company, Philadelphia, 1986, p. 605.
25. Wilkinson, G. T., et al: Possible "orf" (contagious pustular dermatitis, contagious ecthyma of sheep) infection in the dog. Vet. Rec. 87:766, 1970.
26. Willemse, A., and Egberink, H. F.: Transmission of cowpox virus infection from domestic cat to man. Lancet 1:1515, 1985.

7

Fungal Diseases

Cutaneous Mycology

Fungi are omnipresent in our environment. Of the thousands of different fungal species, only a few have the ability to cause disease in animals. The great majority of fungi are either soil organisms or plant pathogens; however, more than 300 species of fungi have been reported to be animal pathogens. A mycosis (pl. mycoses) is a disease caused by a fungus. A dermatophytosis is an infection of the keratinized tissues, nail, hair, and stratum corneum that is caused by a species of *Microsporum*, *Trichophyton*, or *Epidermophyton*. These organisms—dermatophytes—are unique fungi that are able to invade and maintain themselves in keratinized tissues (Fig. 7:1). A dermatomycosis is a fungal infection of hair, nail, or skin that is caused by a nondermatophyte, a fungus not classified in the genera *Microsporum*, *Trichophyton*, or *Epidermophyton*.[29] Dermatophytosis and dermatomycosis are different clinical entities. Fungi, however, are not nearly as common a cause of skin disease as supposed, and many nonspecific, pruritic, and nonpruritic dermatoses are diagnosed as dermatomycoses on the basis of inadequate evidence. Some clinicians use "grass fungus" as a collective term for these problems when in fact contact dermatitis or factors other than fungi are involved. On the other hand, many true fungal infections probably are not diagnosed because of the variability of clinical presentations.

> *Many nonfungal dermatoses are erroneously called "fungal infections."*

GENERAL CHARACTERISTICS OF FUNGI

The kingdom of fungi (Fungi) is recognized as one of the five kingdoms of organisms. The other four kingdoms are bacteria and blue-green algae (Monera), protozoa (Protista), plants (Plantae), and animals (Animalia).[12] Fungi are eukaryotic achlorophyllous organisms that may grow in the form of a yeast (unicellular) or a mold (multicellular-filamentous), or in both forms. Fungal cell walls consist of chitin, chitosan, glucan, and mannan and are used to separate the fungi from the Protista. Unlike plants, fungi do not have chlorophyll. The kingdom of Fungi contains five divisions: Chytridomycota, Zygomycota, Basidiomycota, Ascomycota, and Fungi Imperfecti or Deuteromycota.

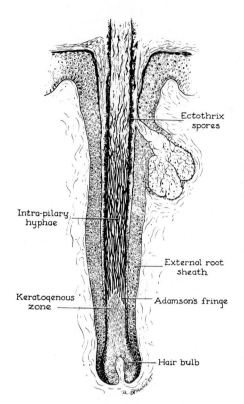

Ectothrix
spores

Intra-pilary
hyphae

Keratogenous
zone

External root
sheath

Adamson's fringe

Hair bulb

Figure 7:1. Diagrammatic representation of an infected hair illustrating the main features of the host-parasite relationship characteristic of dermatophyte infection of haired skin. The fungal filaments do not extend into the bulb of the hair but terminate abruptly in contact with hair matrix cells, which still retain their nuclei. Only the *fully* keratinized portion of the hair shaft is invaded. (From Pillsburg, Shelley, and Kligman: Dermatology. W. B. Saunders, Philadelphia, 1956.)

Fungi have traditionally been identified and classified by their method of producing conidia and spores, by the size, shape, and color of the conidia, and by the type of hyphae and their macroscopic appearance (e.g., by the color and texture of the colony and sometimes by physiologic characteristics.) Therefore, it is important to understand the terminology describing these characteristics. A single vegetative filament of a fungus is a hypha. A number of vegetative filaments are called hyphae, and a mass of hyphae is known as mycelium. Hyphae can be either septate, having divisions between cells, or sparsely septate, having many nuclei within a cell. This latter condition is known as being coenocytic. The term conidium (pl. conidia) should be used only in regard to an asexual propagule or unit that gives rise to genetically identical organisms. A conidiophore is a simple or branched mycelium, bearing conidia or conidiogenous cells. A conidiogenous cell is any fungal cell that gives rise to a conidium. (Modern taxonomists also may use sexual reproduction characteristics and biochemical and immunologic methods for identification.)

There are six major types of conidia: blastoconidia, arthroconidia, annelloconidia, phialoconidia, poroconidia, and aleurioconidia (Table 7:1 and Fig. 7:2). More detailed information about fungal taxonomy can be found in the third edition of this text[75a] or in the text by Chandler and associates.[12]

Changes in the scientific names of the pathogenic fungi, stemming from new taxonomic studies have caused confusion with some of the names that were formerly widely used. Some names have been based on geographic distribution or have been created by the indiscriminate lumping of dissimilar diseases. We will attempt to name diseases based on a single etiologic agent and common usage, tempered by contemporary knowledge of geographic

Table 7–1. MAJOR TYPES OF CONIDIA

Conidia	Characteristics	Example
Blastoconidia	Cells produced by a blowing-out process from the parent cell (usually single cells)	*Candida, Cryptococcus*
Arthroconidia	Cells produced by septation and fragmentation of true hyphae	*Geotrichum*
Annelloconidia	Cells produced as the extruded end of a conidiophore; new conidia form through the scar of each previous conidium	*Scopulariopsis*
Phialoconidia	Cells released from open growing point on conidiogenous cell	*Aspergillus, Penicillium*
Poroconidia	Thick-walled cells developed through pores in wall of conidiophores, often muriform and pigmented	*Alternaria*
Aleurioconidia	Single cells extruded from conidiophore	*Microsporum, Trichopyton*

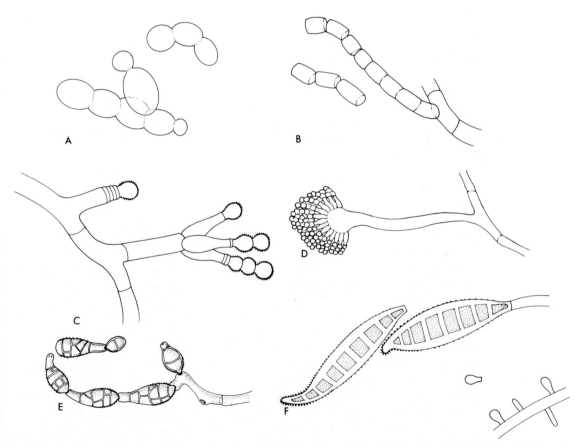

Figure 7:2. Major types of conidia. *A,* Blastoconidia (*Candida*). *B,* Arthroconidia (*Geotrichum*). *C,* Annelloconidia (*Scopulariopsis*). *D,* Phialoconidia (*Penicillium*). *E,* Poroconidia (*Alternaria*). *F,* Aleurioconidia (*Microsporum*).

distribution and current taxonomy. We will divide mycotic diseases into three categories: superficial, subcutaneous, and systemic. The first category contains the most common fungal diseases in veterinary dermatology.

CHARACTERIZATION OF PATHOGENIC FUNGI

Fungi that are pathogenic to plants are distributed throughout all divisions of fungi, but those pathogenic to animals are found primarily in the Fungi Imperfecti and the Ascomycota.[90]

> *Many fungi can become pathogens in immunologically compromised animals.*

The term fungus includes yeasts and molds. A yeast is a unicellular budding fungus that forms blastoconidia, while a mold is a filamentous fungus. Some pathogenic fungi, such as *Histoplasma capsulatum, Coccidioides immitis, Sporothrix schenckii,* and *Blastomyces dermatitidis,* are dimorphic. Dimorphic fungi are capable of existing in two different morphologic forms. For example, at 37°C in enriched media or in vitro *B. dermatitidis* exists as a yeast, but at 30°C it grows as a mold. *C. immitis* is unique because at 37°C or in tissue, spherules containing endospores are formed. Some fungi such as *Aspergillus* form true hyphae in tissue and are a mold at either 30°C or 37°C. Another manifestation of fungal growth in tissue is the presence of granules that are organized masses of hyphae in a crystalline or amorphous matrix. These granules are characteristic of the mycotic infection mycetoma. They are the result of interaction between the host tissue and the fungus.

COMMON FUNGAL CONTAMINANTS

At one time, numerous fungi were thought to be pathogens. Today, with the increased use of broad-spectrum antibiotics, immunosuppressive therapy, and improved mycologic techniques, even many fungi that were considered to be contaminants have, in fact, been found to be pathogenic. The following criteria can be helpful in differentiating a pathogenic from a contaminant fungus: source, number of colonies isolated, species, whether it can be repeatedly isolated, and, most important, the presence of fungal elements in the tissue. A fungus isolated from a normal sterile site such as a biopsy specimen warrants more credence as a pathogen than that same fungus isolated from the surface of the skin, where it may be an airborne contaminant. The number of colonies isolated should influence the decision as to whether an organism is a contaminant or a pathogen. One isolated colony of *Aspergillus* may have resulted from an airborne conidium that floated into a plate, while a petri dish filled with *A. fumigatus* could represent a pathogen. Colonies that are not seen on the streak line of the agar should be considered to be contaminants. Certain species of fungi are definitely recognized as pathogens, however, and if only one colony is isolated, it should be reported. Such organisms include *Blastomyces dermatitidis, Histoplasma capsulatum, Coccidioides immitis,* and *Cryptococcus neoformans.* Another indication of fungal pathogenicity is that the same fungus can be repeatedly isolated from the lesion. In order to confirm that a fungus is a cause of a mycosis, the fungal structures observed in tissue or a direct smear must correlate with the fungus identified in culture.

> *Many different fungi look identical in tissue section; therefore, for a correct diagnosis, a fungus must be cultured and identified.*

Although gross colonies of dermatophytes are never black, brown, or green, the proper identification of organisms in fungal cultures should be made by medical laboratory clinicians who have expertise in such matters. The third edition of this text has more information about the cultural growth of the three common dermatophytes (*M. canis*, *M. gypseum*, and *T. mentagrophytes*) and twelve other commonly isolated fungal contaminants (*Aspergillus, Penicillium, Scopulariopsis, Alternaria, Cladosporium, Fusarium, Candida, Rhodotorula, Geotrichum, Rhizopus, Absidia*, and *Mucor*).[75a] An English study of the normal fungal flora of canine skin found *Cladosporium* and *Alternaria* to be most common. *Mucor* and *Rhizopus* were increasingly common in cultures made from November through the winter, while *Penicillium* was found at all times.[83] There was an increased recovery of *Cladosporium* and *Alternaria* from abnormal skin, compared with normal skin, but a large number of normal animals did not harbor fungi at all.

CULTURE AND EXAMINATION OF FUNGI

> *Fungal culture is mandatory for proper identification of fungi.*

Proper specimen collection, isolation, culture and correct identification are necessary to determine the cause of a fungal infection. Detailed information on these important techniques are given in Chapter Three.

Superficial Mycoses

These are fungal infections that involve superficial layers of the skin, hair, and nails. The organisms may be dermatophytes such as *Microsporum* and *Trichophyton*, which are able to utilize keratin. However, other fungi such as *Candida* and *Malassezia (Pityrosporum)* may also produce superficial mycoses.

DERMATOPHYTOSIS

CAUSE AND PATHOGENESIS

The dermatophytes that most frequently infect animals are *Microsporum* and *Trichophyton*. These genera can be divided into three groups on the basis of natural habitat: geophilic, zoophilic, and anthropophilic. Geophilic dermatophytes, such as *M. gypseum*, normally inhabit the soil in which they decompose keratinous debris. Zoophilic dermatophytes, such as *M. canis*, *M. distortum*, and *T. equinum* have become adapted to animals and only rarely are found in the soil. Anthropophilic dermatophytes, such as *M. audouinii*, have become adapted to humans and will not survive in soil. Zoophilic dermatophytes often cause less inflammatory reaction in animals than geophilic or anthropophilic fungi.

Three fungi cause the great majority of all clinical cases of dermatophytosis in dogs and cats.[77] These are *M. canis*, *M. gypseum*, and *T. mentagrophytes*. Within the United States the incidence and prevalence of dermatophytosis vary with the climate and natural reservoirs. In a hot, humid climate a higher incidence is observed than in a cold, dry climate.

Kaplan and Ivens[50] reported that the seasonal incidence of dermatophytosis in dogs and cats in the United States varies with the species of fungus. The incidence may also depend on the climate and on the amount of time the animal spends outdoors, thus being more exposed to geophilic species. In general, the incidence for dogs in the Northern Hemisphere can be summarized as follows: (1) *M. canis* was high in the period from October to February and low from March to September; (2) *M. gypseum* was high in the period from July to November and low from December to June; (3) *T. mentagrophytes* was present all year, with a peak occurring in November and December. In general, the incidence for cats can be summarized as follows: (1) *M. canis* varied little all year; (2) *M. gypseum* and *T. mentagrophytes* were rarely reported in cats, but a slight increase may occur during the summer and fall months.

Other fungi reported to cause dermatomycoses in cats, dogs, and humans are listed in Table 7:2.

When an animal is exposed to a dermatophyte, an infection may or may not be established. Despite exposure, disease in the form of skin lesions may not result. Fungal organisms only invade hairs in the anagen stage of the hair growth cycle (see Fig. 7:7). A survey of 142 healthy, asymptomatic Belgian dogs yielded eight (5.6 per cent) cultures of dermatophytes, by means of the brush culture technique. Three were *M. canis*, and five were *Trichophyton mentagrophytes*. Yeasts (*C. albicans* and *M. pachydermitis*) were isolated from 2.8 per cent.[104] In New Zealand, 199 asymptomatic cats were sampled with the brush technique and 38 (19 per cent) had dermatophytes isolated from the hair coat. Thirteen of these were *M. canis*, five were *M. cookei*, five were *T. ajelloi*, and fifteen were *T. terrestre*. Several cats had multiple isolates.[113] It often appears that young animals (as well as children) are more susceptible to infection and are more likely to show clinical lesions than are adults. This difference may be caused by biochemical alterations in the skin, skin secretions, especially sebum, the growth and replacement of hair, the physiologic status of the host as related to age, and the development of the ability to manifest an allergic response to fungal organisms and their products. Age appears to increase this type of immune competence.[20] Natural and experimental infections have been shown to incite various forms of hypersensitivity in their hosts and in some instances to stimulate formation of circulating antibodies. There is no correlation between the level of antibody and degree of resistance to reinfection. Complete, lasting immunity to reinfection in the absence of an allergic response has not been achieved by immunization procedures using whole killed dermatophytes or their extracts.

Local factors, such as the mechanical barrier of intact skin and mucous membranes, and the fungistatic activity of sebum and sweat caused by their

Table 7–2. SOME FUNGI REPORTED TO CAUSE DERMATOPHYTOSIS OR DERMATOMYCOSIS IN ANIMALS AND HUMANS*

Fungus	Reservoir	Dog	Cat	Humans
Alternaria spp.†	Soil, organic debris	Rare	Not reported	Rare
Alternaria alternata†	Soil, organic debris	Rare	Not reported	Rare
Aspergillus spp.	Organic debris	Occasional	Not reported	Infrequent, sporadic
Aspergillus deflectus	Organic debris	Rare	Not reported	Not reported
Aspergillus fumigatus	Organic debris, soil	Occasional	Occasional	Rarely reported
Aspergillus niger‡	Organic debris	Rare	Not reported	Reported
Aspergillus terreus	Organic debris	Rare	Not reported	Not reported
Blastomyces dermatitidis	Soil in beaver lodges	Frequent	Reported	Infrequent
Candida spp.	Normal microflora of gastrointestinal tract	Rare	Not reported	Frequent
Candida albicans	Normal microflora of gastrointestinal tract	Rare	Not reported	Relatively common
Candida krusei†	Unknown	Rare	Not reported	Reported
Candida parapsilosis†	Human nails, insect and vegetable refuse	Rare	Not reported	Reported
*Chrysosporium evolceanui**	Soil	Rare	Not reported	Questionable report
Cladosporium spp.	Decaying plants	Not reported	Rare	Rare
Coccidioides immitis	Desert soil	Reported	Rare	Common in endemic areas
Cryptococcus spp.	Pigeon droppings	Occasional	Occasional	Reported
Cryptococcus neoformans	Pigeon droppings	Occasional	Occasional	Reported
Curvularia geniculata	Plant debris	Not reported	Rare	Reported
Drechslera spicifera	Plants, grains	Reported	Rare	Rare
Epidermophyton floccosum‡	Humans	Rare	Not reported	Common
Exophiala jeanselmei‡	Plant debris, soil	Not reported	Rare†	Reported
Geotrichium spp.	Decaying leaves	Not reported	Rare	Rare
Hansenula anomala	Soil and plant debris, grains	Reported	Not reported	Questionable
Histoplasma capsulatum	Soil and quano	Common in endemic areas	Common in endemic areas	Common in endemic areas
Malassezia spp. (*Pityrosporum*)	Skin	Common	Occasional	Reported
Malassezia pachydermatis (*Pityrosporum*)	Skin	Common	Occasional	Not reported
Microsporum audouinii†	Humans	Rare	Rare	Sporadic
Microsporum canis	Cats	Common	Common	Common
Microsporum cookei†	Soil	Rare	Reported	Reported
Microsporum distortum†	Unknown	Rare	Rare	Uncommon
Microsporum gallinae	Poultry	Rare	Rare	Rare
Microsporum gypseum	Soil	Common	Common	Occasional
Microsporum nanum†	Swine	Reported	Not reported	Rare
Microsporum persicolor†	Bank vole	Rare	Not reported	Uncommon
Microsporum vanbreuseghemii	Soil	Rare	Rare	Rare
Moniliella suaveolens	Cheese	Not reported	Rare	Not reported
Oidiodendron kalrai†	Soil, wood	Rare	Not reported	Not reported
Paecilomyces spp.	Soil saprophyte	Rare	Not reported	Rare
Paecilomyces fumosoroseus	Soil saprophyte	Not reported	Rare	Rare
Penicillium martensii	Plant debris	Not reported	Rare	Not reported
Phialophora spp.‡	Plant debris	Not reported	Rare	Reported
Phialophora verrucosa	Soil saprophyte	Not reported	Reported	Rare
Prototheca wickerhamii	Water	Rare	Reported	Reported
Pseudoallescheria boydii	Soil	Rare	Not reported	Reported
Pseudomicrodochium suttonii	Unknown	Rare	Not reported	Not reported
Rhinosporidium seeberi	Water?	Rare	Not reported	Reported
Scopulariopsis brevicaulis	Soil	Rare	Not reported	Reported
Sepedonium spp.†	Soil and fungi	Rare	Not reported	Not reported
Sporothrix schenckii	Soil, vegetation, timber	Rare	Frequent	Sporadic
Stemphylium spp.	Decaying plants	Not reported	Reported	Rare
Trichophyton spp.	Soil, humans, animals	Common	Common	Reported
Trichophyton ajelloi†	Soil	Rare	Not reported	Questionable
Trichophyton equinum var autotrophicum†	Horses	Rare	Not reported	Reported

Table continued on following page

Table 7–2. SOME FUNGI REPORTED TO CAUSE DERMATOPHYTOSIS OR DERMATOMYCOSIS IN ANIMALS AND HUMANS* *Continued*

Fungus	Reservoir	Dog	Cat	Humans
Trichophyton erinacei	Hedgehogs	Rare	Rare	Frequent
Trichophyton megninii†	Man	Rare	Rare	Reported
Trichophyton mentagrophytes	Dogs or rodents	Common	Common	Common
Trichophyton mentagrophytes var. *quinckeanum*†	Mice	Rare	Rare	Not reported
Trichophyton rubrum	Humans	Rare	Rare	Common
Trichophyton schoenleinii†	Humans	Rare	Rare	Common
Trichophyton simii	Soil, small animals	Rare	Not reported	Reported
Trichophyton terrestre	Soil	Rare	Rare	Reported
Trichophyton verrucosum†	Cattle	Rare	Rare	Common
Trichophyton violaceum†	Humans	Rare	Rare	Common
Trichosporon pullulans	Skin saprophyte	Not reported	Rare	Rare

*The references for data in this table are listed at the end of the chapter references.

For an organism to be demonstrated as pathogenic, it should be cultured from skin lesions and fungal elements consistent with the isolated fungus must be observed in tissue sections. Unless otherwise noted, organisms in this table were reported to have met these criteria.

†This fungus was cultured from an apparent case of dermatophytosis or dermatomycosis but not demonstrated in tissues.

‡A fungus presumed to be this organism was demonstrated in tissues from an apparent case of dermatophytosis or dermatomycosis but not confirmed by culture.

fatty acid content are potent deterrents to fungal invasion. Organisms that penetrate these lines of defense elicit an inflammatory response and may be phagocytized by circulating or fixed-tissue phagocytes. The antigen of an invading agent initiates production of specific antibodies and the sensitization of thymus-dependent lymphocytes (T cells). On subsequent exposure to this antigen, the T cells undergo transformation and produce nonantibody lymphocytic factors that direct phagocytosis, promote capillary permeability, cause stimulation and proliferation of unsensitized lymphocytes, and exert a cytotoxic effect.

As there is no correlation between circulating antibodies and protection, it is thought that the cell-mediated immune response is the mainstay of defense of the body against fungal infection. This observation is supported by the frequent complication of fungal infections in patients undergoing immunosuppressive therapy.

The course of the disease may be responsive to therapy, may be responsive but not cured by treatment, or may resolve spontaneously. The last process is a factor possibly overlooked in some claims of merit for certain medications.

Following recovery, varying degrees of resistance to infection have been noted, lasting from a few months to 1½ years at most.[20] This resistance may be a response to an organism of the same or of a different fungal species.

Dermatophytosis has been transmitted by rubbing infected tissue into gently abraded skin, and apparently natural infection is by contact. Contaminated brushes, combs, and clippers may be important fomites. Some fungal elements may remain viable in the dry stage for as long as 5 to 7 years, and *M. canis* may live at least 13 months.[18] Carrier cats may spread infection for short periods, but the real long-term reservoir in a cattery is the cat with minimal clinical lesions.

The zoonotic potential for ringworm (*M. canis*) in cats is serious. In a study of British households containing infected cats, 50 per cent of the in-contact persons contracted ringworm, and in these homes 69 per cent had at least one family member affected (see Fig. 7:9G).[82]

In cats, the majority of dermatophyte infections are caused by *M. canis*. In dogs, *M. canis* is the most frequent cause, followed by *M. gypseum* and *T. mentagrophytes*. However, there is great variation in the proportion in which these three fungi occur in different parts of the country.

SKIN RESPONSE TO DERMATOPHYTES

In mild infections on glabrous skin, the response to dermatophytes is minor and easily missed. Mild hyperplasia of the horny layer may be observed. Fungal growth may be scant, and special stains may be needed to demonstrate fungi. As fungal growth becomes more prolific the entire epidermis may become hyperplastic. These same hyperplastic changes occur in the hair follicles, and the root sheath is well cornified so that the hairs become surrounded by wide collars of keratin and hyphae. The bulge may produce a conical dilation of the opening of the hair follicle, a process that gives a false impression of papillomatous swelling.

Folliculitis is a common finding in dermatophyte infections (Fig. 7:3). Histologic sections of biopsies from cases of folliculitis/furunculosis should always be carefully scrutinized for fungal elements (Fig. 7:4). The reaction in the viable follicle consists of mild congestion and edema of the dermal papilla, together with a mild lymphocytic infiltration. If secondary bacterial infection occurs, microabscesses form in the superficial epidermis, together with a suppurative folliculitis. A localized severe inflammation accompanied by swelling, with a deep boggy ulcerative area exuding pus, is known as a kerion. Dermatophytes usually do not survive in living cells.

Cases of granulomatous subcutaneous dermatophytosis in cats caused by *M. canis* or *Trichophyton* sp. have been reported.[38, 72, 103, 114] The lesions seem to be more common in Persian cats, and there is speculation that they may be

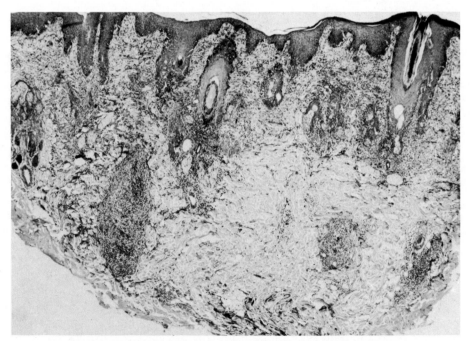

Figure 7:3. Follicularly oriented inflammation in a cat with dermatophytosis.

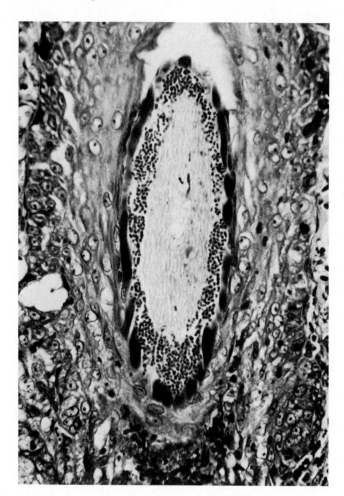

Figure 7:4. *Microsporum canis* in a cat. Note arthroconidia surrounding hair shaft (AOG stain).

associated with altered immune status. Affected tissue is often associated with the amorphous eosinophilic material characteristic of the Splendore-Hoeppli reaction, which is an antigen-antibody reaction to alien fungi in the hypersensitized host. The lesions may be induced by trauma in areas of the skin containing dermatophytes. The process begins as a mycotic folliculitis: a granulomatous folliculitis and furunculosis, progressing to nodular and diffuse granulomatous dermatitis in the deep dermis and subcutis (Fig. 7:5). (See Fig. 7:11*A,B*). The follicle becomes disrupted, and a fragment of infected hair with its fungal elements is displaced into the dermis or subcutis, where a foreign body response is elicited. The hair is resorbed, but the fungal elements remain for a prolonged period (Fig. 7:6). Baxter (in the text by Moschella and co-authors)[74] believes that this is *not* an exception to the rule that dermatophytes grow only in dead tissue. In these cases the fungus usually does not proliferate in the dermis but is passively sequestered and persists for a period of time. The preferred term for this condition is pseudomycetoma.

The invasion of hair by a dermatophyte has been studied extensively (Fig. 7:7).[45] Hair is always invaded in both ectothrix and endothrix infections. The endothrix fungi are those that do not form masses of external conidia. Fungal elements deposited on the skin reach the follicle orifice by the second day; they penetrate the hair shaft by working under the cuticle, lifting it away from the

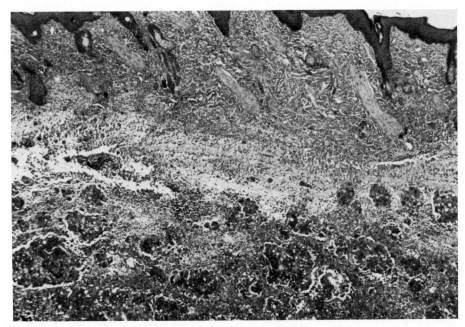

Figure 7:5. Subcutaneous dermatophytosis in a cat (*Trichophyton* sp.). Diffuse panniculitis with tissue grains.

shaft and growing downward. Fungal elements reach the keratogenous zone and form Adamson's fringe by the seventh to eighth day. Growing hair contains carbohydrates, nitrogenous substances, and nucleoprotein derivatives in addition to keratin, and these meet the metabolic needs of the fungus to support

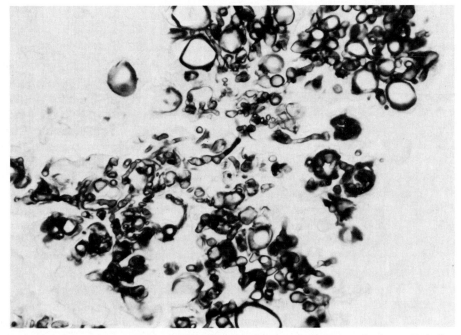

Figure 7:6. Subcutaneous dermatophytosis (*Trichophyton* sp.). Numerous hyphae with bulbous dilatations (GMS stain).

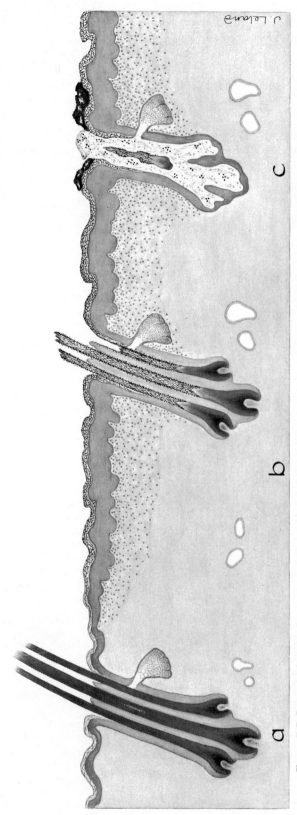

Figure 7:7. Dermatophytosis dermogram. *A*, Normal hair follicles. *B*, There is invasion of the hair follicle by a dermatophyte. Hyphae and arthroconidia can be seen affecting only the keratinized portions of the skin and appendages. There is epidermal hyperplasia and an inflammatory infiltration. The third hair is broken off, but hair roots are intact. Fungi are growing downward on the hair, forming Adamson's fringe—a zone just above the area of keratin synthesis. No fungi can be seen in the living cells of the dermis or epidermis. *C*, There is partial destruction of the hair follicle. Hairs have been lost, a follicular plug has formed, and crusts appear on the epidermal surface. The general histologic picture varies from that of a perivascular dermatitis (hyperplastic, spongiotic) to that of folliculitis or furunculosis.

growth. Fungi do not penetrate the mitotic region of the hair, and when the hair growth terminates, fungal growth terminates and the clinical infection resolves spontaneously. A "patch of ringworm" is a community of more or less independent hair infections, since each follicle is in its own stage of the hair cycle. In addition, for some unknown reason a few hairs are resistant to fungal invasion even while they are growing.[55] Although the shafts of "club" or dead telogen hairs may be invaded by the dermatophyte, the infection does not persist, since the infection is terminated when the hair is lost.

The gross appearance of dermatophytosis varies. There are usually different degrees of scaling, encrustation of epithelial debris, and loss of hair. The hair loss is not permanent unless the follicle is destroyed by inflammation. Usually the hairs become brittle and break off near the skin surface, leaving a short stubby hair shaft that can be seen emerging through scales and crusts.

In the course of some dermatophyte infections, the organisms tend to die in the center of the lesions, and the skin in those areas returns to normal. The organisms at the periphery of the lesion remain active and produce a circular "ringworm" lesion. It has been postulated that the lesion creates an unfavorable site for fungal growth, whereas the fungus at the periphery thrives, and the lesion tends to grow outward in a circular manner. However, the exact mechanism for this circular growth is unknown.

CLINICAL FEATURES

> ### *Dermatophytosis can present a variety of clinical syndromes.*

Many long-haired adult cats are inapparent carriers of dermatophytes. Upon careful inspection they may have minimal lesions that are seen as a patchy alopecia. The affected hairs in these areas may be broken, appearing as short stubble. Barely discernible scaly patches may be seen, but some areas have raised erythematous plaques.

The classic "ringworm" lesion is a rapidly expanding circular patch that may be only 1 to 4 cm in diameter but can expand to any size (Fig. 7:8A–D). The lesions can be oval, irregular, or diffuse in shape (Fig. 7:8C).

Sometimes a generalized form may affect large portions of the body. This is especially common in chronic *M. gypseum* and *T. mentagrophytes* infections (Figs. 7:8G and 7:9A–H). Distribution patterns on the body in these generalized cases are often helpful diagnostically, and typical patterns are seen in Fig. 7:10.

Folliculitis is present in most cases of dermatophytosis. Conical dilation of the hair follicle ostium, or papules and pustules involving the hair follicle, should always raise suspicion of a fungal infection. The area of folliculitis can be local or diffuse and may be associated with any of the syndromes described here.

"Miliary dermatitis" in cats can occasionally be caused by a dermatophyte infection (see Table 9:27). It may appear as a diffuse folliculitis and/or as large areas of scaly epidermis with broken hairs.

A kerion, which has been described as a localized area of acutely inflamed skin that is swollen, boggy and oozing pus (Fig. 7:8B), is a suppurative folliculitis and furunculosis with both fungal and bacterial infections present. These infections may appear as a deep pyoderma, especially if they affect the nose or feet. In dogs, they are often associated with *M. gypseum* and *T. mentagrophytes*.

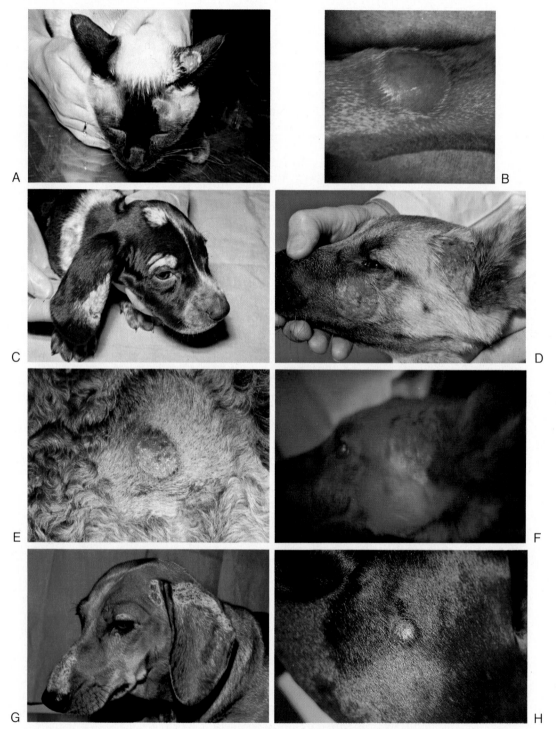

Figure 7:8 *See legend on opposite page*

Pseudomycetoma refers to a cutaneous or subcutaneous nodule(s) that develops as a result of a granulomatous folliculitis and furunculosis caused by a dermatophyte (Fig. 7:11A,B). Seen predominantly in long-haired cats, it is associated with *M. canis* and *Trichophyton* sp.[44, 72, 103, 114]

Onychomycosis is a dermatophyte infection of the nails often caused by *T. mentagrophytes*. The nails are often dry, brittle, and grossly deformed. They may crack, and the shell of hard keratin may separate from the nail bed (see p. 824).

Rarely canine and feline dermatophytosis may be associated with the simultaneous presence of two dermatophytes, such as *M. canis* and *T. mentagrophytes, M. persicolor* and *M. gypseum*, or *T. mentagrophytes* and *T. erinacei*.[9a, 9b, 10b]

DIAGNOSIS

Fungal tests may be useful in diagnosis. These tests are described in detail in Chapter Three.

Wood's light examination for fluorescence causes only certain strains of *M. canis, M. audouinii, M. distortum,* and *T. schoenleinii* to produce a positive yellow-green color. Only about half of *M. canis* infections fluoresce under Wood's light (Fig. 7:8D,F), and other dermatophytes of dogs and cats do not fluoresce. Microscopic examination of hairs (in mineral oil or in potassium hydroxide [KOH] preparation) may demonstrate hyphae and conidia in the hairs or keratin scales (see p. 131). Fungal culture of affected hair and scales is required for definitive diagnosis (see p. 133). Caution is warranted here, since dermatophytes may be cultured from the skin and hair of normal cats and dogs and of those with nonfungal skin diseases. These dermatophytic isolates may reflect a "carrier" state or recent exposure to a contaminated environment (e.g., hunting dogs and *M. gypseum*). Microscopic examination of hairs or skin biopsy and staining with a fungal stain such as periodic acid-Schiff (PAS) or Gomori's methenamine silver (GMS) should be used in combination with fungal culture to confirm any diagnosis of dermatophytosis.

Histopathology. The histopathologic features of dermatophytosis are as variable as the clinical lesions. There is no diagnostic histopathologic appearance that is characteristic of dermatophytosis. The most common histopathologic patterns observed in dermatophytosis are (1) perifolliculitis, folliculitis, and furunculosis (see Fig. 7:3); (2) perivasular dermatitis (spongiotic or hyperplastic) with orthokeratotic or parakeratotic hyperkeratosis of the epidermis and hair follicles; and (3) intraepidermal vesicular (spongiotic) or pustular dermatitis. A rare histopathologic pattern is that of diffuse or nodular dermatitis (suppurative, pyogranulomatous, or granulomatous) with the fungus present as "grains"

Figure 7:8. Dermatophytosis. *A,* Classic "ringworm" lesions in a cat caused by *Microsporum canis. B, M. canis* infection near carpus of Vizula. This is a kerion. It is swollen, red, ulcerated, and infected. Licking has kept the exudate removed. *C, M. canis* infection in a pointer puppy whose littermates were also affected. Note the relative lack of inflammation caused by a zoophilic dermatophyte in a dog. *D,* Side view of German shepherd puppy with two facial lesions caused by *M. canis.* The lesion near the ear fluoresced on Wood's light examination. The lesion near the eye did not. See *F* on this plate. (Courtesy B. R. H. Farrow.) *E, M. canis* infection in a French poodle. The circular, red, slightly elevated plaque became apparent when the crust was removed and the surrounding area was clipped. *F,* Side view of puppy in *D* showing facial lesion anterior to ear fluorescing to Wood's light with the typical green-yellow color. (Courtesy B. R. H. Farrow.) *G, M. gypseum* caused a chronic fungal infection in this dachshund, who apparently contracted the geophilic dermatophyte by rooting in the ground with his nose. Eight months of griseofulvin therapy were required to control this stubborn infection. *H, Microsporum gypseum* kerion. Ulcerated nodule on lateral thorax of a dog.

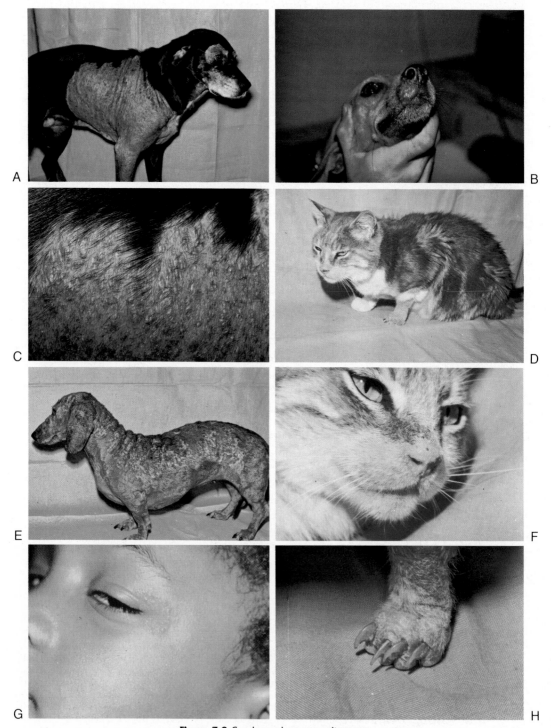

Figure 7:9 *See legend on opposite page*

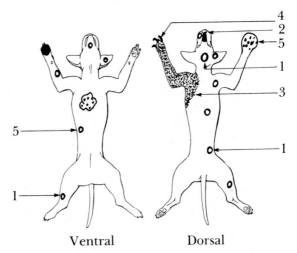

Figure 7:10. Dermatomycoses and dermatophytoses distribution pattern. *1*, Dermatophytosis (*M. canis*). *2*, Dermatophytosis (*M. gypseum*). *3*, Dermatophytosis (*T. mentagrophytes*). *4*, Onychomycosis. *5*, Mycetoma.

Ventral   Dorsal

and hyphae within the dermis or subcutis or both. This is known as pseudomycetoma (see Figs. 7:5 and 7:6).

Septate fungal hyphae and spherical and oval conidia may be present within the stratum corneum, the hair follicles, or in and around the hairs (see Fig. 7:4). The number of fungal elements present is usually inversely proportional to the severity of the inflammatory response. For diagnosis, the histologic examination does not appear to be as discriminating as fungal culture. In feline dermatophytosis, skin biopsy was positive on about 80 per cent of the culturally proven clinical cases (although multiple serial tissue sections were not examined).

Dermatophytes are often visible in the H & E–stained sections but are more readily detected with PAS, GMS, or acid orcein-Giemsa (AOG) stains. Fungi are PAS positive and gram positive.

Differential Diagnosis. Numerous conditions are commonly misdiagnosed as fungal lesions. Some are listed here.

Staphylococcal folliculitis is *by far* the most common cause of ringworm-like lesions in the dog. Seborrheic lesions also frequently mimic the circular lesions of ringworm. Differentiation is made by observing the course of the disease and by evaluating the skin of the entire body, rather than just the individual lesions. Demodicosis, especially in a localized form, also develops circular lesions. A skin scraping quickly differentiates these conditions. Circular abrasions may resemble ringworm lesions. Contact dermatitis of the paws is frequently mistaken for a "fungus" infection. Histiocytomas are solitary well-circumscribed, alopecic, or ulcerated neoplasms of young dogs that may resemble *T. mentagrophytes* or *M. gypseum* kerion reactions (Fig. 7:9B). They are differentiated by negative fungal culture and histologic examination. Epidermal collarettes are characteristically seen in certain skin diseases (especially staph-

Figure 7:9. Dermatophytosis. *A, Trichophyton mentagrophytes* caused this extensive, almost generalized dermatophytosis of two years' duration. Hair loss resulting from the disease—the area was not clipped. *B*, Localized *T. mentagrophytes* lesion (kerion) on nose of young pup. This may resemble a granuloma or a histiocytoma. *C*, Close-up of skin from *A* showing the papular erythematous alopecia. A few pustules and vesicles can be seen in the area. *D, T. mentagrophytes* lesions on a cat. Note the dry, scaly, slightly reddened lesions on the nose and foreleg. *E*, Generalized *T. mentagrophytes* infection complicated by secondary bacterial infection. Note the self-inflicted trauma at the ear margins caused by shaking the head. *F*, Closer view of face lesion of cat in *D*. *G, Microsporum canis* in a child. Annular erythema with papulovesicular margin affecting lateral canthal area. *H*, Closer view of foot lesion of cat in *D*.

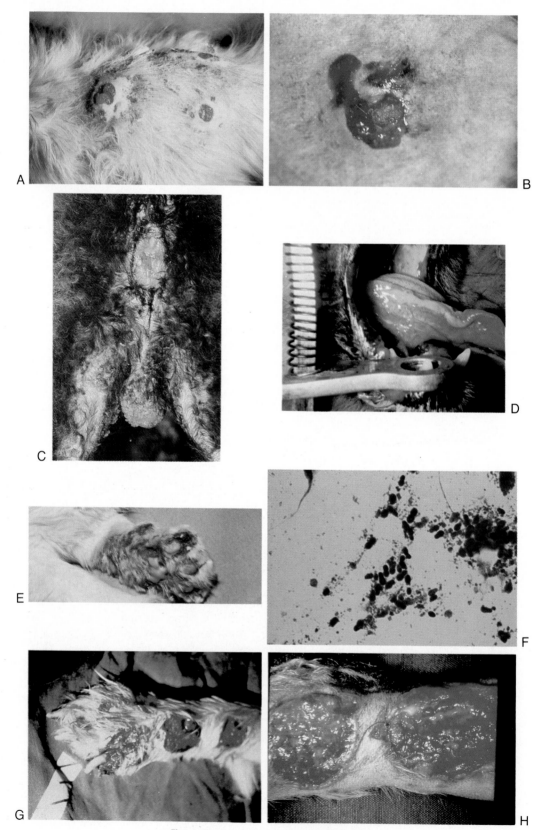

Figure 7:11 *See legend on opposite page*

ylococcal folliculitis) and can be mistaken for dermatophytosis because of their circular configuration. Appropriate cultures and histologic sections with special stains should be diagnostic. Although subcutaneous infections are usually bacterial, infection with *Trichophyton* sp. or *M. canis* has been reported to cause pseudomycetomas (see Fig. 7:11A,B).

Staphylococcal furunculosis, demodicosis, acral lick dermatitis, and certain neoplasms (histiocytoma, mast cell tumor, lymphosarcoma) may resemble a kerion (Figs. 7:8B,H and 7:9B). A suppurative folliculitis with both fungal and bacterial infections is present. Diagnosis is made by appropriate cultures and biopsies.

CLINICAL MANAGEMENT

Dermatophytosis is usually a self-limiting disease, with spontaneous remission occurring within 1 to 3 months. For this reason and because of the expense and possible side-effects associated with systemic griseofulvin therapy (see p. 179), clipping, topical therapy, and appropriate isolation and sanitation may be all that is indicated in most cases.

Griseofulvin is the systemic drug of choice for therapy of chronic, severe or multifocal cases of dermatophytosis. It is also indicated in immunosuppressed patients. The dose of the microcrystalline form (Fulvicin u/f) is 20 to 100 mg/kg of body weight daily.[4, 39, 95] This can be administered daily in food in divided doses. The drug may cause vomiting if given on an empty stomach. Absorption is greatly enhanced if it is administered with a high-fat meal. The drug should be continued until fungal cultures are negative or 2 weeks beyond clinical cure (an average of 4 to 6 weeks). Good results may be obtained with lesser dosage (5 to 10 mg/kg divided daily) of a special microcrystalline polyethylene glycol (PEG) form of griseofulvin.[13] The potential of this formulation to be toxic to cats may be of concern. Bone marrow suppression is occasionally produced, so periodic CBCs should be monitored.[44] In addition, griseofulvin occasionally produces side-effects such as anorexia, vomiting, and diarrhea (see Chapter Four). *The drug is contraindicated during pregnancy because it is teratogenic.* Griseofulvin does *not* reliably eliminate fungal elements from the hair and skin surface in a short period of time; therefore, topical therapy and clipping are *always* indicated.

The affected area of skin should be shaved or clipped to avoid reinfection from infected hairs. Long-haired animals with multiple widespread lesions should receive total body clips. Gentle cleansing with povidone-iodine (Betadine) or chlorhexidine (Nolvasan) shampoo is useful to prevent secondary bacterial infection and for its antifungal effect. Dipping or rinsing with lime-sulfur solution, chlorhexidine solution (15 ml Nolvasan sol/gal water) or captan is highly recommended. A dip prepared from a 1:200 dilution of 45 per cent technical captan is safe for dogs and cats. One or two dips a week can be given

Figure 7:11. Miscellaneous fungal infections. *A,* Ulcerated nodules (pseudomycetoma) due to *Trichophyton* sp. over the back of a cat. (From Scott, D. W.: Feline dermatology 1900–1978: A monograph. J.A.A.H.A. *16:*331, 1980. Courtesy C. Griffin.) *B,* Close-up view of lesion in A. *C,* Candidiasis. Moist, erythematous, eroded, and exudative lesions of the anus and scrotum of a poodle. (From Pichler, M. E., Gross, T. L., et al.: Cutaneous and mucocutaneous candidiasis in a dog. Compend. Cont. Ed. 7:225, 1985.) *D,* Candidiasis: Whitish-gray plaque on the cheek and linear band of affected mucosa on the tongue. (Courtesy N. T. Field.) *E,* Mycetoma in the paw of a cat with characteristic fistulous openings covered with hemorrhagic crusts (see p. 320). *F,* Budding yeast bodies of *Malassezia pachydermitis* in ear smear (Wright-Giemsa stain). *G,* Ulcers due to aspergillosis on the leg of a dog. (Courtesy R. E. W. Halliwell.) *H,* Close-up of lesion in G.

until clinical improvement appears. A 13 per cent solution of thiabendazole (Tresaderm) in water applied three times weekly to cats for several weeks is effective and safe.[41] Recently, a 0.2 per cent enilconazole solution has been very effective for the topical treatment of canine and feline dermatophytosis in Europe.[10a]

Numerous topical fungicidal and fungistatic ointments are in common use. Some of these are keratolytic agents (salicylic acid, undecylenic acid), that remove the keratin in which the fungus grows. Other preparations (Whitfield's ointment) cause inflammation, which interferes with the normal activity of the dermatophytes. Clinicians should use care when applying irritating preparations, as they may encourage secondary pyoderma. These older drugs are less popular now.

Many new, relatively nontoxic and nonirritating preparations are presently available. Tolnaftate preparations (Tinactin) are fungistatic but have *not* been effective in animal dermatophytosis—especially in areas of hairy skin. A 2 per cent topical cream or solution of miconazole nitrate (Micotin, Conofite) is effective for topical use, particularly because of its low toxicity and wide fungicidal spectrum. Clotrimazole (Lotrimin) is a broad-spectrum, fungicidal agent available in a 1 per cent cream or solution that is effective in animal dermatophytoses and candidiasis. Other useful topical agents for local "spot" treatments include chlorhexidine, povidone-iodine, thiabendazole (Tresaderm) or clotrimazole. Topical treatment with a combination of an antifungal imidazole and a corticosteroid enhances the resolution of localized ringworm lesions.[52]

In dermatophyte infections in humans, fungi can be cultured not only from the visible lesion but also from the normal-looking skin, up to 6 cm from the margin of the lesion.[56] This emphasizes the need to extend topical treatments well into the areas of normal skin surrounding obvious lesions.

Ketoconazole (Nizoral) is a water-soluble imidazole derivative that is active in vitro against dermatophytic fungi at concentrations achievable by oral treatment. In vivo studies of dermatophyte-infected guinea pigs showed the oral dosage of the drug to be effective prophylactically and therapeutically.[9] Ketoconazole acts by inhibition only. It has a broad spectrum of activity, but relapses following therapy are not uncommon.[62] The drug is useful in chronic cases of dermatophytosis due to *Trichophyton* infection, but there are reports of some *M. canis* isolates being resistant.[112]

The response to therapy with ketoconazole appears to be independent of the response to other antifungal drugs and associated immune suppression. Length of therapy in human beings varied from 3 days for *Candida* vaginitis to 12 months for onychomycosis.[43] Most superficial mycoses required 2 to 8 weeks of therapy (a mean of 4 weeks).[10a, 62, 100] The drug is absorbed best in an acid medium, so it should be given at mealtime with tomato juice added to the food. Milk and antacids should be withheld. Side-effects include gastric irritation, anorexia, hepatic toxicity, and lightening of the hair coat (see Chapter Four). Rare cardiorespiratory and anaphylactic reactions have been seen.[31] Veterinary dosage for dogs is 5 to 10 mg/kg OD or BID with the higher doses needed for skin infections. For cats, give 5 to 10 mg/kg OD or EOD. Despite apparent clinical cure, medication may have to be continued for 3 to 6 months in some cases to prevent relapse.[35]

Vaccines for fungal infections are highly controversial and of unproven merit.

Onychomycosis is often very difficult to cure. Six to 12 months of griseofulvin or ketoconazole therapy may be required. Surgical declawing may be a practical therapeutic alternative.

Prophylaxis with griseofulvin for exposed animals is effective. High doses of 50 mg/kg daily for 10 to 14 days may be adequate. Infected animals should be isolated from contact with people or pets. Bedding, leashes, and other contaminated equipment should be sterilized or destroyed. *Control measures* in cat colonies have been well documented.[18] Many normal cats were observed to be carriers of dermatophytes. However, the disease is most common in kittens, less so in adult females, and least common in adult males. The infection can be airborne or spread by direct contact. Carrier cats may spread the infection for a short time, but the long-term reservoir is the cat with minimal clinical lesions. Cats in the home can be potent sources of infection to children. Therefore, infected cats may require hospitalization.

An infected cattery should be surveyed by examining each cat carefully with a Wood's light and by culturing skin scrapings and hair from each cat, using Mackenzie's toothbrush technique (see Chapter Three). An on-site cattery inspection by the veterinarian will make his advice more useful. Cats with fluorescent hairs or positive cultures should be isolated and especially segregated in regard to the ventilation system. Animals should be clipped, treated twice weekly with chlorhexidine solution (see earlier discussion), given full doses of griseofulvin for at least 6 weeks, and managed so they do not change cages. Attendants should wear gloves and protective clothes and caps. This disease is a formidable public health problem, and many people who are in contact with active cases, such as cattery and veterinary workers, may be infected. Walls, benches, cages, and so forth should be washed once weekly with iodophor or some other effective cleansing solution. Carried out over a period of weeks, these procedures usually result in satisfactory control. Chlorine solutions (Clorox) are also effective as fungicidal agents on the premises. However, it should be remembered that dermatophytes persist in dry premises for 12 to 52 months.

When new cats are added to a colony they should be examined carefully by Wood's light, cultured by the brush technique, and held in strict isolation for 30 days until culture results are known. Under no circumstances should they be added to the colony unless the tests are negative.

DERMATOMYCOSES

Candidiasis
(Moniliasis)

Candidiasis is a very rare infection of the mucous membrane or skin caused by *Candida* sp.

CAUSE AND PATHOGENESIS

Candida species are yeasts characterized by the formation of blastoconidia, pseudohyphae, and occasionally true hyphae in culture and tissue. *Candida albicans* is considered to be part of the normal microflora of the intestinal tract of warm-blooded animals. Local infection develops with certain predisposing factors, such as excessive moisture, debilitation, and lowered host resistance that result from prolonged use of antibiotics, steroids, or immunosuppressive agents. Yeast infections have not been a serious problem in veterinary medicine, perhaps because the above factors are seldom in effect for prolonged periods of time.

C. albicans is a colonist on normal animals, while other *Candida* species are opportunistic, basically saprophytic yeasts that are found in nature on a variety of substrates. *C. albicans* and *C. parapsilosis* have been shown to produce disease in small animals.[57]

Persistent moisture is a predisposing cause of candidiasis.

CLINICAL FEATURES

These species have a distinct predilection for mucous membranes, areas of mucocutaneous junctions, or areas where moisture may persist and macerate the skin. On mucous membranes the lesions appear as thick white opaque plaques. On skin the lesions are less distinct, and moist, red, eroded areas predominate. Clinical cases of *C. albicans* in dogs have been reported in the perineum, nares, planum nasale, ventral abdomen, scrotum, external ear, nail folds, vagina, and the oral mucosa.[84] Some of the skin lesions can be hyperkeratotic. *C. parapsilosis* was thought to be the cause of moist, red, ulcerative lesions on the base of the tail in one case.[17]

The most common and stubborn site of candidiasis is the oral mucosa (Fig. 7:11D). Oral lesions consist of whitish gray plaques that tend to coalesce into linear bands surrounded by an area of inflamed mucosa. The lesions occur most commonly on the mucous lining of the lips, the cheeks, and the ventral surface of the tongue. White papules are sometimes seen on the dorsal lingual surface. A foul-smelling mucous discharge, mixed with saliva, accompanies the oral lesions. In vaginal lesions a thin, whitish discharge is seen.

Skin lesions are rarely reported; however, they are observed to consist of vesiculopustules covered with brownish crusts. *Candida* may complicate acute otitis externa or pyotraumatic dermatitis ("hot spots"). Schwartzman and associates[94] induced skin lesions experimentally. The acute, oozing red plaques that developed on the macerated suppurative surface of the skin resembled hot spots. Organisms were easily found by direct smears, and if the lesions were dried and exposed to air, the organisms could only be found for 2 days. Candidiasis should be suspected when acute moist lesions develop near mucocutaneous junctions or on hairless areas of the skin (Fig. 7:11C). The course is chronic, and some cases are refractory to treatment.

DIAGNOSIS

Smears of the exudate from typical lesions can be stained with new methylene blue or Diff Quik, or mounted in KOH or in lactophenol cotton blue preparations. Blastoconidia (budding cells) and pseudohyphae may be observed in these preparations. It is important to differentiate them from *Malassezia*. (Fig. 7:11F) Fungal culture is also useful. Most yeasts will grow on Sabouraud's dextrose agar. Some species of yeasts are inhibited by cycloheximide and therefore will not grow on a medium containing this antimicrobial agent. Cultures should be incubated at 30°C. If a 30°C incubator is not available, plates should be incubated at room temperature. Do not incubate cultures at 37°C, because some yeasts will not grow at this temperature. *Candida* species appear as soft, cream-colored colonies within 2 to 7 days. Differentiation of *Candida* species is made by their ability to assimilate and ferment various substrates. The AP1 20C system is a reliable and convenient system for presumptive identification of clinically significant yeasts.[59, 85]

Histopathology. Histopathologically, candidiasis is characterized by perivascular dermatitis (spongiotic or hyperplastic), intraepidermal pustular dermatitis (especially subcorneal), or folliculitis (suppurative). Systemic candidiasis is characterized by necrosis with minimal inflammation. *Candida* species are usually present, in small to large numbers, in the stratum corneum and rarely in the hairs or dermis. The organisms may be seen in histologic sections as blastoconidia (ovoid cells that are often budding and that range from 3 to 5 μm in diameter) (see Fig. 7:2A), as pseudohyphae, and occasionally as hyphae. Usually, *Candida* species are easily visualized in H & E–stained sections but may be highlighted with PAS or GMS stains.

Candida organisms must be demonstrated to be invading tissue to confirm the diagnosis.

Differential Diagnosis. Candidiasis must be distinguished from other ulcerative and gangrenous stomatitides (e.g., chemical, uremic, autoimmune, foreign body, neoplastic); pyotraumatic dermatitis; vulvar fold dermatitis; bacterial or fungal otitis externa; pemphigus vulgaris; bullous pemphigoid; systemic lupus erythematosus; erythema multiforme; epidermotropic lymphosarcoma; and dermatophilosis. These entities can be differentiated by fungal and bacterial cultures and histopathologic sections.

CLINICAL MANAGEMENT

Correction of predisposing causes is fundamental. Correction of immunodeficiency states or avoidance of immunosuppressive drugs may be most helpful. Excessive moisture must be avoided. Nystatin can be applied topically for *Candida* infections with good results. The affected area should be clipped of hair, washed, and dried, and nystatin should be applied topically to the skin or ear canal four times daily. Treatment should be continued after recovery to ensure against relapses. Oral or vulvar infections can be treated with one of the following: gentian violet 1:10,000 in 10 per cent alcohol daily, potassium permanganate 1:3000 in water daily, or nystatin suspension four times daily. Broad-spectrum fungal topical medications such as miconazole (Conofite) or clotrimazole (Lotrimin) are effective. Ketoconazole given orally should be effective.[49] It has been used successfully in systemic candidiasis in neutropenic dogs.[108] In severe unresponsive cases, amphotericin B may be used, but it may be nephrotoxic if administered systemically and should be used by that route only in desperate situations. Response may be seen in a few days in cutaneous, ear, and mucocutaneous infections, but treatment of several weeks is needed for response in cases of onychomycosis, which often relapse. Immunostimulation with levamisole may be of possible benefit in unresponsive cases. Levamisole is given orally in a dose of 2 to 5 mg/kg three times weekly.

Malassezia Infection

Malassezia pachydermatis (Pityrosporum canis) is a yeast that is commonly isolated from the normal and abnormal skin and external ear canals of dogs and cats, but it only rarely produces disease.

CAUSE AND PATHOGENESIS

Malassezia pachydermatis has been isolated from 36 to 57 per cent of normal canine ears. Factors such as ear carriage, age, environment, and frequency of brushing and ear cleaning were not significant in regard to the incidence of the yeast, but there was a possible correlation of incidence to the amount of hair in the ear canal and frequency of bathing. The organism grew better at 37°C, compared with 20°C.[92, 102] Although it is a commensal organism, it might rarely become a secondary invader or pathogen, especially when related to excessive wax production or accumulation of moisture. It is commonly found in the anus, anal sacs, rectum, vagina, and auditory canals.

In the ear canal the organisms are found on the skin surface, but extensive areas of dermatitis have been reported on the trunk where the organisms invaded the epidermis. It is unclear whether the organisms themselves were producing the skin lesions, or if the signs were an id reaction to the yeast.

CLINICAL FEATURES

Mycotic otitis may cause head shaking, ear scratching, excessive aural discharge, pain on manipulation of the ear, and a faint "yeasty" odor.[8]

A generalized seborrheic dermatitis has been reported to be associated with Malassezia organisms that were invading the epidermis.[65] Affected animals were mildly pruritic and had erythematous macules and papules with many irregular white or slate-gray scaly plaques. The lesions were located on the hairy chest wall and in the axillary and inguinal regions. Erythematous, pruritic plaques may also appear on the lips and in skin folds.[23] However, it is unclear whether Malassezia pachydermitis is the primary causative agent of these lesions.

DIAGNOSIS

The organisms are easily collected by skin scrapings of the scaly plaques on the body or by sterile swabs of the waxy exudate in the ear canal. The exudate is smeared on a glass slide, stained with Diff Quik or new methylene blue, and observed for yeast cells (Fig. 7:11F). This genus is distinguished from other genera by the formation of broad phialides (flask-shaped mycelial projections). M. pachydermitis does grow on Sabouraud's dextrose agar at room temperature but grows better at 30 to 35°C. A thin layer of olive oil or vegetable oil on the agar surface may aid isolation.

Histopathologic examination will be useful in demonstrating organisms in the epidermis.

CLINICAL MANAGEMENT

Keeping the affected area dry or, in the case of otitis externa, reducing the pH with vinegar or Domeboro otic drops is helpful. In otitis externa the most important step is identifying and treating the underlying cause, at which point the yeasts will return to normal numbers. Medications that are successful for topical treatment include miconazole, nystatin, thiabendazole, the iodophores, or chlorhexidine. Oral dosage of ketoconazole 10 mg/kg BID for 1 month was successfully used in the seborrheic syndrome.[65]

Trichosporonosis

Trichosporon spp. (*T. beigelii, T. cutaneum, T. pullulans*) are saprophytic yeasts that have been isolated from soil and are presumed to be contaminants from urine and throat cultures. The organisms belong to the family Cryptococcacae and have been reported to cause a cutaneous and a nasal granuloma in two cats. The lesions may appear following a bite, and the infection may be enhanced by immunosuppression resulting from drugs or diseases, such as diabetes mellitus, neoplasms, or FeLV infection. If so, the organism may spread to multiple organs, and can be fatal. There is no known therapy. (See references for Table 7:2).

Subcutaneous Mycoses

Subcutaneous mycoses are fungal infections that have invaded the viable tissues of the skin. These infections are usually acquired by traumatic implantation of organisms that normally exist in soil or vegetation. The lesions are chronic, and in most cases they remain localized. The terminology used in reference to subcutaneous mycoses has been contradictory and confusing. The term phaeohyphomycosis includes subcutaneous and systemic diseases of humans and lower animals caused by fungi that develop in the host tissue in the form of dark-walled septate mycelial elements. Chromoblastomycosis is characterized by sclerotic bodies (chromo bodies, Medlar bodies), which are large, dark-walled cells of 4 to 12 μm in diameter, located in subcutaneous microabscesses. No chromoblastomycosis cases have been confirmed in dogs. Both conditions are mycotic infections characterized by the presence of dematiaceous (pigmented) fungal elements in tissue.

In contrast to phaeohyphomycosis and chromoblastomycosis, a mycetoma is a unique fungal infection marked by granules or grains, tumefaction, and draining sinuses. Mycetomas may be either eumycotic mycetomas or actinomycotic mycetomas. The etiologic agents of eumycotic mycetomas are fungi, whereas actinomycotic mycetomas are caused by members of the *Actinomycetales*, such as *Nocardia*, which are bacteria. Eumycotic mycetomas may be caused by dematiaceous fungi (black-grained mycetomas) or nonpigmented fungi (white-grained mycetomas). Pseudomycetomas have similar lesions, although with subtle microscopic differences in the nature of the granule formation, but they are caused by dermatophytes or bacteria (such as *Staphylococcus* sp.). Terms such as Madura foot, maduromycosis, and maduromycetoma should be discouraged, since they refer to human infections named for a geographic location.

Recently, the term hyolohyphomycosis has been proposed to encompass all opportunistic infections caused by nondematiaceous fungi (as the *aspergilli*), the basic tissue forms of these being in the nature of hyaline hyphal elements that are septate, branched or unbranched, and occasionally toruloid.[66] Another term that creates confusion is phycomycosis. Pythiosis and zygomycosis are now the preferred names for phycomycosis. Members of the genus *Pythium* are properly classified in the kingdom Protista and in the phylum Oomycetes. The class Phycomycetes formally no longer exists. Some members of the class belong to the kingdom Protista, and some belong to the phylum of either Zygomycota or Chytridiomycota. Included in the Zygomycota are the orders Mucorales and Entomophthorales. Some fungi from both orders are pathogenic. The term zygomycosis is now used to include both mucormycosis and ento-mophthoromycosis.

Subcutaneous mycoses and their infective agents include the following:

1. Eumycotic mycetoma (*Pseudoallescheria boydii, Curvularia geniculata*).
2. Phaeohyphomycosis (*Drechslera spicifera, Pseudomicrodochium suttonii, Phialophora verrucosa, Exophiala jeanselmei, Moniliella suaveolens, Stemphylium* sp., *Cladosporium* sp.).
3. Pythiosis (*Pythium* sp.) (formerly Phycomycosis—the organism was called *Hyphomyces destruens*).
4. Protothecosis (*Prototheca wickerhamii*). Protothecosis is usually a systemic disease in dogs and cats. Prototheca have been classified as algae by some taxonomists.
5. Sporotrichosis (*Sporothrix schenckii*). May also be systemic.
6. Rhinosporidiosis (*Rhinosporidium seeberi*).
7. Zygomycosis (*Basidiobolus haptosporus, Conidiobolus coronatus*).

Mycetoma

Mycetomas are rare, chronic, subcutaneous swellings produced by fungi in tissue. The characteristic fistulas produce pus that contains granules or "grains."

CAUSE AND PATHOGENESIS

Mycetoma is a rare trauma-induced disease, often associated with penetrating wounds, that may involve the skin, subcutaneous tissue, fascia, and bone. Mycetomas are usually restricted to one area of the body, usually the abdomen or a foot (see Fig. 7:11E). Etiologic agents of eumycotic mycetoma reported in animals include *Curvularia geniculata, Pseudoallescheria (Allescheria) boydii.*[47] (Occasionally, the actinomycetes *Nocardia asteroides, N. caviae, N. braziliense*, and *Actinomyces* spp. are involved in actinomycotic mycetomas of dogs and cats.) In order to be classified as a mycetoma, the fistulous discharge must contain granules of organized, compact mycelial growth. True granules vary in color, size, shape, and texture. Color may be white, yellow, or black, depending on the particular fungus involved.[81] Usually *C. geniculata* produces black-to-brown granules, whereas *P. boydii* produces white-to-yellow granules. Although only a few confirmed cases of mycetoma have been reported in the United States, there have probably been many undiagnosed cases. Common dermatophyte media that contain inhibitors such as cycloheximide will discourage growth of mycetoma fungi in vitro. The lesions resemble chronic, nonhealing abscesses, and animals with undiagnosed cases of mycetoma may have been euthanized after failure to respond to treatment for a bacterial infection.

CLINICAL FEATURES

> **The triad of swelling, draining fistulas, and granules should suggest a mycetoma.**

At first the foot (or other affected area) is tender, painful, and swollen. At this stage the lesion resembles an early abscess. Soon thereafter, many draining sinuses form, and their openings exude a serous or purulent discharge. Chronic fistulous tracts are established. As some fistulas heal, scar tissue develops and forms the hard tumor-like mass that is characteristic of chronic mycetomas. Hemorrhagic crusts form over some fistulous orifices (see Fig. 7:11E). Finally, the whole area enlarges grotesquely and fails to respond to conservative antibacterial or antifungal treatment. Extension of the disease process into the deeper areas can involve the bones as the fungus penetrates the periosteum.

DIAGNOSIS

> **Use plain Sabouraud's dextrose agar for culturing. Some antimicrobial inhibitors in other agars will discourage growth of mycetoma fungi.**

While the suspicion of mycetoma or pseudomycetoma may arise from the lack of response to antibiotics and drainage, in cases with subcutaneous infection, laboratory work is essential for diagnosis. Occasionally, direct smears are helpful and histopathologic sections may demonstrate fungal elements. However, culture on plain Sabouraud's dextrose agar is essential in order to identify the specific fungal organism. This is sophisticated work that requires the expertise of a trained mycologist.

Histopathology. Eumycotic mycetomas are characterized by diffuse or nodular dermatitis (suppurative, pyogranulomatous, or granulomatous). Fungal elements are present as a "grain" (thallus) within the tissues (Fig. 7:12). The "grains" consist of septate branching hyphae, vesicles, and a cementing matrix. The fungal elements may be pigmented or nonpigmented. Hyphae are often visualized in H & E–stained sections but are highlighted by PAS, GMS, and Gridley stains (Fig. 7:13).

Differential Diagnosis. Abscesses bear a slight resemblance to mycetoma in an early stage, especially in cats (see Fig. 7:11E). However, abscesses respond rapidly to liberal surgical drainage and parenteral antibiotics, whereas mycetomas do not. Fistulas caused by foreign bodies (foxtails, awns, thorns) do not usually have chronic, hard, fibrotic tissue masses. Neoplasms cause swellings and often ulcerate, but they do not form fistulas with granules in the exudate. Atypical mycobacterial granuloma, feline leprosy, and pseudomycetoma should also be considered. Special stains can be useful in demonstrating acid-fast organisms, bacteria, or fungal elements.

CLINICAL MANAGEMENT

Surgical removal of the fibrinous mass is helpful in the early stages. Amputation of the affected paw can be curative, but removing the cosmetically

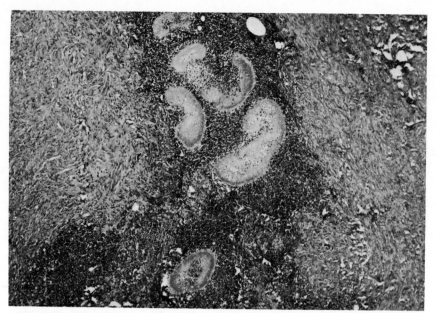

Figure 7:12. Mycetoma in a dog. Note numerous tissue grains within a pyogranuloma.

disfiguring and painful growth is usually a last resort. Ketoconazole has not been promising in therapeutic trials in humans, since it does not penetrate fibrous tissue well. Other antifungal agents are ineffective.

Pseudomycetoma

Pseudomycetoma is a rare, subcutaneous infection caused by a dermatophyte or nonactinomycete bacteria. It appears to be similar superficially to eumycotic

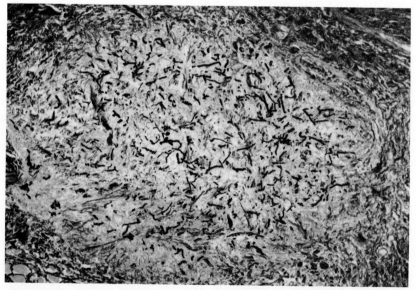

Figure 7:13. Histologic appearance (low power) of a mycetoma caused by *Curvularia geniculata* and reproduced from a section stained with Gomori's methenamine silver. It demonstrates numerous dark fungal fragments, chlamydospores, and hyphae in the center of a necrotic granulomatous reaction. (At this magnification cell types cannot be identified, but multinucleated foreign body giant cells, macrophages, neutrophils, lymphocytes, and plasma cells are present.)

mycetomas, but there are differences in the granules and mycelial aggregates of each condition, and of course identification of the fungal or bacterial organism is diagnostic. *Trichophyton* sp. and *Microsporum* sp. have been identified from several cases of pseudomycetoma in long-haired cats.[103] A more complete discussion is included under dermatophytoses, p. 303. Staphylococci and possibly other nonactinomycete bacteria are rarely the cause of pseudomycetoma (see p. 270).

Phaeohyphomycosis

Phaeohyphomycosis is a rare subcutaneous infection caused by dematiaceous (dark) septated hyphae. This disease differs from mycetomas in that the fungus is not organized into granules. *Drechslera spicifera, Moniella suaveolens, Exophiala jeanselmei, Phialophora verrucosa, Stemphylium* sp., and *Cladosporium* sp. have been isolated from phaeohyphomycosis in cats.[22, 69, 75, 99] Two additional feline cases of phaeohyphomycosis were reported from tissue sections but not confirmed by cultures.[40, 42]

A new organism (*Pseudomicrodochium suttonii*) causing phaeohyphomycosis was isolated from an ear lesion in a dog.[2] In addition, canine cases have been reported to be caused by *D. spicifera* and *Phialemonium obovatum*.[58, 64]

The dematiaceous fungi that cause phaeohyphomycosis can only be differentiated by culture.

CAUSE AND PATHOGENESIS

This rare disease may have been overlooked in the past because special laboratory techniques are required for diagnosis. Phaeohyphomycosis has been caused by fungi such as *D. spicifera, P. verrucosa,* and *P. suttonii. D. spicifera* is the imperfect state of *Cochliobolus spicifer,* a member of the Ascomycota, which is commonly found in soil and can be a plant pathogen. *P. suttonii's* natural habitat is unknown. Other reported cases of phaeohyphomycoses of cats have not been confirmed by isolation of the etiologic agent. It could be speculated that some mycetomas of dogs have actually been phaeohyphomycosis caused by *D. spicifera,* which resembles fungi of the genus *Curvularia* or *Helminthosporium.* The characteristic features of these fungi are their preference for subcutaneous tissue, while the epidermis and the dermis are usually spared, and histologically, their lack of organization in grains. Unlike infection with the systemic fungi such as *Coccidioides immitis,* the internal organs are usually not invaded. Typically, a primary site exists, such as a paw or chest, where the organism is inoculated. A carefully taken history may reveal the primary site. Despite similar onsets of infection, the severity and clinical course vary greatly. Fistulous subcutaneous nodules that fail to respond to antibiotic treatment should be considered as possible phaeohyphomycosis lesions.

CLINICAL FEATURES

The typical case begins with a subcutaneous nodule that gradually enlarges. One or more fistulas form in some of the nodules, exuding a yellow or pink purulent exudate. The lesions may become ulcerated (Figs. 7:14A,B) and are relatively painless when palpated. Lesions are most commonly seen on the distal extremities and the trunk. An excised lesion will often return at the same site.

DIAGNOSIS

Mycotic culture is necessary for diagnosis. Exudates from fistulas or pieces of biopsy tissue are placed on plain Sabouraud's dextrose agar without cyclo-heximide or antibiotics. Cultures should be incubated at 30°C or room temper-ature. *Drechslera spicifera* grows rapidly, and the colonies can reach a 75 mm diameter in 7 days. *Pseudomicrodochium suttonii* grows very slowly and may reach 12 to 13 mm in diameter after 2 weeks. Identification of the organism should be made by a qualified mycologist.

Histopathology. Subcutaneous phaeohyphomycosis is characterized by diffuse or nodular dermatitis (suppurative, pyogranulomatous, or granuloma-tous). Fungal elements are present as pigmented, septate hyphae, with occa-sional pigmented vesicles (Fig. 7:14C). The organisms are best visualized with H & E stain to determine the hyphal color. However, sections stained with PAS and GMS sections help detail the varied morphology of the etiologic agents.

Differential Diagnosis. The differential diagnosis of phaeohyphomycosis includes chronic abscesses and foreign body fistulas. Both entities typically produce an inflammatory exudate and respond to surgical and antibacterial therapy. Feline leprosy is differentiated from phaeohyphomycosis by the identification of numerous acid-fast bacilli demonstrated with Fite-Faraco stain. Differentiation from skin tumors can be made by histology. Mycetomas and pseudomycetomas are differentiated by the characteristic granules in the exu-date, together with cultures and special fungal stains.

CLINICAL MANAGEMENT

Affected tissues are surgically excised, using the same technique as that for malignant neoplasms. With blunt dissection the underlying subcutaneous tissue is completely freed, and all visibly affected tissue is surgically removed. Lesions of the paws are more difficult to treat, and amputation of one or more toes may be required. Recurrences may occur 3 to 6 months after the first surgery. The new granulomatous masses must be excised again.

Systemic fungicides, such as griseofulvin, amphotericin B, or ketoconazole, are reported to be ineffective against phaeohyphomycosis.[16] However, intrale-sional amphotericin B therapy has been reported to be successful in humans,[14] and ketoconazole was effective for the management of phaeohyphomycosis due to *Phialophora* sp. on the paw of a cat.[107] In addition, 5-fluorocytosine and local hyperthermia have been reported to be effective in humans with chro-moblastomycosis and phaeohyphomycosis.[101, 106]

Amphotericin B and fluorocytosine[69] and ketoconazole[99] have been used successfully in two cases in cats. Test culture inhibitions should be made against several drugs to determine potential efficacy. Itraconazole has been effective in human cases.[89]

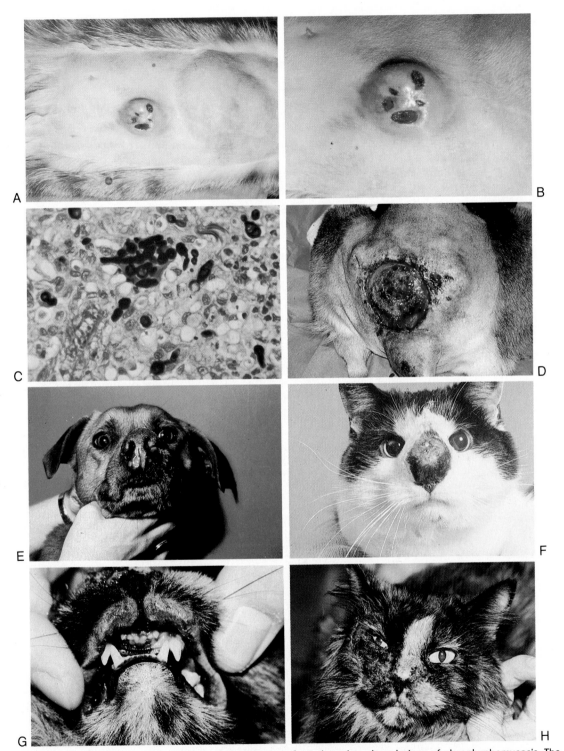

Figure 7:14. Phaeohyphomycosis. *A,* Thorax and abdomen of cat shaved to show lesions of phaeohyphomycosis. The smaller mass had draining fistulas. *B,* Close-up of draining swelling shown in *A. C,* Individual hyphae and a small group of hyphae and chlamydospores of *Drechslera spicifera* dispersed in infected tissue of cat (× 500, Gomori–H & E stain). (Courtesy Mycology Division, Communicable Disease Center, U.S.D.A.) *D,* Ulcerated tumors over dorsal lumbosacral area of a dog with pythiosis. (Courtesy C. Foil.) *E,* Ulcerated nodules on nose of a dog with blastomycosis. (Courtesy J. Brace.) *F,* Feline cryptococcosis. Granulomatous involvement of bridge of nose. *G,* Feline cryptococcosis. Bilateral ulcers of the upper lip. *H,* Facial ulceration in a cat with cryptococcosis.

Pythiosis
(Phycomycosis)

Pythiosis is a rare, poorly responsive fungal disease of the subcutaneous (and gastrointestinal) tissues of dogs.

CAUSE AND PATHOGENESIS

Organisms tentatively identified as *Pythium* sp. (formerly *Hyphomyces destruens*) have been associated with this disease, which is well recognized in horses and has formerly been called phycomycosis. Members of the genus *Pythium* that have aquatic motile zoospores are in the infective stage for plant hosts. Many members of the genus *Pythium* are pathogens of aquatic and semiaquatic plants. The organism affecting horses in some parts of the world has been identified as *Pythium gracile*, but species identification of canine isolates has not been reported.

The disease appears to be restricted to warm climates such as are found in the southeastern United States, especially the Gulf Coast states. It usually occurs in summer or late fall. Affected animals almost always have access to bodies of water that are rich in organic material (standing water), and in vitro, the motile zoospores are chemically attracted to animal hairs. Trauma, even minor excoriations, may be necessary for development of the disease, since it has been a common finding in many of the reported cases.[78] Most of the canine cases have involved young adult, large-breed dogs, possibly because these animals frequent the environment necessary to acquire the infection.[30]

CLINICAL FEATURES

Lesions usually have been present for at least 1 month when the case is presented, and they occur on the nasal portion of the face, the rump, tail or the limbs. They appear as slightly pruritic, poorly defined nodules that soon become ulcerated (Fig. 7:14D). Some lesions become boggy and develop fistulas that drain a serosanguinous or purulent exudate. Older lesions may be marked by multifocal hemorrhagic necrotic ulcers. Some lesions spread rapidly, probably reflecting the tendency of the organism to invade vessels. The "leeches" or "kunkers," (elongated, gritty, coral-like bodies found in the sinus tracts), which characterize pythiosis in horses, are *not* seen in dogs.[30a]

DIAGNOSIS

Only occasionally will cytologic examination of the exudates demonstrate the fungal elements.

Histologic examination of deep biopsy specimens stained with GMS may reveal the characteristic infrequently septate, irregular, branching, broad hyphae. They are not apparent in H & E–stained sections, a characteristic that helps differentiate them from zygomycetes, similar-appearing fungi that do stain with H & E.

Positive diagnosis is made only by culture and identification of the organisms from surgically collected tissues from the center of the lesions.

Histopathology. Histologic lesions are characterized by severe ulcerative pyogranulomatous dermatitis and/or cellulitis. Multifocal areas of necrosis may

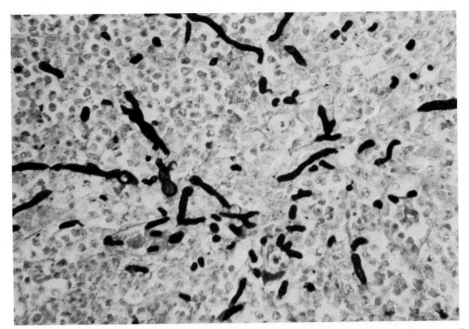

Figure 7:15. Canine pythiosis. Numerous hyphae in a pyogranulomatous dermatitis. (Courtesy C. Foil.)

be infiltrated with neutrophils and macrophages. The discrete granulomas contain eosinophilic cell debris and are surrounded by eosinophils, neutrophils, macrophages, epithelioid cells, and multinucleated giant cells. GMS–stained sections of the granulomas and adjacent thrombosed arteries usually demonstrate numerous broad, nonseptate branching hyphae (Fig. 7:15). The characteristic wide hyphae are 4.5 μm to 5.5 μm in diameter.

Differential Diagnosis. The differential diagnosis should include other fungal and bacterial infections, demodicosis, various neoplasms, and acral lick dermatitis.

CLINICAL MANAGEMENT

The prognosis must be guarded, since aggressive surgical excision, including amputation of the affected extremity, is the only treatment that has been successful.[80] Some cases have resulted in subsequent relapses, and traditional systemic antifungal medications have not been effective. This situation would be expected, however, since *Pythium* organisms probably do not possess the ergosterol-rich cell membrane structure, which is characteristic of true fungi and renders them susceptible to systemic antifungal drugs such as amphotericin B and the imidazoles.

Immunotherapy with transfer factor has not been successful in limited trials.[78]

Protothecosis

Protothecosis is a rare, chronic, nodular granulomatous infection of the subcutaneous tissue that is caused by algae.

CAUSE AND PATHOGENESIS

Prototheca sp. are achloric algae that are thought to be variants of green algae. They are common environmental saprophytes and are rarely associated with disease in animals or humans. To date, *Prototheca wickerhamii* is the only species to be reported in cats and dogs.

CLINICAL FEATURES

Protothecosis has been reported involving the skin of cats and the skin and mucocutaneous ocular tissues of dogs.[15, 33, 51, 71] Lesions may appear on the distal extremities, head, pinna, chest, and nares. They may be small, nonreactive nodules or ulcerated or crusted nodules (granulomas) with a thick, mucoid, yellow-to-pink exudate. Dissemination to the regional lymph nodes may be observed.

DIAGNOSIS

Diagnosis may be confirmed by culturing the organisms on plain Sabouraud's dextrose agar or by specific fluorescent antibody reagents applied to formalin-fixed tissues.

Histopathology. Biopsy specimens reveal a granulomatous or pyogranulomatous dermatitis and/or panniculitis. The organisms are usually present in large numbers as spherical or cresentic sporangia which vary from 2 μm to 20 μm in diameter. They stain poorly or not at all with H & E stain and are best seen with GMS, Gridley's, or PAS preparations of biopsy specimens.

Differential Diagnosis. One should consider bacterial infection, mycetoma, pseudomycetoma, phaeohyphomycosis, sporotrichosis, neoplasms such as histiocytoma, and mastocytoma, feline leprosy, atypical mycobacterial infections, and other systemic mycoses that affect the skin (blastomycosis, histoplasmosis, cryptococcosis).

CLINICAL MANAGEMENT

Nonreactive nodules, in their early stages, can sometimes be removed surgically with success. In later stages they may recur, and no truly successful therapy is known. Amphotericin B has been used successfully in one human case.[67]

Sporotrichosis

Sporotrichosis is an uncommon chronic granulomatous infection caused by the dimorphic fungus *Sporothrix schenckii*.

CAUSE AND PATHOGENESIS

S. schenckii is found in decaying vegetation, humus, and sphagnum moss. The organism gains entrance to its host by wound contamination, especially in puncture wounds from thorns (particularly rose thorns), wood slivers, or bites. Sporotrichosis has been reported in dogs, cats, other animals, and humans (especially farmers and florists). Sporotrichosis should be considered contagious, particularly if there are open wounds that may be contaminated with exudates. The infection has been reported as a real public health concern for practicing veterinarians and their assistants[27, 28] (Fig. 7:16H).Cats with sporotrichosis usually have myriads of fungal organisms and are especially hazardous to human contacts. Skin penetration or the contamination of open wounds is not necessary for transmission.[26, 27] Always wear rubber gloves and wash thoroughly with fungicidal antiseptics (chlorhexidine or povidone-iodine) after handling infected cats. The geographic distribution of *Sporothrix schenckii* is universal, but the fungus is most common along the coastal regions and river valleys of the southern United States, or in countries with similar climates. As a dimorphic fungus, it is a yeast in tissues and on medium at 37°C but a mold on Sabouraud's dextrose agar at 25 to 30°C.

CLINICAL FEATURES

Sporotrichosis occurs in three clinical syndromes: the cutaneous-lymphatic, cutaneous, and disseminated.

In the *Cutaneous-lymphatic* form, lesions occur as round, firm nodules at the point of entry, with the infection progressing to the subcutaneous tissues and lymphatic system. Tender nodules and lymph nodes may become ulcerative and often discharge a thick, brown-red exudate.

The *cutaneous form* is a primary infection of the skin that remains localized. Lesions are diffusely scattered, circular with raised borders, ulcerated, non-painful, and alopecic (Fig. 7:16A,B). They may appear as multiple firm nodules that spread slowly and do not respond to vigorous antibacterial therapy (Fig. 7:16C). Cats often have ulcerated lesions of the face (Fig. 7:16D–G). Another skin form presents a verrucous appearance, with well-demarcated round or oval alopecic lesions covered with small scales and bordered by microabscesses.[97]

Either form may be associated with the *disseminated form*, in which many deep tissues are infected.[53] This is more common in cats than dogs.[3, 5] The organism rarely invades bone, lung, liver, spleen, kidneys, testes, or the gastrointestinal and central nervous systems.

The incubation period is approximately 1 month.[7] The course is usually chronic and prolonged. Symptomatic or antibacterial treatments are futile. With proper sodium iodide therapy, nondisseminated forms typically respond promptly and dramatically with complete resolution.

DIAGNOSIS

Direct culture from purulent material or biopsy specimens is reliable, and organisms grow readily on either Sabouraud's dextrose agar at 30°C or brain-heart infusion agar at 37°C. Because of the small numbers of yeast cells in the lesions, direct examination of material in smears rarely detects the fungus.

S. schenckii grows as a mold forming two types of conidia. *S. schenckii* has the ability to grow as a mold at room temperature and as a yeast at 37°C or in the tissues. However, other closely related genera and species are also dimorphic. For this reason dimorphism cannot be used as a final identification characteristic. A qualified mycologist should identify the cultures.

Mouse inoculation using 0.2 ml of a dense mycelial suspension injected intratesticularly produces a purulent orchitis, and examination of the exudate reveals cigar-shaped and oval blastoconidia. Direct smears of lesions in dogs

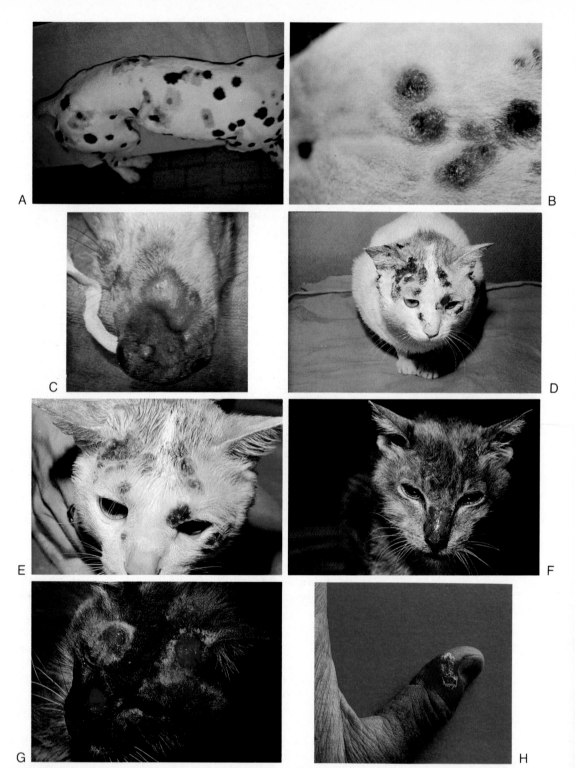

Figure 7:16. Sporotrichosis. *A*, General view of Dalmatian dog with cutaneous lesions of sporotrichosis. Note the diffusely scattered but focal nature of the dorsally located lesions (hair has been clipped around each lesion). *B*, Closer view of the dorsum of the head of the patient in *A*. The lesions are glistening, and slightly crusted and have very well-defined, slightly raised borders. *C*, The multiple nodular lesions on the nose of this collie were firm, painful, and not ulcerated, and well demarcated. This patient has additional lesions on the lower eyelids, and all responded promptly to iodide therapy after many months of negative results with other forms of treatment. *D*, Multiple ulcers and crusts on the face of a cat with sporotrichosis. *E*, Close-up of cat in *D*. *F*, Facial ulcers in a cat with sporotrichosis. *G*, Close-up of cat in *F*. *H*, Sporotrichosis lesion on veterinarian's thumb (G.H.M.).

330

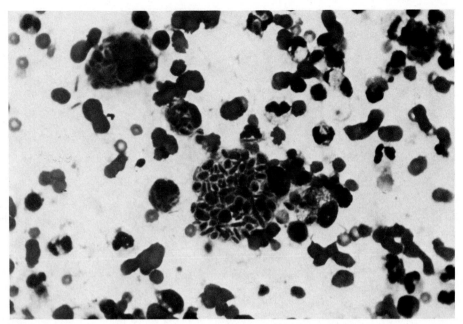

Figure 7:17. Feline sporotrichosis. Numerous yeast and cigar bodies in a macrophage. (Courtesy J. M. MacDonald.)

and humans are of limited value because of the paucity of organisms. Organisms are usually abundant in cats (Fig. 7:17).

Fluorescent antibody techniques using fluorescein-labeled rabbit antiglobulin, specific for *S. schenckii*, applied to exudates from lesions may be a sensitive test but requires sophisticated laboratory equipment. Fungal cells are seen as brightly fluorescent bodies against a dark background.

An indirect immunoperoxidase staining method applied to 4 per cent formaldehyde-fixed tissues localizes *S. schenckii* and *C. neoformans* in tissue specimens in 24 hours.[91]

Histopathology. Histopathology of sporotrichosis is characterized by early perivascular dermatitis (spongiotic or hyperplastic) and later by diffuse or nodular dermatitis (suppurative, pyogranulomatous, or granulomatous) (Fig. 7:18). Intraepidermal microabscesses and pseudocarcinomatous epidermal hyperplasia may be seen. *S. schenckii* is present as round-to-oval cells producing buds that range from 3 to 6 μm in diameter. The classic "cigar bodies" (4 to 8 μm in length, 1 to 2 μm in diameter) are less commonly observed (Fig. 7:19). Except in feline tissue, *S. schenckii* is often impossible to find in histologic sections, even with special stains such as PAS and GMS. Asteroid bodies that are the result of antigen-antibody complexes formed from the fungal cell wall may be seen. However, this host-parasite interaction is not unique to *S. schenckii*.

Differential Diagnosis. Sporotrichosis should be differentiated from chronic ulcers and granulomas caused by other agents that affect skin. Mycoses such as histoplasmosis, blastomycosis, cryptococcosis, phaeohyphomycosis, mycetoma, pseudomycetoma, and dermatophytosis can be identified by fungal culture and by histopathology. Fungal stains may be helpful. Histologic sections of feline leprosy lesions stained with Fite-Faraco reveal numerous acid-fast bacilli. Skin tumors such as histiocytomas and mastocytomas can be diagnosed by histologic sections stained by H & E or toluidine blue. Pyodermas should be identified by bacterial cultures and routine histologic sections.

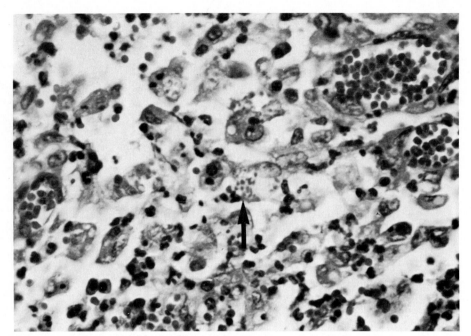

Figure 7:18. Feline sporotrichosis. Pyogranulomatous dermatitis with intracellular yeast and cigar bodies (arrow).

CLINICAL MANAGEMENT

It is helpful to determine the focus of infection that initiated the lesion, (e.g., rose thorns, wood slivers from kennel doors, bedding of sphagnum moss), in order to prevent reinfection.

Nondisseminated forms usually respond well to oral dosages of inorganic

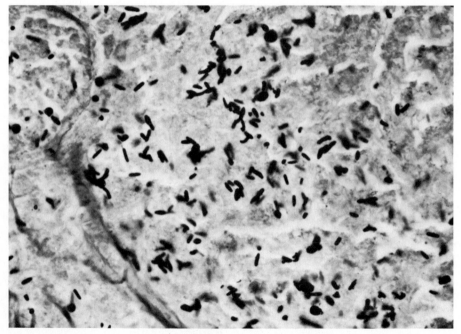

Figure 7:19. Canine sporotrichosis. Numerous yeast and cigar bodies (GMS stain).

iodides, and the prognosis is good. One author (Scott) has recommended 20 per cent sodium iodide (NaI) given orally to dogs at a dose of 0.2 ml/kg of body weight (40 mg/kg) two to three times daily.[95] The solution has a palatable sweet taste compared with potassium iodide (KI) and is well absorbed. Response may be noted within 1 week, but treatment should be continued for 30 days after apparent "cure" to prevent relapse. Others have obtained good results using a similar dosage of KI.[21] Cats are particularly susceptible to iodism. An oral dose of NaI, 20 mg/kg once daily or BID, is recommended. If dogs and cats show signs of iodism (see p. 179), the drug should be stopped and reinstituted at a lower dose when side-effects disappear. The rationale for iodide therapy is not clear, since the fungus will grow in 10 per cent KI, and no concentrations of iodide have been demonstrated at the site of infection. Possibly, the iodide augments the natural resistance of the host in some small but vitally necessary way. A defect or complete lack of the natural immunologic process may explain why some cases disseminate and respond poorly to treatment.

Hot packs, applied to superficial local lesions two to three times daily to produce local hyperthermia, or hot water soaking have been beneficial adjunctive therapy in human cases.

The disseminated form does not usually respond well to iodide therapy alone, but successful results have been reported following systemic use of amphotericin B, which probably provides the greatest hope for animals, too; however, the potential toxicity and the difficulty of dosage must be considered before therapy is initiated. Vandevelde and colleagues[105] used 5-fluorocytosine in humans and laboratory animals in an oral dosage, which may cause neutropenia, hepatic dysfunction, and a scrotal dermatitis. Some organisms rapidly develop resistance to 5-fluorocytosine. The combination of amphotericin B and 5-fluorocytosine may be used as a desperation measure. The combination reduces potential toxicities but may not be any more effective than amphotericin B alone.

Ketoconazole and NaI have been used concurrently to treat feline sporotrichosis successfully. Both drugs have potential toxicity for cats, so the dosage must be adjusted carefully.[10, 27] With ketoconazole, medication should be started at 10 mg/kg BID, and the dose doubled weekly until response or toxicity results. (See Chapter 4, p. 179.)

Systemic Mycoses

Systemic mycoses are fungal infections of internal organs that may disseminate secondarily to the skin. Fungi that cause systemic mycoses exist in soil or vegetation and only rarely are pathogens. In endemic regions, many animals are exposed to fungi causing systemic infections without developing clinical disease.

When the skin is involved, fistulas or nodules called infectious granulomas are produced. These infections are usually not contagious, since the animal inhales or contacts conidia from a specific ecologic niche. The systemic mycoses will be discussed only briefly here, and the reader is referred to texts on mycology and infectious diseases for additional information. Fungi that cause systemic mycoses are divided into primary and secondary pathogens.

Primary pathogens are organisms that are able to invade a normal healthy host. Clinical diseases ranging from asymptomatic to severe infections may result from inhalation of conidia.

Primary Pathogen	Usual Habitat
Blastomyces dermatitidis	Humid, organically enriched soils (beaver lodges)
Coccidioides immitis	Soil of semiarid areas
Histoplasma capsulatum	Soil contaminated by feces of birds, bats, and poultry

Secondary pathogens may be found in animals or the environment, but they initiate infection only when the resistance of the host is compromised.

Secondary Pathogen	Usual Habitat
Aspergillus spp.	Vegetation and soil
Candida spp.	Gastrointestinal and reproductive tract
Cryptococcus neoformans	Soil and pigeon droppings
Mucor spp.	Vegetation and soil
Paecilomyces spp.	Soil

Blastomycosis

Blastomycosis is a chronic granulomatous, suppurative, systemic infection caused by the dimorphic fungus *Blastomyces dermatitidis*.

The organism has been isolated from organically enriched soil (i.e., beaver lodges).[54] Incidence of the disease is highest in the Ohio and Mississippi River basin states. It is more common in dogs than in cats.[34] *B. dermatitidis* can invade any tissue and thus can produce diverse clinical syndromes.[11] Usually the fungus enters the respiratory system, but multisystemic involvement is common, and in addition to the lungs it especially favors ocular, osseous, and integumentary tissue. About 40 per cent of dogs with blastomycosis have skin involvement.[24] This can occur by external invasion or internal dissemination.

Skin lesions vary greatly in character, but typically they occur as chronic, ulcerated, granulomatous papules and nodules of 0.5 cm to 10.0 cm in size, or as draining tracts (Fig. 7:14E), which exude a seropurulent exudate. They may involve head, legs, chest, and scrotum. Regional lymphadenopathy is often dramatic.[61]

Diagnosis is usually made by microscopic identification of the organism in exudate or tissue from an infected site. Cytologic examination of fresh smears of exudate or tissue aspirates from lesions or enlarged lymph nodes (stained with Diff Quik) will commonly make the diagnosis. If organisms are not abundant, special stains (PAS or Gridley's) may be useful in making them stand out. The organisms are refractile, spherical, double-walled, yeastlike bodies that are 8 to 20 μm in diameter (Fig. 7:20). They are located extracellularly and they may or may not be budding.[86] Agar-gel immunodiffusion test for systemic fungi (not specific for blastomycosis, however), histologic examination, and fungal culture of a tissue specimen or biopsy may also be diagnostic. Histologic examination of cutaneous biopsy sections are characterized by pseudocarcinomatous hyperplasia, intraepidermal and dermal abscesses, chronic pyogranulomatous to granulomatous dermatitis and, of course, identification of the typical yeast cells of *B. dermatitidis*. The dimorphic organism is a broad-based yeast in tissues or in cultures at 37°C and a mold at 20°C.

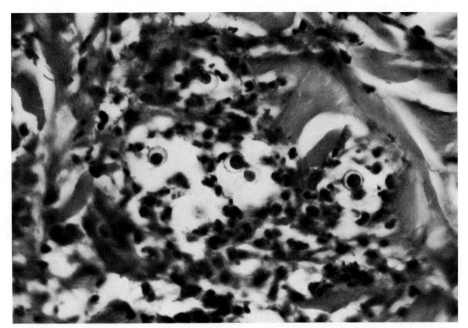

Figure 7:20. Canine blastomycosis. Large, round, thick-walled yeast bodies (H & E stain).

Differential diagnosis should include pyoderma resulting from bacterial, fungal, or parasitic causes; immune-mediated diseases; foreign body granuloma; neoplasms; and other deep fungal diseases (histoplasmosis, cryptococcosis, sporotrichosis, coccidioidomycosis, and aspergillosis).

Clinical management can be approached with guarded optimism. Although blastomycosis is not highly contagious, some zoonotic concern is warranted. Humans have contracted the disease by inoculation from dog bites and from injury sustained during a necropsy.[37, 48]

Treatment must be prolonged, and at present it should be started with amphotericin B for an initial rapid effect and continued with ketoconazole for long-term outpatient therapy. Dunbar has used ketoconazole alone in a dosage of 30 mg/kg orally once daily for 2 months with good results in three of four dogs treated for generalized blastomycosis.[25] (See dosage details in Chapter 4, p. 179.)

Coccidioidomycosis

Coccidioidomycosis is a fungal disease endemic to desert areas such as the southwestern United States. It is caused by *Coccidioides immitis*, a thick-walled spherule that reproduces by endosporulation.[32] The disease is asymptomatic in many individuals but produces serious multisystemic lesions in others. In rare cases where there are skin lesions, the infection may be only incidental. However, primary skin invasion has been reported.[109] Lesions may appear as abscesses, draining fistulas, or granulomas. Diagnosis is made by identification of the characteristic spherules in exudates, in histologic sections. The organisms appear as, round, double-walled structures 10 to 80 μm in diameter with endospores (Fig. 7:21). With PAS stain, the spherule wall is not stained but the endospores are bright red. Diagnosis can also be made by an exudate culture,

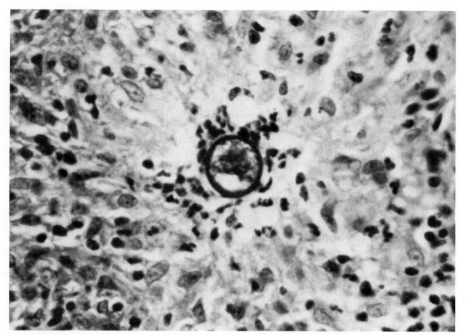

Figure 7:21. Canine coccidioidomycosis. *Coccidioides immitis* spherule in center of pyogranuloma (PAS stain).

but this is dangerous; consequently, the material should be placed on Sabouraud's agar and sent to laboratories equipped to handle such hazardous materials.

Treatment is with amphotericin B or ketoconazole.[6, 110] (See also Chapter 4, Dermatologic Therapy, p. 179.)

Histoplasmosis

Histoplasmosis is a ubiquitous disease that has an especially high incidence in river valleys of the southern and midwestern United States. It is caused by *Histoplasma capsulatum,* a dimorphic fungus that grows naturally in soils enriched with bird and bat droppings. Yeast forms of the organism appear in the cytoplasm of cells of the reticuloendothelial system as delicate budding, spherical or egg-shaped bodies 2 to 4 μm in diameter (Fig. 7:22). A clear artifactual space may appear within the cells on H & E–stained sections, presenting the false appearance of a capsule.[6]

In the rare cases of skin involvement, the lesions consist of firm nodules that may ulcerate. Amphotericin B or ketoconazole may be successful in treatment of some cases.[44]

Aspergillosis

Aspergillus sp. is ubiquitous in soil and vegetation and infests small animals only as an opportunist. It has low pathogenicity for skin and mucous membranes, and infections are usually associated with immune deficiency states or long-term administration of immunodepressant drugs. This fungus causes disseminated disease in dogs and cats.[19, 44]

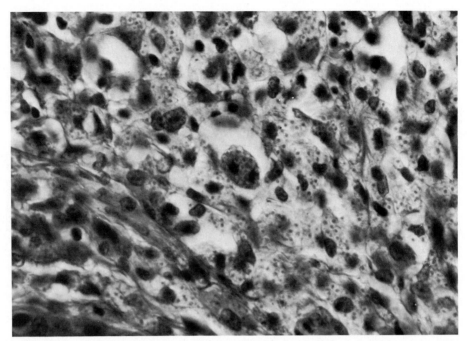

Figure 7:22. Canine histoplasmosis. Numerous small, intracellular yeast bodies in a granuloma (H & E stain).

The organism stains well with H & E, but Gridley's stain may best show the characteristic septate hyphae (4 μ in diameter) which branch repeatedly in the same direction.[87] *A. fumigatus, A. niger, A. terreus,* and *A. deflectus* are the species affecting small animals.[19, 46]

Clinically the mucocutaneous areas of the eyelids and nares may be eroded (See Fig. 19:5). Skin lesions vary from small areas of erythema and pruritus[44] to thick-walled abscesses, granulomas, or ulcers (Fig. 7:11*G,H*). Aspergillosis may also cause rhinitis and sinusitis[60, 111] and may be the cause of significant dermal and pulmonary allergies in humans.[44]

Diagnosis is made by histopathology and culture from infected tissues. Sections from affected lesions are characterized by diffuse and nodular dermatitis (suppurative, pyogranulomatous, or granulomatous) or by necrosis with minimal inflammation (Fig. 7:23). Organisms are usually seen easily with special fungal stains (Fig. 7:24).

Clinical management can be difficult. Prognosis for disseminated cases is poor. *In vitro* sensitivity testing of organisms is recommended to guide therapy. Amphotericin B and 5-fluorocytosine are usually the best choices for systemic therapy.[44] Strains that are resistant to the latter drug develop readily, however.[104] (See also Chapter 4, p. 181.) Topical therapy with enilconazole nose drops has been highly effective for nasal aspergillosis.[98]

Cryptococcosis

Cryptococcosis is caused by *Cryptococcus neoformans*, a ubiquitous yeastlike fungus that is usually a saprophyte. It is isolated from soil contaminated by pigeon droppings but has been cultured from a variety of locations, such as the intestinal tract and skin of normal animals. The organism is an opportunist,

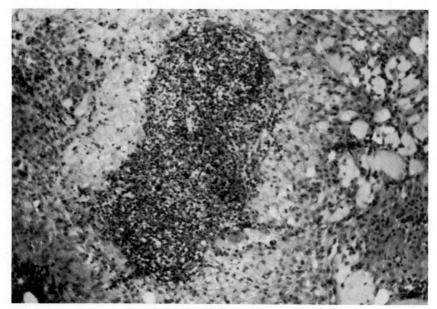

Figure 7:23. Aspergillosis in a dog. Note pyogranulomatous dermatitis. (Courtesy R. E. W. Halliwell.)

which may become established in animals that are debilitated or immunode-pressed by drugs, such as corticosteroids or cancer chemotherapy agents, or by diseases that produce immunodepression, such as FeLV, lymphosarcoma, leukemia, canine distemper, diabetes mellitus, and hypervitaminosis A.

Infections are contracted from the environment, and the disease is more common in geographic areas with warm, humid climates such as northern Australia and the southeastern United States. The portal of entry is usually the

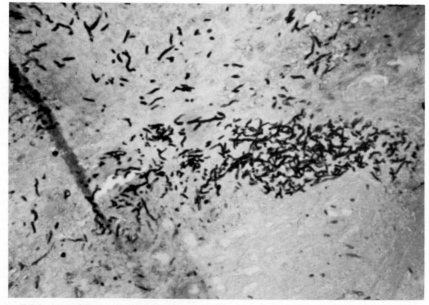

Figure 7:24. Aspergillosis in a dog. Note branching fungal hyphae within dermal pyogranuloma (GMS stain). (Courtesy R. E. W. Halliwell.)

upper respiratory system with hematogenous or lymphogenous spread to other systems including the skin.

The organisms in yeast form appear as round or oval thin-walled cells surrounded by a mucinous capsule of variable thickness, which forms a clear or refractile halo (Fig. 7:25). The cells are 2.0 to 8.0 μm in the laboratory, but as large as 15 μm in tissue sections. They reproduce by budding. There are four distinct serotypes (A, B, C, and D), which vary in pathogenicity. Type A is prevalent in the United States. *C. neoformans* was long considered to exist exclusively as a yeast, but it has now been shown to have a sexual reproductive phase and therefore is classified as a basidiomycete bearing the name *Filobasidiella neoformans*. The mycelial form does not produce clinical disease.

Clinical signs involving the skin are usually most common on the head (Fig. 7:14F–H). The lesions may be rapidly growing, firm papules and nodules (0.1 to 1.0 cm in diameter) in the dermis or subcutis. The nodules often ulcerate and leave a granular surface covered with serous exudate. They frequently form crust and the lesions may heal. Other lesions may be fluctuant or abscess-like. Lesions may be single or numerous and widely distributed over the body. Regional lymphadenopathy may be present. The incidence in cats is higher than in dogs, perhaps because cats are more closely associated with pigeons and pigeon lofts. It is the most frequently diagnosed systemic mycosis of cats.[44]

Diagnosis is made by smears of exudate stained by new methylene blue, Diff Quik, or India ink, in which the halo around the cells stands out well, or by histologic examination of biopsy tissue. Identification of the organism by culture on Sabouraud's dextrose agar (plain) is definitive. Serologic tests, especially indirect fluorescent antibody and latex agglutination tests, are useful in supporting the diagnosis and monitoring the course of the disease.[44]

The histologic appearance may be cystic (Fig. 7:26) and surprisingly acellular, or it may be pyogranulomatous to granulomatous (Fig. 7:27). Organ-

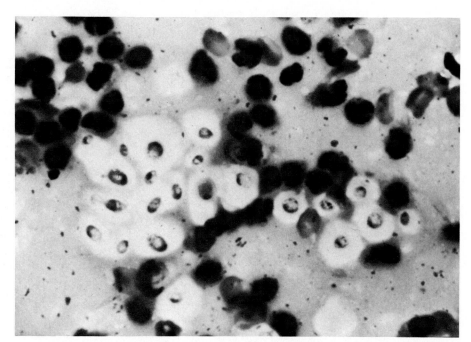

Figure 7:25. Canine cryptococcosis. Encapsulated yeast bodies in direct smear (NMB stain).

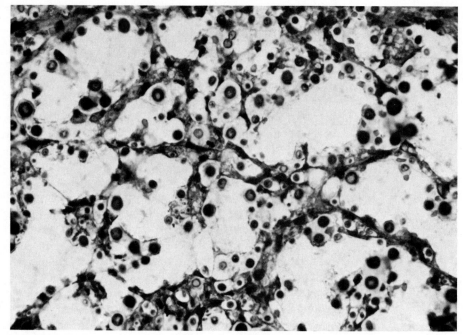

Figure 7:26. Feline cryptococcosis. Numerous encapsulated yeast bodies on a cystic background (Mucicarmine stain).

isms are always numerous. Mucicarmine is the most useful special stain, as it stains the cell capsule.

Clinical management is difficult since the prognosis is guarded at best. If the diagnosis is made early and single or discrete lesions can be removed surgically, the treatment may be successful. However, concurrent therapy with ketoconazole is recommended, and one should be alert to possible recurrence.

Previous drug treatments with amphotericin B or 5-fluorocytosine or combinations of the two have shown generally unsatisfactory results.[44] Ketoconazole alone or in combination with surgical excision has been much more successful. At a dosage of 10 mg/kg or more, once or twice daily for 2 to 8 months, cutaneous cases in many cats and dogs have resolved satisfactorily.[70, 76, 81, 93] The latex agglutination test for detecting cryptococcal capsular antigen can be used not only to facilitate diagnosis but also to monitor response to therapy.[76]

Paecilomycosis

Paecilomycosis is a rare, chronic disease caused by an opportunistic fungus, *Paecilomyces* sp. The organism usually is a saprophyte on soil or decaying vegetation but has been pathogenic to several species of animals including humans. Illness occurred in individuals who were debilitated or immunosuppressed. Disease manifestations developed slowly and were protracted. A cat developed an ulcerated nodule of 1.0 cm in diameter on a paw, which was caused by *P. fumosorseus*.[28] A German shepherd with chronic otitis externa resulting from *Paecilomyces* sp. developed otitis interna and general systemic involvement that was particularly noted in the brain, liver, and abdominal lymph nodes.[79] The ear canals were hypertrophied and ulcerated, and smears of the waxy exudate showed large numbers of yeastlike organisms.

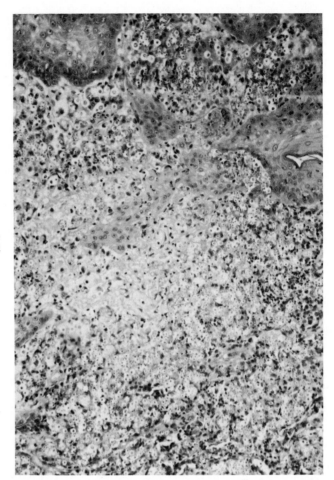

Figure 7:27. Feline cryptococcosis. Numerous encapsulated yeast bodies in pyogranuloma (H & E stain).

Needle aspirates of the granulomatous mass on the cat's paw were highly cellular and consisted of epithelioid cells, neutrophils, and numerous pseudohyphae and yeastlike structures. The pseudohyphae were thick, branched, and septate, and the yeast forms were 3- to 6-μm thin-walled oval structures that somewhat resembled the yeast form of *Histoplasma capsulatum*. Histopathologic examination of the mass from the paw revealed a multifocal pyogranulomatous dermatitis with infiltration into the dermis and subcutis. Variably sized yeastlike structures and pseudohyphae were seen. They stained with H & E and PAS stains.

The prognosis for paecilomycosis is poor. Radical surgical excision followed by prolonged high-dosage treatment with ketoconazole has been ineffective.

References

1. Ackerman, B. A.: Histologic Diagnosis of Inflammatory Skin Diseases. Lee & Febiger, Philadelphia, 1978.
2. Ajello, L., and Padhye, A. A.: Phaeohyphomycosis in a dog caused by *Pseudomicrodochium suttonii* sp. Mycotaxon 12:3, 1980.
3. Anderson, N. V., Ivoghli, D., Moore, W. E., and Leipold, H. W.: Cutaneous sporotrichosis in a cat: a case report. J.A.A.H.A. 9:526, 1973.
4. Artis, W. M., Odle, B. M., and Jones, H. E.: Griseofulvin-resistant dermatophytosis correlates with *in vitro* resistance. Arch. Dermatol. 117:16, 1981.
5. Attleberger, M. H.: Subcutaneous and opportunistic mycoses, the deep mycoses, and actinomycetes. *In* Kirk, R. W., (ed.): Current Veterinary Therapy VII. W. B. Saunders Company, Philadelphia, 1980.

6. Attleberger, M. H.: Subcutaneous and opportunistic mycoses; systemic mycoses; and actinomycosis, nocardiosis, and dermatophilosis. In Kirk, R. W., (ed.): Current Veterinary Therapy VIII, W. B. Saunders Company, Philadelphia, 1983.

7. Barbee, W. C., Evert, A., and Davidson, E. M.: Animal model of human disease: sporotrichosis. Am. J. Pathol. 86:281, 1977.

8. Baxter, M.: Pityrosporum pachydermatis in pendulous and erect ears of dogs. (Correspondence) N. Z. Vet. J. 24:69, 1976.

9. Borelli, D., et al.: Ketoconazole, an oral antifungal: laboratory and clinical assessment of imidazole drugs. Postgrad. Med. J. 55:657, 1979.

9a. Bourdeau, P., et al: Dermatite generalisee du chien due a une infection mixte a Microsporum persicolor et a Microsporum gypseum. Point Vet. 14:69, 1982.

9b. Bourdeau, P. and Chermette, R.: Dermatite localisee du chien due a une infection mixte Trichophyton mentagrophytes et Trichophyton erinacei. Point Vet. 19:619, 1987.

10. Burke, M. J., Graves, G. F., et al.: Successful treatment of cutaneolymphatic sporotrichosis in a cat with ketoconazole and sodium iodide. J.A.A.H.A. 19:542, 1983.

10a. Bussieras, J., et al: Le traitement des teignes des carnivores domestiques au moyen de derivatives recents de l'imidazole. Pract. Med. Chirurg Anim. Comp. 19:152, 1984.

10b. Bussieras, J., et al: Dermatite generalisee du chien, due a une infection mixte par Microsporum canis et par Trichophyton mentagrophytes. Point Vet. 13:43, 1982.

11. Carlton, W. W.: A case of blastomycosis in a dog with pulmonary, cutaneous and ocular lesions. J.A.A.H.A. 10:586, 1974.

12. Chandler, F. W., Kaplan, W., Ajello, L.: Histopathology of Mycotic Diseases. Year Book Medical Publishers, Chicago, 1980.

13. Chester, D. K.: Superficial fungal infections of the skin. Compend. Cont. Ed. 1:910, 1979.

14. Clark, R. F.: Chromoblastomycosis of the ear. Successful intralesional therapy with amphotericin B. Cutis 24:326, 1979.

15. Coloe, P. J.: Prototheconis in a cat. J.A.V.M.A. 180:78, 1982.

16. Cucé, L. C., Wroclawski, E. K., and Sampaio, S. A.: Treatment of paracoccidioidomycosis, candidiasis, chromomycosis, lobomycosis, and mycetoma with ketoconazole. Int. J. Dermatol. 19:405, 1980.

17. Dale, J. E.: Canine dermatosis caused by Candida parapsilosis. Vet. Med. (S.A.C.) 67:548, 1972.

18. Dawson, C. E., and Noodle, B. M.: The treatment of Microsporum canis ringworm in a cat colony. J. Small Anim. Pract. 9:613, 1968.

19. Day, M. J., Penhale, W. J., et al.: Disseminated aspergillosis in dogs. Aust. Vet. J. 63:55, 1986.

20. De Lameter, E. D.: Experimental studies with dermatophytes. IV. Influence of age on the allergic response in experimental ringworm in the guinea pig. J. Invest. Dermatol. 5:423, 1942.

21. Dion, W. M., and Speckman, G.: Canine otitis externa caused by fungus Sporothrix schenckii. Can. Vet. J. 19:40, 1978.

22. Dion, W. M., Pukay, B. P., and Bundza, A.: Feline cutaneous Phaeohyphomycosis caused by Phialophora verrucosa. Can. Vet. J. 23:48, 1982.

23. Dufort, R.: Pityrosporon canis as a cause of canine chronic dermatitis. Vet. Med. (S.A.C.) 78:1055, 1983.

24. Dunbar, M.: Canine blastomycosis. Derm. Reps. 1:1, 1982.

25. Dunbar, M., Pyle, R. L., et al.: Treatment of canine blastomycosis with ketoconazole. J.A.V.M.A. 182:156, 1983.

26. Dunstan, R. W., Langham, R. F., et al.: Feline sporotrichosis: a report of five cases with transmission to humans. J. Am. Acad. Dermatol. 15:37, 1986.

27. Dunstan, R. W., Reimann, K. A., et al.: Feline sporotrichosis. J.A.V.M.A. 189:880, 1986.

28. Elliott, G. S., Whitney, M. S., et al.: Antemortem diagnosis of paecilomycosis in a cat. J.A.V.M.A. 184:93, 1984.

29. Emmons, C. W., Binford, C. H., Utz, J. P., and Kwon-Chung, K. J.: Medical Mycology. Lea & Febiger, Philadelphia, 1977.

30. English, P. B., and Frost, A. J.: Phycomycosis in a dog. Aust. Vet. J. 61:291, 1984.

30a. Fadok, V. A. Granulomatous dermatitis in dogs and cats. Sem. Vet. Med. Surg. 2:186, 1987.

31. Fainstein, V., and Bodey, G. P.: Cardiorespiratory toxicity due to miconazole. Ann. Intern. Med. 93:432, 1980.

32. Fiese, M. J.: Coccidioidomycosis. C. C. Thomas, Springfield, Illinois, 1958.

33. Finnie, J. W., and Coloe, P. J.: Cutaneous protothecosis in a cat. Aust. Vet. J. 57:307, 1981.

34. Foil, C. S.: Personal communication, 1987.

35. Foil, C. S.: Antifungal agents in dermatology. In Kirk, R. W., (ed.): Current Veterinary Therapy IX. W. B. Saunders Company, Philadelphia, 1986, p. 560.

36. Gillespie, J. H., and Timoney, J. F.: Hagan and Bruner's Infectious Diseases of Domestic Animals. 7th ed. Cornell University Press, Ithaca, 1981.

37. Gnann, J. W., Bressler, G. S., et al.: Human blastomycosis after a dog bite. Ann. Intern. Med. 98:48, 1983.

38. Griffen, C.: Personal communication, 1982.

39. Harris, P. A., and Riegelman, S.: Metabolism of griseofulvin in dogs. J. Pharm. Sci. 58:93, 1969.

40. Haschek, W. M., and Kasali, O. B.: A case of cutaneous feline phaeohyphomycosis caused by Phialophora gougerotti. Cornell Vet. 67:467, 1977.

41. Heymann, L. D.: Thiabendazole treatment of ringworm in a cat. Mod. Vet. Pract., 545, June 1986.

42. Hill, J. R., Migaki, J., and Phemister, R. D.: Phaeomycotic granuloma in a cat. Vet. Pathol. 15:559, 1978.

43. Holmberg, K., Liden, S., (eds.): Diagnosis and treatment of local mycoses. Acta Derm. Venereol. [Suppl.] (Stockh.) 121:13, 1986.

44. Holzworth, J.: Diseases of the Cat. Vol. I. W. B. Saunders Company, Philadelphia, 1987.

45. Hutton, R. D., Kerbs, S., and Yee, K.: Scanning electron microscopy of experimental Trichophyton mentagrophyte infections in guinea pig skin. Infect. Immun. 21:247, 1978.

46. Jang, S. S., Dorr, T. E., et al.: Aspergillus deflectus infection in four dogs. J. Med. Vet. Mycol. 24:95, 1986.

47. Jang, S. S., and Popp, J. A.: Eumycotic mycetoma in a dog caused by Allescheria boydii. J.A.V.M.A. 157:1071, 1970.

48. Jaspers, R. H.: Transmission of blastomyces from animals to man. J.A.V.M.A. 164:8, 1974.

49. Jones, H. E., Simpson, J. G., and Artis, W. M.: Oral ketoconazole: an effective safe treatment for dermatophytosis. Arch. Dermatol. 117:129, 1981.

50. Kaplan, W., and Ivens, M. S.: Observations on seasonal variations in incidence of ringworm in dogs and cats in the U.S.A. Sabouraudia 1:91, 1961.

51. Kaplan, W., et al.: Prototheconis in a cat: first recorded case. Sabouraudia 14:281, 1976.

52. Katz, H. I., Bard, J., et al.: SCH 370 (clotrimazole-betamethasone diprorionate) cream in patients with tinea cruris or tinea corporus. Cutis 34:183, 1984.

53. Kier, A. B., Mann, P. C., and Wagner, J. E.:

Disseminated sporotrichosis in a cat. J.A.V.M.A. *175*:202, 1979.

54. Klein, B. S., Vergeront, J. M., et al.: Isolation of *Blastomyces dermatitides* in soil associated with a large outbreak of blastomycosis in Wisconsin. New Engl. J. Med. *314*:529, 1986.

55. Kligman, A. M.: Pathophysiology of ringworm infections in animals with skin infections. J. Invest. Dermatol. *27*:171, 1956.

56. Knudsen, E. A.: The real extent of dermatophyte infection. Br. J. Dermatol. *92*:413, 1975.

57. Kral, F., and Uscavage, J. P.: Cutaneous candidiasis in a dog. J.A.V.M.A. *136*:612, 1960.

58. Kwochka, K. W., Mays, M. B. C., et al.: Canine phaeohyphomycosis caused by *Drechslera spicifera*: A case report and literature review. J.A.A.H.A. *20*:625, 1984.

59. Land, G. A.: Evaluation of the New Apl 20C strip for yeast identification against a conventional method. J. Clin. Microbiol. *10*:357, 1979.

60. Lane, J. G., Clayton-Jones, D. G., Thoday, K. L., and Thomsett, L. R.: The diagnosis and successful treatment of an *Aspergillus fumigatus* of the frontal sinus and nasal chamber of a dog. J. Small Anim. Pract. *15*:79, 1974.

61. Legendre, A., Walker, M., Buyukmichi, N., and Stevens, R.: Canine blastomycosis: a review of 47 clinical cases. J.A.V.M.A. *178*:163, 1981.

62. Legendre, A., and Steltz, M.: A multi-center, double-blind comparison of ketoconazole and griseofulvin in the treatment of infections due to dermatophytes. Rev. Infect. Dis. *2*:586, 1980.

63. Leuka, D. C., and Kainer, R. A.: Hyperthermia in therapy of dermatomycosis of dog and cats. Vet. Med. (S.A.C.) *76*:658, 1981.

64. Lomax, L. G., Cole, J. R., et al.: Osteolytic phaeohyphomycosis in a German shepherd dog caused by *Phialemonium obovatum*. J. Clin. Microbiol. *23*:987, 1986.

65. Mason, K. V.: Generalized dermatitis associated with *Malassezia pachydermatis* in three dogs. Proceedings, annual meeting Am. Acad. Vet. Derm. Phoenix, 1987, p. 35.

66. Matsuda, T., and Matsumoto, T.: Disseminated hyolohyphomycosis in a leukemic patient. Arch. Dermatol. *122*:1171, 1986.

67. Mayhall, C. G., et al.: Cutaneous prototheccosis. Successful treatment with amphotericin B. Arch. Dermatol. *112*:1749, 1976.

68. McGinnis, M. R.: Laboratory Handbook of Medical Mycology. Academic Press, Inc., New York, 1980.

69. McKenzie, R. A., Connole, M. D., et al.: Subcutaneous phaeohyphomycosis caused by *Monilialla suaveolens* in two cats. Vet. Pathol. *21*:582, 1984.

70. Medleau, L., Hall, E. J., et al.: Cutaneous cryptococcosis in three cats. J.A.V.M.A. *187*:169, 1985.

71. Migaki, G., et al.: Canine prototheccosis: review of the literature and report of an additional case. J.A.V.M.A. *181*:794, 1982.

72. Miller, W. H., Goldschmidt, M.: Mycetomas in the cat caused by a dermatophyte—a case report. J.A.A.H.A. *22*:255, 1986.

73. Moriello, K. A.: Ketoconazole: clinical pharmacology and therapeutic recommendations. J.A.V.M.A. *188*:303, 1986.

74. Moschella, S. L., Pillsbury, D. M., and Hurley, H. J.: *Dermatology*. W. B. Saunders Company, Philadelphia, 1975, pp. 655–656.

75. Muller, G. H., Kaplan, W., Ajello, L., and Padhye, A. A.: Phaeohyphomycosis caused by *Drechslera spicifera* in a cat. J.A.V.M.A. *166*:150, 1975.

75a. Muller, G. H., Kirk, R. W., and Scott, D. W.: Small Animal Dermatology. 3rd ed. W. B. Saunders Company, Philadelphia, 1984.

76. Noxon, J. O., Monroe, W. E., et al.: Ketoconazole therapy in canine and feline cryptococcosis. J.A.A.H.A. *22*:179, 1986.

77. O'Neill, C. S.: Feline dermatophytosis. Part I. Carnation. Res. Dig. *18*:1, 1982.

78. O'Neill, C. S., Short, B. G., et al.: A report of subcutaneous pythiosis in five dogs and a review of the etiologic agent *Pythium* spp., J.A.A.H.A. *•20*:959, 1984.

79. Patterson, J. M., Rosendal, S., et al.: A case of disseminated paeocilomycosis in a cat. J.A.V.M.A. *19*:569, 1983.

80. Pavletic, M. M., and MacIntire, D.: Phycomycosis of the axilla and inner brachium in a dog: Surgical excision and reconstruction with a thoracodorsal axial pattern flap. J.A.V.M.A. *180*:1197, 1982.

81. Pentlarge, V. W., and Martin, R. A.: Treatment of cryptococcosis in three cats using ketoconazole. J.A.V.M.A. *188*:508, 1985.

82. Pepin, G. A., and Oxenham, M.: Zoonotic dermatophytosis (ringworm). Vet. Rec. *25*:110, 1986.

83. Philpot, C. M., and Berry, A. P.: The normal fungal flora of dogs. Mycopathologia *87*:155, 1984.

84. Pichler, M. E., Gross, T. L., et al.: Cutaneous and mucocutaneous candidiasis in a dog. Comp. Cont. Ed. *7*:225, 1985.

85. Pinello, C. B., Naudo, P. J., and D'Amato, R. F.: Development of an interpretative system for the identification of yeasts. Species *2*:1, 1978.

86. Pyle, R. L., et al.: Canine blastomycosis. Compend. Cont. Ed. *3*:963, 1981.

87. Raper, K. B., and Fennel, D. I.: The Genus, Aspergillus. Robert E. Krieger Publishing Company, New York, 1973.

88. Read, S. I., and Sperling, L. C.: Feline sporotrichosis: transmission to man. Arch. Dermatol. *118*:429, 1982.

89. Restrepo, A., Robleto, J., et al.: Itraconazole therapy in lymphangitic and cutaneous sporotrichosis. Arch. Dermatol. *122*:413, 1986.

90. Rippon, J. W.: Medical Mycology, The Pathogenic Fungi and the Pathogenic Actinomycetes. W. B. Saunders Company, Philadelphia, 1982.

91. Russell, B., Beckett, J. H., and Jacobs, P. H.: Immunoperoxidase localization of *Sporothrix schenckii* and *Cryptococcus neoformans*. Arch. Dermatol. *115*:433, 1979.

92. Sanguinetti, V., Tampieri, M. P., et al.: A survey of 120 isolates of *Malassezia pachydermatis*. Mycopathologia *85*:93, 1984.

93. Schulman, J.: Ketoconazole for successful treatment of cryptococcosis in a cat. J.A.V.M.A. *187*:508, 1985.

94. Schwartzman, R. M., Deubler, M. J., and Dice, P. F.: Experimentally induced monilia (*Candida albicans*) in the dog. J. Small Anim. Pract. *6*:327, 1965.

95. Scott, D. W., Bentinck-Smith, J., and Haggerty, G. F.: Sporotrichosis in three dogs. Cornell Vet. *64*:416, 1974.

96. Scott, D. W.: Feline dermatology 1900–1978: Monograph. J.A.A.H.A. *16*:331, 1980.

97. Scott, D. W.: Sporotrichosis. *In* Kirk, R. W., (ed.): Current Veterinary Therapy V. W. B. Saunders Company, Philadelphia, 1974.

98. Sharpe, N.: Personal communication, 1987.

99. Sousa, C. A., Ihrke, P. J., et al.: Subcutaneous phaeohyphomycosis (*Stemphillium* sp. and *Cladosporium* sp. infections) in a cat. J.A.V.M.A. *185*:673, 1984.

100. Symoens, J., et al.: An evaluation of two years of clinical experience with ketoconazole. Rev. Infect. Dis. *2*:674, 1980.

101. Tagami, H., et al.: Topical heat therapy for cutaneous chromomycosis. Arch. Dermatol. *115*:740, 1979.

102. Trettian, A. L.: The role of *Malassezia pachydermatis* in the external ear canal of normal dogs. Proceedings, annual meeting Am. Acad. Vet. Derm. Phoenix, 1987, p. 26.
103. Tuttle, P. A., and Chandler, F. W.: Deep dermatophytosis in a cat. J.A.V.M.A. *183*:1106, 1983.
104. Van Cutsem, J., De Keyser, F., et al.: Survey of fungal isolates from alopecia and asymptomatic dogs. Vet. Rec. *116*:568, 1985.
105. Vandevelde, A. G., Mauceri, A. A., and Johnson, J. E.: 5-Fluorocystosine in the treatment of mycotic infections. Ann. Intern. Med. *77*:43, 1972.
106. Vitto, J., et al.: Chromomycosis. Successful treatment with 5-fluorocystosine. J. Cutan. Pathol. *6*:77, 1979.
107. Walton, D. K.: Personal communication, 1982.
108. Weber, M. J., Keppen, M., et al.: Treatment of systemic candidiasis in neutropenic dogs with ketoconazole. Exp. Hematol. *13*:791, 1985.
109. Wolf, A. M.: Primary cutaneous coccidioidomycosis in a dog and a cat. J.A.V.M.A. *174*:504, 1979.
110. Wolfe, A. M., and Poppagianis, D.: Canine coccidioidomycosis: treatment with a new antifungal agent, ketoconazole. Calif. Vet. *5*:25, 1981.
111. Wood, G. L., et al.: Disseminated aspergillosis in a dog. J.A.V.M.A. *172*:704, 1978.
112. Woodard, D. C.: Ketoconazole therapy for *Microsporum* spp. dermatophytes in cats. Fel. Pract. *13*:28, 1983.
113. Woodgyer, A. J.: Asymptomatic carriage of dermatophytes by cats. N. Z. Vet. J. *25*:67, 1977.
114. Yager, J. A., and Wilcock, B. P.: Mycetoma-like granuloma in a cat caused by *Microsporum canis*. J. Comp. Path. *96*:171, 1986.

References for Table 7–2

Alternaria species

Bone, W. J., and Jackson, W. F.: Pathogenic fungi in dermatitis incidence in two small animal practices in Florida. Vet. Med. (S.A.C.) *66*:140, 1971.

Alternaria alternata

Dogvich, N. A.: Ekema Spiny Sobak-Mikolicheskoe Zabolevanie. (Spinal eczema in dogs: a fungal disease). Veterinariya *39*:31, 1962.
Dogvich, N. A.: Kvaprosu Ob Epidermofitii Sobak. Veterinariya *41*:37, 1965.

Aspergillus species

Grono, L. R., and Frost, A. J.: Otitis externa in the dog: the microbiology of the normal and affected external ear canal. Aust. Vet. J. *45*:420, 1969.
Otto, E. F.: Aspergillosis in the frontal sinus of a dog. J.A.V.M.A. *156*:1903, 1970.

Aspergillus deflectus

Jang, S. S., Dorr, T. E., et al.: *Aspergillus deflectus* infections in four dogs. J. Am. Vet. Mycol. *24*:94, 1986.

Aspergillus fumigatus

Garbolino, F., Gevry, J., et al.: Rhinite necrossante aspergillaire. (Necrotic rhinitis caused by *Aspergillus*). Rev. Med. Vet. *129*:581, 585, 1978.
Lane, J. G., Clayton-Jones, D. G., et al.: Diagnosis and successful treatment of *Aspergillus fumigatus* infection of the frontal sinuses and nasal chambers of dogs. J. Small Anim. Pract. *15*:79, 1974.
Rudolph, R., Kupper, W., et al.: Mycotic rhinitis caused by *Aspergillus fumigatus* fresenius in dogs: diagnosis and differential diagnosis with special reference to radiography. Berl. Much. Tierärtl. Wschr. *87*:87, 1974.

Aspergillus niger

Lapcevic, E., and Ciric, V.: Aspergiloza Kao Uzrocnik Zapaljenja Spoljasnjeg Kanala Pasa. (Aspergillosis as the cause of otitis externa in dogs). (Vet. Fac. Belgrade) Vet. Glas. *17*:105, 1963.

Aspergillus terreus

Day, M. H., Penhale, W. J., et al.: Disseminated aspergillosis in dogs. Aust. Vet. J. *63*:55, 1986.

Blastomyces dermatitidis

Legendre, A. M., Walker, M., et al.: Canine blastomycosis: a review of 47 clinical cases. J.A.V.M.A. *178*:1163, 1981.

Candida albicans

Kral, F., and Uscavage, J. P.: Cutaneous candidiasis in a dog. J.A.V.M.A. *136*:612, 1960.
Webster, F. L., Whyard, B. H., et al.: Treatment of otitis externa in the dog with Gentocin otic. Can. Vet. J. *15*:176, 1974.

Candida krusei

Dufait, R.: Over Enkele Gevallen Van Dermatitis Bij de Hond, Toegeschreven Ann Gistceilen (genus *Candida* en *Pityrosporum*). (Some cases of canine dermatitis probably due to yeasts [*Candida* and *Pityrosporum*]). Vlaams Diergeneesk. Tijdsch. *44*:92, 1975.

Candida parapsilosis

Dale, J. E.: Canine dermatosis caused by *C. parapsilosis*. Vet. Med. (S.A.C.) *67*:548, 1972.

Chrysosporium evolceanui

Hazsig, M., Vries, G. A., et al.: *Chrysosporium evolceanui* from pathologically changed dog's skin. Veterinarski Arhiv. *45*:209, 1974.
Cladosporium species (see reference under *Stemphylium* species)

Coccidioides immitis

Wolf, A. M.: Primary cutaneous coccidioidomycosis in a dog and a cat. J.A.V.M.A. *174*:504, 1979.

Cryptococcus species

Brown, R. J., Nowlin, C. L., et al.: Dermal cryptococcosis in a cat. Mod. Vet. Pract. *59*:447, 1978.
Humphrey, J. D., Fordham, A., et al.: Cryptococcosis in a cat in Papua, New Guinea. Aust. Vet. J. *53*:197, 1977.

Cryptococcus neoformans

Howell, J. McC., and Allan, D.: A case of cryptococcosis in the cat. J. Comp. Pathol. Ther. *74*:415, 1964.
Trautwein, G., and Nielson, S. W.: Cryptococcosis in two cats, a dog, and a mink. J.A.V.M.A. *140*:437, 1962.

Curvularia geniculata

Bridges, C. H.: Maduromycotic mycetomas in animals: *Curvularia geniculata* as an etiologic agent. Am. J. Pathol. *33*:411, 1957.

Brodey, R. S., et al.: Mycetoma in a dog. J.A.V.M.A. *151*:442, 1967.

Drechslera spicifera

Kwochka, K. W., Calderwood-Mays, M. B., et al.: Canine phaeohyphomycosis caused by *Drechslera spicifera*: a case report and literature review. J.A.A.H.A. *20*:625, 1984.

Muller, G. H., Kaplan, W., et al.: Phaeohyphomycosis caused by *Drechslera spicifera* in a cat. J.A.V.M.A. *166*:150, 1975.

Epidermophyton floccosum

Boro, B. R., et al.: Ringworm in animals due to *Epidermophyton floccosum*. Vet. Rec. *107*:491, 1980.

Terreni, A. A., Gregg, W. B., et al.: *Epidermophyton floccosum* infection in a dog from the United States. Sabouraudia *23*:141, 1985.

Exophialia jeanselmei

Haschek, W. M., and Kasali, O. B.: A case of cutaneous feline phaeohyphomycosis caused by *Phialophora gougerotti*. Cornell Vet. *67*:467, 1977.

Geotrichium species

Holzworth, J., Blouin, P., et al.: Mycotic diseases. In: Holzworth, J., (ed.): Diseases of the Cat. Medicine and Surgery. W. B. Saunders Company, Philadelphia, 1987, Chapter 9.

Hansenula anomala

Joly, S.: As Leveduras e a Antibios. (Yeast and antibiosis). Mycopath. Mycol. Appl. *33*:269, 1967.

Histoplasma capsulatum

Gabbert, N., et al.: Disseminated histoplasmosis in three cats. J.A.A.H.A. *13*:46, 1977.

Noxon, J. O., Digilio, K., et al.: Disseminated histoplasmosis in a cat: successful treatment with ketoconazole. J.A.V.M.A. *181*:817, 1982.

Kable, S., Koschmann, J. R., et al.: Endemic canine and feline histoplasmosis in El Paso, Texas. J. Med. Vet. Mycol. *24*:41, 1986.

Malassezia species

Fraser, G.: The fungal flora of the canine ear. J. Comp. Pathol. *71*:1, 1961.

Malassezia pachydermatis

Dufait, R.: *Pityrosporum canis* as the cause of canine chronic dermatitis. Vet. Med. (S.A.C.) *78*:1055, 1983.

Smith, J. M.: The association of yeast with chronic otitis externa in the dog. Aust. Vet. J. *44*:413, 1968.

Microsporum audouinii

Kaplan, W., Georg, K. K., et al.: Recent developments in animal ringworm and their public health implication. Ann. N.Y. Acad. Sci. *70*:639, 1958.

Microsporum canis

Kaplan, W., and Ivens, M. S.: Observations on the seasonal variations in incidence of ringworm in dogs and cats in the United States. Sabouraudia *1*:91, 1961.

Menges, R. W., and Georg, L. K.: Observations of feline ringworm caused by *Microsporum canis* and its public health significance. Proceedings, annual meeting Am. Vet. Med. Assoc., 1955, p. 571.

Microsporum cookei

Ajello, L.: A new *Microsporum* and its occurrence in soil and animals. Mycologia *51*:62, 1959.

Quaite, R. A., and Lutwyche, P.: *Microsporum cookei* as the suspected cause of ringworm in a dog. Vet. Rec. *109*:311, 1981.

Scott, D. W.: Feline dermatology 1900–1980: Monograph. J.A.A.H.A. *16*:331, 1980.

Microsporum distortum

Kaplan, W., Georg, L. K., et al.: Isolation of *Microsporum distortum* from animals in the United States. J. Invest. Dermatol. *28*:449, 1957.

Microsporum gallinae

Dvořák, J., and Otčenášek, M.: Geophilic, zoophilic, and anthrophilic dermatophytes. A review. Mycopath. Mycol. Appl. *23*:294, 1964.

Microsporum gypseum

Kaplan, W., Georg, L. K., et al.: Ringworm in cats caused by *Microsporum gypseum*. Vet. Med. *52*:347, 1957.

Menges, R. W., and Georg, L. K.: Canine ringworm caused by *Microsporum gypseum*. Cornell Vet. *47*:91, 1957.

Microsporum nanum

Carman, M. G., Rush-Munro, F. M., et al.: Dermatophytes isolated from domestic and feral animals. N. Z. Vet. J. *27*:136, 143, 1979.

Muhammed, S. I.: The isolation of *M. nanum* from a dog with skin lesions. Vet. Rec. *95*:573, 1974.

Microsporum persicolor

Bourdeau, P.: Quel est votre diagnostic? Point Vet. *19*:665, 1987.

Microsporum vanbreuseghemii

Georg, L. K., Ajello, L., et al.: A new species of *Microsporum* pathogenic to man and animals. Sabouraudia *1*:189, 1962.

Moniliella suaveolens

McKenzie, R. A., Connole, M. D., et al.: Subcutaneous phaeohyphomycosis caused by *Moniliella suaveolens* in two cats. Vet. Pathol. *21*:582, 1984.

Oidiodendron kalrai

Tewari, R. P., and Macpherson, C. R.: Pathogenicity and neurological effects of *Oidiodendron kalrai* for mice. J. Bacteriol. *95*:1130, 1968.

Paecilomyces species

Patterson, J. M., Rosendal, S., et al.: A case of disseminated paecilomycosis in the dog. J.A.A.H.A. *19*:569, 1983.

Paecilomyces fumosoroseus

Elliott, G. S., Whitney, M. S., et al.: Antemortem diagnosis of paecilomycosis in a cat. J.A.V.M.A. *184*:93, 1984.

Penicillium martensii

Senser, F.: *Penicillium martensii* Biourge als Erreger Einer. (*Penicillium Martensii* Biourge as a cause of a fungal infection). Mycose. Zentlb. Bakt. Parasilkde I (org.) *200*:519, 1966.

Phialophora species

Hill, J. R., Migaki, G., et al.: Phaeomycotic granuloma in a cat. Vet. Pathol. *15*:559, 1978.

Dion, W. M., Pukay, B. P., et al.: Feline cutaneous phaeohyphomycosis caused by *Phialophora verrucosa*. Can. Vet. J. *23*:48, 1982.

Phialophora verrucosa

McKeever, P. J., Caywood, D. D., et al.: Chromomycosis in a cat: successful medical therapy. J.A.A.H.A. *19*:533, 1983.

Prototheca species

Euzeby, J.: The laboratory diagnosis of cutaneous and subcutaneous mycoses in animals. Folia Veterinaria Latina 7:111, 1977.

Prototheca wickerhamii

Coloe, P. J., and Allison, J. F.: Protothecosis in a cat. J.A.V.M.A. 180:78, 1982.

Kaplan, W., et al.: Protothecosis in a cat: first recorded case. Sabouraudia 14:281, 1976.

Sudman, M. S., Majka, J. A., et al.: Primary mucocutaneous protothecosis in a dog. J.A.V.M.A. 163:1372, 1973.

Pseudoallescheria boydii

Kurtz, H. J., Finco, D. R., et al.: Maduromycosis (Allescheria boydii) in a dog. J.A.V.M.A. 157:917, 1970.

McGinnis, J. R., Padhye, A. A., et al.: Pseudoallescheria negroni et fischer 1943 and its later synonym Petriellidium malloch 1970. Mycotaxon, 1982.

Siebold, H. R.: Mycetoma in a dog. J.A.V.M.A. 127:444, 1955.

Pseudomicrodochium suttonii

Ajello, L., Padhye, A. A., et al.: Phaeohyphomycosis in a dog caused by Pseudomicrodochium suttonii. Mycotaxon 12:131, 1980.

Rhinosporidium seeberi

Mayer, J. H., and Diaz, B. E.: Primer caso de Rhinosporidiosis Rhinosporidium seeberi en Canis familiaris. (First case of rhinosporidiosis in the dog). Ann. Inst. Med. Region (Resistencia) 4:2, 1954.

Scopulariopsis brevicaulis

Hubálek, Z., and Balcaříkova, A.: Vorkommen von Aspergillen und Scopulariopsiden in den Hautlasionen der Huastiere. (Occurrence of Aspergillus and Scopulariopsis in skin lesions of domestic animals). Mykosen 12:611, 1969.

Sepedonium species

Tewari, R. P.: U.P. Coll. Vet. Sci. and Animal Husbandry, Mathura, India): Studies on some mycotic infections of domestic animals and poultry. Agra Univ. J. Res. (Sci.) 12:163, 1963.

Sporothrix schenckii

Dion, W. M., and Speckmann, G.: Canine otitis externa caused by the fungus Sporothrix schenckii. Can. Vet. J. 19:44, 1978.

Kier, A. B., Mann, P. C., et al.: Disseminated sporotrichosis in a cat. J.A.V.M.A. 175:202, 1979.

Stemphylium species and Cladosporium species

Sousa, C. A., Ihrke, P. J., et al.: Subcutaneous phaeohyphomycosis (Stemphylium species and Cladosporium species infections) in a cat. J.A.V.M.A. 185:673, 1984.

Trichophyton species

Bostelmann, R. W.: Trichophyton infection in antarctic sledge dogs. Vet. Rec. 98:425, 1976.

Trichophyton ajelloi

Kaplan, W., Georg, L. K., et al.: Recent developments in animal ringworm and their public health implication. Ann. N.Y. Acad. Sci. 70:636, 1958.

Trichophyton equinum

Rebell, G., and Taplin, D.: Dermatophytes: Their recognition and identification. University of Miami Press, Coral Gables, Florida, 1974.

Trichophyton equinum var. autotrophicum

(See Microsporum nanum)

Trichophyton erinacei

Ainsworth, G. C., and Austwick, K. C.: Fungal Diseases of Animals. Commonwealth Agricultural Bureau. Farnham Royal, England, 1973.

Trichophyton megninii

(See T. quinckeanum)

Trichophyton mentagrophytes

Georg, L. K., Roberts, C. S., et al.: Trichophyton mentagrophytes infections in dogs and cats. J.A.V.M.A. 130:427, 1957.

La Touche, C. J., and Forster, R. A.: Chronic infection in a cat due to Trichophyton mentagrophytes (Robin) Blanchard. Sabouraudia 3:11, 1963.

Trichophyton quinckeanum

Dvořák, J., and Otčenášek, M.: Geophilic, zoophilic, and anthropophilic dermatophytes: a review. Mycopath. Mycol. Appl. 23:294, 1964.

Trichophyton rubrum

Chabraborty, A. N., Ghosh, S., et al.: Isolation of Trichophyton rubrum Castellani Sabouraud 1911 from animals. Can. J. Comp. Med. 18:436, 1954.

Kaplan, W., and Gump, R. H.: Ringworm in a dog caused by Trichophyton rubrum. Vet. Med. 53:139, 1958.

Kushida, T.: An additional case of canine dermatophytosis. Jpn. J. Vet. Sci. 41:77, 1979.

Trichophyton schoenleinii

Kral, F.: Skin diseases. Adv. Vet. Sci. 7:183, 1962.

Trichophyton simii

Tewari, R. P.: Trichophyton simii infections in chickens, dogs, and man in India. Mycopath. Mycol. Appl. 39:293, 1969.

Trichophyton terrestre

Connole, M. D.: Keratinophilic fungi in cats and dogs. Sabouraudia 4:45, 1965.

Gentles, J. C., Dawson, C. O., et al.: Keratinophilic fungi in cats and dogs II. Sabouraudia 4:171, 1965.

Scott, D. W., Kirk, R. W., et al.: Dermatophytosis due to Trichophyton terrestre infection in a dog and cat. J.A.A.H.A. 16:53, 1980.

Trichophyton verrucosum

(See T. quinckeanum)

Trichophyton violaceum

(See T. quinckeanum)

Trichosporon pullulans

Doster, A. R., Erickson, E. D., et al.: Trichosporonosis in two cats. J.A.V.M.A. 190:1184, 1987.

Green, C. E., Miller, D. M., et al.: Trichosporon infection in a cat. J.A.V.M.A. 187:946, 1985.

CHAPTER

8

Cutaneous Parasitology

Animal skin is exposed to attack by many kinds of animal parasites. Each species has a particular effect on the skin; the effect can be mild, such as in the case of the isolated fly or mosquito bite, or severe, such as in the case of generalized demodicosis or canine scabies. Although the reaction of the skin to the infestation may be slight, the common parasitisms must be considered here because the dermatologist is the logical consultant in such cases.

When ectoparasites serve as vectors or intermediate hosts of bacterial, rickettsial, or parasitic diseases they become more important than when they produce only their own effect. A severe local or systemic reaction may result when toxins are injected into the skin (tick paralysis). The larvae of some parasites live in wounds or on macerated skin to produce a condition known as myiasis. The most serious dermatologic concern develops when the dermatosis produced by parasites living in or on the skin produces irritation and sensitization.

Some parasites live on the skin (*Cheyletiella* mites and biting lice), subsisting on the debris and exudates that are produced on its surface. Others live on the skin but periodically penetrate its surface to draw nourishment from blood and tissue fluids (fleas, sucking lice, and ticks). Still others live within the skin for at least part of their life cycle, producing more severe cutaneous effects (demodectic and sarcoptic mites).

The reaction of the skin to these insults varies from trivial to lethal but usually includes inflammation, edema, and an attempt to localize the "foreign body," toxin, or excretory products of the parasite. These secretions are often allergenic and cause itching and burning sensations.

Although many kinds of parasites affect animals, we will discuss only those in the following list, which includes the important skin parasites of dogs and cats in North America (Table 8:1).

Helminth Parasites

ANCYLOSTOMIASIS AND UNCINARIASIS
(Hookworm Dermatitis)

The larvae of *Ancylostoma braziliense, A. caninum,* and *Uncinaria stenocephala* cause a characteristic skin lesion in humans that is called "creeping eruption." The skin lesions that these larvae produce in the dog or cat are not as severe, since these animals are their specific hosts. The skin lesions often are incidental to completion of the normal life cycle of the parasite, with the larvae quickly

347

Table 8–1. COMMON SKIN PARASITES

Helminth parasites
  Pelodera strongyloides
  Strongyloides stercoralis
  Anatrichosoma sp.
  Ancylostoma caninum and *A. braziliense* (hookworm dermatitis)
  Uncinaria stenocephala (hookworm dermatitis)
  Dirofilaria immitis
  Schistosoma cercariae
  Dracunculus insignis (D. medinensis)

Arthropod parasites
  Arachnida
    Acarina
      Argasid ticks (soft)
        Otobius megnini (spinous ear tick)
      Ixodid ticks (hard)
        Rhipicephalus sanguineus (brown dog tick)
        Dermacentor variabilis (American dog tick)
        Ixodes spp.
        Amblyomma spp.
      Dermanyssus gallinae (poultry mite)
      Walchia americana
      Trombicula alfreddugèsi (chigger mites)*
      Euschongastia latchmani
      Bryobia praetiosa
      Trombicula autumnalis
      Trombicula sarcina
      Lynxacarus radovsky
      Otodectes cynotis (ear mites)
      Cheyletiella yasguri, C. blakei, C. parasitovorax
      Demodex canis (demodicosis)
      Demodex cati
      Demodex sp. (cat mite)
      Sarcoptes scabiei (var. *canis*) (canine scabies)
      Notoedres cati (feline scabies)
      Spiders
  Insecta
    Phthiraptera (lice)
      Linognathus setosus (sucking louse of dogs)
      Trichodectes canis (biting louse of dogs)
      Felicola subrostratus (biting louse of cats)
      Heterodoxus spiniger (biting louse of dogs, warm climates only)
    Siphonaptera (fleas)
      Ctenocephalides felis (cat flea)
      Ctenocephalides canis (dog flea)
      Echidnophaga gallinacea (sticktight flea)
      Pulex irritans (human flea)
    Diptera (flies)
      Cuterebra maculata (skin bots)
      Calliphorids (blow flies)
      Sarcophagids (flesh flies)
      Stomoxys calcitrans (stable fly)
      Miscellaneous (mosquitoes, black flies, and so on)
    Hymenoptera (bees, wasps, hornets)

*Chiggers belong to the genus *Trombicula*. In veterinary literature one sees the names *Eutrombicula* and *Neotrombicula* used. Each is the term for a subgenus.

abandoning the skin and proceeding to other parts of the body. Although percutaneous entry can lead to completion of the life cycle, larvae penetrating by this route rarely mature.[89] The larvae are present on the grass and in the soil of runs and paddocks during the spring and summer in cool climates, and animals exposed to them become infected. Thus, the disease is essentially one of kenneled dogs on grass or earth runs that have poor sanitation.[9]

Cutaneous lesions seem to be more prevalent in areas with predominant infestation with *U. stenocephala* (Ireland, parts of England and the United States), although animals with ancylostomiasis may also have skin lesions. *U. stenocephala* produces a marked dermatitis on skin penetration but rarely completes its life cycle by this route. It is insignificant as a blood sucker compared with *A. braziliense* or *A. caninum.*[7] The latter can complete its life cycle via skin penetration.

Hookworm dermatitis has been produced by natural and experimental infestations with *U. stenocephala.*[9, 22, 129] In both types of cases, similar clinical and histologic lesions were produced. The third-stage larvae enter the dog's skin on areas of the body that frequently contact the ground. The larvae approach the skin up a temperature gradient to a peak at the animal's approximate body temperature. They primarily enter at an area of desquamation on the skin, although a few may use hair follicles. Entry into the horny layer parallels the skin surface, and there is little evidence of enzymatic activity. The larvae are thought simply to exert pressure by undulating activity, the forward movement being achieved by pushing back against rigid keratinized cells. This route follows the line of least resistance through the outer layers.[84] Once they are through the epidermis, the dermis appears to cause little hindrance to the migrating larvae. After larvae pass through tissue, the cells reunite and there is little lasting evidence of their passage.[84] Some other species of hookworm larvae do cause loss of integrity of the epidermis as they penetrate it.

Clinical signs of hookworm dermatitis are initially red papules on those parts of the body in frequent contact with the ground. Later these areas become uniformly erythematous, and then thickened and alopecic. The feet are especially affected (Fig. 8:1). However, the skin of the sternum, ventral abdomen, and tail; pubic and preputial surfaces; and the lateral and posterior aspects of the feet and legs may be involved too. Skin over the bony prominences of the elbows, hocks, and ischial tuberosities may have more obvious lesions owing

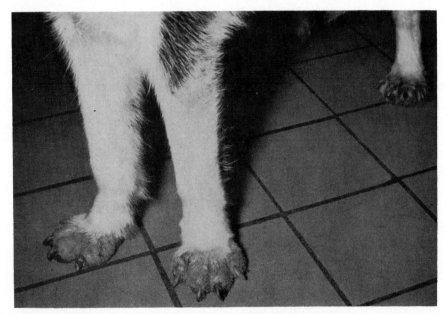

Figure 8:1. Hookworm dermatitis. A Siberian husky confined to a dirt-based run and affected with *Ancylostoma caninum* shows lesions of chronic hookworm dermatitis on all four feet. There is alopecia, erythema, swelling, and crusting.

to the thickened skin and hair loss. The interdigital webs may be erythematous and the feet may be swollen, painful, and hot. The footpads become spongy and soft, especially at the pad margins where the tissue can be readily grooved and often stripped from the underlying dermis. The chronic inflammation causes the claws to grow rapidly and to appear deformed. They may be friable and may break off, leaving thick, tapered stumps. Arthritis of the interphalangeal joints may be present too.[7] Pruritus is mild but evident, especially during initial larval penetration, as licking and chewing at the feet are observed.

Histopathology reveals varying degrees of perivascular dermatitis (hyperplastic, spongiotic) with eosinophils and neutrophils. The epidermis may contain recent larval migration tracts, which may occasionally be traced into the dermis as linear tracts of neutrophils and eosinophils. Larvae are rarely found, but if present are surrounded by clusters of neutrophils, eosinophils, and mononuclear cells. Hypersensitivity has been suggested as a cause of the lesions.[121]

Diagnosis can be made with reasonable certainty by observation of the clinical signs, a positive fecal examination for hookworm eggs, and a history of poor housing and sanitation. Differential diagnosis may be complicated by a coincidental infection with hookworms. Ectoparasitisms such as the following should be considered: fleas; sarcoptic, otodectic, and demodectic mange; and contact dermatitis and intradermal penetration by parasites such as strongyloides and schistosomal agents. Most can be diagnosed by a combination of history, physical examination, and skin scrapings or skin biopsy.

Treatment should emphasize cleaning the premises, frequent removal of feces, and generally improved hygiene, combined with appropriate routine anthelminthic treatment to all dogs in the kennel. Dry, paved runs or periodic treatment of dirt or gravel runs with 10 pounds of borax per 100 square feet of run may be helpful, but borax or salt will kill vegetation. Attention to measures designed to improve foot health are important, so toenails should be kept trimmed short to improve foot conformation and help to alleviate joint stress. The paws should be kept clean and dry. Exercising dogs on new clean pasture is beneficial too.

PELODERA DERMATITIS
(Rhabditis, Rhabditic Dermatitis)

Pelodera dermatitis is a local erythematous, nonseasonal pruritic dermatitis caused by a cutaneous infestation of the larvae of *Pelodera strongyloides*.

In regard to *cause and pathogenesis*, under filthy conditions the larvae of the free-living nematode *P. strongyloides* may invade the skin of dogs. The adult parasites have a direct life cycle and live in damp soil or decaying organic material such as rice hulls, straw, or marsh hay that has been stored in contact with the ground for many months. The larvae may invade the skin of animals that comes in contact with contaminated soil or hay.[132] The larvae are about 600 μm long (Fig. 8:2) and may be found in skin scrapings from affected skin or in the associated bedding. In histologic sections, larvae and some parthenogenetic females may be found in the hair follicles where a typical folliculitis is present.

Pasyk[105] described pelodera dermatitis in an 11-year-old girl who slept with a pet dog that also had the condition. The larvae invaded the epidermis and

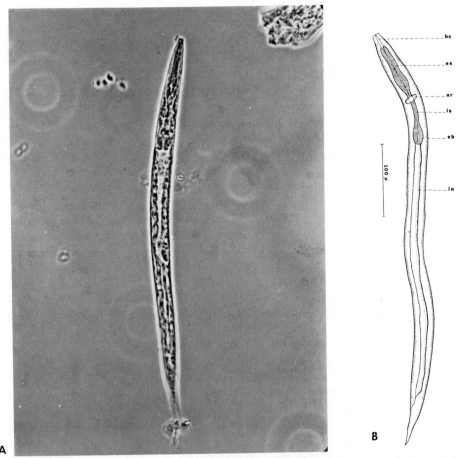

Figure 8:2. *A,* Larva of the free-living nematode, *Pelodera strongyloides.* (Courtesy Jay R. Georgi.) *B,* Larva of *Pelodera strongyloides:* bc = Buccal capsule; es = esophagus; nr = nerve ring; is = isthmus; eb = esophageal bulb; in = intestine. (From Willers, W. B.: *Pelodera strongyloides* in association with canine dermatitis in Wisconsin. J.A.V.M.A. *156:*319, 1970.)

hair follicles, and the inflammatory infiltrate of mononuclear and eosinophilic cells surrounded necrotic hair follicles and extended to capillaries and venules of the upper dermis. It was noted that the child might have contracted the infestation from the dog, but it seems more reasonable that both individuals were infested from the usual environmental sources. Harmon[59] and Smith and colleagues[131] report that human skin infections with larval nematodes can be contracted from dogs with *Ancylostoma braziliense, Ancylostoma caninum, Uncinaria stenocephala, Gnathostoma spinigerum,* and *Strongyloides stercoralis* as well as *Pelodera strongyloides.*

Clinical features of pelodera dermatitis include a distribution of skin lesions that typically involves areas that contact the ground—feet, legs, perineum, lower abdomen and chest, and under tail (Figs. 8:3*A* to *C* and 8:4).[19a, 143] The affected skin is erythematous and partially to completely alopecic, and there are multiple papules that later develop to crusts, scales, and secondary infection from the constant scratching (Fig. 8:3*D*). Pruritus varies from mild to intense.

In *diagnosis,* skin scrapings readily reveal small, motile nematode larvae (625 to 650 μm in length). The history of typical bedding and intense pruritus together with the skin scrapings should be diagnostic, but differential rule-outs

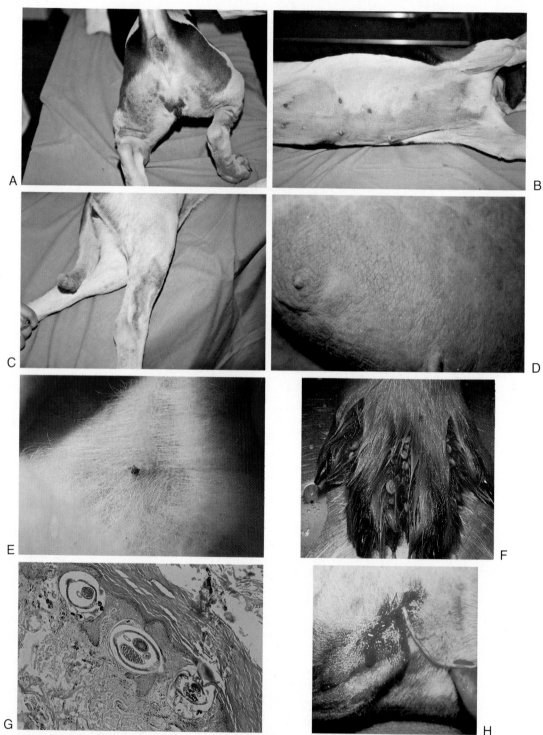

Figure 8:3. Pelodera dermatitis. *A,* Rear legs and hind quarters of beagle with pelodera dermatitis. The involved areas are alopecic and erythematous. *B,* Ventral chest and abdomen of patient in *A.* Bloody areas are sites of skin scrapings. *C,* Lateral hock and thigh of patient in *A. D,* Close view of skin of patient in *A* showing intense erythema, multiple papules, and alopecia. *E,* Tick bite. Erythematous nodule with tick attached. (Courtesy W. H. Miller, Jr.) *F,* Tick infestation. Pododermatitis in a dog associated with numerous interdigital ticks. (Courtesy W. H. Miller, Jr.) *G,* Anatrichosomiasis. Nematode segments within the epidermis of a cat's footpad. *H,* Dracunculosis. Ulcerated skin lesion of English pointer's neck with female adult emerging from fistula. (Courtesy G. G. Doering.)

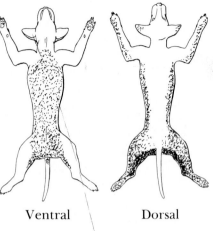

Ventral   Dorsal

Figure 8:4. Pelodera dermatitis distribution pattern. Affected areas are those that normally contact the ground when the dog is sitting or lying down—the chest, the abdomen (ventral and lateral sides), the feet, the sides and backs of the legs, and the perineum. There are alopecia and multiple erythematous papules.

include hookworm dermatitis, dirofilariasis, and strongyloidiasis (all on the basis of the larval findings). Skin lesions grossly may be suggestive of contact dermatitis, bacterial folliculitis dermatophytosis, demodicosis, or scabies.

Skin biopsy reveals varying degrees of perifolliculitis, folliculitis, and furunculosis (Fig. 8:5). Nematode segment are present within hair follicles and dermal pyogranulomas. Eosinophils are numerous.

Treatment is simple and effective. Complete removal and destruction of bedding are mandatory. Beds, kennels, or cages should be thoroughly washed and sprayed with an insecticide such as malathion or diazinon. The bedding should be replaced with cedar or other wood shavings, cloth, or shredded paper. The patient should be bathed with a warm water shampoo to soften and remove crusts and then with a parasiticidal dip, as for scabies[66] (see p.

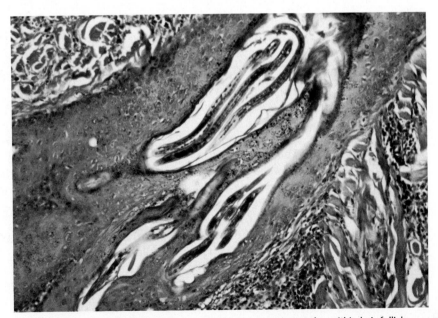

Figure 8:5. Pelodera dermatitis in a dog. Numerous nematodes within hair follicle.

404). This should be repeated at least twice at weekly intervals. This procedure usually results in prompt relief of itching and rapid healing. In a few cases, prednisolone may be given for a few days to help stop the self-trauma due to pruritus; and systemic antibiotics may be indicated for severe secondary pyoderma. The infestation is self-limiting and will resolve spontaneously once the animals are removed from the source of contamination.[132]

STRONGYLOIDES STERCORALIS–LIKE INFECTION

Malone and colleagues[83] in a single report, described an apparently rare helminth similar to *Strongyloides stercoralis* that was isolated from the ileum and jejunum of five of ten Boston terriers in a kennel. Three weeks after a new pup was placed in the kennel, 6-month-old puppies developed mucoid, blood-flecked feces, anemia, general lymphadenopathy, and focal dermatitis. The hair was rough, dull, and dry, and crusted lesions of 1 cm in diameter were on the tail, distal rear legs, the ventral trunk, and other areas of ground and body contact. Some pups had a severe, hemorrhagic pododermatitis. The dogs were housed in outdoor pens with concrete and shaded grassy areas. Fecal samples contained large embryonated and unembryonated ova (80 by 35 μm) and first-stage larvae (200 μm). The ova were larger than those of *S. stercoralis* (normally 55 by 32 μm), and this parasite usually sheds only first-stage larvae in the feces.

When feces were cultured for 18 hours, free-living adults and third-stage larvae were produced.

Treatment with thiabendazole, 11.4 mg/kg once daily orally, was given for 5 days. This was repeated once for a second 5-day course, and all clinical signs resolved after the second treatment. Interestingly, after the second day of thiabendazole therapy, large numbers of adult strongyloides parasites were found in the feces.

ANATRICHOSOMIASIS

Anatrichosomiasis is a type of larval migrans caused by the nematode *Anatrichosoma cutaneum*, which produces blisters on the hands and feet of monkeys and humans in Africa. A case has been reported in a 13-year-old South African cat caused by a *Anatrichosoma* sp. worm.[122] The cat presented for lameness with necrosis, sloughing, and ulceration of the footpads of all four feet. Treatment was not attempted and the cat was euthanized. Histopathologic findings included superficial perivascular dermatitis with numerous worms and bioperculate eggs located in necrotic migratory tracts within the epidermis (Fig. 8:3G). Female worms averaging 42 mm in length were identified only as *Anatrichosoma* sp.[122]

A female, 5-month-old boxer was found to be passing double-operculated eggs in its feces. Similar eggs were obtained from skin scrapings taken from a raised, flaking, erythematous nodule on the dorsal midline in the lumbar region. The nodule was removed surgically, and the eggs from the scraping and the nematode segments found in histologic sections were identified as an *Anatrichosoma* sp.[62a]

SCHISTOSOMIASIS
(Schistosome Dermatitis)

Schistosome cercariae of ducks, shore birds, voles, mice, or muskrat (natural hosts) penetrate the skin of humans, or other warm-blooded animals that are abnormal hosts, and produce a pruritic dermatitis.

Schistosome eggs are shed in the feces of the natural host. The miracidia hatch within 20 minutes and must either find a mollusk (snail) host within 12 hours or die. They form sporocysts in the mollusk and hatch in 5 weeks as cercaria. These are shed into water but also die in 24 hours unless they reach a warm-blooded natural host. Once there, they go to the liver and the intestinal wall, where eggs are laid and passed in the feces.[64] These parasites are trematodes: *Trichobilharzia ocellata, T. stagmicolae,* and *T. physellae* infest waterfowl of the Great Lakes area, while *Austrobilharzia variglandis* afflicts ducks and terns in Florida and Hawaii.[132] In humans the condition has been called swimmer's itch, clam digger's itch, and rice paddy itch. These conditions occur because the cercariae penetrate the skin of the abnormal host and produce clinical disease. Although skin exposed to infested bodies of water from spring to fall may become infected, animals are more apt to be swimming and the cercariae are much more numerous in the water on bright warm days of midsummer; thus, infection is most common then. At the time of penetration, the cercariae produce macules and wheals that last 15 to 20 hours. These later develop into papules and, after 2 to 4 days, into vesicles. These stages are intensely pruritic. They are often confused with mosquito, chigger, or flea bites. Healing takes place in 5 to 7 days, as the cercariae are walled off by an acute inflammatory reaction with infiltration of neutrophils, lymphocytes, and eosinophils. Some humans with the condition have only one strong reaction and on subsequent exposures seem immune, but most individuals experience increasingly severe reactions on each re-exposure.

Local treatment of the skin is not effective except with palliative antipruritic lotions. Control measures should primarily emphasize staying out of the water. Actions such as removing water vegetation that encourages snail populations or killing the mollusks by adding dilute copper sulfate solution to small ponds are of limited value. The authors are not aware of documented cases of canine schistosomiasis in the literature but have seen dogs that had signs and a history suggestive of the problem.

DRACUNCULOSIS

Dracunculus insignis is a parasite of dogs and wild carnivores of North America.[35, 68, 104a] *D. medinensis* (guinea worm) affects human beings, cats, and other animals in Asia and Africa. *D. insignis* has been reported to affect the dog, racoon, mink, fox, otter, and skunk.[35] The intermediate host is a *Cyclops* (a crustacean) that is ingested from contaminated water by the host. The larvae develop in the host over a period of 8 to 12 months. The adults develop in the subcutaneous tissue of the abdomen and limbs. Usually a nodule (2.5-cm diameter) forms, and eventually a fistula develops (Fig. 8:6). Just before the fistula opens, the host may show urticaria, itching, and a slight fever. When the host enters cool water the female worm is stimulated to release larvae (Fig. 8:7), which escape

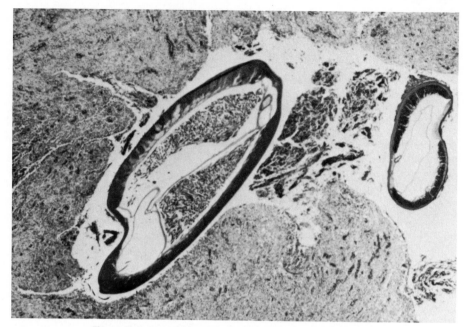

Figure 8:6. Dracunculosis. Nematode segments in an abscess.

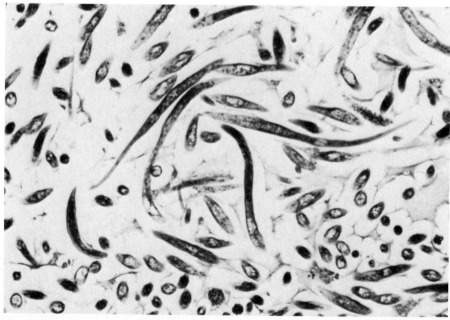

Figure 8:7. Dracunculosis. Characteristic larvae (enlargement of section from the adult nematode segments as seen in Figure 8:6).

through the cutaneous fistula. Some may enter the blood, but they can be distinguished from *Dirofilaria* and *Dipetalonema* larvae by the long tapered tails. One can also apply cold water to the fistula to stimulate the female and then make a smear of the exudate to identify the larvae.

Clinical features are chronic single to multiple nodules on the limbs, head, or abdomen that eventually ulcerate and do not heal (see Fig. 8:3H). The lesions are often painful and pruritic.[110, 147] The adult parasites (female, 17 by 70 cm; male 17 by 22 cm) may occasionally be seen in fistulae. Exfoliative cytology may reveal neutrophils, eosinophils, and macrophages as well as larvae (about 500 μm length). Histologic examination of an excised lesion reveals a pseudocyst containing adult and larval nematodes and surrounded by fibrosis and eosinophilic pyogranulomatous inflammation.[104a]

Treatment, classically, is to gently remove the worm by *carefully* winding it up on a stick over a period of several days. Subsequently, healing of the fistula is prompt.[132] However, the nodule may be excised surgically.[68] Soulsby[132] suggests that large doses of diethylcarbamazine, or thiabendazole for 2 or 3 days, will kill both adults and larvae, while Subrahmanyam and associates[135] used metronidazole (Flagyl) in a dog at doses of 200 mg BID for 10 days with apparent success. Thiabendazole, metronidazole, and niridazole are effective for reducing the severity of the clinical signs, favoring spontaneous expulsion of the worms, and facilitating extraction.[104a]

Control measures depend on improving contaminated water supplies. After a period of time the incidence decreases and the disease dies out. It can be prevented also by drinking only water that is passed through a very fine filter.

DIROFILARIASIS
(Heartworm Dermatitis)

The larvae of *Dirofilaria immitis* are found in the blood and occasionally in the subcutaneous tissues. Scott and Vaughn have reported four dogs with clinical, histopathologic, and therapeutic observations that suggest their dermatologic syndrome might be associated with a hypersensitivity reaction to *D. immitis* microfilaria.[120, 125] McKee,[86] Carmichael and Bell,[26] and others have reported pustular eruptions, pruritic ulcerative dermatitis, and nodular ulcerative lesions in dogs with filariasis, but a cause-and-effect relation was not demonstrated. *D. immitis* was also found in a cutaneous granuloma on the leg of a cat.[123a]

In the cases reported by Scott, mature, large-breed dogs had several-month histories of chronic, nonresponsive skin lesions. All exhibited chronic, ulcerated, multifocal nodules that involved the head (lips, pinna, nose), trunk, and proximal extremities (see Fig. 9:34A,B). The dogs were otherwise healthy. Differential diagnoses included acral lick dermatitis, sporotrichosis, dermatophytosis, mycetoma, actinomycosis, and neoplasia. Numerous injectable and oral glucocorticoids, ointments, antibiotics (including griseofulvin), shampoos, and sedatives had been used in the dogs without effect.

Skin scrapings failed to reveal parasites, and cultures failed to grow bacteria and fungi. Blood samples contained microfilariae in three cases and no microfilariae in one case (occult filariasis).

Histopathology revealed varying degrees of angiocentric pyogranulomatous dermatitis (see Figs. 9:35, 9:36). Microfilarial segments were present intravascularly and extravascularly within the granulomatous dermal nodules.[125] Eosinophils varied in number from few to many.

Many of the blood vessels in the central areas of the lesions contained microfilariae, but none of the deep dermal or subcutaneous vessels outside the lesions showed cellular infiltrates or microfilariae. Special stains showed no microbial agents. The enzyme-linked immunosorbent assay (ELISA) test for antiadult *D. immitis* antibodies was positive in the dog with occult filariasis.

Three dogs were treated with the standard heartworm protocol of thiacetarsamide and dithiazanine.[120] One case was treated with thiacetarsamide and ivermectin.[125] In each case the skin lesions healed completely within 5 to 8 weeks after completion of therapy. The dogs have remained well for a 2- to 3-year follow-up period. Many of the findings reported are consistent with filarial dermatitis in other species (elaeophoriasis, stephanofilariasis, and onchocerciasis).

Arthropod Parasites

ARACHNIDS

Arachnids differ from insects in the absence of wings, the presence of four pairs of legs in adults, and fusion of the head and thorax. With ticks and mites, the head, thorax, and abdomen are fused so that they have lost their external signs of segmentation. The mouthparts and their base together are called the gnathosoma or capitulum. The rest of the parasite consists of fused elements of the head along with the thorax and abdomen, together called the idiosoma. There are separate sexes.

Parasitic Ticks

Ticks differ from mites in their larger size, the hairless or short-haired leathery body, exposed armed hypostome, and the presence of a pair of spiracles near the coxae of the fourth pair of legs. Most are not host specific. Ticks are divided into argasid or soft ticks and ixodid or hard ticks. The argasid are more primitive and less often parasitic, produce fewer progeny, and infest the premises occupied by their hosts. Ixodid ticks are more specialized and highly parasitic, produce more progeny, and infest the open country frequented by their hosts.[92]

ARGASID (SOFT) TICKS

These are more commonly parasites of birds and are found frequently in warmer climates. In regions in which they are endemic, however, they may infest all types of wild and domestic animals. They have no dorsal plate, the sexes are similar, the capitulum is not visible dorsally, and the spiracles lie in front of the third pair of unspurred coxae. Ticks of this class seldom travel far from their lairs and are often nocturnal feeders. Only one species will be discussed.

Spinous Ear Tick. This tick (*Otobius megnini*) is found in the external ear canal of dogs and cats, but its range is limited to the southern United States, especially the Southwest. The larvae and nymphs infest the ear canal of the host, producing acute otitis externa, pain, and occasional convulsions. Often the ear canals become packed with immature ticks, but in some cases only a few are found. The life cycle is described in Figure 8:8. Adults are fiddle-shaped with a constriction in the middle, but they are not spiny and do not

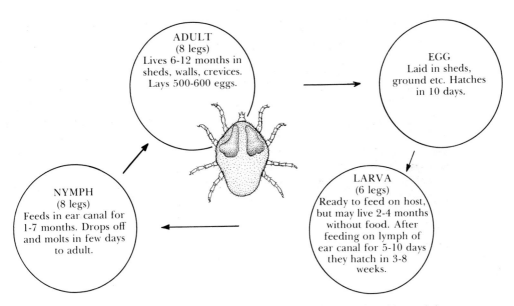

Figure 8:8. Life cycle of *Otobius megnini* (spinous ear tick) (5 to 12 months).

feed, since they are not parasitic. The larvae, engorged on lymph from the ear canal, are yellow or pink. They are about 0.3 cm and spherical, with three pairs of minute legs. The nymphs, which also inhabit the ear canal, are bluish gray with four pairs of yellow legs (Fig. 8:9). They are widest in the middle, and the skin has numerous sharp spines.

Damage from spinous ear ticks results from the loss of blood and lymph. In addition, severe irritation and secondary otitis cause vigorous head shaking and scratching.

Treatment involves mechanical removal of ticks with forceps, spraying or dipping the coat with insecticidal materials such as pyrethroids or malathion, and treatment of the otitis externa with antibiotic-corticosteroid lotions such as Panalog, Liquichlor, or Tresaderm.

Reinfestation is a problem, so destruction of the lairs or nests of the ticks is important. Spraying the sheds, grounds, woodpiles, and other "homesites" with 0.25 per cent malathion, dioxathion 0.5 per cent solution, or chlorpyrifos (Vet-Kem Yard and Kennel Spray) may be effective. Repeat application as necessary, since complete eradication is difficult.

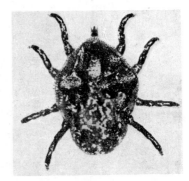

Figure 8:9. Nymph of *Otobius megnini*, the spinous ear tick. (From Lapage, G.: Monnig's Veterinary Helminthology and Entomology. 5th ed. The Williams & Wilkins Company, Baltimore, 1962.)

IXODID (HARD) TICKS

Hard ticks possess a chitinous shield, the scutum, which covers the dorsal surface of the male and the anterior dorsal part of the female. The capitulum is visible dorsally at the anterior end, and its base is important taxonomically. The sexes are dissimilar, although both are bloodsuckers. It is beyond the scope of this text to identify ticks specifically, but because *Rhipicephalus sanguineus* (in comparison with *Dermacentor*) can reproduce easily in buildings and thus presents special control problems, a few key features for identifying genera are described (Figs. 8:10 and 8:11).

Rhipicephalus is recognized by the vase-shaped base of the capitulum, by elongated spiracles, and in the male by triangular adanal plates. The fourth coxae are no larger than the other three.

Dermacentor ticks are characterized by the very large fourth coxae, the rectangular base of the capitulum, and the ornate scutum.

The general life cycle of ixodid ticks is given in Figure 8:12, although each species may vary slightly in some details. Generally, completion of the life cycle requires three hosts, preferably animals of varied size, for the larva, nymph, and adult, although some species pass through all stages on the same mammal. If the complicated life cycle is interrupted, the tick can survive for long periods or hibernate through the winter. Although the life cycle is usually completed in a single year, it may be extended for 2 or 3 years.

While off the host, these ticks infest ground that is covered with small bushes and shrubs. They resist cold but are susceptible to strong sunlight, desiccation, and excessive rainfall. They do require a moist environment.

Common Species of Ixodid Ticks Affecting Dogs and Cats

Rhipicephalus sanguineus. The brown dog tick is widely distributed in North America and is the primary tick problem in many sections of the United States, because it can survive indoors, owing to its low moisture requirements, and can complete its life cycle with only one animal as host. Although its principal host is the dog, it is found on other canine and feline species, rabbits, horses, and humans. It requires three distinct hosts (but perhaps the same

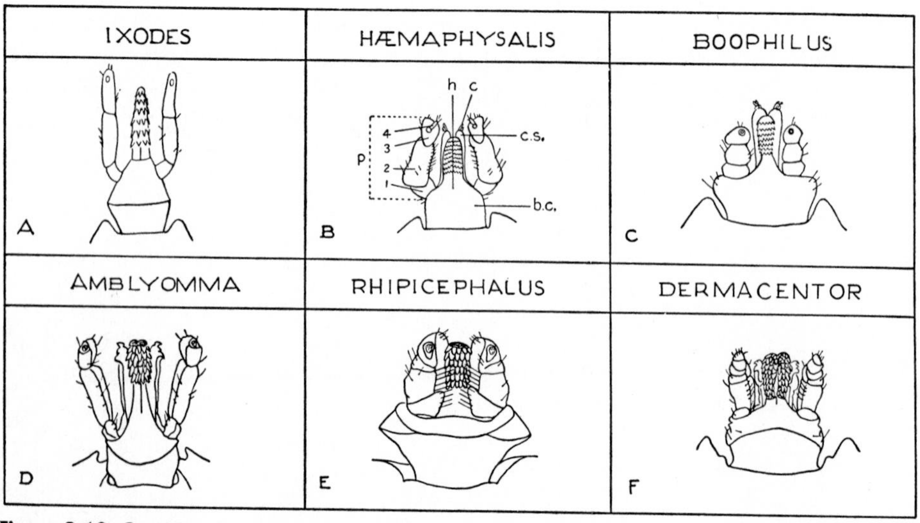

Figure 8:10. Capitula of various genera of hard ticks, ventral view: b.c. = basis capituli, c = chelicera, c.s. = sheath of chelicera, h = haustellum, p = pedipalps. (From Belding, D. L.: Textbook of Parasitology. Appleton-Century-Crofts, New York, 1965.)

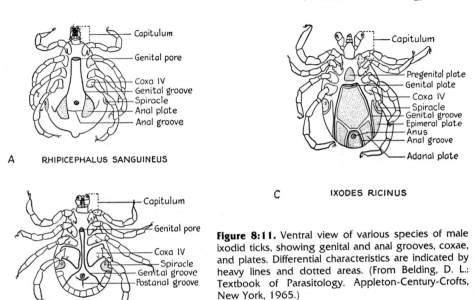

Figure 8:11. Ventral view of various species of male ixodid ticks, showing genital and anal grooves, coxae, and plates. Differential characteristics are indicated by heavy lines and dotted areas. (From Belding, D. L.: Textbook of Parasitology. Appleton-Century-Crofts, New York, 1965.)

animal) in its life cycle. It can transmit babesiosis and anaplasmosis, *Ehrlichia canis* and *Francisella tularensis,* and can cause tick paralysis.

Dermacentor variabilis. The American dog tick is also widely distributed in North America but is especially common along the Atlantic coast in areas of shrub and beach grass. The principal host of the adult tick is the dog, but humans, domestic animals, and large fur-bearing mammals may be attacked. The principal host of the immature tick is the field mouse, but other small rodents or larger mammals may be infested. It spreads Rocky Mountain spotted fever, St. Louis encephalitis, tularemia, and anaplasmosis and causes tick paralysis.

Other Ticks That May Affect Dogs and Cats. These include *Dermacentor*

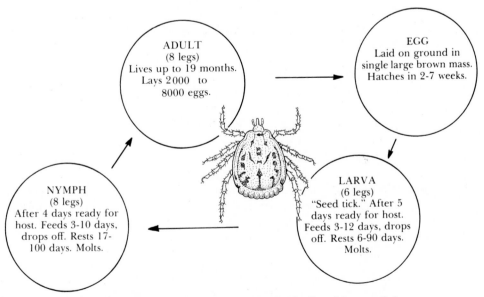

Figure 8:12. Life cycle of ixodid (hard) ticks (2 to 24+ months).

andersoni (Rocky Mountain wood tick), *Dermacentor occidentalis* (Pacific or West Coast tick), *Ixodes scapularis* (black-legged tick), *Amblyomma maculatum* (Gulf Coast tick), and *Amblyomma americanum* (Lone Star tick).

DAMAGE FROM TICKS

Ticks injure animals by the irritation of their bites, by "hypersensitivity" reactions (see p. 490), by serving as vectors for bacterial, rickettsial, viral, and protozoan diseases, and by producing tick paralysis through their poisonous secretions (Fig. 8:3E,F).

Tick paralysis has been produced by 12 ixodid species including *Dermacentor variabilis* and is seen in many hosts including dogs and cats. The paralysis is caused by a protein toxin produced by the salivary glands of the tick. It may be elaborated by ovarian function, as it is associated with egg production. Individual ticks vary in their toxin-producing capacity, although those attached near the spine and neck seem to produce a more severe intoxication. The toxin affects the lower motor neurons of the spinal cord and cranial nerves and produces a progressive ascending flaccid paralysis.[11, 67]

TREATMENT AND CONTROL OF TICKS

In cases of tick paralysis, rapid recovery follows mechanical removal of the complete tick or ticks. When animals are infested by small numbers of ticks, picking them off the host is often simple and easy. An effective method is to soak the tick in alcohol, grasp the head parts at the surface of the skin gently with a 5-inch curved Crile "mosquito" hemostat, and apply firm traction. Ticks are commonly found in the ears and between the toes. The collected ticks should be burned or soaked in alcohol until dead. Under no conditions should ticks be removed from animals by soaking them in gasoline or kerosene, or by applying a lighted cigarette—the consequences to the skin are too severe.

With heavy or persisting infestations the dog may be treated topically with 4 per cent malathion powder or 0.5 per cent solution. Chlorpyrifos (Dursban) may be used effectively on the dog or the premises. Because of susceptibility to most topical insecticides, cats should be treated only with powders of methoxychlor (2 per cent), pyrethrin (1 per cent), or carbaryl (5 per cent) or malathion dips.

Infestations of *Rhipicephalus sanguineus* in houses and kennels can often be controlled or eliminated by repeated spraying of woodwork, crawl spaces, pipe clearances, and cracks with chlorfenvinphos (Dermaton Dip). *In severe cases, commercial exterminators should be employed.*

Outdoor control measures can help limit ticks by controlling their hosts and by destroying or treating vegetation. The population of wild rodent hosts can be reduced by trapping or poisoning. Their habitat can be destroyed by cutting and burning brush and grass, by cultivating land, and by rotating pastures. In urban areas, grass and shrubbed areas can be treated with toxaphene, diazinon, or dieldrin dusts (or sprays) applied at the rate recommended by the label. They are applied in the spring and repeated once during midsummer.

Parasitic Mites

Mites are members of the order Acarina. They are smaller than ticks and do not have a leathery covering; the hypostome may be unarmed, and some mites have spiracles on the cephalothorax. Parasitic mites are chiefly ectoparasites of the skin, mucous membranes, or feathers, but a few are endoparasites. They are distributed worldwide, and they infest plants and animals, cause direct injury to animals, and spread disease. Because of their prevalence and clinical importance, four parasitic mites—*Cheyletiella* spp., *Demodex* spp., *Sarcoptes scabiei* (var. *canis*), and *Notoedres cati*—and the diseases they cause are discussed in depth beginning on p. 369.

DERMANYSSUS GALLINAE (POULTRY MITE)

This mite attacks poultry, wild and cage birds, dogs, and cats, as well as humans. It is called the red mite but is only red when engorged with blood. At other times it is white, gray, or black (Fig. 8:13A). The engorged adult, which is the largest form, is only 1.1 mm in size (Fig. 8:14). It lives in nests and cracks in cages or houses and after a meal of blood lays up to seven eggs at a time. They hatch to six-legged nymphs that do not feed. After 48 hours these molt to eight-legged protonymphs that feed and molt, 48 hours later, to deutonymphs. These also feed and molt 48 hours later to adults. The whole cycle takes only 7 days under ideal conditions, but without feeding opportunities it may last 5 months.

This mite affects dogs and cats only rarely and almost accidently. Wild birds nesting in the eaves of houses have mites, which may enter open windows and affect people and animals living there.[21] Ramsay and Mason[108] found such large numbers of mites covering a dog's body that the small grayish white mites crawling on the hair resembled the dandruff of cheyletiellosis. In that case itching was not severe. Most cases are associated with pets that have access to chicken houses or live in recently converted poultry quarters. Clinical signs include erythema and papulocrustous, intensively pruritic eruptions, especially over the back and extremities (see Fig. 8:13B). Diagnosis is made by finding the mites in skin scrapings. Almost any insecticidal bath, dip, or spray will eliminate the mites, but the affected premises that initiated the infection should be treated to prevent reinfestation.

LYNXACARUS RADOVSKY (CAT FUR MITE)

These small mites are endemic in Australia and Hawaii and have been reported in Florida.[54] They have elongated bodies, 430 to 520 μm in length, and flaplike sternal extensions. These contain the first two legs, which grasp the hair of the host (Fig. 8:15). All the legs have terminal suckers. Because all fur mites are generally alike, a competent parasitologist is needed for accurate species identification.

These mites are not highly contagious. Bowman[20] reported only one of fourteen cats in a group to be affected. Usually there is little itching. The mites attach to the hair and give a "salt and pepper" appearance to the dull and dirty coat. Although hair is easily epilated, the skin either is normal or has widespread papulocrustous eruption. Mites usually congregate along the topline attached to the terminal parts of the hair. However, they may occasionally be found all over the body. Diagnosis is made by skin scrapings or acetate tape impression to isolate mites. Treatment with insecticidal sprays or dips, or lime-sulfur dips weekly is usually adequate therapy.

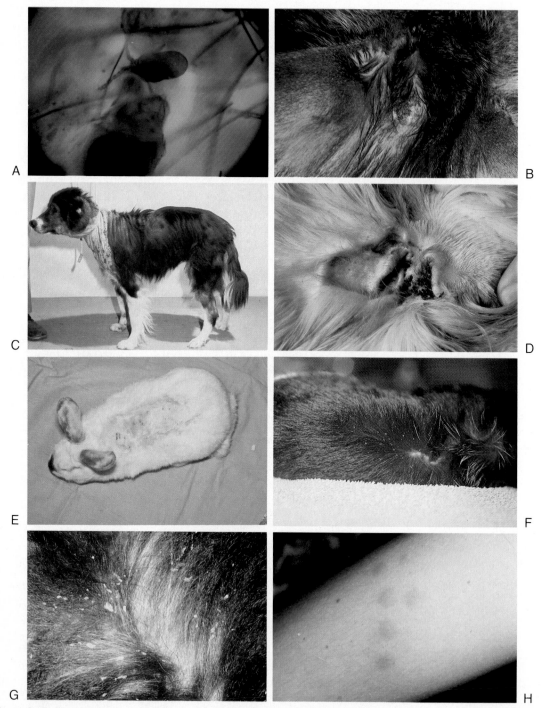

Figure 8:13. Parasitic mites. *A, Dermanyssus gallinae* poultry mite adult. *B,* Erosion, crusts, and excoriations on head of cat infested with *Dermanyssus gallinae*. *C,* Dog with severe case of generalized otodectic mange. *D,* Dark brown, waxy exudate and crusts in the ear of a dog with *Otodectes cynotis*. (Courtesy R. L. Collinson.) *E,* Rabbit with shoulders and back clipped to show scaly lesions of cheyletiella dermatitis. *F,* Scaling over the dorsum of a cat with cheyletiellosis. (Cat is lying on its side on a green towel.) *G, Cheyletiella* infestation in dog. The white specks are "walking dandruff." *H,* Papular urticaria of human skin due to *Cheyletiella blakei* bites.

Figure 8:14. *Dermanyssus gallinae* (De-geer). Left, dorsal view of female; right, ventral view of female. (From Lapage, G.: Monnig's Veterinary Helminthology and Entomology. 5th ed. The Williams & Wilkins Company, Baltimore, 1962.)

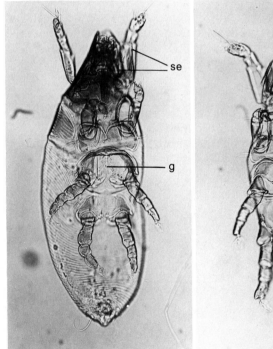

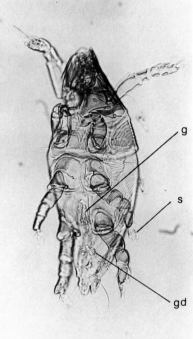

Figure 8:15. *Lynxacarus radovsky*, female in ventral view: se = sternal extensions; g = genitalia. Body length = 515 μm. *B, Lynxacarus radovsky*, male in ventral view: g = genitalia; s = sucker; gd = genital disc. Body length = 430 μm. (From Bowman, W. L., and Domrow, R.: The cat-fur mite in Australia. Austral. Vet. J. *54*:403, 1978. Photographs by R. Wilson.)

TROMBICULIDIASIS (CHIGGERS, HARVEST MITES)

Although 20 of about 700 species of chigger mites can cause disease, only two are reported here.

Trombicula (Eutrombicula) Alfreddugesi (North American Chigger), and Trombicula (Neotrombicula) Autumnalis. The adult form is a scavenger living on decaying vegetable material. It is orange-red, is about the size of the head of a pin, and lives about 10 months, producing probably one generation per year. The eggs are laid in moist ground and hatch to six-legged red larvae that are parasitic and feed on animals. They drop to the ground and become nymphs, and finally adults (Fig. 8:16). The entire cycle is complete in 50 to 70 days, but adult females may live longer than a year. They are usually found in ground–skin contact areas like the legs, feet, head, ears, and ventrum. Signs are variable. The bite usually produces severe irritation and an intensely pruritic papulocrustous eruption, but it may also cause nonpruritic pustules and crusts. Secondary scaling and alopecia may appear. Mites may be found in and around the ears of cats but are easily distinguished from *Otodectes* (ear mites) by their intense orange-red color and because they adhere tightly to the skin.[23, 53, 58, 79] However, when removed from the host for microscopic examination, they should be placed in mineral oil immediately or they will jump away.

> *Diagnosis is made by finding the bright orange mite on the lesion. However, since it stays on the host for only 3 to 15 days, it may be gone when the patient is examined.*

Chiggers are seasonal in summer and fall and are especially common in the central United States. Affected patients have a history of environmental contact in woods and fields. Skin biopsy reveals varying degrees of superficial perivascular dermatitis (spongiotic hyperplastic) in which eosinophils are numerous.

Treatment is successful with one or two parasiticidal dips (Paramite) and with thiabendazole drops (Tresaderm) applied to the ear canals.[53] Patients must be kept from contaminated areas to prevent reinfestation. Systemic corticosteroids administered for 2 to 3 days will help relieve the intense itching.

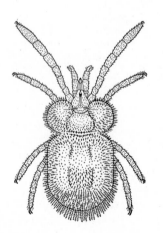

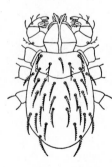

Figure 8:16. *A, T. alfreddugesi* (North American chigger) adult; *B, T. alfreddugesi* larva, dorsal view (legs omitted). (From Belding, D. L.: Textbook of Parasitology. Appleton-Century-Crofts, New York, 1965.)

X 20   X 100

Walchia Americana. This is a chigger mite that has been reported to be common in squirrels and small rodents in the southwestern and eastern United States and has been reported in one cat.[79] The larvae live on the surface of the skin. Their salivary secretions allow them to feed on tissue liquids of the host. A walled-off channel is formed on the skin surface as a host reaction that attempts to isolate the parasite. The larvae detach and enter decaying wood for a quiet period. Active nymphs emerge and forage, become quiet again as they pass through the imagochrysalis stage, and then emerge as adults. These feed principally on the Collembolla insect (spring tail). The adults lay many eggs, which hatch to parasitic larvae. Some chiggers have a special liking for certain body locations on the host. The mite prefers the ventrum, but is also found on the ears and back.

In the cat reported by Lowenstine and colleagues,[79] the lesions were on the ventral trunk, medial surface of the legs, and the interdigital spaces. Lesions could be palpated, but the hair needed to be parted carefully to see them easily. There was nodular thickened skin, and the surface was cracked and scaly, with moist, serous-yellow exudate. The paws were swollen and the claws were cracked. The cat shook its feet as if it had stepped into something noxious. Close inspection revealed nonpruritic papules (0.1 to 0.3 cm) with a few wheals and flares. Skin scrapes produced few mites, but a skin biopsy contained many mites.

Histopathology reveals varying degrees of intraepidermal pustular-to-vesicular dermatitis. Hyperkeratosis is marked, and mite segments are seen within the epidermis. Eosinophils and mast cells are numerous.

Treatment with insecticidal powders for the mites and broad-spectrum antibiotics for the secondary infection produced a good response in 10 days.

OTODECTES CYNOTIS (EAR MITES)

Otodectes cynotis is a psoroptid mite that does not burrow but lives on the surface of the skin. Adult mites are large, white, and freely moving. The anus is terminal, they have four pairs of legs, and all except the rudimentary fourth pair of the female extend beyond the body margin. All legs of the male bear short, unjointed stalks (pedicles) with suckers, which are also present on the first two pairs of legs of the females.

The life cycle lasts 3 weeks (Fig. 8:17). The egg is laid with a cement that sticks it to the substrate. After a 4-day incubation, it hatches to produce the six-legged larva. At this point, the larva feeds actively for 3 to 10 days, rests 10 to 30 hours, and hatches to the protonymph, which has eight legs, although the last pair are very small. After a simple active and resting stage, the protonymph molts into the deutonymph. The deutonymph is usually approached by the adult male (Fig. 8:18), and the two become attached (end to end) by the pair of dorsal posterior suckers on the body of the nymph and those on the rear legs of the adult male. If a male adult is produced from the deutonymph, the attachment has no physiologic significance; however, if a female emerges, copulation occurs at that moment, and the female will become egg bearing. Females that are not attached, and thereby do not permit copulation at the moment of ecdysis, do not lay eggs. Sexual dimorphism occurs only in the adult form. The first four legs of all stages bear unjointed, short stalks and suckers, but only the adult males have suckers on the rear legs.

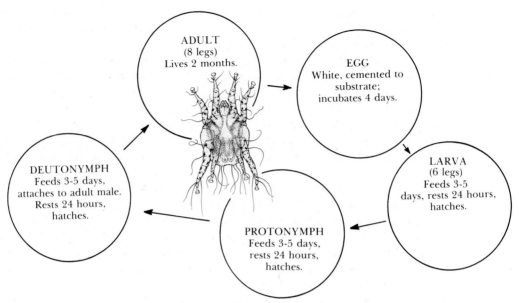

Figure 8:17. Life cycle of *Otodectes cynotis* (three weeks).

The mites feed on epidermal debris and tissue fluid from the superficial epidermis. In this way the host is exposed to, and immunized against, mite antigen.[106, 137] There is no delayed hypersensitivity, but a reaginic antibody develops early in the disease and precipitating antibodies later in its course.

Mites cause intense irritation and thick, reddish brown crusts in the ears of dogs and cats (Fig. 8:13*D*). The ears become filled with a mixture of loose crusts and cerumen. Lesions may be restricted to the external ear canal, but mites are commonly found on other areas of the body, especially on the neck, rump, and tail.[16a, 121] Some cases closely resemble flea bite hypersensitivity (Fig. 8:13*C*). Other conditions to be ruled out include pediculosis, pelodera derma-

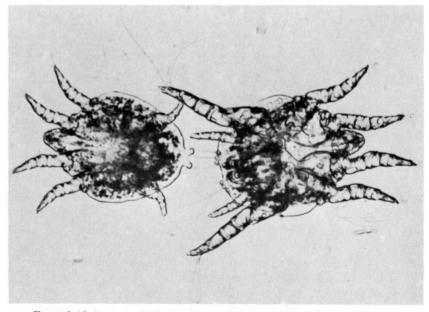

Figure 8:18. Larger male *Otodectes cynotis* mite approaching a deutonymph.

titis, scabies, chiggers, and allergic dermatitis. Ear mites are highly contagious and especially prevalent in the young. Many species of carnivores can be infested, as the mites are not host specific.

Harwick[60] describes human lesions and Larkin and Gaillard[78] state that the mites may live in the premises for months. Weisbroth and colleagues[138] noted very little effect from attempts at control using dichlorvos (Vapona) flea collars.

Control of mites is especially difficult in kennel or cattery situations, where multiple animals are found together. Suggestions for flea control (see p. 416) are also appropriate here. Thorough cleaning and insecticidal treatment of the premises, using residual materials such as diazinon or malathion, are desirable. These procedures should be combined with complete treatment of all parts of every animal in contact, using appropriate flea sprays, powders, or dips. This is the most important part of therapy. Repeat weekly for 4 weeks.

Local treatment of the ears is of course important. Many miticidal agents are available commercially, but the authors prefer one part rotenone in oil (Canex) diluted with three parts mineral oil. The ears are gently cleaned, and the oil mixture is applied twice weekly; later, once weekly is effective. Treat 2 weeks beyond the point of apparent clinical cure.

One or two subcutaneous injections of 200 to 400 µg/kg ivermectin is reported to cure otodectic mange in dogs[145] and in cats.[16, 47] All animals were cured, and no side-effects resulted. This drug form is not approved for use in dogs and cats in the United States. Amitraz (Mitaban) is highly effective when applied as ear drops twice weekly. The solution is 1 ml of stock Mitaban with 33 ml of mineral oil. Although it is not approved for cats in the United States, Bussieras and Chermette[25] use 0.5 per cent amitraz in 50 per cent propylene glycol in the ears and apply an entire body wash of 500 ppm as the initial treatment.

Ear mites in rabbits are usually caused by *Psoroptes cuniculi*. Affected ears often have thick cores of dry crusted material that may adhere to the lining of the ear canal. This material should be softened with mineral oil for 12 to 24 hours. It can then be removed with less trauma, and the mites in the ear can be treated as described for *Otodectes cynotis*.

HOUSEDUST MITES

These mites are known to be agents that are allergenic to human beings, and it is probable that they affect dogs too. Over 1000 mites have been found per gram of dust in 34 per cent of houses examined.[2] The most common mite is *Dermatophagoides pteronyssimus*, but *Cheyletus eruditus* and *Tyrophagus farinae* were also found. It is possible that these mites are associated with asthma or papular urticaria in humans.[2] Positive results of intradermal tests for *Dermatophagoides* spp. were obtained in 30 per cent of patients, whereas all controls were negative. These mites may be associated with allergic dermatitis in dogs that react positively to housedust allergen tests. *Dermatophagoides* and *Otodectes* mites may effectively cross react and produce allergy in humans.[78] Both types of mites have been shown to live in houses for months, and as a result the public health significance of "ear mites" assumes new significance.

CHEYLETIELLA
("Walking Dandruff")

Cheyletiella dermatitis is a mild, nonsuppurative mite-induced dermatitis produced by *Cheyletiella* spp. living on the surface of the skin.

Cause and Pathogenesis. *Cheyletiella* mites are large mites that affect cats, dogs, rabbits, and humans.[128] The disease is common but often unrecognized in humans, and the three species of mites may go freely to various host species.[3, 29] In general, *C. yasguri* is considered the species found in dogs; *C. blakei,* the species in cats; and *C. parasitovorax,* the species in rabbits. However, there is still confusion in the literature concerning absolute host specificity. Most outbreaks previously reported in dogs were probably *C. yasguri* rather than *C. parasitovorax.*[107] Cats usually have *C. parasitovorax* or *C. blakei* (a species that varies only slightly), and *C. yasguri* is found in cats only accidently, when a dog in the household is affected.[45, 52] *C. yasguri* usually affects humans transiently. Foxx and Ewing[46] were able to use *C. yasguri* in experimental studies involving rabbits and dogs, which suggests that it does not have extreme host specificity. Their excellent report of the morphologic features, behavior, and life history of *C. yasguri* is recommended for further details about the mite (see also Table 8:2). Niiyama and Ohbayashi[95] discuss the morphologic details of *C. blakei.*

The large mites (385 μm) have four pairs of legs bearing combs instead of claws (Fig. 8:19). The most diagnostic feature of *Cheyletiella* spp. is the accessory mouthparts or palpi that terminate in prominent hooks (Fig. 8:20). The heart-shaped sensory organ on genu I is diagnostic of *C. yasguri,* the cone-shaped sensory organ is diagnostic of *C. blakei,* and the global sensory organ is diagnostic of *C. parasitovorax* (Fig. 8:19).

The mites usually do not burrow but live in the keratin layer of the epidermis and are not associated with hair follicles. They move about rapidly in pseudotunnels in dermal debris but periodically attach themselves firmly to the epidermis, pierce the skin with their stylelike chelicerae, and become engorged with a clear colorless fluid.[46]

The ova are smaller than louse nits and are attached to hairs by fine fibrillar strands. In contrast, louse eggs are cemented firmly to the host's hairs (Fig. 8:21).

Cheyletiella mites are not predacious on other mites. The entire life cycle (Fig. 8:22) is completed on one host; the mite is an obligate parasite, as larvae,

Table 8–2. DIFFERENTIATION OF CHEYLETIELLA SPECIES*

C. yasguri	C. parasitovorax	C. blakei
One large, dorsal trapezoid propodosoma shield and two small, round plates.	Only one large dorsal shield.	
Tips of first row of setae (bristles) of the hysterosoma do not reach insertion point of second row.	Tips of first row of setae (bristles) extend clearly over the insertion point of second row of setae of the hysterosome.	Female: hysterosome shield absent.
Of the four setae of the second row, the outer, plumose (feathered) setae are only slightly longer than the inner, simple (smooth) ones.	Of the four setae of the second row, the outer, plumose (feathered) setae are three times as long as the inner, simple (smooth) ones.	Male: simple, long, saber-like setae.
A heart-shaped sense organ is on the genu I (Fig. 8–20).	An egg-shaped or global sense organ is on the genu I.	A conical sense organ is on the genu I.

*Modified from Foxx, T. S., and Ewing, S. A.: Morphologic features, behavior and life history of *Cheyletiella yasguri.* Am. J. Vet. Res. *30:*269, 1969; and Rack, G.: *Cheyletiella yasguri,* 1965, ein fakultativ menschenpathogener Parasit des Hundes. Z. Parasitenkd. *36:*321, 1971.

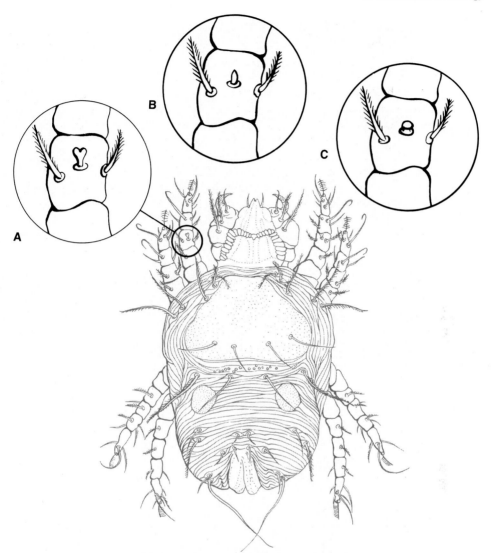

Figure 8:19. Artist's sketch of adult female *Cheyletiella yasguri mite*, showing characteristic saddle-shaped body and diagnostic hooks of the accessory mouth parts. Insert *A* shows the heart-shaped sense organ on genu I that typifies *C. yasguri; B* shows the conical sense organ on genu I that typifies *C. blakei; C* shows the global sense organ on genu I that typifies *C. parasitovorax.*

nymphs, and adult males die within 48 hours after leaving the host. Adult females are more hardy and may live free of their host for up to 10 days if carefully refrigerated.[29, 46] Stein has reported seeing *Cheyletiella* mites crawling in and out of the nostrils of cats, and thus has added a new twist to the epidemiology and therapy of the disease.[133]

The mites are highly contagious, especially between young host animals, but humans may be affected too. Severe problems are often found in litters or in pet shops where sanitation practices are poor. Adult dogs and cats are usually only lightly infected, even when in direct contact with infected puppies and kittens, and very few mites or eggs can be demonstrated in debris from their coats. Both dogs and cats may be a source of human infection.[52] In one survey, 27 of 41 catteries that had problems with a pruritic dermatitis had cheyletiellosis.[103] In 20 per cent of the cases, human cases were found too. *C.*

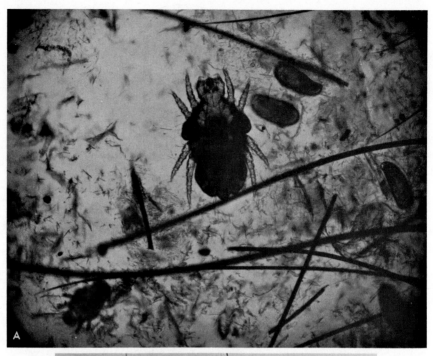

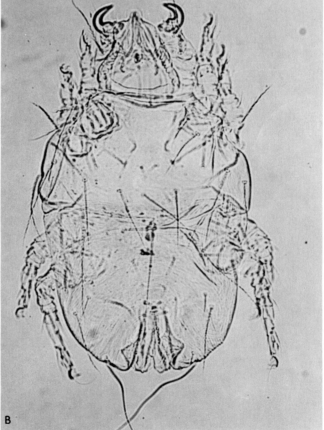

Figure 8:20. *A, Cheyletiella yasguri* adult, larva, and eggs from skin scraping (low power). *B, Cheyletiella yasguri* adult mite showing the diagnostic hooks of the accessory mouthparts.

Figure 8:21. Comparison of eggs attached to hair. Left—*Cheyletiella* egg. Small, attached at one end by filaments. Right—louse egg. Large, adhering closely to hair along most of its length.

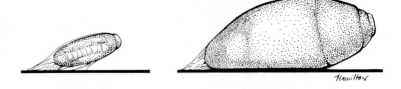

blakei was isolated in all cases. Cheyletiella infestation often causes a mild feline dermatosis but probably should be of more concern as a cause of human parasitic dermatitis transmissable from cats.[95]

There is no doubt that the public health aspects of this parasite are important, since frequent contact with infected animals may produce an uncomfortable skin disease in humans. Human infestations vary in severity, but after direct contact with infested animals has occurred, grouped, erythematous macules form on the arms, trunk, and buttocks (see Fig. 8:13*H*). These rapidly develop a central papule that becomes vesicular and then pustular, finally rupturing to produce a yellow crusted lesion that is frequently excoriated because of the intense pruritus. Although the lesions are severely inflamed, they are well demarcated from surrounding skin. Older lesions have an area of central necrosis, which is highly diagnostic. Constant animal contact is usually needed to maintain human infections. With no further infestation,

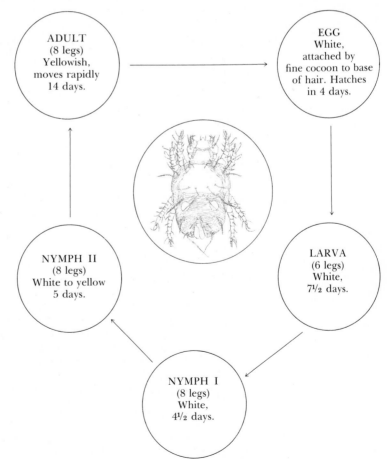

Figure 8:22. Suggested life cycle of *Cheyletiella yasguri.*

ADULT
(8 legs)
Yellowish,
moves rapidly
14 days.

EGG
White,
attached by
fine cocoon to base
of hair. Hatches
in 4 days.

NYMPH II
(8 legs)
White to yellow
5 days.

LARVA
(6 legs)
White,
7½ days.

NYMPH I
(8 legs)
White,
4½ days.

lesions subside in 3 weeks. One of the authors (G.H.M.) knows of a case in which a heavily infested Welsh corgi slept in the same bed with its owner, who claims to have had no itching or visible lesions.

> **Simple scurfy dandruff with or without pruritus in young puppies is highly suggestive of Cheyletiella dermatitis.**

The course of the infection is chronic, affecting otherwise healthy individuals for many months. Infestation is most severe and generalized in 2- to 8-week-old puppies. Older individuals may be almost asymptomatic carriers.

In rabbits, early concentrations of mites are found in the scapular area (see Fig. 8:13E), but on puppies they are usually found in the rump region. These spread over the back and head, but eventually much of the body is affected. Cats tend to have milder, more diffuse lesions, although the back is most frequently involved (Figs. 8:13F and 8:23). Often, they are remarkably free of pruritus. The cat's daily licking and washing probably remove many mites, and as a result they may be hard to find. Affected animals have excessively scurfy, slightly oily coats. The white (or yellowish) mites and eggs together with the keratin scales produced by the epidermal reaction cause an appearance of severe "dandruff" in either cats or dogs (see Fig. 8:13G). With the exception of the scaling, there is remarkably little skin reaction per se in many animals, and in some cases the animal is an asymptomatic carrier. Occasionally, cats will develop a widespread papulocrustous eruption.[87]

Cats with *C. blakei* in a large cattery infestation had discrete dried red-yellow exudate, patchy crusts, and thick scabs over much of their bodies.[103] Even these cases, however, had predominant lesions of a fine, powdery dandruff.

Diagnosis. Careful inspection of the "scurfy" skin with a high-power magnifying loupe usually reveals moving, white opaque mites. An acetate tape impression is a fine technique for collecting mites (see p. 121). One can also brush the epidermal dermis from the hair and skin onto a sheet of clean paper or plastic, or use mineral oil on a scalpel and make a regular skin scraping. In long-haired or dense-coated animals, clipping the area to be scraped is very

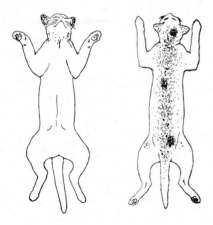

Figure 8:23. *Cheyletiella.* Multiple white dandruff-like flakes are seen in the hair coat over the dorsal spine and head. There may be local dense accumulations that almost look crusty. There usually are few primary skin lesions or alopecia. The pattern is same for dog or cat.

Ventral   Dorsal

helpful. Deep scrapings (to bleeding) are not necessary. The debris is collected and examined under a dissecting microscope for diagnosis of typical mites (see Fig. 8:20). Multiple skin scrapings in cats, combing with a fine flea comb, KOH digestion, and further microscopic examination may be necessary for definitive diagnosis in some cases.

Ova and adult mites have been found in fecal flotation samples.[29] The large eggs (230 by 100 μm) are often embryonated and 3 to 4 times as large as hookworm eggs.

In the differential diagnosis, one should consider other mite infestations (*Otodectes cynotis, Sarcoptes scabiei, Notoedres cati, Dermanyssus gallinae,* and *Eutrombicula alfreddugesi*), which can be differentiated by microscopic inspection of the mites. Pediculosis and flea infestations can be differentiated by identifying the parasite, and *Pelodera strongyloides* can be diagnosed by skin scrapings. Canine flea bite hypersensitivity can be distinguished by severe pruritus, which is not usually present in *Cheyletiella* infestations. Canine and feline flea allergy dermatitis must be considered and can be diagnosed by history, clinical signs, and evidence of fleas.

Idiopathic seborrhea is rare in young animals and would produce negative skin scrapings. Seborrhea in young animals may be associated with endoparasitism and poor nutrition as well as cheyletiellosis. When cheyletiellosis produces a widespread papulocrusteous dermatitic eruption in cats, the differential diagnosis is lengthy (see Table 9:27).

Histopathology reveals varying degrees of superficial perivascular dermatitis (hyperplastic, spongiotic). Mite segments are occasionally found within the hyperkeratotic stratum corneum (Fig. 8:24). Eosinophils vary in number, from few to many.

Treatment. These mites are easily destroyed by most insecticides. Many cases are probably "cured" without diagnosis when the owner treats the itchy pet with flea powder or a flea shampoo such as Mycodex with carbaryl. Thorough treatment of all animals on the premises is necessary. Malathion,

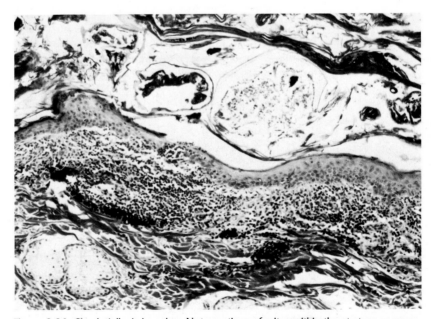

Figure 8:24. Cheyletiellosis in a dog. Note sections of mites within the stratum corneum.

lime sulfur, pyrethroids, or carbaryl will be effective for dogs. Pyrethrins, carbaryl powders, or lime-sulfur dips may be used safely on cats or rabbits. Treatment should be repeated three times at weekly intervals. Recently ivermectin (300 μg/kg given subcutaneously and repeated in 2 to 3 weeks) was found to be very effective for the treatment of canine and feline cheyletiellosis.[104b]

Although mites usually do not live more than 48 hours when they are off the host,[29] a few may live for as long as 10 days; therefore a strong effort should be made to physically clean the premises, improve sanitation practices, and spray the area thoroughly at least once with a good residual insecticide.

All new animals should be carefully inspected and dusted or sprayed with an insecticide before being added to colony-housed animal facilities.

CANINE DEMODICOSIS
(Demodectic Mange, Follicular Mange, Red Mange)

Demodicosis is an inflammatory parasitic skin disease of dogs characterized by the presence of larger-than-normal numbers of demodectic mites. The initial proliferation of mites may be due to a genetic or immunologic disorder.

Cause and Pathogenesis

The Parasite. The mite, *Demodex canis* (Leydig, 1859), is part of the normal fauna of canine skin and is present in very small numbers in most healthy dogs. The skin of dogs with demodicosis, however, is ecologically favorable to the reproduction and growth of demodectic mites. They seize this opportunity to colonize the hair follicles and populate the skin by the thousands. The resulting alopecia and erythema are known as demodicosis. The entire life cycle of the mite is spent on the skin.[115] The parasite resides within the hair follicles and rarely the sebaceous glands, where it subsists by feeding on cells, sebum, and epidermal debris.

Four stages of *D. canis* may be demonstrated in skin scrapings (Fig. 8:25). Fusiform eggs hatch into small, six-legged larvae, which molt into eight-legged nymphs and then into eight-legged adults (Fig. 8:26).[100] The male adult measures 40 by 250 μm and the female, 40 by 300 μm. Mites (all stages) may be found in the lymph nodes, intestinal wall, spleen, liver, kidney, urinary bladder, lung, thyroid, blood, urine, and feces. However, mites found in these extracutaneous sites are usually dead and degenerate, and represent simple

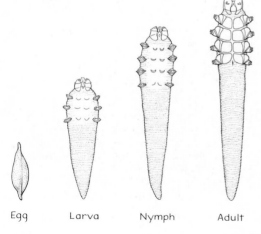

Figure 8:25. Adult and immature forms of *Demodex canis.*

Egg   Larva   Nymph   Adult

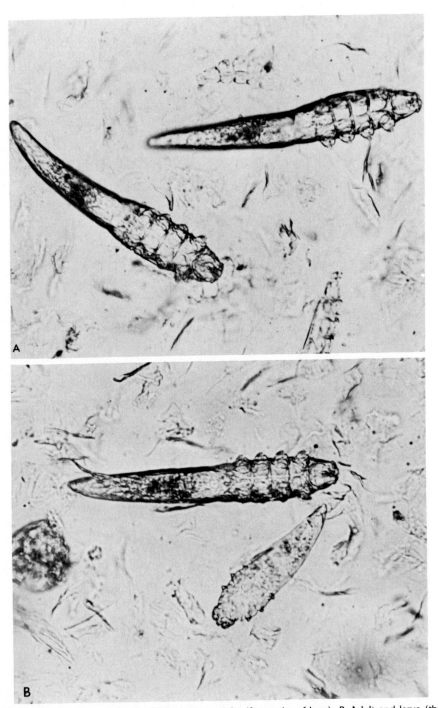

Figure 8:26. *Demodex canis* (× 500). *A*, Two adults (four pairs of legs). *B*, Adult and larva (three pairs of stubby legs). *C*, Nymph (four pairs of stubby legs). *D*, Egg (arrow). *E*, Adult *Demodex cati* in skin scraping. It is similar to *D. canis* except for a somewhat slimmer abdomen. (Courtesy J. Georgi.) *F*, *D. cati* ovum in skin scraping. It is slim and oval rather than spindle-shaped. (Courtesy J. Georgi.) *G, H*, Unnamed adult demodicid and ovum in skin scraping from cat. This mite is morphologically similar to *Demodex criceti*, which is found on hamsters. Note blunt, rounded abdomen.

Illustration continued on following page

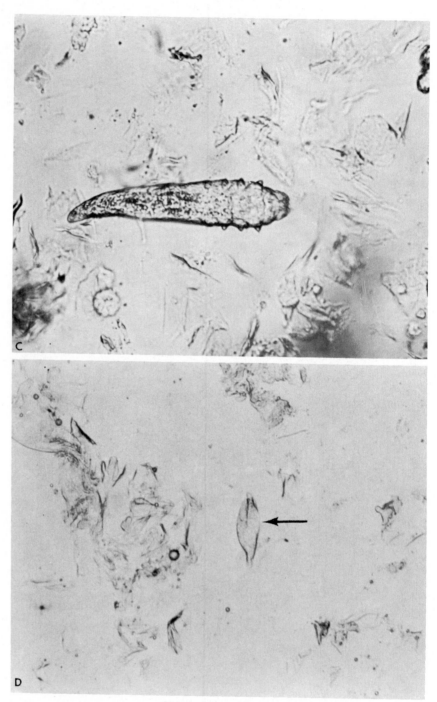

Figure 8:26 *Continued*

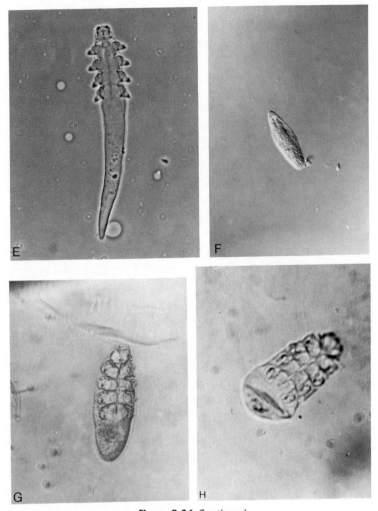

Figure 8:26 *Continued*

drainage to these areas via the blood stream or lymphatics. Thus, Sako and Yamane[113] found that 76 per cent of the dogs with generalized demodicosis that were examined had mites in their superficial and deep lymph nodes, but the numbers were small compared with those in the skin, and the percentage of adults, nymphs, larvae, and eggs were the same.

Transmission. D. canis is a normal resident of canine skin. Transmission occurs by direct contact from the bitch to nursing neonates during the first 2 or 3 days of neonatal life.[49] Mites may be demonstrated in the hair follicles of puppies by the time they are 16 hours old. The mites are first observed on the muzzle of the puppies, which emphasizes the importance of direct contact and nursing. Attempts to transmit the disease by feeding dogs mites, by administering mites intraperitoneally or intratracheally, or by placing diseased animals in direct contact with non-neonatal healthy animals have failed.[114, 123] When puppies were taken by cesarean section and raised away from the infected bitch, they did not harbor mites, indicating that in utero transmission does not occur.[98, 123] Similarly, mites cannot be demonstrated in stillborn puppies.[114]

Sako[115] found the thermotactic zone of *D. canis* to be between 16 and 41°C. Movement of the mites ceased at environmental temperatures below 15°C. Under various laboratory and artificial conditions, mites could live away from dogs for as long as 37 days.[115] However, these mites lost their ability to infect (invade the hair follicles of) dogs. On a more practical note, once on the surface of the skin, mites are rapidly killed by desiccation in 45 to 60 minutes at 20°C and a relative humidity of 40 per cent.[99]

Types of Demodicosis. Two types of demodicosis are generally recognized: localized and generalized. The course and prognosis of the two types are vastly different.

Localized demodicosis occurs as one or more small, circumscribed, erythematous, scaly nonpruritic-to-pruritic areas of alopecia, most commonly on the face and forelegs (Fig. 8:27). The course is benign and most cases usually resolve spontaneously.

Generalized demodicosis covers large areas of the body, but especially the head and legs. It can be further divided into (1) juvenile onset (3 to 12 months), (2) adult onset (usually over five years), and (3) chronic demodectic pododermatitis (pododemodicosis).

Most cases of generalized demodicosis start as local lesions in young dogs. If lesions do not undergo spontaneous remission or receive adequate treatment, the patient carries the disease into adulthood. A careful case history should reveal the date of onset.

Adult-onset generalized demodicosis is rare, but when it occurs it can be as serious as the juvenile form. It has been observed to start in dogs as old as 14 years. Internal disease or malignant neoplasia is often diagnosed in adult-onset demodicosis patients within a year of the onset of the generalized demodectic lesions. In these cases, the dog has tolerated and controlled the demodectic mites as part of its normal cutaneous fauna for years. If resistance of the host decreases, the mites suddenly multiply by the thousands. One can speculate that some internal diseases may cause immunosuppression or otherwise lower the dog's capacity to control the number of mites, and adult-onset demodicosis occurs. Owners need to be warned that even if the generalized demodicosis is cured, the dog must be observed carefully for major systemic illnesses and malignant neoplasia.

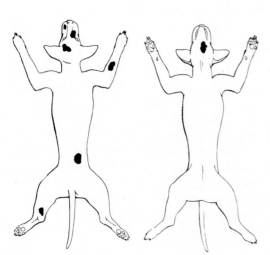

Figure 8:27. Localized demodicosis distribution pattern.

> *Adult-onset demodicosis is often followed by cancer or internal disease.*

In pododemodicosis, the disease is confined to the paws. This can occur as a result of generalized demodicosis, in which the lesions heal everywhere except on the paws. The foot can also be involved, especially in Old English sheepdogs, without generalized lesions having been observed previously. The digital, interdigital, and plantar involvements are almost always complicated by secondary bacterial infections (Fig. 8:31F,H).

> *A skin scraping for demodectic mites MUST be made in all skin diseases of the feet and in all pyodermas and seborrheas.*

Demodicosis may occasionally occur as an erythematous, ceruminous otitis externa. Microscopic examination of ear wax or scrapings of the external ear canal reveal numerous demodectic mites.

Certain breeds seem to be predisposed to generalized demodicosis. Four long-haired breeds in this category are the Old English sheepdog, the collie, the Afghan hound, and the German shepherd. Adult-onset demodicosis occurs in cocker spaniels in larger numbers than would be expected. The following short-coated breeds also seem to be predisposed: Staffordshire terriers, pit bull terriers, Doberman pinschers, Dalmations, Great Danes, English bulldogs, Boston terriers, dachshunds, Chihuahuas, boxers, pugs, Chinese Shar Pei, beagles, and pointers. Short-haired breeds and brachiocephalic breeds top the list of those susceptible. Demodicosis is extremely rare in poodles. Purebred dogs have a much higher incidence than do mongrels.[119]

A hereditary predisposition has been observed regularly in breeding kennels. Certain breeders can predict which litters will develop the disease. In an affected litter, all or some of the siblings develop generalized demodicosis. Elimination of affected or "carrier" dogs (both parents and siblings) from a breeding program greatly reduces or eliminates the incidence of demodicosis in that population of dogs. By following this strict culling program, some kennels have virtually eliminated the disease from their line of breeding.

> *The tendency to develop generalized demodicosis seems to be hereditary.*

Other predisposing factors suggested for demodicosis include age, short hair, poor nutrition, estrus, parturition, stress, endoparasites, and debilitating diseases. Most of these factors are difficult to evaluate and many are highly unlikely. Length of hair coat, size and activity of sebaceous glands, sex, hypothyroidism, and biotin deficiency have been shown to have no effect on the development or progression of demodicosis.[123] In fact, the great majority of clinical cases are seen in purebred dogs that are on excellent diets and otherwise in generally good condition.

Immunology of Demodicosis

Scott[119] has summarized the immune aspects of demodicosis as follows:

Recently, much attention has been given to the link between the major histocompatibility complex (and presumably the immune response gene) in humans and certain disease states, such as pemphigus vulgaris, atopic disease, diabetes mellitus, and dermatitis herpetiformis. This fascinating field of immunogenetics is in its infancy in veterinary medicine. Preliminary results of D–LA typing in normal dogs and dogs with demodicosis indicate that there may be a link,[55] again pointing to the importance of genetics and the immune response. It is likely that such immunogenetics would explain the association of factor VII deficiency in beagles (autosomal incomplete dominant inheritance) and a reported apparent predisposition to demodicosis.[34]

That the immune response plays a vital role in the development of demodicosis is irrefutable. Demodicosis has been produced in dogs with antilymphocyte serum,[123] azathioprine,[104] and long-term, high-dosage corticosteroids.[118] In addition, the authors have seen the sudden onset of demodicosis in the older dog, which is unlikely to be genetically determined. In these instances, underlying diseases of potentially immunosuppressive nature have been discovered, i.e., malignant neoplasia, liver disease, hyperadrenocorticism, dirofilariasis. Correction of these underlying conditions, where possible, has resulted in resolution of the demodicosis. It is interesting to speculate on the role of the known natural decline in cell-mediated immune responsiveness of the older canine patient in demodicosis of the older dog.

Studies of immunocompetence in canine demodicosis have been directed at nonspecific immunity, humoral immunity (B cell), and cell-mediated immunity (T cell).

Nonspecific Immunity. Nonspecific immunity in canine demodicosis has been studied only from the standpoint of the neutrophil. No absolute deficiences of neutrophils or abnormalities in neutrophil morphology have been observed.[123, 124] Two indices of neutrophil function—the nitroblue tetrazolium dye reduction test and the bactericidal assay—have been normal in the dogs examined by one of the authors (D.W.S.). Other aspects of nonspecific immunity, such as serum complement, have not been studied.

Humoral Immunity. Dogs with generalized demodicosis, when injected with a novel antigen such as Aleutian mink disease virus, develop antibody titers that are quantitatively similar to those developed in normal dogs.[31] In addition, the patients with demodicosis who were examined by Scott have had normal titers against canine distemper and infectious canine hepatitis viruses. Unvaccinated dogs with generalized demodicosis also develop normal antibody titers when vaccinated with canine distemper–infectious canine hepatitis vaccine.

Scott also observed that plasma cells (derived from B lymphocytes) are present in normal or (more commonly) elevated numbers in various tissues (skin, bone marrow, lymph nodes, spleen, blood) of dogs with demodicosis. Examination of lymph node and spleen from dogs with demodicosis has revealed no hypocellularity (rather, *hyper*cellularity) of B-cell areas.

Cellulose acetate serum protein electrophoresis in dogs with generalized demodicosis has revealed consistent elevations in the α_2- and β-globulin fractions.[123] Elevations in the γ-globulin fraction have been less consistent, and have usually accompanied secondary deep pyoderma. The significance of these nonspecific changes is not known.

Direct immunofluorescence testing was used to study skin biopsies from dogs with demodicosis and from specific-pathogen–free dogs. The numbers of cutaneous mast cells with demonstrable IgE were identical in the two groups of dogs.[61]

Thus, no evidence of humoral immunodeficiency has been gathered in dogs with generalized demodicosis. In fact, their B-cell responses appear to be excessive.

In view of the state of T-cell suppression known to exist in dogs with chronic generalized demodicosis (to be discussed), this overactivity of the B-cell system may be the result of loss of suppressor T-cell function, as is seen in systemic lupus erythematosus.

Cellular Immunity. Dogs with chronic generalized demodicosis have severely depressed T-cell responses, as measured by in vitro lymphocytic blastogenesis (IVLB) to various mitogens (phytohemagglutinin, concanavalin A, pokeweed mitogen).[31, 32, 63, 123, 124] As these dogs rarely have lymphopenia[123, 124] and have no hypocellularity of the T-cell areas of lymph nodes and spleen, this T-cell defect would appear to be suppression, rather than deficiency. Therapeutic eradication of the mites results in restoration of T-cell function.[123, 124] Thus, the demonstrated T-cell suppression is associated with the large population of mites.

When the suppressed cells from dogs with demodicosis are washed and cultured in a medium that is free of autologous serum, IVLB responses are normal.[31, 32, 63, 124] In addition, when normal dog lymphocytes are cultured with the serum from dogs that have generalized demodicosis and depressed IVLB responses, the IVLB responses in normal cells are suppressed.[63, 124] Thus, the T-cell suppression is associated with a humoral immunosuppressive factor. Hirsh and associates[63] demonstrated that this serum factor is not cortisol. This serum immunosuppressive factor also disappears as the mites are eradicated, indicating that it, too, is associated with the large number of mites.[63, 117, 124] The immunosuppressive factor appears to be in the B-globulin fraction of serum.[73]

Corbett and colleagues[31, 32] employed a lymphocyte membrane fluorescence technique, using rabbit antidog whole globulin, and found that the lymphocytes from dogs with generalized demodicosis exhibited a greater than twofold increase in the number of fluorescing cells, compared with normal dog lymphocytes. Similar results were obtained with rabbit anti-dog IgG. When the lymphocytes from dogs with generalized demodicosis were trypsinized and reincubated for 24 hours, they exhibited a 50 per cent decrease in number of fluorescing cells, and a 20 per cent increase in IVLB responses. These results could suggest that the serum immunosuppressive factor is serum immunoglobulin or antigen-antibody complex.

These findings indicate that chronic generalized demodicosis is accompanied by a state of severe T-cell suppression. However, both the T-cell suppression and the serum immunosuppressive factor disappear when the mites are eradicated. Thus, the demonstrated immunodeficiency state is *secondary* to the disease and *is not* the *cause* of the disease. This is confirmed by the fact that dogs with localized demodicosis and early generalized demodicosis have normal IVLB responses and no serum immunosuppressive factor.[31, 124]

Barta and associates[12] studied lymphocyte function in a limited number of dogs with uncomplicated demodicosis, with demodicosis complicated by pyoderma and with pyoderma alone. There was a good correlation between the extent of pyoderma (with or without demodicosis) and the degree of suppression of lymphocyte blastogenesis caused by serum from each dog. None of three dogs with uncomplicated demodicosis had detectable suppression of blastogenesis by the serum. These workers concluded that the suppressive factor in the serum was a consequence of pyoderma and not the mites. However, few cases were studied and absolute numbers of mites were not considered, a factor that might have an influence on the degree of suppression. (Complicated cases are usually teeming with mites, while uncomplicated cases characteristically have fewer mites in less extensive areas of the body.) Further investigation of this observation is necessary.

Results of intradermal skin testing have shown that dogs have depressed delayed-type hypersensitivity responses to phytohemagglutinin and concanavalin A[62, 123] and dinitrochlorobenzene.[32] Intradermal skin tests with phytohemagglutinin were used to identify Doberman pinscher puppies that were predisposed to demodicosis.[140] Of special interest is the finding that dogs with generalized demodicosis fail to respond to intradermal challenge with a crude demodex antigen, whereas normal dogs and dogs that spontaneously recover from demodicosis have good delayed-type hypersensitivity responses.[14, 31, 32]

Consideration of the above findings—the genetic predilection, the unresponsiveness to demodex mite antigen, the secondary T-cell suppression by a serum immunosuppressive factor associated with the large number of mites, and the hyper-responsive B-cell system—suggests an attractive hypothesis on the pathomechanism of generalized demodicosis in most dogs:

> *Generalized demodicosis is the manifestation of a hereditary, specific T-cell defect for* **Demodex canis**, *wherein the mite is allowed to multiply to large numbers and induce a humoral substance (mite antigen-antibody complex?) that causes generalized T-cell suppression (cell-mediated immunodeficiency).*

Clinical Features

Localized Demodicosis. A patch of skin develops mild erythema and partial alopecia. Pruritus may or may not be present, and the area may be covered with fine silvery scales. One to several squamous patches can be present (Fig. 8:27). The most common site is the face, especially the periocular area and the commissures of the mouth (Fig. 8:28A). Next, in order of occurrence, are the forelegs. More rarely, one or more patches are seen on the trunk or rear legs. Most cases occur at 3 to 6 months of age and heal spontaneously without treatment, but a few early cases (up to 10 per cent) progress to the generalized form.[76] When the disease is controlled, hair will begin to regrow within 30 days. Subsequently, recurrences are rare because the skin has apparently become a less favorable habitat for the rapid reproduction of mites or the immunocompetence of the host has returned to normal.

Generalized Demodicosis. Although localized demodicosis is a mild clinical disease, generalized demodicosis is one of the most severe canine skin diseases; it can terminate fatally. The disease begins as a localized case, but instead of improving it becomes worse. Numerous lesions appear on the head, legs, and trunk (Fig. 8:29). Each macule gets larger, and some coalesce to form patches (see Fig. 8:31E). Mites developing in the hair follicle produce a folliculitis (Fig. 8:30). Peripheral lymphadenopathy is marked. When secondary pyoderma complicates these lesions, edema and crusting elevate the patches into plaques. Deep folliculitis develops, and exudates are produced and form thick crusts (Figs. 8:28B and 8:31A,B,E). Bacteria thrive under these crusts and in the follicles. Coagulase-positive *Staphylococcus intermedius* is the most common

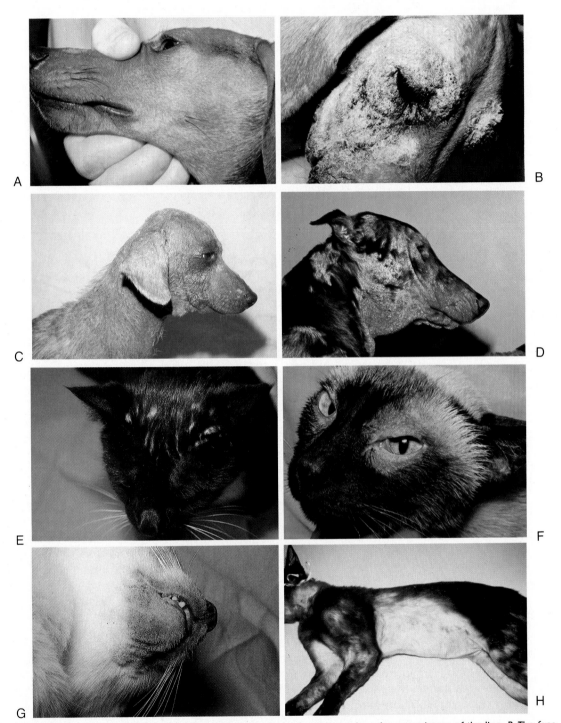

Figure 8:28. Demodicosis. *A,* Localized demodicosis. A single alopecic patch at the commissure of the lips. *B,* The face of a dachshund with chronic pyogenic demodicosis. *C,* Crossbred dog with classic chronic generalized demodicosis. Note hyperpigmentation. *D,* A nine-month-old Doberman pinscher whose once beautiful face is disfigured by the effects of the disease. The loose fold of skin at the throat containing numerous pustules is characteristic. *E,* Feline demodicosis. Alopecia and scaling of forehead and ears. *F,* Demodicosis in a cat. Only the eyelids and periocular area are affected. Infections with *Demodex cati* are usually mild. *G,* Feline demodicosis. Alopecia and hyperpigmentation of chin and lips. *H,* Bilaterally symmetric alopecia in a cat with generalized demodicosis. (Courtesy B. Stein.)

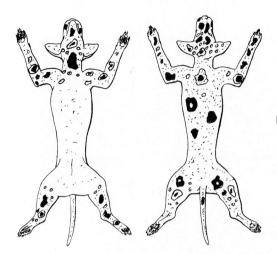

Figure 8:29. Generalized demodicosis distribution pattern.

bacterial organism to complicate generalized demodicosis. *Pseudomonas aeruginosa* causes severe pyogenic complications and is especially refractory when it occurs with demodectic pododermatitis. *Proteus mirabilis* is another serious secondary bacterial invader in generalized demodectic mange.

After several months, the chronically infected skin is covered with crusted, pyogenic, hemorrhagic, and follicular-furuncular lesions (Figs. 8:28*D* and 8:31*B,E*). The abdomen is least affected, perhaps because fewer hair follicles are in that area. Numerous lesions are concentrated on the head and neck, and involvement may be severe. Many owners elect euthanasia for their pets at this stage.

Pododemodicosis. Demodicosis can be present on the feet of dogs without generalized lesions. The case history reveals whether the dog once had generalized demodicosis that healed, all except the foot lesions, or whether the paws were the only part of the body ever affected. The digital and interdigital lesions are especially susceptible to secondary pyodermas (Fig. 8:31*F,H*). In some individuals, pododemodicosis can be chronic and extremely resistant to therapy. The pain and edema is especially distressing to large dogs such as Great Danes, Newfoundlands, St. Bernards, or Old English sheepdogs.

In summary, one dog can progress through the following stages: localized demodicosis, generalized demodicosis, generalized pyogenic demodicosis, and/or chronic pyogenic pododemodicosis.

Diagnosis

Skin scrapings, properly made and interpreted, are diagnostic of demodicosis. The affected skin should be squeezed to help extrude the mites from the hair follicles, and skin scrapings should be deep and extensive. Diagnosis is made either by the demonstration of large numbers of adult mites or by finding an increased ratio of immature forms (ova, larvae, and nymphs) to adults. The demonstration of an occasional adult mite in skin scrapings is consistent with a diagnosis of normal skin, *not* demodicosis. It would seem that skin scraping is a straightforward, easy laboratory procedure; however, every year the authors continue to receive cases on referral that were somehow negative on scraping and were misdiagnosed. *Adequate skin scrapings are mandatory in all cases of canine pyoderma and seborrhea complex.* When negative skin scrapings are obtained from a Shar Pei or from a dog with interdigital pyoderma, a skin biopsy specimen should be examined before demodicosis is ruled out.

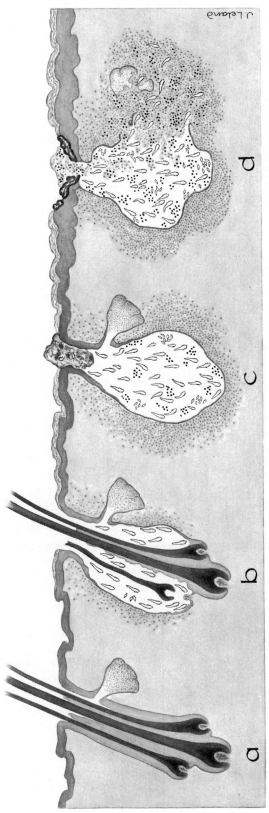

Figure 8:30. Demodicosis dermogram. *a,* Normal multiple hair follicle with sebaceous gland. *b,* Localized demodicosis. One hair follicle is shown with a small colony of *Demodex canis.* A few eggs are seen, and one accessory hair is degenerating and partly broken. A very mild perifollicular infiltrate develops as the follicle dilates. *c,* Pustule formation in *generalized pyogenic demodicosis* (folliculitis). The hairs are gone, and a comedo consisting of keratin, sebum, debris, and dead mites plugs the follicular orifice. The ballooning hair follicle accommodates the expanding mite colony, which is packed with numerous adult mites, immature forms, and eggs. The clusters of black dots represent *staphylococci* that have invaded the hair follicle. *d,* The ballooned hair follicle ruptures and transforms into a pustule and later into an intradermal abscess (furunculosis). (Figure 8:28G shows many gross lesions in this stage.) The sebaceous gland disintegrates. At this stage there is exudation through the follicular orifice. Some abscesses break through the epidermis separately. The epidermis is acanthotic, hyperkeratotic, and crusted. Thousands of similar lesions produce the clinical appearance of generalized pustular demodicosis.

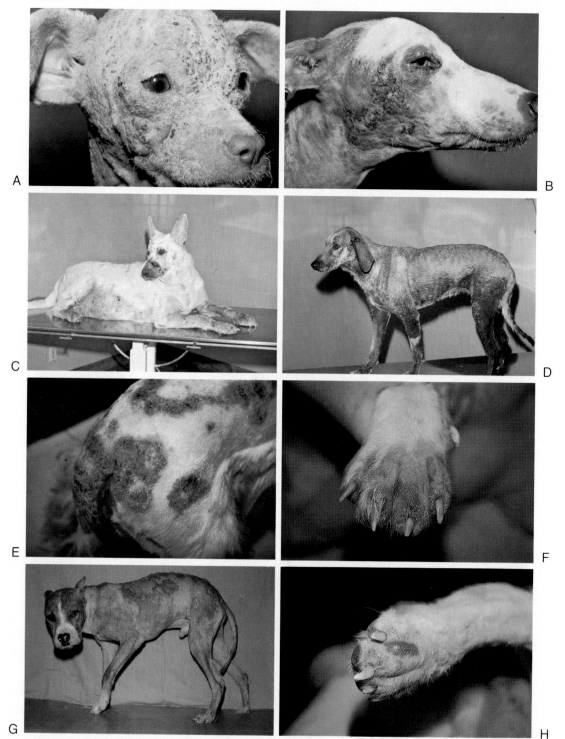

Figure 8:31. Demodicosis. *A,* Chihuahua showing extensive erythema, alopecia, and crusting typical of generalized demodicosis with pyoderma. *B,* Whippet with acute pyoderma of face, lips, and eyelids secondary to generalized demodicosis. *C,* Typical distribution of lesions of face and extremities in generalized demodicosis. *D,* Hound-cross with chronic generalized demodicosis. *E,* Well-demarcated, alopecic crusted patches of generalized demodicosis with pyoderma on the rump of a West Highland white terrier. These lesions are not easily recognized unless the hair is clipped away. *F,* Canine pododemodicosis. Erythema, alopecia, hyperpigmentation of a paw. *G,* Pit bull terrier–cross with chronic generalized demodicosis and typical distribution pattern. *H,* Canine pododemodicosis. Pododermatitis and one large hemorrhagic bulla (*Proteus* sp. furuncle).

388

Evaluation of the hemogram of dogs with generalized demodicosis has shown that over 50 per cent of these dogs have a normocytic or normochronic, nonregenerative anemia. This is consistent with chronic disease and infection, and certainly is not specific for generalized demodicosis. In addition, over 50 per cent of dogs with generalized demodicosis may have low baseline levels of serum thyroxine (T_4) and triiodothyronine (T_3). Thyroid-stimulating hormone (TSH) response tests in these dogs are usually normal, and the patients are *not* hypothyroid. The low T_4/T_3 baseline levels are secondary to the chronic dermatitis (see euthyroid sick syndrome p. 578).

Histopathology. Skin biopsy reveals varying degrees of perifolliculitis, folliculitis, and furunculosis.[119, 124] Affected follicles are filled with demodectic mites, keratinous debris, and variable numbers and types of inflammatory cells. Secondary bacterial infection (intraepidermal pustular dermatitis, folliculitis-furunculosis) is common (Figs. 8:32 and 8:33).

Dogs with localized demodicosis or generalized demodicosis that spontaneously regresses usually have perifollicular and periglandular cellular reactions that include numerous lymphoid cells. Dogs with generalized demodicosis and secondary cell-mediated immunosuppression exhibit two histopathologic stages: a stage of minimal-to-absent cellular response, in which mites are confined to hair follicles; and a stage of extensive cellular response, in which follicular rupture occurs and mites are released into the dermis to act as foreign bodies.

Differential Diagnosis. Since skin scrapings easily reveal mites in cases of demodicosis, the disease is seldom confused with others. However, it is important to remember that a few mites (usually without eggs or immature forms) can be found in some normal skin or in skin scrapings from animals with other diseases. This is especially true of scrapings made on dogs' faces.

Generalized pyoderma may resemble demodicosis, and every folliculitis case should be suspect. Dermatophytosis resembles patches of localized,

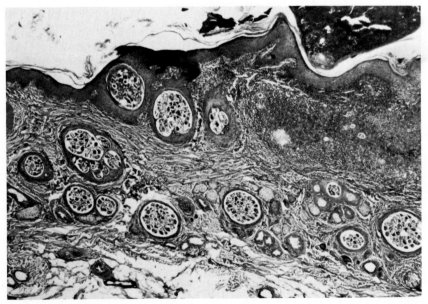

Figure 8:32. Demodicosis in a dog. Note hair follicles containing numerous mite segments and a pyogranuloma due to follicular rupture in the upper right.

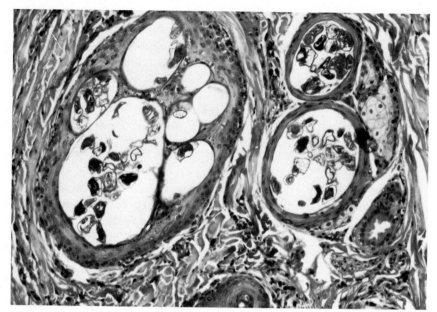

Figure 8:33. Demodicosis in a dog. Note numerous mite segments within hair follicles.

squamous demodicosis. Differentiation is made by skin scrapings, KOH preparations, mycotic culture, and Wood's light. Superficial abrasions in young
dogs sometimes resemble the erythematous patches of localized demodicosis.
Conversely, demodicosis may be mistaken for abrasions. Acne on the face of
young dogs sometimes resembles pustular demodicosis, and certain demodectic
pustules on the abdomen and inside surface of the thighs resemble canine acne
lesions. Differentiation can be made by examination of skin scrapings or by
biopsy. Contact dermatitis exhibits erythematous papules that occasionally
resemble pustular demodicosis. Localized seborrheic dermatitis may closely
resemble squamous demodicosis. Pemphigus complex and dermatomyositis
facial lesions can also mimic demodicosis.

Clinical Management

Localized Demodicosis. This is a mild disease that usually heals spontaneously in a few weeks. One study showed no difference in healing, between
treated and untreated cases.[119] There is no evidence that treatment of localized
demodicosis prevents generalization in cases so destined. If the clinician
believes that some form of topical treatment is indicated, a mild rotenone
ointment (Goodwinol ointment), lindane and benzyl benzoate lotion, or benzoyl
peroxide gel (OxyDex Gel, Pyoben Gel) can be gently massaged into the
alopecic area once a day. The medication should be rubbed in the direction of
the hair growth so that as few as possible hairs are pulled out. The owner
should be informed that rubbing will remove hairs and to expect the alopecic
area to be larger after a few treatments. This will not affect the outcome of the
disease, as the lesions only *appear* to be getting larger. It is important to check
the general health status of the dog at this time, paying special attention to
diet, endoparasite problems, and vaccination needs. Amitraz is *not* a rational
treatment for localized demodicosis when 90 per cent of the cases will clear
spontaneously. Do not risk developing resistant mites.

At a return visit 4 weeks later, the veterinarian can determine if there is
any indication of generalized demodicosis. The skin scraping at the beginning

of localized demodicosis often reveals numerous live adult mites and immature forms. After 4 weeks of treatment, skin scrapings from healing cases should show fewer mites, fewer immature forms, and sometimes no live mites. If the lesions are spreading and the mite count (including the ratio of immature to adult) is high, the dog should be treated for generalized demodicosis. Regional or generalized lymphadenopathy is a poor prognostic finding and often foretells generalized demodicosis.

Many drugs receive credit for demodicosis cures that in reality are spontaneous recoveries.

Generalized Demodicosis. This serious disease is difficult to treat. The owner of the afflicted dog must be made aware of this and informed of the estimated length and cost of treatment, as well as the prognosis for a clinical cure. Euthanasia, commonly resorted to in the past, is rarely necessary if a dedicated owner will use modern remedies. This does not mean that treatment is easy or foolproof, but 94 per cent of the cases of one author (G.H.M.) recovered completely. Most of the remaining cases could be controlled, almost lesion-free, with monthly or bimonthly maintenance treatments. Many owners accept this regimen as an acceptable price for salvaging their pet's lives.

A discussion of euthanasia before outlining the treatment may seem strange, but it is necessary because the prognosis of generalized demodicosis has improved dramatically in the past 5 years. First, approximately 30 to 50 per cent of all dogs with generalized demodicosis under 1 year of age recover spontaneously with or without treatment. Early treatment is desirable but does not seem to influence spontaneous recovery. To euthanize 6- to 12-month-old dogs because they have severe generalized demodicosis is unwarranted, since many of them will recover spontaneously if secondary pyodermas and seborrheas are controlled and the general health status is good. Dogs over 2 years of age or with adult-onset generalized demodicosis have a much less favorable prognosis. The disease can often be controlled but not always cured.

Amitraz has made the treatment of generalized demodicosis much easier. The drug is diamide, N^1 (2,4-dimethylphenyl)–N–[[(2,4-dimethylphenyl) imino]methyl]–N–methylmethanidamide. It is marketed in the United States as Mitaban. Slightly different formulations of amitraz are presently marketed in England as Ectodex Dog Wash or Taktic, which are reported to be highly potent acaricides.[24, 25, 38] One of the authors (G.H.M.) has investigated this drug since 1977 and has used it on over 400 dogs with generalized demodicosis.[94] None had localized demodicosis, and many were in extremely advanced stages of the disease (see Figs. 8:32 and 8:33). Over 86 per cent of all cases completely recovered with only four to eight topical treatments. The remaining 14 per cent were kept in good condition by periodic maintenance treatments every 2, 4, or 8 weeks. Many of these dogs, also, may eventually achieve permanent cure.

To achieve maximum results with amitraz as formulated for use in the United States, it is imperative to follow this protocol:

1. Clip the dog's entire hair coat to allow the aqueous solution to contact the skin better and attain excellent skin coverage.

2. Remove all crusts. In some cases, tranquilization or anesthesia is necessary, because some crusts adhere tightly and removal without anesthesia would be painful.

3. Apply protective ophthalmic ointment to the eyes. Wash the entire dog with a medicated shampoo designed to kill bacteria and remove scales and exudates (Betadine, Nolvasan, Sebbafon, pHisoderm, or LyTar). Soaking in a whirlpool bath or a gentle stream of water is beneficial. Even though the skin may appear raw and irritated after the above procedures, the medication now will have optimum contact with the affected skin. Gently dry the dog with a towel. Alternatively, the cleansing preparation can be done the day before treatment.

4. Apply amitraz solution (Mitaban) by wetting and sponging. The solution must be applied to the entire body—to normal as well as to affected areas of skin. Although the solution is not irritating, *it is mandatory for persons applying amitraz to wear protective gloves and work in a well-ventilated area*. Amitraz causes a transitory sedative effect for 12 to 24 hours, especially after the first treatment, but has no other apparent side-effects. Owners should be warned to expect the mild sedation in treated dogs. One of the authors (D.W.S.) has seen two dogs with severe generalized demodicosis develop severe edema associated with pain and pyrexia in areas of affected skin within a few hours after being dipped with amitraz. This persisted for 2 to 4 days. One dog was euthanized after 48 hours, while the other dog recovered with symptomatic therapy. In the dog that recovered, subsequent dips with amitraz did not produce side-effects.

Healing begins immediately as the mites are killed and new hair grows rapidly. In 4 to 10 weeks, the new hair coat is glossy and normal. If there is pododemodicosis, the paws can be immersed in a small pan containing amitraz solution and gently massaged to facilitate penetration. Do not rinse. The medication should remain on the skin for 2 weeks. Although about half the drug is retained in the skin for 2 weeks, some may be lost if the dog gets wet or swims.[127] In this case, a new application may be given before the next treatment is due.

5. Blow dry the dog.

6. Although it is not necessary to repeat clipping and shampooing before each treatment, it makes sense to remove any new crusts before each treatment. As a general rule, a thorough bath the day *before* each treatment will speed penetration of the amitraz and avoid dilution resulting from the dog being too wet from a same-day bath.

7. Continue the amitraz applications every 2 weeks until two successive biweekly skin scrapings fail to reveal live demodectic mites.

8. Four weeks after the last treatment, the dog should be returned for re-evaluation. This should include multiple skin scrapings from the most severely affected lesions. Relapses are not common but occur in about 10 per cent of the cases. In dogs with disease that relapses, the above protocol is repeated. Estrus and pregnancy can trigger a relapse; therefore, all recovered females should be spayed. The procedure is also highly recommended to eliminate this heritable disease from the breeding program. *Do not use recovered animals as breeders.*

The preceding description outlines the protocol to be followed using the product approved by the FDA for use in the United States. It is applied in a concentration of 250 ppm. While it seems that this drug is undoubtedly the most effective treatment available today, there is still world-wide debate concerning the best way to use it and the prognosis for cure. Scott and Walton treated 17 dogs with generalized demodicosis, and although six responded initially, all relapsed within 10 months.[126] White and Stannard,[139] and Kwochka and coworkers[77] reported slightly over 50 per cent cures in a series of animals followed for 3 years. Kwochka had much better results in a second series of patients by doubling the frequency of treatment to once weekly. Bussieras,[25] who has used the drug for 7 years, believes it is an exceptionally effective and safe treatment for generalized demodicosis if applied weekly by sponging on the entire body at concentrations of 500 to 1000 ppm (frequency and levels not FDA approved in the United States). Thus, it seems that the concentration of the drug and the frequency of application have much to do with successful treatment. It is also apparent that some dogs respond clinically but are never clear of the mites and must be treated regularly every 2 to 4 weeks for the rest of their lives to remain well. This possibility should be explained to owners before treatment starts, but not with such emphasis as to encourage euthanasia. If regular long-term therapy is necessary, it may be a happier solution than euthanasia. Recently a polyvinyl collar impregnated with 9 per cent amitraz was reported to be effective for the treatment of canine demodicosis.[47a] As the majority of the treated dogs were 1 year of age or less and had localized demodicosis, the results must be interpreted cautiously.

Ivermectin, 400 μg/kg administered subcutaneously, once weekly for 8 weeks, has been shown to be without benefit for demodicosis.[126]

Vitamin E given orally at 200 mg per dog, five times daily for 6 weeks, was reported to cause improvement in 141 of 143 dogs with generalized demodicosis. The dogs were found to have vitamin E serum levels significantly lower than normal, and vitamin E deficiency is known to suppress lymphocyte function.[41] These therapeutic results were not duplicated in another trial.[91]

Antibacterial therapy. When pustules (folliculitis-furunculitis) are present in generalized demodicosis, attention must be directed to the secondary bacterial infection. By far, the most common organism is coagulase-positive *Staphylococcus intermedius*, usually a penicillinase producer (see p. 245). The cephalosporins, erythromycin, lincomycin, oxacillin, and chloramphenicol are often effective (see p. 247). Bactericidal antibiotics are preferable in these immunosuppressed dogs. Cases complicated by *Pseudomonas aeruginosa* are particularly serious and may be fatal. Gentamicin or injectable carbenicillin offers the best therapy for infections caused by *P. aeruginosa*. Penicillin, ampicillin, sulfonamides, and tetracyclines are seldom useful for any of the secondary bacterial dermatoses.

Bacterial complications of demodicosis are benefited during the early treatment stages by daily whirlpool baths with a dilute antiseptic solution of povidone-iodine (Betadine), chlorine, or chlorhexidine (Nolvasan) (see p. 151).

Under no circumstances should systemic corticosteroids be used in cases of generalized demodicosis.

Corticosteroids are contraindicated in patients with demodicosis, since these dogs are immunosuppressed.

In general, hormonal therapy is of no benefit. Thyroid hormone is without effect, unless the patient is truly hypothyroid. Estrogens may decrease sebum and, theoretically, may decrease the mites' food supply, whereas androgens do the opposite and are always contraindicated. These theoretic statements have no clinical application, however. Levamisole and thiabendazole are immunostimulants that have no clinically beneficial effect on generalized demodicosis.

Basically, dogs over 2 years of age are treated using the same procedure as for younger animals, but a longer treatment period may be necessary. Although adult-onset generalized demodicosis is rare, it does occur. The sudden susceptibility to a mite that has been present for years indicates that the dog's resistance has failed. In at least half of all adult-onset cases an internal disease or malignant neoplasm will appear within 6 to 12 months.[90, 119] Long-term immunosuppressive therapy (glucocorticoids, cytotoxic drugs, topical nitrogen mustard) may precipitate demodicosis in adult dogs.

When generalized demodicosis develops in older dogs, internal disease or malignant neoplasms often develop within 1 year.

The owner should be warned of that possibility. General physical examinations with appropriate laboratory work should be given to all dogs with adult-onset demodicosis at the time of diagnosis and repeated at least every 6 months thereafter.

It is strongly recommended not to breed dogs that have recovered from general demodicosis or those that have produced affected pups. It is clear that the tendency to develop this disease is inherited. *The American Academy of Veterinary Dermatology recommends neutering all dogs who have had generalized demodicosis, so that the incidence of the disease is decreased and not perpetuated.*

Advise breeders not to use previously infected or carrier animals for breeding.

FELINE DEMODICOSIS

Feline demodicosis is caused by (1) *Demodex cati* and (2) a species of *Demodex* that has not yet been named.[30, 93]

D. cati is much like *Demodex canis*, with minor taxonomic differences (Fig. 8:26E). The ova are slim and oval (Fig. 8:26F) rather than spindle shaped, and all immature life stages are narrower in *D. cati* than in *D. canis*. It is a rare disease that usually affects the eyelids, periocular area, head, and neck (Fig. 8:28F,G).[50] Lesions are variably pruritic and consist of patchy erythema, scaling, crusting, and alopecia. It is the localized type of demodicosis and is usually self-limiting. Feline demodicosis may also occur as a ceruminous otitis externa.[121] A mild ointment containing rotenone (such as Goodwinol) can be used in treatment on the erythematous, alopecic patches.

Generalized feline demodicosis is very rare and never as severe as the canine form.[141] Cases may be more common in purebred Siamese and Burmese cats.[134] The mites are found primarily on the head, but they may spread from there to the neck and legs. A few lesions may extend to the trunk. The lesions consist of circumscribed macules and patches with alopecia, scaling, erythema, hyperpigmentation, and crusting. Some cats develop generalized lesions. Pruritus is variable. Always make skin scrapings from scaly and pigmented patches on the skin of cats. In two cases, large numbers of mites were found in scrapings of the ear canal of healthy cats.[33] Generalized demodicosis due to D. cati is usually associated with underlying disease: diabetes mellitus,[99, 139a] feline leukemia virus infection, and systemic lupus erythematosus.[87a, 121] One case had raised exudative lesions on the lips and chin.[5] Mites and a staphylococcus were obtained, and the cat had a marked lymphopenia associated with long-term therapy for a respiratory infection. D. cati was isolated from nose lesions in a litter of snow leopards.[42] Although the data are scarce for such a rare disease, clinicians should be aware of its possible association with serious systemic disease. Histologic examination reveals varying degrees of perifolliculitis and folliculitis, with mites in hair follicles, or mild superficial perivascular dermatitis with mites found in surface keratin.

A few cases were reported of animals that recovered in a short time spontaneously or as a result of such mild remedies as topical lime-sulfur dips, carbaryl shampoos, malathion dips, or rotenone in mineral oil (Canex and mineral oil). The apparent ease with which generalized demodicosis can be treated in cats may be explained by the often superficial location of mites in the skin of cats as compared with that in the skin of dogs. Recently, weekly dips with 250 ppm of amitraz have been effective for the treatment of feline demodicosis.[81a]

The other species of mite causing feline demodicosis is unnamed but bears a close taxonomic resemblance to Demodex criceti, which is found in the epidermal pits in the stratum corneum of hamsters.[85, 101] The mites affecting cats are shorter and have broad, blunted abdomens (Fig. 8:26G), unlike the slim, elongated abdomens of D. cati.[30, 142] They are very superficially located and only inhabit the stratum corneum. Skin scrapings of affected skin usually reveal numerous mites.

The clinical signs with the unnamed Demodex sp. may be suggestive of feline scabies, with severe pruritus; alopecic, scaly, excoriated, and crusted lesions are seen, often concentrated on the head, neck, and elbows (Fig. 8:28E). Other cases have multifocal erythema and hyperpigmentation with broken, stubby hairs located on the proximal rear legs, flanks, and ventral abdomen. Some are cases of symmetric alopecia with or without scaling, which mimics feline symmetric alopecia, psychogenic alopecia, or hypersensitivity reactions (Fig. 8:28H).

Histologically, minimal inflammation is observed. The epidermis may be irregularly acanthotic and hyperkeratotic, with mites in the stratum corneum. No mites are found in the hair follicles.

Differential diagnosis of the second type of feline demodicosis must include all feline dermatoses that are associated with excessive grooming such as psychogenic alopecia and dermatitis. It also should include dermatophytosis, feline symmetric alopecia, atopy, food hypersensitivity, feline scabies, contact dermatitis, flea bite hypersensitivity, seborrheic dermatitis and the demodicosis caused by D. cati. Careful skin scrapings are of paramount importance in the work-up for each of these conditions in order to make a proper diagnosis.

The prognosis is favorable, as cases usually respond to simple treatments such as three dips with a solution of malathion or lime-sulfur at weekly intervals. Cats with demodicosis caused by the unnamed mite are usually otherwise healthy.

CANINE SCABIES
(Sarcoptic Mange)

Canine scabies is a nonseasonal, intensely pruritic, transmissible infestation of the skin of dogs caused by the mite *Sarcoptes scabiei* var. *canis*.

Cause and Pathogenesis. The causative mite belongs to the family Sarcoptidae, as does *Notoedres cati*, the cause of feline scabies. Because these mites have much in common, their 17- to 21-day life cycles are presented together (Fig. 8:34). Copulation of adults occurs in a molting pocket on the surface of the skin. The fertilized female excavates a burrow through the horny layer of the skin at a rate of 2 to 3 mm/day and lays eggs in the tunnel behind her (Fig. 8:35). The eggs hatch as larvae and burrow to the surface of the skin, where they travel about feeding and eventually resting in a molting pocket. Nymphs also wander about the skin, but they may stay in the molting pocket until they are mature. Mites prefer skin with little hair, so they are most common on the ears, elbows, abdomen, and hocks. As the disease spreads and hair is lost, they may eventually colonize large areas of the host's body. The entire life cycle may be complete in only 3 weeks.

Adult mites are small (200 to 400 μm), oval, and white with two pairs of short legs anteriorly that bear long unjointed stalks with suckers (Fig. 8:36). The stalks are of medium length in *Notoedres cati* (Fig. 8:37). Two pairs of posterior legs are rudimentary and do not extend beyond the border of the body. The posterior legs carry long bristles, not suckers, although the fourth pair of legs of the male have suckers. The anus of *Sarcoptes canis* is terminal, whereas that of *N. cati* has a dorsal location—an important point of differentiation.

Sarcoptes scabiei var. *canis* mites primarily affect dogs, since they are fairly host specific. However, they can attack other hosts (cat, fox, humans) for periods of time.[37, 60A]

The mites will affect humans who have close contact with infected dogs, and it is possible that the human variety affects dogs.[102] This may explain the

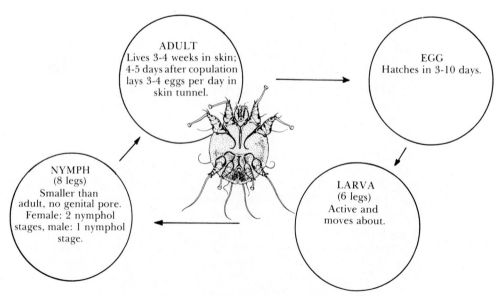

Figure 8:34. Life cycle of sarcoptid mites (17 to 21 days).

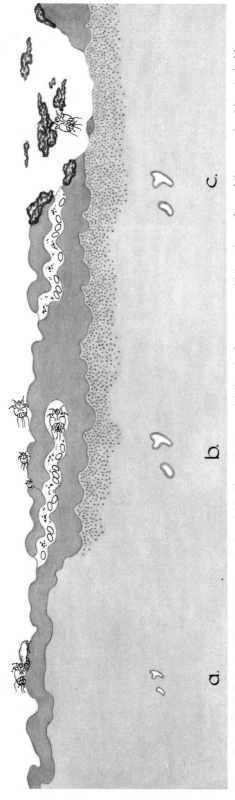

Figure 8:35. Canine scabies dermogram. *a*, An adult male contacts an adult female *Sarcoptes scabiei* on the surface of the normal epidermis. *b*, After mating, the gravid female burrows into the epidermis and tunnels at a rate of about 2 mm per day, leaving behind her ova and fecal pellets. As the eggs hatch, the larvae bore to the surface and form epidermal molting pockets. After molting they emerge as nymphs. The mites' activity causes the skin to react with acanthosis, hyperkeratosis, vascular dilatation, and cellular infiltration of the upper dermis. *c*, Intense pruritus causes self-inflicted excoriations. The mite's burrow is opened by the trauma of scratching, and the female mite is exposed and dies. Loss of mites from this process may be the reason that skin scrapings of abraded tissue fail to reveal mites. Eggs and fecal debris that remain in the burrow continue to cause pruritus, however. Oozing exudates coagulate to form crusts on the surface of the lesion.

disagreement concerning the length of time humans may be infected. Reactions in humans occur within 24 hours after brief direct exposure and are characterized by pruritic papules on the trunk and arms (Fig. 8:38A,B).[130] Pruritus is severe, especially when the skin is warm—as it is in bed at night. Mites burrow but usually remain on the aberrant host for only a few days. The lesions regress spontaneously in 12 to 14 days, if only a few mites were transmitted and contact with affected dogs is terminated. However, with many mites and prolonged repeated contact, the human lesions persist for long periods. Variations in the above syndrome have been reported in which patients did not develop lesions until 3 to 4 days after exposure.[96] This may represent a hypersensitivity reaction, and patients reacting more quickly may have been sensitized previously. In one case, lesions continued to spread for several weeks after animal contacts were removed.[96] Skin scrapings revealed mites and mite eggs, one of which later hatched. In this case the skin lesions were typical of canine scabies in humans, and the mites came from a positive case of canine scabies; thus it would appear that the mite was able to propagate in the human host. (One can speculate, in view of the unusual course, about whether this might have been a case in which human scabies in the dog was returned to its natural host.) There is one report, however, of a child with Norwegian scabies caused by *Sarcoptes scabiei* var. *canis*.[82] Similar mites were found on three dogs in the household and on all other members of the family.

Canine *Sarcoptes* mites can live on human beings for at least 6 days and produce ova during that time.[75] Itching started within 2 hours of experimental implantation of mites, so it is concluded that hypersensitivity was not a factor.[75]

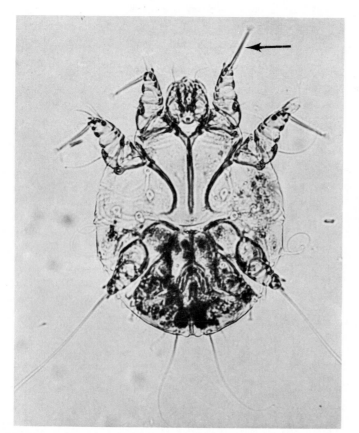

Figure 8:36. Adult *Sarcoptes scabiei* (var. *canis*). Note the long unjointed stalks and suckers.

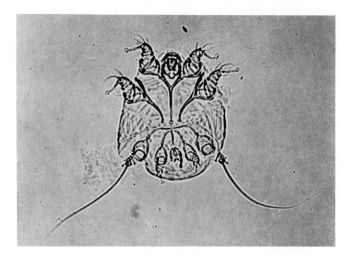

Figure 8:37. Adult *Notoedres cati.* Note the medium length stalks, the striated integument, and the lack of a terminally located anus. The mite is smaller than *Sarcoptes scabiei* (var. *canis*).

In general, human infestations clear spontaneously when the affected dog is removed from contact. The mites are very susceptible to drying and live only a few days off the host. Scabies is highly contagious, and it spreads readily by direct contact. Hospital cages or kennels should be thoroughly cleaned, dried, and sprayed with an insecticide before new animals are placed in them. Animals of all ages, sexes, and breeds are equally susceptible, but artificial age bias may exist for susceptibility of younger dogs due to habitat situations.

Clinical Features. The distribution pattern of canine scabies (Fig. 8:39) typically involves the ventral portions of the abdomen, chest, and legs. The ears and elbows, favorite habitats of mites, are almost always affected and are premier places for obtaining diagnostic scrapings (Figs. 8:38D,F, and 8:40A,B). However, some animals have no ear lesions. The disease spreads rapidly until the entire body may be affected. Alopecia is present, and early skin lesions are characteristic. These are pruritic, reddish papulocrustous eruptions (Fig. 8:38D). Typically, they have thick yellowish crusts, and the intense and constant itching soon produces extensive excoriation. Bleeding, hemorrhagic crusts, and secondary bacterial infection soon follow (Fig. 8:40A,B). These patients are miserable because they are constantly scratching themselves. Itching is thought to be more severe in warm environments (e.g., indoors or by the stove). Anderson[4] reports on a patient that has been on long-term corticosteroid therapy. Variable pruritus and multiple crusts with great numbers of mites were observed. The dog was anemic and had enlarged lymph nodes, a leukocytosis, and a normal number of eosinophils.

Lesions appear shortly after exposure to an affected dog. They spread rather quickly and, unless treated, may progress to involve the entire dog. The course may last weeks or years. Unfortunately, it is often misdiagnosed as an "allergy" and treated only with corticosteroids. In long-term cases hyperpigmentation of the affected skin is common. Most patients also have a general lymphadenopathy.

Canine scabies is a commonly missed dermatologic diagnosis. If you suspect it, treat it.

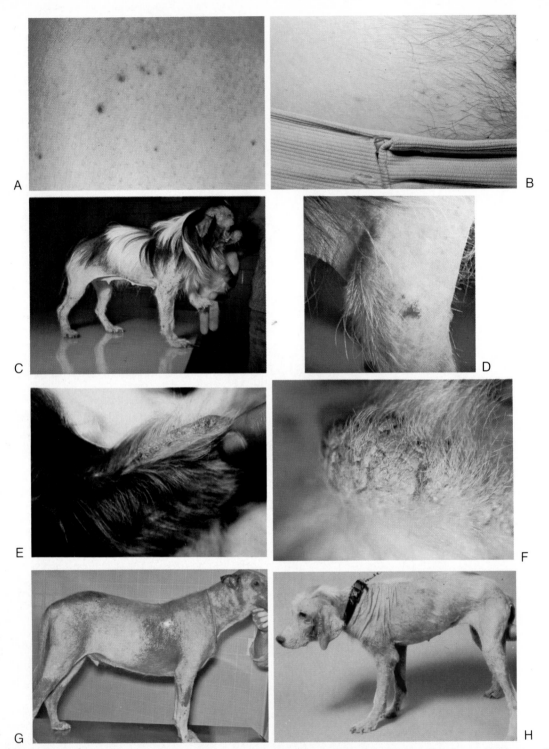

Figure 8:38. Canine scabies. *A*, Crusted papules on human skin (forearm), the typical lesion of canine scabies in man. *B*, Erythematous papules above the belt line characterize the temporary invasions of human skin by *Sarcoptes scabiei* (var. *canis*). *C*, Canine scabies four weeks after onset in Japanese spaniel. Fourteen dogs in a kennel were affected. This illustrates the typical distribution pattern. *D*, Closer view of same patient as in *C*, showing area on elbow where diagnostic skin scraping was made. The typical papular "rash" is well illustrated in this view. *E*, Ear margin showing characteristic grayish yellow crusts on affected skin. *F*, Crusted lesions on the elbow that are typical of a chronic case. *G*, Clipped collie responding to treatment shows hyperpigmented reactions (black) in areas of chronic lesions of canine scabies. *H*, Generalized erythema and alopecia of dog with extensive scabies.

400

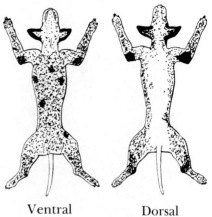

Ventral   Dorsal

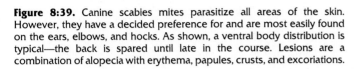

Figure 8:39. Canine scabies mites parasitize all areas of the skin. However, they have a decided preference for and are most easily found on the ears, elbows, and hocks. As shown, a ventral body distribution is typical—the back is spared until late in the course. Lesions are a combination of alopecia with erythema, papules, crusts, and excoriations.

Many clinicians rub the dog's ear flap on itself. In cases with ear lesions the hind leg scratch reflex will be stimulated. This is a sign suggestive of sarcoptic mange.

Scabies incognito is a puzzling syndrome of canine scabies that occurs in meticulously groomed, pampered dogs. They scratch incessantly and have few, if any, real lesions other than mild erythema and occasional excoriations. They are often treated for an "allergy" with systemic corticosteroids but without benefit. These dogs have had scabies ever since they came in contact with an infected dog or environment, but mites are not found in skin scrapings. Thorough grooming may have removed superficial mites and crusts, so only a few mites remain—enough to cause pruritus, but too few to find. These dogs respond rapidly and dramatically to proper antiscabies therapy.

Diagnosis. Sarcoptic mites are difficult to find, and therefore multiple deep scrapings are indicated. For scraping, choose skin sites that have not been excoriated. In these areas look for red, raised papules with yellowish crusts on top (Fig. 8:40*B*). Look for lesion on the ears and elbows, since these are areas preferred by the mites, and make 10 to 15 extensive scrapings. Collect large amounts of material, spread on slides with mineral oil and carefully examine every field. One mite or its dark brown oval fecal pellets are diagnostic (Fig. 8:40*C,D*). In about one-half of the cases, no mites will be found,[102] but if the clinical features are suggestive, make a presumptive diagnosis of canine scabies and treat for that disease. One of the best diagnostic aids is the prompt response to therapy. Other laboratory aids are of less significance, but a few patients will have mites in the feces, and a few will be diagnosed from skin biopsies. A hemogram may reveal eosinophilia and/or nonregenerative anemia.

Histologic examination may be useful but rarely is conclusive, unless actual mites are seen in the biopsy. Always select an active papule, undisturbed by excoriation, as the biopsy specimen. Mites may be found in the superficial epidermis and the stratum corneum. Histopathology reveals varying degrees of superficial perivascular dermatitis (hyperplastic, spongiotic). Mite segments are found rarely within the superficial epidermis (Fig. 8:41). A suggestive histopathologic clue is the presence of focal areas of epidermal edema, exocytosis, degeneration, and necrosis ("nibbles") (Fig. 8:42). Eosinophils vary in number, from few to many. Focal parakeratotic hyperkeratosis is often pronounced.

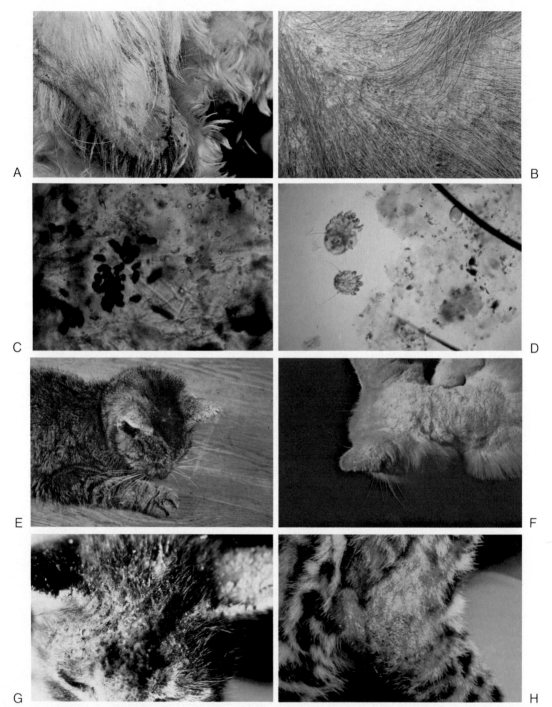

Figure 8:40. Canine scabies: *A,* Margin of the ear (pinna) is a characteristic site. *B,* Grayish crusts on the body mimic seborrheic dermatitis. Hemorrhagic area is from skin scraping (positive). *C, Sarcoptes scabiei* fecal pellets, a diagnostic clue. *D, Sarcoptes scabiei* mites, an egg, and brown fecal pellets. Feline scabies: *E,* Dry, crusted lesions on the edges of the ears and face are typical of feline scabies. *F,* Thickened skin with dry, adherent crusts shown on an area clipped of hair for better visualization. *G,* Severe crusting of face and ears. (Courtesy Dr. Lennox.) *H,* Dry, crusted gray lesions on the skin of the elbow of an ocelot.

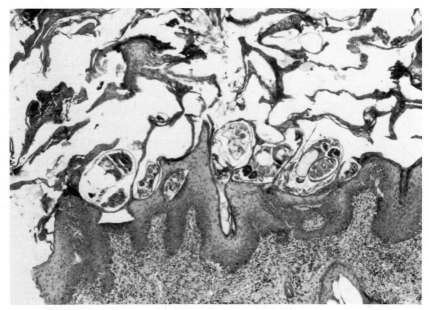

Figure 8:41. Canine scabies. Note mite segments within stratum corneum.

Differential diagnosis should include contact dermatitis, atopy or food hypersensitivity, pelodera dermatitis, pediculosis, cheyletiellosis, otodectic dermatitis, dermatophytosis, seborrheic dermatitis, generalized pyoderma or folliculitis, and bacterial hypersensitivity. Any one of these dermatoses at a particular stage might resemble scabies. Failure to find mites should not eliminate that diagnosis, although doing so is a common mistake. Many such cases are erroneously treated as an allergy. Careful history, physical examina-

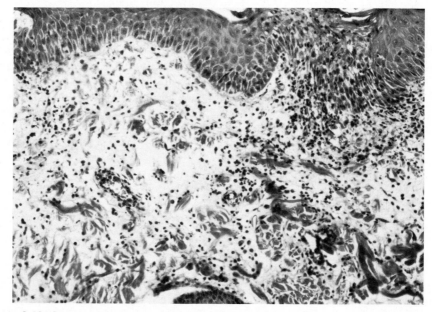

Figure 8:42. Canine scabies. Hyperplastic perivascular dermatitis with focal epidermal necrosis and exocytosis ("nibbles").

tion, or appropriate cultures, biopsy, and scrapings, and especially response to acaricidal dips, usually will satisfactorily resolve the diagnostic problem.

Treatment. The mites must be eradicated. Treatment should be started as soon as the diagnosis is made. This disease is highly contagious in a kennel or hospital! Hair should always be clipped and the patient bathed in an antiseborrheic shampoo to remove crusts and other debris. Then an acaricidal dip should be applied thoroughly and allowed to soak every inch of the skin surface. Spot treatment is ineffective. Particular care should be taken around the ears and eyes; skin in those regions is often severely infected, yet delicate and easily irritated by parasiticidal dips. Systemic corticosteroids in full "antiallergic" doses (1.0 mg/kg prednisone or prednisolone daily) for 2 to 3 days are useful to provide relief from scratching and to stop self-mutilation until the mites are eliminated. Amitraz (Mitaban) has been advocated as an effective miticide, if used three times at 2-week intervals,[43, 44] although it is not licensed for this use in the United States. Other parasiticidal dips such as chlordane and lindane can be used at weekly intervals for 4 to 12 weeks or until 2 weeks after clinical remission, with good results. Organophosphate resistance is an increasing problem in the United States and is the rule in Sweden.[1] Commercial lime-sulfur orchard spray solution is especially safe and effective. It has no residual effect but is miticidal, antifungal, antibacterial, and antipruritic. The last property may be helpful in these cases. The lime-sulfur should be applied warm in a 2 to 3 per cent solution after a cleansing bath and repeated weekly *at least* four times, no matter how rapid and complete the apparent recovery. Some scabies cases may respond dramatically in 24 to 48 hours after the first treatment. This continues so that in 7 to 10 days the lesions are healing nicely. In some cases the pruritus continues for 3 to 4 weeks after therapy has been instituted, probably as a result of hypersensitivity. Therapy should not be stopped too early, because it may take months for a complete response to occur. Treatment is not completed until the last egg has hatched and the last mite has been killed.

A single subcutaneous injection of 200 to 400 µg ivermectin was reported to cure canine scabies.[127a, 145] However, this treatment should be repeated in 2 weeks. Ivermectin is not approved by the FDA for use in the United States for canine scabies. It should *never* be used for collies or Shetland sheep dogs.

In scabies cases, it is important to *treat all animals in contact* or on the premises, as some may be asymptomatic carriers. Although the mites are easily killed by drying when they are off the host a few days, the environment should be cleaned and parasiticidal sprays should be used on kennels, shipping boxes, harnesses, collars, and brushes. Most human lesions derived from canine exposure resolve spontaneously within 4 weeks after the dogs are treated adequately.

FELINE SCABIES
(Notoedric Mange)

Feline scabies is a contagious parasitic disease of cats caused by *Notoedres cati*.

Cause and Pathogenesis. *Notoedres cati* primarily attacks cats but may also infect foxes, dogs, and rabbits. It causes transient lesions in humans.[136] The mites are obligate parasites that survive off the host for only a few days. The disease is highly contagious by direct contact and characteristically affects whole litters and both sexes of adult cats. Affected animals have large numbers of mites, which are easily found on skin scrapings.[65] Notoedric mange appears in epizootics; it is rarely diagnosed in some parts of the country but is endemic and common in a few local areas. It was very common in the 1940s. Perhaps the incidence will increase sometime in the future as the cycle turns up again.

The mite belongs to the family Sarcoptidae, and since its basic life cycle and structure are very similar to that of canine scabies, the two are discussed together on page 396. The main features of taxonomic differentiation for the clinician are that *Notoedres cati* mites are smaller than *Sarcoptes canis* and have medium-length unjointed sucker-bearing stalks on their legs. They also have more body striations and, most important, have a dorsal anus, as compared with the terminal anus of *Sarcoptes*.[51] The abundant mites are much easier to find on skin scrapings than they are in cases of *S. canis*. One city cat with scabies was observed from which one of the authors (R.W.K.) has identified *S. canis* mites. Hawkins and coworkers[60a] have reported a similar case.

Feline scabies is highly contagious and intensely pruritic.

Clinical Features. The distribution is typical (Fig. 8:43). Lesions first appear at the medial proximal edge of the pinna of the ear (Fig. 8:40E). They spread rapidly to the upper ear, face, eyelids, and neck. They also extend to the feet and perineum. This probably results from the cat's habits of washing and of sleeping in a curled position.

Female mites burrow into the horny layer of the epidermis between hair follicles. These burrows appear on the skin surface in the center of minute papules. The skin soon becomes thickened, wrinkled, and folded and later is covered with dense, tightly adhering, yellow-to-gray crusts (Figs. 8:40E to *H*). There is partial alopecia in affected areas. Intense pruritus develops, and the excoriations produced by scratching become secondarily infected. As the disease progresses, the hair loss and skin lesions spread until large areas of the body are involved. Peripheral lymphadenopathy is usually present.

Diagnosis. The distribution of lesions, intense pruritus, and identification of mites are diagnostic features. The differential diagnosis should rule out

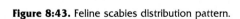
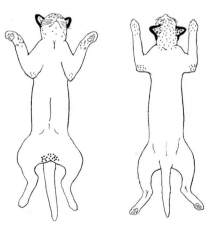

Figure 8:43. Feline scabies distribution pattern.

Otodectes infection, dermatophytosis, cheyletiellosis, pediculosis, atopy, food hypersensitivity, pemphigus foliaceus or erythematosus, systemic lupus erythematosus, and fight wounds of the head and ears. These diagnoses are eliminated by skin scrapings, food exclusion, and a proper history.

Histopathology reveals varying degrees of superficial perivascular dermatitis (hyperplastic, spongiotic). Mite segments may be found within the superficial epidermis (Fig. 8:44). Eosinophils vary in number, from few to many. Focal parakeratotic hyperkeratosis is usually pronounced.

Treatment. Most parasiticidal agents are contraindicated because of extreme toxicity to cats. Sulfur in various forms is usually safe. With the cat under sedation, the hair is clipped from affected areas. The cat is bathed in warm water and soap to loosen scales and debris. A 2.5 per cent warm water solution of commercial lime-sulfur solution (orchard spray) should be applied and allowed to dry on the skin. A slightly better-smelling and cosmetically less objectionable, but less effective, lime-sulfur dip is now commercially available (Lym Dyp). The lime-sulfur dip is repeated 10 and 20 days later. Additional dips should be made until 2 weeks after complete cure. All cats on the premises must be treated, since cats in preclinical stages of the disease might be carriers. The response to treatment is usually rapid and complete, if all cats are thoroughly treated and re-exposure is prevented. Malathion dips are also effective and relatively safe. Wilkinson has reported a single application of 0.025 per cent amitraz to be effective in the treatment of notoedric mange in

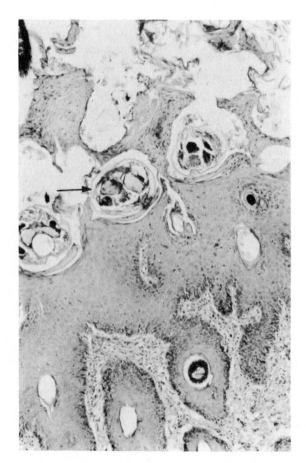

Figure 8:44. Histopathologic section of cat skin with three *Notoedres cati* mites in the stratum corneum. The arrow points to the central mite. Note extensive acanthosis, hyperkeratosis, parakeratosis, prominent rete ridges, and infiltration of inflammatory cells in the superficial dermis. (Courtesy B. Bagnall.)

cats.[141] Bigler and associates treated 17 cats with ivermectin (1.0 mg/kg given subcutaneously). All cats were cured by a single injection, and there were no side-effects.[16] Amitraz and ivermectin are *not* approved for use on cats in the United States.

Spiders

Spiders are arachnids that inhabit woodpiles, old buildings, and refuse areas. The four species of spiders that are medically important in the United States are the black widow (*Latrodectus mactans*), the red-legged widow (*Latrodectus bishopi*), the brown recluse (*Loxosceles reclusa*), and the common brown spider (*Loxosceles unicolor*).[144]

Spider bites occur most commonly on the forelegs and face. Bites of spiders of the genus *Latrodectus* (the widows) initially consist of two small puncture marks with local erythema. The local reaction may develop into granulomatous nodules within a few days. Bites of spiders of the genus Loxosceles (the brown spiders) initially appear as puncture marks surrounded by local erythema.[15] Within a few hours they become vesicular and very painful. The next day the lesions turn black and become necrotic, and a large indolent ulcer develops.

Systemic reactions to spider bites may be severe. They may be manifested by salivation, nausea and diarrhea, ataxia and convulsions, or paralysis, any of which occur within 6 to 48 hours.

Although spider bites are rarely recognized and reported, they are probably underdiagnosed in veterinary medicine.[88] Diagnosis should be based on history and the physical examination. Recommended early bite wound therapy includes local infusion with 2 per cent lidocaine and triamcinolone acetonide.[97] Systemic support with analgesics, calcium gluconate, and epinepherine and glucocorticosteroids may be needed. In the case of bites of *Latrodectus* spp., the local infusion of 1.0 ml of antivenin is recommended.[97] Chronic nonhealing ulcers may take months to heal and may be best treated by surgical excision.

Spiders can be controlled by cleaning up woodpiles and outdoor sites; by eliminating scattered debris; and by spraying insecticides under appliances, in cupboards, in cracks in basement and attic floors, and outdoors under eaves and in window wells and woodpiles. The most effective insecticides are Baygon 1.1 per cent, dichlorvos (DDVP) 0.5 per cent, Diazinon 0.5 per cent, Dursban 0.5 per cent, or Ficam 0.25 per cent. Application should be repeated every 2 to 3 weeks as needed.[72, 144]

INSECTS

The numerous species of insects play important roles in the health of animals as vectors of disease and as irritants to the skin. The head of insects bears appendages and sensory organs, such as antennae and simple or compound eyes. The structure of the masticatory mouthparts varies depending on the feeding habits. The thorax typically carries two pairs of wings and three pairs of legs. The abdomen is segmented and terminates in the male hypopygium or the female ovipositor. The body is encased in hard chitinous plates connected by flexible membranes. The life cycles of insects are of three types: direct development, incomplete metamorphosis, or complete metamorphosis. In the first type, the newly hatched insect is a small replica of the adult. Incomplete metamorphosis occurs in primitive insects, and the larvae differ from adults size, proportion, and lack of wings. Complete metamorphosis is found in more specialized species, the wormlike larva differing from the adult in regard to feeding habits. After several molts, it pupates and emerges as an adult. The larva and pupa possess characteristic hairs, bristles, and appendages, which are of taxonomic importance. The durations of adult pupal and larval stages vary with the species and the environment.

Pediculosis

Pediculosis is infestation with lice.

Cause and Pathogenesis. Lice are small, degenerate, dorsoventrally flattened, wingless insects that do not undergo true metamorphosis. The eyes are reduced or absent, and each leg bears one or two claws. There is one pair of spiracles on the mesothorax, and usually six pairs on the abdomen. Lice are host specific and spend their entire life on their host. They survive only a few days if separated from the host. Lice are spread by direct contact or by contaminated brushes and combs. The operculated white eggs (nits) are cemented firmly to the hairs of the host. In contrast, cheyletiella ova are smaller and loosely attached to the hair shafts (see Fig. 8:21). The nymph hatches from the egg, undergoes three ecdyses (molting), and becomes the adult (Fig. 8:45). The entire cycle lasts 14 to 21 days.

Lice are divided into two suborders: Anoplura, or sucking lice, and Mallophaga, or biting lice.

Anoplura. These have mouthparts adapted for sucking the blood of the host. With heavy infestations, they produce sufficient anemia to cause weakness, and some animals become distraught and ill-tempered because of the chronic irritation. The only species found commonly on dogs is *Linognathus setosus* (Figs. 8:46A and 8:47C).

Mallophaga. These so-called biting lice feed on epithelial debris and hair, but some species also have mouthparts adapted for drawing blood from their

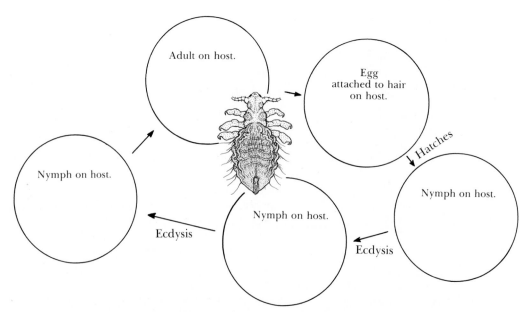

Figure 8:45. Life cycle of the louse (14 to 21 days).

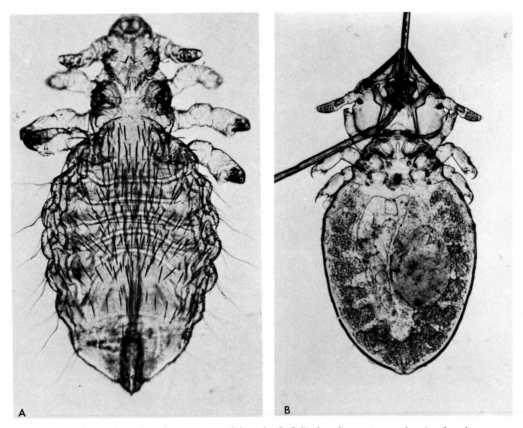

Figure 8:46. *A, Linognathus setosus*, adult male. *B, Felicola subrostrata*, egg-bearing female.

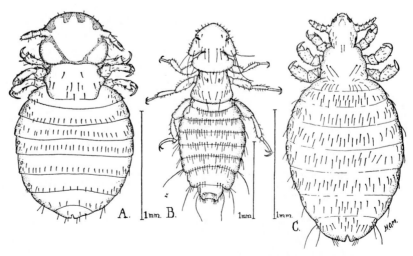

Figure 8:47. Dog lice. *A, Trichodectes canis. B, Heterodoxus spiniger, C, Linognathus setosus.* (From Lapage, G.: Monnig's Veterinary Helminthology and Entomology. 5th ed. The Williams & Wilkins Company, Baltimore, 1962.)

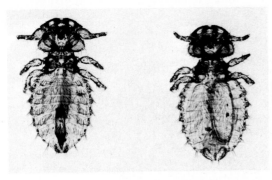

Figure 8:48. *Trichodectes canis.* Male (left); egg-bearing female (right).

hosts. Since they are very active, they may cause more irritation than do sucking lice, and rubbing by their host may cause alopecia. *Trichodectes canis* (Figs. 8:47*A* and 8:48), is the common biting louse of dogs. It may act as the intermediate host of the dog tapeworm, *D. caninum. Felicola subrostratus* infests cats (Figs. 8:46*B* and 8:49) and may either be asymptomatic or cause severe pruritus with dermatitis and hair loss on the back. *Heterodoxus spiniger* may be found on dogs in warm climates only (Fig. 8:47*B*). A single case of *Phthirus pubis* (human pubic louse) infesting a dog has been reported. The dog, which had no clinical signs, slept in the bed of its owner, who was infested with the louse.[48]

Lice are relatively host specific and spend all their lives on the host. This makes control easier.

Clinical Features. Lice can be highly irritating to the host and can cause intense itching. They accumulate under mats of hair and around the ears and body openings. Sucking lice produce anemia and severe debilitation. Sucking lice do not move rapidly and are easily seen and caught (see Fig. 8:56*H*). Biting lice, however, move rapidly and may be difficult to find and capture.

Lice produce few direct lesions, but excoriations and secondary dermatitis from scratching may be severe. Pediculosis may look like miliary dermatitis in cats and like flea bite hypersensitivity in dogs. Papules and crusts may be found. Debilitated, anemic, and frustrated patients often are ill-tempered and

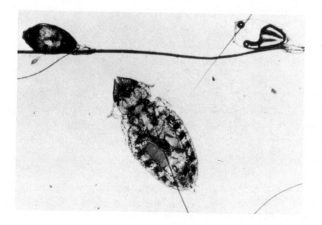

Figure 8:49. *Felicola subrostrata,* egg-bearing female. Intact egg on left; empty case on right.

difficult to handle. The patient's coat is often dirty, matted, and ill-kempt, as this is a disease of neglect often associated with overcrowding and poor sanitation. The animal has a "mousy" odor, especially when wet.

In some cases, animals are asymptomatic carriers or have only seborrhea sicca with variable pruritus. Pediculosis is often more prevalent in the winter months, perhaps owing to the growth of longer, heavier hair coats and closer contact among animals. In addition, the high ambient and skin surface temperature during summer can be lethal to lice.

Pediculosis is a rare diagnosis in most veterinary practices. Lice are easily killed by common flea shampoos, sprays, or powders; consequently, owners usually eliminate these parasites with routine grooming care. More insecticidal shampoos are used today than were used many years ago, and louse infestation has decreased proportionately.

Diagnosis. Diagnosis is made by physical examination to find and identify the lice (Figs. 8:46 and 8:49). See page 129 for a description of the acetate tape impression method of immobilizing lice for identification.

Differential diagnosis of pediculosis should include seborrhea, scabies, flea bite hypersensitivity, miliary dermatitis, cheyletiellosis, and *Dermanyssus, Lynxacarus,* or *Trombicula* infestations. Skin scrapings and acetate tape examinations should resolve any diagnostic questions.

Treatment. All affected animals and others in close association with them should be treated. Thick mats and hair tags should be clipped away. After a regular soap and water shampoo, the animal should be soaked or sprayed thoroughly with a good insecticide. Lice are susceptible to almost all parasiticidal agents.

Cats. Use pyrethrin or carbamate shampoos. After being dried, cats can be sprayed or dusted with products containing pyrethrins and carbaryl (Sevin). Treatment should be repeated within 10 to 14 days, because not all the nits may be killed and any that remain will have hatched by that time. Two per cent lime-sulfur dips are also effective but smelly.

Dogs. Stronger medications with residual action can be used on dogs, although lice are easily killed with the preceding preparations. Bathing with a shampoo containing synergized pyrethrin or a pyrethroid is effective. Dogs can then be dipped in 0.25 per cent dichlorovinyl dimethyl phosphate (DDVP) or 5 per cent carbaryl (Sevin) as a follow-up treatment. A second or third treatment in 10 to 14 days is recommended. These treatments are usually highly effective.

Histopathology reveals varying degrees of superficial perivascular dermatitis (hyperplastic, spongiotic).[121] Eosinophils are usually prominent.

Severely anemic and depressed patients with extreme parasite infestations may go into shock and die following vigorous treatment. It is best to transfuse blood, provide a high-protein diet, and reduce the number of parasites with carbaryl or other powders first. More complete treatment as just outlined can be given several days later.

It is advisable to thoroughly clean bedding, the premises, and grooming implements at least once, even though lice do not live when they are off the host.

Fleas

Fleas are small, brown, wingless insects with laterally compressed bodies (Fig. 8:50). Males are smaller than females, and the chitinous head bears antennae,

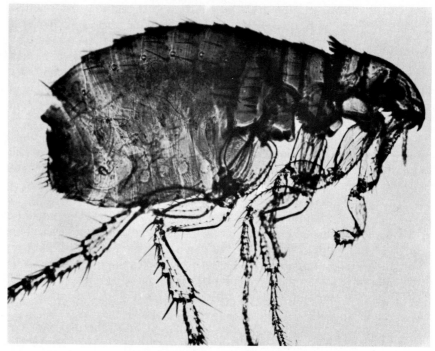

Figure 8:50. *Ctenocephalides felis* adult.

eyes, combs, and suctorial mouthparts (Figs. 8:51 and 8:53C, D). The prothoracic and genal combs are useful taxonomically. Each segment of the three-sectioned thorax bears a pair of powerful legs terminating in two curved claws. The structure adapts fleas for the purpose of powerful jumping, which enables them to transfer from host to host.

Fleas develop by complete metamorphosis (Fig. 8:52). The eggs, which are ovoid, white, and glistening, are laid on the premises in cracks of buildings or

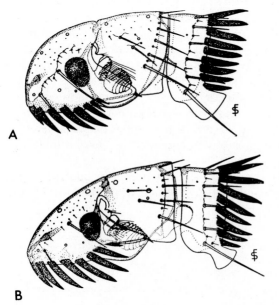

Figure 8:51. *A, Ctenocephalides canis,* female. Head and pronotum showing one of the antennae and the genal and pronotal combs. *B, Ctenocephalides felis,* female. Head and pronotum showing one of the antennae and the genal and pronotal combs. (From Lapage, G.: Veterinary Parasitology, 2nd ed. Charles C Thomas, Springfield, Ill., 1967.)

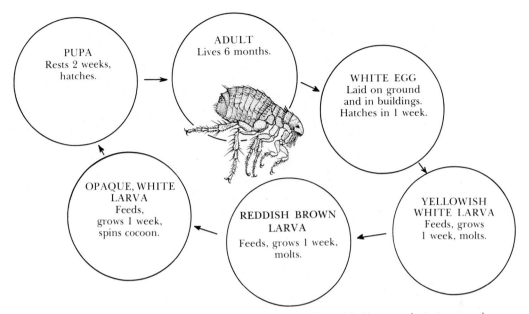

Figure 8:52. Life cycle of *Ctenocephalides felis* (three weeks to two years).

on damp ground (Figs. 8:53*E* and 9:30). Those that are laid on the host soon fall off, since they are not sticky. The female lays only 3 to 18 eggs at one time, but with frequent blood meals and frequent copulation she may lay several hundred in her life span of 1 year. Adult fleas separated from the host live only 1 to 2 months. Cat and dog fleas do not adapt well to altitudes higher than 5000 feet. However, small rodent fleas thrive in a dry climate and at even higher altitudes. Fleas lay more eggs when the temperature reaches the range of 65°F to 80°F and when the humidity is high (70 per cent). After incubation of 2 to 12 days, the egg hatches into the larva—an active white bristled worm with chewing mouthparts. They ingest fecal blood casts from adult fleas and thus may develop a reddish tinge. The posterior end has two hooked processes called anal struts, which are used for locomotion. These distinguish a flea larva from that of a dipterous insect. Larvae grow and molt twice over a period of 9 to 200 days. The third molt produces an opaque white larva that becomes quiescent and spins a loose, whitish gray cocoon, inside which it pupates for 7 days to 1 year. The adult flea breaks out of the cocoon and looks for a host on which to feed. Details of the flea life cycle are illustrated in color in Figure 8:53.

Echidnophaga gallinacea, the sticktight poultry flea (Fig. 8:54), is found in warm climates. It also attacks dogs and cats. Adult fleas of the species are active at first, but during copulation the female attaches herself to the skin of the host's face (see Fig. 8:56*G*, p. 420). She does not move rapidly but burrows into the skin and forms an ulcerated nodule in which she lays her eggs. The eggs hatch on the host, but the larvae fall off and the life cycle of about 1 month is completed as described for other fleas.

In reporting on *E. gallinacea* infections in dogs, Kalkofen and Greenberg[70] have emphasized the importance of premises formerly occupied by fowl as a potent and prolonged source of infestation of dogs. These fleas may be found clustered around the eyes, between the toes, on the scrotum, and on sparsely haired underparts. They respond to standard methods of flea control.

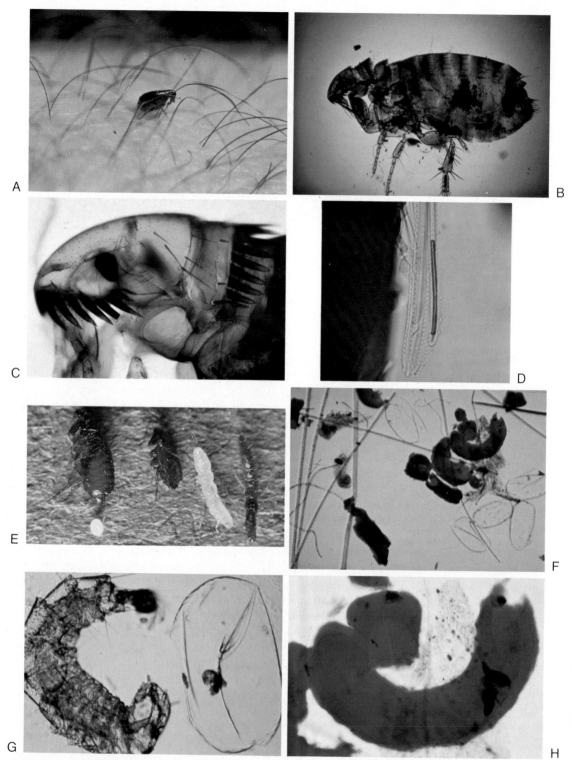

Figure 8:53. *Ctenocephalides felis.* *A,* Adult flea (*Ctenocephalides felis*) on human skin. *B,* Adult female flea (*Ctenocephalides felis*). *C, Ctenocephalides felis* head and pronotum showing one antenna and the genal and pronotal combs. *D,* Sucking mouthparts: Epipharynx half-filled with blood and lacinia or piercing stylets. *E,* Stages of life cycle (from left to right): Adult female with egg, adult male, mature larva ready to pupate (white), young larvae after first blood meal (red). The pupa is not illustrated. *F,* Empty flea egg cases (lower right), young yellow-white larvae (upper left) and blood fecal crusts from adult fleas to be used as larval food. *G,* Just hatched, yellow-white larva and its empty egg case. *H,* Closer view of red, bloody, fecal crusts illustrated in *F.*

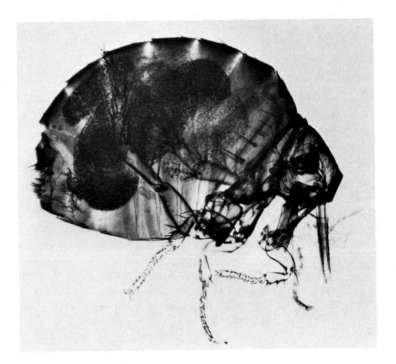

Figure 8:54. *Echidnophaga gallinacea* (sticktight flea) adult.

Pulex irritans, the flea that infects humans (Fig. 8:55), is not commonly recognized by veterinarians as a problem of pet animals. Kalkofen and Greenberg[69] have shown that in the southeastern United States it may even be the most frequently encountered species of fleas on dogs. It is transmitted more readily from dogs to humans and may persist longer on humans than do *Ctenocephalides* spp. In many cases, however, *P. irritans* preferred the dog as a host, when given the choice. This flea may be of additional public health significance, because it may be a vector for plague (*Yersinia pestis*).

Fleas produce severe skin irritation because of their frequent bites. The itching induces self-mutilation by the host. Flea saliva is highly antigenic in some individuals and produces an allergic dermatitis[57] (see p. 482). Fleas may be mechanical vectors of many diseases and are important vectors of *Pasteurella* infections. The cat and dog fleas (*C. felis* and *C. canis*) are also intermediate hosts of the dog tapeworm (*Diplidium caninum*). The sticktight flea produces special skin lesions of the face, in addition to the effects mentioned above.

Without question, *C. felis* is the common flea of dogs and cats in most areas of the United States, with *C. canis* being found only occasionally. Sticktight fleas are rare. The human flea *Pulex irritans* and the rat flea *Leptopsylla segnis* may also attack dogs, cats, and humans. Bites on humans tend to be focused

Figure 8:55. *Pulex irritans*, the human flea (× 17). *A*, female; *B*, male. (From Herns, W. B., and James, M. T.: Medical Entomology, 5th ed. New York, Copyright 1961 by The Macmillan Company.)

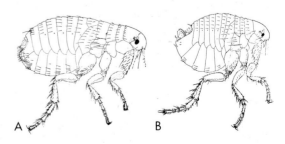

A   B

on the lower legs and trunk, and some people are more susceptible to flea bites than others. The lesions are multiple red papules that are intensely pruritic.

FLEA CONTROL

The Premises. Because fleas spend only short periods on their host, the major effort for flea control must be directed to the premises where the eggs, larvae, pupae, and some adults congregate.[17] Damp, cool floors—especially those of dirt, sand, or concrete—and cracks and crevices are favorite areas for flea development.

> *The major effort for flea control must be directed at the premises.*

Because some stages of the flea's life cycle persist for months, chemicals with residual action are needed, and they must be repeated periodically.[80] In severe cases it is wise to obtain the services of a professional exterminator. This is desirable even in cold climates where fleas tend to be a seasonal problem. Once hard frosts have eliminated the fleas outdoors the attack can be concentrated indoors, and with careful planning and the use of effective insecticides the flea battle can be won—at least until warm weather arrives again.[18] Some commercial exterminators use bendiocarb or ficam; but the premises can also be effectively treated with insecticides such as malathion (4 per cent dust, 0.05 to 0.5 per cent spray), dioxathion (Delnav) 5 per cent, dichlorvos (DDVP) 1 per cent, chlorpyrifos (Dursban) 0.5 per cent, or methylcarbamate powder 5 per cent. Methoprene and fenoxycarb are insect growth regulators that prevent fourth instar larvae from undergoing metamorphosis into adults. Since these compounds act on the immature flea and not the adults, they should be used in conjunction with a fast-acting adulticide. Foggers are helpful for short-term use on active fleas but have no residual action. They are also expensive, and because of their large droplet size they do not penetrate rugs and fail to reach areas under beds or chairs or in closets. The effect of foggers is enhanced when combined with a residual spray applied to the problem areas cited above. Use of both foggers *and* sprays containing pyrethrin, methoprene, and chlorpyrifos appears to provide effective, long-lasting control of fleas in the house (Siphotrol Products, Vet Kem). Trials conducted under field conditions demonstrated that aerosol and pressurized-spray formulations of fenoxycarb and methoprene had at least 60-day activity.[102a] Microencapsulation extends the effective life of many insecticides and allows long-term control of emerging adults (Sectrol and Duratrol Products, 3M Company). Trials conducted under field conditions demonstrated that propetamphos spray or microencapsulated diazinon provided excellent flea control for at least 60 days.[102a] Products used in the home should be tested for possible staining before application. The vacuum cleaner can be a real aid in removing eggs and immature forms of the flea, especially when vacuuming is preceded by the application of flea powders. Special attention should be given to cracks and corners. It is important to remember to empty and burn the vacuum contents; otherwise the cleaner only serves as an incubator, releasing more fleas to the environment as they hatch. Flea collars or other sources of volatile insecticides should not be placed in the vacuum bag, as such products will be dissipated into the environment, with possible toxic effects to people.

The Animal Host. Treatment of *all* contact animal hosts must be coordinated with treatment of the premises.[81] A most effective treatment is bathing with a simple flea shampoo (containing pyrethrin, lindane, or carbamate) followed by a dip in a dilute solution of a residual insecticide that is allowed to dry on the skin. The patient then must be sprayed or dusted with flea medication once or twice weekly to maintain control. In some animals, sprays or powders alone may be preferable. Sprays containing pyrethrins and carbaryl as well as powders with carbaryl (Sevin) are usually effective for dogs or cats over 4 weeks old. These can also be applied to the pet's bedding with favorable results. Powders tend to leave a dust over clothing and furniture, but they stick well in the coat. While sprays avoid the mess, the hissing of the spray upsets some animals, especially cats. Either can best be applied if the pet's head and eyes are covered with a towel and the material is applied while the hair is being ruffled to allow the material to penetrate deeply into the coat. The fingers can then be used to spread the material through the coat and around the head and ears. Application should be repeated after grooming or bathing, or even after severe wetting of the coat from rain or swimming.

In the experience of many animal owners and clinicians, flea collars have not lived up to their advertised claims. All collars begin to lose activity after 3 weeks.[109] Collars containing chlorpyrifos seem to be effective longer; however, collars or medallions are only aids that will kill some fleas, but not control them. They give a false sense of security to owners, who then often neglect the really important aspects of a total control program. Collars can cause contact irritation in certain individuals, so they must be observed carefully for untoward effects.

Flea collars containing dichlorvos (Vapona) tend to release more medication in hot dry environments, and toxicity has been reported in cats within 5 to 15 days after application of a collar.[39] Signs were prominent in Siamese cats and included salivation, diarrhea, ataxia, aplastic anemia, and a focal dermatitis (see p. 774). In experimental use (hot, dry climate, poor ventilation, close confinement), cervical dermatitis, ataxia, and depression were seen in 74, 42, and 10 per cent, respectively, of cats wearing dichlorvos collars.[13]

In the experience of the authors and others,[139b] electronic flea collars have been ineffective in the control of fleas.

Flea repellents have long been added as an extra organic ingredient to sprays and powders. Recently, sprays have been introduced for over-the-counter sales as "flea repellents." They appear promising but have not been available long enough for critical evaluation. Skin-So-Soft bath oil (Avon) has been shown to produce significant but not complete effects as a flea repellent on dogs.[40] There are no clinical or experimental data to show that thiamine, brewer's yeast, or garlic are effective flea repellents.[56, 121]

Dichlorvos fly strips can be useful in flea control. They can be suspended several feet above the cat or dog bed to bathe the area constantly in dichlorvos vapors. Thus, there is a continuous effect on the premises, and the animal is constantly treated while in the area, without any contact toxicity. If the dog has a house outdoors, one-half of the strip can be attached to the *underside* (inside) of the roof and one-half placed under the floor. Treatment is obtained without contact. This fly strip system is also effective for control of several other ectoparasites and insects, and it keeps the premises treated, even when the patient is away—a real boon.

Systemic insecticides have also been advocated for flea control. Some clinicians use much larger doses than recommended here and claim superior in efficacy.[27] (See p. 181). For dogs only, agents such as cythioate (Proban), 3 mg/kg every 3 to 4 days orally, or fenthion (Pro-Spot), 8 mg/kg applied to the skin surface every 14 days, may kill fleas that have ingested blood,[19] but by then the flea saliva has been injected and the potential for flea bite hypersensitivity has not been averted. Thus, these products, too, are only a part of a complete flea control program.

Much is said about fleas developing "resistance" to insecticidal materials. This is true to some extent, but the problem is undoubtedly viewed out of context by owners who de-flea their pets and return them to an infested environment; there, of course, they pick up more fleas. Perhaps the most effective test is to catch some live fleas and put them in a jar with the insecticide—it is amazing how rapidly they die. This is a point to use in emphasizing the necessity of total environmental control. Most resistant fleas are from areas where the premises cannot adequately be treated or where large populations of fleas exist all the year, as in many tropical or sunbelt regions. The resistant nature of fleas from the southeastern United States, specifically Florida, is proven.[116] In this region, numerous insecticides are used in an attempt to control fleas and other insects. It is surmised that constant exposure to insecticides causes selection for survival of fleas having gene complements that code for enhanced detoxification capabilities.[116]

Recent studies have demonstrated that cat fleas from different regions of the United States do indeed show different patterns of insecticide resistance.[35a, 72a, 116a] A Kentucky strain of cat flea was quite susceptible to propetamphos and diazinon, but more resistant to chlorpyrifos.[116a] In a comparison of insecticide activity against California and Florida strains of cat fleas,[35a] (1) chlorpyrifos was the most effective against both strains, (2) the Florida strain was much more resistant to malathion, carbaryl and bendiocarb, and (3) the California strain was more resistant to propoxur. Such studies indicate that clinicians need to be aware of regional differences in insecticide efficacy, and that the field strain of flea being used for testing flea control products will likely influence the results obtained.

Summary of Flea Control. A summary of flea control can be outlined as follows:

A. The home
   1. Vacuum and/or mop all floors to remove eggs, larvae, and pupae.
   2. Thoroughly wash or destroy all pet bedding.
   3. Employ a commercial exterminator *or* use combination of foggers and sprays with insecticides and insect growth regulator, or microencapsulated insecticides (pyrethrins).
   4. Repeat treatment monthly until controlled, then every 4 months.
B. The outdoors: Spray outdoor areas frequented by pets with diazinon or chlorpyrifos. Repeat every 2 to 3 weeks, as needed.
C. The pet (the least important step)
   1. Remove all pets from the premises during treatment.
   2. Bathe pets, using pyrethrin shampoo.
   3. Rinse well and dip with synthetic pyrethroid or organic phosphate dip.
   4. Maintain residual insecticidal effect by regularly (at least weekly) dusting or spraying with carbaryl, malathion, and pyrethrins, singly or in combination.
      Further information about insecticidal treatments is provided in Chapter Four, Dermatologic Therapy.

Diptera (Flies)

Medically, flies form a most important order of arthropods, as they transmit, or are intermediate hosts for, many bacterial, viral, protozoan, and helminth disease agents. However, their effects on skin are minor and are limited to bites (mosquitoes, stable flies, black flies, and deer flies) and to myiasis.

The reaction to insect bites varies, since some individuals are less attractive or less susceptible to certain flies. The local lesion is a sensitivity reaction that may become less severe with repeated exposures. The systemic reaction to injected antigen, however, often increases with repeated exposures (e.g., to bee and mosquito antigens), and severe local edema (see Fig. 8:58) or anaphylaxis may develop.

The primary lesion is a wheal or papule around a bleeding point (Fig. 8:56C,D). The reaction may be transient or may persist for weeks. In the latter case a pseudocarcinomatous hyperplasia develops, with scaling and alopecia. A perivascular or diffuse dermal infiltrate of eosinophils, plasma cells, and lymphocytes may be present.

Fly Dermatitis. Adult male and female flies (*Stomoxys calcitrans*) are peculiarly adapted for attacking the skin of the host and sucking blood. The rasping teeth and blades of the labella tear open the skin, and the labella and whole proboscis are plunged into the wound to suck blood. The entire action is highly irritating to the host and conducive to spreading disease.

The flies usually attack the face or ears of dogs. The multiple bites are commonly found on the tips of the ears (Fig. 8:56A) or at the folded edge of the skin in dogs whose ears are tipped over (such as shelties, collies and others (Fig. 8:56B). Erythema and hemorrhagic crusts, caused by oozing serum and blood, are typical lesions. Afflicted dogs are always housed outdoors, and often confined so that they cannot escape the fly attacks.

Ordinary fly repellents, fly or flea spray, or pastes made of flea powder applied to the affected skin help to prevent repeated bites. Many flea sprays and powders contain complex organic compounds as repellents. They are known as MKG 11 or MKG 326. In addition, diethyltoluamide ("DEET"), present in mosquito repellents for people (Cutter's and OFF), may be effective if applied sparingly to the hair near the body areas that are attractive to flies. Flea repellent sprays have been introduced recently for over-the-counter sales. They appear to be promising but have not been available long enough for thorough evaluation. The patient should be housed indoors during the day, if possible, until the lesions heal. Topical medications such as antibiotic corticosteroid (Panalog) ointment may be beneficial. Affected skin should be kept clean and dry.

The source of the flies should be investigated, and straw piles, manure pits, and other likely areas can be sprayed with an insecticide (dichlorvos [Vaponal], diazinon, carbamate, or malathion) every 3 weeks to help decrease the fly population.

Black flies (*Simuliidae* species) are tiny biting flies that reproduce in shaded areas with running water. They are seasonal in early spring and summer but during that time cause severe reaction in people and animals alike. Their bites are concentrated on hairless areas like the abdomen, head, ears, and legs (Fig. 8:56D). The lesions are intensely pruritic papules, crusts, and ulcers, with hemorrhage and severe excoriation that result in circumscribed areas of necrosis. Horsefly (*Tabanus*), deer fly (*Chrysops*), and mosquito bites tend to be less reactive than black fly bites, but they are all diagnosed, managed, and prevented in the same way as described for stable flies.

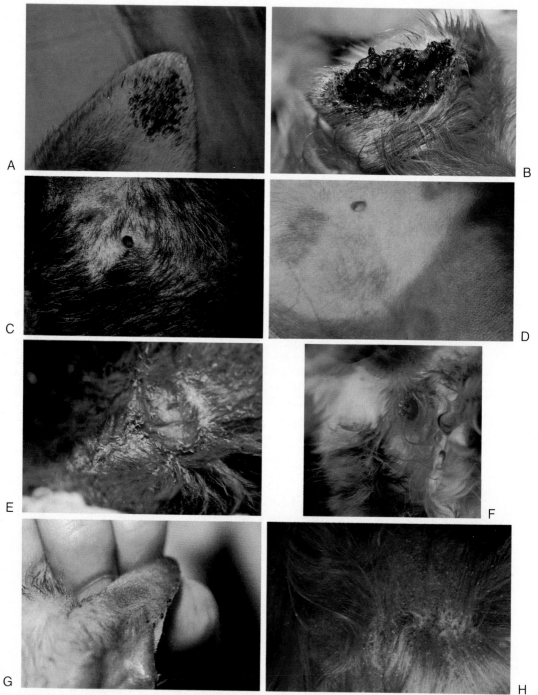

Figure 8:56. *A*, Fly dermatitis on a German shepherd's pinna. Hemorrhagic crusts form from oozing blood and serum that result from the rasping mouth parts of stable flies (*Stomoxys calcitrans*). *B*, Collie with folded ear shows extensive fly bite lesions at fold of ear with secondary pyoderma. *C*, Multiple erythematous flea bites on dog's abdomen. Note flea just below dark nipple. *D*, Multiple ecchymotic black fly bites on glabrous skin of canine abdomen. *E*, Myiasis. Moist exudative skin lesions attract flies. Note many white fly larvae on surface of skin and hair. *F*, Cuterebra fistula in the neck of a Persian kitten. Larva is present in opening of fistula. *G*, Sticktight fleas on the pinna of a cat. (Courtesy G. A. Kunkle.) *H*, Trunk of Irish setter with *Linognathus setosus*. Nits and adults can be seen among the hairs.

Myiasis. The adult forms of many dipterous flies place eggs on the wet, warm skin of debilitated weakened animals with draining wounds or urine-soaked coats (Fig. 8:56E). However, animals that are attractive are not equally so at all stages to all flies. As the skin breaks down and liquifies, it becomes attractive to other flies, and in some cases the initial larval infestation modifies the habitat to further attract a second or third species. Calliphorids (blow flies) and sarcophagids (flesh flies) are most common in small animal myiasis. True screwworms, *Cochliomyia hominovorax*, have been eliminated from large areas of North America. They are obligate parasites of living tissue and are never common in dogs and cats. Specific identification is not important in the treatment of most myiasis cases. However, larvae can be kept until adult flies develop, or the posterior aspect of the larvae can be examined for posterior spiracles and stigmal plates that are taxonomically significant.

The larvae found in cutaneous myiasis are highly destructive and produce lesions over extensive areas with "punched out" round holes in the skin. These may coalesce to form broad defects with scalloped margins. The larvae may be found under the skin and in the tissues. Favorite locations are around the nose, eyes, mouth, anus, and genitalia, or adjacent to neglected wounds. Myiasis is always a disease of neglect.

Treatment requires clipping hair away from the lesions and cleaning them with a detergent material such as povidone-iodine (Betadine). The larvae must be meticulously removed from deep crevices and from under the skin. Nitrofurazone or other topical antibiotics should be applied to the wound, and the rest of the coat should be sprayed with an appropriate insecticide, such as 0.25 per cent malathion solution. Daily routine wound care is necessary, and the patient should be housed in screened, fly-free quarters. Usually healing is rapid and complete, but one should also be concerned about the original cause. Fecal or urinary incontinence, a continually wet coat, fold dermatoses, or constant salivation or lacrimation, together with poor hygiene, sets up the potential for myiasis. These underlying factors must be corrected as a primary part of therapy.

Cuterebra Species. Adult *Cuterebra* flies are large and beelike with vestigial mouthparts, but they neither bite nor feed. They are not directly attracted to a host species but oviposit on stones or vegetation near the entrance to the burrows or nests of animals to which they are probably attracted at night. Animals become infested as they pass through areas contaminated with the eggs of *Cuterebra* spp. Larvae enter the body via natural body openings, by skin penetration, or by ingestion as the animal grooms contaminated fur.[6, 51] The natural hosts are usually rabbits and other rodents, and in these animals the parasites exhibit host and site specificity.[71] Rabbit *Cuterebra* are less host specific and are the species that usually affect young cats and dogs.

Since cats and dogs are abnormal hosts, the larvae undergo aberrant migrations and have been reported in the brain, pharynx, nostrils, and eyelids. Typical cases involving the skin are usually localized to the regions of the head, neck, or trunk. Cases usually occur in late summer or fall when the larvae enlarge and produce a swelling of 1 cm in diameter, which develops a fistula (Fig. 8:56F).

Treatment involves incising or spreading the fistulous opening and extracting the "grub" by means of a mosquito forceps. Care should be taken to avoid crushing the larva, as retained parts may produce allergic or irritant reactions. The infected wound should be treated, but healing will be slow.

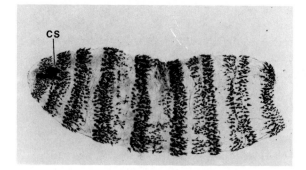

Figure 8:57. Wholemount of cleared *Cuterebra* sp. second instar larva. Note darkly pigmented cephalopharyngeal skeleton (CS) and rows of spines. Posterior spiracular segments have been removed (× 13). (From Kazocos, K. R., et al.: *Cuterebra* species as a cause of pharyngeal myiasis in cats. J.A.A.H.A. *16*:773, 1980.)

Identification is usually possible, since the second instar larvae are 5 to 10 mm long and cream to gray in color, with 10 to 12 visible body segments, the first 8 to 10 of which are encircled by three to four rows of scattered dark spines and spinules (Fig. 8:57). They have well-developed cranial mouth hooks, but no head capsule or legs. Molting occurs and the third instar is the dark, thick, heavily spined larva the clinician sees in the subcutaneous or submucosal pocket (Fig. 8:56*F*).

Hymenoptera (Bees, Wasps, Hornets)

These venomous insects are not parasitic. They possess membranous wings and mouthparts for chewing, sucking and licking. The ovipositor of the female is adapted for stinging. She has paired venom glands that express a toxin during the sting. When bees and certain wasps sting, the tip of the abdomen and the whole poison apparatus breaks off and remains in the wound. The gland may continue to express poison, so the "stinger" should be removed from the skin as soon as possible. Other wasps and hornets may sting repeatedly, since they remain intact. Local redness, edema, and inflammation soon develop (Fig. 8:58), and in some animals severe anaphylaxis occurs. If cardiac and respiratory impairment result, the patient may die.

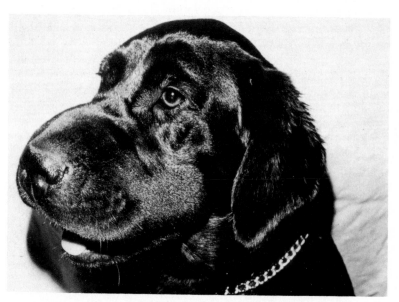

Figure 8:58. Bee sting. The local edema, pain, and redness on the nose of this Labrador retriever disappeared within three hours after systemic corticosteroid therapy.

The stinger should be removed, if it can be located. In severe cases with anaphylaxis, epinepherine should be given intramuscularly, and glucocorticoids intravenously. With urticaria, epinepherine or large doses of prednisolone followed by a rapid-acting antihistamine should be administered systemically. Hot compresses may relieve local pain. Subsequent bites or multiple bites make the reaction more severe.

References

1. Adolphsson, A.: Personal communication, 1982.
2. Alexander, J. O'D.: Mites and skin disease. Clin. Med. 79:14, 1979.
3. Alexander, M. M., and Ihrke, P. J.: Cheyletiella dermatitis in small animal practice: a review. Calif. Vet. 36:9, 1982.
4. Anderson, R. K.: Canine scabies. Compend. Cont. Ed. 1:687, 1979.
5. Bailey, R. G., and Thompson, R. C.: Demodectic mange in a cat. Aust. Vet. J. 57:49, 1981.
6. Baird, C. R.: Development of Cuterebra ruficrus (Diptera: Cuterebridae) in six species of rabbits and rodents with a morphological comparison of C. ruficrus and C. jellisoni third instars. J. Med. Ent. 9:81, 1972.
7. Baker, K. P.: Clinical aspects of hookworm dermatitis. Vet. Dermatol. Newsl. 6:69, 1981.
8. Baker, K. P.: Studies on the tissue response to the genus Demodex. Vet. Dermatol. Newsl. 4:16, 1979.
9. Baker, K. P., and Grimes, T. D.: Cutaneous lesions in dogs associated with hookworm infestation. Vet. Rec. 87:376, 1970.
10. Barr, M.: Propylene glycol: a solvent-vehicle of increased importance in dermatology. Am. J. Pharmacol. 137:107, 1965.
11. Barsanti, J. A.: Botulism, tick paralysis and acute polyradiculoneuritis. In Kirk, R. W., (ed.): Current Veterinary Therapy VII. W. B. Saunders Company, Philadelphia, 1980.
12. Barta, O., Waltman, C., et al.: Lymphocyte transformation suppression caused by pyoderma—failure to demonstrate it in uncomplicated demodectic mange. Comp. Immunol. Microbiol. Infect. Dis. 6:9, 1983.
13. Bell, T. G., et al.: Ataxia, depression, and dermatitis associated with use of dichlorvos-impregnated collars in the laboratory cat. J.A.V.M.A. 168:579, 1975.
14. Bell, T. G., and Farris, R. A.: A discourse and proposal on the genesis of generalized demodectic mange: a theory of production of lesions through an immunosuppressive mechanism. West. Vet. 1:21, 1973.
15. Berger, R. S.: The unremarkable brown recluse spider bite. J.A.M.A. 225:1109, 1973.
16. Bigler, B., et al.: Este erfolgversprechende Ergebnisse in der Behandlung von Notoedres cati mit Ivermectin. Schweiz. Arch. Tierheilkd. 126:365, 1984.
16a. Bilger, D., and Drion, M.: Dermatite a Otodectes cynotis. Point Vet. 16:92, 1984.
17. Bledsoe, B., Fadok, V. A., et al.: Current therapy and new developments in indoor flea control. J.A.A.H.A. 18:415, 1982.
18. Bowen, J. M.: Ctenocephalides (flea) pharmacology. Georgia Vet. 30:6, 1978.
19. Bowen, P. M., and Caldwell, N. J.: Use of cythioate to control external parasites on cats and dogs. Vet. Med. (S.A.C.) 77:79, 1982.
19a. Bourdeau, P.: Cas de dermatite a rhabitides (Pelodera strongyloides) chez un chien. Point Vet. 16:5, 1984.
20. Bowman, W. L.: The cat fur mite (Lynxacarus rhadovsky) in Australia. Aust. Vet. J. 54:403, 1978.
21. Brockis, D. C.: Mite infestations (letter). Vet. Rec. 107:315, 1980.
22. Buelke, D. L.: Hookworm dermatitis. J.A.V.M.A. 148:735, 1971.
23. Bullmore, C. C., Weiss, M. E., et al.: Feline trombiculosis. Feline Pract. 6:36, 1976.
24. Bussieras, J.: Le traitement de la demodecie du chien par l'amitraz. Rec. Med. Vet. 155:685, 1979.
25. Bussieras, J., and Chermette, R.: Amitraz and canine demodicosis. J.A.A.H.A. 22:779, 1986.
26. Carmichael, J., and Bell, F. R.: Filariasis in dogs in Uganda. J.S. Afr. Vet. Assoc. 14:12, 1943.
27. Carr, S. H.: Clinical observations on the topical use of fenthion. Canine Pract. F:69, 1980.
28. Charlesworth, E. N., and Johnson, J. L.: An epidemic of canine scabies in man. Arch. Dermatol. 110:574, 1974.
29. Cohen, S. R.: Cheyletiella dermatitis (in rabbit, cat, dog, man). Arch. Dermatol. 116:435, 1980.
30. Conroy, J. D., Healey, M. C., et al.: New Demodex sp. infesting a cat: a case report. J.A.A.H.A. 18:405, 1982.
31. Corbett, R., et al.: Cellular immune responsiveness in dogs with demodectic mange. Transplant. Proc. 7:557, 1975.
32. Corbett, R. B., et al.: The cell-mediated immune response: its inhibition and in vitro reversal in dogs with demodectic mange. Fed. Proc. 35:589, 1976.
33. Desch, C., and Nutting, W. B.: Demodex cati, Hirst, 1919: a redescription. Cornell Vet. 69:280, 1979.
34. Dodds, J.: Bleeding disorders: their importance in everyday practice. Proceedings, A.A.H.A. 44:147, 1977.
35. Doering, G. G.: Dracunculus insignis in dogs. Presented at the American Academy of Veterinary Dermatology Annual Meeting, Boston, April 30, 1977.
35a. El-Gassar, L. M., et al.: Insecticide resistance in the cat flea. J. Econ. Entomol. 79:132, 1986.
36. Fadok, V. A.: Miscellaneous parasites of the skin (Part I). Compend. Cont. Ed. 2:707, 782, 1980.
37. Fain, A.: Epidemiological problems of scabies. Int. J. Dermatol. 17:20, 1978.
38. Farmer, H., and Seawright, A. A.: The use of amitraz (N1(2,4-dimethylphenyl)–N–[[(2,4-dimethylphenyl)imino]methyl]–N– methylmethanimidamide) in demodicosis in dogs. Aust. Vet. J. 56:537, 1980.
39. Farrell, R. K., Bill, T. G., et al.: Toxicity of flea collars. J.A.V.M.A. 166:1054, 1975.
40. Fehrer, S. L., and Halliwell, R. E.: Effectiveness of Avon's Skin-So-Soft as a flea repellent on dogs. J.A.A.H.A. 23:217, 1987.
41. Figueiredo, C.: Vitamin E serum contents, erythrocyte and lymphocyte counts, PCV and hemo-

globin determination in normal dogs, dogs with scabies and dogs with demodicosis. Proceedings, Am. Acad. Vet. Derm. Orlando, 1985.

42. Fletcher, K. C.: Demodicosis in a group of juvenile snow leopards. J.A.V.M.A. 177:896, 1980.

43. Folz, S. D.: Canine scabies (Sarcoptes scabiei infestation). Compend. Cont. Ed. 6:176, 1984.

44. Folz, S. D., Krotzer, D. D., et al.: Evaluation of a sponge-on therapy for canine scabies. J. Vet. Pharmacol. Ther. 7:29, 1984.

45. Fox, J. G., and Hewes, K.: Cheyletiella infestation in cats. J.A.V.M.A. 169:332, 1976.

46. Foxx, T. S., and Ewing, S. A.: Morphologic features, behavior and life history of Cheyletiella yasguri. Am. J. Vet. Res. 30:269, 1969.

47. Franc, M., et al.: Essai de traitment de l'otacriase du chat par les invermectines. Revue Med. Vet. 136:683, 1985.

47a. Franc, M., and Soubeyroux, H.: Le traitement de la demodecie du chien par un collier a 9% amitraz. Rev. Med. Vet. 137:583, 1986.

48. Frye, F. L., and Furman, D. P.: Phthiriasis in a dog. J.A.V.M.A. 152:1113, 1968.

49. Gaafer, S. M., and Greve, J.: Natural transmission of Demodex canis in dogs. J.A.V.M.A. 148:1043, 1966.

50. Gabbert, N., and Feldman, B. F.: A case report—feline demodex. Feline Pract. 6:32, 1976.

51. Georgi, J.: Parasitology for Veterinarians. 4th ed. W. B. Saunders Company, Philadelphia, 1985.

52. Gething, M. A.: Cheyletiella infestation of the cat. The Vet. Ann. J. Bristol, England, 1973.

53. Greene, R. T., Scheidt, V. J., et al.: Trombiculiasis in a cat. J.A.V.M.A. 188:1054, 1986.

54. Greve, J. H., and Gerrish, R. R.: Fur mites (Lynxacarus) from cats in Florida. Feline Pract. 11:28, 1981.

55. Halliwell, R. E. W.: Personal communication, University of Florida, 1977.

56. Halliwell, R. E. W.: Ineffectiveness of thiamine (vitamin B_1) as a flea-repellent in dogs. J.A.A.H.A. 18:423, 1982.

57. Halliwell, R. E. W.: Flea allergy dermatitis. In Kirk, R. W., (ed.): Current Veterinary Therapy VIII. W. B. Saunders Company, Philadelphia, 1983.

58. Hardison, J. L.: A case of Eutrombicula alfreddugesi (chiggers) in a cat. Vet. Med. (S.A.C.) 72:47, 1977.

59. Harmon, R. R. M.: Parasites, worms and protozoa. In Rook, A., William, D. S., and Ebling, E. J. G., (eds.): Textbook of Dermatology. Blackwell Scientific Publications, Oxford, 1979.

60. Harwick, R. P.: Lesions caused by canine ear mites. Arch. Dermatol. 114:130, 1978.

60a. Hawkins, J. A., McDonald, R. K., et al.: Sarcoptes scabei infestation in a cat. J.A.V.M.A. 190:1572, 1987.

61. Healy, M. C., and Gaafar, S. M.: Demonstration of reaginic antibody (IgE) in canine demodectic mange: an immunofluorescent study. Vet. Parasitol. 3:107, 1977a.

62. Healy, M. C., and Gaafar, S. M.: Immunodeficiency in canine demodectic mange. II. Skin reactions to phytohemagglutinin and concanavalin A. Vet. Parasitol. 3:133, 1977b.

62a. Hendrix, C. M., Blagburn, B. L., et al.: Anatrichosoma sp. infection in a dog. J.A.V.M.A. 191:984, 1987.

63. Hirsh, D. C., et al.: Suppression of in vitro lymphocyte transformation by serum from dogs with generalized demodicosis. Am. J. Vet. Res. 36:1591, 1975.

64. Hoeffler, D. F.: Swimmer's itch. Cutis 19:461, 1977.

65. Holzworth, J.: Notoedric mange of cats. In Kirk, R. W., (ed.): Current Veterinary Therapy III. W. B. Saunders Company, Philadelphia, 1968.

66. Horton, M. L.: Rhabditic dermatitis in dogs. Mod. Vet. Pract. 61:158, 1980.

67. Ilkiw, J. E.: Tick paralysis in Australia. In Kirk, R. W., (ed.): Current Veterinary Therapy VII. W. B. Saunders Company, Philadelphia, 1980.

68. Johnson, G. C.: Dracunculus insignis in the dog. J.A.V.M.A. 165:533, 1974.

69. Kalkofen, U. P., and Greenberg, J.: Public health aspects of Pulex irritans infestations in dogs. J.A.V.M.A. 165:903, 1974.

70. Kalkofen, U. P., and Greenberg, J.: Echidnophaga gallinacea infestations in dogs. J.A.V.M.A. 165:447, 1974.

71. Kazocos, K. R., et al.: Cuterebra species as a cause of pharyngeal myiasis in cats. J.A.A.H.A. 16:773, 1980.

72. King, L. E.: Spider bites. Arch. Dermatol. 123:41, 1987.

72a. Koehler, P. G., et al.: Residual efficacy of insecticides applied to carpet for control of cat fleas. J. Econ. Entomol. 79:1036, 1986.

73. Krawiec, D. R., and Gaafar, S. M.: Studies on immunology of demodicosis. J.A.A.H.A. 16:669, 1980.

74. Kristensen, S., Haarlov, N., et al.: A study of skin diseases of dogs and cats. IV. Patterns of flea infestations in dogs and cats in Denmark. Nord. Vet. Med. 30:401, 1978.

75. Kummel, B.: Case presentation. Am. Acad. Vet. Derm. annual meeting, Atlanta, April, 1981.

76. Kwochka, K. W.: Canine demodicosis. In Kirk, R. W., (ed.): Current Veterinary Therapy IX. 531. W. B. Saunders Company, Philadelphia, 1986.

77. Kwochka, K. W., Kunkle, G. A., et al.: The efficacy of amitraz for generalized demodicosis in dogs: A study of two concentrations and frequencies of application. Compend. Cont. Ed. Pract. Vet. 2:334, 1980.

78. Larkin, A. D., and Gaillard, G. E.: Mites in cat ears, a source of cross antigenicity with house dust mites. Preliminary report. Ann. Allergy, 46:301, 1981.

79. Lowenstine, L. J., Carpenter, J. L., et al.: Trombiculosis in a cat. J.A.V.M.A. 175:289, 1979.

80. MacDonald, J., and Miller, T. A.: Dynamics of natural flea infestation and evaluation of a control program. Canine Pract. 11:7, 1984.

81. MacDonald, J. M., and Miller, T. A.: Parasiticide therapy in small animal dermatology. In Kirk, R. W., (ed.): Current Veterinary Therapy IX. W. B. Saunders Company, Philadelphia, 1986.

81a. Maillard, R.: Quel est votre diagnostic? Point Vet. 19:569, 1987.

82. Maldonado, R. R., Tamayo, L., et al.: Norwegian scabies due to Sarcoptes scabiei var. canis. Arch. Dermatol. 113:1733, 1977.

83. Malone, J. B., et al.: Strongyloides stercoralis–like infection in a dog. J.A.V.M.A. 176:130, 1980.

84. Matthews, B. E.: Mechanics of skin penetration by hookworm larvae. Vet. Derm. Newsl. 6:75, 1981.

85. McDougal, B. J., and Novak, C. P.: Feline demodicosis caused by an unnamed demodex mite. Compend. Sm. Anim. Cont. Ed. 8:820, 1986.

86. McKee, A. J.: Microfilaria found in the skin. Vet. Med. 33:115, 1938.

87. McKeever, F. J., and Allen, S. K.: Dermatitis associated with Cheyletiella infestation in cats. J.A.V.M.A. 174:718, 1979.

87a. Medleau, L., et al.: Demodicosis in cats. J.A.A.H.A. 24:85, 1988.

88. Meerdink, G. L.: Bites and stings of venomous animals. In Kirk, R. W., (ed.): Current Veterinary Therapy VIII. W. B. Saunders Company, Philadelphia, 1983.

89. Miller, T. A.: Vaccination against hookworm diseases. Adv. Parasitol. 9:153, 1971.

90. Miller, W. H.: Canine demodicosis. Compend. Cont. Ed. 2:334, 1980.

91. Miller, W. H.: Personal communication, 1987.

92. Moriello, K. A.: Common ectoparasites of the dog. Part I, Fleas and Ticks Canine Pract. 14:7, 1987.

93. Muller, G. H.: Feline demodicosis. In Kirk, R. W., (ed.): Current Veterinary Therapy VIII. W. B. Saunders Company, Philadelphia, 1983.

94. Muller, G. H.: Demodicosis treatment with Mitaban liquid concentrate (amitraz). J.A.A.H.A. 19:435, 1983.

95. Niiyama, M., and Ohbayashi, M.: Cheyletiella blakei in a cat. Jpn. J. Vet. Sci. 41:395, 1979.

96. Norins, A. L.: Canine scabies in children. Am. J. Dis. Child. 117:239, 1969.

97. Northway, R. B.: A therapeutic approach to venomous spider bites. Vet. Med. 80:38, 1985.

98. Nutting, W. B.: Hair follicle mites (Acari: Demodicidae) of man. Int. J. Dermatol. 15:79, 1976.

99. Nutting, W. B.: Hair follicle mites (Demodex spp.) of medical and veterinary concern. Cornell Vet. 66:214, 1976.

100. Nutting, W. B., and Desch, C. E.: Demodex canis: redescription and reevaluation. Cornell Vet. 68:139, 1978.

101. Nutting, W. B.: Demodex creciti, notes on its biology. J. Parasitol. 44:328, 1958.

102. Orkin, M., et al.: Scabies and Pediculosis. J. B. Lippincott Company, Philadelphia, 1977.

102a. Osbrink, W. L. A., et al.: Distribution and control of cat fleas in homes in Southern California. J. Econ. Entomol. 79:135, 1986.

103. Ottenshot, T. R. F., and Gil, D.: Cheyletiellosis in long-haired cats. Tijdschr Diergeneeskd 103:1104, 1978.

104. Owen, L. N.: Transplantation of canine osteosarcoma. Eur. J. Cancer 5:615, 1969.

104a. Panciera, D. L., and Stockham, S. L.: Dracunulus insignia infection in a dog. J.A.V.M.A. 192:76, 1988.

104b. Paradis, M., and Villeneuve, A.: Efficacy of ivermectin against Cheyletiella yasguri infestation in dogs. Can. Vet. J. 1988 (in press).

105. Pasyk, K.: Dermatitis rhabditidosa in an 11-year-old girl. Br. J. Dermatol. 98:107, 1978.

106. Powell, M. B., Weisbroth, S. H., et al.: Reaginic hypersensitivity in Otodectes cynotis infestation of cats and mode of mite feeding. Am. J. Vet. Res. 41:877, 1980.

107. Rack, G.: Cheyletiella yasquri, 1965 ein fakultativ menschenpathogener Parasit des Hundes. Z. Parasitenkd. 36:321, 1971.

108. Ramsay, G. W., and Mason, P. C.: Chicken mite (D. gallinae) infesting a dog. N.Z. Vet. J. 23:155, 1975.

109. Randall, W. F., Bradley, R. E., et al.: Field evaluation of antiflea collars for initial and residual efficacy in dogs. Vet. Med. (S.A.C.) 75:606, 1980.

110. Rash, D. M., and Benzon, S. P.: Dracunculosis in a dog. Mod. Vet. Pract. 62:701, 1981.

111. Reedy, L. M.: Common parasitic problems in small animal dermatology. J.A.V.M.A. 188:362, 1986.

112. Rosser, E.: Comments on transmission of demodectic mites. Am. Anim. Hosp. Assoc. 54th Annual Meeting, Phoenix, March, 1987.

113. Sako, S., and Yamane, O.: Studies on the canine demodicosis. II. The significance of presence of the parasite in lymphatic glands of affected dogs. Jpn. J. Parasitol. 11:93, 1962.

114. Sako, S., and Yamane, O.: Studies on the canine demodicosis. III. Examination of the oral-internal infection, intrauterine infection, and infection through respiratory tract. Jpn. J. Parasitol. 11:499, 1962.

115. Sako, S.: Studies on the canine demodicosis. IV. Experimental infection of Demodex folliculorum var. canis to dogs. Trans. Tottori Soc. Agri. Sci. 17:45, 1964.

116. Schick, M. P., and Schick, R. O.: Understanding and implementing safe and effective flea control. J.A.A.H.A. 22:421, 1986.

116a. Schwinghammer, K. A., et al.: Comparative toxicity of ten insecticides against the cat flea, Ctenocephalides felis. J. Med. Entomol. 22:512, 1985.

117. Scott, D. W.: Further studies on the immunologic and therapeutic aspects of canine demodicosis. J.A.V.M.A. 167:855, 1975.

118. Scott, D. W.: Demodicosis (demodectic mange, follicular mange, red mange) In Kirk, R. W., (ed.): Current Veterinary Therapy VI. W. B. Saunders Company, Philadelphia, 1977.

119. Scott, D. W.: Canine demodicosis. Vet. Clin. North Am. (Small Anim. Pract.) 9:79, 1979.

120. Scott, D. W.: Nodular skin disease associated with dirofilaria immitis infection in the dog. Cornell Vet. 69:233, 1979.

121. Scott, D. W.: Feline dermatology 1900–1978: a monograph. J.A.A.H.A. 16:331, 1980.

122. Scott, D. W.: Feline dermatology 1979–1982: Introspective retrospections. J.A.A.H.A. 20:537, 1984.

123. Scott, D. W., Farrow, B. R. H., et al.: Studies on the therapeutic and immunologic aspects of generalized demodectic mange in the dog. J.A.A.H.A. 10:233, 1974.

123a. Scott, D. W.: The skin. In Holzworth, J. (ed.): Diseases of the Cat: Medicine & Surgery. W. B. Saunders Company, Philadelphia, 1987, p. 619.

124. Scott, D. W., Schultz, R. D., et al.: Further studies on the therapeutic and immunologic aspects of generalized demodectic mange in the dog. J.A.A.H.A. 12:203, 1976.

125. Scott, D. W., and Vaughn, T. C.: Papulonodular dermatitis in a dog with occult filariasis. Comp. Anim. Pract. 1 p. 31, March 1987.

126. Scott, D. W., and Walton, D. K.: Experiences with the use of amitraz and ivermectin for the treatment of generalized demodicosis in dogs. J.A.A.H.A. 21:535, 1985.

127. Shirk, M. A.: Therapy of demodicosis. Presentation at Am. Acad. Vet. Dermatol. meeting at A.A.H.A. Annual Meeting, Atlanta, April, 1981.

127a. Singh, J., and Gill, B. S.: Invermectin treatment of sarcoptic mange in dogs. Mod. Vet. Pract. 68:437, 1987.

128. Smiley, R. L.: A review of the family Cheyletiellidae (Acarina). Ann. Entomol. Soc. Am. 63:1056, 1970.

129. Smith, B. L., and Elliott, D. C.: Canine pedal dermatitis due to percutaneous Uncinaria stenocephala infection. N.Z. Vet. J. 17:235, 1969.

130. Smith, E. B., and Claypoole, T. F.: Canine scabies in dogs and humans. J.A.M.A. 199:94, 1967.

131. Smith, J. D., Goette, D. K., et al.: Larva currens; cutaneous strongyloides. Arch. Dermatol. 112:1161, 1976.

132. Soulsby, E. J. L.: Helminths, Arthropods and Protozoa of Domesticated Animals. 7th ed. Lee & Febiger, Philadelphia, 1982.

133. Stein, B.: Personal communication, 1982.

134. Stogdale, L., and Moore, D. J.: Feline demodicosis. J.A.A.H.A. 18:427, 1982.

135. Subrahmanyam, B., Rami-Reddy, Y., et al.: Dracunculus medinesis (guinea worm) infestation in a dog and its therapy with Flagyl. Indian Vet. J. 53:637, 1976.

136. Thomsett, L. R.: Mite infestations of man contracted from dogs and cats. Br. Med. J. 3:93, 1968.

137. Weisbroth, S. H., Powell, M. B., et al.: Immunopathology of naturally-occurring otodectic otoa-

cariasis in the domestic cat. J.A.V.M.A. *165*:1088, 1974.

138. Weisbroth, S. H., Wilhelmsen, C., and Powell, M. B.: Efficacy of Vapona-containing flea collars for control of otodectes mites. Cornell Vet. *64*:549, 1979.

139. White, S. D., and Stannard, A. A.: Canine demodicosis. *In* Kirk, R. W., (ed.): Current Veterinary Therapy VIII, W. B. Saunders Company, Philadelphia, 1983.

139a. White, S. D., et al.: Generalized demodicosis associated with diabetes mellitus in two cats. J.A.V.M.A. *191*:448, 1987.

139b. Whiteley, H. E.: Five flea-control programs for cats. Vet. Med. *82*:1022, 1987.

140. Wilkie, B. N., Markham, R. J. F., et al.: Deficient cutaneous response to PHA-P in healthy puppies from a kennel with a high prevalence of demodicosis. Can. J. Comp. Med. *43*:415, 1979.

141. Wilkinson, G. T.: An overview of feline skin disease. Australia Proc. Univ. Sydney Post-Grad Comm. Vet. Sci. *57*:277, 1981.

142. Wilkinson, G. T.: Demodicosis in a cat due to a new mite species. Feline Pract. *13*:32, 1983.

143. Willers, W. B.: Pelodera strongyloides in association with canine dermatitis in Wisconsin. J.A.V.M.A. *156*:319, 1970.

144. Wong, R. C., Hughes, S. E., et al.: Spider bites (in depth review). Arch. Dermatol. *123*:98, 1987.

145. Yazwinski, T. A., et al.: Efficacy of ivermectin against *Sarcoptes scabiei* and *Otodectes cynotis* infestations of dogs. Vet. Med. (S.A.C.) *76*:1749, 1981.

9

Immunologic Diseases

Cutaneous Immunology

Because of the incredible expansion of knowledge in basic and clinical immunology, it has become impossible to keep up with new information related to clinical immunodermatologic problems. An adequate review of this information is decidedly beyond the scope of this chapter. For the practitioner, student, and academician interested in details, a plethora of basic and clinical immunology texts, as well as in-depth dermatology texts, is available.[49, 62, 96, 149, 162, 171, 212, 217a, 227] In this section we will confine ourselves to a brief overview of basic and clinical immunodermatology.

The immune system and its inflammatory limb are complex models of biologic activity and interaction. There is a tendency to dissect the immune response into its individual components and to discuss them as autonomous functional units. However, immune responses are delicately interwoven and interdependent, and manipulation of one component influences all others (Fig. 9:1).

CUTANEOUS INFLAMMATION

Inflammation may be defined as the changes occurring in living tissue when it is injured, provided that the injury is not severe enough to immediately kill all the cells.[227] Inflammatory changes include both the processes of tissue damage induced by the initial stimulus and those induced by the autologous changes occurring after the initial stimulus. The intensity and duration of the inflammation are controlled, to some extent, by the nature of the stimulus and the severity of the damage.

Regardless of the injurious agent or the area involved, the inflammatory response is characterized by a certain number of tissue adjustments that involve mainly blood vessels and fluid and other cellular components of the blood, as well as the surrounding connective tissue. Thus, very similar findings may accompany the inflammatory response of the skin to bacteria, fungi, parasites, heat, cold, radiation, chemicals, mechanical trauma, or allergens.

To the clinician, cutaneous inflammation may be characterized by (1) *redness* (rubor) due to vasodilation, (2) *swelling* (tumor) due to increased capillary permeability resulting in edema, (3) *heat* (calor) due to increased blood flow, and (4) *pain* (dolor) or *pruritus*, or both, due to involvement of peripheral nerve fibers.

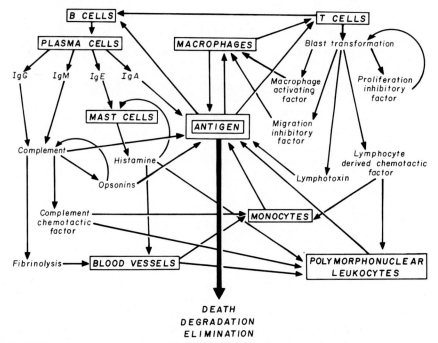

Figure 9:1. The immune system—a complex system of interrelated components. Activity of one component often affects others. (From Dahl, M. V.: Clinical Immunodermatology. Year Book Medical Publishers, Inc., Chicago, 1981.)

OVERVIEW OF THE IMMUNE SYSTEM

The immune response results from an integrated sequence of events involving antigens, lymphocytes, antibodies, lymphokines, mediator substances, and effector cells operating under genetic and physiologic controls to protect the host from harmful agents and to remove dead or injured tissue. Sometimes the immune response misfunctions by under-responding or over-responding. Under-response predisposes one to infections and hinders the elimination of noxious substances. Over-response produces excessive inflammation and may lead to autoimmunity. Both under-response and over-response can lead to dermatologic disease. Age, nutrition, and stress can have profound effects on the immune response.[48, 54, 175, 180, 213a]

Cells Involved in the Immune Response

Lymphocytes are classically divided into two main types: B cells (bursa or bone-marrow derived) and T cells (thymus dependent) (see Fig. 9:1).

B cells are characterized by possessing surface immunoglobulins, Fc receptors, and C3b receptors. B cells differentiate into *plasma cells*, which produce the immunoglobulins, IgG, IgM, IgA, and IgE (Table 9:1), and they are responsible for humoral (antibody) immunity. The humoral immune system is instrumental in initiating immune and inflammatory responses. It is under genetic control and also under positive and negative feedback control systems that modulate the amount of response. Humoral immunity provides primary defense against invading bacteria and neutralization activity against circulating viruses. A model for a spontaneous condition in animals that is similar to

Table 9:1. BASIC CHARACTERISTICS OF IMMUNOGLOBULIN CLASSES IN DOGS AND CATS

Property	IgG	IgM	IgA	Ige*
Usual sedimentation coefficient	7S	19S	11S	8S
Molecular weight	180,000 d	900,000 d	360,000 d	200,000 d
Electrophoretic mobility	γ	β	$\beta-\gamma$	$\beta-\gamma$
Characteristic heavy-chain antigen	γ	μ	α	ϵ
Major site of synthesis	Spleen and nodes	Spleen and nodes	Intestine	Intestine
Subclasses	Dog (IgG_1, IgG_{2a}, IgG_{2b}, IgG_{2c}) Cat (IgG_1, IgG_2)	—	—	—

*IgE has not been demonstrated in the cat.

selective IgA deficiency in humans has been described in beagles.[60] The condition appeared to be hereditary and was characterized by recurrent superficial staphylococcal folliculitis and suppurative otitis externa, in association with severe IgA deficiency. A similar IgA deficiency syndrome has been described in Shar Pei with respiratory disease and an atopic-like dermatosis.[138a] Relative serum IgA deficiency has also been reported as a breed abnormality in German shepherds.[242] However, no disease associations were mentioned.

T cells are responsible for cell-mediated immunity. Among the many functions attributable to T cells are the following: (1) helping B cells make antibody (T-helper) cells, (2) suppressing B-cell antibody production (T-suppressor cells), (3) directly damaging "target" cells, (4) mediating delayed hypersensitivity reactions, (5) suppressing delayed hypersensitivity reactions mediated by other T cells, (6) modulating the inflammatory response with lymphokines, (7) inducing graft rejection, and (8) producing graft-versus-host reactions. Cell-mediated immunity is specifically geared to defend against organisms that are intracellular or otherwise hidden from circulating or humoral factors (intracellular viruses, fungi, *Mycobacteria*, and parasites). T cells seem to play a central role in orchestrating the immune response. They can force B cells to make greater or lesser quantities of antibodies, or they can reduce cell-mediated immune reactions. T cells are able to elaborate lymphokines that amplify or dampen phagocytic activity, collagen production, vascular permeability and coagulation phenomena. They can kill microorganisms and other cells, or they can recruit effector cells to perform this function. T-cell function is known to be suppressed by numerous infections (staphylococcal pyoderma, demodicosis, blastomycosis, canine distemper, feline leukemia virus infection), cancers, and drugs.[20, 149, 227] A sex-linked (male) combined immunodeficiency disease has been reported in basset hounds.[60a, 83a] Affected pups were lymphopenic, hypoglobulinemic, stunted, and unthrifty. They had severe pyoderma, stomatitis, and otitis, and they rapidly succumbed to viral infections (especially canine distemper) before 4 months of age.

Monocytes and *macrophages* (the mononuclear phagocyte system) have critical phagocytic, secretory, and antigen-processing functions (Table 9:2). Mononuclear phagocytes are necessary for processing antigen to initiate im-

Table 9:2. MONOCYTE-MACROPHAGE FUNCTIONS

1. Antigen Processing

2. Phagocytosis

Ingestion of microorganisms
Ingestion of insoluble particles
Killing of antibody-coated cells
Wound débridement
Dead cells and remnant digestion

3. Secretion

Enzymes

Lysozyme
Neutral proteases
Plasminogen activator
Collagenase
Elastase
Leukokinins
Acid hydrolases
Proteases
Lipases
Deoxyribonucleases
Phosphatases
Glucosidases
Sulfatases

Complement Components
C1, C2, C3, C4, C5
All components of alternate pathway

Enzyme Inhibitors
Plasmin inhibitors
Alpha$_2$-macroglobulin

Binding Proteins
Transferrin
Fibronectin

Endogenous Pyrogens

Reactive metabolites of oxygen
Superoxide
Hydrogen peroxide
Hydroxyl radical
Singlet oxygen

Bioactive lipids
Prostaglandins
Thromboxanes
Leukotrienes
Platelet activating factors

Monokines
Neutrophil chemotactic factor
Lymphocyte activating factors
Lymphocyte suppressor factors
Colony stimulating factor
Alpha interferon
Fibroblast stimulating factors
Fibroblast suppressor factors
Interleukin 1

mune responses and for secreting biologically active substances that mediate the immune and inflammatory response.

Neutrophils, as their major role, have the function of containing infection (Table 9:3). However, owing to their numerous chemoattractants (Table 9:4) and intracellular products (Table 9:5), they are omnipresent participants in virtually all immune and inflammatory reactions. Neutrophil dysfunctions have been described in dogs with pyoderma and generalized demodicosis,[119, 120] but are likely secondary to the skin disease. Hereditary (autosomal recessive)

Table 9:3. NEUTROPHIL FUNCTIONS

Phagocytosis (after opsonization)
Killing
   Nonoxidative (lysozyme, elastase, proteases)
   Oxidative (H_2O_2, singlet oxygen, hydroxyl radical, superoxide)
Degranulation
Chemotaxis
Modulation of inflammation
Inhibit fibroblast chemotaxis

Table 9:4. CHEMOATTRACTANTS FOR NEUTROPHILS

Bacterial products
C5a (derived from complement activation; tissue, virus, and bacterial enzymes cleave C5)
C3a
C567
Kallikrein
Denatured protein
Lymphokines
Monokines
Neutrophil chemotactic factor (NCF) from mast cells
Eosinophil chemotactic factor of anaphylaxis (ECF–A) from mast cells
Lipid chemotactic factors (HETE, etc.) from mast cells
Lysosomal proteases
Collagen breakdown products
Fibrin breakdown products
Plasminogen activator
Prostaglandins
Leukotrienes
Immune complexes

intracellular killing defects have been demonstrated in neutrophils from Irish setters with recurrent bacterial infections (canine granulocytopathy syndrome)[83a, 161] and in gray collies with cyclic hematopoiesis (see p. 710).

Eosinophils, effector cells in hypersensitivity reactions, also participate in the downgrading of inflammation (Tables 9:6 and 9:7).[153a] They are also phagocytic (immune complexes, mast cell granules, aggregated immunoglobulins, and certain bacteria and fungi). Eosinophils also play a unique role in the defense of the host against extracellular parasitic infection.

Basophils are effector cells in hypersensitivity reactions (containing histamine and other inflammatory mediators, similar to mast cells) and are involved in cutaneous basophil hypersensitivity, a T cell–controlled reaction, which is important in host responses to various ectoparasites.

Table 9:5. NEUTROPHIL PRODUCTS

Antimicrobial Enzymes
  Lysozyme
  Myeloperoxidase

Proteases
  Collagenase
  Collagenolytic proteinase
  Elastase
  Cathepsin G
  Leukokinins

Hydrolases
  Cathepsin B
  Cathepsin D
  N-acetyl-β-glucosaminidase
  β-glycerophosphatase
  β-glucuronidase

Others
  Lactoferrin
  Eosinophil chemotactic factor
  Leukotrienes
  Pyrogen
  Prostaglandins
  Thromboxanes

Table 9:6. EOSINOPHIL PRODUCTS AND THEIR FUNCTIONS

Substance	Function
Acid phosphatase	Unknown
Arylsulfatase	Inactivates leukotrienes
Cationic protein	Inactivates heparin
Collagenase	Lyses collagen
Histaminase	Degrades histamine
Hydrogen peroxide	Cytotoxic
Kininase	Inactivates kinins
Leukotrienes	Proinflammatory
Major basic protein	Cytotoxic
Peroxidase	Stimulates mast cell secretion
Phospholipase	Inactivates platelet activating factor (PAF)
Plasminogen	Lyses fibrin
Prostaglandins	Inhibit mast cell degranulation
Pyrogen	Produces fever
Zinc	Inhibits mast cell degranulation

Table 9:7. CHEMOATTRACTANTS FOR EOSINOPHILS

Factor	Source
Histamine	Mast cells
Eosinophil chemotactic factor of anaphylaxis (ECF–A)	Mast cells, neutrophils
Eosinophil stimulation promoter (ESP)	T lymphocytes
Immune complexes	—
C5a	Complement
C567	Complement
Hydroxyeicosatetraenoic acid (HETE)	Platelets, mast cells, arachidonic acid
Leukotrienes	Mast cells, mononuclear cells, polymorphonuclear cells, keratinocytes

Table 9:8. MAST CELL PRODUCTS AND THEIR ACTIONS

Mediator	Action
Histamine	Smooth muscle contraction, increased vascular permeability, elevation of cyclic AMP, enhancement or inhibition of chemotaxis
Leukotrienes	Smooth muscle contraction, increased vascular permeability, chemotaxis of neutrophils, eosinophils, monocytes, and fibroblasts; epidermal hyperplasia
Platelet activating factor (PAF)	Increased vascular permeability, platelet and neutrophil activation
Eosinophil chemotactic factor of anaphylaxis (ECF–A)	Chemoattraction of eosinophils and neutrophils
Neutrophil chemotactic factor (NCF)	Chemoattraction of neutrophils
Lipid chemotactic factors (HETE, etc.)	Chemoattraction of eosinophils, neutrophils, and monocytes
Heparin	Anticoagulation, inhibition of complement activation, inhibition of proteolytic enzymes
Proteolytic enzymes	Proteolysis and hydrolysis

Langerhans' cells are located in the epidermis. They are cells of the monocyte-macrophage series, the primary function of which is presentation of antigens to lymphocytes. The role of the Langerhans' cell in the mammalian epidermis is probably to process antigens absorbed through the skin.

Mast cells are believed to be of monocytogenous origin.[153] These cells serve as repositories for numerous inflammatory mediator substances, including histamine, leukotrienes, eosinophil chemotactic factor of anaphylaxis, and proteolytic enzymes (Table 9:8).[108a, 227] The major role of mast cells is probably the recruitment of eosinophils and neutrophils, immunoglobulins, and complement from the circulation. The actions of mast cell mediators can be divided into three broad categories: (1) to increase vascular permeability and contract smooth muscle, (2) to be chemotactic for or to activate other mediators, and (3) to modulate the release of other mediators. Mast cells may be divided morphologically and functionally into type I (atypical, mucosal) and type II (typical, connective tissue) cells.[20a, 20b, 26b] "Mucosal" and "connective tissue" are misleading terms, as both types occur in mucosa and connective tissue. This heterogeneity of mast cells has been demonstrated in dog skin.[20a, 20b] The skin of atopic dogs contains at least two subsets of mast cells that are distinguished in the following ways: (1) histologically by metachromatic staining properties in different fixatives, and (2) functionally, by response to antigen in vivo.

Mediator Substances

The changes observed in inflammation are mediated by substances derived from the plasma, from cells of the damaged tissue, and from infiltrating leukocytes. The interactions between cells and soluble mediators determine the inflammatory response. Some mediators augment inflammation, while others suppress it. Some mediators antagonize or destroy other mediators, whereas others amplify or generate other mediators. All mediators and cells normally act together in a harmonious fashion to maintain homeostasis and to protect the host against infectious agents and other noxious substances.

A current summary of inflammatory mediator substances and their biologic actions are listed and cross-referenced in Table 9:9. It is important to note that *histamine* appears to be a minor mediator of pruritus and cutaneous inflammation in dogs and cats, as antihistamines are often ineffective for controlling pruritic and inflammatory dermatoses in these species. *Proteolytic enzymes* appear to be the important pruritogenic mediators in dogs and cats.

Interestingly, histamine has two types of effects on hypersensitivity reactions: "proinflammatory" and "anti-inflammatory." The proinflammatory effects of histamine (see Table 9:8) are mediated through histamine$_1$ (H$_1$) receptors and resultant decreases in intracellular cyclic adenosine monophosphate (AMP) (Fig. 9:2). The anti-inflammatory effects of histamine (inhibition of inflammatory mediator substances release from mast cells, neutrophils, lymphocytes, and monocyte-macrophages) are mediated through H$_2$ receptors and resultant increases in cyclic AMP. Canine and feline blood vessels have been reported to possess both H$_1$ and H$_2$ receptors.[20a]

Complement is a series of several plasma proteins that induce and influence immunologic and inflammatory events (Table 9:10).[5, 82] The critical step in the generation of biologic activities from the complement proteins is the cleavage of C3. There are two pathways for the cleavage of C3 (the classic and the alternative [properdin]), a pathway to amplify C3 cleavage, and an effector

Table 9:9. INFLAMMATORY MEDIATORY SUBSTANCES AND THEIR ACTIONS

Mediator	Action
Histamine	See Table 9:8
Serotonin	Smooth muscle contraction, increased vascular permeability
Leukotrienes	See Table 9:8
ECF–A	See Table 9:8
NCF	See Table 9:8
PAF	See Table 9:8
Heparin	See Table 9:8
Prostaglandins	Increased vascular permeability, potentiate itch and pain, modulate cyclic AMP and the release of other mediators
Thromboxanes	Increased vascular permeability, potentiate itch and pain, modulate cyclic AMP and the release of other mediators
Neutrophil proteases	Proteolysis and hydrolysis
Monocyte-macrophage proteases	Proteolysis and hydrolysis
Mast cell proteases	Proteolysis and hydrolysis
Eosinophil proteases	Proteolysis and hydrolysis
Lymphokines	See Table 9:12
Monokines	See Table 9:12
Kallikrein and kinins	Smooth muscle contraction, increased vascular permeability, pain, neutrophil chemotaxis
Complement	See Table 9:10
Fibrin breakdown products (fibrinopeptides)	Increased vascular permeability, neutrophil chemotaxis

sequence. The biologic activities attributed to various complement components are listed in Table 9:11. In dogs, hemolytic complement levels were reported to be decreased with enteropathies, hepatopathies, systemic lupus erythematosus, and systemic glucocorticoid therapy.[139, 140] A genetically determined (autosomal recessive) deficiency of C3 has been reported in Brittany spaniels that have recurrent bacterial skin infections and sepsis.[83a, 253]

Immune complexes are a heterogenous group of immunoreactants formed by the noncovalent union of antigen and antibody.[225, 257] Many factors influence the formation, immunochemistry, biology, and clearance of these reactants. Circulating immune complexes influence both the afferent and efferent limbs of the immune response and can mediate tissue damage in certain pathologic states. Circulating immune complexes can be measured by a number of generally unavailable techniques, including C1q-binding assay, solid-phase C1q assay, conglutinin, and Raji cell assays. Circulating immune complexes have been detected in numerous human dermatoses and probably play an important role in the pathogenesis of systemic lupus erythematosus and vasculitis. Circulating immune complexes have been demonstrated in 6 per cent of a normal dog population, in contrast to 25 per cent of a population of sick dogs,[224] and in numerous conditions such as diabetes mellitus, hypothyroidism, arthropathies, nephropathies, neuropathies, mycotic and parasitic infections, systemic and discoid lupus erythematosus, cutaneous vasculitis, generalized demodicosis, and pyoderma.[53, 158, 224]

Lymphokines and *monokines* are proteins produced by activated T lymphocytes and monocyte-macrophages. More than 30 cytokines have been described, but it is not clear whether each has a unique function or if a given cytokine may perform several different functions. In any case, cytokines play a key role in inducing and modulating inflammatory reactions, especially in

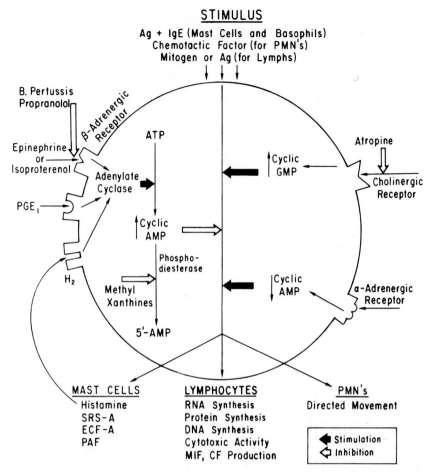

Figure 9:2. Diagrammatic representation of pathways by which pharmacologic mediators might act on mast cell, lymphocyte, and PMN leukocyte membrane receptors to alter intracellular cyclic nucleotides, which in turn may either enhance or inhibit the function of those cells. Abbreviations include the following: Ag = antigen, PGE_1 = prostaglandin E_1, SRS—A = slow-reacting substance of anaphylaxis, ECF—A = eosinophil chemotactic factor of anaphylaxis, PAF = platelet activating factor, MIF = migration inhibitor factor, CF = chemotactic factor. (From Hanifin, J. M., and Lobitz, W. C.: Newer concepts of atopic dermatitis. Arch. Dermatol. *113*:663, 1977.)

Table 9:10. COMPLEMENT FUNCTIONS

Causes cell lysis
Kills certain bacteria and protozoa
Chemoattracts neutrophils, eosinophils, and monocyte-macrophages
Attaches antigens to phagocytes (immune adherence)
Opsonizes microorganisms and particles
Neutralizes certain viruses
Induces mast cell degranulation (anaphylatoxins)
Produces kinins
Activates clotting and fibrinolysis
Modulates inflammation by feedback mechanisms and interplay with inhibitors
Interacts with B lymphocytes
Mediates lysosome release

Table 9:11. BIOLOGIC ACTIONS OF COMPLEMENT COMPONENTS

Factor	Action
C2-derived peptide (C-kinin)	Increased vascular permeability
C3a	Anaphylatoxin (releases mediators from mast cells); chemotactic to neutrophils, eosinophils, and monocyte-macrophages
C3b	Immune adherence, enhanced phagocytosis, secretion of lysosomal enzymes
C5a	Anaphylatoxin; chemotactic to neutrophils and monocyte-macrophages; secretion of lysosomal enzymes
C567	Chemotactic to neutrophils, eosinophils, and monocyte-macrophages
C5-9	Lysis of membranes

cell-mediated immune reactions and delayed-type hypersensitivity reactions (Table 9:12). Recently, it was recommended that the various cytokines be gathered into three major groups: (1) interleukin 1 (lymphocyte blastogenic factor, antibody production–enhancing factor, endogenous pyrogen, fibroblast stimulation factor, etc.) produced by macrophages, keratinocytes, and Langerhans' cells, (2) interleukin 2 (T-cell growth factor, thymocyte-activating factor, thymocyte-stimulating factor, etc.) produced by T cells, and (3) interleukin 3 (T-cell and mast cell growth factor) produced by T cells.[49, 125, 217a, 227]

Prostaglandins and *leukotrienes*, playing a central role, often act synergistically with other mediators, both in the expression of the efferent limb of immune-based inflammatory responses and in acute inflammatory responses when specific immunity does not play a primary role.[52] Prostaglandins and leukotrienes are produced by most, if not all, cells participating in the afferent and efferent limbs of the immune system as well as by keratinocytes, fibroblasts, and endothelial cells. Their formation depends on the deacylation of arachidonic acid from cellular phospholipids, catalyzed by the activity of various phospholipases, and the subsequent utilization of arachidonic acid by cyclo-oxygenase and various lipoxygenase enzymes. Cyclo-oxygenase converts free arachidonic acid to the endoperoxides that serve as precursors of the thromboxanes as well

Table 9:12. LYMPHOKINES AND MONOKINES AND THEIR FUNCTIONS

Lymphokine	Function
Migration inhibition factor (MIF)	Inhibits macrophage movement
Leukocyte inhibition factor (LIF)	Inhibits neutrophil movement
Macrophage activating factor	Increases macrophage adherence, phagocytosis, and protein synthesis
Lymphocyte-derived chemotactic factor	Chemotactic to monocytes
Eosinophil stimulation promoter (ESP)	Chemotactic to eosinophils
Skin reactive factor	Induces vascular permeability
Transfer factor	Educates unsensitized lymphocytes
Interferon	Defense against virus, modulates lymphocyte and macrophage functions
Lymphocyte blastogenic factor	Recruits unsensitized lymphocytes
Antibody production enhancing factor	Increases antibody production
Antibody production suppressing factor	Decreases antibody production
Proliferation inhibitor factor	Inhibits cell division of various cells
Lymphotoxin	Cytotoxic for various cells
Fibroblast stimulation factor	Increases collagen production
Lymph node permeability factor	Induces vascular permeability
Interleukin 2	Initiates and maintains T lymphocyte proliferation
Interleukin 1	Stimulates T-cell and B-cell activity; pyrogen

as the various prostaglandins and prostacyclin. The lipoxygenases form hydro-peroxy-eicosatetraenoic acids (HPETEs), which are further metabolized to the hydroxy-eicosatetraenoic acids (HETEs) and leukotrienes. These arachidonic acid oxygenation products have numerous complex effects on the inflammatory response (Tables 9:8 and 9:9) and are currently the focus of much pathogenetic and therapeutic research.

THE ROLE OF CYCLIC NUCLEOTIDES IN INFLAMMATION

Szentivanyi proposed the β-adrenergic theory of atopic disease in 1968. He suggested that the heightened sensitivity of atopic human beings to various pharmacologic agents could be due to a blockage of β-adrenergic receptors in tissues. Since that time, there has been an explosion of investigative effort in the field of the cyclic nucleotides.[139, 217a] In brief, the cyclic nucleotides, cyclic AMP and cyclic guanosine monophosphate (GMP), appear to serve as the intracellular effectors of a variety of cellular events. They are viewed as exerting opposing influences in a number of systems.

A number of pharmacologic agents are known to act via various cell receptors to influence intracellular levels of cyclic AMP and cyclic GMP (see Fig. 9:2). In general, substances that elevate intracellular cyclic AMP levels (β-adrenergic drugs, prostaglandin E, methylxanthines, histamine, and other mediator substances) or reduce intracellular cyclic GMP levels (anticholinergic drugs) tend to stabilize the cells (lymphocytes, monocyte-macrophages, neutrophils, mast cells) and inhibit the release of various inflammatory mediators. On the other hand, substances that reduce cyclic AMP levels (α-adrenergic drugs) or elevate cyclic GMP levels (cholinergic drugs, ascorbic acid, estrogen, levamisole) tend to labilize the cells and promote the release of inflammatory mediators. Further studies in the area of cyclic nucleotides and biologic regulation may produce significant advances in the areas of disease pathomechanism and control of immunologic inflammation.

THE MAJOR HISTOCOMPATIBILITY COMPLEX AND SKIN DISEASE

The major histocompatibility complex (MHC) is a chromosomal region that contains several genes that are important in the determination of cell surface antigens.[93, 94, 228] These antigens are glycoproteins on the cell surface of nucleated cells that aid in the recognition of "self" and "nonself." Three classes of genes are located within the MHC: (1) class I genes code for antigens that provoke graft rejection, (2) class II genes (immune response genes) code for antigens that regulate an animal's ability to mount an immune response, and (3) class III genes code for some complement components.

The collective name given to the genes of the MHC depends on the species of animal: dog leukocyte antigens (DLA), cat leukocyte antigens (CLA). Class I antigens are serologically defined and measured in vitro using a microlymphocytotoxicity assay. Class II antigens are lymphocyte defined and measured in vitro by the mixed lymphocyte culture.

In humans, many dermatoses have been related to certain human leukocyte antigen (HLA) types.[11, 49] Future studies in dogs and cats may be useful for gaining insight in regard to the inheritance and early detection of dermatoses, as well as for the breeding of disease-resistant animals.[228]

TYPES OF HYPERSENSITIVITY REACTIONS

Immunology is the science that permits the study of the mechanisms that preserve the biologic identity of animal organisms, or the self from the nonself. This function is carried out by a process characterized by two outstanding features: specificity and memory. If this process is effective, it is correctly called "allergy." When it is protective, this specific, effective immunologic response is called "immunity." If this response is injurious, it is called "hypersensitivity." In practice, the terms "allergy" and "hypersensitivity" are inappropriately used interchangeably.

Clinical hypersensitivity disorders have been divided by Gell and Coombs, on an immunopathologic basis, into four types.

Type I: immediate (anaphylactic)

Type II: cytotoxic

Type III: immune complex

Type IV: cell mediated (delayed)

Clearly, this scheme is oversimplified because of the complex inter-relationships that exist among the several occurrences that constitute an inflammatory response. In most pathologic events, immunologically initiated responses will almost certainly involve multiple components of the inflammatory process. Realization that this is a simplistic approach to immunopathology has provoked other investigators to modify the original scheme of Gell and Coombs, often to a seemingly hopeless degree of hair splitting.[220] In this section we will briefly examine the classic Gell and Coombs classification of hypersensitivity disorders, because (1) it is applicable to discussions on cutaneous hypersensitivity diseases, and (2) it is still the immunopathologic scheme used by most authors and by major immunologic and dermatologic texts.[49, 62, 149, 162, 171, 212, 217a, 227]

Type I (anaphylactic, immediate) hypersensitivity reactions are classically described as those involving genetic predilection, reaginic antibody (IgE) production, and mast cell degranulation. A genetically programmed individual inhales (or possibly ingests or absorbs percutaneously) a complete antigen (e.g., ragweed pollen) and responds by producing a unique antibody (reagin, IgE). IgE is homocytotropic and avidly binds membrane receptors on tissue mast cells and blood basophils. When the eliciting antigen comes in contact with the specific reaginic antibody, a number of inflammatory mediator substances are released and cause tissue damage. It is important to note that older terms like "reaginic," "homocytotropic," or "skin-sensitizing" antibodies are *not* strictly synonymous with IgE, as subclasses of IgG may also mediate type I hypersensitivity reactions. Examples of type I hypersensitivity reactions in dogs and cats include urticaria, angioedema, anaphylaxis, atopy, food hypersensitivity, flea bite hypersensitivity, and drug eruption.

Classic type I hypersensitivity reactions appear within minutes of challenge and abate within 30 to 60 minutes.[108a] Recently, *late-phase immediate hypersensitivity reactions* have been recognized and studied.[11a, 104, 108a, 122] The onset of these mast cell–dependent reactions occurs 4 to 8 hours after challenge (neutrophils and eosinophils found histologically) and persist up to 24 hours (mononuclear cells predominate histologically). These late-phase reactions can be reproduced with intradermal injections of leukotrienes, kallikrein, or platelet-activating factor (PAF). Although late-phase reactions to the intradermal injection of allergens have been recorded in atopic dogs,[20b] the clinical importance of late-phase reactions remains to be defined in dogs and cats.

Type II (cytotoxic) hypersensitivity reactions are characterized by the binding of antibody (IgG or IgM), with or without complement, to complete antigens on body tissues. This binding of antibody, with or without complement, results in cytotoxicity or cytolysis. Examples of type II hypersensitivity reactions in dogs and cats include pemphigus, pemphigoid, cold agglutinin disease, and drug eruption.

Type III (immune complex) hypersensitivity reactions are characterized by the deposition of circulating antigen-antibody complexes (in slight antigen excess) in blood vessel walls. These immune complexes (usually containing IgG or IgM) then fix complement, which attracts neutrophils. Proteolytic and hydrolytic enzymes released from the infiltrating neutrophils produce tissue damage. Type I hypersensitivity reactions and histamine release may be important in the initiation of immune complex deposition. Examples of type III hypersensitivity reactions in dogs and cats include lupus erythematosus, leukocytoclastic vasculitis, drug eruption, and bacterial hypersensitivity.

Type IV (cell-mediated, delayed) hypersensitivity reactions classically do not involve antibody-mediated injury. An incomplete antigen (hapten) interacts with a tissue protein (e.g., collagen) to form a complete antigen. This complete antigen is processed by monocyte-macrophages or Langerhans' cells (in contact hypersensitivity), whereupon it "sensitizes" T lymphocytes. These sensitized T lymphocytes respond to further antigenic challenge by releasing lymphokines that produce tissue damage. It has been suggested that the term "cell mediated" is an unfortunate misnomer for this type of immunologic reaction, as it is no more or less cell mediated than antibody-dependent reactions that are ultimately due to the participation of a lymphocyte or plasma cell. Examples of type IV hypersensitivity reactions in dogs and cats include contact hypersensitivity, flea bite hypersensitivity, and drug eruption.

Types I, II, and III hypersensitivity reactions together form the "immediate" hypersensitivity reactions. They are all antibody mediated, and thus there is only a short delay (from minutes to a few hours) before their tissue-damaging effects become apparent. Type IV hypersensitivity is the "delayed" hypersensitivity reaction. It is *not* antibody mediated, and it classically requires 24 to 72 hours before becoming detectable.

DERMATOHISTOPATHOLOGIC FINDINGS IN HYPERSENSITIVITY DISORDERS

An unfortunate tendency exists in medical writing to suggest that the type of hypersensitivity reaction involved in a cutaneous disorder can reliably be inferred from the histologic examination of skin biopsy specimens. This is simply not true. As a result of the multiplicity of mediators and chemoattractants associated with inflammatory cells, there is a great overlap of cytologic characteristics of the various hypersensitivity reactions. The difficulty in identifying the type of reaction is further complicated by the duration of the dermatosis, secondary changes (excoriation, infection), and any therapy rendered.

Thus, in a type I hypersensitivity reaction, one might expect eosinophils and mast cells to be prominent. However, in both dogs and humans, two allegedly classic examples of type I hypersensitivity—atopy and urticaria—are characterized by neutrophilic and/or mononuclear cell inflammatory infiltrates, with mast cells variably altered and eosinophils rarely seen.[124, 187a] On the other hand, eosinophils may be prominent in ectoparasite- or endoparasite-related dermatoses and furunculosis, while the number of mast cells may be increased in many nonimmunologic chronic dermatoses, cutaneous neoplasms, and fibroplasia.

Another example would be contact hypersensitivity, the alleged prototype of cutaneous type IV hypersensitivity. One would expect to find lymphohistiocytic cells predominating. However, the histopathologic findings in contact hypersensitivity are pleomorphic, variable, and nondiagnostic, with eosinophils, neutrophils, mast cells, and basophils varying in their numbers and frequency (see p. 469).[124, 127, 139]

Skin biopsy is unquestionably a valuable diagnostic aid. In selected cases, it may allow the clinician to identify the type of hypersensitivity reaction involved in the dermatosis in question. Three "giants" in the field of dermatohistopathology have summarized the situation in an excellent fashion:

> The student must realize that he sees one fleeting moment in the pathologic process fixed, and that each section is a random two-dimensional sample of a three-dimensional organ and may not be representative of all the changes present in the biopsy specimen.[155]
> A biopsy *in parte*, like a snapshot, records a partial truth, that is, one perception of an event at a moment in its history.[2]

SELECTED LABORATORY TESTS IN IMMUNODERMATOLOGY

Several laboratory tests are used in the evaluation of patients with suspected immunologic dermatoses. A review of all such tests is beyond the scope of this chapter, and the reader is referred to several excellent references.[49, 62, 65, 149, 162, 171, 212, 217a, 227] Only the most commonly used, readily available, or potentially useful of these tests are mentioned here.

Intradermal Skin Testing

Intradermal skin testing is most commonly used for the diagnosis of canine and feline atopy, flea bite hypersensitivity, and canine bacterial hypersensitivity. Intradermal skin testing is not usually used in human atopic dermatitis. Details on procedures and interpretation are found on pages 454 and 455, respectively.

In humans, intradermal skin testing with various "recall" antigens (trichophytin, candidin, streptokinase-streptodornase, mumps, and so on) and T-cell mitogens (phytohemagglutinin, concanavalin A) has successfully been used to assess cell-mediated (T-lymphocyte) immunocompetence.[49, 62, 65, 162, 171, 212, 217a] Such procedures have been largely unsuccessful, to date, in testing skin of dogs and cats.[139, 149, 227]

Patch Testing

Patch testing is the only way to definitively diagnose contact hypersensitivity (see p. 466). This procedure is not standardized for dogs and cats and is fraught with numerous technical and interpretational pitfalls.[127, 217a]

Radioallergosorbent Test (RAST)

The radioallergosorbent test (RAST) measures the amount of antigen-specific IgE in the serum of a patient.[49, 86, 217a] The RAST offers some *advantages* over skin testing in the diagnosis of atopy: (1) it presents no patient risk, (2) results are quantitative, (3) it is convenient for the patient, (4) allergens are stable in solid-phase state, and (5) it is preferable to skin testing in patients with widespread dermatitis. Among the *disadvantages* of RAST are (1) expense, (2) lack of widespread availability, (3) poor correlation with clinical hypersensitivity to several allergens, (4) relatively lower sensitivity of RAST, as compared with skin testing, and (5) frequent false positives and false negatives.[4, 86, 92, 139, 217a] It is unlikely that RAST will ever replace intradermal skin testing for the diagnosis and management of atopy. An ELISA test is also available (see p. 458).

Immunofluorescence Testing of Tissue and Serum

Immunofluorescence testing has become an invaluable supplement to clinical and histologic examination in the diagnosis and understanding of many dermatologic disorders.[22, 23, 49, 193, 194, 206, 217a] However, these tests are fraught with numerous procedural and interpretational pitfalls, including method of specimen handling, choice of substrates used, method of substrate handling, specificity of conjugates, fluorescein-protein-antibody concentrations, and unitage of conjugates. An in-depth discussion of these factors is beyond the scope of this chapter, and the reader is referred to Beutner and colleagues[22, 23] for details. Animals should not be given systemic glucocorticoids for at least 3 weeks prior to testing, if possible.[206]

Direct Immunofluorescence Testing (DIT)

Direct immunofluorescence testing (DIT) refers to the examination of tissues (skin and mucosa, lesional and normal) for various immunoreactants (immunoglobulins, complement components).[22, 23] It is imperative that primary lesions (vesicles, bullae, pustules) and perilesional tissue be examined.[206] In the case of bullous disorders, this may require the frequent (every 2 to 4 hours) examination of a patient for several days, until a primary lesion appears.

Lesions are carefully removed by means of punch biopsy or by careful scalpel excision. At present, quick-freezing and a special transport medium are the most widely used methods for handling specimens for DIT. Formalin fixation may destroy the antigenicity of deposited immunoreactants and should not be used. *Quick-freezing* involves snap freezing specimens in isopentane at $-160°C$ and holding them at $-70°C$ in an ultralow-temperature freezer until testing. This procedure is impractical for the practitioner.

The other method of handling and processing specimens for DIT requires the use of *special preservative solution* (Michel's fixative) that allows easy transport of biopsy specimens to the laboratory. The formula for Michel's fixative is shown in Table 9:13. The results of studies of tissues processed by quick-freezing and of those kept in Michel's fixative for a period of from several days to 2 weeks are comparable.[35, 139] Studies in dogs and cats suggest that specimens may reliably be preserved in Michel's fixative for at least 7 to 14 days,[139] and in some instances specimens have successfully been preserved for 4 to 8 years.[101] The pH of Michel's fixative must be carefully maintained at 7.0 to 7.2 to ensure accurate results.[206]

Specimens that are quick-frozen or preserved in Michel's fixative are *not* satisfactory for routine histologic examination, and separate biopsy samples should be preserved in formalin for dermatohistopathology. Specimens for DIT can also be satisfactorily preserved overnight in sterile physiologic saline.

Table 9:13. MICHEL'S FIXATIVE

1. *Preparation of Buffer:* Add 2.5 ml of 1 M potassium citrate buffer (pH 7.0), 5 ml of 0.1 M MgSO$_4$, and 5 ml of 0.1 M N-ethylmaleimide to 87.5 ml of distilled water. Adjust the final mixture to pH 7.0 to 7.2 with 1 M KOH.

2. *Preparation of Fixative:* Dissolve 55 g of (NH$_4$)$_2$SO$_4$ in 100 ml of buffer. The final composition of the fixative is as follows:

(NH$_4$)$_2$SO$_4$	3.12 M
N-ethylmaleimide	0.005 M
MgSO$_4$	0.005 M
Citrate	0.025 M

3. *Procedure for Use:*
   a. Place tissue biopsy into fixative.
   b. Do not freeze before putting in fixative.
   c. On receipt of laboratory of tissue in fixative, biopsy should be washed three times for 10 minutes in the buffer and frozen at −70°C.

DIT has been shown to be reliable for the diagnosis of pemphigus, pemphigoid, and lupus erythematosus.[206, 207] All forms of pemphigus are characterized by the intercellular deposition of immunoglobulin (usually IgG) and occasionally of complement (C3) (Fig. 9:3). In addition, pemphigus erythematosus may involve concurrent deposition of immunoreactants at the basement membrane zone (Fig. 9:4).

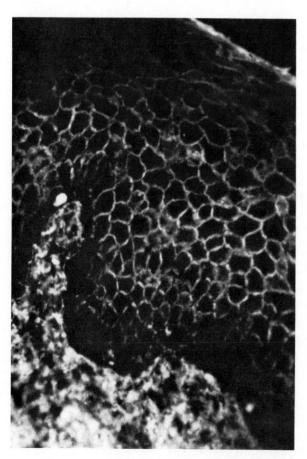

Figure 9:3. Canine pemphigus vulgaris. Direct immunofluorescence testing reveals host IgG within the intercellular spaces of epidermis. (From Scott, D. W., and Lewis, R. M.: Pemphigus and pemphigoid in a dog and man: comparative aspects. J. Am. Acad. Dermatol. 5:148, 1981.)

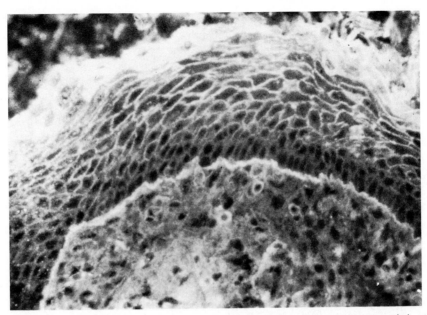

Figure 9:4. Canine pemphigus erythematosus. Direct immunofluorescence testing reveals host IgG within the intercellular spaces of epidermis and along the basement membrane zone. (From Scott, D. W., and Lewis, R. M.: Pemphigus and pemphigoid in a dog and man: comparative aspects. J. Am. Acad. Dermatol. 5:148, 1981.)

Pemphigoid (see p. 513) and lupus erythematosus (see p. 517) are characterized by the deposition of immunoreactants at the basement membrane zone. (Fig. 9:5). Some cases of pemphigoid and lupus erythematosus are characterized by the deposition of only IgM or IgA,[206, 207] a fact that emphasizes the need to test for several immunoreactants.

In humans, a distinction between systemic and discoid lupus erythematosus can often be made by comparing the results of DIT in lesional skin versus normal, non–sun-exposed skin.[22, 23] Immunoreactants may be deposited at the basement membrane zone in normal, sun-exposed skin in up to 60 per cent of the patients with systemic lupus erythematosus, while this is rare in discoid lupus erythematosus. This comparison is probably not valid in the hairy dog and cat. DIT of normal skin has usually been negative in dogs with systemic and discoid lupus erythematosus.[189, 190]

The deposition of immunoreactants in the intercellular spaces or at the basement membrane zone can occur in diseases other than pemphigus, pemphigoid, and lupus erythematosus.[58, 102, 113, 207, 237, 238, 255] *Intercellular* deposition of immunoreactants has been seen in dogs with staphylococcal folliculitis, vasculitis, systemic lupus erythematosus, and mycosis fungoides.[176, 207] Patchy, focal deposition of immunoreactants in the intercellular spaces appears to be fairly common when the epidermis is edematous, and it represents the intercellular percolation of immunoglobulins. *Basement membrane zone* deposition of immunoreactants has been seen in linear IgA dermatosis, vasculitis, drug eruption, staphylococcal folliculitis, dermatophytosis, and the Vogt-Koyanagi-Harada–like syndrome.[176, 207] In addition, immunoglobulin, especially IgM, may be demonstrated at the basement membrane zone of normal canine footpad and nasal epithelium, and of normal human skin.[70, 193, 194, 255] In summary, the results of direct immunofluorescence testing must always be cautiously interpreted in light of the clinical and histopathologic findings in a patient.[121, 207, 240]

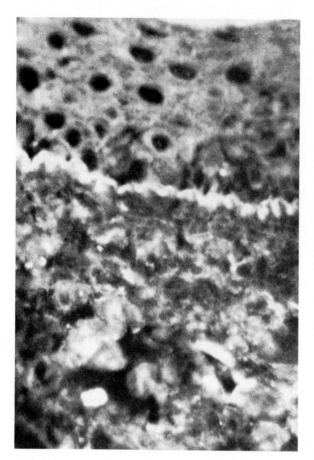

Figure 9:5. Canine bullous pemphigoid. Direct immunofluorescence testing reveals host IgG deposited at the basement membrane zone. (From Scott, D. W., Manning, T. O., Smith, C. A., and Lewis, R. M.: Observations on the immunopathology and therapy of canine pemphigus and pemphigoid. J.A.V.M.A. *180*:48, 1982.)

Figure 9:6. Canine cutaneous vasculitis. Direct immunofluorescence testing reveals host IgG within blood vessel walls.

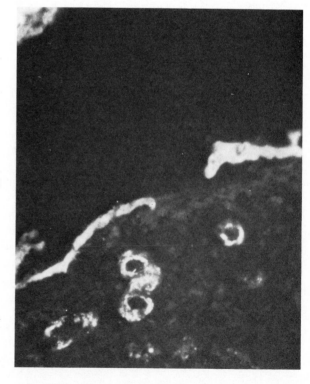

DIT has also been used to study cutaneous vasculitis (see p. 533).[22, 23, 139, 207] Immunoglobulin or complement, or both, may be demonstrated in vessel walls (Fig. 9:6) and occasionally at the basement membrane zone, in both the neutrophilic and lymphocytic forms of cutaneous vasculitis. However, DIT is usually not needed and is not particularly useful for diagnosis. Furthermore, if DIT is performed, this must be done within the first 4 hours after lesion formation. The mere demonstration of immunoreactants in vessel walls does not confirm their pathogenicity.

In summary, direct immunofluorescence testing is influenced by many factors. Fluorescence may be positive "falsely" in many diseases, and may be negative falsely in the immune-mediated disorders.[79e, 206, 207] Direct immunofluorescence findings must always be evaluated in view of the historical, clinical and histopathologic findings.

Indirect Immunofluorescence Testing (IIT)

Indirect immunofluorescence testing refers to the examination of serum for various autoantibodies.[22, 23, 207] About 5 to 10 ml of blood without anticoagulants should be collected. Serum is separated from the clot and sent to the laboratory at ambient or frozen temperatures. The substrate of choice for IIT has not been established in animals or humans. Serum samples are applied to species-specific stratified squamous epithelium (tongue, buccal mucosa, esophagus). Everything from species-specific skin, lip, tongue, and esophagus to monkey esophagus, guinea pig esophagus, rabbit esophagus, monkey lip and guinea pig lip and esophagus has been used as substrate for IIT, with no single substrate yielding consistently superior results.[22, 23, 33, 99, 211] Whichever substrate is chosen, the tissue should be quick-frozen within minutes after collection and stored for no longer than 10 to 14 days.

IIT has been used for the detection of pemphigus (anti-intercellular substance of keratinocytes) and pemphigoid (anti–basement membrane zone of stratified squamous epithelium) antibodies. Although IIT is reported to be positive in up to 90 per cent of human beings with active pemphigus and in 40 to 70 per cent of those with bullous pemphigoid, circulating autoantibodies may be absent in the presence of active disease or present in the absence of disease. In addition, it has been reported that human pemphigus and pemphigoid antibodies cannot reliably be depended on as a guide to therapy or prognosis and that the detection of these autoantibodies is fraught with difficulties (technical problems with procedures, prozones, and substrate selection; immune complexes; need for multiple serum samples). Finally, pemphigus-like antibodies (to be distinguished from true pemphigus antibodies by their failure to bind to a substrate in vivo) are present in patients with a great variety of conditions (burn patients; skin transplant patients; patients with drug eruptions; pemphigoid, dermatophytosis, and other dermatoses; and normal human beings).

IIT is usually negative in canine and feline pemphigus and in canine pemphigoid.[133, 207] In addition, pemphigus-like antibody has been demonstrated in dogs with generalized demodicosis and erythema multiforme, indicating not only that IIT is rarely positive in true canine pemphigus but that it may be positive in nonpemphigus diseases (at similar titers).[207] In one study[71] pemphigus-like antibodies were detected in 68 per cent of cats with indolent ulcer of the lip. The validity of these findings has been questioned,[208] and studies conducted more recently have failed to demonstrate in cats either pemphigus-like antibodies or true pemphigus antibodies.[194] It may be that (1) all pemphigus and pemphigoid antibodies are bound to substrate in vivo, (2) these autoantibodies are often bound in circulating immune complexes, or (3) present veterinary technology is inadequate.[95, 133, 191, 204]

ANTINUCLEAR ANTIBODY TEST

Antinuclear antibodies (ANAs) are a heretogeneous population of antibodies directed against multiple nuclear antigens.[23, 40, 49, 123] ANAs are not species specific, and consequently any source of nuclear material can be used for the test. However, the antisera (anti-immunoglobulins) used in this indirect immunofluorescence test *must* be species specific. In addition, as ANA can be represented by any immunoglobulin class, antisera should be polyvalent.

ANA tests are most commonly performed on rat liver sections or imprints. Rat liver stored at −70°C or less may be kept for 4 weeks. Reliable, reproducible ANA tests depend on a careful definition of test methods, including substrate antigens and reagents. Unfortunately, there is no standardized, universally accepted ANA test. Because of this, the incidence and titers of ANA reported in healthy individuals and diseased patients may vary markedly from one laboratory to another. This lack of standardization makes it impossible to compare ANA test results from one laboratory with results reported from a different laboratory.

ANA tests are most commonly done to help confirm a diagnosis of systemic lupus erythematosus (see p. 519). It must be remembered, however, that ANA may be found in many disease states, during therapy with certain drugs (e.g., griseofulvin, hydralazine, oral contraceptives, penicillin, phenytoin, procainamide, sulfonamides, tetracyclines), and in normal individuals.[23, 40, 123] Examples of disorders of dogs and cats in which ANA have been detected include systemic and discoid lupus erythematosus, lymphocytic thyroiditis, pemphigus vulgaris, pemphigus erythematosus, bullous pemphigoid, rheumatoid arthritis, autoimmune hemolytic anemia, idiopathic thrombocytopenia, drug eruption, endocarditis, various cancers, feline leukemia virus infection, feline infectious peritonitis, heartworm disease, cholangiohepatitis, staphylococcal folliculitis, canine scabies, actinomycosis, nocardiosis, pneumonia, plasma cell pododermatitis, Vogt-Koyanagi-Harada–like syndrome, and generalized demodicosis.[106, 139, 208, 214]

Antinuclear antibodies, as well as anticytoplasmic antibodies, have been used in human medicine to help define various diseases and disease subsets.[40, 49, 123] Emphasis is placed on immunofluorescence patterns and titers. Criticisms of such categorization include the following: (1) the tests are not standardized, (2) different investigators mean different things when using similar terms, (3) patterns can change depending on antibody titers, (4) not all substrates are created equally, (5) observer bias is considerable, and (6) different internal antigens may yield similar immunofluorescence patterns. Investigations of the nature and specificity of antinuclear antibodies in dogs and cats have failed to show any significance of pattern or titer.[106, 182, 208, 214]

Immunoperoxidase Methodology

Formalin-fixed, paraffin-embedded skin may be examined for the presence of immunoreactants using immunoperoxidase methods.[83b, 137, 222] Advantages of these techniques include the following: (1) routinely fixed and prepared tissues can be used for both conventional light microscopy and immunohistologic study, and (2) immunofluorescence equipment is not needed. However, the enhanced sensitivity of immunoperoxidase methodology results in reduced specificity. Intercellular and basement membrane–bound immunoreactants are frequently found in nonautoimmune inflammatory skin disorders, a situation requiring confirmatory histopathology and clinical findings before an accurate interpretation can be made.

Hypersensitivity Disorders

URTICARIA AND ANGIOEDEMA
(Hives)

Urticaria and angioedema are variably pruritic, edematous skin disorders, which are immunologic or nonimmunologic in nature. They are uncommon in the dog and rare in the cat.

CAUSE AND PATHOGENESIS

Urticaria and angioedema can result from many stimuli, both immunologic and nonimmunologic (Table 9:14).[49, 62, 139] Immunologic mechanisms include type I and III hypersensitivity reactions. Nonimmunologic factors that may precipitate or intensify urticaria and angioedema include physical forces (pressure, sunlight, heat, exercise), psychologic "stresses," genetic abnormalities, and various drugs and chemicals (aspirin, narcotics, foods, food additives). Atopic humans have an increased incidence of urticaria and angioedema, but no such predilection has been reported in dogs and cats. Factors reported to have caused urticaria and angioedema are listed in Table 9:15.

CLINICAL FEATURES

No age, breed, or sex predilections have been reported for urticaria and angioedema in dogs and cats. Clinical signs may be acute (most common) or chronic. In humans, acute urticaria and angioedema are empirically defined as episodes lasting less than 6 weeks, while those lasting several weeks or longer are referred to as chronic. Urticarial reactions are characterized by localized or generalized wheals, which may or may not be pruritic and may or may not

Table 9:14. ETIOLOGIC FACTORS IN URTICARIA AND ANGIOEDEMA

Drugs	Genetic abnormalities
Foods	Physical agents
Inhalants	Dermatographism
Infections and infestations	Pressure
Insect or arthropod stings and bites	Cold
Penetrants and contactants	Heat
Internal diseases (especially connective tissue diseases, malignancies)	Cholinergic
	Solar
Psychogenic factors	Vibration
	Water

Table 9:15. FACTORS REPORTED TO HAVE CAUSED URTICARIA AND ANGIOEDEMA IN DOGS AND CATS

Foods
Drugs (penicillin, ampicillin, tetracycline, vitamin K, propylthiouracil, amitraz, doxorubicin, radiocontrast agents)
Antisera, bacterins, and vaccines (panleukopenia, leptospirosis, distemper-hepatitis, rabies, feline leukemia)
Stinging and biting insects (bee, hornet, mosquito, black fly, spider, ant)
Allergenic extracts*
Blood transfusions
Plants (nettle, buttercup)
Intestinal parasites (ascarids, hookworms, tapeworms)
Infections (staphylococcal pyoderma, canine distemper)*
Sunlight*
Excessive heat or cold*
Estrus*
Dermatographism*
Atopy*
Psychogenic factors*

*Reported in dogs only.

exhibit serum leakage or hemorrhage (Figs. 9:7 and 9:8). Characteristically, the wheals are evanescent lesions, with each lesion persisting less than 24 hours. Urticarial lesions may occasionally assume bizarre patterns (serpiginous, linear, arciform, annular, papular). Angioedematous reactions are characterized by localized or generalized large, edematous swellings, which may or may not be pruritic and exhibit serum leakage or hemorrhage.

DIAGNOSIS

The *differential diagnosis* includes folliculitis, cellulitis, vasculitis, erythema multiforme, lymphoreticular neoplasia, and mast cell tumor. Staphylococcal

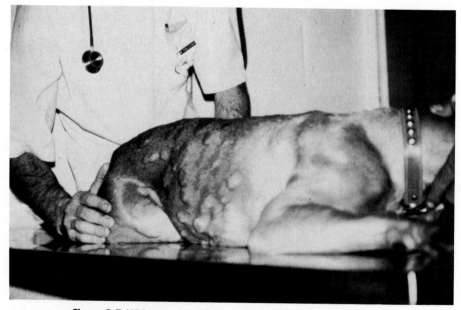

Figure 9:7. Widespread urticaria in a dog with food hypersensitivity.

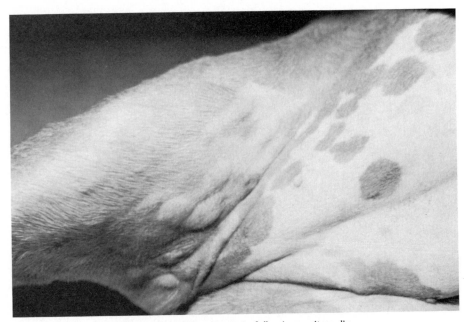

Figure 9:8. Urticaria in groin following amitraz dip.

folliculitis is the most common cause of misdiagnosed "urticaria" in dogs. *Definitive diagnosis* is based on history, physical examination, and pursuit of the etiologic factors listed in Table 9:14. A specific etiologic diagnosis can usually be made in acute cases, but chronic urticaria and angioedema are extremely frustrating diagnostic challenges, with 75 to 80 per cent of such cases in human patients defying specific etiologic diagnosis.

Histopathology. Skin biopsy shows a variable, nondiagnostic pattern, from simple vascular dilatation and edema in the superficial and middle dermis to pure superficial perivascular dermatitis with varying numbers of mononuclear cells, neutrophils, mast cells, and eosinophils (uncommon) to leukocytoclastic vasculitis. Direct immunofluorescence testing of urticarial lesions in humans is usually negative, but occasionally reveals immunoglobulin or complement, or both, in blood vessel walls (especially when the histologic reaction is vasculitic).

CLINICAL MANAGEMENT

The prognosis for urticarial reactions is favorable, as general health is not usually affected. The prognosis for angioedema varies with severity and location. Angioedematous reactions involving the nasal passages, pharynx, and larynx may be fatal.

Therapy includes (1) elimination and avoidance of known etiologic factors, and (2) treatment of symptoms with epinephrine (epinephrine 1:1000 at 0.1 to 0.5 ml subcutaneously or intramuscularly) or glucocorticoids (prednisolone or prednisone at 2 mg/kg, given orally, intramuscularly, or intravenously), or both. Antihistamines are not useful in the treatment of existing urticaria and angioedema but may be useful in the prevention of future reactions or in the management of chronic cases.

ATOPY

(Atopic Dermatitis, Atopic Disease, Allergic Inhalant Dermatitis)

Atopy is a common, genetically programmed, pruritic dermatitis of dogs and cats, in which the patient becomes sensitized to predominantly inhaled environmental antigens.

CAUSE AND PATHOGENESIS

Strong breed predilections, familial involvement, and limited breeding trials have demonstrated that canine atopy is genetically programmed.[139, 161a, 184, 187a] The exact mode of inheritance is unknown, and a pilot study failed to demonstrate any clear-cut relationship between dog leukocyte-antigen typing and canine atopy. In cats, familial involvement also suggests genetic programming.[202]

Canine atopy has been classified as a type I hypersensitivity reaction. Genetically predisposed dogs inhale, and possibly ingest or absorb percutaneously, various allergens that provoke allergen-specific IgE production. IgE fixes to tissue mast cells, especially in the skin (the primary target organ of canine atopy). When mast cell–fixed IgE reacts with its specific allergen or allergens, mast cell degranulation and release of many pharmacologically active compounds (see p. 433) ensue. Canine IgE is (1) not precipitated in the presence of antigen, (2) inactivated at 56°C, (3) not complement fixing, (4) antigenically similar to human IgE, and (5) capable of passively transferring atopic sensitivities to normal dogs by Prausnitz-Küstner (P-K) testing.[85, 139]

However, the role of IgE in the pathogenesis of atopy remains unclear. In human atopy the following are observed: (1) 20 per cent of the patients have normal or low serum IgE levels; (2) atopy has been recognized in patients with agammaglobulinemia; and (3) abnormally increased serum IgE levels generally do not fluctuate consistently during exacerbations, remissions, or treatment.[92, 139] Additionally, in neither humans nor dogs does the positive skin test that detects the presence of allergen-specific IgE produce the type of skin lesion seen with the clinical disease. Recently, Willemse and colleagues[251, 252] were unable to detect IgE in dogs with naturally occurring atopy, or in dogs experimentally sensitized to DNCP and *Toxocara canis* eggs: this resulted in spite of their use of the rabbit antidog IgE serum originally utilized by Halliwell and coworkers.[85] However, Willemse and associates consistently demonstrated a reaginic antibody, confirmed by passive cutaneous anaphylaxis (PCA) and P-K testing in the IgGd subclass. This is similar to the situation in some humans and laboratory animals, and would suggest that (1) immunoglobulins other than the classic IgE may be involved in the pathogenesis of atopy, or that (2) elevated IgE/IgGd levels are simply an epiphenomenon, a coincident feature of disordered cell regulation in atopy rather than an essential pathogenic factor.[92, 105, 234, 251, 252] Thus, recent attention has focused on the β-adrenergic blockade theory of allergy and on T-cell function.

Studies in a basenji-greyhound model of atopy have revealed the following: (1) airway hypersensitivity to methacholine, citric acid, and leukotrienes, (2) elevated blood histamine and leukotriene levels after antigen challenge, (3) blunted cyclic AMP response to β-adrenergic agents, (4) adenylate cyclase activities and β-adrenergic receptor numbers and affinities similar to those of normal dogs, and (5) elevated levels of phosphodiesterase.[32, 45, 95a] These studies suggest that the blunted cyclic AMP responses in atopic dogs are due to increased phosphodiesterase activity, rather than to defects in the β-adrenergic receptor–adenylate cyclase system.

Ample clinicopathologic and therapeutic evidence of the existence of atopy in cats is now available.[131, 160, 202] However, definitive laboratory documentation, including the characterization of the reaginic antibody involved (IgE? IgG?), has not been accomplished.

Katz has recently introduced the concept of "allergic breakthrough."[108] Normally, according to this concept, IgE antibody production is maintained at a low magnitude following sensitization because of the existence of a normal suppressive, or "damping," mechanism that exists specifically to limit the quantity of IgE antibodies produced during any particular response. If any one of a number of possible perturbations (respiratory viral infections, hormonal fluctuations) disturbs this damping mechanism in such a way as to diminish the overall damping capabilities to a sufficiently low level, and if when the damping threshold is lowered the individual becomes sensitized to one or more allergenic substances, the unfortunate juxtaposition in time can result in allergic breakthrough. This means that the quantity of IgE antibody produced for the particular allergen rises into the allergic zone, thereby leading to the development of allergic symptomatology. Interestingly, one study in dogs has related season of birth to allergic symptomatology.[233] Fifty-six per cent of the atopic dogs studied were born during the onset of pollen seasons, as compared with 24 per cent of the control dogs.

Atopic human beings demonstrate (1) increased percentage carrier states and actual numbers of *Staphylococcus aureus* in both lesional and normal skin; and (2) various immunodeficiency states relative to suppression of lymphocyte and neutrophil functions.[92] It is not known whether similar situations exist in canine and feline atopy, but such alterations in microbial flora and immunologic reactivity may explain the predilection of atopic dogs for secondary pyoderma.

The average serum histamine concentration in atopic dogs was reported to be 1.46 ng/ml, *lower* than that found in normal dogs (3.66 ng/ml).[161b] In the same study, the average response of the serum histamine concentration of atopic dogs to nasal aerosols of antigens that had given positive results on intradermal skin testing was 0.98 ng/ml (pre–antigenic exposure) to 2.70 ng/ml (10 to 20 minutes post-exposure). Nasal exposure to antigens that did *not* give positive reactions on intradermal skin testing resulted in average values of 0.76 ng/ml pre-exposure and 1.48 ng/ml post-exposure.[161b]

CLINICAL FEATURES

Atopy is the second most common hypersensitivity skin disorder of dogs and cats, probably accounting for 8 to 10 per cent of the skin disorders in these species.[139, 202]

Certain breeds are known to have a predilection for canine atopy, including Cairn terriers, West Highland white terriers, Scottish terriers, Lhasa Apsos, wire-haired fox terriers, Dalmatians, pugs, Irish setters, Boston terriers, Golden retrievers, boxers, English setters, Labrador retrievers, and miniature schnauzers.[143, 174, 187a, 233, 234, 249a] Canine atopy is seen more commonly in females than in males.[77, 174, 187a, 233, 234] No breed or sex predilections have been reported for feline atopy.

> **Onset of atopy usually occurs between 1 and 3 years of age.**

The age of onset of clinical signs in atopic dogs varies from 6 months to 7 years, with about 70 per cent of the dogs first manifesting clinical signs between 1 and 3 years of age.[77, 143, 187a, 249a] An exception to this general rule would be the Shar Pei breed, wherein the signs of atopy may begin as early as 3 months of age. Clinical signs may initially be seasonal or nonseasonal, depending on the allergens involved. About 80 per cent of all atopic dogs eventually have nonseasonal clinical signs.[44, 77, 143, 187a, 249a] About 80 per cent of the atopic dogs initially manifest clinical signs in the period from spring to fall, while about 20 per cent begin in winter.[202]

In cats, clinical signs may be seasonal or nonseasonal, and 75 per cent of the animals initially manifest clinical signs between 6 months and 2 years of age.[202]

> **Pruritus is the outstanding clinical sign in canine atopy. Primary skin lesions, in the absence of secondary infection, are not commonly seen.**

The skin lesions seen in atopic dogs are usually those associated with self-trauma, secondary pyoderma, and secondary seborrheic skin disease.[143, 184, 187a, 249a] Primary skin lesions, other than those associated with secondary pyoderma, are rarely seen. Pruritus and resultant skin lesions usually involve the face, feet, and ventrum, or some combination thereof (Fig. 9:9). Generalized cutaneous involvement may eventually be present in about 40 per cent of the dogs. Chronic inflammation and pruritus produces variable degrees of hyperpigmentation, lichenification, alopecia, and salivary staining of the hair coat. Atopic otitis externa and conjunctivitis may be present in about 50 per cent of the dogs.[143, 187a, 249a] Secondary pyoderma (folliculitis, furunculosis, pyotraumatic dermatitis) and seborrheic skin disease may be present in about 33 per cent and 12 per cent, respectively, of atopic dogs.[143, 187a, 249a] Hyperhidrosis may be present in 10 to 20 per cent of the atopic dogs.

Noncutaneous clinical signs reported to occur occasionally in atopic dogs include rhinitis, asthma, cataracts, urinary and gastrointestinal disorders, and hormonal hypersensitivity.[143, 187a] Atopic female dogs may exhibit irregular estrus cycles, low conception rates, and a high incidence of pseudopregnancy.[187a]

The cutaneous manifestations of feline atopy are remarkable, but frustrating due to their variability.[131, 160, 196, 208] Cutaneous syndromes associated with feline atopy may include (1) facial pruritus, with or without lesions, (2) pruritic ears with or without lesions, (3) a widespread pruritic papulocrustous dermatitis ("miliary dermatitis"; see p. 485), (4) indolent ulcer, eosinophilic plaque, or eosinophilic granuloma (see p. 561), (5) symmetric alopecia, and (6) generalized pruritus, with or without lesions. These remarkably diverse disease manifestations may appear in various combinations in the same cat. Perhaps the most frustrating manifestation of feline atopy is symmetric alopecia without skin lesions. In many instances, owners of these cats will deny that the cats are pruritic. It must be remembered that many cats are reclusive groomers and scratchers and that their owners truly may never observe these behaviors.

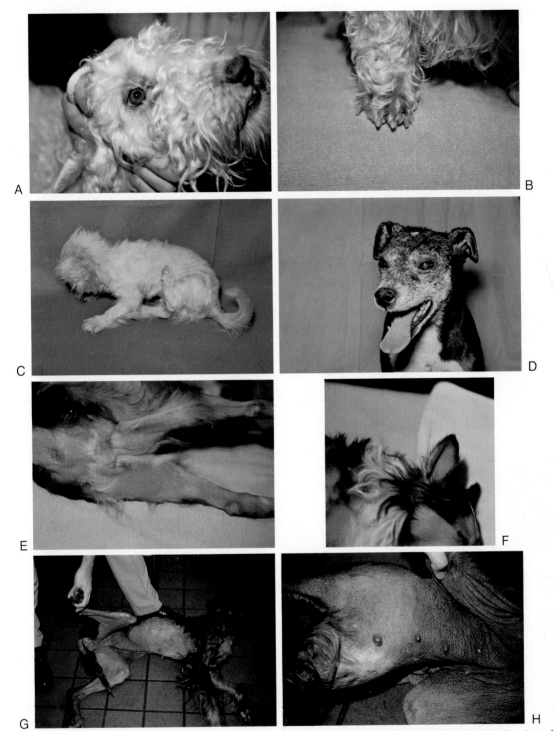

Figure 9:9. Atopic disease. *A*, Face rubbing causes erythema, while eye and nasal discharges cause rust discoloration of surrounding white hairs. *B*, Paw licking results in rust-colored digital hairs. *C*, White dog showing general erythema and intense itching. *D*, Face of terrier with atopy whose skin has dry crusts, erythema, and excoriations from scratching. *E*, Alopecia and severe erythema of perineum and rear legs. *F*, Alopecia and erythema inside pinna of dog with atopy. *G*, Alopecia, hyperpigmentation and lichenification of abdomen, inner legs, and ventral chest, and nipple enlargement due to chronic inflammation and pruritus in an atopic dog. *H*, Close-up of *G*.

These cats are usually misdiagnosed as having endocrine disorders. The first step in successful management of these symmetrically alopecic cats is to determine whether their hair is falling out or is being pulled out. If the hairs are easily epilated and they taper to normal distal ends, it can be concluded that they are falling out (endocrine, telogen/anagen defluxion, feline symmetric alopecia). However, if the hairs are not easily epilated and are broken off at the distal ends, they are being chewed, licked, or scratched off (as in cases of atopy, food hypersensitivity, flea bite hypersensitivity, psychogenic alopecia). When in doubt, an Elizabethan collar can be put on the cat for 3 to 4 weeks to observe the course of the hair loss. In addition, fecal examination may reveal large quantities of hair in cats that are licking excessively. Atopic cats may develop moderate to marked peripheral lymphadenopathy.[202]

DIAGNOSIS

The *differential diagnosis* is variable and lengthy, because canine atopy syndromes predominantly consist of a pruritic facial dermatitis, a pruritic pododermatitis, a pruritic otitis externa, a pruritic ventral dermatitis, or a pruritic generalized dermatitis. Some of the more common differentials include flea bite hypersensitivity, food hypersensitivity, contact dermatitis (primary irritant or hypersensitivity), scabies, intestinal parasite hypersensitivity, folliculitis, *Pelodera* dermatitis, and hookworm dermatitis. In the cat, the differential diagnosis includes the various causes of widespread pruritic papulocrustous dermatitis (see p. 485), symmetric alopecia (see p. 701), and indolent ulcer, eosinophilic plaque, or eosinophilic granuloma (see p. 561).

The diagnosis is based on history, physical examination, ruling out other differentials, and intradermal skin testing. Peripheral and tissue eosinophilia are rare in atopic *dogs*, unless the dogs have concurrent ectoparasitisms or endoparasitisms.[187a, 248] However, atopic *cats* frequently have peripheral and tissue eosinophilia.[202]

Intradermal Skin Testing. A tentative diagnosis of canine and feline atopy can be made on the basis of history, clinical signs, and laboratory rule-outs. A definitive diagnosis of atopy and revelation of the allergens involved can only be made with intradermal skin testing.

Clinicians must skin test one to two dogs or cats weekly to develop the expertise needed for good results.

Unfortunately, virtually no attempts have been made to standardize intradermal skin testing procedures in dogs and cats. Thus, one is faced with choosing among skin testing regimens that differ in test allergen concentrations (250 to 1500 protein nitrogen units [PNU]/ml), allergen volumes injected (0.02 to 0.1 ml/allergen), test reading intervals (once to several times over the course of 24 hours), and determination of a positive reaction.[139, 143, 187a] The intradermal skin test is thought to be superior to the scratch and prick tests.

In general, the recommended aqueous test allergen concentration is 1000 PNU/ml or 1:1000 weight/volume (w/v). As the allergenic fraction of antigen is always protein, the use of PNU (measurement of protein content) is preferable to w/v (measurement of actual amount of pollen, dust, etc.).[26, 87, 247, 258] Recently, "histamine equivalent units" or "histamine reactive values" have been used and are proposed as a more uniform measurement of the biologic activity of allergens.[26, 247] Some authors[12, 13, 139, 143] have reported that house dust, mold mixes, cattle hair, wool, and feathers often produce irritant reactions, and should be used at 250 to 500 PNU/ml. Other data do not support these reports but show that tobacco and cat dander frequently cause false-positive reactions.[187a]

A positive skin test reaction (a "2-plus" or greater reaction) is often defined as a wheal that is at least 3 mm larger in diameter than the saline control reaction.[139] However, one report concluded that the use of such a grading system would have greatly increased the number of clearly false-positive skin test reactions.[187a]

In hyposensitization, correlate skin test results with history to select the antigens for treatment.

Allergen Selection. Skin test allergen selection is an important subject. There is such a great regional variation in floral allergens that it is important to know what pollinates in *your* particular locale. Consultations with local physician allergists, botany departments, pollen centers, and allergen firms, in addition to national pollen charts, are essential.[139, 142]

It is important to select allergens from a reputable drug firm and to purchase from only one firm, if possible. Tremendous unresolved problems surround the standardization of allergenic extracts, including standards for raw material collection, methods of measuring the purity of raw materials, techniques for identifying many substances, a variety of methods of manufacturing, and determination of allergen stability and potency.[139, 173, 258] Bioactivity of commercial products varies from 10- to 1000-fold, and no relationship was found between bioactivity and concentrations declared in PNU or w/v.[26, 258]

Testing with allergen *mixes* is undesirable.[139, 143, 187a] Such mixes frequently result in false-negative reactions (individual allergens within the mix are in a concentration too dilute for testing) and also fail to include many important pollen and mold allergens. For these reasons, skin testing with commercial "regional" allergen kits is unsatisfactory. Allergens commonly reported to be important in dogs and cats include house dust, human dander, feathers, kapok, molds, weeds, grasses, and trees.[44, 143, 160, 164a, 174, 187a, 202, 234, 249a] Most animals are multisensitive.[143, 164a, 184, 187a, 202] Recently *Acarus siro* (a storage mite found in poorly dried and stored cereals) antigen was reported to cause positive skin test reactions in 75 per cent of the atopic dogs tested.[235]

It is essential to remember that a positive skin test reaction means *only* that the patient has skin sensitizing antibody. It does not necessarily mean that the patient has clinical allergy to the allergen(s) injected. Thus, it is essential that "positive" skin test reactions be interpreted in light of the patient's history. By the same token, a negative skin test does not necessarily mean that the patient is not atopic. Ten to 30 per cent of the otherwise classic atopic dogs may have negative skin tests.[44, 164a, 187a, 234, 249a] This probably reflects failure (by limiting the number of test allergens used) to challenge dogs with the appropriate allergens, or the intervention of various factors known to produce false-negative reactions (see p. 456).

Table 9:16. REASONS FOR FALSE-POSITIVE INTRADERMAL SKIN TEST REACTIONS

1. Irritant test allergens (especially those containing glycerin; also some house dust, feather, wool, mold, and food preparations)
2. Contaminated test allergens (bacteria, fungi)
3. Skin sensitizing antibody only (prior clinical or present subclinical sensitivity)
4. Poor technique (traumatic placement of needle; dull or burred needle; too large a volume injected; air injected)
5. Substances that cause nonimmunologic histamine release (narcotics)
6. "Irritable" skin (large reactions seen to *all* injected substances, including saline control)
7. Dermatographism

> *Learn about false-positive and false-negative reactions in intradermal skin testing.*

Many factors may lead to false-positive or false-negative skin test reactions in dogs (see Tables 9:16 and 9:17).[12, 13, 139, 143] These factors must be carefully considered when skin testing is performed. The most common cause of negative skin test reactions is the recent administration of certain drugs: glucocorticoids, antihistamines, progestagens. There are *no* reliable withdrawal times for these drugs. The testability of the patient can *only* be determined by histamine responsiveness (see later discussion). In humans, it has been reported that (1) positive skin test reactions may persist long after clinical hypersensitivity has disappeared, (2) skin test reactions may be positive for years before clinical allergy develops, and (3) up to 50 per cent of the general population may have positive skin test reactions to one or more allergens. Similar information is not available for dogs, although available data suggest that positive skin test reactions in nonatopic dogs and cats are rare.[13, 24, 177, 184, 187a] Studies of intradermal skin test reactions in normal dogs have revealed the following: (1) no breed differences, (2) no age differences, or decreased reactivity with increasing age, (3) no sex differences, or increased reactivity of females to some allergens, (4) decreased reactivity to some allergens with increasing hair coat pigmentation,

Table 9:17. REASONS FOR FALSE-NEGATIVE INTRADERMAL SKIN TEST REACTIONS

1. Subcutaneous injections
2. Too little allergen
   a. Testing with mixes
   b. Outdated allergens
   c. Allergens too dilute (1000 PNU/ml recommended)
   d. Too small volume of allergen injected
3. Drug interference
   a. Glucocorticoids
   b. Antihistamines
   c. Tranquilizers
   d. Progestational compounds
   e. Any drug that lowers blood pressure significantly
4. Anergy (testing during peak of hypersensitivity reaction)
5. Inherent host factors
   a. Estrus, pseudopregnancy
   b. Severe stress (systemic disease, fright, struggling)
6. Endoparasitism or ectoparasitism? ("blocking" of mast cells with antiparasitic IgE?)
7. Off-season testing (testing more than one to two months after clinical signs have disappeared)
8. Histamine "hyporeactivity"

(5) decreased reactivity to histamine in hospitalized dogs compared with normal household dogs (stress related?), and (6) weekly intradermal injections of allergens resulting in multiple positive reactions to allergens that originally tested negative (usually within 8 weeks).[13, 177, 249a]

Make sure the patient is testable and the owner is cooperative.

Clearly, intradermal skin testing is not a procedure to be taken lightly. It requires keen attention to details and possible pitfalls, together with experience and lots of practice. Clinicians who cannot skin test dogs and cats on a weekly or biweekly basis will probably be unhappy with the results. However, in experienced hands, the intradermal skin test is a powerful tool in the diagnosis and management of canine and feline atopy. Where possible, difficult cases should be referred to clinicians who specialize in this subject.

Procedure. A commonly used procedure for intradermal skin testing is as follows:

1. Make sure the patient is testable! One-twentieth (0.05) to one-tenth (0.1) ml of 1:100,000 histamine phosphate is injected intradermally. A wheal 15 to 20 mm in diameter should be present at 15 to 30 minutes after injection. If the histamine wheal is small to absent, postpone intradermal skin testing and test the animal with histamine on a weekly basis until the expected reaction is seen.

2. Preferably, hold the animal in lateral recumbency for testing. Make the animal comfortable on a blanket with a towel over its head. If this is impossible, the dog may be immobilized with a short-acting barbiturate, with or without gas anesthesia. It has been shown that xylazine hydrochloride (Rompun) and atropine sulfate are also satisfactory patient relaxants for skin testing.[13, 139]

3. The skin over the lateral thorax is the preferred test site. Because different areas of skin vary in responsiveness, the site used should be consistent from patient to patient. Gently clip the hair with a No. 40 blade, using *no* chemical preparation to clean the test site. Use a felt-tipped pen to mark each injection site. Place injection sites at least 2.5 cm apart, avoiding dermatitic areas.

4. Using a 26- to 27-gauge 3/8-inch needle attached to a 1-ml disposable syringe, carefully inject, intradermally, 0.05 ml of each test allergen (1000 PNU/ml). In addition, inject intradermally 0.05 ml of saline or diluent control ("negative" control) and 0.05 ml of 1:100,000 histamine phosphate ("positive" control). Read the test sites at 15 and 30 minutes. Prevent the animal from traumatizing the test area.

5. By convention, a "2-plus" or greater reaction is considered to be potentially significant and must be carefully correlated with the patient's history. With experience positive reactions may be "guesstimated" by visual inspection. However, it is strongly recommended that the novice *measure* the diameter of each wheal in millimeters. A positive skin test reaction may then be objectively defined as a wheal having a diameter that is equal to or larger than that halfway between the saline and histamine controls.

The size of positive skin test reactions does *not* necessarily correlate with their clinical importance. Systemic reactions (anaphylaxis) to intradermal skin testing are extremely rare in dogs and cats. Delayed skin test site reactions (24 to 48 hours after injection) are rarely seen, and are of unknown significance.

Intradermal skin testing is being performed with increasing frequency in cats.[131, 160, 202] In general, the protocol for dogs and cats is the same. Cats may be restrained physically, in a cat bag, or with 5 to 10 mg/kg ketamine given intramuscularly. Some interpretational differences exist for cats, however. Feline wheals tend to be small, flat, poorly circumscribed, nonerythematous, and often better felt than seen. In addition, skin test reactivity usually peaks between 5 and 15 minutes following injection. Studies on skin test reactivity in normal cats found occasional positive reactions in normal cats, and increased reactivity in young animals and animals with dark hair coats.[24]

Two other laboratory tests have been used in humans and dogs to evaluate the atopic patient: the radioimmunosorbent test (RIST), and the radioallergosorbent test (RAST). RIST measures total serum IgE, and RAST measures allergen-specific serum IgE. In general, these tests are of limited benefit in both species.[86, 92, 139, 251] In dogs, total serum IgE levels are very much higher than those in human beings, with the mean level in normal dogs reported to be 198.9 µg/ml, which is similar to that found in atopic dogs.[86, 91, 184] The highest serum IgE levels are found in dogs with endoparasitism. The value of RAST (see p. 440) as a diagnostic tool in human and canine atopy is controversial, since comparisons between positive RAST, positive skin tests, and various provocative measures have not always shown good agreement.[79d, 86, 92, 139] It is unlikely that RAST will ever replace skin testing for the diagnosis of canine, feline, or human atopy.

In the United States, two serological tests have recently been marketed to veterinarians for the diagnosis and treatment of canine atopy: a radioallergosorbent test (RAST) and an enzyme-linked immunoabsorbent assay (ELISA).[79d] A pilot study designed to assess the reproducibility and agreement with results of intradermal skin testing of these two serological tests revealed significant problems with reproducibility and false-positive reactions.[79d]

Although the discrepancies in both the RAST and the intradermal skin test may be explained by numerous difficulties in technique, sensitivity, and so forth, they may also be seen as supporting the proposal that immediate skin test reactivity and the presence of allergen-specific antibodies are no more than secondary features of atopy.[252a] Because of these difficulties, the concept of major and minor diagnostic features has been introduced in an attempt to provide consistency in the diagnosis of atopy in dogs and humans.[252a, 252b] For dogs, the following criteria have been proposed:

A. At least three of the following *major* features should be present:
   1. Pruritus
   2. Facial and/or digital involvement
   3. Lichenification of the flexor surface of the tarsus or the extensor surface of the carpus
   4. Chronic or chronically relapsing dermatitis
   5. An individual or familial history of atopy
   6. A breed predilection
B. At least 3 of the following *minor* features should also be present:
   1. Onset of signs before 3 years of age
   2. Facial erythema and cheilitis
   3. Bacterial conjunctivitis
   4. A superficial staphylococcal pyoderma
   5. Hyperhidrosis
   6. Immediate skin test reactivity to inhalant allergens

7. Elevated allergen-specific IgGd
8. Elevated allergen-specific IgE

Histopathology. Skin biopsy of atopic dogs reveals variable degrees of superficial perivascular dermatitis (pure, spongiotic, hyperplastic) with mononuclear cells or neutrophils usually predominating (Figs. 9:10, 9:11, and 9:12).[187a] Similar dermal changes of a milder degree may be seen in clinically normal skin. Histopathologic findings consistent with secondary pyoderma (suppurative folliculitis, perifolliculitis, intraepidermal pustular dermatitis) are commonly seen in biopsies of atopic canine skin.

Skin biopsy of atopic cats reveals variable degrees of superficial perivascular dermatitis, wherein eosinophils are frequently an important inflammatory cell.[202] Atopic cats manifesting indolent ulcer, eosinophilic plaque, or eosinophilic granuloma will have histopathologic changes typical of these entities (see p. 561–564).

CLINICAL MANAGEMENT

Prognostically, the atopic dog and cat have about an 80 per cent chance of developing nonseasonal disease. Natural desensitization is extremely rare.

Before discussing the details of therapy, it is imperative to mention the concept of "hypersensitivity threshold."[139, 144] A certain allergenic load from many sources may be tolerated by an individual without any disease manifestations, but a small increase in that load (one or more allergens) may push him over the threshold and initiate clinical signs. Equally important when considering the cause of dermatologic disorders is the concept of "summation of effect"; for example, a subclinical hypersensitivity in combination with a flea infestation, a mild pyoderma, or a dry environment may produce marked discomfort, which could be absent if any one disorder existed alone. Thus, it is very important to evaluate all possible contributions to the clinical signs in "allergic" dogs and cats.

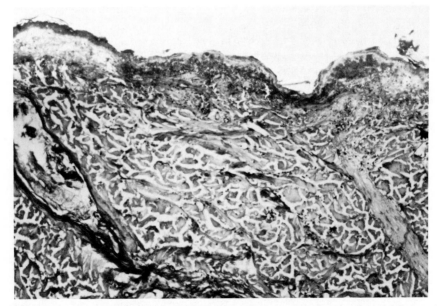

Figure 9:10. Canine atopy. Focal erosion and ulceration (excoriation) with minimal inflammation. (From Scott, D. W.: Observations on canine atopy. J.A.A.H.A. *17*:91, 1981.)

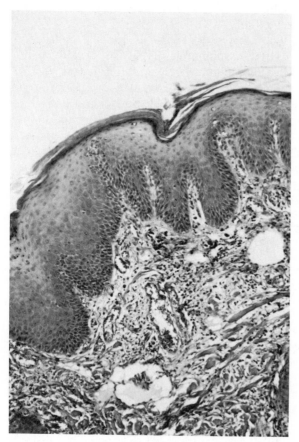

Figure 9:11. Canine atopy. Hyperplastic perivascular dermatitis. (From Scott, D. W.: Observations on canine atopy. J.A.A.H.A. *17*:91, 1981.)

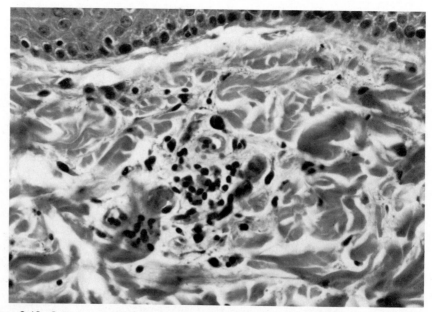

Figure 9:12. Canine atopy. Perivascular accumulation of mononuclear cells. (From Scott, D. W.: Observations on canine atopy. J.A.A.H.A. *17*:91, 1981.)

Therapy for atopy includes various combinations of avoidance, hyposensitization, and systemic antipruritic drugs.[144, 187a, 202]

Avoidance. Avoidance of allergens is not always possible or practical. However, some patients may greatly benefit from avoidance of confirmed allergens such as feathers (pillows, birds), cats (dander), newsprint (newspaper), and tobacco smoke.[187a] Such manipulations and benefits would not be as accurate without identification of the offending allergen(s) by skin testing.

Systemic Glucocorticoids. Systemic glucocorticoids are usually very effective for the management of atopy. Prednisolone or prednisone is administered orally (1 mg/kg SID for dogs, 2 mg/kg SID for cats) for 5 to 10 days, and then on an alternate-day regimen (see p. 203) as needed. This schedule is relatively safe compared with long-acting corticosteroids. Some animals become less and less responsive to glucocorticoids with the passage of time. It must be remembered that the response to systemic glucocorticoids is not an all-or-none phenomenon (see p. 198). When animals have undesirable side-effects or poor responses to one glucocorticoid, another glucocorticoid may successfully be substituted. In such situations, oral methylprednisolone, triamcinolone, or dexamethasone may be tried. However, the latter two drugs are not well suited to alternate-day therapy. In cats, methylprednisolone acetate (20 mg/cat, subcutaneously) is often effective (see p. 202). However, injections should *never* be repeated more often than every 2 to 3 months.

Hyposensitization. Hyposensitization (immunotherapy) is indicated in animals in which avoidance of antigens is impossible and in which the necessary regimens of glucocorticoids or other antipruritic drugs are unsatisfactory or contraindicated. Although hyposensitization has been reported to be effective in 50 to 80 per cent of the atopic dogs and cats treated,[44, 77, 131, 139, 144, 160, 202, 249] virtually no attempts have been made to standardize hyposensitization regimens in the dog or to scientifically compare their merits. Thus, published regimens vary in the form of allergen used (aqueous, alum precipitated, propylene glycol suspended, glycerinated), the number of injections given, the dose of allergen administered, and the route of administration (subcutaneously, intramuscularly, intradermally). A double-blind study of hyposensitization in atopic dogs (alum-precipitated allergens versus placebo) found a 59 per cent improvement with the vaccine, and a 21 per cent improvement with a placebo.[249] Immediate skin test reactivity disappeared in dogs that responded well.

The mechanism of action of hyposensitization is unclear. Various hypotheses include (1) humoral desensitization (reduced levels of IgE), (2) cellular desensitization (reduced reactivity of mast cells and basophils), (3) immunization (induction of "blocking antibody"), (4) tolerization (generation of allergen-specific suppressor cells), or (5) some combination thereof.[139, 144, 249]

Three forms of allergens have been used for hyposensitizing atopic dogs.[139] *Aqueous allergens*, which are rapidly absorbed, necessitate smaller doses, and require multiple, frequent injections, constitute the type that is most commonly used today.[116, 131, 139, 144, 160] *Alum-precipitated allergens* are intermediate in action between the aqueous and emulsion allergens. They are more slowly absorbed than the aqueous allergens; as a result, larger doses, fewer and less frequent injections, and more rapid hyposensitization are possible. Concern has been expressed about the possible carcinogenicity of alum precipitates, and these are increasingly less available today. *Emulsion allergens* (aqueous allergens in propylene glycol, glycerin, or mineral oil) are the most slowly absorbed, allowing the largest doses, the least number of injections, and the most rapid

Table 9:18. HYPOSENSITIZATION SCHEDULE FOR AQUEOUS ALLERGENS*

Injection No.	Day No.	Vial 1† (100 to 200 PNU/ml)	Vial 2 (1000 to 2000 PNU/ml)	Vial 3 (10,000 to 20,000 PNU/ml)
1	1	0.1 ml		
2	2	0.2 ml		
3	4	0.4 ml		
4	6	0.8 ml		
5	8	1.0 ml		
6	10		0.1 ml	
7	12		0.2 ml	
8	14		0.4 ml	
9	16		0.8 ml	
10	18		1.0 ml	
11	20			0.1 ml
12	22			0.2 ml
13	24			0.4 ml
14	26			0.8 ml
15	28			1.0 ml
16	38			1.0 ml
17	48‡			1.0 ml

*Injections are given subcutaneously.
†Protein nitrogen unit (PNU) value of each vial represents the *total* of *all* allergens used.
‡Thereafter, repeat injections (1.0 ml) every 20 to 40 days, as needed.

hyposensitization. Sample hyposensitization regimens utilizing these three forms of allergens are presented in Tables 9:18 to 9:20. By convention, no more than 10 allergens have been used at once for hyposensitization.[144, 187a] In animals with multiple sensitivities (e.g., 20 to 30) considerable detective work and good fortune are required to be able to select the 10 "most important" allergens related to their atopic disease. Recently, success has safely been achieved with the inclusion of up to 30 or more allergens in aqueous vaccines for atopic dogs.[144]

Depending on which form of allergen is being utilized, a beneficial response may be seen as early as 1 month or as late as 1 year after hyposensitization is begun. "Booster" injections of allergens are administered as needed (when clinical signs first begin to reappear), and, depending on the form of allergens involved and the vaccine protocol being used, boosters may be needed every 3 weeks to 6 months. Experience with the patient allows the owner and the

Table 9:19. HYPOSENSITIZATION SCHEDULE FOR ALUM-PRECIPITATED ALLERGENS*

Injection No.	Week No.	Dose in PNU†
1	1	100
2	2	200
3	3	400
4	5	800
5	8	1500
6	12	2000
7	16	3000
8	20	6000
9‡	24	10,000

*Injections are given subcutaneously.
†Dose is per allergen.
‡Thereafter, repeat injections (10,000 PNU each allergen) every 1 to 6 months, as needed.

Table 9:20. HYPOSENSITIZATION SCHEDULE FOR EMULSION ALLERGENS*

Injection No.	Week No.	Dose in PNU†
1	1	10,000
2	3	12,500
3	5	15,000
4	9	17,500
5‡	13	20,000

*Aqueous allergens are mixed with sterile propylene glycol or sterile 50 per cent glycerine at a ratio of 4 parts allergen to 1 part adjuvant. Injections are given subcutaneously.
†Dose is per allergen.
‡Thereafter, repeat injections (20,000 PNU each allergen) as needed.

veterinarian to predict how long the patient will be asymptomatic following booster injections. Boosters are then administered shortly before clinical signs would be expected to flare up. Intervals between boosters may vary at different times of the year. In general, atopic dogs and cats require lifetime administration of vaccine. There is no indication that breed, sex, age, or duration of clinical signs affect the success of hyposensitization.[77, 144, 187a, 249] Most authors report that the likelihood of successful hyposensitization is greater in animals with fewer positive reactions.[77, 144, 187a]

Adverse reactions to hyposensitization are rare in dogs and cats, and they include (1) intensification of clinical signs for a few hours to a few days, (2) local reactions (edema with or without pain and/or pruritus) at injection sites, and (3) anaphylaxis.[139, 144, 249] Adverse reactions are treated according to symptom. Intensification of clinical signs may indicate that the animal's maximum tolerance dose of allergens has been exceeded and that the final hyposensitizing dose achieved needs to be lowered. In humans, most studies on the possible long-term adverse effects of hyposensitization have failed to demonstrate any clinical or immunologic abnormalities. However, one study of 20 consecutive human patients with polyarteritis nodosa revealed that in six patients the onset of vasculitic symptoms coincided with hyposensitization for atopy.[139]

In the severely affected, nonseasonal atopic dog and cat, it may be necessary to control the symptoms with systemic glucocorticoids during hyposensitization. As long as prednisolone or prednisone doses are kept as low as possible and administered on an alternate-day basis (see p. 203), hyposensitization can still be successful.[144, 187a]

Nonsteroidal Drugs. A number of other drugs have been used to treat canine and feline atopy, with little or no documentation of benefit. These include (1) antihistamines, (2) antiseratonins (cyproheptadine, methysergide), (3) aspirin, (4) orgotein (metalloprotein, nonsteroidal anti-inflammatory), (5) phenothiazine tranquilizers, (6) barbiturates, (7) megadoses of vitamin C, and (8) megadoses of vitamin E.[139, 144] A recent study[210] of nonsteroidal antipruritic agents in dogs with hypersensitivity skin disease found the following drugs to be effective: (1) eicosapentaenoic acid–containing product (Dermcaps, 1 capsule/ 9.1 kg orally SID in 11 per cent of dogs), (2) chlorpheniramine (4 mg/dog orally TID in 9.0% per cent of dogs), (3) diphenhydramine (2 mg/kg orally TID in 6.5 per cent of dogs), and (4) hydroxyzine (2 mg/kg orally TID in 6.5 per cent of dogs). More importantly, if these drugs were all tried separately in the same dog, the chance of one being effective for the dog was 40 per cent. Aspirin (25 mg/kg orally TID), vitamin E (400 IU orally BID) and zinc methionine (Zinpro,

1 tablet/9.1 kg orally SID) are rarely effective.[135b, 210] See page 189 for detailed discussions of these drugs.

In atopic cats, chlorpheniramine (2 mg/cat orally BID) is often effective.[135, 211]

In atopic human patients, hyposensitization, antihistamines, transfer factor, and levamisole have rarely been beneficial.[64, 105, 139, 210] The combined use of H_1- and H_2-blocking antihistamines was reported to be no more efficacious than the use of H_1 blockers alone in both dogs and humans.[64, 135b] Additionally, the use of H_2 blockers alone often *increased* the level of pruritus.[64] Evening primrose oil (γ-linolenic acid, linoleic acid) was initially touted as a beneficial oral medication for atopic humans.[256] However, further studies failed to document this claim.[18, 215]

Tolerization. Recently, tolerization has been pursued as a therapeutic approach for atopic diseases.[25] It has been shown that conjugating allergens with isologous alphaglobulins, the copolymer of D-glutamic acid or D-lysine, or polyethylene glycol results in nonimmunogenic products that suppress allergen-specific IgE synthesis, presumably by inducing allergen-specific suppressor T lymphocytes. Further work in this area is awaited with great interest.

CONTACT HYPERSENSITIVITY
(Allergic Contact Dermatitis)

Contact hypersensitivity is a rare, variably pruritic, maculopapular dermatitis of dogs and cats, usually affecting sparsely haired skin in "contact" areas.

CAUSE AND PATHOGENESIS

Few reports of naturally occurring contact hypersensitivity in dogs and cats were documented by patch testing. Thus, most of the literature and data on naturally occurring "allergic contact dermatitis" in dogs and cats are of dubious validity and value.

In most instances, contact hypersensitivity represents a type IV hypersensitivity reaction (see p. 438).[49, 62, 127, 139, 147, 172a, 225a] Increased concentrations of arachidonic acid, prostaglandin E_2, and leukotriene B_4 were found in the skin of humans with contact hypersensitivity, but not in the skin of humans with primary irritant contact dermatitis.[19] In humans, contact hypersensitivity can also be due to type I hypersensitivity reaction (contact urticaria).[62, 127] This type of contact hypersensitivity has *not* been reported in dogs and cats.

Experimental attempts to induce contact hypersensitivity in dogs and cats have given inconsistent results. Nobreus and colleagues[148] using a modified "maximization technique" of intradermal and topical sensitization, successfully sensitized dogs to dinitrochlorobenzene. They showed that the sensitization could be transferred to normal dogs with thoracic duct lymphocytes and that sensitization could be suppressed with antilymphocyte serum. Krawiec and Gaafar[114] successfully sensitized dogs to dinitrochlorobenzene with intradermal and topical challenge. Schultz and Adams[181] reported that helminth antigens, tissue antigens, viral antigens, bacterial antigens, fungal antigens, protein antigens, dinitrochlorobenzene, and mitogens had been used experimentally and clinically in dogs and cats to elicit delayed-type hypersensitivity responses in the skin, with limited reproducibility or irreproducible results. Schultz and

Maguire[179] induced delayed-type hypersensitivity in normal cats with dinitro-chlorobenzene. Kunkle and Gross[117] reported a beautifully documented case of naturally occurring contact hypersensitivity to *Tradescantia fluminensis* (wandering Jew plant) in a dog.

It can be concluded from the above investigations that contact hypersensitivity *can* be induced in dogs and cats, but only with difficulty and inconsistent results, as compared with tests on humans and guinea pigs.

CLINICAL FEATURES

Naturally occurring contact hypersensitivity was reported to account for about 1 to 5 per cent of all canine dermatoses[225a, 236, 250] and to be rare in cats.[187] Walton[236] reported that over 20 per cent of his cases of canine contact hypersensitivity occurred in yellow Labrador retrievers. In a study of 22 cases (confirmed by closed patch testing) of contact hypersensitivity in dogs in Denmark,[225a] 50 per cent of the dogs were German shepherds, whereas this breed accounted for only 16 per cent of the purebred registered dogs.

In humans (1) much variation in susceptibility to contact sensitization has been observed, (2) distinct trends toward genetic clustering have been recognized, (3) individuals sensitized to one substance are more likely to become sensitized to another, and (4) males have a higher sensitization rate than females.[62, 127]

Although contact hypersensitivity can be produced in dogs after a 3- to 5-week sensitization period, the sensitization period for dogs and cats with contact hypersensitivity is usually in excess of 2 years, in over 70 per cent of the cases.[225a, 236] Substances reported to cause naturally occurring "allergic contact dermatitis" in dogs and cats are listed in Table 9:21. Again, virtually none of these has been well documented with patch testing. In the Danish study, confirmed contact hypersensitivity to the following substances was documented: thiuram mix, cobalt chloride, nickel sulfate, quinoline mix, colophony, black rubber mix, wood alcohols, epoxy resin, balsam of Peru, carba mix, formaldehyde, fragrance mix, ethylene diamine, primin, wood tar, and naphthyl mix.[225a]

Clinical signs of contact hypersensitivity include varying degrees of dermatitis, which tend to be confined to hairless or sparsely haired areas of skin

Table 9:21. SUBSTANCES REPORTED TO CAUSE NATURALLY OCCURRING "ALLERGIC CONTACT DERMATITIS" IN DOGS AND CATS

Substance Category	Examples
Plants	Pollens and resins (grasses, trees, weeds), jasmine blossoms, poison ivy, poison oak, wandering Jew
Medications	Topicals, neomycin, tetracaine and other "caines," soaps, shampoos (especially those containing tars and creosols), petrolatum, lanolin, disinfectants, insecticides (shampoos, dips, sprays, flea and tick collars and medallions)
Highly chlorinated water	
Home furnishings	Fibers (wool, nylon, synthetics), dyes, mordants, finishes, polishes, cleansers, rubber and plastic products, detergents, cat litter, collars (leather, metal)

in "contact" regions; ventral aspect of paws (*not* pads), ventral abdomen, tail, thorax, and neck as well as scrotum, point of the chin, perineum, and pinnae (Figs. 9:13, 9:14, and 9:16A to D). If the allergen is in a topical medicament or in liquid, aerosol, or powder form, cutaneous reactions may also be seen in haired areas as well (Fig. 9:15). Reactions to rubber or plastic dishes and chew toys are usually confined to the lips and nose (Fig. 9:16C). Skin lesions may include various combinations of erythema, macules, papules, plaques, hyperpigmentation or hypopigmentation, excoriations, and lichenification (Fig. 9:16B). Secondary pyoderma or seborrheic skin disease, or both, may be present. Pruritus varies, from mild to intense. Contact hypersensitivities may be seasonal or nonseasonal depending on the allergens involved. In multiple dog or cat households, involvement of a single animal would suggest hypersensitivity, while clinical signs in multiple animals would point to irritant reactions.

DIAGNOSIS

The differential diagnosis includes primary irritant contact dermatitis, atopy, food hypersensitivity, canine scabies, pelodera dermatitis, hookworm dermatitis, and staphylococcal folliculitis.

Definitive diagnosis is based on history, physical examination, provocative exposure, and patch testing. Provocative exposure involves avoiding contact with suspected allergenic substances for 7 to 10 days at a time.[117, 139, 236] The animal is then re-exposed to these substances, one at a time, and observed for an exacerbation of the dermatosis over a 7- to 10-day period. Provocative exposure is time consuming, requires a patient, dedicated owner, and is frequently impossible to undertake. Additionally, provocative exposure does *not* reliably distinguish between hypersensitivity and irritant skin reactions.

The *patch test* is the method for documenting contact hypersensitivity.[62, 117, 127, 225a, 236, 250] In the classic closed patch test, the test substance(s) is applied to a piece of cloth or soft paper that is then placed directly on intact skin, covered with an impermeable substance and affixed to the skin with tape. After 48 hours the patch(es) is removed and the condition of the underlying skin examined.

Owing to (1) the logistic problems of applying and securing patch testing substances to dogs and cats, and (2) the absence of commercially available patch testing kits that have been developed for or shown to be valid in dogs

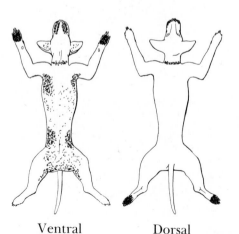

Figure 9:13. Allergic contact dermatitis distribution pattern.

Ventral   Dorsal

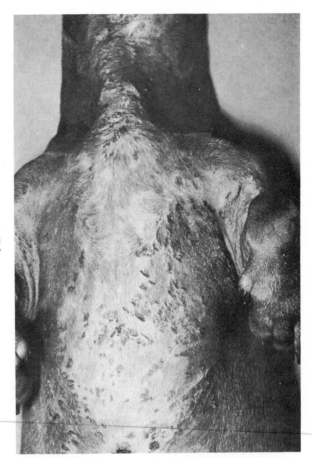

Figure 9:14. Poison oak dermatitis on the ventral surface of the neck, chest, and abdomen of a dachshund. (Chest and neck shown.) Vesicles form first but are soon ruptured by the dog, leaving an erythematous, scaly dermatitis.

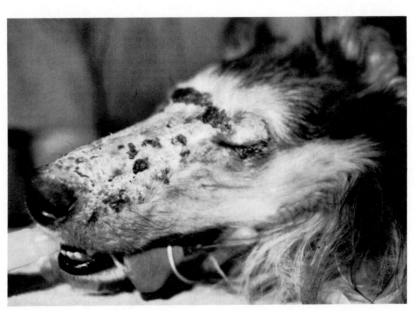

Figure 9:15. Contact dermatitis due to nystatin (Panolog) on the bridge of the nose of a dog.

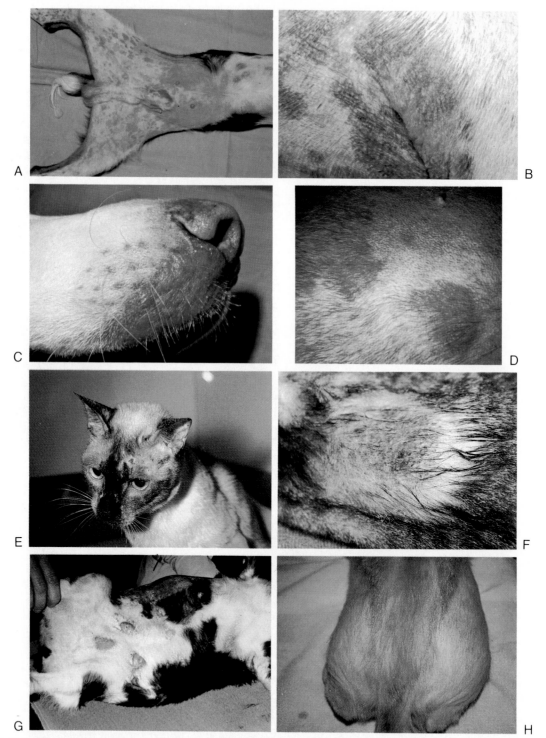

Figure 9:16. Allergic contact dermatitis. *A*, Allergic contact dermatitis affecting the glabrous skin with papules and patches of erythema. *B*, Axilla of affected dog shows erythema and papules—the primary lesions. *C*, Plastic dish dermatitis. The erythematous patch on the lip and alopecia are caused by contact with a plastic dish during eating. Note partial depigmentation of the tip of the nose. *D*, Patchy reaction resulting from contact with pigmented nylon carpeting (German short-haired pointer). *E*, Feline atopy. Facial excoriations. *F*, Feline atopy. Papulocrustous and excoriated dermatitis on the back. *G*, Feline atopy. Multiple eosinophilic plaques on abdomen. *H*, Feline atopy. Symmetric hypotrichosis over rump.

and cats, patch testing is rarely done. Walton[236] recommended "open" patch testing in the dog and listed suggested allergen concentrations and vehicles for canine patch testing. In open patch testing, the allergen(s) is merely rubbed into a suitably marked test site of normal skin, and the test site(s) is then examined daily over a 5-day period. Walton[236] reported that positive patch test reactions were apparent after 1 to 5 days. Positive patch test reactions in dogs are much less inflammatory than those seen in human beings and guinea pigs, and usually consist of mild erythema and edema, and variable degrees of pruritus. In the Danish study, 63 per cent of the affected dogs were monosensitive, and 23 per cent were sensitive to two allergens.[225a]

Until patch testing becomes standardized for dogs and cats, the diagnosis of contact hypersensitivity will remain elusive. For now, closed patch testing with suspected allergens in their natural state is probably the most sensible way to proceed. The dorsolateral thorax is gently clipped, and suspected allergens are applied to the skin, taped in place, and secured under a body bandage. The test materials are removed in 48 hours, and the test sites are observed for the following 3 to 5 days. Substances eliciting positive reactions should be tested on normal animals to make sure that they are not irritants. The pitfalls of patch testing and its interpretation are many, and the interested reader is referred to other texts[62, 127, 225a] for details.

Histopathology. Skin biopsy in canine and feline contact hypersensitivity is nondiagnostic. In experimentally induced contact hypersensitivity in dogs and cats, skin biopsy revealed varying degrees of superficial perivascular dermatitis with mononuclear cells predominating.[114, 117, 179] However, in other attempts to induce type IV hypersensitivity reactions in dog and cat skin, biopsies revealed varying degrees of superficial perivascular dermatitis in which neutrophils prevailed.[181] In naturally occurring contact hypersensitivity of dogs, cats, and human beings, skin biopsy is nondiagnostic, showing varying degrees of superficial perivascular dermatitis (spongiotic, hyperplastic) wherein neutrophils or mononuclear cells may predominate.[62, 127, 139, 225a] No significant differences are found in the number of mononuclear inflammatory cells or in their subclasses in skin from humans with allergic or primary irritant contact dermatitis.[159] Histopathologic findings consistent with secondary pyoderma or seborrheic skin disease, or both, may be present.

CLINICAL MANAGEMENT

The prognosis for contact hypersensitivity is good. Therapy of contact hypersensitivity in dogs and cats may include avoidance of allergens or the use of glucocorticoids. Avoidance of allergens is preferable but may be impossible, depending on the nature of the substances or if they cannot be identified. In such instances, glucocorticoids are very effective. Some animals can be managed with topical glucocorticoids alone (see p. 198). Other animals require systemic glucocorticoids. Prednisolone or prednisone may be administered orally at 1 mg/kg SID for 5 to 7 days, and then on an alternate-day regimen as needed (see p. 202).

Hyposensitization to certain contactants has been shown to be possible in humans.[62, 127, 225a] However, such hyposensitization is usually limited and temporary. In general, attempts to hyposensitize human beings, dogs, and cats to contactants have been totally unsuccessful.[62, 127, 139, 225a, 236]

FOOD HYPERSENSITIVITY
(Food Allergy)

Food hypersensitivity is an uncommon, nonseasonal, pruritic skin disorder of dogs and cats that is associated with presumed hypersensitivity reactions to antigenic material in the diet.

CAUSE AND PATHOGENESIS

Diet has long been recognized as a cause of hypersensitivity-like skin reactions in dogs, cats, and human beings. Although the pathomechanism of food hypersensitivity is unclear, type I hypersensitivity reactions are well documented in humans, and type III and IV reactions have been suspected.[16, 108a, 139, 217a] "Immediate" (within minutes to hours) and "delayed" (within several hours to days) reactions to foods have also been seen in the dog and cat.[14, 139, 202, 245] It has been estimated that food hypersensitivity accounts for (1) as many as 1 per cent of all canine and feline dermatoses in a general practice and (2) about 10 per cent of all canine allergic skin diseases (excluding parasitic allergy).[14, 139] Food hypersensitivity is the third most common hypersensitivity skin disease in dogs and cats, after flea bite hypersensitivity and atopy.

No age, breed, or sex predilections have been reported for canine and feline food hypersensitivity. Although it is always important to seek a dietary change that may have preceded the dermatosis, about 70 per cent of the affected animals have been eating the offending diet for over 2 years.[14, 139]

CLINICAL FEATURES

Food hypersensitivity can mimic numerous cutaneous syndromes (Table 9:22). It is obvious, based on this table, that there is no classic set of cutaneous signs that are pathognomonic for food hypersensitivity in the dog and cat. A variety of primary and secondary skin lesions are seen in food allergy. These include papules, plaques, pustules, wheals, erythema, ulcers, excoriation, scales, and crusts (Fig. 9:17). In general, the major complaint is pruritus; the pruritus is nonseasonal and often poorly responsive to glucocorticoids.

Table 9:22. DERMATOSES THAT FOOD HYPERSENSITIVITY CAN MIMIC IN DOGS AND CATS

Dog	Cat
Atopy	Widespread papulocrustous dermatitis (so-called miliary dermatitis)
Scabies	
Flea bite hypersensitivity	Facial dermatitis, pruritic (e.g., atopy, scabies)
Folliculitis, generalized, pruritic	Pruritus, generalized
Seborrheic skin disease, pruritic	Urticaria and angioedema
Recurrent pyotraumatic dermatitis	Seborrheic skin disease, pruritic
Urticaria and angioedema	Eosinophilic plaque
Otitis externa, pruritic	Indolent ulcer
Pruritus, generalized	Eosinophilic granuloma
	Psychogenic alopecia
	Otitis externa, pruritic

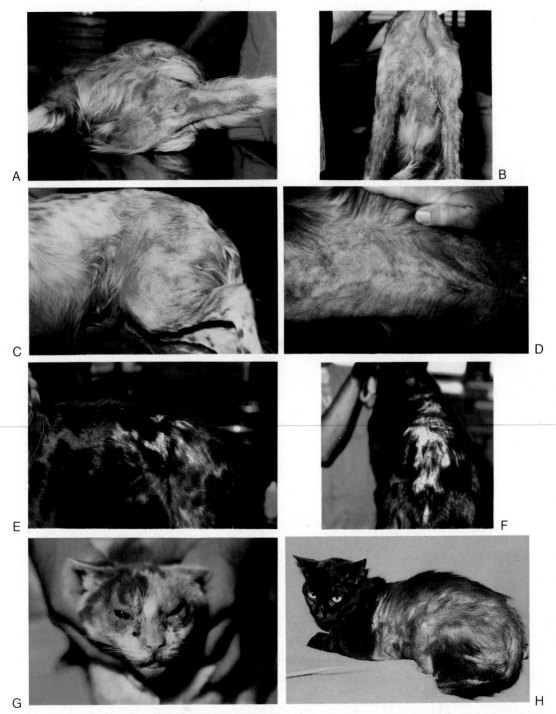

Figure 9:17. Food hypersensitivity. *A*, Erythema and alopecia over the perineum, ventral tail, and caudal thighs of a dog with food hypersensitivity. *B*, Severe erythema and alopecia over the ventral neck and chest and the front legs of a dog with food hypersensitivity. *C*, Erythema and alopecia over the lateral thighs of a dog with food hypersensitivity. *D*, Linear excoriations on the abdomen and ventral thorax of a dog with food hypersensitivity. *E*, Alopecia and scaling over the rump and flank of a dog with food hypersensitivity. *F*, Alopecia and scaling over the dorsal lumbosacral area of a dog with food hypersensitivity. *G*, Facial erythema, edema, and excoriation in a cat with food hypersensitivity. (From Scott, D. W.: Feline dermatology 1900–1978: a monograph. J.A.A.H.A. *16:*331, 1980.) *H*, Hypotrichosis of trunk and rump due to hair pulling in a cat with food hypersensitivity.

> **In food hypersensitivity, the pruritus is often poorly responsive to glucocorticoids.**

Pruritic bilateral otitis externa and secondary seborrheic skin disease and/or pyoderma are commonly seen in conjunction with food hypersensitivity. Concurrent gastrointestinal disturbances (vomiting, diarrhea, colic) have been reported in 10 to 15 per cent of the canine and feline cases. Cats with severe food hypersensitivity may have moderate to marked peripheral lymphadenopathy.[202] Concurrent respiratory disturbances (asthma) or seizures are rare.[139] In humans, the noncutaneous symptoms associated with food hypersensitivity are numerous ("tension-fatigue syndrome"), and malaise and dullness have been observed in dogs and cats.

DIAGNOSIS

The differential diagnosis in dogs includes atopy, drug hypersensitivity, flea bite hypersensitivity, pediculosis, intestinal parasite hypersensitivity, scabies, seborrheic skin disease, and folliculitis. In the cat, the differential diagnosis includes atopy, flea bite hypersensitivity, drug hypersensitivity, intestinal parasite hypersensitivity, cheyletiellosis, pediculosis, scabies, trombiculidiasis, folliculitis, and psychogenic alopecia. At present, the definitive diagnosis of food hypersensitivity in dogs and cats is reliably made only on the basis of elimination diets and test meal investigations. The animals are fed a "hypoallergenic" diet for 21 days. Hypoallergenic diets must be individualized for each patient, based on careful dietary history. The objectives of the diet are (1) to feed the animals dietary substances that they are not commonly exposed to, and (2) to feed the animals a diet that is free of additives (colorings, flavorings, preservatives). Switching from one commercial diet to another, or the use of Prescription Diet d/d (Hill's), is *not* satisfactory. Frequently used components of a hypoallergenic diet include lamb, fileted white fish, tuna fish canned in water, rabbit, venison, turkey, rice, and potatoes, pending the dietary history.[14, 139, 245] The major clinical sign being evaluated during the elimination diet is the pruritus. The level of pruritus should markedly decrease, often within the first 3 to 7 days, but occasionally not until 21 days. The diagnosis is then *confirmed* by feeding the animal its normal diet and seeing the dermatosis exacerbate within 7 days.

Little information is available on the dietary items responsible for food hypersensitivity in dogs and cats, because few owners are willing to separate a diet into its components and to feed each item individually in order to identify the responsible allergen. Evidence, to date, suggests that most dogs and cats are sensitive to a single dietary substance and that beef, dairy products, wheat, and soy are the most common offenders.[14] Table 9:23 lists dietary items reported to have caused food hypersensitivity in dogs and cats.

Routine laboratory tests are not useful in diagnosing canine and feline food hypersensitivity. Blood or tissue eosinophilia are rare in the dog, but common in the cat.[14, 132, 139, 202] Prick, scratch, and intradermal skin testing with food allergens in dogs and cats with food hypersensitivity are of no benefit. Numerous factors may influence the applicability of whole food extracts for skin testing, including the effects of cooking, processing, digestion, metabolism, additives, and contaminants on the original whole food substance. Attempts

Table 9:23. DIETARY ITEMS REPORTED TO CAUSE FOOD HYPERSENSITIVITY IN DOGS AND CATS

Dog		Cat	
Cow's milk	Wheat	Cow's milk	Fish (variety)
Beef	Corn	Beef	Eggs
Mutton	Soy	Mutton	Canned foods
Pork	Rice flour	Pork	Dry foods
Chicken	Potatoes	Chicken	Cod-liver oil
Rabbit	Kidney beans	Rabbit	Benzoic acid
Horse meat	Canned foods	Horse meat	
Fish (variety)	Dog biscuits		
Eggs	Dog foods (including		
Oatmeal	Prescription Diet d/d)		
	Artificial food additives		

to diagnose food hypersensitivity by blood samples (leukocytotoxicity, permanent elimination of toxins, RAST) are unreliable in dogs, cats, and humans.[16, 57, 131a, 208, 211]

Histopathology. Skin biopsy reflects the variability of the gross morphology of skin lesions, and is usually characterized by varying degrees of superficial perivascular dermatitis (pure, spongiotic, hyperplastic) with neutrophils or mononuclear cells usually predominating in dogs, but with eosinophils frequently seen in cats.[139, 202] Food-hypersensitive cats that present with indolent ulcers, eosinophilic plaques, or eosinophilic granulomas have dermatohistopathologic findings consistent with these lesions (see p. 563). Secondary suppurative changes (intraepidermal pustular dermatitis, perifolliculitis, folliculitis), are frequently seen (Fig. 9:18).

CLINICAL MANAGEMENT

The prognosis for food hypersensitivity is usually good. Therapy of food hypersensitivity consists of avoiding offending foods or using systemic gluco-

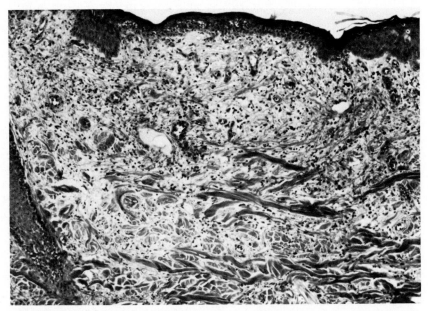

Figure 9:18. Canine food hypersensitivity dermatitis. Hyperplastic perivascular dermatitis.

corticoids. "Hypoallergenic" diets are formulated by adding single foodstuffs to the diet, one at a time, and evaluating each item for 7 days. In this way, a tolerable, varied diet can usually be achieved over the course of 4 to 6 months. Such diets need to be balanced with vitamin, mineral, and fatty acid supplements. In cats, a source of dietary taurine is also essential, and this may be supplied in the form of ½ tsp of clam juice mixed with the food daily. As a compromise, animals can be provoked daily, for 7 days at a time, with each of major food groups (beef, dairy products, wheat, soy) to determine whether one of these groups exacerbates the condition.[14] Based on the information obtained from this provocation, a commercial food that does not contain the offending substance(s) can be selected. Prescription Diet d/d (Hill's) can also be tried for dogs and cats, although some cats will not eat it. It has been reported that food hypersensitivities in dogs and cats rarely involve multiple allergens and that naturally occurring hyposensitization rarely occurs. Rarely, animals develop further dietary hypersensitivities and require re-evaluation by test meals.

When hypoallergenic diets are not feasible, systemic glucocorticoids or antihistamines may be used to suppress clinical signs. However, food hypersensitivity is often poorly responsive to these drugs. In humans, oral cromoglycate has produced variable results in the management of food hypersensitivity.[16, 78] To date, this drug has not been evaluated in animals.

DRUG ERUPTION
(Drug Allergy, Dermatitis Medicamentosa)

Drug eruption in dogs and cats is a rare, variably pruritic, and pleomorphic cutaneous or mucocutaneous reaction to a drug in dogs and cats.

CAUSE AND PATHOGENESIS

Drugs responsible for skin eruptions may be administered orally, topically, or by injection or inhalation. The incidence of drug eruption in dogs and cats is unknown but is reported to occur in up to 15 per cent of all hospitalized human patients.

Adverse drug reactions may be divided into two major groups: (1) *predictable*, usually dose-dependent and related to the pharmacologic actions of the drugs, or (2) *unpredictable*, often dose-independent and related to the individual's immunologic response (hypersensitivity) or to genetic differences in susceptibility of patients (idiosyncracy or intolerance), which are often related to metabolic or enzymatic deficiencies.[55, 254] Many cutaneous effects of certain drugs are predictable. For instance, many of the anticancer or immunosuppressive drugs can cause alopecia, purpura, poor wound healing, and increased susceptibility to infection through their effects on cellular biology (see Table 9:25).[30] Drug hypersensitivities are believed to involve type I, II, III, and IV reactions. Human patients with systemic lupus erythematosus and atopy are thought to be predisposed to drug eruption, but no such observations have been made for the dog and cat.

CLINICAL FEATURES

Any drug may cause an eruption (Tables 9:24 and 9:25), and no specific type of reaction results from any one drug. Thus, drug eruption can mimic

Table 9:24. DRUGS REPORTED TO CAUSE CUTANEOUS HYPERSENSITIVITY-LIKE REACTIONS IN DOGS AND CATS[74, 94a, 128, 129, 139, 167a, 187, 196, 208, 230]

Dog	Cat
Acetylpromazine	Ampicillin
Ampicillin	Aurothioglucose
Aurothioglucose	Cephaloridine
Bacterins	Dichlorvos
Benzoyl peroxide	FeLV antiserum
Cephalexin	Gentamicin
Chloramphenicol	Griseofulvin
Coal tar	Hetacillin
Cyclosporine	Penicillin
Dapsone	Propylthiouracil
Diethylcarbamazine	Sulfonamides
Doxorubicin	Tetracycline
5-Fluorocytosine	Vaccines
Gentamicin	Various otic preparations (especially Tresaderm
Griseofulvin	and chlorinated hydrocarbon-containing
Levamisole	miticides)
Lime sulfur	
Neomycin	
Penicillin	
Phenytoin	
Prednisolone	
Primidone	
Quinidine	
Streptomycin	
Sulfonamides	
Synthetic estrogens	
Tetracaine	
Tetracycline	
Thiabendazole	
Thiacetarsamide	
Thyroid extract	
Triamcinolone	
Vaccines	
Various otic preparations (especially	
Tresaderm and Unitop)	

virtually any dermatosis (Table 9:26 and Figs. 9:19 to 9:22). No breed, age, or sex predilections have been reported for canine and feline drug eruption. The most common drugs recognized to produce drug hypersensitivity–like reactions are the sulfonamides (especially Tribrissen) and the penicillins (especially

Table 9:25. DRUGS REPORTED TO CAUSE CUTANEOUS SIDE-EFFECTS IN DOGS AND CATS[17, 219, 224a, 243]

Drug	Side-Effects
Azathioprine	Alopecia, pyoderma, demodicosis
Bleomycin	Ulceration at pressure points and onychomadesis
Chlorambucil	Alopecia, hyperpigmentation
Cyclophosphamide	Alopecia, pyoderma
Cyclosporine	Hirsutism, papillomatosis, lymphoplasmacytoid dermatosis
Doxorubicin	Flushing and pruritus (acute), and symmetric alopecia and hyperpigmentation (chronic)
Glucocorticoids	Cushingoid changes
Hydroxyurea	Alopecia
Isotretinoin	Mucocutaneous erythema and crusting
Mechlorethamine	Demodicosis

Table 9:26. MORPHOLOGIC FORMS OF CUTANEOUS DRUG HYPERSENSITIVITIES IN DOGS AND CATS

Erythema multiforme	Toxic epidermal necrolysis
Erythroderma	Urticaria and angioedema
Exfoliative dermatitis	Vesicobullous dermatitis (pemphigus- or
Fixed drug eruption	pemphigoid-like)
Papular dermatitis	Otitis externa
Purpura	

ampicillin, amoxicillin).[55, 211, 254] Erythema multiforme and toxic epidermal necrolysis have been most commonly seen with Tribrissen, cephalexins, and levamisole administration.[207, 211, 230] Diethylcarbamazine and 5-fluorocytosine have been associated with fixed drug eruption on the scrotum of male dogs.[129, 211] A hypersensitivity reaction (probably type III) associated with Tribrissen administration (probably sulfadiazine related) has been recognized in Doberman pinschers (genetically programmed?).[74] Cyclosporine has been reported to cause a lymphoplasmacytoid dermatitis with malignant features (usually a solitary plaque or nodule) in dogs.[166, 167]

Because drug eruption can mimic so many different dermatoses, it is imperative to have an accurate knowledge of the medications given to any patient with an obscure dermatosis.

> *Drug eruptions are often pruritic, and usually poorly responsive to systemic glucocorticoids.*

Drug eruption may occur after a drug has been given for days or years, or a few days after drug therapy is stopped. At present, the only reliable test for

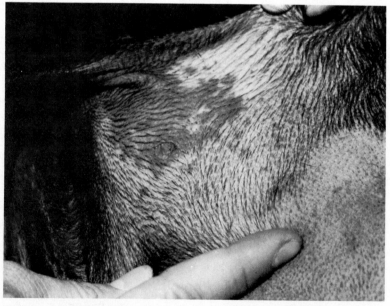

Figure 9:19. Drug eruption (chloramphenicol) in a dog. Petechiae and ecchymoses in the axilla.

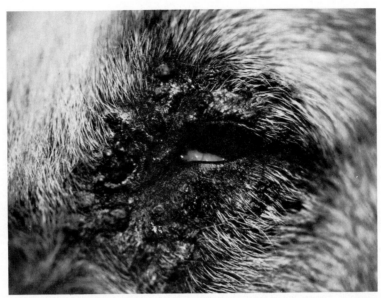

Figure 9:20. Periocular alopecia, erosion, and crusting in a dog with drug eruption (triple sulfa). (From Scott, D. W., Barrett, R. E., and Tangorra, L.: Drug eruption associated with sulfonamide treatment of vertebral osteomyelitis in a dog. J.A.V.M.A. *168*:1111, 1976.)

the diagnosis of drug eruption is to withdraw the drug and watch for disappearance of the eruption (usually 10 to 14 days). However, drug eruptions may occasionally persist for weeks to months after the offending drug is stopped. Purposeful readministration of the offending drug to determine whether the eruption will be reproduced is undesirable and may be dangerous.

DIAGNOSIS

The *differential diagnosis* is complex, as drug eruption may mimic virtually any dermatosis. In general, there are no specific or characteristic laboratory

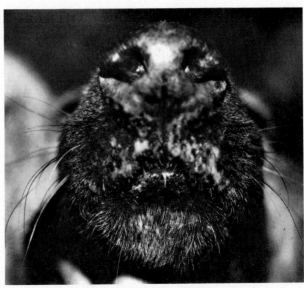

Figure 9:21. Erythema, depigmentation, erosion, and crusting on the muzzle of a dog with drug eruption (triple sulfa).

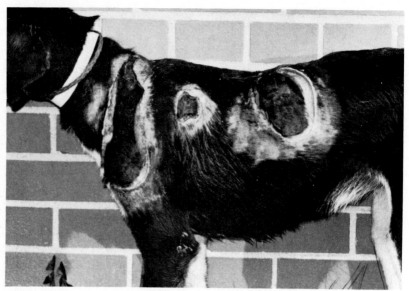

Figure 9:22. Drug eruption (Keflex) in a dog. Focal areas of epidermal necrosis and resultant ulceration.

findings that indicate drug eruption. Results of in vivo and in vitro immunologic tests have usually been disappointing.

Helpful criteria for distinguishing drug hypersensitivity include the following: (1) hypersensitivity occurs in a minority of patients receiving the drug, (2) observed manifestations do not resemble known pharmacologic actions of the drugs, (3) prior exposure to drug may have been tolerated without adverse effects, (4) reaction conforms to manifestations generally acknowledged as demonstrating hypersensitivity, (5) reaction is reproduced by administration of

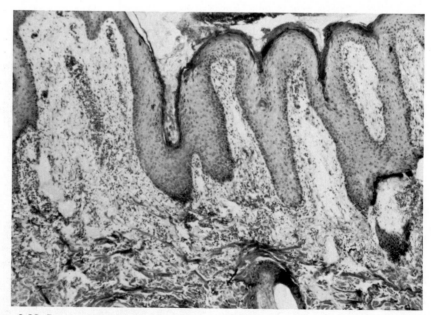

Figure 9:23. Drug eruption (triple sulfa) in a dog. Hyperplastic perivascular dermatitis. (From Scott, D. W., Barrett, R. E., and Tangorra, L.: Drug eruption associated with sulfonamide treatment of vertebral osteomyelitis in a dog. J.A.V.M.A. *168*:1111, 1976.)

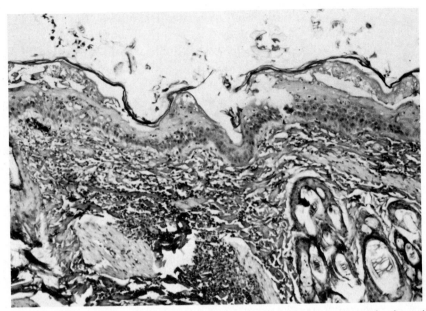

Figure 9:24. Drug eruption (penicillin) in a cat. Epidermal necrosis and perivascular dermatitis.

small doses of the drugs, or cross-reacting drugs, (6) resolution occurs within several days after drug is discontinued.

Just as the clinical morphology of drug eruptions varies greatly, so do the histologic findings. *Histologic* patterns recognized with cutaneous drug eruptions include perivascular dermatitis (pure, spongiotic, hyperplastic), interface dermatitis (hydropic, lichenoid), intraepidermal vesiculopustular dermatitis, and subepidermal vesicular dermatitis (Figs. 9:23, 9:24, and 9:25). Eosinophils are rarely seen.

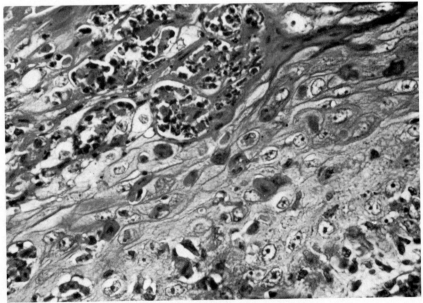

Figure 9:25. Drug eruption (Keflex) in a dog. Necrosis of individual keratinocytes and epidermal microabscesses.

Direct immunofluorescence testing in drug eruptions may reveal immunoreactants deposited in a variety of nondiagnostic patterns, especially in the walls of blood vessels and at the basement membrane zone.[72, 176, 211]

CLINICAL MANAGEMENT

The prognosis for drug eruption is usually good, unless other organ systems are involved. Therapy of drug eruption includes (1) discontinuing the offending drug, (2) treating symptoms with topical and systemic medications, as indicated, and (3) avoiding chemically related drugs. Drug eruptions may be poorly responsive to glucocorticoids.

HORMONAL HYPERSENSITIVITY

Hormonal hypersensitivity is a rare, pruritic, papulocrustous dermatitis of dogs and humans, associated with hypersensitivity reactions to sex hormones.[62, 139]

CAUSE AND PATHOGENESIS

Although the pathomechanism of the dermatitis is unknown, results of intradermal skin testing in dogs and humans suggest that type I and IV hypersensitivity reactions to endogenous progesterone, estrogen, or testosterone are involved.

CLINICAL FEATURES

No age or breed predilections have been reported. However, over 90 per cent of the reported cases have occurred in intact females. Affected females often have a history of repeated pseudopregnancy or irregular estral cycles or both. Dermatologic signs include a pruritic, erythematous, often papulocrustous eruption that usually begins in the perineal, genital, and caudomedial thigh regions, is bilaterally symmetric, and progresses cranially (Fig. 9:26). The feet, face, and ears are commonly affected in chronic cases. Enlargement of the vulva and nipples is often seen (Figs. 9:27 and 9:28). In female dogs, the dermatologic signs usually coincide initially with estrus or pseudopregnancy, or both, but tend to become more severe and protracted with each episode until the dog may have some degree of pruritic dermatitis at all times. In male dogs, dermatologic signs are nonseasonal.

DIAGNOSIS

The *differential diagnosis* includes flea bite hypersensitivity, food hypersensitivity, atopy, drug hypersensitivity, intestinal parasite hypersensitivity, folliculitis, and ovarian imbalance type I. *Definitive diagnosis* is made by history, physical examination, intradermal skin testing, and response to therapy. Intradermal skin testing is performed with aqueous progesterone (0.025 mg), estrogen (0.0125 mg), and testosterone (0.05 mg), and the skin is observed for immediate and delayed hypersensitivity reactions. Histopathology is nondiagnostic, revealing varying degrees of superficial perivascular dermatitis (pure, spongiotic, hyperplastic) with neutrophils or mononuclear cells predominating.

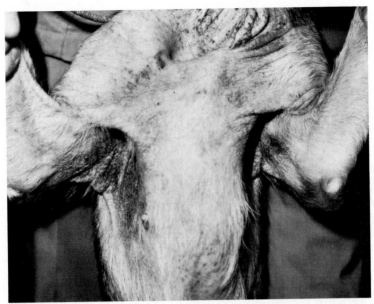

Figure 9:26. Canine hormonal hypersensitivity. Traumatic and inflammatory alopecia, hyperpigmentation, and lichenification of ventral neck and chest, axillae, and medial forelimbs.

CLINICAL MANAGEMENT

The prognosis for hormonal hypersensitivity is favorable if neutering can be performed. Therapy includes (1) ovariohysterectomy or castration and (2) treatment of symptoms with topical and systemic medicaments, as indicated. Response to neutering is dramatic, with marked improvement occurring within 5 to 10 days. Response to systemic glucocorticoids is usually unsatisfactory. In female dogs, response to repositol testosterone (1.0 mg/kg intramuscularly) is a useful presurgical diagnostic aid, with dramatic relief of pruritus occurring within 7 days. Perhaps antiandrogens (e.g., certain progestogens) could be used in a similar manner in male dogs, but this possibility is unproven.

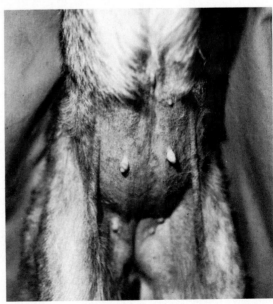

Figure 9:27. Canine hormonal hypersensitivity. Traumatic and inflammatory alopecia with gynecomastia.

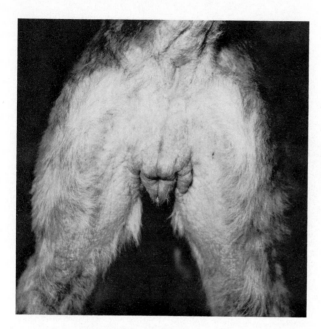

Figure 9:28. Canine hormonal hypersensitivity. Inflammatory and traumatic alopecia with lichenification and vulvar enlargement.

PARASITIC HYPERSENSITIVITY

Flea Bite Hypersensitivity
(Flea Allergy Dermatitis)

Flea bite hypersensitivity is a pruritic, papulocrustous dermatitis in animals that become sensitized to allergenic material(s) in flea saliva. It is *the* most common hypersensitivity skin disorder in dogs and cats.

CAUSE AND PATHOGENESIS

The etiopathogenesis of flea bite hypersensitivity has been most extensively studied in the guinea pig.[139] Flea saliva contains several potentially antigenic substances, including polypeptides, amino acids, aromatic compounds, and fluorescent materials. Gel filtration of flea saliva revealed that allergens were present in a high molecular weight fraction (about 4000 to 10,000 daltons) and in a highly fluorescent aromatic fraction (less than 1000 daltons). When flea saliva alone was injected intradermally or intraperitoneally into guinea pigs, sensitization did not occur. This result demonstrated that the allergenic substance(s) was a hapten. Induction of hypersensitivity was independent of the number of fleas biting or the dose of flea extract, and sensitization was systemic. It was also shown that dermal collagen appeared to be the cutaneous adjuvant for one or more flea saliva haptens.

A predictable sequence of sensitization for flea bite hypersensitivity in guinea pigs has been demonstrated:

Stage I—induction
Stage II—delayed-type hypersensitivity
Stage III—delayed and immediate types of hypersensitivity
Stage IV—immediate-type hypersensitivity
Stage V—nonreactivity

Thus, flea bite hypersensitivity in the guinea pig involves both type I and IV hypersensitivity reactions. It was also demonstrated that *Ctenocephalides felis*, *Pulex irritans*, and *P. simulans* shared one or more antigens and that guinea pigs and human beings sensitized to one type of flea reacted to all species.

Most dogs and cats that are flea saliva hypersensitive have immediate skin test reactions to the intradermal injection of flea antigen, indicating a type I hypersensitivity reaction and an antigen with a molecular weight of 5000 to 10,000 daltons (nonhaptenic).[87–90, 118, 202] Flea hypersensitive dogs also usually have delayed skin test reactions indicating a type IV hypersensitivity reaction (haptenic). Delayed skin test reactions have *not* been reported in flea hypersensitive cats.[118, 138, 202] The orderly sequence of flea sensitivity that develops in guinea pigs does not occur in dogs and cats,[89, 90] and dogs and cats rarely, if ever, achieve natural desensitization.[139] Other experimental aspects of skin testing and dermatohistopathology in dogs with flea bite hypersensitivity have suggested that late-phase immediate hypersensitivity (IgE) reactions (see p. 438) and cutaneous basophil hypersensitivity reactions may play a role in the pathogenesis of skin lesions.[80, 89, 90, 91b] It is likely that animals do *not* develop skin lesions as a result of flea infestation, unless they are flea hypersensitive.

Studies on intradermal skin test reactions to flea antigen and on the serum levels of antiflea IgE and IgG in experimentally maintained dogs, as well as in dogs kept as pets or in animal shelters, have indicated that dogs continually exposed to fleas either fail to develop flea bite hypersensitivity or develop it later and to a lesser degree.[89–91] This observation suggests that continually exposed dogs may become partially or completely immunologically tolerant. It also suggests that if a dog has an abundance of fleas and no evidence of a hypersensitivity reaction, it might be prudent to refrain from introducing a diligent flea-control program.[89]

Whereas up to 40 per cent of the normal dog and cat populations in flea-endemic areas may have positive intradermal skin test reactions to flea antigen,[89–91, 138] up to 80 per cent of the atopic dogs in the same area may be positive. This suggests that the atopic state may predispose dogs to developing flea bite hypersensitivity.

CLINICAL FEATURES

No breed or sex predilections are apparent. Although dogs and cats may develop flea bite hypersensitivity at any age, it is rare for clinical signs to develop in animals less than 6 months of age. The most common age of onset is 3 to 5 years.

Canine and feline flea bite hypersensitivity is characterized by a pruritic, papulocrustous dermatitis (Fig. 9:29). Lesions are typically confined to the dorsal lumbosacral area, caudomedial thighs, ventral abdomen, flanks, and neck (Fig. 9:30). The typical distribution pattern is illustrated in Figures 9:31 and 9:32. This cutaneous reaction is particularly common in cats and may be caused by a number of specific diseases (Table 9:27). Generalized cutaneous signs may be present in severely hypersensitive animals. Pyotraumatic dermatitis ("hot spots"), secondary pyoderma, alopecia, and secondary seborrhea are not uncommon. Flea hypersensitive cats may also present with (1) symmetric alopecia (little or no dermatitis) or (2) indolent ulcer, eosinophilic plaque, eosinophilic granuloma, or some combination of these three lesions (see p. 561).[202] Cats with flea bite hypersensitivity may develop moderate-to-marked

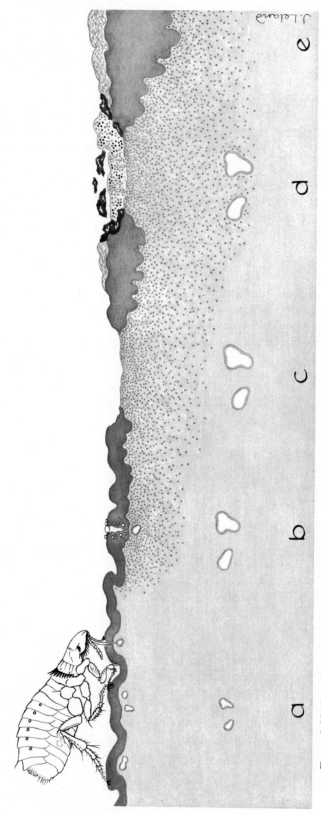

Figure 9:29. Flea allergy dermatitis dermogram. *A,* A flea feeds on normal skin by penetrating the epidermis with its sharply toothed laciniae. Without entering the puncture wound, the flea sucks up blood along a tube formed by the labrum-epipharynx and the laciniae. Saliva enters the wound during this blood sucking process. *B,* A saliva-filled puncture wound remains in the skin, and in animals hypersensitized to flea saliva an antibody-antigen reaction takes place (immediate type). *C,* Excoriation with dermal inflammatory infiltration results from self-inflicted trauma. *D,* Acute moist dermatitis develops on an excoriated lesion. There is superficial bacterial infection with massive dermal inflammation, exudation, and crust formation. *E,* Chronic flea allergy dermatitis causes thickening of the skin with acanthosis, hyperkeratosis, and lichenification. The thickened epidermis presents a formidable obstacle to future penetrations of the skin by the flea's mouthparts.

peripheral lymphadenopathy.[202] Flea bite hypersensitivity is usually distinctly seasonal (summer and fall) in areas of the world with cold winters. In warm climates or where household infestation persists, flea bite hypersensitivity may be nonseasonal, although clinical signs are still usually more severe in summer and fall.

DIAGNOSIS

The differential diagnosis in the dog includes food hypersensitivity, atopy, drug hypersensitivity, intestinal parasite hypersensitivity, and folliculitis. In the cat, the differential diagnosis includes the diseases listed in Table 9:27.

Definitive diagnosis is based on history, physical examination, intradermal skin testing with flea antigen, and response to therapy. The morphology and distribution of the skin lesions are very suggestive. The presence of fleas or flea dirt is also a helpful finding. However, realizing that (1) fleas spend most of their life *off* of the host and (2) recent bathing or dipping will have removed fleas and flea dirt, the inability to demonstrate fleas or flea dirt on the animal in *no way* precludes the diagnosis.

Blood eosinophilia is often present in dogs and cats with flea bite hypersensitivity.[139, 202] Skin biopsy is nondiagnostic, revealing varying degrees of superficial perivascular dermatitis (pure, spongiotic, hyperplastic), with eosinophils often being a predominant cell type.[80, 139, 202] In addition, eosinophilic intraepidermal microabscesses in association with epidermal edema and necrosis may be seen (Fig. 9:33). Histopathologic findings consistent with secondary pyoderma (suppurative folliculitis, intraepidermal pustular dermatitis) are common. Cats presenting with clinical lesions of indolent ulcer, eosinophilic plaque, and eosinophilic granuloma have dermatohistopathologic findings consistent with those entities (see p. 561–564).

Older reports on the use of intradermal skin testing for the diagnosis of flea bite hypersensitivity were contradictory and inconclusive, owing to many procedural differences.[139] Glycerinated antigens should *not* be used, as primary

---

Table 9:27. DIFFERENTIAL DIAGNOSIS OF WIDESPREAD PAPULOCRUSTOUS DERMATITIS ("MILIARY DERMATITIS") IN THE CAT

Hypersensitivity reactions
  Flea bite hypersensitivity
  Atopy
  Food hypersensitivity
  Drug hypersensitivity
  Intestinal parasite hypersensitivity
  Feline hypereosinophilic syndrome

Ectoparasitisms
  Cheyletiellosis
  Otodectic mange
  Trombiculidiasis
  Cat fur mite
  Pediculosis

Infections
  Dermatophytosis
  Staphylococcal folliculitis

Dietary imbalances
  Biotin deficiency
  Fatty acid deficiency

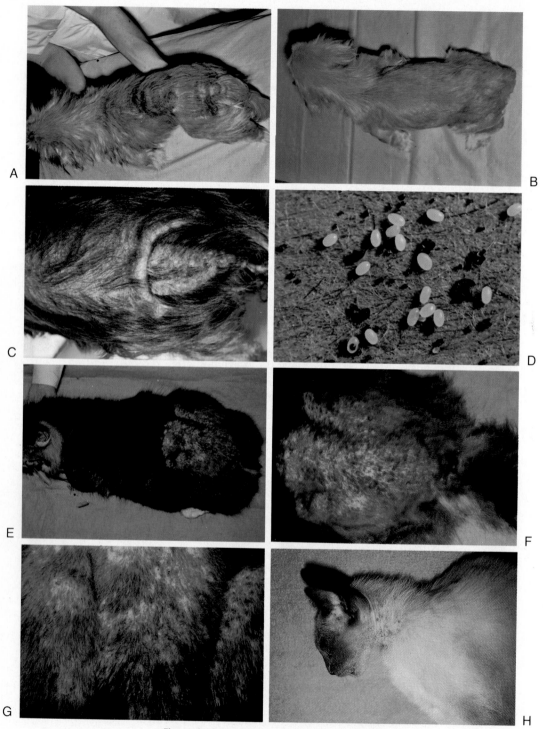

Figure 9:30 *See legend on opposite page*

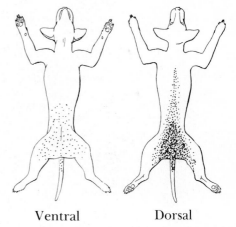

Figure 9:31. Flea allergy dermatitis (canine) distribution pattern.

Ventral   Dorsal

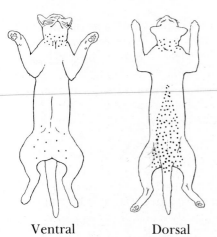

Figure 9:32. Flea allergy dermatitis (feline) distribution pattern.

Ventral   Dorsal

Figure 9:30. *Flea allergy dermatitis (canine). A,* Chronic flea allergy dermatitis in a Pekingese, showing alopecia, hyperpigmentation, and lichenification on the lower back and tail base. *B,* Same dog as in *A.* Hair has regrown completely after eight months of treatment consisting exclusively of flea eradication. *C,* After many seasons of affliction, area of the lower back and tail becomes hairless, thickened, gray, and folded. *D,* Macrophotograph of white flea eggs and dark brown flea fecal crusts on a piece of blue paper. Newly hatched flea larvae find the available fecal crusts a handy source of food. *Flea allergy dermatitis (feline). E,* Numerous miliary lesions clustered on the back of this cat. Area has been clipped in *E, F, G,* and *H* to expose lesion. *F,* Closer view of the lower back of *E.* Note crusts and erosions. *G,* The individual miliary lesions are shallow excoriations covered with a small brown crust. Some crusts have been removed to show the lesion's base. *H,* Other common sites of the papulocrustous dermatitis of flea bite hypersensitivity are the neck and throat.

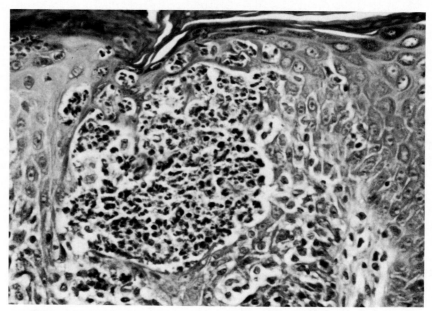

Figure 9:33. Canine flea allergy dermatitis. Epidermal eosinophilic microabscess.

irritant and false-positive reactions are produced in dogs and cats. In the United States, one commercial aqueous flea antigen (Flea Antigen, Greer Laboratories) has emerged as a very reliable product.[87-90, 118, 138, 202] This product is injected intradermally (0.05 ml of 1:1000 w/v aqueous solution), along with positive (histamine) and negative (saline) controls (see p. 457), and skin reactions are read at 15 and 30 minutes and at 24 and 48 hours. About 80 per cent of flea hypersensitive dogs have both immediate and delayed reactions, whereas the other 20 per cent have one or the other. Only immediate reactions have been seen in cats. Intradermal skin testing has also been found to be reliable for the diagnosis of flea bite hypersensitivity in dogs in France.[43] It is essential to remember that a positive immediate skin test reaction *only* means that the patient has skin sensitizing antibody. It does not necessarily mean that the patient has clinical allergy. Thus, although virtually all flea hypersensitive dogs and cats have positive skin test reactions to flea antigen, so does a portion of the normal dog and cat population. Current or recent drug administration (especially glucocorticoids and progestagens) is a frequent cause of false-negative skin tests (see p. 456).

CLINICAL MANAGEMENT

In general, flea bite hypersensitivity in dogs and cats tends to worsen as the animals age. Clinical signs begin a little earlier in the season, persist a little longer, and tend to become progressively more severe. Naturally occurring desensitization is apparently rare.

Therapy of flea bite hypersensitivity may include flea control (see p. 416), systemic glucocorticoids, and hyposensitization. Flea control and systemic glucocorticoids are usually quite effective for the management of short- or long-term flea bite hypersensitivity in colder climates, but less so in subtropical to tropical climates. Prednisolone or prednisone is given orally at 1 mg/kg SID for dogs and 2 mg/kg SID for cats, for 5 to 7 days and then in an alternate-day regimen (see p. 203), as needed. Where glucocorticoids are unsatisfactory, flea hypersensitive dogs may respond to antihistamines (chlorpheniramine 4 mg TID orally; diphenhydramine 2 mg/kg TID orally; hydroxyzine 2 mg/kg TID orally) or an eicosapentaenoic acid–containing product (Derm Caps, 1 capsule/ 9.1 kg SID orally).[210] In cats, chlorpheniramine (2 to 4 mg BID orally) is a particularly useful antihistamine.[135, 211] Of course, the single most effective therapy would be separating the fleas from the pet or eliminating the fleas. This involves concentrating extermination efforts on the indoor and outdoor premises. Employing a skillful commercial exterminator is often the most effective way of controlling fleas and is highly recommended.

The following are additional facts about flea control on dogs and cats:

1. Flea shampoos have almost no residual actions. The active ingredient is rinsed off.

2. Thiamine, brewer's yeast, garlic, and sulfur do not have repellent action.

3. Flea collars have little or no value for flea control in many parts of the country.

4. Systemic antiflea agents are effective, but do not kill the flea until *after* it has injected flea saliva; thus, they are of minimal benefit to the patient with flea hypersensitivity.

5. Flea control on the premises with foggers and residual sprays is effective and highly recommended.

The reader is referred to page 416 for details on flea control.

The efficacy of hyposensitization in canine and feline flea bite hypersensitivity is still controversial. Enthusiastic proponents and outspoken critics abound.[139, 208] However, recent double-blind controlled studies in dogs[84] and cats[118] have shown that hyposensitization with aqueous whole flea antigens in flea bite hypersensitivity is rarely effective, as well as being expensive and time consuming. However, results of hyposensitization with an alum-precipitated whole flea antigen in dogs with flea bite hypersensitivity suggested that a double-blind, long-term cross-over study should be conducted to assess the clinical efficacy of this protocol.[172b]

Based on current available information, treatment of canine and feline flea bite hypersensitivity with presently available commercial whole flea extracts should be viewed as a "last ditch" therapeutic effort having a slim chance of success. In such instances, one could try any of the whole flea extracts—Flea Antigen, Hollister-Stier Laboratories; Flea Antigen, Haver-Lockhart Laboratories; Flea Antigen, Center Laboratories; Flea Antigen, Greer Laboratories; and Whole Flea Extract, Nelco Laboratories—given 0.5 to 1.0 ml intradermally, once weekly, to effect (6 to 12 weeks). If results were successful, booster injections could be administered as needed (every 1 to 3 months).

Canine Scabies
(Sarcoptic Mange)

Hypersensitivity appears to play a considerable role in canine and human scabies.[62, 139] In both species, dermatologic changes are often completely out of proportion to the number of mites present, and pruritus and dermatitis can continue for days to weeks after the mites are destroyed with miticidal agents. In the dog, other evidence suggesting the importance of hypersensitivity includes (1) presence of asymptomatic carriers, (2) rare concurrent proteinuria, and (3) rare concurrent immune complex glomerulonephritis.

Additional evidence for immunologic participation in the pathogenesis of human scabies includes (1) accelerated clinical response to fewer mites upon reinfestation, (2) partial immunity if cured after sensitization has occurred, (3) lower serum IgA levels in scabietic patients as compared with noninfested controls, (4) positive skin test reactions to scabies antigen in scabietic patients but not in noninfested controls, (5) increased incidence of circulating immune complexes in scabietic patients, (6) positive Prausnitz-Küstner testing with serum from scabietic patients and scabies-mite antigen in normal individuals, and (7) deposition of IgG, IgM, and C3 at the basement membrane zone and within dermal blood vessel walls on direct immunofluorescence testing of scabietic skin.

For further details on canine scabies, see page 396.

Otodectic Acariasis
(Ear Mites)

Hypersensitivity appears to play a role in some cases of otodectic acariasis in cats. Clinically, cats occasionally develop a widespread, pruritic, papulocrustous dermatitis associated with *Otodectes cynotis* infestation.[202] Immunologically, passive cutaneous anaphylaxis reactions to *O. cynotis* antigen were reported in cats with experimentally induced ear mite infestations, demonstrating the existence of reaginic antibody in cats.[156]

Tick Bite Hypersensitivity

Cutaneous hypersensitivity reactions to tick bites have been recognized in dogs and humans.[62, 126, 139] The proposed pathomechanism of these reactions involves type III and type IV hypersensitivity responses. No age, breed, or sex predilections have been reported.

Cutaneous hypersensitivity reactions to tick bites in dogs and cats may be characterized by (1) focal areas of necrosis and ulceration, (2) nodules that may or may not be erythematous, pruritic, and ulcerated, and (3) pruritic pododermatitis. Diagnosis is based on history and physical examination.

Skin biopsy may reveal leukocytoclastic vasculitis with hemorrhage, necrosis, and ulceration (type III reaction), or nodular-to-diffuse dermatitis due to granulomatous or pyogranulomatous inflammation (type IV reaction), often with numerous eosinophils and lymphoid hyperplasia. Tick mouthparts are seldom found in biopsy specimens.

Therapy includes tick removal and control. Surgical excision or glucocorticoids are effective for severe or persistent reactions.

Intestinal Parasite Hypersensitivity

Various intestinal parasites (ascarids, *Coccidia*, hookworms, tapeworms, whipworms) of dogs, cats, and humans may rarely be associated with pruritic dermatoses.[62, 139] The pathomechanism of these dermatoses is unknown, but a type I hypersensitivity reaction is likely. Although the pathomechanism is unknown, a clear relationship between the parasite and the dermatosis is established, since (1) eliminating the parasites cures the dermatosis and (2) reinfestation with the parasite reproduces it.

Clinical signs include (1) generalized or multifocal pruritic, papulocrustous dermatitis, (2) pruritic seborrheic skin disease, (3) pruritic urticaria, or (4) pruritus without skin lesions. Other signs referable to intestinal parasitism may or may not be present. No age, breed, or sex predilections have been reported.

Diagnosis is made by history, physical examination, fecal examinations, and response to therapy. Skin biopsy is nondiagnostic, revealing varying degrees of superficial perivascular dermatitis (pure, spongiotic, hyperplastic), often with small-to-large numbers of eosinophils.

Therapy includes (1) elimination of the parasites and (2) treatment of symptoms with topical (shampoos, soaks) and systemic medicaments (gluco-corticoids), as indicated.

Dirofilariasis
(Heartworm)

Numerous rare skin disorders associated with *Dirofilaria immitis* infection have been described in dogs.[87, 205] The pathomechanism of these skin disorders is unknown, although a hypersensitivity to *D. immitis* microfilariae has been suggested. No age, breed, or sex predilections have been reported.

Cutaneous syndromes reported in association with dirofilariasis in dogs include (1) a pruritic, ulcerative nodular dermatitis of the head, trunk, and limbs; (2) a pruritic papulocrustous dermatitis resembling canine scabies; (3) a pruritic ulcerative dermatitis of the head and limbs; (4) an erythematous, alopecic dermatitis of the chest and limbs; and (5) seborrheic skin disease (Figs. 9:34*A, B*).

Diagnosis is based on history, physical examination, demonstrating *D. immitis* microfilariae in peripheral blood and in skin biopsies, ruling out other possible causes of the dermatosis, and response to therapy for dirofilariasis. Most dogs with dirofilariasis have peripheral eosinophilia and serum hyper-gammaglobulinemia.[36] About 50 per cent of affected dogs also have peripheral basophilia. In about 20 per cent of the dogs with dirofilariasis, microfilariae cannot be demonstrated in peripheral blood (occult dirofilariasis), owing to an immune-mediated reaction against microfilarial antigen. Various enzyme-linked immunosorbent assay (ELISA) methodologies for the detection of adult *D. immitis*–associated antigens (Filarochek, Mallinckrodt; Dirochek, Synbiotics; ClinEase-CH, Norden; CITE, Agri Tech Systems) are very useful for the detection of occult dirofilariasis.[37]

Histologic examination of the nodular form of cutaneous dirofilariasis reveals superficial and deep perivascular to nodular dermatitis.[46, 205] Eosinophils are numerous. Pyogranulomas may be situated perivascularly, with microfilariae present intravascularly (Fig. 9:35), or interstitially surrounding extravascular microfilariae (Fig. 9:36).

Therapy consists of (1) thiacetarsamide (Caparsolate Sodium) at 2.2 mg/kg intravenously BID for 2 consecutive days, for adult *D. immitis*, and (2) dithia-zanine (Dizan) at 7 to 11 mg/kg orally SID for 7 to 10 days; *or* levamisole (Levasole) at 10 to 11 mg/kg orally SID for 7 to 14 days (*not* approved for this use in the United States); *or* ivermectin (Ivomec) at 50 μg/kg orally once (*not* approved for this use in the United States) for microfilarial *D. immitis*.[38] The nodular form of cutaneous dirofilariasis heals within 5 to 8 weeks after the completion of microfilaricidal therapy. Prevention is accomplished with the use of diethylcarbamazine (Caricide) at 6.5 mg/kg orally SID or ivermectin (Heart Guard) at 6 μg/kg orally once a month.[38]

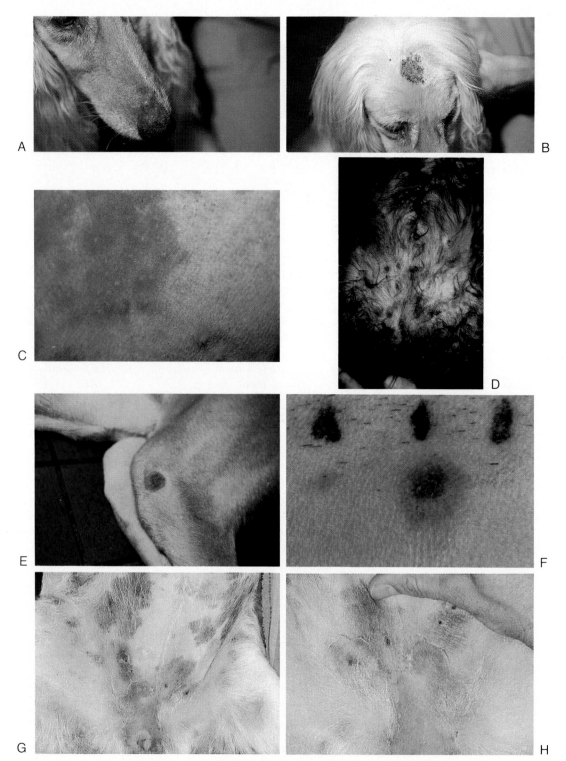

Figure 9:34 *See legend on the opposite page*

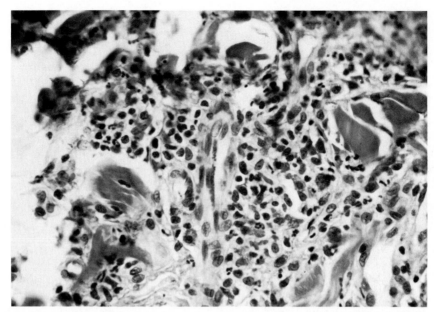

Figure 9:35. Canine dirofilariasis. Perivascular pyogranuloma with microfilarial segment within blood vessel.

BACTERIAL HYPERSENSITIVITY
(Staphylococcal Hypersensitivity)

Bacterial hypersensitivity is a rare, severely pruritic, pustular dermatitis in dogs, associated with a presumed hypersensitivity reaction to staphylococcal antigen.

CAUSE AND PATHOGENESIS

In humans, bacterial antigens are thought to elicit types I, II, III, and IV hypersensitivity reactions in the skin.[62, 139] The pathomechanism of bacterial hypersensitivity in dogs is unclear, although evidence supporting the existence of a type III, and perhaps a type I, hypersensitivity reaction has been reported.[91a, 157, 186]

Figure 9:34. *A*, Erythematous papules on bridge of nose of a dog with cutaneous dirofilariasis. *B*, Ulcerated, crusted nodule on head of a dog with cutaneous dirofilariasis. *C*, Multiple erythematous pustules on the abdomen of a dog with bacterial hypersensitivity. (From Scott, D. W., MacDonald, J. M., and Schultz, R. D.: Staphylococcal hypersensitivity in the dog. J.A.A.H.A. *14:*766, 1978.) *D*, Multiple hemorrhagic bullae on the abdomen of a dog with bacterial hypersensitivity. *E*, Annular erythematous plaque with central hyperpigmentation on the stifle of a dog with bacterial hypersensitivity. (From Scott, D. W., MacDonald, J. M., and Schultz, R. D.: Staphylococcal hypersensitivity in the dog. J.A.A.H.A. *14:*766, 1978.) *F*, Hemorrhagic bulla skin test reaction 48 hours after the intradermal injection of *Staphylococcus aureus* bacterin-toxoid (Staphoid A–B) in a dog with bacterial hypersensitivity. (From Scott, D. W., MacDonald, J. M., and Schultz, R. D.: Staphylococcal hypersensitivity in the dog. J.A.A.H.A. *14:*766, 1978.) *G*, Canine sterile eosinophilic pustulosis. Pustules and annular erosions on abdomen. *H*, Close up of dog in *G*. Annular erosion with epidermal collarettes.

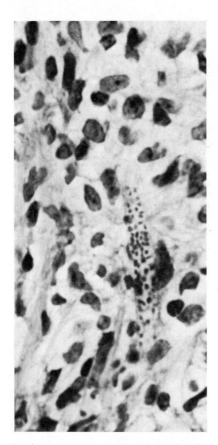

Figure 9:36. Canine cutaneous dirofilariasis. Extravascular microfilaria within granuloma.

CLINICAL FEATURES

Clinical signs associated with canine bacterial hypersensitivity include intense pruritus in conjunction with a superficial or deep pustular and/or seborrheic dermatitis. Erythematous pustules and hemorrhagic bullae are seen with bacterial hypersensitivity (Fig. 9:34C,D). "Target" or "bull's-eye" lesions (annular or arciform areas of central erythema and/or hyperpigmentation, alopecia, and scaling) that spread peripherally and often coalesce are very common but nondiagnostic (Fig. 9:34E). Helpful historical clues may include prior pyogenic infection, poor or incomplete response to systemic glucocorticoids, and rapid response to appropriate systemic antibiotics. Relapse after cessation of short-term antibiotic therapy is common.

Approximately 50 to 80 per cent of the dogs have concurrent diseases that appear to predispose them to, or intensify, the bacterial hypersensitivity.[157, 186] Examples of such diseases include seborrheic skin disease, hypothyroidism, other hypersensitivities (atopy, food hypersensitivity, flea bite hypersensitivity), and foci of chronic infection (anal sacculitis, gingivitis, tonsillitis, otitis externa).

DIAGNOSIS

The differential diagnosis includes ruling out bacterial folliculitis, demodicosis, dermatophytosis, seborrheic skin disease, subcorneal pustular dermatosis, sterile eosinophilic pustulosis, pemphigus foliaceus, systemic lupus erythematosus, atopy, food hypersensitivity, scabies, and flea bite hypersensitivity.

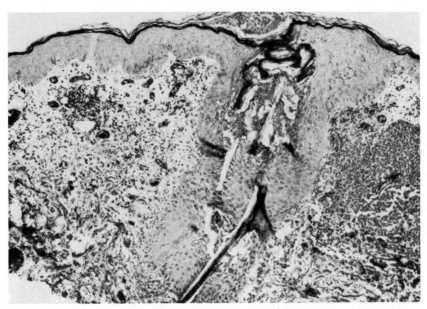

Figure 9:37. Bacterial hypersensitivity in a dog. Folliculitis with marked vascular dilatation and extravasation of erythrocytes. (From Scott, D. V., MacDonald, J. M., and Schultz, R. D.: Staphylococcal hypersensitivity in the dog. J.A.A.H.A. *14:*766, 1978.)

Definitive diagnosis is based on history, physical examination, bacterial culture, skin biopsy, and intradermal skin testing. All reported cases of canine bacterial hypersensitivity have had pure cultures of either coagulase-positive *Staphylococcus* sp. (most cases) or coagulase-negative *Staphylococcus* sp. (rare cases).

Histopathology. Skin biopsy reveals varying degrees of vasculitis and intraepidermal pustular dermatitis or folliculitis-furunculosis (Figs. 9:37, 9:38,

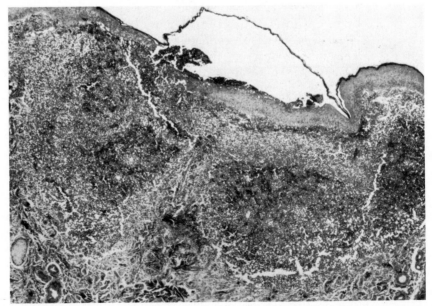

Figure 9:38. Bacterial hypersensitivity in a dog. Subepidermal hemorrhagic bulla. (From Scott, D. W., MacDonald, J. M., and Schultz, R. D.: Staphylococcal hypersensitivity in the dog. J.A.A.H.A. *14:*766, 1978.)

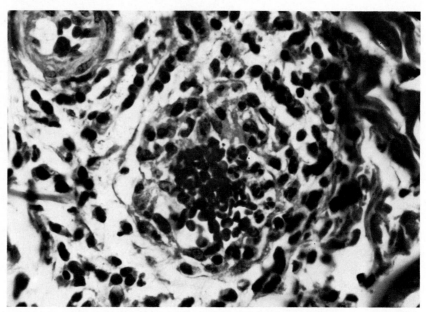

Figure 9:39. Canine bacterial hypersensitivity. Mixed-cell (neutrophils, mononuclear cells) vasculitis with endothelial swelling and degeneration or vacuolization of vessel wall. (From Scott, D. W., MacDonald, J. M., and Schultz, R. D.: Staphylococcal hypersensitivity in the dog. J.A.A.H.A. *14*:766, 1978.)

and 9:39).[46, 186] The vasculitis is usually mixed (neutrophils and mononuclear cells), and significant leukocytoclasis and fibrinoid degeneration are uncommon.

Intradermal Skin Testing. Intradermal skin testing with a staphylococcal cell wall–toxoid product (Staphoid A–B) has been useful for diagnosing canine bacterial hypersensitivity.[157, 186] The product is diluted with an equal volume of sterile saline, and 0.1 ml of the mixture is injected intradermally. Virtually all dogs, normal or dermatitic from *any* cause, will develop an immediate wheal and flare reaction that persists for 12 to 18 hours and appears to be irritant in nature. However, at 24 to 72 hours after injection, dogs with bacterial hypersensitivity develop erythematous, indurated, oozing, pruritic reactions that may turn red-purple, necrose, and ulcerate (Arthus reaction) (Fig. 9:34F). Diagnostic skin testing with bacterial antigens presents problems resulting from a lack of uniformity of staphylococcal antigens, the complex antigenic structure of staphylococci and their metabolites, and various nonimmunologic cutaneous reactions.[139]

CLINICAL MANAGEMENT

Treatment of canine bacterial hypersensitivity may vary, depending on the existence of concurrent diseases and the age of the dog. In those cases in which an underlying disease can be detected and successfully managed, a 3- to 8-week course of appropriate systemic antibiotics is often curative. In cases in which no underlying disease can be detected but the dog is less than 1 year of age, the above course of antibiotic therapy may still be curative.

However, when no underlying disease can be detected and the dog is over 1 year of age, the idiopathic bacterial hypersensitivity will probably have to be managed for life with repeated antibiotic or biologic therapy. Biologic therapy is preferred, as repeated antibiotic therapy usually leads to increasing bacterial

Table 9:28. SCHEDULE FOR THE BIOLOGIC THERAPY OF CANINE BACTERIAL HYPERSENSITIVITY, USING STAPHOID A–B 50:50 WITH SALINE*

Day	Intradermal Dose in ml	Subcutaneous Dose in ml
1	0.10	0.15
2	0.10	0.40
3	0.10	0.65
4	0.10	0.90
5	0.10	1.15
12	0.10	1.40
19	0.10	1.65
26	0.10	1.90

*See also Table 4:45, page 185.

drug resistance, increasing drug expense, and euthanasia. Biologic therapy with Staphoid A–B has been reported to be successful in up to 67 to 88 per cent of the mature dogs with idiopathic bacterial hypersensitivity.[157, 186] The product is diluted with an equal volume of sterile saline and injected intradermally and subcutaneously, as indicated in Table 9:28. Initially, the cutaneous reaction to the intradermal portion of the therapy is pronounced and resembles that seen with diagnostic testing. This intradermal reaction abates as the dog responds. Uncommonly, dogs develop severe reactions to the subcutaneous portion of the therapy—localized angioedema to generalized pruritus with or without urticaria—for a few hours or up to 1 to 2 days. At this point, the subcutaneous portion of the therapy is permanently discontinued. If the dog responds well to biologic therapy, booster injections are administered as needed, usually every 1 to 3 months. Other bacterial vaccines that may be tried include Staphage Lysate and Lysigin (see p. 186). When biologic therapy is unsuccessful, the therapy of choice for recurrent bacterial hypersensitivity is chronic, once-a-day antibiotic administration (see p. 268).

FUNGAL HYPERSENSITIVITY

Cutaneous hypersensitivity reactions to fungi are thought to be important in humans, but the importance of such reactions in dogs and cats is unknown.[62, 139] Hypersensitivity to *Candida albicans* infections has been suspected in some cases of paronychia and gingivitis in dogs and cats, in which the tissue response was out of proportion to the degree of infection found. Fungal kerions are thought to represent hypersensitivity reactions to dermatophytes. Hypersensitivity reactions have been suspected in the pruritic widespread papulocrustous eruptions in cats associated with *Microsporum canis* infections.

Autoimmune Disorders

The major level of control of the autoreactive clones of lymphocytes is suppression by suppressor T cells that are specific for those clones.[76, 183, 227] The development of autoimmune diseases is a reflection of a lack of control or a bypass of the normal control mechanisms. The possible defects that cause deregulation of the controlled autoreactive clones include (1) polyclonal B cell activation, (2) suppressor T-cell bypass, (3) suppressor T-cell dysfunction, (4) increased helper T-cell function, (5) autoantigen modification, (6) cross-reacting antigens, (7) inappropriate interleukin 2 production, and (8) idiotype–anti-idiotype imbalance.[1, 76, 115, 183, 227] In addition, there is sexual dimorphism in the immune response, with female sex hormones tending to accelerate immune responses and male sex hormones tending to suppress responses.[8, 81]

Autoimmune diseases represent robust and inappropriate immune reactions arising out of a background of immunodefectiveness and immune dysregulation. For years, the only approach to therapy has been generalized and nonspecific immunosuppression with powerful and toxic drugs. This is an infant field attempting to use more specific immunomodulation as a new treatment to restore immune balance and to turn off autoreactivity.[183, 223] The therapeutic modalities under investigation include (1) specific deletion or suppression of autoreactive lymphocytes (monoclonal antibodies; monoclonal anti-idiotype antibodies; attenuation with T cell lines), (2) general biologic approaches (sex hormone modulation; dietary manipulation; total lymphoid irradiation), and (3) new pharmacologic approaches (thymic hormones, immunomodulating drugs [levamisole, imuthiol, isoprinosine], cyclosporine). It is unknown whether these immunopharmacologic approaches will ultimately be successful.

PEMPHIGUS

The pemphigus complex is a group of uncommon autoimmune diseases described in humans, dogs, and cats. They are vesiculobullous-to-pustular, erosive-to-ulcerative disorders of the skin that may also affect the mucous membranes.

CAUSE AND PATHOGENESIS

Pemphigus is characterized histologically by intraepidermal acantholysis, and immunologically by the presence of an autoantibody ("pemphigus antibody") to the glycocalyx of keratinocytes. Pemphigus antigens are heterogeneous (12 to 160 kD), present in all mammalian and avian skin, and associated with desmosomal and nondesmosomal cell membrane areas.[49, 75, 112, 216] Recent work has suggested that the pemphigus vulgaris and pemphigus foliaceus antigens are different molecules.[112, 154, 216] Pemphigus vulgaris and pemphigus foliaceus antibodies from human patients reproduce their respective clinical, histopathologic, and immunopathologic syndromes, when injected into neonatal mice.[56, 164] The proposed pathomechanism of blister formation in pemphigus includes (1) the binding of pemphigus antibody at the glycocalyx of keratinocytes, (2) internalization of the pemphigus antibody and fusion of the antibody with intracellular lysomes, and (3) resultant activation and release of a keratinocyte proteolytic enzyme ("pemphigus acantholytic factor"), which diffuses into the extracellular space and hydrolyzes the glycocalyx. The resultant loss of intercellular cohesion leads to acantholysis and blister formation within the epidermis (Fig. 9:40). The pemphigus antibody–induced acantholysis is *not* dependent on complement or inflammatory cells. Pemphigus, thus, represents a type II hypersensitivity reaction.

Other factors thought to be involved in the pathogenesis of some cases of pemphigus include drug provocation (especially penicillamine and phenylbutazone), ultraviolet light, and emotional upset.[7, 62, 139, 191, 232]

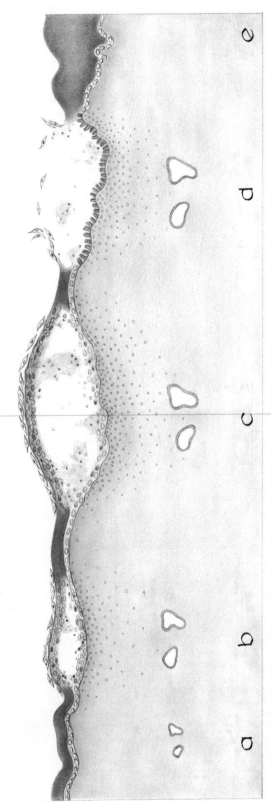

Figure 9:40. Pemphigus vulgaris dermogram. *A*, Normal skin. *B*, Small suprabasilar cleft causing a small vesicle. An inflammatory infiltrate is beginning to form under the affected basal layer. *C*, Larger suprabasilar cleft is causing a large vesicle. The epidermis below the suprabasilar cleft is becoming acanthotic, and the inflammatory infiltrate is increasing. The suprabasilar cleft contains fluid and a slight amount of cellular debris. *D*, The vesicle has ruptured, leaving an ulcerated epidermis with exposure of the basal layer that contains characteristic "tombstone" cells. Remnants of the eroded epidermis form a keratin rim. *E*, After healing with systemic corticosteroids, the epidermis is acanthotic for a short period of time.

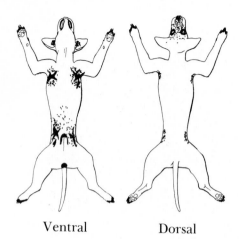

Ventral   Dorsal

Figure 9:41. Canine pemphigus distribution pattern.

Pemphigus is uncommon in dogs and cats. It accounts for about 0.3 per cent of all canine and feline skin disorders seen at the New York State College of Veterinary Medicine.

CLINICAL FEATURES

Pemphigus Vulgaris. Pemphigus vulgaris has been reported in dogs and cats and is the second most common type.[79b, 191, 206, 221] No age, breed, or sex predilections have been reported. Pemphigus vulgaris is a vesiculobullous erosive-to-ulcerative disorder that may affect the oral cavity, mucocutaneous junctions (lips, nostrils, eyelids, prepuce, vulva, anus), skin, or any combination thereof (Fig. 9:41). About 90 per cent of the animals have oral cavity lesions at the time of diagnosis, and oral cavity involvement is the initial sign in about 50 per cent. Cutaneous lesions occur most commonly in the axillae and groin. Dogs with this distribution of lesions may previously have been misdiagnosed as having "hidradenitis suppurativia." Onychomadesis may be seen. Pemphigus vulgaris limited to the skin is rare. (Fig. 9:42A, B).

> *Ninety per cent of dogs and cats with pemphigus vulgaris have oral lesions.*

Figure 9:42. Pemphigus complex. *A,* Ulceration of the lips, chin, and nasal philtrum of a cat with pemphigus vulgaris. (From Manning, T. O., Scott, D. W., Smith, C. A., and Lewis, R. M.: Pemphigus diseases in the feline: seven case reports and discussion. J.A.A.H.A. *18*:432, 1982.) *B,* Ulceration of the hard and soft palate of a cat with pemphigus vulgaris. (From Manning, T. O., Scott, D. W., Smith, C. A., and Lewis, R. M.: Pemphigus diseases in the feline: seven case reports and discussion. J.A.A.H.A. In press.) *C,* Multiple crusted, erythematous plaques over the dorsum of a dog with pemphigus vegetans. (From Scott, D. W.: Pemphigus vegetans in a dog. Cornell Vet. *67*:374, 1977.) *D,* Multiple crusted, erythematous plaques over the dorsum and side of a dog with pemphigus vegetans. (From Scott, D. W.: Pemphigus vegetans in a dog. Cornell Vet. *67*:374, 1977.) *E,* Multifocal areas of alopecia, crusting, and hyperpigmentation in a dog with pemphigus foliaceus. (From Manning, T. O., Scott, D. W., Kruth, S. A., Sozanski, M., and Lewis, R. M.: Three cases of canine pemphigus foliaceus, and observations on chrysotherapy. J.A.A.H.A. *16*:189, 1980.) *F,* Alopecia, crusting, and scaling on the side of a dog with pemphigus foliaceus. *G,* Facial scaling, crusting, and alopecia in a dog with pemphigus foliaceus. *H,* Feline pemphigus foliaceus. Erythema, erosion, crusting, and alopecia of pinna.

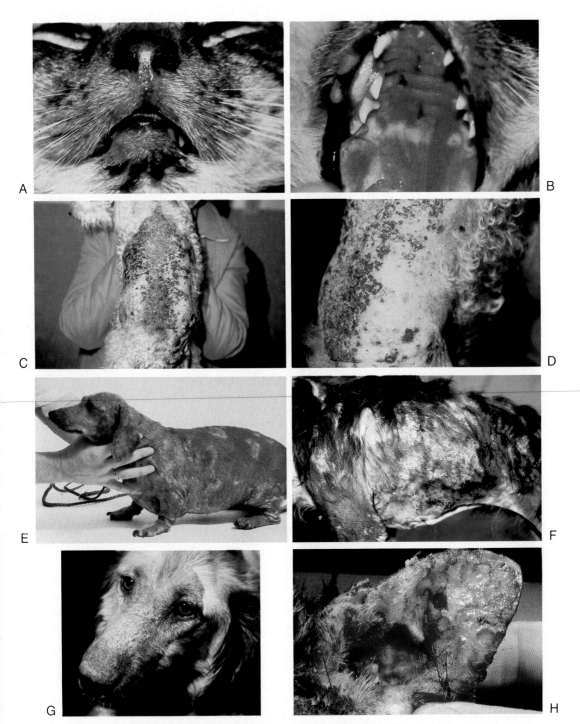

Figure 9:42 *See legend on the opposite page*

Due to the thinness of canine and feline epidermis, vesicles and bullae are fragile and transient. Thus, clinical lesions usually include erosions and ulcers bordered by epidermal collarettes, and the Nikolsky sign may be present (Fig. 9:43). Pruritus and pain are variable, and secondary pyoderma and lymphadenopathy may be present. Severely affected animals may be anorectic, depressed, or febrile.

Results of routine laboratory determinations (hemogram, serum chemistries, urinalysis, serum protein electrophoresis) are nondiagnostic, often revealing mild-to-moderate leukocytosis and neutrophilia, mild nonregenerative anemia, mild hypoalbuminemia, and mild-to-moderate elevations of $alpha_2$, beta, and gamma globulins.

Pemphigus Vegetans. Pemphigus vegetans has been reported in the dog, but is extremely rare.[79b, 206] No age, breed, or sex predilections are apparent. Pemphigus vegetans is a vesiculopustular disorder that evolves into verrucous vegetations and papillomatous proliferations, which ooze and are studded with pustules (Fig. 9:42C, D). The Nikolsky sign may be present. Pruritus and pain are variable, and the dogs are usually otherwise healthy. Pemphigus vegetans is thought to represent a more benign or abortive form of pemphigus vulgaris in an animal that has more "resistance" to the disease.

Pemphigus Foliaceus. Pemphigus foliaceus has been reported in dogs and cats and is the most common type.[34, 79b, 99, 191, 206, 221] No age or sex predilections have been reported. In dogs, Akitas, chow chows, dachshunds, bearded collies, Newfoundlands, Doberman pinschers, and Schipperkes may be predisposed.[99, 206] Pemphigus foliaceus is characterized by vesiculobullous or pustular dermatitis. Mucocutaneous orientation is uncommon, and oral cavity involvement is rare. The primary lesions are transient, so presenting lesions usually consist of erythema, oozing, crusts, scales, alopecia, and erosions bordered by epidermal collarettes (Fig. 9:42E to H). The Nikolsky sign may be present. Pemphigus foliaceus usually begins on the face and ears; it commonly involves the feet, footpads (villous hyperkeratosis or "hard pad"), and groin and becomes multifocal or generalized within 6 months in many animals (Fig. 9:44A, B). Some dogs and cats with pemphigus foliaceus present with only footpad lesions and may be lame.[15, 100, 206] Paronychia and involvement of the nipples are commonly seen in cats. Nasal depigmentation may result in photodermatitis (see pemphigus erythematosus). Pruritus and pain are variable, and secondary pyoderma and peripheral lymphadenopathy may be present. Severely affected animals may be anorectic, depressed, or febrile.

Pemphigus foliaceus seldom has oral or mucocutaneous lesions but often has footpad hyperkeratosis.

Figure 9:43. Canine pemphigus vulgaris. *A,* Large eroded, ulcerated patches in the axillary and inguinal areas. *B,* Preputial ulcers in a dog with pemphigus. (Courtesy, E. Feldman.) *C,* Canine pemphigus vulgaris. Ulceration of oral mucosa and lips. *D,* Canine pemphigus vulgaris. Annular ulcers with collarettes near anus. *E,* Canine pemphigus vulgaris. Ulceration of vulva. *F,* Highly erythematous, ulcerated plaque typical of the cutaneous lesions of untreated canine pemphigus vulgaris. *G,* Canine pemphigus vulgaris. Axillary ulceration. *H,* Intercellular fluorescence of the intercellular space substance using indirect immunofluorescent staining technique. (Courtesy, A. V. Cox and B. V. Russell.)

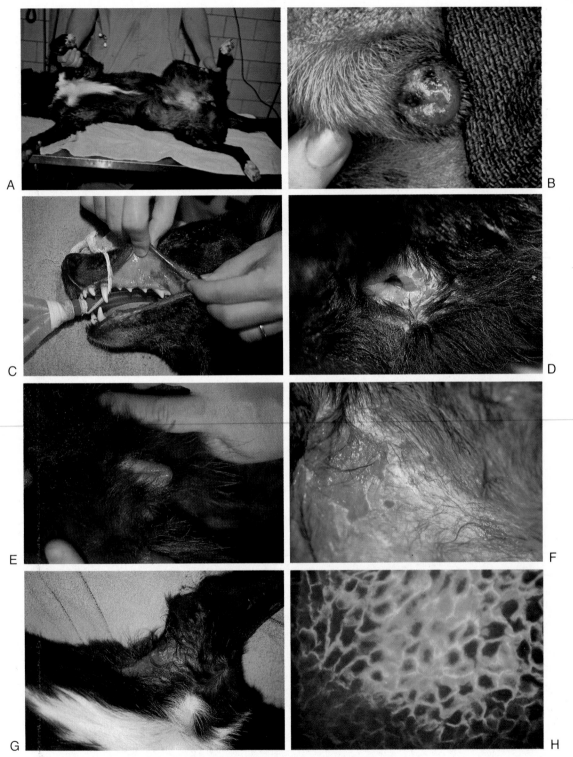

Figure 9:43. *See legend on opposite page*

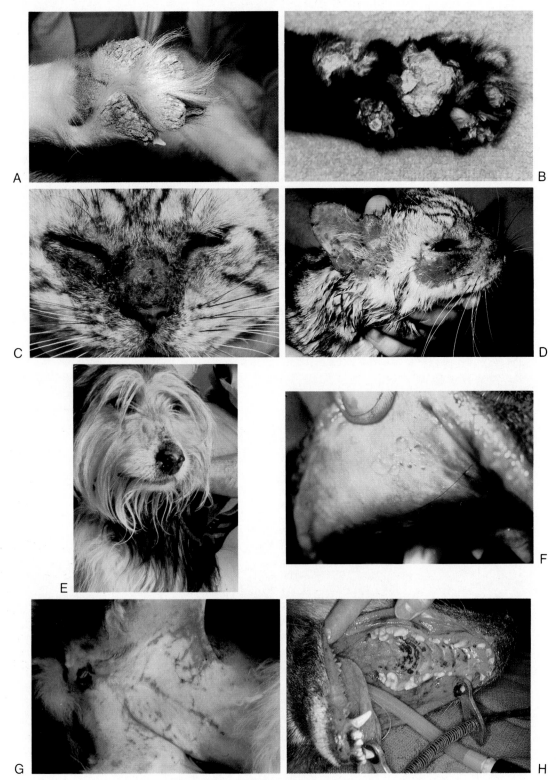

Figure 9:44 *See legend on the opposite page*

Results of routine laboratory examinations (hemogram, serum chemistries, urinalysis, serum protein electrophoresis) are nondiagnostic, often revealing mild-to-moderate leukocytosis and neutrophilia, mild-to-moderate nonregenerative anemia, mild hypoalbuminemia, and mild-to-moderate elevations of alpha$_2$, beta, and gamma globulins. Eosinophilia is occasionally found.

Pemphigus Erythematosus. Pemphigus erythematosus has been reported in dogs and cats.[21, 192, 206] No age or sex predilections are known. In dogs, collies and German shepherds may be predisposed.[206] Pemphigus erythematosus is characterized by a vesiculobullous or pustular dermatitis of the face and ears. As the primary lesions are transient, dogs and cats have erythema, oozing crusts, scales, alopecia, and erosions bordered by epidermal collarettes (Fig. 9:44C,D). The Nikolsky sign may be present. Pruritus and pain are variable. The nose frequently becomes depigmented, whereupon photodermatitis becomes an aggravating factor (Fig. 9:44E). If the nasal region is primarily involved, the condition is often worse in sunny weather and the dog may be misdiagnosed as having "nasal solar dermatitis (collie nose)". Oral cavity involvement has not been reported, and affected animals are usually otherwise healthy. Occasional animals have isolated skin lesions distant from the face and ears, such as on the paws. Pemphigus erythematosus is thought to represent a more benign form of pemphigus foliaceus. Some workers have also suggested it may represent a crossover syndrome between pemphigus and lupus erythematosus.

DIAGNOSIS

Nasal depigmentation can be a diagnostic dilemma.

The differential diagnosis of *pemphigus vulgaris* includes bullous pemphigoid, systemic lupus erythematosus, erythema multiforme, toxic epidermal necrolysis, drug eruption, mycosis fungoides, lymphoreticular neoplasia, candidiasis, and the numerous causes of canine and feline ulcerative stomatitis. The differential diagnosis of *pemphigus vegetans* includes bacterial and fungal granulomas, and cutaneous neoplasia (especially lymphoreticular neoplasia, mastocytoma, and papilloma or fibropapilloma). The differential diagnosis of *pemphigus foliaceus* and *pemphigus erythematosus* includes bacterial folliculitis, dermatophytosis, demodicosis, dermatophilosis, seborrheic skin disease, lupus erythematosus, subcorneal pustular dermatosis, sterile eosinophilic pustulosis,

---

Figure 9:44. Pemphigus complex and bullous pemphigoid. *A*, Hyperkeratosis of the footpads in a dog with pemphigus foliaceus. *B*, Hyperkeratosis of the footpads in a cat with pemphigus foliaceus. *C*, Facial alopecia and crusting in a cat with pemphigus erythematosus. (From Scott, D. W., Miller, W. H., Lewis, R. M., Manning, T. O., and Smith, C. A.: Pemphigus erythematosus in the dog and cat. J.A.A.H.A. *16*:815, 1980.) *D*, Erythema, alopecia, erosion, and crusting of the face and ear of a cat with pemphigus erythematosus. (From Scott, D. W., Miller, W. H., Lewis, R. M., Manning, T. O., and Smith, C. A.: Pemphigus erythematosus in the dog and cat. J.A.A.H.A. *16*:815, 1980.) *E*, Nasal erythema, ulceration, crusting, and depigmentation in a dog with pemphigus erythematosus. *F*, Bullae on the labial mucosa of a dog with bullous pemphigoid. (From Scott, D. W., and Lewis, R. M.: Pemphigus and pemphigoid in dog and man: comparative aspects. Am. Acad. Dermatol. 5:148, 1981.) *G*, Ulceration in the groin of a dog with bullous pemphigoid. *H*, Canine bullous pemphigoid. Severe oral ulceration.

linear IgA dermatosis, zinc-responsive dermatitis, dermatomyositis, and lymphoreticular neoplasia.

The definitive diagnosis of pemphigus is based on history, physical examination, direct smears, skin (or mucosal) biopsy, and immunofluorescence testing. Microscopic examination of direct smears from intact vesicles or pustules or from recent erosions often reveals numerous neutrophils (nondegenerate), occasionally numerous eosinophils, few-to-no bacteria (especially intracellularly), and numerous acantholytic keratinocytes (see Fig. 9:53).[191, 206] Occasional acantholytic keratinocytes may be seen in any suppurative condition, but when present in clusters or large numbers in several microscopic fields they are strongly indicative of pemphigus.

Histopathology. Skin biopsy may be diagnostic or strongly supportive in pemphigus.[191, 206] Intact vesicles, bullae, or pustules are essential. Because these lesions are so fragile and transient, it may be necessary to hospitalize the animal so that it can be carefully scrutinized every 2 to 4 hours for the presence of primary lesions. When a bullous lesion is observed, it must be biopsied immediately. Multiple biopsies and serial sections will greatly increase the chances of demonstrating diagnostic histologic changes. In addition, because canine and feline blisters usually fill rapidly with leukocytes, they are usually grossly and microscopically pustular, thus confusing clinician and pathologist alike.

Pemphigus vulgaris is characterized by suprabasilar acantholysis with resultant cleft and vesicle formation (Fig. 9:45). Basal epidermal cells remain attached to the basement membrane zone like a row of "tombstones" (Fig. 9:46). *Pemphigus vegetans* is characterized by epidermal hyperplasia, papillomatosis, and intraepidermal microabscesses that contain predominantly eosinophils and acantholytic keratinocytes (Figs. 9:47 to 9:49). *Pemphigus foliaceus and pemphigus erythematosus* are characterized by intragranular or subcorneal acantholysis with resultant cleft and vesicle or pustule formation (Figs. 9:50 to 9:54). Within the vesicle or pustule, cells from the stratum granulosum may be seen attached to the overlying stratum corneum (granular cell "cling-ons") (Fig. 9:55). Either neutrophils or eosinophils may predominate within the vesicle or pustule.

Other helpful histopathologic findings that may be seen in canine and feline pemphigus include (1) a lichenoid cellular infiltrate (mononuclear cells, plasma cells, neutrophils), (2) eosinophilic exocytosis and microabscess formation within the epidermis or follicular outer root sheath or both (pemphigus foliaceus, erythematosus, and vegetans) (Fig. 9:48), (3) involvement of the follicular outer root sheath in the suprabasilar, intraepidermal, intragranular, or subcorneal acantholytic process, and (4) acantholytic, dyskeratotic granular epidermal cells ("grains") at the surface of erosions (pemphigus foliaceus and erythematosus) (Fig. 9:54).

Electron microscopic examination of canine and human pemphigus lesions has suggested that dissolution of the intercellular cement substance is the initial pathologic change, followed by the retraction of tonofilaments, disappearance of desmosomes, and acantholysis.[7, 191]

Direct immunofluorescence testing (see p. 441) reveals the diffuse intercellular deposition of immunoglobulin (usually IgG), and occasionally complement, within the epidermis or mucosa in 50 to 90 per cent of the patients.[7, 99, 206, 240] The variability in positive results reflects differences in laboratory techniques, lesion selection, previous or current glucocorticoid therapy, and possibly other

Text continued on page 512

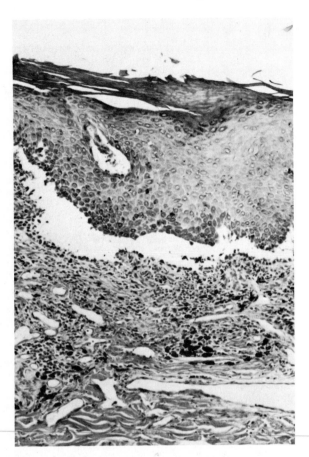

Figure 9:45. Canine pemphigus vulgaris. Suprabasilar acantholysis and cleft formation. (From Scott, D. W., Manning, T. O., Smith, C. A., and Lewis, R. M.: Pemphigus vulgaris without mucosal or mucocutaneous involvement in two dogs. J.A.A.H.A. *18*:401, 1982.)

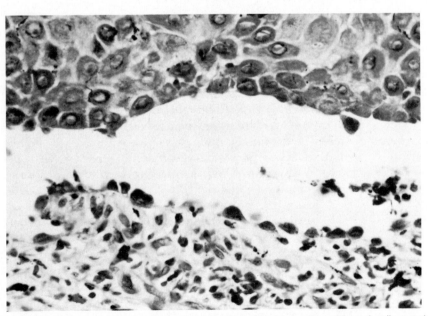

Figure 9:46. Canine pemphigus vulgaris. Suprabasilar cleft with basilar epidermal cells remaining attached to the dermis like a row of "tombstones." (From Scott, D. W., Manning, T. O., Smith, C. A., and Lewis, R. M.: Pemphigus vulgaris without mucosal or mucocutaneous involvement in two dogs. J.A.A.H.A. *18*:401, 1982.)

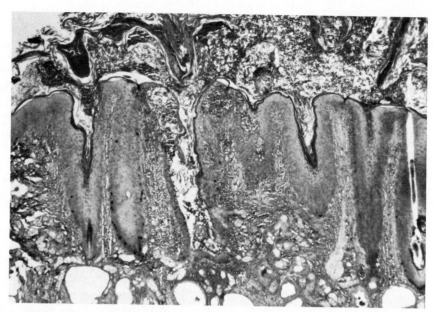

Figure 9:47. Canine pemphigus vegetans. Papillated epidermal hyperplasia, hyperkeratosis, papillomatosis, and several intraepidermal microabscesses. (From Scott, D. W.: Pemphigus vegetans in a dog. Cornell Vet. *67*:374, 1977.)

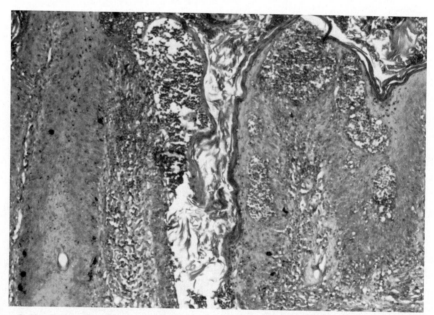

Figure 9:48. Canine pemphigus vegetans. Seven intraepidermal eosinophilic microabscesses. (From Scott, D. W., and Lewis, R. M.: Pemphigus and pemphigoid in dog and man: comparative aspects. J. Am. Acad. Dermatol. *5*:148, 1981.)

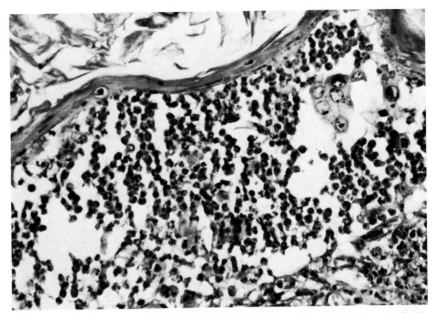

Figure 9:49. Canine pemphigus vegetans. Intraepidermal microabscess containing predominantly eosinophils and a few acantholytic keratinocytes. (From Scott, D. W.: Pemphigus vegetans in a dog. Cornell Vet. *67*:374, 1977.)

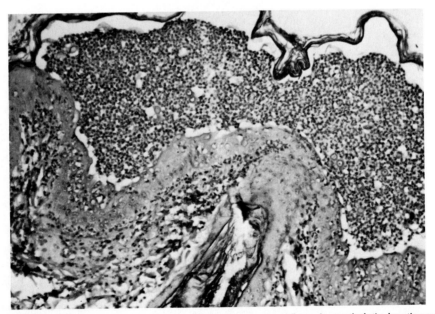

Figure 9:50. Canine pemphigus foliaceus. Numerous neutrophils and acantholytic keratinocytes within a subcorneal pustule. (From Scott, D. W., and Lewis, R. M.: Pemphigus and pemphigoid in dog and man: comparative aspects. J. Am. Acad. Dermatol. *5*:148, 1981.)

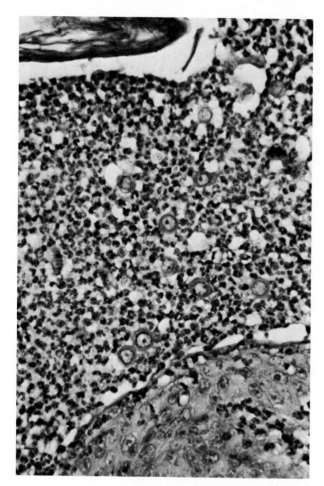

Figure 9:51. Canine pemphigus foliaceus. Numerous acanthocytes within subcorneal pustule.

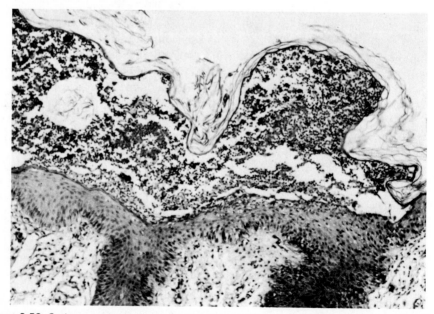

Figure 9:52. Canine pemphigus erythematosus. Subcorneal pustule containing numerous neutrophils and acantholytic keratinocytes. (From Scott, D. W., Miller, W. H., Lewis, R. M., Manning, T. O., and Smith, C. A.: Pemphigus erythematosus in the dog and cat. J.A.A.H.A. *16*:815, 1980.)

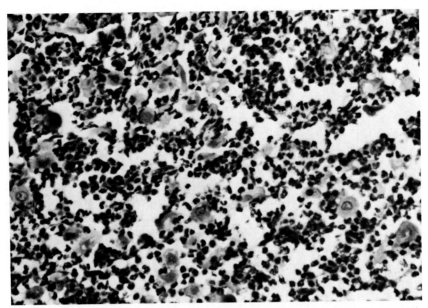

Figure 9:53. Canine pemphigus erythematosus. Close-up of numerous neutrophils and acantholytic keratinocytes within a subcorneal pustule. (From Scott, D. W., Miller, W. H., Lewis, R. M., Manning, T. O., and Smith, C. A.: Pemphigus erythematosus in the dog and cat. J.A.A.H.A. *16*:815, 1980.)

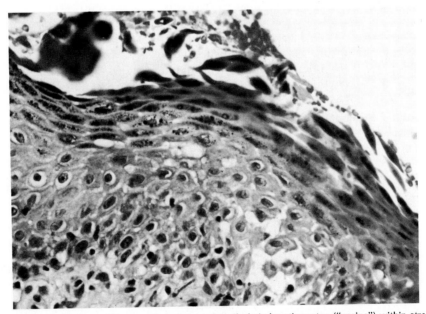

Figure 9:54. Canine pemphigus erythematosus. Acantholytic keratinocytes ("grains") within stratum granulosum at the surface of an erosion. (From Scott, D. W., and Lewis, R. M.: Pemphigus and pemphigoid in dog and man: comparative aspects. J. Am. Acad. Dermatol. 5:148, 1981.)

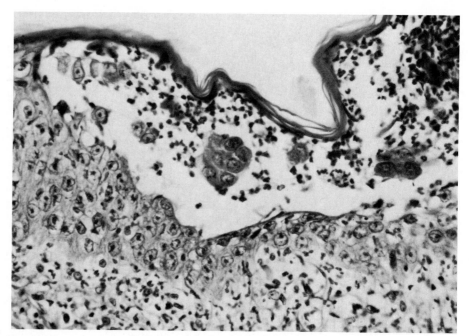

Figure 9:55. Feline pemphigus foliaceus. Subcorneal vesicopustule with acanthocytes and "cling-ons."

factors. In addition, immunoreactants may be found in the intercellular spaces of skin and oral mucosa in other conditions (see p. 445). It is important to sample intact vesicles and pustules and perilesional tissue. *Indirect immunofluorescence testing* (see p. 445) is rarely positive in canine and feline pemphigus. In pemphigus erythematosus, direct immunofluorescence testing often reveals the deposition of immunoglobulin, with or without complement, at the basement membrane zone in addition to the intercellular spaces of the epidermis (see p. 441). These patients usually have positive antinuclear antibody (ANA) results as well, thus prompting some workers to contemplate the existence of a crossover syndrome between pemphigus and lupus erythematosus.

CLINICAL MANAGEMENT

The prognosis for canine pemphigus appears to vary with the form and severity of the disease.[99, 191, 206] The natural course of untreated cases is unclear. Veterinarians have long recognized refractory mucocutaneous erosive or ulcerative disorders and severe exfoliative dermatoses that have resulted in the death or euthanasia of affected dogs and cats. Retrospectively, many of those dogs may have had pemphigus vulgaris or foliaceus. Based on the small numbers of cases documented in the veterinary literature, (1) pemphigus vulgaris appears to be a severe disease that is often fatal unless treated, (2) pemphigus foliaceus is less severe but without therapy may be fatal, and (3) pemphigus erythematosus and vegetans are usually benign disorders that rarely produce systemic signs.

Therapy of canine and feline pemphigus is often difficult, requiring large doses of systemic glucocorticoids, with or without other potent immunomodulating drugs. Side-effects are common, varying from mild to severe, and close physical and hematologic monitoring of the patient is critical. Additionally, therapy must usually be maintained for prolonged periods of time, if not for life. Thus, the therapeutic regimen must be individualized for each patient, and owner education is essential.

Large doses of systemic glucocorticoids (2.2 to 4.4 mg/kg prednisolone or prednisone, given orally SID for dogs, and 4.4 to 6.6 mg/kg given orally SID for cats) are usually listed as the initial treatment of choice for pemphigus.[99, 191, 206] In many instances, however, glucocorticoid therapy is unsuccessful, or intolerable side-effects develop. In general, glucocorticoids are satisfactory in only about 50 per cent of the dogs and cats with pemphigus.[34, 99, 191, 206]

When systemic glucocorticoids are unsatisfactory, the addition or substitution of other immunomodulating drugs may allow significant reduction or termination of glucocorticoid dosage, and superior management.[191, 206] Drugs that may be useful include (1) azathioprine (Imuran) 2.2 mg/kg, orally SID, then every 48 hours (*dogs*), (2) chlorambucil (Leukeran) 0.1 to 0.2 mg/kg, orally SID, then every 48 hours, (3) dapsone 1 mg/kg, orally TID, then as needed (*dogs*), (4) aurothioglucose (Solganol) (see p. 192), (5) cyclosporine 15 to 27 mg/kg/day, orally.[79b, 99, 150, 167, 191, 206, 221] The reader is referred to Chapter 4, Dermatologic Therapy, for discussions of these immunomodulating drugs. Azathioprine should be used very cautiously in cats, as even small doses (1 mg/kg orally every 48 hours) may produce fatal leukopenia and/or thrombocytopenia.[34, 208] Recently glucocorticoid pulse therapy (11 mg/kg methylprednisolone sodium succinate given intravenously during a 1-hour period for 3 consecutive days) was used to induce remissions in cases of canine pemphigus (see p. 202).[245a]

In animals in which significant nasal depigmentation has occurred, and photodermatitis has become an aggravating factor, photoprotection is an important therapeutic adjunct.[191, 206] Avoidance of sunlight between 8:00 AM and 5:00 PM is helpful. The use of sunscreens containing para-aminobenzoic acid with high sun-protective factor values (15 or greater) is mandatory. Sunscreens should be applied 1 to 2 hours before sun exposure is anticipated and reapplied every 3 to 4 hours.

BULLOUS PEMPHIGOID

Bullous pemphigoid is a rare autoimmune vesiculobullous, ulcerative disorder of skin or oral mucosa, or both, that has been reported in dogs and humans.

CAUSE AND PATHOGENESIS

Bullous pemphigoid is characterized histologically by subepidermal vesicle formation and immunologically by the presence of an autoantibody ("pemphigoid antibody") against antigen at the basement membrane zone of skin and mucosa.[6, 49, 111, 204] The bullous pemphigoid antigen (220 to 240 kD) is present in all mammalian and avian skin, and is associated with hemidesmosomes of epidermal basal cells and the upper portion of the underlying lamina lucida. The proposed pathomechanism of blister formation in bullous pemphigoid includes (1) the binding of complement-fixing pemphigoid antibody at the basement membrane zone, (2) complement fixation, and (3) chemoattraction of neutrophils and eosinophils, whose release of proteolytic enzymes may disrupt dermoepidermal cohesion, resulting in dermoepidermal separation and vesicle formation. Human pemphigoid antibodies, when injected into rabbit cornea or guinea pig skin, produce locally the clinical, histologic, and immunopathologic features of bullous pemphigoid.[6]

Other factors thought to be involved in the pathogenesis of some cases of bullous pemphigoid include drug provocation (especially sulfonamides, penicillins, furosemide), and ultraviolet light.[6, 111, 128, 204, 232]

Bullous pemphigoid is rare in dogs, accounting for about 0.1 per cent of all canine skin disorders seen at the New York State College of Veterinary Medicine.

CLINICAL FEATURES

Canine bullous pemphigoid has no reported age or sex predilections. However, collies and, perhaps, Doberman pinschers appear to be breeds that are predisposed to the development of bullous pemphigoid.[9, 47, 79b, 204, 244] Bullous pemphigoid is a vesiculobullous, ulcerative disorder that may affect the oral cavity, mucocutaneous junctions, skin, or any combination thereof (see Figs. 9:44F to H). About 80 per cent of the dogs have oral cavity lesions at the time of diagnosis. Oral cavity involvement has been recognized either after or at the same time as the cutaneous signs and rarely as the initial event. Cutaneous lesions occur most commonly in the axillae and groin. Dogs with this distribution of lesions may previously have been misdiagnosed as "hidradenitis suppurativa." Paronychia, onychomadesis, or footpad ulceration may be seen. An insidious, chronic, clinically benign form of cutaneous bullous pemphigoid has been recognized in dogs, with lesions confined to the axillae, groin, or isolated mucocutaneous areas such as the anus and prepuce. However, most cases are more severe and widespread, and they are often clinically indistinguishable from pemphigus vulgaris. Clinical variants seen in humans—cicatricial pemphigoid (mucosal and Brunsting-Perry types), vesicular pemphigoid (pemphigoid herpetiformis), pemphigoid vegetans, pemphigoid nodularis, and erythrodermic pemphigoid—have not been recognized in dogs.[6, 204]

Vesicles and bullae are often fragile and transient. Thus, clinical lesions usually include ulcers bordered by epidermal collarettes. The pseudo-Nikolsky sign may be present. Pruritus and pain are variable, and secondary pyoderma is common. Severely affected dogs may be anorectic, depressed, or febrile, and may die, owing to fluid/electrolyte/protein imbalances and septicemia.

Results of routine laboratory determinations (hemogram, serum chemistries, urinalyses, serum protein electrophoresis) are nonspecific, often revealing mild-to-moderate leukocytosis and neutrophilia, mild nonregenerative anemia, mild hypoalbuminemia, and mild-to-moderate elevations of alpha$_2$, beta, and gamma globulins.[204] Peripheral eosinophilia is rare.[206]

DIAGNOSIS

The differential diagnosis includes pemphigus vulgaris, systemic lupus erythematosus, erythema multiforme, toxic epidermal necrolysis, drug eruption, mycosis fungoides, lymphoreticular neoplasia, candidiasis, and the numerous causes of canine ulcerative stomatitis.

Definitive diagnosis of bullous pemphigoid is based on history, physical examination, skin (or mucosal) biopsy, and immunofluorescence testing. Microscopic examination of direct smears from intact vesicles, bullae, or recent ulcers do *not* reveal acantholytic keratinocytes. Skin biopsy may be diagnostic or strongly supportive in bullous pemphigoid. Intact vesicles or bullae are essential, and because of their transient nature it may be necessary to hospitalize the dog so that it can be carefully scrutinized every 2 to 4 hours for the presence of primary lesions. Multiple biopsies and serial sections will greatly increase the chances of demonstrating diagnostic histologic changes.

Bullous pemphigoid is characterized *histologically* by subepidermal cleft and vesicle formation (Fig. 9:56).[204, 206] Acantholysis is *not* seen. Inflammatory infiltrates vary from mild and perivascular to marked and lichenoid (Figs. 9:56 and 9:57). Neutrophils and mononuclear cells usually predominate. Tissue eosinophilia is rare. Subepidermal vacuolar alteration appears to be the earliest prevesicle histopathologic finding (Fig. 9:58).

Electron microscopic examination of pemphigoid lesions has revealed the following: smudging, thickening, and interruption of the basement membrane zone; fragmentation and disappearance of anchoring fibrils, anchoring filaments, and hemidesmosomes; basal cell degeneration; and separation occurring between the basal cell membrane and the basal lamina (lamina lucida).[6, 204]

Direct immunofluorescence testing (see p. 441) reveals a linear deposition of immunoglobulin, and usually complement, at the basement membrane zone of skin or mucosa in 50 to 90 per cent of patients.[6, 204, 206, 240] C3 is the most commonly demonstrated immunoreactant. It would appear to be important to test with all classes of immunoglobulins, as in some dogs results will be positive for only IgM or IgA. It is important to sample intact vesicles and bullae, and perilesional tissue. *Indirect immunofluorescence testing* (see p. 445) is usually negative in canine bullous pemphigoid.

CLINICAL MANAGEMENT

The prognosis for canine bullous pemphigoid appears to vary with the clinical form. The natural course of untreated cases is unclear. Veterinarians

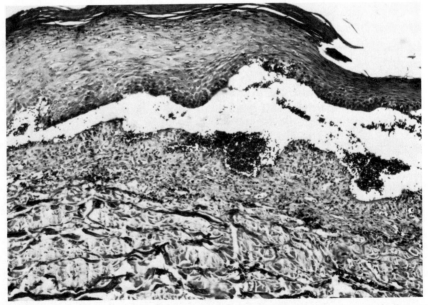

Figure 9:56. Canine bullous pemphigoid. Subepidermal vesicle and lichenoid band of inflammatory cells. (From Scott, D. W., and Lewis, R. M.: Pemphigus and pemphigoid in dog and man: comparative aspects. J. Am. Acad. Dermatol. 5:148, 1981.)

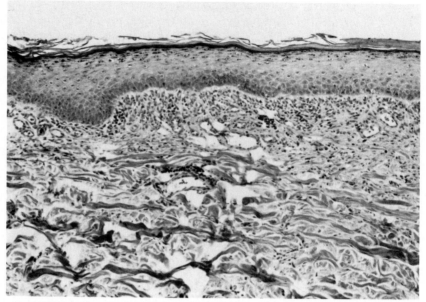

Figure 9:57. Canine bullous pemphigoid. Subepidermal vacuolar alteration and lichenoid band of inflammatory cells.

have long recognized refractory mucocutaneous ulcerative disorders that resulted in the death or euthanasia of affected dogs. Retrospectively, many of these dogs may have had bullous pemphigoid. Based on the small number of cases documented in the veterinary literature, canine bullous pemphigoid is usually a severe disease. Although it is often fatal unless treated, it may occasionally be a relatively benign, localized cutaneous disorder.[204, 206]

Therapy of canine bullous pemphigoid is often difficult, requiring large doses of systemic glucocorticoids, with or without other potent immunomod-

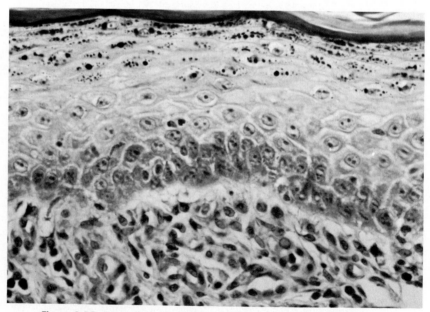

Figure 9:58. Canine bullous pemphigoid. Subepidermal vacuolar alteration.

ulating drugs. Side-effects are common, varying from mild to severe, and close physical and hematologic monitoring of the patient is critical. Additionally, therapy usually must be maintained for prolonged periods of time if not for life. Thus, the therapeutic regimen must be individualized for each patient, and owner education is essential.

> **Treatment with systemic corticosteroids was ineffective in nearly half the cases of bullous pemphigoid.**

Mild cases of canine bullous pemphigoid may be successfully managed with topical glucocorticoids or relatively low doses of systemic glucocorticoids (2.2 mg/kg prednisolone or prednisone, orally, SID), and therapy may occasionally even be terminated.[204] However, most cases require aggressive chemotherapy.[204, 206] In one study of nine dogs with bullous pemphigoid,[204] the following observations were made: (1) 1.0 mg/kg prednisolone, given orally, BID was ineffective for controlling the disease, and (2) 3.0 mg/kg prednisolone, given orally, BID was effective for controlling the disease. However, at the larger dose, two of the nine dogs were euthanized because of unacceptable side-effects, and another two died after 7 to 10 days of therapy (acute pancreatitis). Thus, systemic glucocorticoids were unsatisfactory for treatment in four of nine dogs (44 per cent).

When systemic glucocorticoids are unsatisfactory for treatment, the addition or substitution of other immunomodulating drugs may allow significant reduction or termination of glucocorticoid dosage, and superior patient management.[6, 204] Drugs that may be useful include (1) azathioprine (Imuran) 2.2 mg/kg, orally, SID, then every other day, (2) chlorambucil (Leukeran) 0.1 mg/kg, orally, SID, then every 48 hours, (3) dapsone, 1 mg/kg, given orally, TID, then as needed, (4) 6-mercaptopurine, 2.2 mg/kg, orally, SID, then every other day, or (5) aurothioglucose (chrysotherapy using Solganol). The reader is referred to Chapter 4 for discussions on these immunomodulating drugs.

Recently, both tetracycline and erythromycin have been reported to be beneficial in the treatment of bullous pemphigoid in humans.[226] It is thought that the benefit derived from these drugs is related to their ability to inhibit neutrophil chemotaxis and random migration.

Because (1) cutaneous lesions of bullous pemphigoid in humans can be induced by exposure to ultraviolet light, and (2) canine bullous pemphigoid may worsen with exposure to ultraviolet light, it may be prudent to avoid direct exposure to sunlight between 8:00 AM and 5:00 PM[204, 244]

SYSTEMIC LUPUS ERYTHEMATOSUS

Systemic lupus erythematosus is an uncommon multisystemic autoimmune disorder of dogs, cats, and humans.

CAUSE AND PATHOGENESIS

The etiology of systemic lupus erythematosus appears to be multifactorial, with genetic predilection, immunologic disorder (suppressor T-cell deficiency;

B-cell hyperactivity; deficiencies of complement components), viral infection, and hormonal and ultraviolet light modulation all playing a role.[5, 40, 49] B-cell hyperactivity results in a plethora of autoantibodies formed against numerous body constituents. In humans, a number of drugs (especially procainamide, hydralazine, isoniazid, and several anticonvulsants) are known to precipitate or exacerbate systemic lupus erythematosus.[40, 232] Vaccination with a modified live virus product containing distemper, hepatitis, parainfluenza, and parvovirus antigens was suspected to have precipitated systemic lupus erythematosus in a dog.[3] Tissue damage in systemic lupus erythematosus appears to be due to a type III hypersensitivity reaction. The New Zealand Black and the F_1 hybrid of the New Zealand Black and New Zealand White mouse develop a lupus-like disease that has many similarities to systemic lupus erythematosus in humans.[40, 66, 67]

In the dog, the serologic abnormalities associated with spontaneous canine systemic lupus erythematosus can be transmitted both to normal dogs and to mice by means of cell-free extracts, thus suggesting an infective agent.[139, 213] However, none of these dogs, as yet, has developed overt systemic lupus erythematosus, indicating that other factors are involved in the pathogenesis of the clinical entity. It has been reported that dogs with systemic lupus erythematosus have lower levels of circulating thymic factors than do normal dogs, which is analogous to the situation in humans.[136a, 139]

In a colony of dogs obtained by the mating of a male and female, each having SLE, the F_1 generation had no clinical signs; with subsequent breeding a few dogs in the F_2 generation were affected; and clinical signs were frequent and marked in the F_3 generation.[136a] Affected dogs had depressed suppressor cell activity.

The pathogenesis of skin lesions in systemic lupus erythematosus is unclear. Four characteristics of cutaneous lupus erythematosus are (1) photosensitivity, (2) keratinocyte damage, (3) lymphohistiocytic infiltration, and (4) autoantibody deposition or production.[10, 40, 66, 67] Skin lesions may be induced with ultraviolet light exposure. However, infusion of antinuclear antibodies does not produce skin lesions, and immune complexes appear at the basement membrane zone *after* dermatohistopathologic changes appear. A current hypothesis for the pathogenesis of skin lesions is as follows: (1) ultraviolet light penetrating to the level of epidermal basal cells induces, on the keratinocyte surface, the expression of antigens previously found only in the nucleus or cytoplasm; (2) specific autoantibodies to these antigens that are present in plasma and in tissue fluid bathing the epidermis attach to keratinocytes and induce antibody-dependent cytotoxicity of keratinocytes; and (3) injured keratinocytes release interleukin 2 and other lymphocyte attractants, which account for the resultant lymphohistiocytic infiltrate.[10, 40, 238] Immunopathologic studies of cutaneous and oral mucosal lupus erythematosus lesions in humans have revealed a predominance of helper T cells and macrophages, and a near absence of B cells and Langerhans' cells.[10, 237] In humans, retroviral antigen has been demonstrated at the basement membrane zone of skin lesions, and evidence has been presented suggesting that the immune deposits are complement activating and may be functional and involved in the inflammatory response.[68, 69, 139]

No age or sex predilections are apparent in canine and feline systemic lupus erythematosus.[207] In dogs, the collie, Shetland sheepdog, and German shepherd appear to be predisposed.[107, 207]

CLINICAL FEATURES

The clinical signs associated with systemic lupus erythematosus are varied and changeable. Because of this phenomenal clinical variability and ability to mimic numerous diseases, systemic lupus erythematosus has been called the "great imitator." Polyarthritis, fever, proteinuria, anemia, skin disease, and oral ulcers are the most common abnormalities in dogs.[189, 207, 213] Other syndromes reported in association with canine systemic lupus erythematosus include pericarditis, polymyositis, myocarditis, pneumonitis, peripheral lymphadenopathy, splenomegaly, pleuritis, neurologic disorders (seizures, meningitis, myelitis, psychoses, polyneuropathy), and lymphedema. In the cat, skin lesions, persistent skin infections, fever, peripheral lymphadenopathy, hemolytic anemia, and glomerulonephritis have been reported in association with systemic lupus erythematosus.[207]

The cutaneous manifestations of canine and feline systemic lupus erythematosus are extremely diverse and include seborrheic skin disease, cutaneous or mucocutaneous vesiculobullous disorders, footpad ulcers and hyperkeratosis, discoid lupus erythematosus, refractory secondary pyodermas, panniculitis (lupus profundus), and nasal dermatitis ("collie nose" or "nasal solar dermatitis") (Fig. 9:59A to H). Skin lesions may be multifocal or generalized and commonly involve the face, ears, and distal limbs. They may be exacerbated by exposure to sunlight. Pruritus is variable and scarring is common.

DIAGNOSIS

The differential diagnosis of cutaneous systemic lupus erythematosus is lengthy, owing to the varied and changeable cutaneous manifestations of the disorder. Typical rule-outs include seborrheic skin disease, dermatophytosis, bacterial folliculitis, demodicosis, food hypersensitivity, scabies, pemphigus vulgaris, bullous pemphigoid, discoid lupus erythematosus, erythema multiforme, toxic epidermal necrolysis, mycosis fungoides, candidiasis, and lymphoreticular neoplasia.

The definitive diagnosis of systemic lupus erythematosus is often one of the most challenging tasks in medicine. The disease is so variable in its clinicopathologic presentations that any dogmatic diagnostic categorization is impossible. The clinicopathologic abnormalities that are demonstrated depend on the organ system(s) involved and may include anemia (nonregenerative or hemolytic) with or without a positive direct Coombs' test, thrombocytopenia with or without a positive platelet-factor-3 test, leukopenia or leukocytosis, proteinuria, hypergammaglobulinemia (polyclonal), and sterile synovial exudate obtained by arthrocentesis. The lupus erythematosus (LE) cell test may be positive in up to 60 per cent of the patients, but it is variable from day to day, is steroid labile, and lacks sensitivity and specificity. The assay has been discontinued in many of the leading laboratories in human medicine (Fig. 9:60).[40, 107, 123, 189]

The antinuclear antibody (ANA) test is presently considered the most specific and sensitive serologic test for systemic lupus erythematosus.[40, 107, 189] The ANA test is positive in up to 90 per cent of the cases of active systemic lupus erythematosus. Great caution is warranted in the interpretation of ANA test results. In general, results from different laboratories cannot be compared. It is important to record the titer (and compare it with normals for the *same*

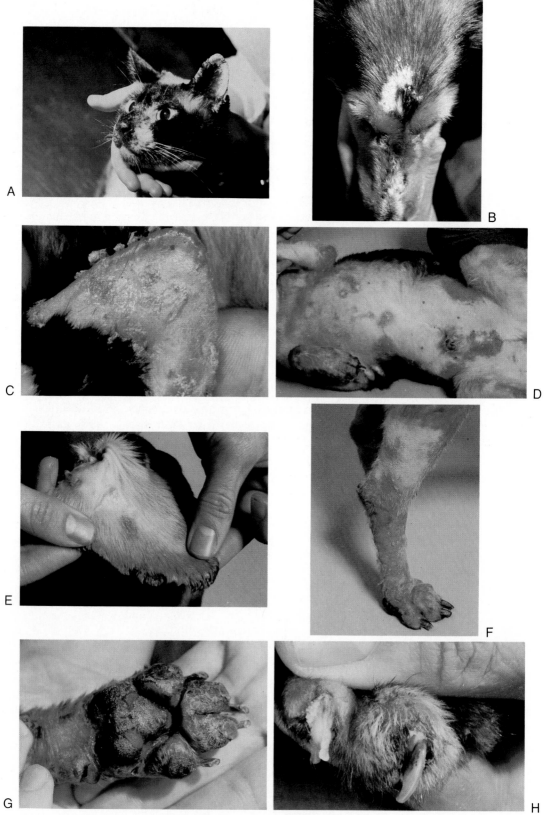

Figure 9:59 *See legend on the opposite page*

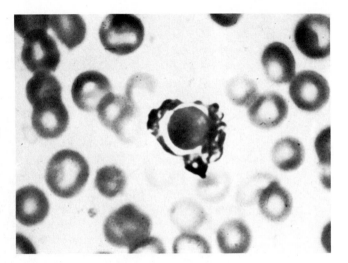

Figure 9:60. L.E. cell test, A neutrophil containing homogeneous nuclear material.

laboratory) and the pattern of nuclear fluorescence (Fig. 9:61). The rim (ring, peripheral) pattern is the one most commonly seen in systemic lupus erythematosus, but titers and patterns appear to have little or no specificity in dogs and cats (see p. 446). There is no clear, constant correlation between clinical disease activity and positive ANA.[136a, 189]

Preparations of the protozoan *Crithidia luciliae* have become commercially available for assaying patient sera for antibodies against native deoxyribonucleic acid (DNA).[40] Large surveys employing this substrate in dogs and cats have not been reported, although preliminary reports indicate that it is rarely positive in dogs with systemic lupus erythematosus and in those with positive ANA,[136a, 139] which suggests that dogs rarely form antibodies against native DNA. In addition, recent studies challenge the purity of *C. luciliae*.[151] The standard Farr test (radioimmunoassay) for the measurement of anti–native DNA antibodies in humans is unsatisfactory in dogs, resulting in numerous false positives.[189]

About 10 per cent of human patients with systemic lupus erythematosus are ANA–negative.[40] These patients have unique anticytoplasmic antibodies (anti-Ro), which are not detected when traditional ANA test substrates (mouse or rat liver) are employed, and, as a result, special substrates (calf thymus, normal human lymphocytes, human epithelial tissue culture line) are needed. The importance of this autoantibody system in dogs and cats is unknown.

Figure 9:59. *A*, Alopecia, erythema, crusting, and depigmentation of the face and ear of a cat with systemic lupus erythematosus. (From Scott, D. W., Haupt, K. H., et al.: A glucocorticoid-responsive dermatitis in cats, resembling systemic lupus erythematosus in man. J.A.A.H.A. *15*:157, 1979.) *B*, Patchy alopecia and scaling on the head and bridge of the nose in a dog with systemic lupus erythematosus. (Courtesy W. H. Miller, Jr.) *C*, Erythema, alopecia, ulceration, and crusting on the pinna of a cat with systemic lupus erythematosus. (From Scott, D. W., Haupt, K. H., et al.: A glucocorticoid-responsive dermatitis in cats, resembling systemic lupus erythematosus in man. J.A.A.H.A. *15*:157, 1979.) *D*, Bullae and ulcers on the ventrum of a dog with systemic lupus erythematosus. *E*, Necrosis of the margin of the pinna in a dog with systemic lupus erythematosus. *F*, Erythema, alopecia, and ulceration of the hind leg of a dog with systemic lupus erythematosus. *G*, Ulcerated footpads of a dog with systemic lupus erythematosus. *H*, Bacterial paronychia in a cat with systemic lupus erythematosus. (From Scott, D. W., Haupt, K. H., et al.: A glucocorticoid-responsive dermatitis in cats, resembling systemic lupus erythematosus in man. J.A.A.H.A. *15*:157, 1979.)

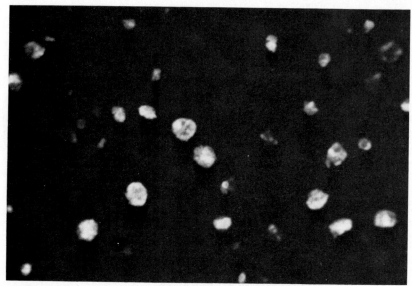

Figure 9:61. ANA test. Diffuse nuclear fluorescence from a cat with systemic lupus erythematosus.

However, it could explain the negative ANA results occasionally obtained in dogs with systemic lupus erythematosus.[189]

Recently, investigators have attempted to better understand lupus erythematosus in humans by studying subsets of patients on the basis of one clinical characteristic (or a set of them), histopathologic or immunopathologic findings, or serologic studies.[40] The use of this subset approach may allow the clinician to gain insight into prognosis, improved therapy, or presumed pathogenesis. Currently, three subsets for cutaneous lupus erythematosus are recognized: (1) chronic cutaneous (discoid) lupus erythematosus, (2) subacute cutaneous lupus erythematosus, and (3) acute cutaneous lupus erythematosus. The applicability of such subsets to the canine and feline diseases is presently unknown.

The *dermatohistopathologic changes* in systemic lupus erythematosus vary with the type of gross morphologic lesions and may be nondiagnostic.[40, 124, 189, 207] The most characteristic finding is interface dermatitis (hydropic or lichenoid or both), which may involve hair follicle outer root sheaths (Figs. 9:62 to 9:65). Other common findings include subepidermal vacuolar alteration ("subepidermal bubblies"), focal thickening of the basement membrane zone, and myxedema. Uncommon findings include intrabasal to subepidermal vesicles, leukocytoclastic vasculitis, and lupus erythematosus panniculitis (see p. 831). In humans, these changes are often not present until the skin lesions are at least 6 weeks old.

Direct immunofluorescence testing reveals the deposition of immunoglobulin or complement or both at the basement membrane zone, often known as a positive "lupus band," in 50 to 90 per cent of the patients.[40, 189, 207] The variability in positive results reflects differences in laboratory techniques, lesion selection (age and activity of lesion), previous or current glucocorticoid therapy, and possibly other factors. In addition, immunoreactants may be found at the basement membrane zone of skin in *many* other conditions (see p. 443). In dogs, C3 is the most commonly detected immunoreactant, with IgA and IgM being the most commonly detected immunoglobulins.[207] In humans, it is often

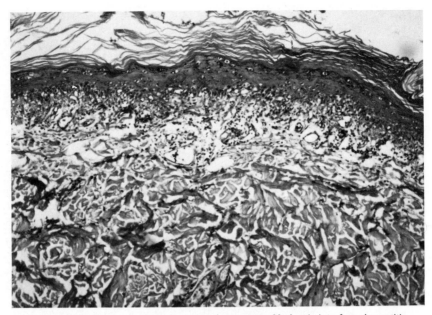

Figure 9:62. Canine systemic lupus erythematosus. Hydropic interface dermatitis.

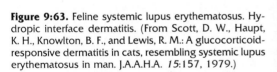

Figure 9:63. Feline systemic lupus erythematosus. Hydropic interface dermatitis. (From Scott, D. W., Haupt, K. H., Knowlton, B. F., and Lewis, R. M.: A glucocorticoid-responsive dermatitis in cats, resembling systemic lupus erythematosus in man. J.A.A.H.A. 15:157, 1979.)

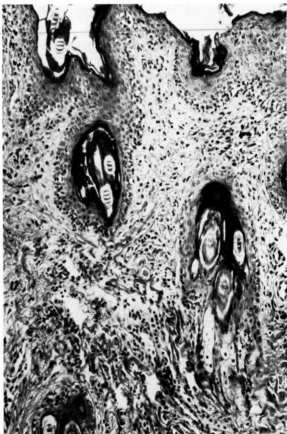

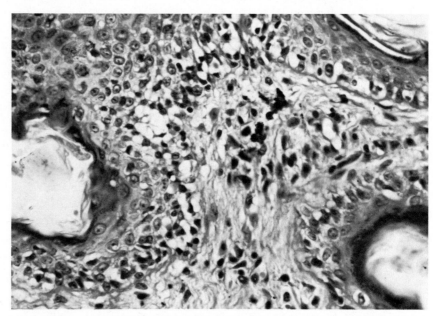

Figure 9:64. Feline systemic lupus erythematosus. Hydropic degeneration of epidermal basal cells. (From Scott, D. W., Haupt, K. H., Knowlton, B. F., and Lewis, R. M.: A glucocorticoid-responsive dermatitis in cats, resembling systemic lupus erythematosus in man. J.A.A.H.A. *15*:157, 1979.)

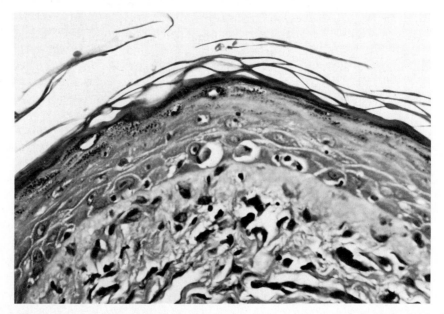

Figure 9:65. Canine systemic lupus erythematosis. Two large, round civatte (colloid) bodies in the stratum basale epidermis can be seen in the center of the photograph.

possible to distinguish between systemic lupus erythematosus and discoid lupus erythematosus on the basis of direct immunofluorescence testing of lesional and sun-exposed normal skin. In human patients with systemic lupus erythematosus, sun-exposed normal skin may have a positive "lupus band" in up to 60 per cent of the cases, whereas this rarely occurs in discoid lupus erythematosus.[40] This criterion is of no value in the hairy dog and cat, wherein normal skin is usually negative.[189, 213] Also, it is recommended that (1) biopsies not be taken from edematous lesions (only about 47 per cent of such lesions are positive), (2) biopsies be taken from lesions over 1 month old (only about 30 per cent are positive if less than 1 month old), (3) skin with telangiectases not be biopsied (17 per cent of such lesions are positive, regardless of their etiology), and (4) all glucocorticoid and immunomodulating therapy be terminated, if possible, 3 weeks prior to biopsy.[23, 189]

Electron microscopy reveals that immunoreactants are deposited below the basal lamina (lamina densa), in association with degenerative changes in epidermal basal cells and the basement membrane zone.[40, 41, 124]

Because no single laboratory test is diagnostic for systemic lupus erythematosus, a number of groups have produced sets of classification criteria for making the diagnosis.[40, 189] Although such criteria have acknowledged validity in humans, there is no such validation of criteria for dogs and cats. The veterinarian must rely on the recognition of multisystemic disease (especially joint, skin, kidney, oral mucosa, hematopoietic system), positive ANA, and confirmatory histopathologic and immunopathologic findings in involved skin and oral mucosa or both.[189]

CLINICAL MANAGEMENT

The prognosis in systemic lupus erythematosus is generally unpredictable.[40, 189, 207, 213] In the dog, it appears that patients with joint, skin or muscle disease respond more reliably to medication, and are maintained in relatively long periods of clinical remission. On the other hand, dogs with hemolytic anemia or thrombocytopenia or both often do not respond satisfactorily to systemic glucocorticoids and require other immunomodulating drugs or splenectomy or both. Animals with glomerulonephritis regularly developed progressive renal failure in spite of therapy.

Therapy of systemic lupus erythematosus must be individualized. The initial agent of choice is probably large doses of systemic glucocorticoids (2.2 to 4.4 mg/kg prednisolone or prednisone given orally, SID).[189, 207, 213] When systemic glucocorticoids are unsatisfactory, other immunomodulating drugs may be useful: (1) azathioprine (Imuran) given orally at 2.2 mg/kg SID, then every other day, or (2) chlorambucil (Leukeran) given orally at 0.2 mg/kg SID, then every other day (for *dog*).[189, 213] Splenectomy may be needed for patients with severe hemolytic anemia or thrombocytopenia or both.

Levamisole (Levasole) given at 2.5 mg/kg every 48 hours has occasionally been beneficial in dogs and humans with systemic lupus erythematosus.[189] *Chrysotherapy* (injectable aurothioglucose, oral auranofin) has occasionally been used to reduce glucocorticoid requirements in dogs but would be contraindicated in patients with renal disease.[189, 239] *Aspirin* has occasionally been effective in the management of dogs and humans.[40, 189] Other drugs used in human patients—dapsone, antiandrogens, antimalarials, colchicine or arachidonic acid analogs—are of undetermined benefit to dogs and cats.[40, 103, 217] Recently, *plasmapheresis* has been used to enhance initial response to chemotherapy in dogs and humans with severe systemic lupus erythematosus.[6, 130] This technique, presently used as a research tool, is hazardous and expensive.

Prognostically, it may be stated that (1) over 40 per cent of the dogs with systemic lupus erythematosus are dead within 1 year after the diagnosis is made, either as a result of natural (renal disease, septicemia) or drug-induced causes, or owing to euthanasia; (2) dogs that respond well to therapy often do so with glucocorticoids alone and often go into long-term remission on alternate-morning therapy; and (3) some dogs, having been controlled well with therapy for several months, remain in prolonged drug-free remission.[189, 213]

Several reports have recently shown that people in close contact with dogs having systemic lupus erythematosus or high-titer ANA have no increased clinical or serologic evidence of systemic lupus erythematosus when compared with nonexposed human beings.[189, 213]

DISCOID LUPUS ERYTHEMATOSUS
(Cutaneous Lupus Erythematosus)

Discoid lupus erythematosus is an uncommon autoimmune dermatitis of dogs that is usually confined to the face.

CAUSE AND PATHOGENESIS

Discoid lupus erythematosus is thought to be a benign variant of systemic lupus erythematosus, in which systemic involvement is absent and the disorder is confined to the skin. In humans, it has been demonstrated that the lymphocytes infiltrating skin lesions of discoid and systemic lupus erythematosus are predominantly T cells, and that T helper cells predominate in discoid lupus, while T suppressor cells predominate in systemic lupus.[110]

CLINICAL FEATURES

In the dog, no age predilection has been reported. However, females and collies, German shepherds, Shetland sheepdogs, and Siberian huskies demonstrate predilection.[190, 207, 213] A recent report from France indicated that males, German shepherds, collies, Brittany spaniels, and German shorthaired pointers were predisposed.[148a]

Clinical signs of canine discoid lupus erythematosus initially include depigmentation, erythema, and scaling of the nose (Fig. 9:66A,B). A helpful early change is the conversion of the normally rough, cobblestone-like architecture of the nasal planum into a smooth surface. Erosion, ulceration, and crusting commonly develop, and the disorder often spreads up the bridge of the nose. Less frequently, lesions may be seen periocularly, on the ears, on the distal limbs, and on the genitals. The lips may also be involved, and small punctate ulcers may be seen in the oral cavity (Fig. 9:66C). Occasional dogs present with only lesions of both pinnae or with nasodigital hyperkeratosis.[190, 192] Pruritus and pain are variable. Scarring and variable degrees of permanent leukoderma are common.

Discoid lupus erythematosus in dogs is frequently exacerbated or precipitated by exposure to ultraviolet light. Thus, canine discoid lupus is frequently

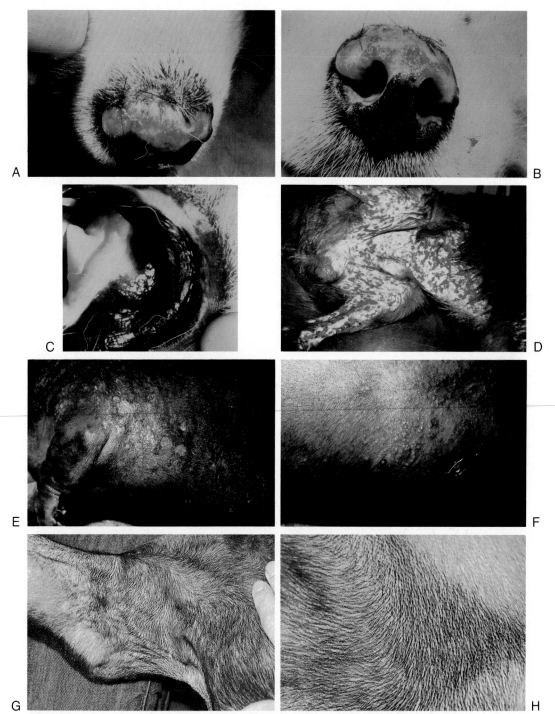

Figure 9:66. *A,* Nasal erythema, ulceration, and depigmentation in a dog with discoid lupus erythematosus. (From Walton, D. K., Scott, D. W., et al.: Canine discoid lupus erythematosus. J.A.A.H.A. *17*:851, 1981.) *B,* Frontal view of nose of dog in *A. C,* Depigmentation of the lip in a dog with discoid lupus erythematosus. (From Walton, D. K., Scott, D. W., et al.: Canine discoid lupus erythematosus. J.A.A.H.A. *17*:851, 1981.) *D,* Severe ulceration of the ventrum, medial thighs, and scrotum of a dog with toxic epidermal necrolysis. (Courtesy G. T. Wilkinson.) *E,* Ulcers and necrotic (black) skin on the side of a dog with toxic epidermal necrolysis. *F,* Vesicles on the abdomen of a dog with toxic epidermal necrolysis. *G,* Canine erythema multiforme. Annular and serpiginous erythema in axilla. *H,* Canine erythema multiforme. Serpiginous erythema.

more severe in the summer and in parts of the world with sunny climates. It is very likely that the disorder previously referred to as "nasal solar dermatitis," or "collie nose," included many dogs with discoid lupus erythematosus, systemic lupus erythematosus, pemphigus foliaceus, and pemphigus erythematosus. Squamous cell carcinomas are known to develop rarely in chronic discoid lupus erythematosus skin lesions.

DIAGNOSIS

The differential diagnosis includes demodicosis, dermatophytosis, dermatophilosis, bacterial folliculitis, pemphigus erythematosus, pemphigus foliaceus, drug eruption, mycosis fungoides, dermatomyositis, contact dermatitis in response to plastic or rubber, vitiligo, Vogt-Koyanagi-Harada–like syndrome, and systemic lupus erythematosus.

Definitive diagnosis of canine discoid lupus erythematosus is based on history, physical examination, skin biopsy, and immunopathology. Routine laboratory determinations (hemogram, serum chemistries, urinalysis, serum protein electrophoresis) are usually unremarkable. The ANA and LE cell tests are almost always negative.

Histopathology. Skin biopsy reveals an interface dermatitis (hydropic or lichenoid or both) (Fig. 9:67).[190, 207] Focal hydropic degeneration of basal epidermal cells, pigmentary incontinence, focal thickening of the basement membrane zone (Fig. 9:68), Civatte (colloid) bodies (Fig. 9:65), and marked accumulations of mononuclear cells and plasma cells around dermal vessels and appendages are important histopathologic features of discoid lupus erythematosus. Dermal mucinosis of variable degrees is also a frequent feature of canine discoid lupus erythematosus.[165]

Direct immunofluorescence testing reveals deposition of immunoglobulin or

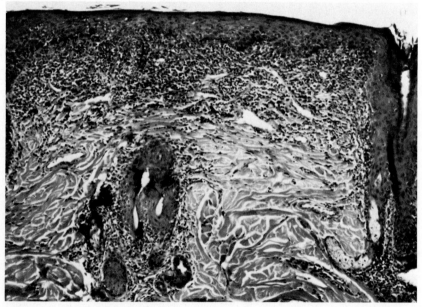

Figure 9:67. Canine discoid lupus erythematosus. Lichenoid interface dermatitis. (From Scott, D. W., Manning, T. O., Smith, C. A., and Lewis, R. M.: Linear IgA dermatoses in the dog. Cornell Vet 72:394, 1982.)

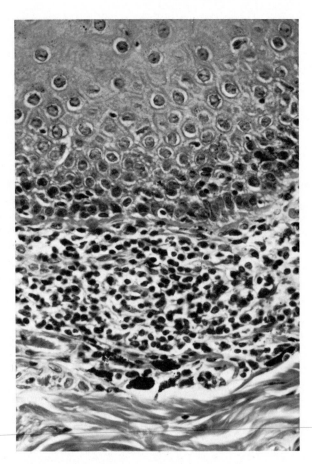

Figure 9:68. Canine discoid lupus erythematosus. Lichenoid interface dermatitis with thickening of the basement membrane zone. (From Walton, D. K., Scott, D. W., Smith, C. A., and Lewis, R. M.: Canine discoid lupus erythematosus. J.A.A.H.A. *17*:851, 1981.)

complement or both at the basement membrane zone.[148a, 207] In dogs, C3 is the most commonly demonstrated immunoreactant.[207] It would appear to be important to test for individual immunoglobulin classes, as either IgG, IgM, or IgA may be the only demonstrable immunoglobulin.[207] In humans, it is recommended that (1) edematous lesions not be biopsied (only about 47 per cent of such lesions are positive), (2) telangiectatic areas *not* be biopsied (about 17 per cent of the telangiectatic skin lesions of *any* dermatosis are positive), and (3) lesions less than 1 month old *not* be biopsied (only about 30 per cent of such lesions are positive). Additionally, in humans, discoid lupus may often be distinguished from systemic lupus with direct immunofluorescence testing of lesional and normal *sun-exposed* skin. Normal sun-exposed skin from human patients with discoid lupus is rarely positive, whereas it may be positive in up to 60 per cent of the patients with systemic lupus.[40] This criterion is of dubious value in the dog (unless it is bald!).[190] Indirect immunofluorescence testing is negative in discoid lupus erythematosus.

CLINICAL MANAGEMENT

The prognosis for discoid lupus erythematosus is usually good.[148a, 190, 207] Therapy will probably need to be continued for life, and marked depigmentation predisposes to sunburn and possible squamous cell carcinoma.

Therapy of canine discoid lupus erythematosus must be appropriate to the individual.[79, 79b, 148a, 190, 207, 213] Mild cases may be controlled by and *all* cases benefit from avoidance of exposure to intense sunlight (from 8:00 AM to 5:00 PM), the use of topical sunscreens, and the use of topical glucocorticoids (see p. 168). For more severe or refractory cases, systemic drugs may be added to the treatment regimen. Systemic glucocorticoids (2.2 mg/kg prednisolone or prednisone, given orally SID) are often effective. In cases in which systemic glucocorticoids are contraindicated or unsatisfactory, vitamin E (400 to 800 IU dl-α-tocopherol acetate, given orally BID) may be effective. Vitamin E appears to have a 1- to 2-month lag phase before its benefit is recognized clinically, and systemic glucocorticoids may be used concurrently during this period. Vitamin E should be administered 2 hours before or after feeding. In humans, discoid lupus erythematosus is often responsive to antimalarial drugs (chloroquine [Aralen]; hydroxychloroquine [Plaquenil], quinacrine [Atabrine]).[40, 62] These drugs may be useful in the dog, as well, but dosage, efficacy, and toxicity need to be carefully evaluated (see p. 195).[139] Other drugs occasionally found to be beneficial in humans include retinoids, dapsone, and gold (oral or injectable).[40, 50, 62, 145] The usefulness of these compounds in dogs is presently unknown.

COLD AGGLUTININ DISEASE
(Cold Hemagglutinin Disease, Cryopathic Hemolytic Anemia)

CAUSE AND PATHOGENESIS

Cryoglobulins and cryofibrinogens are proteins that can be precipitated from serum and plasma, respectively, by cooling.[62, 139] Cryoglobulins have been classified into three types according to their characteristics: (1) type I cryoglobulins are composed solely of monoclonal immunoglobulins or free light chains (Bence Jones proteins) and are most frequently associated with lymphoproliferative disorders; (2) type II cryoglobulins are composed of monoclonal and polyclonal immunoglobulins and are most frequently associated with autoimmune and connective tissue diseases; and (3) type III cryoglobulins are composed of polyclonal immunoglobulins and are seen with infections, autoimmune disorders, and connective tissue diseases. Cutaneous signs associated with cryoglobulins and cryofibrinogens are due to vascular insufficiency (obstruction, stasis, spasm, thrombosis).

CLINICAL FEATURES

Cold agglutinin disease has been rarely reported to cause skin disease in dogs and cats.[139, 146, 178, 208] Cold agglutinin disease is an autoimmune disorder associated with cold-reacting (usually IgM) erythrocyte autoantibodies. The cryopathic autoantibody is most active at colder temperatures (0 to 4°C) but has a wide range of thermal activity (0 to 30°C). Cold agglutinin disease represents a type II hypersensitivity reaction and has been associated with idiopathy and lead poisoning in dogs, and with upper respiratory infection in cats.

Clinical signs of cold agglutinin disease are variable and relate to either anemia or intracapillary cold hemagglutination or both. Skin lesions include erythema, purpura, acrocyanosis, necrosis, and ulceration. Skin lesions generally involve the extremities (paw, ears, nose, tip of tail) and are precipitated or exacerbated by exposure to cold (Fig. 9:69A).

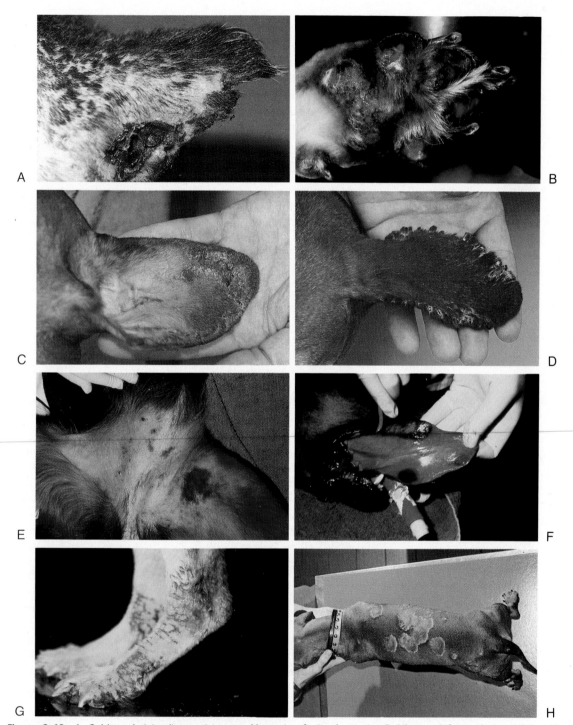

Figure 9:69. *A,* Cold agglutinin disease in a cat. Necrosis of pinnal margin. *B,* Ulcerated footpads in a dog with leukocytoclastic vasculitis. *C,* Cutaneous vasculitis in a dog. Necrosis and ulceration tracing pinnal vasculature. *D,* Cutaneous vasculitis in a dog. Scalloping of pinnal margin due to necrosis and scarring. *E,* Cutaneous vasculitis in a dog. Purpura on the abdomen and medial thigh. *F,* Punctate ulcers on the tongue of a dog with leukocytoclastic vasculitis. *G,* Ulceration of the hind leg and footpads in a dog with toxic epidermal necrolysis. *H,* Canine linear IgA dermatosis. Annular, coalescing areas of alopecia, scaling, crusting, and hyperpigmentation.

DIAGNOSIS

The differential diagnosis includes systemic lupus erythematosus, vasculitis, dermatomyositis, disseminated intravascular coagulation, and frostbite.

Definitive diagnosis of cold agglutinin disease is made by history, physical examination, and demonstrating significant titers of cold agglutinins. In vitro autohemagglutination of blood at room temperature can be diagnostic for cold-reacting autoantibodies. Blood in heparin or ethylenediaminetetra-acetic acid (EDTA) is allowed to cool on a slide, thus permitting the autoagglutination to be readily visible macroscopically. The reaction can be accentuated by cooling the blood to 0°C, or reversed by warming the blood to 37°C. Doubtful cases can be confirmed via Coombs' test if the complete test is performed at 4°C and the Coombs reagent has activity against IgM. Caution in interpretation of the "cold" Coombs' test is warranted, as normal dogs and cats may have titers up to 1:100.

Histopathology. Skin biopsy usually reveals necrosis, ulceration, and often secondary suppurative changes. Fortuitously, some sections may show thrombotic-to-necrotic blood vessels or blood vessels containing an amorphous eosinophilic substance consisting largely of precipitated cryoglobulin.[124]

CLINICAL MANAGEMENT

The prognosis for cold agglutinin disease will vary with the underlying cause. Therapy of cold agglutinin disease includes (1) correction of the underlying cause, if possible, (2) avoidance of cold, and (3) immunosuppressive drug regimens (glucocorticoids, azathioprine, etc.).

GRAFT-VERSUS-HOST DISEASE

Graft-versus-host disease is a well-recognized result of bone marrow transplantation in dogs and humans.[27, 62, 93, 218] The disease occurs whenever lymphoid cells from an immunocompetent donor are introduced into a histoincompatible recipient that is incapable of rejecting them. It is generally accepted that the disease results from donor T-cell responses to recipient transplantation antigens.

In dogs and humans, a bone marrow graft from a donor genetically identical for major histocompatibility complex is followed by significant graft-versus-host disease in about 50 per cent of recipients, despite postgraft immunosuppressive therapy. The principal target organs are the skin, liver, and intestinal tract. In dogs, *acute* graft-versus-host disease develops about 2 weeks after grafting and is characterized by erythroderma, jaundice, diarrhea, and gram-negative infections. *Chronic* graft-versus-host disease develops about 3 to 4 months after grafting and is characterized by exfoliative erythroderma, ulcerative dermatitis, ascites, and gram-positive infections.

Diagnosis is based on history, physical examination, and skin biopsy. Histopathologic findings in *acute* graft-versus-host disease include varying degrees of interface dermatitis (hydropic or lichenoid) with "satellite cell necrosis."[27, 93, 124] In *chronic* graft-versus-host disease, one finds variable sclerodermoid and/or poikilodermatous changes.

Therapy of graft-versus-host disease with various combinations of systemic gluocorticoids, azathioprine, cyclosporine, methotrexate, and antithymocyte serum have been only partially and unpredictably effective.

Immune-Mediated Disorders

VASCULITIS
(Angiitis)

Cutaneous vasculitis is an uncommon disorder in dogs, cats, and humans that is characterized by purpura, necrosis, and ulceration of the extremities.

CAUSES AND PATHOGENESIS

Vasculitides are classified histologically into neutrophilic, lymphocytic, granulomatous, and mixed forms, and the neutrophilic forms may be leukocytoclastic (neutrophil nuclei undergo karyorrhexis, resulting in "nuclear dust") or nonleukocytoclastic.[49, 62, 63, 73, 124, 172, 207] It has been postulated that differences in membrane receptors for immunoglobulin and complement on leukocytes may account for the different histologic appearance of neutrophilic and lymphocytic vasculitides. The pathomechanism of most cutaneous vasculitides is assumed to involve type III hypersensitivity reactions. Type I hypersensitivity reactions may be important in the initiation of immune complex deposition in blood vessel walls.

Cutaneous vasculitis may be associated with coexisting disease (infections, malignancies, connective tissue disorders such as lupus erythematosus) or precipitating factors (drugs), or it may be idiopathic (about 50 per cent of all cases).[40, 62, 73, 96, 172, 207] Focal cutaneous vasculitic reactions at the site of rabies vaccination have been described in dogs and cats.[176, 246] Reactions were characterized by roughly annular areas of variable alopecia, erythema, scaling, and hyperpigmentation overlying an indurated dermis and subcutis. The caudal or lateral thigh was typically involved (Fig. 9:70). The lesions generally appeared 1 to 6 months following vaccination and persisted for months to years.

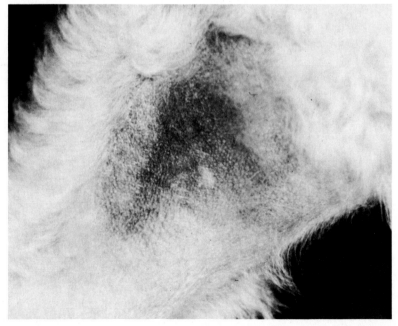

Figure 9:70. Alopecic, hyperpigmented plaque on caudomedial thigh due to postvaccinal vasculitis.

CLINICAL FEATURES

Cutaneous signs of vasculitis usually include palpable purpura, hemorrhagic bullae, necrosis, and "punched-out" ulcers, especially involving the extremities (paws, pinnae, lips, tail, and oral mucosa), and may clearly be associated with vascular pathways (Fig. 9:69*B* to *F*). The lesions may or may not be painful. Constitutional signs may be present, including anorexia, depression, and pyrexia. Pitting edema of extremities, polyarthropathy, and myopathy have been reported in dogs.[158] Any age, breed, or sex may be affected, but dachshunds and Rottweilers may be predisposed.[207]

A *proliferative thrombovascular necrosis* has been recognized in dogs.[79a] The etiology is unknown, and there are no apparent age, breed, or sex predilections. Lesions begin on the apex margins of the pinnae and spread along the concave surface. An elongated necrotic ulcer is at the center of the lesions. There is often a thickened, scaly, hyperpigmented zone surrounding the ulcers. The lesions are wedge shaped, with the wide base at the pinnae apex. As the ulcer enlarges, the older areas undergo complete necrosis, resulting in a deformed pinnal margin.

DIAGNOSIS

The differential diagnosis includes systemic lupus erythematosus, cold agglutinin disease, frostbite, disseminated intravascular coagulation, and lymphoreticular neoplasia. Definitive diagnosis is based on history, physical examination, and skin biopsy. Histopathology reveals varying degrees of neutrophilic and/or lymphocytic vasculitis (Fig. 9:71), possibly reflecting the age of the lesions and the types of immune reactants. Fibrinoid necrosis may or may not be present. Involvement of deep dermal vessels may suggest systemic disease.[172] When the deep vasculature is affected, necrosis of appendages and subcutaneous fat may be seen. The lesions most likely to show diagnostic changes are those from 8 to 24 hours old. Once the diagnosis of cutaneous vasculitis has been established, it is imperative that underlying etiologic factors be sought and eliminated (Table 9:29). Cutaneous vasculitis has been reported in dogs with systemic lupus erythematosus, rheumatoid arthritis, polyarteritis nodosa, Rocky Mountain spotted fever, or staphylococcal hypersensitivity, and as an idiopathic occurrence.[59, 139, 158, 207] In addition, lymphocytic vasculitis has been recognized in a dog with ampicillin drug eruption and in a dog with severe flea bite hypersensitivity.[139] Proliferative thrombovascular necrosis is characterized by arteriolar proliferation, sclerosis, hyalin degeneration, and eventually thrombosis.[79a] No inflammatory vasculitis is recognized.

Direct immunofluorescence testing may demonstrate immunoglobulin or complement, or both, in vessel walls and occasionally at the basement membrane zone in both the neutrophilic and lymphocytic forms of cutaneous vasculitis.[62, 158, 207] However, direct immunofluorescence is usually not needed, is not particularly useful for diagnosis, and, if it is performed, must be done within the first 4 hours after lesion formation. Studies in humans have shown that the intradermal injection of 0.02 ml of a histamine phosphate solution into the skin of patients with active cutaneous vasculitis was a reliable method for demonstrating the deposition of immune reactants, with direct immunofluorescence testing of the injection site performed 4 hours after injection.[139]

Dogs with active vasculitis may have increased levels of circulating immune complexes, decreased levels of serum complement, and hypergammaglobulinemia.[158]

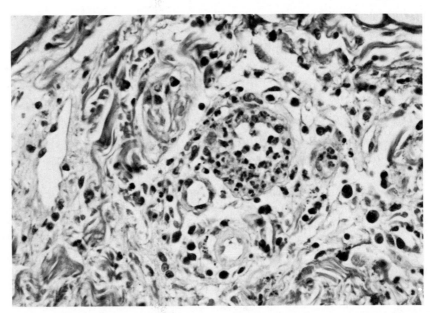

Figure 9:71. Canine cutaneous leukocytoclastic vasculitis. Degeneration of blood vessel wall with leukocytoclasis and "nuclear dust" formation. (From Manning, T. O., and Scott, D. W.: Cutaneous vasculitis in a dog. J.A.A.H.A. *16*:61, 1980.)

CLINICAL MANAGEMENT

It is difficult to predict the course of the disease in any individual case. A single episode lasting a few weeks may occur, or the disorder may be chronic or recurrent. The outcome depends on the extent of internal organ involvement (especially renal and neurologic) and the underlying or precipitating factor(s).

Treatment of vasculitis includes (1) correction of the underlying cause and (2) immunomodulatory drug treatment.[62, 207] In some cases, systemic prednisone or prednisolone (2 to 4 mg/kg/day orally) is effective.[62, 158, 207] For other cases that are refractory to glucocorticoids, sulfones such as dapsone (1 mg/kg TID orally) or sulfasalazine (20 to 40 mg/kg TID orally) may be effective (see p. 194).[59, 63, 207] Cyclophosphamide has been useful in some patients,[62, 158] and colchicine is often beneficial in humans.[39] In some cases, therapy can be stopped after 4 to 6 months of treatment. Other patients require long-term maintenance therapy with reduced drug doses and reduced frequencies of administration (see p. 195). Proliferative thrombovascular necrosis is slowly progressive and unresponsive to all medical therapies that have been tried.[79a] The current treatment of choice is partial surgical removal of the pinna. Relapses have occurred only when attempts were made to save as much tissue as possible.

Table 9:29. ETIOLOGIC FACTORS IN CUTANEOUS VASCULITIS

Infections (bacterial, mycobacterial, fungal, viral, rickettsial)
Injection of foreign proteins (sera, vaccines, hyposensitization)
Chemicals (insecticides, fungicides, petroleum products)
Drugs (antibiotics)
Other diseases (systemic lupus erythematosus, rheumatoid arthritis, ulcerative colitis, malignancies)

ERYTHEMA MULTIFORME

Erythema multiforme is an uncommon acute, usually self-limited eruption of the skin or mucous membranes, or both, characterized by distinctive gross lesions and a diagnostic sequence of pathologic changes.

CAUSE AND PATHOGENESIS

Despite recognition of multiple etiologic and triggering causes, the pathogenesis of erythema multiforme is not fully understood. It is currently considered to be a hypersensitivity reaction and has been associated with infections, drugs, neoplasia, and "connective tissue" diseases.[74a, 97, 98, 207] In humans, direct immunofluorescence testing reveals immunoreactants (especially C3 and IgM) at the basement membrane zone and, in about 50 per cent of the cases, in the walls of superficial dermal blood vessels.[61, 97] In addition, circulating immune complexes are often present. Erythema multiforme has been recognized in dogs in association with infections (staphylococcal folliculitis, anal sacculitis), drug therapy (aureothioglucose, cephalexin, chloramphenicol, diethylcarbamazine, gentamicin, levamisole, l-thyroxine, trimethoprim-sulfadiazine), and idiopathy.[74b, 201, 207, 230] In cats, erythema multiforme has been reported in association with drug therapy (penicillin, aurothioglucose).[207]

CLINICAL SIGNS

Prodromal or concurrent clinical signs may reflect the underlying cause. As the name "multiforme" implies, the skin lesions are variable, but are usually characterized by an acute, rather symmetric onset of (1) erythematous macules or slightly elevated papules that spread peripherally and clear centrally, producing annular ("target") or arciform patterns, (2) urticarial plaques, (3) vesicles and bullae, or (4) some combination thereof (Fig. 9:66G, H). The lesions and patients with maculopapular eruptions are usually asymptomatic (erythema multiforme minor). Occasionally, animals become systemically ill (fever, depression, anorexia) and have rather extensive vesiculobullous and ulcerative lesions of the mucocutaneous areas, oral mucosa, conjunctiva, pinnae, axillae and groin (erythema multiforme major, Stevens-Johnson syndrome).[29] Characteristically, in the maculopapular and urticarial forms of erythema multiforme, the overlying skin and hair coat are normal.

DIAGNOSIS

The differential diagnosis includes bacterial folliculitis, dermatophytosis, demodicosis, urticaria, and other vesicular and pustular disorders. *Maculopapular* lesions are characterized histologically by hydropic interface dermatitis with prominent single-cell necrosis of keratinocytes and satellitosis of lymphocytes and macrophages. Rarely, a dense lichenoid inflammatory infiltrate is seen. *Urticarial* lesions are characterized by hydropic interface dermatitis and striking dermal edema (Fig. 9:72). Dermal collagen fibers become vertically oriented and attenuated, presenting a weblike appearance ("gossamer collagen") (Fig. 9:73). *Vesiculobullous* lesions are characterized by segmental full-thickness coagulation necrosis of epithelium (Fig. 9:74). A superficial perivascular accumulation of predominantly lymphohistiocytic cells is typical, and

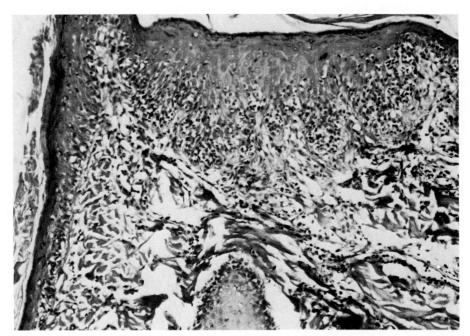

Figure 9:72. Canine erythema multiforme. Hydropic interface dermatitis.

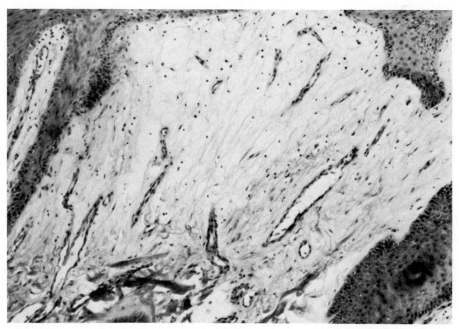

Figure 9:73. Canine erythema multiforme. Marked dermal edema with vertical stretching of collagen fibers ("gossamer collagen").

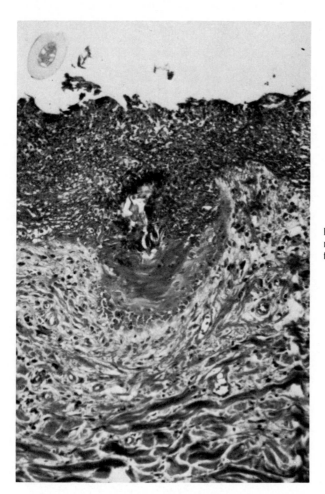

Figure 9:74. Canine erythema multiforme. Full-thickness coagulation necrosis of epidermis, involving hair follicle outer root sheath.

subepidermal cleft and vesicle formation may occur, owing to separation of the necrotic epithelium from the underlying connective tissue at the basement membrane zone. Definitive diagnosis is made by history and physical examination, laboratory rule-outs, and skin biopsy. Skin biopsy findings vary with the gross morphology of the lesions.[207] The maculopapular form of erythema multiforme is characterized by *lack* of surface pathology (lack of scale, crust, oozing, hair loss). The urticarial form of erythema multiforme is characterized by the *persistence* of urticarial lesions, as opposed to the evanescent nature of the wheals in true urticaria.

CLINICAL MANAGEMENT

Erythema multiforme may run a mild course, spontaneously regressing within a few weeks. An underlying cause should be sought and corrected, whenever possible, which will also result in spontaneous resolution of the erythema multiforme. Severe vesiculobullous cases of erythema multiforme require supportive care and an exhaustive search for underlying causes. The usefulness of systemic glucocorticoids and other immunomodulating drugs in erythema multiforme is controversial, and severe vesiculobullous eruptions are usually poorly responsive to these drugs.[74a, 211]

TOXIC EPIDERMAL NECROLYSIS

Toxic epidermal necrolysis is a rare, variably painful, vesiculobullous and ulcerative disorder of skin and oral mucosa in dogs, cats, and human beings.

CAUSE AND PATHOGENESIS

Toxic epidermal necrolysis has been temporally associated with drugs (50 per cent of the cases), toxins, infections, malignancies, and other systemic disorders (Table 9:30).[51, 150a, 152, 207, 230] Some cases are idiopathic. Although the pathomechanism of toxic epidermal necrolysis is unknown, histopathologic and immunopathologic studies suggest an epitheliotropic lymphocyte-macrophage-mediated immunologic insult.[134, 169, 170]

CLINICAL FEATURES

Clinically, toxic epidermal necrolysis is usually characterized by an acute onset of constitutional signs (pyrexia, anorexia, lethargy, depression) and a multifocal or generalized vesiculobullous disease (Fig. 9:66F, p. 527). Vesicles and bullae, necrosis, and resultant ulcers with epidermal collarettes may be found anywhere in the skin and often involve the oral mucosa, mucocutaneous junctions, and footpads (Figs. 9:66D to F and 9:69G, pp. 527 and 531). Nikolsky's sign is usually present. Cutaneous pain is usually moderate to marked. There are no apparent age, breed, or sex predilections.

DIAGNOSIS

The differential diagnosis includes pemphigus vulgaris, bullous pemphigoid, systemic lupus erythematosus, erythema multiforme, and lymphoreticular neoplasia.

Definitive diagnosis is based on history, physical examination, and skin biopsy. A hemogram usually reveals neutropenia or neutrophilia.[51, 207] In humans, persistent neutropenia portends a fatal outcome.[241]

Histopathology. Histopathologic findings in toxic epidermal necrolysis are identical, regardless of underlying cause, and include hydropic degeneration of basal epidermal cells, full-thickness coagulation necrosis of the epidermis, and minimal dermal inflammation ("silent dermis") (Fig. 9:75).[152, 207] Dermoepidermal separation results in subepidermal vesicles (Fig. 9:76). The periodic

Table 9:30. ETIOLOGIC FACTORS ASSOCIATED WITH TOXIC EPIDERMAL NECROLYSIS IN DOGS AND CATS

Dog	Cat
Bacterial endocarditis	FeLV antiserum (caprine)
Myeloproliferative disease	Cephaloridine
Cholangiohepatitis	Ampicillin
Hepatic necrosis	Hetacillin
Splenic fibrosarcoma	Idiopathic
Levamisole	
Cephalexin	
Idiopathic	
5-Fluorocytosine	

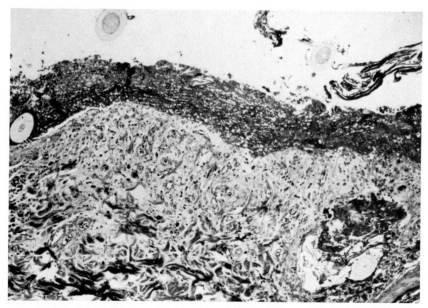

Figure 9:75. Canine toxic epidermal necrolysis (associated with staphylococcal endocarditis). Full-thickness epidermal necrosis with minimal inflammation. (From Scott, D. W., Halliwell, R. E. W., Goldschmidt, M. H., and DiBartola, S.: Toxic epidermal necrolysis in two dogs and a cat. J.A.A.H.A. *15*:271, 1979.)

acid-Schiff (PAS)–positive basement membrane zone, when present, is usually located at the floor of the vesicles. It must be emphasized that toxic epidermal necrolysis is not usually the definitive diagnosis. It is imperative to remember that toxic epidermal necrolysis is only a cutaneous reaction pattern, and every attempt must be made to find the underlying cause.

Direct and indirect immunofluorescence testing are usually negative.[134, 152, 207, 241]

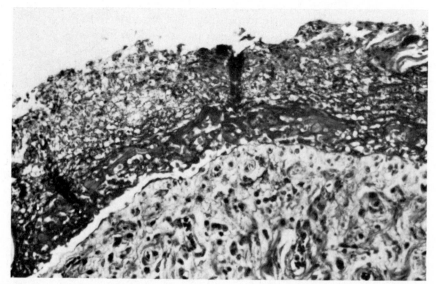

Figure 9:76. Canine toxic epidermal necrolysis (staphylococcal endocarditis). Full-thickness epidermal necrosis with subepidermal cleft formation. (From Scott, D. W., Halliwell, R. E. W., Goldschmidt, M. H., and DiBartola, S.: Toxic epidermal necrolysis in two dogs and a cat. J.A.A.H.A. *15*:271, 1979.)

CLINICAL MANAGEMENT

The prognosis for toxic epidermal necrolysis is guarded to poor, pending identification of the underlying cause, with a 20 to 50 per cent mortality rate in humans. The mortality is greatest in idiopathic cases, wherein a precipitating factor cannot be recognized and specifically corrected. The sequelae and prognosis are similar to those of a massive second-degree burn, owing to fluid, electrolyte, and colloid losses and to secondary infections that compound the loss of epidermal barrier function.

Treatment includes (1) correction of the underlying cause and (2) symptomatic and supportive measures (fluids, antibiotics, topicals, and so on). The use of systemic glucocorticoids is controversial, most investigators believing that these drugs are at best not helpful, and at worst detrimental.[152, 241] Recovery (pending underlying cause) usually occurs in 2 to 3 weeks.

LINEAR IgA DERMATOSIS

Linear IgA dermatosis is a very rare idiopathic, sterile superficial pustular dermatosis of dachshunds, characterized histologically by subcorneal pustules and immunologically by the deposition of IgA at the basement membrane zone of affected skin.[207] It is not analogous to a similarly named dermatosis of humans.[23]

Clinically, linear IgA dermatosis is characterized by a multifocal-to-generalized pustular dermatitis. The trunk is typically involved. Secondary skin lesions include annular areas of alopecia, erosion, epidermal collarettes, hyperpigmentation, scaling, and crusting (Fig. 9:69H, p. 531). Pruritus is minimal to absent, and the dogs are otherwise healthy. All cases to date have been recognized in adult dachshunds of either sex.

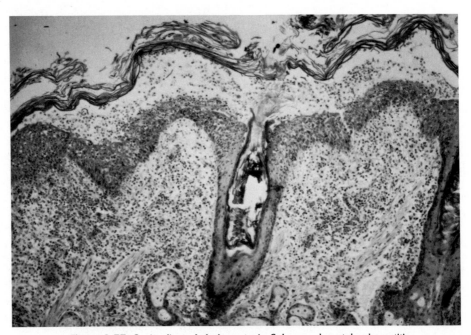

Figure 9:77. Canine linear IgA dermatosis. Subcorneal pustular dermatitis.

The differential diagnosis includes bacterial folliculitis, dermatophytosis, demodicosis, pemphigus foliaceus, systemic lupus erythematosus, and subcorneal pustular dermatosis. Diagnosis is based on culture (negative), skin biopsy (intraepidermal pustular dermatitis, with numerous neutrophils and minimal acantholysis) (Fig. 9:77), and direct immunofluorescence testing (IgA deposited at the basement membrane zone).

Therapy consists of large doses of prednisolone or prednisone (2.2 to 4.4 mg/kg SID, orally, then alternate-day steroid regimens) or dapsone (1 mg/kg orally, TID, then as needed). Interestingly, glucocorticoids may work in one case and not another. The same is true of dapsone. See pages 194 and 198 for discussions of glucocorticoid and dapsone therapy.

Other Immunologic Dermatoses

CUTANEOUS DEPIGMENTATION AND UVEITIS IN DOGS
(Vogt-Koyanagi-Harada–like syndrome)

Cutaneous depigmentation and uveitis is a rare, idiopathic syndrome of concurrent granulomatous uveitis and leukoderma in dogs.

CAUSE AND PATHOGENESIS

The cause of this syndrome is unknown. The syndrome has many similarities to the Vogt-Koyanagi-Harada syndrome in humans, which is currently thought to represent an autoimmune disorder.[42, 62, 109] In humans, cell-mediated hypersensitivity to melanin has been demonstrated.

CLINICAL FEATURES

In humans, the Vogt-Koyanagi-Harada syndrome has three phases: (1) a *meningoencephalitic* phase with prodromata of fever, malaise, headache, tinnitus, nausea, and vomiting, (2) an *ophthalmic* phase with photophobia, uveitis, decreased visual acuity, and potential blindness, and (3) a *dermatologic* phase with poliosis (90 per cent of the cases), alopecia (73 per cent), and vitiligo (63 per cent).[62] The dermatologic signs are usually symmetric, especially involving the head, neck, and eyelids, and they usually mark the convalescent stage when the uveitis begins to abate. The pigmentary changes tend to be permanent.

In dogs, the similar syndrome is usually characterized by the concurrent acute onset of uveitis and depigmentation of the nose, lips, eyelids, and occasionally the footpads and anus (Fig. 9:78A, B).[42, 58a, 62, 135a, 163, 207] In most cases, there is no visible inflammation of the depigmented skin. However,

Figure 9:78. *A,* Canine Vogt-Koyanagi-Harada–like syndrome. Depigmentation of nose, muzzle, and periocular skin. *B,* Canine Vogt-Koyanagi-Harada–like syndrome. Depigmentation of lips. *C,* Feline plasma cell pododermatitis. Swollen footpads. *D,* Feline plasma cell pododermatitis. Swollen footpad with cross-hatched white striae. *E,* Feline polychondritis. Swollen, violaceous pinna. *F,* Canine sterile pyogranuloma. Erythematous nodules bordering footpads. *G,* Canine sterile pyogranuloma. Erythematous nodules bordering nostrils. *H,* Canine sterile pyogranuloma. Multiple erythematosus, ulcerated, crusted papules around eye.

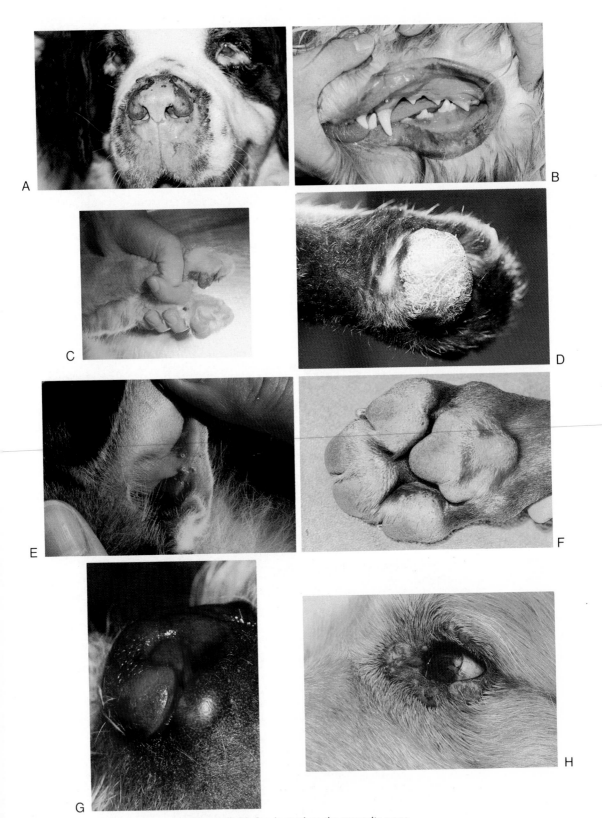

Figure 9:78 *See legend on the opposite page*

occasionally, perhaps associated with exposure to sunlight (photodermatitis), depigmented areas may manifest varying degrees of erythema, erosion, ulceration, and crusting. Patchy leukotrichia may be present in the areas surrounding the cutaneous depigmentation. Rarely, leukoderma and leukotrichia may be widespread. Clinicopathologic evidence of a meningoencephalitic phase is rarely seen in dogs. There are no apparent age or sex predilections, but Akitas, Samoyeds, and Siberian huskies may be predisposed to the syndrome.

DIAGNOSIS

The definitive diagnosis is based on history, physical examination, and skin biopsy. Histopathologic findings in biopsies taken from early skin lesions are characterized by lichenoid interface dermatitis, wherein large histiocytes are a major cellular component (Figs. 9:79 and 9:80).[197] Pigmentary incontinence is pronounced, but hydropic degeneration of epidermal basal cells is often minimal. Skin biopsies taken from chronically depigmented areas may reveal only hypomelanosis. Histopathologic findings in the eye include granulomatous panuveitis and retinitis. Direct and indirect immunofluorescence testing is usually negative.

CLINICAL MANAGEMENT

Early treatment with topical and systemic glucocorticoids (e.g., prednisone or prednisolone given orally at 2.2 mg/kg SID) is indicated in order to prevent blindness.[62, 207] If treated early, variable degrees of cutaneous repigmentation (sometimes complete) usually occur. Dogs usually require chronic alternate-morning oral glucocorticoid therapy (e.g., 0.25 to 1.1 mg/kg prednisone or prednisolone) to prevent recurrence.[207]

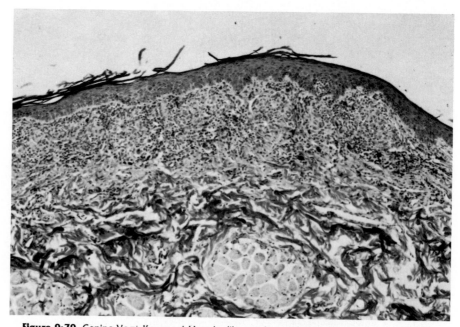

Figure 9:79. Canine Vogt-Koyanagi-Harada–like syndrome. Lichenoid interface dermatitis.

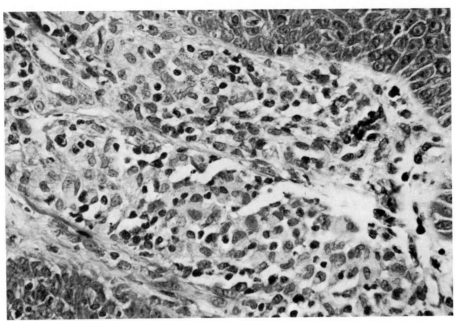

Figure 9:80. Close-up of Figure 9:79. Numerous histocytes in lichenoid band.

RELAPSING POLYCHONDRITIS

In humans, relapsing polychondritis is a rare systemic disease characterized by inflammation and destruction involving both articular and nonarticular cartilagenous structures.[62] It is often classified among the immune-mediated diseases because of similarities to rheumatoid arthritis and lupus erythematosus, as well as its favorable response to immunomodulatory therapy.

Humans with acute disease usually present with swollen, erythematous, and tender ears or nose. Later, affected areas become soft and flabby. Systemic signs may or may not be present. Diagnosis is based on history, physical examination, biopsy, and increased urinary excretion of acid mucopolysaccharides. The disease usually responds to systemic glucocorticoids or dapsone.

A single adult cat has been reported which presented with a history of swollen, erythematous, painful ears.[208] When examined, the pinnae were swollen and meaty, violaceous, and curled and deformed (Fig. 9:78E). Biopsies revealed lymphoplasmacytic inflammation, loss of cartilage basophilia, and cartilage necrosis (Figs. 9:81, 9:82). The clinicopathologic findings were consistent with a diagnosis of relapsing polychondritis. However, the cat was lost to follow up before further diagnostic or therapeutic investigations could be performed.

IMMUNOPROLIFERATIVE ENTEROPATHY OF BASENJI DOGS

Immunoproliferative enteropathy of Basenjis is characterized by chronic intractable diarrhea, progressive emaciation, and gastropathy.[28, 29] An autosomal recessive inheritance of the condition has been hypothesized. A similar disease exists in humans.

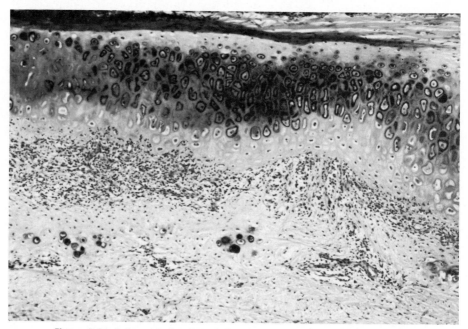

Figure 9:81. Feline polychondritis. Inflammation and necrosis of ear cartilage.

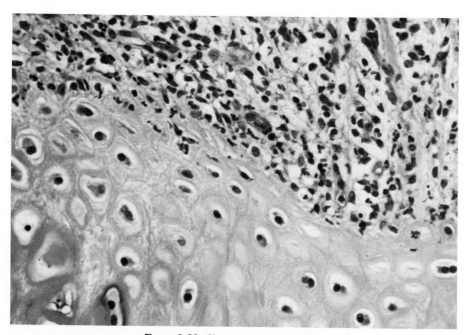

Figure 9:82. Close-up of Figure 9:81.

Basenjis of either sex and a wide age range are affected. Skin lesions are variable and may consist of alopecia, hyperpigmentation, hyperkeratosis, and marginal necrosis and ulceration of the pinna, or a symmetric alopecia of the ventrum. The hair coat is often dry and dull.

Diagnosis is based on history, physical examination, and laboratory testing. Most affected dogs have serum hypergammaglobulinemia. Some dogs are hypothyroid based on thyroid-stimulating hormone (TSH) stimulation tests. Intestinal biopsy reveals lymphoplasmacytic enteritis.

Dermatohistopathologic findings are nondiagnostic. Alopecic skin is characterized by endocrinopathic changes, probably reflecting hypothyroidism. Dermatitic pinnae are characterized by ulcerative perivascular dermatitis, necrosis, and changes consistent with secondary bacterial infection. Although the clinical appearance of the pinnae is suggestive of a vasculopathy, histologic evidence of vessel disease has not been reported.

Therapy is provided according to symptoms and is often disappointing. Genetic counseling, avoidance of stress, and high-quality commercial diets are indicated. Systemic glucocorticoids may be beneficial.

FELINE PLASMA CELL PODODERMATITIS

Plasma cell pododermatitis is a rare cutaneous disorder of cats.[196, 208] The cause and pathogenesis of this disorder are unknown. However, the tissue plasmacytosis, the consistent hypergammaglobulinemia, and the beneficial response to immunomodulating drugs suggest an immune-mediated pathogenesis. In addition, some cases have recurred on a seasonal basis, suggesting an allergic basis. No age, breed, or sex predilections are apparent.

Clinically, plasma cell pododermatitis begins as a soft, nonpainful swelling of multiple footpads on multiple paws (Fig. 9:78C). The central metacarpal or metatarsal pads are usually affected. Lightly pigmented pads may take on a violaceous hue. The surface of affected pads is crosshatched with white scaly striae (Fig. 9:78D). Affected pads feel mushy. The cats are usually otherwise healthy. In some cases, one or more pads may become ulcerated, which occasionally results in pain, lameness, and regional lymphadenopathy.

A minority of cats with plasma cell pododermatitis also have plasma cell stomatitis, which is characterized by ulceroproliferative gingivitis and symmetric vegetative plaques at the palatine arches.[196] In addition, an occasional cat will have immune-mediated glomerulonephritis or renal amyloidosis.[208]

Differential diagnosis includes infectious or sterile granulomas and pyogranulomas, or neoplasia. Definitive diagnosis is based on history, physical examination, aspiration cytology, culture, and biopsy. Neutrophilia and lymphocytosis may be seen, and hypergammaglobulinemia is typical. Carefully performed cultures are negative. Aspiration cytology reveals numerous plasma cells with lesser numbers of lymphocytes and neutrophils. Antinuclear antibody tests are occasionally positive,[196, 208] and direct immunofluorescence testing rarely reveals immunoglobulin at the basement membrane zone.[196, 208] However, these latter two immunologic findings are nondiagnostic.

Histopathology. Early lesions, on footpads or oral mucosa, are characterized by superficial and deep perivascular dermatitis or stomatitis, with plasma cells predominating. Later lesions are characterized by diffuse plasmacytic dermatitis or stomatitis (Fig. 9:83).[196] Many plasma cells contain Russell's bodies.

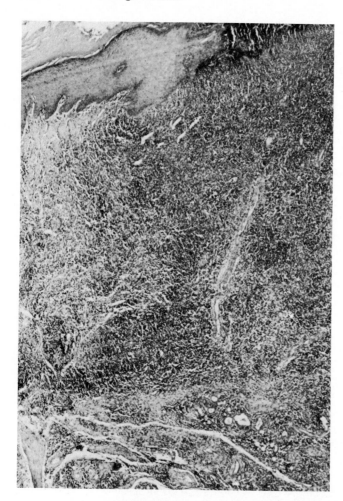

Figure 9:83. Feline plasma cell pododermatitis. Diffuse plasmacytic dermatitis.

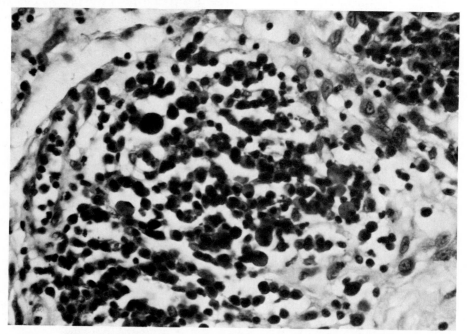

Figure 9:84. Feline plasma cell pododermatitis. Numerous plasma cells.

Variable numbers of neutrophils will be present, reflecting the absence or presence of ulceration and secondary infection (Fig. 9:84). Rarely, a leukocytoclastic vasculitis is also present.

The therapy of choice is not clear. Because plasma cell pododermatitis (1) is usually asymptomatic, and (2) often spontaneously regresses, treatment may not be indicated in most cases. Where treatment is necessary, both large doses of systemic glucocorticoid (prednisone or prednisolone given orally at 4.4 mg/ kg SID) or chrysotherapy (see p. 192) may be effective.

LICHENOID DERMATOSES

Lichenoid dermatoses are rare idiopathic skin disorders of dogs and cats.[31, 197, 198, 211a] The clinical and histopathologic features of these dermatoses suggest an immune-mediated pathomechanism. There are no apparent age, breed, or sex predilections.

Lichenoid dermatoses are characterized by the usually asymptomatic, symmetric onset of grouped, angular, flat-topped papules that develop a scaly to markedly hyperkeratotic surface (Fig. 9:85A to F). Lesions may coalesce to form hyperkeratotic, alopecic plaques. Lesions may occur anywhere. Affected animals are usually otherwise healthy.

Differential diagnosis includes staphylococcal folliculitis, dermatophytosis, demodicosis, and various granulomatous and neoplastic conditions. Definitive diagnosis is based on history, physical examination, laboratory rule-outs, and skin biopsy. Carefully performed cultures are negative. Skin biopsy reveals hyperkeratotic and hyperplastic lichenoid and hydropic interface dermatosis (Fig. 9:86). The inflammatory infiltrate is characteristically lymphoplasmacytic. If intraepidermal pustular dermatitis or suppurative folliculitis or both are present, one should suspect a lichenoid tissue reaction in response to staphylococcal infection.[197] Such cases respond to appropriate systemic antibiotic therapy.

The prognosis for canine and feline idiopathic lichenoid dermatoses appears to be good.[31, 197, 198] All cases have undergone spontaneous remission after a course of 6 months to 2 years. No form of therapy has been shown to be beneficial.

STERILE EOSINOPHILIC PUSTULOSIS

Sterile eosinophilic pustulosis is a rare idiopathic dermatosis of dogs.[195, 209] The peripheral eosinophilia, sterile tissue eosinophilia, and responsiveness to systemic glucocorticoids that characterize this syndrome suggest that it may be immune mediated. However, intradermal skin testing, hypoallergenic diets, and immunopathologic studies have not been helpful in elucidating the etiopathogenesis. No apparent age, breed, or sex predilections exist.

The onset of clinical signs is often acute, and the distribution of lesions is multifocal or generalized. Pruritic, erythematous, follicular and nonfollicular papules and pustules evolve into annular erosions with epidermal collarettes (Fig. 9:34G to H, see p. 492). Peripheral spread, central healing, and hyperpigmentation of lesions result in numerous target lesions. Although most dogs are otherwise healthy, fever, anorexia, depression, and peripheral lymphadenopathy may be present.

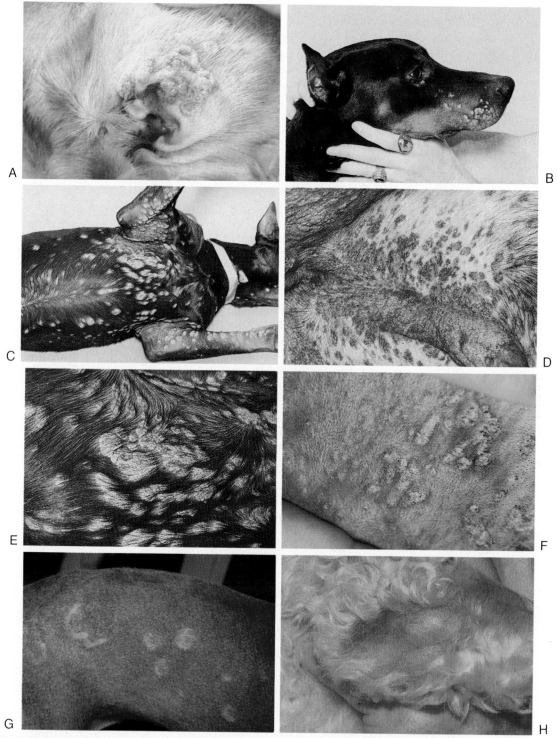

Figure 9:85. *A,* Idiopathic lichenoid dermatitis in a dog. Hyperkeratotic, yellowish lichenoid papules on the pinna. *B,* Idiopathic lichenoid dermatitis in a dog. Lichenoid papules on a face. *C,* Same dog as in *B.* Lichenoid papules and plaques on chest and forelegs. *D,* Same dog as in *B* and *C.* Hyperpigmented lichenoid papules on prepuce and inguinal skin. *E,* Same dog as in *B, C,* and *D.* Lichenoid papules and plaques on chest. *F,* Idiopathic lichenoid dermatitis in a cat. Lichenoid papules and plaques on chest (area has been clipped). *G,* Canine granulomatous sebaceous adenitis. Annular and arciform areas of alopecia and scaling. (Courtesy W. H. Miller, Jr.) *H,* Canine morphea. Alopecic, shiny plaque on lateral elbow.

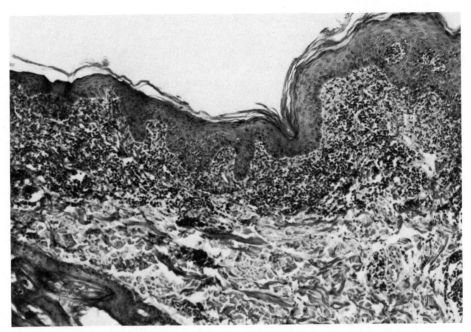

Figure 9:86. Canine idiopathic lichenoid dermatitis. Lichenoid interface dermatitis.

Differential diagnosis includes staphylococcal folliculitis, dermatophytosis, demodicosis, pemphigus foliaceus, and subcorneal pustular dermatosis. Definitive diagnosis is based on history, physical examination, hemogram, direct smears, cultures, and skin biopsy. Most dogs have peripheral eosinophilia (up to 5.6 thou/ml). Direct smears reveal numerous eosinophils, nondegenerative neutrophils, occasional acanthocytes, and no microorganisms. Carefully performed cultures are negative. Biopsy reveals intraepidermal eosinophilic pustular dermatitis and eosinophilic folliculitis and furunculosis (Fig. 9:87). Flame

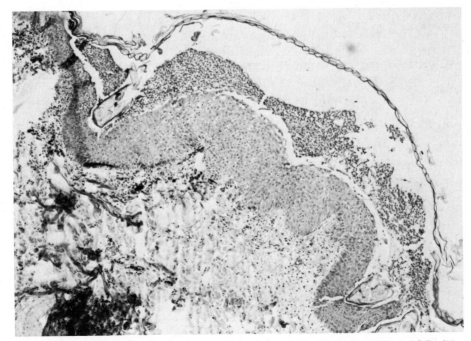

Figure 9:87. Canine sterile eosinophilic pustulosis. Subcorneal pustular dermatitis and folliculitis.

figures are occasionally seen in the surrounding dermis. Direct and indirect immunofluorescence testing is negative. Serum alpha$_2$, beta, and gamma globulins may be elevated.

Most dogs respond well to systemic glucocorticoids (prednisone or prednisolone given orally at 2.2 to 4.4 mg/kg SID) within 5 to 10 days. However, stopping treatment consistently results in relapses. Thus, long-term alternate-morning therapy is indicated, and cure is unlikely.

FELINE HYPEREOSINOPHILIC SYNDROME

The hypereosinophilic syndrome is a rare disorder of cats.[96, 199] It is characterized by a persistent idiopathic eosinophilia associated with a diffuse infiltration of various organs by mature eosinophils. The etiopathogenesis of this syndrome is unknown but is believed to be immune-mediated. There are no apparent age, breed, or sex predilections.

Tissue infiltration with mature eosinophils results in multisystemic organ dysfunction. The bone marrow, lymph nodes, liver, spleen, and gastrointestinal tract are typically involved. Rarely, affected cats may have a dermatosis characterized by generalized maculopapular erythema, severe pruritus, and marked excoriation (Fig. 9:88A, B).

Diagnosis is based on history, physical examination, laboratory rule-outs, and skin biopsy. Moderate to marked peripheral eosinophilia (up to 27.0 thou/ml) is characteristic. Direct smears of skin lesions reveal a predominance of eosinophils and basophils. Skin biopsy reveals variable degrees of superficial and deep perivascular dermatitis, with eosinophils predominating.

The prognosis is poor, as most cases fail to respond to large doses of glucocorticoids.

STERILE GRANULOMA/PYOGRANULOMA

Sterile granulomatous to pyogranulomatous skin disease is rather common in the dog but very rare in cats.[47, 135a, 139] The cause and pathogenesis are unknown. The characteristic granulomatous histopathology, absence of microbial agents and foreign material, and good response to systemic glucocorticoids suggest an immune-mediated pathogenesis. The disorder may occur in dogs of all ages, breeds, and sexes, but collies, Weimaraners, Great Danes, English bulldogs, boxers, golden retrievers, Doberman pinschers, and dachshunds may be predisposed.

Lesions are usually multiple and typically affect the head, pinnae, and paws. Firm, nonpainful, nonpruritic, 0.5 to 5 cm diameter dermal papules,

Figure 9:88. Eosinophilic dermatoses. *A*, Feline hypereosinophilic syndrome. Erythema and excoriation of face and pinna. *B*, Same cat as in *A*. Erythema, alopecia, and excoriation over the back. *C*, Eosinophilic plaque in scattered patches on the cat's abdomen and chest. Hair has been clipped away. Lesions are well demarcated, red, moist, and raised and have been licked incessantly. *D*, Eosinophilic plaque with extensive involvement of the abdomen. Note multiple raised, firm, red, and moist lesions. There is excessive licking at this stage. *E*, Feline eosinophilic plaque. Diffuse eosinophilic dermatitis. *F*, Canine eosinophilic granuloma. Erythematous papules and nodules on abdomen. *G*, Canine eosinophilic granuloma. Ulcerated nodule on prepuce. *H*, Canine eosinophilic granuloma. Ulcerated nodule on foot. (Courtesy of C. E. Griffen.)

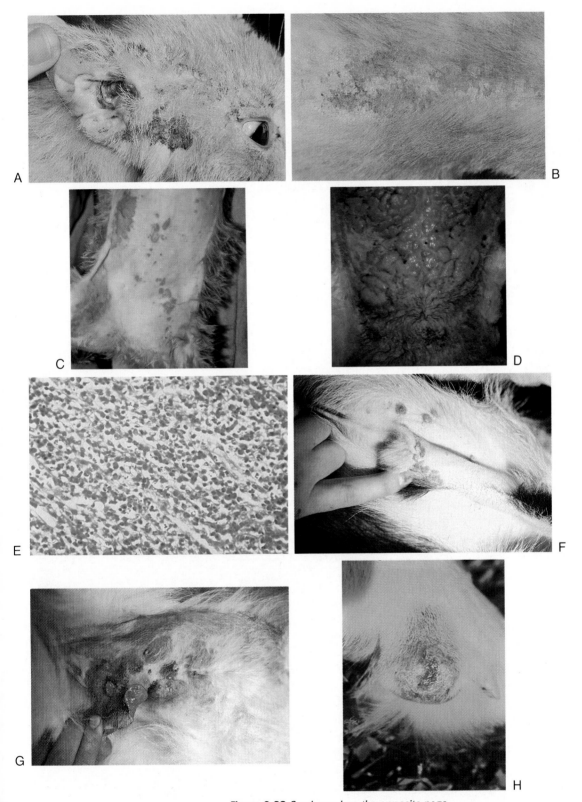

Figure 9:88 *See legend on the opposite page*

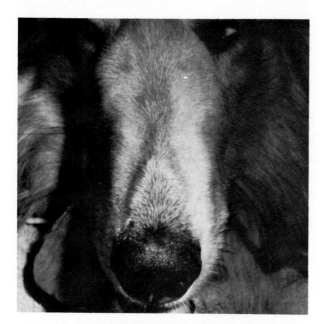

Figure 9:89. Canine idiopathic sterile granuloma. Nodules and plaques on the bridge of the nose.

plaques, and nodules are found (Figs. 9:89, 9:78F, G, p. 543). The lesions may become alopecic, ulcerated, and secondarily infected (Fig. 9:78H). Animals are usually otherwise healthy.

Differential diagnosis includes other granulomatous and pyogranulomatous (bacterial, mycotic, foreign body) and neoplastic disorders. Definitive diagnosis is based on history, physical examination, cultures, and biopsy. Cultures are best made from tissue taken by aseptic surgical biopsy techniques, whereupon they are negative. Biopsy reveals a nodular-to-diffuse granulomatous-to-pyogranulomatous dermatitis. Early lesions show a characteristic vertical orientation

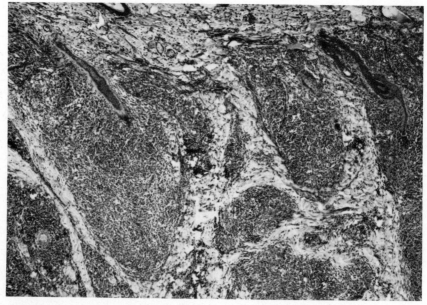

Figure 9:90. Canine idiopathic sterile granuloma. Granulomatous dermatitis that tends to "track" appendages (AOG stain).

of oblong (sausage-shaped) perifollicular granulomas or pyogranulomas, which track but do not initially involve the hair follicles (Fig. 9:90). Special stains and polarization reveal no microorganisms or foreign material.

One of the authors (D.W.S.) has seen a very small number of dogs with widespread papules, plaques, and nodules that were sterile and glucocorticoid responsive. Histologically, these lesions were characterized by nodular sarcoidal granulomatous inflammation. These cases somewhat resembled human sarcoidosis, an immune-mediated granulomatous disease.[49]

Therapy may consist of surgical excision of solitary lesions, where feasible, or systemic glucocorticoids where multiple lesions are present or surgery is impractical. Prednisone or prednisolone are administered orally at 2.2 to 4.4 mg/kg SID until the lesions have regressed (7 to 14 days). Most animals will then require prolonged alternate-morning glucocorticoid therapy. Occasionally, dogs will be unresponsive to glucocorticoids or will become refractory after variable periods of remission. Azathioprine (Imuran) is very useful in such cases[211] and is administered orally at 2.2 mg/kg SID until remission, then on alternate days (see p. 187). The oral administration of sodium iodide also has been reported to be useful in such cases.[58b]

GRANULOMATOUS SEBACEOUS ADENITIS

Granulomatous sebaceous adenitis is a rare idiopathic dermatosis of dogs.[168, 203] The granulomatous histopathology, negative cultures, and response to large doses of systemic glucocorticoids if treated early suggest an immune-mediated assault on sebaceous glands.

There is no apparent sex predilection, and the disorder tends to appear in young adult to middle-aged dogs. Although many breeds may be affected,

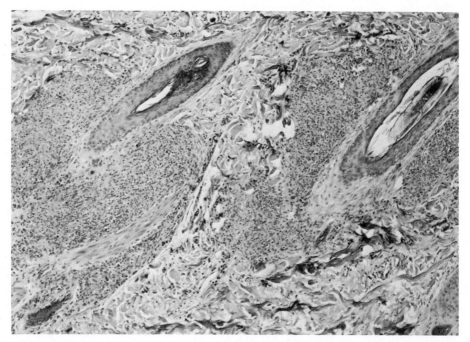

Figure 9:91. Sebaceous adenitis. Perifollicular granulomas where sebaceous glands should be.

there appear to be breed predilections for Vizslas, Akitas, Samoyeds, and black or apricot standard poodles.

In short-coated dogs, such as the Vizsla, lesions begin as generally annular areas of scaling and alopecia which tend to enlarge peripherally, become polycyclic, and occasionally coalesce (Fig. 9:85G, p. 550). Lesions are multiple, most commonly seen on the trunk, and usually asymptomatic.

In longer-coated dogs, lesions begin as diffuse facial or truncal "follicular seborrhea" (yellowish to brownish keratosebaceous casts at follicular openings and adherent to hair shafts). The hair coat becomes progressively thinned, brittle, and covered with keratosebaceous casts. Severe, chronic cases often have medically refractory seborrhea sicca and suffer recurrent bouts of staphylococcal pyoderma.

Differential diagnosis includes demodicosis, dermatophytosis, staphylococcal folliculitis, endocrinopathies, and seborrheic skin disease. Definitive diagnosis is based on history, physical examination, and biopsy. Carefully performed cultures are negative. Skin biopsies reveal variable degrees of granulomatous sebaceous adenitis. Animals with chronic cases exhibit hyperkeratosis, a variable superficial perivascular dermatitis, and a complete absence of sebaceous glands (Figs. 9:91 and 9:92).

Prognosis for recovery is generally poor. Early cases with histologically visible sebaceous glands may respond to large doses of systemic glucocorticoids

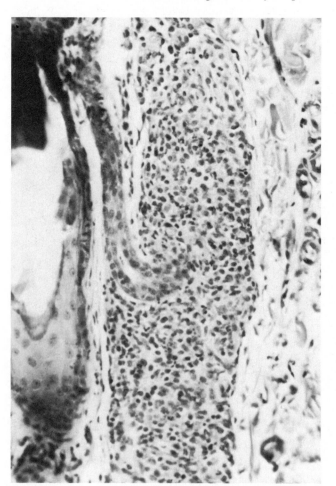

Figure 9:92. Canine granulomatous sebaceous adenitis. Sebaceous duct exiting a granuloma.

(prednisone or prednisolone, 2.2 mg/kg orally SID, then as needed). Chronic cases with no remaining viable sebaceous cells generally do not respond. These dogs can be helped with antiseborrheic shampoos and emollient rinses, but response to treatment is always partial and generally unsatisfactory. A once-daily total body spraying with 75 per cent propylene glycol in water has been reported to be helpful.[79c] Recently, isotretinoin (1 mg/kg SID orally) was reported to be effective in a Vizsla and standard poodles,[217b] and ineffective in Samoyeds and standard poodles.[79c]

CANINE LOCALIZED SCLERODERMA
(Morphea)

Localized scleroderma is a rare disease of dogs.[200] In humans, the etiopathogenesis of localized scleroderma is unknown.[62] Three predominant theories on pathogenesis have emerged: (1) the vascular theory (early endothelial injury, perivascular fibrosis, hypoxia, abnormal vascular reactivity), (2) the abnormal collagen metabolism theory (increased production of collagen, reduced collagenase activity), and (3) the immunologic theory (humoral and cell-mediated autoimmunity). In dogs, no age, breed, or sex predilections are apparent.

Canine localized scleroderma is characterized by asymptomatic, well-demarcated, sclerotic plaques that are alopecic, smooth, and shiny (Fig. 9:85*H*, p. 550). Lesions tend to be linear and occur on the trunk and limbs. Affected dogs are otherwise healthy.

Diagnosis is based on history, physical examination, and skin biopsy. Histopathologically, a fibrosing dermatitis is seen. The overlying epidermis is unremarkable (Fig. 9:93). The entire dermis and subcutis are replaced by collagenous tissue (Fig. 9:94). The normally loose-weave, fine-fibered appearance of the superficial dermis is replaced by dense collagen bundles. Piloseba

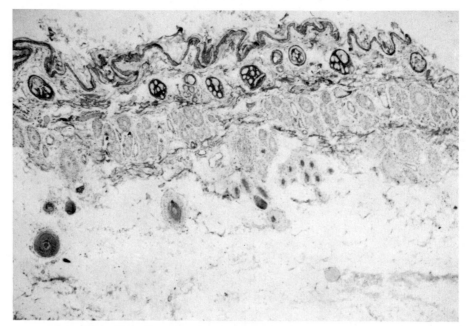

Figure 9:93. Canine morphea. Normal skin peripheral to lesion.

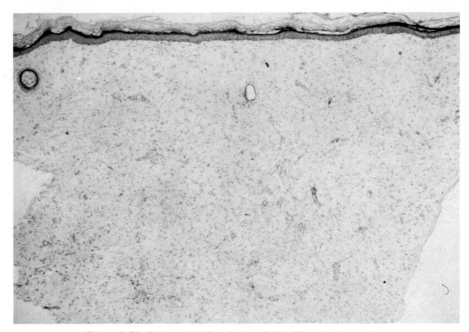

Figure 9:94. Canine morphea. Lesional skin. Fibrosing dermatitis.

ceous units are essentially absent. A mild superficial and deep perivascular accumulation of lymphohistiocytic cells is present (Fig. 9:95).

The prognosis appears to be good, with spontaneous remission occurring over a course of several weeks.[200] In humans, no forms of topical or systemic therapy are known to be of regular benefit to patients with localized scleroderma.

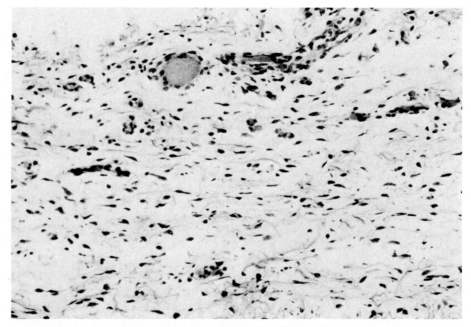

Figure 9:95. Canine morphea. Perivascular accumulation of lymphoid cells within subcutaneous fat.

ALOPECIA AREATA

Alopecia areata is a rare disorder of dogs and cats, characterized by patches of noninflammatory hair loss.

CAUSE AND PATHOGENESIS

Alopecia areata is of unknown cause and unclear pathogenesis.[136, 141] Genetic, endocrine, and psychologic factors have been thought to play a role in humans with alopecia areata. In addition, the following observations in humans with alopecia areata have suggested that this disorder may have an immune-mediated basis: (1) accumulations of lymphoid cells around hair bulbs during the active phase of the disease, (2) occasional association of alopecia areata with other immune-mediated diseases, (3) increased incidence of various autoantibodies in alopecia areata, (4) decreased numbers of circulating T cells, and (5) the deposition of C3 or IgG and IgM or both at the basement membrane zone of the hair follicles in lesional and normal scalp by direct immunofluorescence testing.[62, 124, 136, 141]

CLINICAL FEATURES

In dogs and cats, alopecia areata is characterized by focal or multifocal patches of asymptomatic, noninflammatory alopecia.[47, 83, 139] There are no apparent age, breed, or sex predilections. The alopecic areas are usually well circumscribed, and the exposed skin appears normal (Fig. 9:96). Chronically

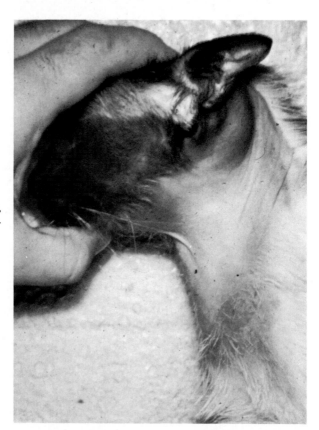

Figure 9:96. Alopecia areata. Well-circumscribed, noninflammatory alopecia of neck. (Courtesy J. D. Conroy.)

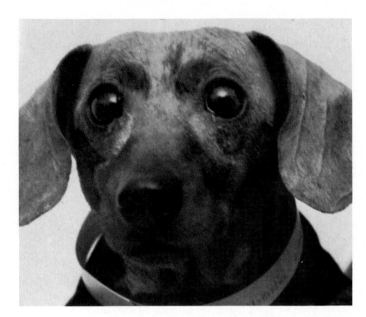

Figure 9:97. Alopecia areata in a dachshund. Alopecia of pinnae and around eyes.

alopecic areas may become variably hyperpigmented. Lesions may occur anywhere, especially the head, neck, and trunk, and are usually asymmetric (Fig. 9:97). "Exclamation point" hairs may be seen near the margin of enlarging lesions. These are short, stubby hairs with frayed, fractured, pigmented distal ends. The shafts undulate or gradually taper. Occasionally alopecia areata may be confined to the dark-haired areas of multicolored hair coats.

DIAGNOSIS

The differential diagnosis includes dermatophytosis, demodicosis, staphylococcal folliculitis, psychogenic alopecia, and endocrinopathies. Definitive diagnosis is based on the insidious onset of asymptomatic, noninflammatory alopecia and on skin biopsy.

Histopathology. The characteristic early histopathologic findings include a peribulbar accumulation of lymphocytes, histiocytes, and plasma cells ("swarm of bees," lymphoplasmacytic perifolliculitis). However, this early change may be difficult to demonstrate, requiring multiple biopsies from the advancing edge of early lesions. Later, the histopathologic findings consist of a predominance of catagen and telogen hair follicles, as well as follicular atrophy. Chronic lesions may show complete absence of hair follicles and a fibrous tract associated with orphaned apocrine and sebaceous glands and arrector pili muscles.

CLINICAL MANAGEMENT

The prognosis for alopecia areata in humans is usually good, with most patients making a complete recovery within 3 to 5 years, with or without therapy. Although topical, intralesional, or systemic glucocorticoids are often recommended for the treatment of alopecia areata in humans, dogs, and cats, there is no clear evidence that they are beneficial.[141, 229] The biologic behavior of alopecia areata in dogs and cats is unclear. One of the authors (D.W.S.) has seen a few dogs spontaneously recover after a course of 6 months to 2 years. Initial hair regrowth is often a color lighter than normal (leukotrichia).

FELINE INDOLENT ULCER
(Eosinophilic Ulcer, Rodent Ulcer)

Indolent ulcer is a common cutaneous and oral mucosal lesion of cats. The cause and pathogenesis of these lesions are not always known. However, several observations suggest that many, if not all, cases of feline indolent ulcer are associated with a hypersensitivity response, some of these cases being as follows: (1) occcurrence of these lesions in cats with documented flea bite hypersensitivity, atopy, or food hypersensitivity, wherein the course of the lesions parallels the course of the underlying hypersensitivity; (2) seasonal recurrence (flea bite hypersensitivity, atopy) of many of the lesions; (3) spontaneous remission of even chronic, medically refractory lesions when affected cats are hospitalized or moved to a new environment; and (4) beneficial response of these lesions to glucocorticoids and, where appropriate, hyposensitization, hypoallergenic diet, or flea control.[131, 160, 187, 196, 202]

Clinically, most indolent ulcers occur unilaterally on the upper lip (Fig. 9:98*A, B*). However, lesions also occur in the oral cavity, in other areas of the skin, and bilaterally (Fig. 9:98*C, H*). The lesions are usually well circumscribed, red-brown, alopecic, and glistening and possess a raised border. Pruritus and pain are rare. Peripheral lymphadenopathy may be present. There are no age or breed predilections, but females may be predisposed. Lip ulcers appear to be precancerous and may undergo malignant transformation into squamous cell carcinoma. Cats with indolent ulcers may also have eosinophilic plaques or eosinophilic granulomas or both.

Differential diagnosis includes infectious ulcers (bacterial, fungal, feline leukemia virus (FeLV)–associated), trauma, and neoplasia (squamous cell carcinoma, mast cell tumor, lymphosarcoma). Carefully performed cultures are negative. Biopsy is nondiagnostic, revealing hyperplastic, ulcerated, superficial perivascular dermatitis, with neutrophils and mononuclear cells usually predominating, and fibrosing dermatitis (Fig. 9:99). Blood eosinophilia and tissue eosinophilia are rare. Chronic, recurrent, increasingly medically refractory cases should be evaluated for underlying flea bite hypersensitivity (see p. 482), atopy (see p. 450), and food hypersensitivity (see p. 470).

Therapy with systemic glucocorticoids is often effective. Prednisone or prednisolone are given orally at 4.4 mg/kg SID until lesions are healed. Alternatively, methylprednisolone acetate (Depo-Medrol) may be given subcutaneously at 20 mg/cat every 2 weeks until lesions are healed. Recurrent lesions may be managed with alternate-evening oral prednisone or prednisolone (see p. 203) or repeated subcutaneous injections of methylprednisolone (*never* more frequently than every 2 months). Medically refractory lesions should be evaluated for underlying hypersensitivity disorders, and managed appropriately. Other methods of treatment reported to be occasionally successful in feline indolent ulcer include radiotherapy, cryosurgery, laser therapy, surgical excision, mixed bacterial vaccines, and immunomodulating drugs such as levamisole, thiabendazole, and aurothioglucose (Solganal).[126a, 126b, 187] Progestational compounds, such as megestrol acetate (Ovaban, Megace) or medroxyprogesterone acetate (Depo-Provera), have also been effective in many cases of feline indolent ulcer. However, because of the side effects resulting from these drugs, they are *not* recommended (see p. 209).

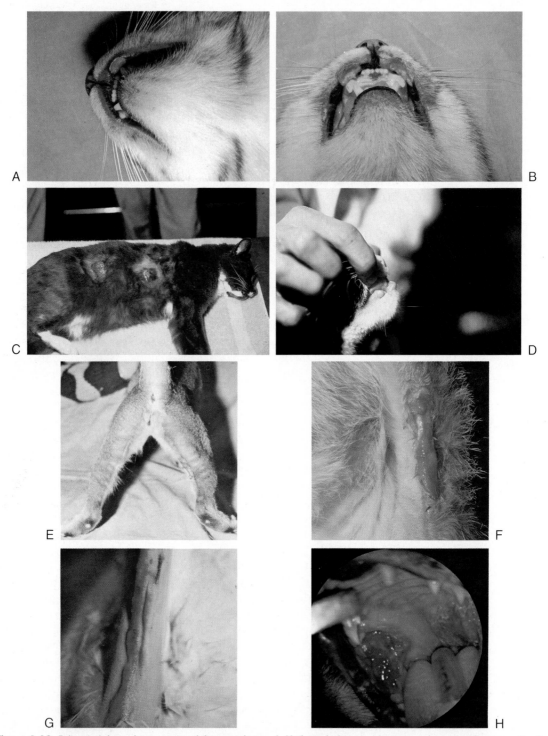

Figure 9:98. Feline indolent ulcer—eosinophilic granuloma. *A,* Unilateral ulcerated lesion on the upper lip opposite the lower canine tooth (indolent ulcer). *B,* Bilateral indolent ulcers that are chronic and necrotic. *C,* Indolent ulcers on the body of a cat. *D,* Eosinophilic granuloma on lip of a cat in area often favored by an indolent ulcer. *E,* Abyssinian cat with eosinophilic granuloma in typical location on posterior thigh. *F,* Same cat as in *E* with the lesion clipped. The lesion is thin and cordlike but very firm. The ulceration is not a common finding. *G,* Typical eosinophilic granuloma on a white cat's rear leg with hair clipped away. The firm cordlike masses are slightly pink and not ulcerated, painful, or pruritic. *H,* Indolent ulcer bilaterally located at the angles of the jaw behind the last molars. A metal mouth gag and plastic endotracheal tube can be seen. The ulcerated lesions have a fibronecrotic surface. Radiation therapy caused prompt remission.

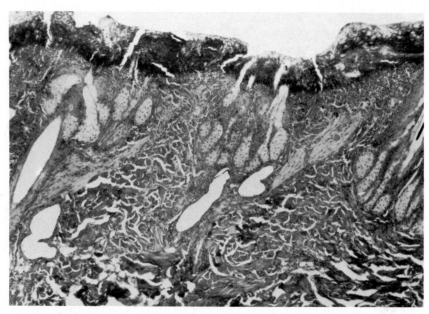

Figure 9:99. Histologic section of indolent ulcer (eosinophilic ulcer). There is surface ulceration with fibrin covering the necrotic surface, and a dense mononuclear cellular infiltrate in the dermis. Note the ulcerative perivascular dermatitis. (From Scott, D. W.: Feline dermatology 1900–1978: a monograph, J.A.A.H.A. *16*:331, 1980.)

FELINE EOSINOPHILIC PLAQUE

Eosinophilic plaque is a common cutaneous lesion of cats. The cause and pathogenesis of these lesions are not always known. However, several observations suggest that many, if not all, cases of feline eosinophilic plaque are associated with underlying hypersensitivity responses such as flea bite hypersensitivity, atopy, or food hypersensitivity (see feline indolent ulcer).[131, 160, 187, 196, 202]

Clinically, most eosinophilic plaques occur on the abdomen and medial thighs (see Fig. 9:88C, D, p. 553). Lesions may be single or multiple, and may also occur in the oral cavity or in other areas of the skin. Eosinophilic plaques are well circumscribed, raised, round to oval, red, oozing, often ulcerated, and 0.5 to 7 cm in diameter. Pruritus is usually severe. Peripheral lymphadenopathy may be present. Cats with eosinophilic plaque may also have indolent ulcers or eosinophilic granulomas or both. There are no age or breed predilections, but females may be predisposed.

Differential diagnosis includes infectious granulomas (bacterial, fungal) and neoplasia (mast cell tumor, lymphosarcoma). Carefully performed cultures are negative. Biopsy reveals hyperplastic superficial and deep perivascular dermatitis with eosinophilia, to diffuse eosinophilic dermatitis (Fig. 9:88E, p. 553). Diffuse spongiosis which involves hair follicle outer root sheaths, and eosinophilic microvesicles and microabscesses may be seen. Due to the large numbers of mast cells commonly present in eosinophilic plaques, close inspection of mast cell morphology and tendency of mast cells to form nodules is in order to distinguish this condition from mast cell tumor. Blood and tissue eosinophilia are constant.

Methods of treatment are as described for feline indolent ulcer.

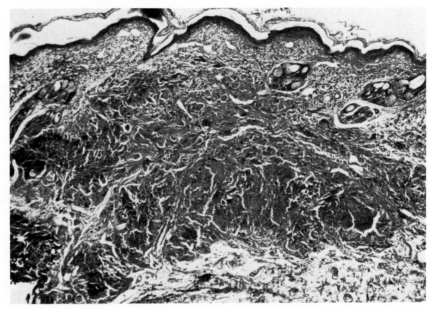

Figure 9:100. Feline eosinophilic granuloma. Granulomatous dermatitis associated with collagen degeneration. (From Scott, D. W.: Feline dermatology 1900–1978: a monograph, J.A.A.H.A. *16*:331, 1980.)

FELINE EOSINOPHILIC GRANULOMA
(Linear Granuloma)

Eosinophilic granuloma is a common cutaneous and oral mucosal lesion of cats. The cause and pathogenesis of these lesions are not always known. However several observations suggest that many, if not all, cases of feline eosinophilic granuloma are associated with underlying hypersensitivity responses such as flea bite hypersensitivity, atopy, or food hypersensitivity (see Feline Indolent Ulcer).[131, 160, 187, 196, 202]

Clinically, most eosinophilic granulomas occur on the caudal thighs, the face, and in the oral cavity. On the caudal thigh, the lesions are usually well-circumscribed, raised, firm, yellowish-to-pink plaques with a distinctive linear configuration ("linear granuloma") (Fig. 9:98*E* to *G*). They are often discovered accidentally, as they are usually nonpruritic. Lesions on the face and in the oral cavity have a papular-to-nodular configuration (Fig. 9:98*H*). Eosinophilic granuloma is the most common cause of lower lip swellings and nodules ("pouting cats") and asymptomatic swollen chins ("fat chinned cats," feline chin edema) in the cat (Fig. 9:98*D*). When the surface of eosinophilic granulomas is eroded or ulcerated, a characteristic speckling with pinpoint white foci (corresponding to foci of collagen degeneration) may be seen. Peripheral lymphadenopathy may be present. Cats with eosinophilic granuloma may also have indolent ulcers or eosinophilic plaques or both. There are no age or breed predilections, but females may be predisposed.

Differential diagnosis includes infectious granulomas (bacterial, fungal) and neoplasia. Biopsy reveals nodular-to-diffuse granulomatous dermatitis with multifocal areas of collagen degeneration (Fig. 9:100). Eosinophils and multi-nucleated histiocytic giant cells are common (Fig. 9:101). Flame figures may be seen. Older lesions are characterized by palisading granuloma formation around

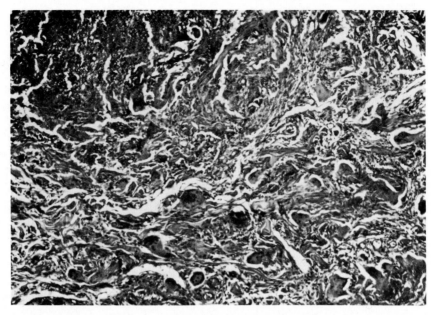

Figure 9:101. Feline eosinophilic granuloma. Granulomatous dermatitis associated with collagen degeneration and foreign body giant cells. (High-power view of Fig. 9:100.)

the foci of degenerate collagen. Blood eosinophilia may be seen, especially with oral lesions. Carefully performed cultures are negative.

Methods of treatment are as described for feline indolent ulcer. Interestingly, many eosinophilic granulomas occurring in cats less than 1 year of age spontaneously regress over a period of 3 to 5 months.

CANINE EOSINOPHILIC GRANULOMA

Eosinophilic granulomas are rare, idiopathic nodular-to-plaquelike lesions associated with collagen degeneration in the oral cavity and skin of dogs.

CAUSE AND PATHOGENESIS

The cause of cutaneous granulomas associated with collagen degeneration is poorly understood.[81a, 188] In humans, occasional cases have been reported following insect bites, tuberculin tests, and other forms of trauma. Proposed pathomechanisms include vasculitis, microangiopathy, disorder of fibrinolysis, disorder of phagocytic function, disorder of catabolic enzyme release, and cell-mediated immune response. In dogs, no antecedent trauma or diseases have been recognized, and cultures for bacteria, fungi, and viruses are negative. Macerated tissue from lesions produces no lesions in dogs into which it is injected. The tissue eosinophilia, occasional blood eosinophilia, and glucocorticoid responsiveness of the lesions have prompted speculation on a hypersensitivity state. Additionally, the tendency of the oral form of the disease to occur in Siberian huskies has suggested a genetic basis for the disease. Some authors have reported the seasonal recurrence of cutaneous eosinophilic granulomas in dogs.[58b]

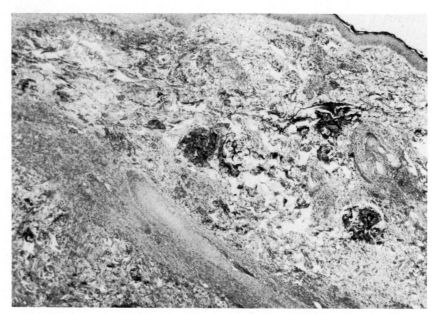

Figure 9:102. Canine eosinophilic granuloma. Granulomatous dermatitis associated with collagen degeneration.

CLINICAL FEATURES

Although any age, breed, or sex of dog may be affected, eosinophilic granulomas occur most commonly in dogs less than 3 years of age (80 per cent of cases), Siberian huskies (76 per cent), and males (72 per cent). Eosinophilic granulomas occur most commonly in the oral cavity as ulcerated palatine plaques and vegetative lingual masses. The vegetative lingual masses often have a greenish brown hue. Less commonly, they occur as multiple cutaneous papules, nodules, and plaques, over the ventral abdomen, prepuce, and flanks (see Fig. 9:88F to H, p. 552). The cutaneous lesions are usually nonpruritic and nonpainful, and the dogs are otherwise healthy. Rarely, solitary lesions occur in the external ear canal.[211]

DIAGNOSIS

Differential diagnosis includes granulomatous and neoplastic disorders. Diagnosis is based on biopsy. Characteristic histopathologic findings include variable-size foci of collagen degeneration, eosinophilic and histiocytic cellular infiltration, and palisading granulomas (Figs. 9:102 and 9:103). Flame figures may be seen. Properly performed cultures are negative, and blood eosinophilia is occasionally seen.

CLINICAL MANAGEMENT

Canine eosinophilic granulomas are usually very glucocorticoid responsive. Seventy-eight per cent of the cases were treated with prednisolone or prednisone orally (0.5 to 2.2 mg/kg/day), their lesions regressed within 10 to 20 days, and no further therapy was needed. Some lesions undergo spontaneous remission.

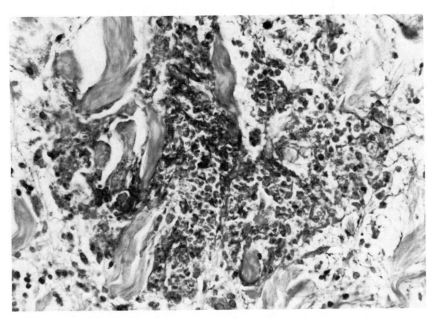

Figure 9:103. Canine eosinophilic granuloma. Focal collagen degeneration and accumulation of eosinophils.

AMYLOIDOSIS

Amyloidosis is a generic term that signifies the abnormal extracellular deposition of one of a family of unrelated proteins that share certain characteristic staining properties and ultrastructural features.[27a, 62, 124] Amyloidosis is not a single disease entity, and amyloid may accumulate as a result of a variety of different pathogenetic mechanisms.

Although the pathogenesis of amyloidosis is unclear, it is morphologically related to cells of the mononuclear phagocytic system, plasma cells, and keratinocytes. Functional studies suggest that such cells play at least a partial role in the genesis of amyloidosis.

Cutaneous amyloidosis associated with a monoclonal gammopathy was reported in an adult female Cocker spaniel.[185] Cutaneous hemorrhage could be induced by flicking the abdominal skin briskly with one's finger or by removing hair. If the skin was traumatized severely, blood oozed through the skin within seconds and clotted immediately. Skin biopsy revealed an amorphous, homogeneous, eosinophilic superficial dermis. The walls of blood vessels in the involved area were thickened by deposition of the homogeneous eosinophilic material. The material was congo red–positive, and a green birefringence of the material was seen in congo red–stained sections examined with polarized light. A monoclonal serum IgG paraprotein was found. No treatment was given, and the dog remained unchanged for 14 months.

References

1. Abdou, N. I.: The idiotype–anti-idiotype network in human autoimmunity. J. Clin. Immunol. 5:365, 1985.
2. Ackerman, A. B.: Histologic Diagnosis of Inflammatory Skin Diseases. Lea & Febiger, Philadelphia, 1978.
3. Ackerman, L., and Bargman, H.: Postvaccinal signs suggestive of systemic lupus erythematosus in a dog. Mod. Vet. Pract. 66:867, 1985.
4. Adkinson, N. F.: The radioallergosorbent test in 1981—limitations and refinements. J. Allergy Clin. Immunol. 67:87, 1981.

5. Agnello, V.: Lupus diseases associated with hereditary and acquired deficiencies of complement. Springer Sem. Immunopathol. 9:161, 1986.

6. Ahmed, A. R.: Bullous pemphigoid. Clin. Dermatol. 5:1987.

7. Ahmed, A. R.: Pemphigus. Clin. Dermatol. 1:1983.

8. Ahmed, S. A., et al.: Sex hormones, immune responses, and autoimmune diseases. Am. J. Pathol. 121:531, 1985.

9. Alhaidari, Z., and Ortonne, J. P.: La pemphigoide bulleuse canine: cas clinique. Point Vet. 16:41, 1984.

10. Andrews, B. S., et al.: Immunopathology of cutaneous lupus erythematosus defined by murine monoclonal abnormalities. J. Am. Acad. Dermatol. 15:474, 1986.

11. Arnett, F. C.: HLA and genetic predisposition to lupus erythematosus and other dermatologic disorders. J. Am. Acad. Dermatol. 13:472, 1985.

11a. Atkins, P. C., and Zweiman, B.: The IgE–mediated late-phase skin response—unraveling the enigma. J. Allergy Clin. Immunol. 79:12, 1987.

12. August, J. R.: The intradermal test as a diagnostic aid for canine atopic disease. J. Am. Anim. Hosp. Assoc. 18:164, 1982.

13. August, J. R.: The reaction of canine skin to the intradermal injection of allergenic extracts. J. Am. Med. Hosp. Assoc. 18:157, 1982.

14. August, J. R.: Dietary hypersensitivity in dogs: Cutaneous manifestations, diagnosis, and management. Compend. Cont. Ed. 7:469, 1985.

15. August, J. R., and Chickering, W. R.: Pemphigus foliaceus causing lameness in four dogs. Compend. Cont. Ed. 7:894, 1985.

16. Bahna, S. L., and Furukawa, C. T.: Food allergy: Diagnosis and treatment. Ann. Allergy 512:574, 1983.

17. Baker, J. R., et al.: Pathological effects of bleomycin in the skin of dogs and monkeys. Toxicol. Appl. Pharmacol. 25:190, 1973.

18. Bamford, J. T. M., et al.: Atopic eczema unresponsive to evening primrose oil (linoleic and α-linoleinic acids). J. Am. Acad. Dermatol. 13:959, 1985.

19. Barr, R. M., et al.: Levels of arachidonic acid and its metabolites in the skin in human allergic and irritant contact dermatitis. Brit. J. Dermatol. 111:23, 1984.

20. Barta, O.: Serum's lymphocyte immunoregulatory factors (slif). Vet. Immunol. Immunopathol. 4:279, 1983.

20a. Becker, A. B., et al.: Mast cell heterogeneity in dog skin. Anat. Rec. 213:477, 1985.

20b. Becker, A. B., et al.: Cutaneous mast cell heterogeneity: Response to allergy in atopic dogs. J. Allergy Clin. Immunol. 78:937, 1986.

21. Bennett, D., et al.: Two cases of pemphigus erythematosus (the Senear-Usher syndrome) in the dog. J. Small Anim. Pract. 26:219, 1985.

22. Beutner, E. H., et al.: Immunofluorescence tests. Int. J. Dermatol. 24:405, 1985.

23. Beutner, E. H., et al.: Immunopathology of the Skin III. Churchill Livingstone, New York, 1987.

24. Bevier, D. E.: The reaction of feline skin to the intradermal injection of allergenic extracts and passive cutaneous anaphylaxis using serum from skin test positive cats. Proceedings, Ann. Meet. Am. Acad. Vet. Dermatol. and Am. Coll. Vet. Dermatol., 1987.

25. Bjorksten, B., and Ahlstedt, S.: Relevance of animal models for studies for immune regulation of atopic allergy. Allergy 39:317, 1984.

26. Bjorksten, F., et al.: Assay of the biologic activity of allergen skin test preparations. J. Allergy Clin. Immunol. 73:324, 1984.

26a. Black, J. W., et al.: Definition and antagonism of histamine H_2-receptors. Nature (London) 236:385, 1972.

26b. Bos, J. D., and Kapsenberg, M. L.: The skin immune system. Immunol. Today 7:235, 1986.

27. Breathnach, S. M.: Current understanding of the aetiology and clinical implications of cutaneous graft-versus-host disease. Brit. J. Dermatol. 114:139, 1986.

27a. Breathnach, S. M.: Amyloid and amyloidosis. J. Am. Acad. Dermatol. 18:1, 1988.

28. Breitschwerdt, E. B., et al.: Clinical and laboratory characterization of Basenjis with immunoproliferative small intestinal disease. Am. J. Vet. Res. 45:267, 1984.

29. Breitschwerdt, E. B.: Immunoproliferative enteropathy of Basenjis. Proceedings, Kal. Kan. Symp. 8:111, 1984.

30. Bronner, A. K., and Hood, A. F.: Cutaneous complications of chemotherapeutic agents. J. Am. Acad. Dermatol. 9:645, 1983.

31. Buerger, R. G., and Scott, D. W.: Lichenoid dermatitis in a cat: A case report. J. Am. Anim. Hosp. Assoc. 24:55, 1988.

32. Butler, J. M., et al.: Pruritic dermatitis in asthmatic Basenji-Greyhound dogs: A model for human atopic dermatitis. J. Am. Acad. Dermatol. 8:33, 1983.

33. Bystryn, J. C., and Sabdinski, M.: Effect of substrate on indirect immunofluorescence tests for intercellular and basement membrane zone antibodies. J. Am. Acad. Dermatol. 15:973, 1986.

34. Caciolo, P. L., et al.: Pemphigus foliaceus in eight cats and results of induction therapy using azathioprine. J. Am. Anim. Hosp. Assoc. 20:571, 1984.

35. Caciolo, P. L., et al.: Michel's medium as a preservative for immunofluorescent staining of cutaneous biopsy specimens in dogs and cats. Am. J. Vet. Res. 45:128, 1984.

36. Calvert, C. A.: Confirming a diagnosis of heartworm infection in dogs. Vet. Med. 82:232, 1987.

37. Calvert, C. A.: The best tests for evaluating the heartworm-infected dog. Vet. Med. 82:238, 1987.

38. Calvert, C. A.: Treating for heartworm disease and its complications; preventing infection whenever possible. Vet. Med. 82:254, 1987.

39. Callen, J. P.: Colchicine is effective in controlling chronic cutaneous vasculitis. J. Am. Acad. Dermatol. 13:193, 1985.

40. Callen, J. P.: Lupus erythematosus. Clin. Dermatol. 3:1985.

41. Camisa, C., and Sharma, H. M.: Vesicobullous systemic lupus erythematosus. Report of two cases and a review of the literature. J. Am. Acad. Dermatol. 9:924, 1983.

42. Campbell, K. L., et al: Generalized leukoderma and poliosis following uveitis in a dog. J. Am. Anim. Hosp. Assoc. 22:121, 1986.

43. Carlotti, D.: Diagnostic de la dermatite par allergie aux piqures de puce (DAPP) chez le chien. Interet des intradermoreactions. Prat. Med. Chirurg. Anim. Comp. 20:41, 1985.

44. Carlotti, D.: La dermatite atopique du chien. Point Vet. 17:5, 1985.

45. Chan, S. C., et al: Elevated leukocyte phosphodiesterase as a basis for depressed cyclic adenosine monophosphate responses in the Basenji greyhound dog model of asthma. J. Allergy Clin. Immunol. 76:148, 1985.

46. Conroy, J. D.: An overview of immune-mediated mucocutaneous diseases of the dog and cat. I. Diseases based on allergic reactions. Am. J. Dermatopathol. 5:505, 1983.

47. Conroy, J. D.: An overview of immune-mediated mucocutaneous diseases of the dog and cat. II.

Other diseases based on immunologic mechanisms. Am. J. Dermatopathol. 5:595, 1983.

48. Corman, L. C.: The relationship between nutrition, infection, and immunity. Med. Clin. North Am. 69:519, 1985.

49. Dahl, M. V.: Immunodermatology II. Year Book Medical Publishers, Chicago, 1988.

50. Dalziel, K., et al: Treatment of chronic discoid lupus erythematosus with an oral gold compound (auranofin). Brit. J. Dermatol. 115:211, 1986.

51. Daniel, G. B., and Patterson, J. S.: Toxic epidermal necrolysis: a case report. J. Am. Anim. Hosp. Assoc. 21:631, 1985.

52. Davies, P., et al: The role of arachidonic acid oxygenation products in pain and inflammation. Ann. Rev. Immunol. 2:335, 1984.

53. DeBoer, D. J., et al: Circulating immune complex concentrations in selected cases of skin disease in dogs. Am. J. Vet. Res. 49:143, 1988.

54. Delafuente, J. C.: Immunosenescence. Med. Clin. North Am. 69:475, 1985.

55. De Swarte, R. D.: Drug allergy—problems and strategies. J. Allergy Clin. Immunol. 74:209, 1984.

56. Diaz, L. A., et al: Human pemphigus autoantibodies are pathogenic to squamous epithelium. Ann. N. Y. Acad. Sci. 475:181, 1986.

57. Donahue, R. E., and Schultz, K. T.: Food allergy testing. Vet. Allergist, Fall 1983.

58. Duschet, P., et al: Erythromelanoderma with eosinophilic spongiosis and epidermal intercellular antibodies. Differentiation from pemphigus. J. Cut. Pathol. 13:40, 1986.

58a. Fabries, L.: Syndrome "VKH" chez le chien. Au sujet de deux cas cliniques. Prat. Med. Chirurg. Anim. Comp. 19:393, 1984.

58b. Fadok, V. A.: Granulomatous dermatitis in dogs and cats. Semin. Vet. Med. Surg. 2:186, 1987.

59. Fadok, V. A., and Barrie, J.: Sulfasalazine responsive vasculitis in the dog: a case report. J. Am. Anim. Hosp. Assoc. 20:161, 1984.

60. Felsburg, P. J., et al: Selective IgA deficiency in the dog. Clin. Immunol. Immunopathol. 36:297, 1985.

60a. Felsburg, P. J., et al.: A canine model for variable, combined immunodeficiency. Clin. Res. 30:347A, 1982.

61. Finan, M. C., and Schroeter, A. L.: Cutaneous immunofluorescence study of erythema multiforme: correlation with light microscopic patterns and etiologic agents. J. Am. Acad. Dermatol. 10:497, 1984.

62. Fitzpatrick, T. B., et al: Dermatology in General Medicine III. McGraw-Hill Book Company, New York, 1986.

63. Fredenberg, M. F., and Malkinson, F. D.: Sulfone therapy in the treatment of leukocytoclastic vasculitis. J. Am. Acad. Dermatol. 16:772, 1987.

64. Frosch, P. J., et al: A double blind trial of H_1 and H_2 receptor antagonists in the treatment of atopic dermatitis. Arch. Dermatol. Res. 276:36, 1984.

65. Fudenberg, H. H., et al: Basic and Clinical Immunology III. Lange Medical Publications, Los Altos, 1980.

66. Furukawa, F., et al: Dermatopathological studies on skin lesions of MRL mice. Arch. Dermatol. Res. 276:186, 1984.

67. Furukawa, F., et al: Genetic studies on the skin lupus band test in New Zealand mice. Clin. Exp. Immunol. 59:146, 1985.

68. Gammon, W. R., et al: Complement-activating immune deposits in systemic lupus erythematosus skin. J. Invest. Dermatol. 81:14, 1983.

69. Gammon, W. R., et al: Evidence supporting a role for immune complex–mediated inflammation in the pathogenesis of bullous lesions of systemic lupus erythematosus. J. Invest. Dermatol. 81:320, 1983.

70. Garthwaite, G., et al: Location of immunoglobulins and complement (C3) at the surface and within the skin of dogs. J. Comp. Pathol. 93:185, 1983.

71. Gelberg, H. B., et al: Antiepithelial autoantibodies associated with the feline eosinophilic granuloma complex. Am. J. Vet. Res. 46:263, 1985.

72. Gibson, L. E., et al: Direct immunofluorescence for the study of cutaneous drug eruptions. Acta Dermatovenereol. 66:39, 1986.

73. Gibson, L. E., and Winkelmann, R. K.: Cutaneous granulomatous vasculitis: its relationship to systemic disease. J. Am. Acad. Dermatol. 14:492, 1986.

74. Giger, U., et al: Sulfadiazine-induced allergy in six Doberman pinschers. J. Am. Vet. Med. Assoc. 186:479, 1985.

74a. Goldberg, G. N.: Erythema multiforme. Controversies and recent advances. Adv. Dermatol. 2:73, 1987.

74b. Goldschmidt, M. H., and Wolfsdorf, K.: Erythema multiforme—a retrospective study of 14 cases in the dog. Ann. Meet. Am. Acad. Vet. Dermatol. and Am. Coll. Vet. Dermatol., 1988.

75. Gorbsky, G., et al: Desmosomal antigens are not recognized by the majority of pemphigus autoimmune sera. J. Invest. Dermatol. 80:475, 1983.

76. Gorman, N. T., and Werner, L. L.: Immune-mediated diseases of the dog and cat. I. Basic concepts and the systemic immune-mediated diseases. Brit. Vet. J. 142:395, 1986.

77. Gosselin, Y., et al: Intradermoreaction and hyposensitization in canine atopy. Can. Vet. J. 24:101, 1983.

78. Graham, P., et al: A study of hypoallergenic diets and oral sodium cromoglycate in the management of atopic eczema. Brit. J. Dermatol. 110:457, 1984.

79. Griffin, C. E.: Nasal dermatitis. Dermatol. Rep. 2:1, 1983.

79a. Griffin, C.: Pinnal diseases. The Complete Manual of Ear Care. Solvay Veterinary, Inc., 1986, p. 21.

79b. Griffin, C. E.: Diagnosis and management of primary autoimmune skin disease: a review. Semin. Vet. Med. Surg. 2:173, 1987.

79c. Griffin, C. E.: Common dermatoses of the Akita, Shar-Pei and Chow Chow. Ann. Meet. Am. Acad. Vet. Dermatol. and Am. Coll. Vet. Dermatol., 1988.

79d. Griffin, C. E.: RAST and ELISA testing in canine atopy. In Kirk, R. W. (ed.): Current Veterinary Therapy X. W. B. Saunders Company, Philadelphia (in press).

79e. Griffin, C. E., and Rosenkrantz, W. S.: Direct immunofluorescence testing: a comparison of two laboratories in the diagnosis of canine immune-mediated skin disease. Semin. Vet. Med. Surg. 2:202, 1987.

80. Gross, T. L., and Halliwell, R. E. W.: Lesions of experimental flea bite hypersensitivity in the dog. Vet. Pathol. 22:78, 1985.

81. Grossman, C. J.: Regulation of the immune response by sex steroids. Endocr. Rev. 5:435, 1984.

81a. Guaguere, E., and Magnol, J. P.: Granulomes eosinophiliques buccaux chez un Chow-Chow. Pract. Med. Chirurg. Anim. Comp. 21:309, 1986.

82. Guenthor, L. C.: Inherited disorders of complement. J. Am. Acad. Dermatol. 9:815, 1983.

83. Guernsey, G. E.: Alopecia areata in a dog. Can. Vet. J. 26:403, 1985.

83a. Gilford, W. G.: Primary immunodeficiency diseases of dogs and cats. Compend. Cont. Ed. 9:641, 1987.

83b. Haines, D. M., et al.: Avidin-biotin-peroxidase complex immunohistochemistry to detect immunoglobulin in formalin fixed skin biopsies in canine autoimmune skin diseases. Can. J. Vet. Res. 51:104, 1987.

84. Halliwell, R. E. W.: Hyposensitization in the treatment of flea-bite hypersensitivity: results of a double-blind study. J. Am. Anim. Hosp. Assoc. 17:249, 1981.

85. Halliwell, R. E. W., et al: Physiochemical properties of canine IgE. Transplant. Proc. 7:537, 1975.

86. Halliwell, R. E. W., and Kunkle, G. A.: The radioallergosorbent test in the diagnosis of canine atopic disease. J. Allergy Clin. Immunol. 62:236, 1978.

87. Halliwell, R. E. W.: Immunology and dermatology. Aust. Vet. Practit. 13:177, 1983.

88. Halliwell, R. E. W.: Flea allergy dermatitis. Current Veterinary Therapy VIII. W. B. Saunders Company, Philadelphia, 1983, p. 496.

89. Halliwell, R. E. W.: Factors in the development of flea-bite allergy. Vet. Med. 79:1273, 1984.

90. Halliwell, R. E. W.: Flea allergy: pathogenesis, therapy, and flea control. Proceedings, A. A. H. A. 52:145, 1985.

91. Halliwell, R. E. W., and Longino, S. J.: IgE and IgG antibodies to flea antigen in differing dog populations. Vet. Immunol. Immunopathol. 8:215, 1985.

91a. Halliwell, R. E. W.: Levels of IgE and IgG antibody to staphylococcal antigens in normal dogs and dogs with recurrent pyoderma. Proceedings, Ann. Meet. Am. Acad. Vet. Dermatol. and Am. Coll. Vet. Dermatol., 1987.

91b. Halliwell, R. E. W., and Schemmer, K. R.: The role of basophils in the immunopathogenesis of hypersensitivity to fleas (Ctenocephalides felis) in dogs. Vet. Immunol. Immunopathol. 15:203, 1987.

92. Hanifin, J. E., et al: Atopy and atopic dermatitis. J. Am. Acad. Dermatol. 15:703, 1986.

93. Harris, C. K., et al: Bone marrow transplantation in the dog. Compend. Cont. Ed. 8:337, 1986.

94. Haskins, M. E., et al: Bone marrow transplantation in the cat. Transplantation 37:634, 1984.

94a. Hendricks, P. M.: Dermatitis associated with the use of primidone in a dog. J. Am. Vet. Med. Assoc. 191:237, 1987.

95. Herrmann, K., et al: Detection of antibodies after immune complex splitting in serum of patients with bullous pemphigoid and systemic lupus erythematosus. Brit. J. Dermatol. 99:635, 1978.

95a. Hirshman, C. A., et al: Elevated mononuclear leukocyte phosphodiesterase in allergic dogs with and without airway hyperresponsiveness. J. All. Clin. Immunol. 79:46, 1987.

96. Holzworth, J.: Diseases of the Cat. Medicine and Surgery. W. B. Saunders Company, Philadelphia, 1987.

97. Howland, W. W., et al: Erythema multiforme: clinical, histopathologic, and immunologic study. J. Am. Acad. Dermatol. 10:438, 1984.

98. Huff, J. C., et al: Erythema multiforme: a critical review of characteristics, diagnostic criteria, and causes. J. Am. Acad. Dermatol. 8:763, 1983.

99. Ihrke, P. J., et al: Pemphigus foliaceus in dogs: a review of 37 cases. J. Am. Vet. Med. Assoc. 186:59, 1985.

100. Ihrke, P. J., et al: Pemphigus foliaceus of the footpads in three dogs. J. Am. Vet. Med. Assoc. 186:67, 1985.

101. Ihrke, P. J., et al: The longevity of immunoglobulin preservation in canine skin utilizing Michel's fixative. Vet. Immunol. Immunopathol. 9:161, 1985.

102. Jacobs, M. I., et al: Variability of the lupus band test. Arch. Dermatol. 119:883, 1983.

103. Jungers, P., et al: Hormonal modulation in systemic lupus erythematosus. Arthritis Rheum. 28:1243, 1985.

104. Kaliner, M., and Lemanske, R.: Inflammatory responses to mast cell granules. Fed. Proc. 43:2846, 1984.

105. Kang, K., et al: Thymopoietin pentapeptide (TP-5) improves clinical parameters and lymphocyte subpopulations in atopic dermatitis. J. Am. Acad. Dermatol. 8:372, 1983.

106. Kass, P. H., et al: Application of the log-linear model in the prediction of the antinuclear antibody test in the dog. Am. J. Vet. Res. 46:2336, 1985.

107. Kass, P. H., et al: Application of the log-linear and logistic regression models in the prediction of systemic lupus erythematosus in the dog. Am. J. Vet. Res. 46:2340, 1985.

108. Katz, D. H.: Regulation of the IgE system: experimental and clinical aspects. Allergy 39:81, 1984.

108a. Keahey, T. M., et al: Immediate hypersensitivity. J. Am. Acad. Dermatol. 17:826, 1987.

109. Kern, T. J., et al: Uveitis associated with poliosis and vitiligo in six dogs. J. Am. Vet. Med. Assoc. 187:408, 1985.

110. Kohchiyama, A., et al: T-cell subsets in lesions of systemic and discoid lupus erythematosus. J. Cut. Pathol. 12:493, 1985.

111. Korman, N.: Bullous pemphigoid. J. Am. Acad. Dermatol. 16:907, 1987.

112. Koulu, L., et al: Human autoantibodies against a desmosomal core protein in pemphigus foliaceus. J. Exp. Med. 160:1509, 1984.

113. Krasnig, S. A., et al: Intercellular complement C3 binding in normal skin of patients without pemphigus. J. Am. Acad. Dermatol. 14:52, 1986.

114. Krawiec, D. R., and Gafaar, S. M.: A comparative study of allergic and primary irritant contact dermatitis with dinitrochlorobenzene (DNCB) in dogs. J. Invest. Dermatol. 65:248, 1975.

115. Kromer, G., et al: Is autoimmunity a side-effect of interleukin 2 production? Immunol. Today 7:199, 1986.

116. Kunkle, G. A.: The treatment of canine atopic disease. Current Veterinary Therapy VII. W. B. Saunders Company., Philadelphia, 1980, p. 453.

117. Kunkle, G. A., and Gross, T. L.: Allergic contact dermatitis to Tradescantia fluminensis (wandering Jew) in a dog. Compend. Cont. Ed. 5:925, 1983.

118. Kunkle, G. A., and Milcarsky, J.: Double-blind flea hyposensitization in cats. J. Am. Vet. Med. Assoc. 186:677, 1985.

119. Latimer, K. S., et al: A transient deficit in neutrophilic chemotaxis in a dog with recurrent staphylococcal pyoderma. Vet. Pathol. 19:223, 1982.

120. Latimer, K. S., et al: Neutrophil movement in selected canine skin diseases. Am. J. Vet. Res. 44:601, 1983.

121. Lazaro-Medina, A., et al: Limitations in the diagnosis of vesiculobullous diseases. Am. J. Dermatopathol. 5:7, 1983.

122. Lemanske, R. F., and Kaliner, M. A.: Late phase allergic reactions. Int. J. Dermatol. 22:401, 1983.

123. Lerner, E. A., and Lerner, M. R.: Whither the ANA? Arch. Dermatol. 123:358, 1987.

124. Lever, W. F., and Schaumburg-Lever, G.: Histopathology of the Skin VI. J. B. Lippincott Company, Philadelphia, 1983.

125. Lisby, G., et al: Interleukin 1. A new mediator in dermatology. Int. J. Dermatol. 26:8, 1987.

126. MacDonald, J. M.: Ectoparasites. In Kirk R. W. (ed.): Current Veterinary Therapy VIII. W. B. Saunders Company, Philadelphia, 1983, p. 488.

126a. MacEwen, E. G., and Hess, P. W.: Evaluation of effect of immunomodulation on the feline eosinophilic granuloma complex. J.A.A.H.A. 23:519, 1987.

126b. Manning, T. O., et al.: Three cases of feline eosinophilic granuloma complex (eosinophilic ulcer) and observations on laser therapy. Semin. Vet. Med. Surg. 2:206, 1987.

127. Marzulli, F. N., and Maibach, H. I.: Dermatotoxicology and Pharmacology. John Wiley & Sons, New York, 1978.

128. Mason, K. V.: Subepidermal bullous drug eruption resembling bullous pemphigoid in a dog. J. Am. Vet. Med. Assoc. 190:881, 1987.

129. Mason, K. V.: Two cases of a fixed drug eruption on the scrotum caused by diethylcarbamazine. Proceedings, Ann. Meet. Am. Acad. Vet. Dermatol. and Am. Coll. Vet. Dermatol., 1986.

130. Matus, R. E., et al: Plasmapheresis in five dogs with systemic immune-mediated disease. J. Am. Vet. Med. Assoc. 187:595, 1985.

131. McDougal, B. J.: Allergy testing and hyposensitization for 3 common feline dermatoses. Mod. Vet. Pract. 67:629, 1986.

131a. McDougal, B. J.: Correlation of results of the radioallergosorbent test and provocative testing in 20 dogs with food allergy. Proceedings, Ann. Meet. Am. Acad. Vet. Dermatol. and Am. Coll. Vet. Dermatol., 1987.

132. Medleau, L., et al: Food hypersensitivity in a cat. J. Am. Vet. Med. Assoc. 189:692, 1986.

133. Medleau, L., et al: Complement immunofluorescence in sera of dogs with pemphigus foliaceus. Am. J. Vet. Res. 48:486, 1987.

134. Merot, Y., and Saurat, J. H.: Clues to pathogenesis of toxic epidermal necrolysis. Int. J. Dermatol. 24:165, 1985.

135. Miller, W. H.: Personal communication, 1987.

135a. Miller, W. H.: Facial dermatoses. Proceedings, Am. Anim. Hosp. Assoc. 53:162, 1986.

135b. Miller, W. H.: Nonsteroidal anti-inflammatory agents in the management of canine and feline pruritus. In Kirk, R. W. (ed.). Current Veterinary Therapy X. W. B. Saunders Company, Philadelphia (in press).

136. Mitchell, J., and Krull, E. A.: Alopecia areata: pathogenesis and treatment. J. Am. Acad. Dermatol. 11:763, 1984.

136a. Monier, J. C., et al: Systemic lupus erythematosus in a colony of dogs. Am. J. Vet. Res. 49:46, 1988.

137. Moore, F. M., et al: Localization of immunoglobulins and complement by the peroxidase antiperoxidase method in autoimmune and non-autoimmune canine dermatopathies. Vet. Immunol. Immunopathol. 14:1, 1987.

138. Moriello, K. A.: Incidence of positive flea antigen reactions in normal Florida cats. Proceedings, Ann. Meet. Am. Acad. Vet Dermatol. and Am. Coll. Vet. Dermatol., 1985.

138a. Moroff, S. D., et al: IgA deficiency in Shar-Pei dogs. Vet. Immunol. Immunopathol. 13:181, 1986.

139. Muller, G. H., et al: Small Animal Dermatology III. W. B. Saunders Company, Philadelphia, 1983.

140. Muller-Peddinghaus, R., et al: Klinische Bedeutung des Serumkomplements bei huuden. Zbl. Vet. Med. A. 30:698, 1983.

141. Nelson, D. A., and Spielvogal, R. L.: Alopecia areata. Int. J. Dermatol. 24:26, 1985.

142. Nesbitt, G. H., et al: Aeroallergens. Compend. Cont. Ed. 6:63, 1984.

143. Nesbitt, G. H., et al: Canine atopy. Part I. Etiology and diagnosis. Compend. Cont. Ed. 6:73, 1984.

144. Nesbitt, G. H., et al: Canine atopy. Part II. Management. Compend. Cont. Ed. 6:264, 1984.

145. Newton, R. C., et al: Mechanism-oriented assessment of isotretnoin in chronic or subacute cutaneous lupus erythematosus. Arch. Dermatol. 122:170, 1986.

146. Niemand, S., et al: Kalteagglutinin-krankheit bei einer Katze. Kleintierpraxis 30:259, 1985.

147. Nishioka, K.: Allergic contact dermatitis. Int. J. Dermatol. 24:1, 1985.

148. Nobreus, N., et al: Induction of dinitrochlorobenzene contact sensitivity in dogs. Monog. Allergy 8:100, 1974.

148a. Olivry, T., et al.: Le lupus erythemateux discoide du chien. A propos de 22 observations. Pract. Med. Chirung. Anim. Comp. 22:205, 1987.

149. Olsen, R. G., and Krakowka, S.: Immunology and Immunopathology of Domestic Animals. Charles C Thomas; Springfield, 1979.

150. Olynyk, G. P., and Guthrie, B. J.: Canine pemphigus vulgaris treated with gold salt therapy. Can. Vet. J. 25:168, 1984.

150a. Panciera, D. L., and Bevier, D.: Management of cryptococcosis and toxic epidermal necrolysis in a dog. J.A.V.M.A. 191:1125, 1987.

151. Parodi, A., and Rebora, A.: Iatrogenic false-positive Crithidia luciliae immunofluorescence test. J. Am. Acad. Dermatol. 14:678, 1986.

152. Parsons, J. M.: Management of toxic epidermal necrolysis. Cutis 38:305, 1985.

153. Parwaresch, M. R., et al: Tissue mast cells in health and disease. Pathol. Res. Pract. 179:439, 1985.

153a. Peters, M. S.: The eosinophil. Adv. Dermatol. 2:129, 1987.

154. Peterson, L. L., and Wuepper, K. D.: Isolation and purification of a pemphigus vulgaris antigen from human epidermis. J. Clin. Invest. 73:1113, 1984.

155. Pinkus, H., and Mehregan, A. H.: A Guide to Dermatohistopathology II. Appleton-Century-Crofts, New York, 1976.

156. Powell, M. A., et al: Reaginic hypersensitivity in Otodectes cynotis infestation of cats and mode of mite feeding. Am. J. Vet. Res. 41:877, 1980.

157. Pukay, B. P.: Treatment of canine bacterial hypersensitivity by hyposensitization with Staphylococcus aureus bacterin-toxoid. J. Am. Anim. Hosp. Assoc. 21:479, 1985.

158. Randell, M. G., and Hurvitz, A. I.: Immune-mediated vasculitis in five dogs. J. Am. Vet. Med. Assoc. 183:207, 1983.

159. Ranki, A., et al: T and B lymphcytes, macrophages, and Langerhans' cells during the course of contact allergic and irritant skin reactions in man. Acta Dermatol. Venereol. (Stockh.) 63:376, 1983.

160. Reedy, L. M.: Results of allergy testing and hyposensitization in selected feline skin diseases. J. Am. Anim. Hosp. Assoc. 18:618, 1982.

161. Renshaw, H. W., and Davis, W. C.: Canine granulocytopathy syndrome: An inherited disorder of leukocyte function. Am. J. Pathol. 95:731, 1979.

161a. Rhodes, K. H., et al.: Comparative aspects of canine and human atopic dermatitis. Semin. Vet. Med. Surg. 2:166, 1987.

161b. Rhodes, K. H., et al: Investigation into the immunopathogenesis of canine atopy. Semin. Vet. Med. Surg. 2:199, 1987.

162. Roitt, I. M.: Essential Immunology IV. J. B. Lippincott Company, Philadelphia, 1981.

163. Romatowski, J.: A uveodermatological syndrome in an Akita dog. J. Am. Anim. Hosp. Assoc. 21:777, 1985.

164. Roscoe, J. T., et al: Brazilian pemphigus foliaceus autoantibodies are pathogenic to BALB/c mice by passive transfer. J. Invest. Dermatol. 85:538, 1985.

164a. Rosenhagen, D., and Hoffmann, G.: Zum Intrakutantest beim Hund-ein Uberblick uber 112 Falle. Kleintierpraxis 31:131, 1986.

165. Rosenkrantz, W. S., et al: Histopathological evaluation of acid mucopolysaccharide (mucin) in canine discoid lupus erythematosus. J. Am. Anim. Hosp. Assoc. 22:577, 1986.

166. Rosenkrantz, W. S., et al: Clinical evaluation of cyclosporine in animal models with cutaneous immune mediated disease. Proceedings, Ann. Meet. Am. Acad. Vet. Dermatol. and Am. Coll. Vet. Dermatol., 1986.

167. Rosenkrantz, W. S., et al: Cyclosporine and cutaneous immune-mediated disease. J. Am. Acad. Dermatol. 14:1088, 1986.

167a. Rosenthal, R. C., and Dworkis, A. S.: Adverse reactions to Leukocell®. J.A.A.H.A. 23:515, 1987.

168. Rosser, E. J., et al: Sebaceous adenitis with hyperkeratosis in the standard poodle: A discussion of 10 cases. J. Am. Anim. Hosp. Assoc. 23:341, 1987.

169. Roujeau, J. C., et al: Lymphopenia and abnormal balance of T-lymphocyte subpopulations in toxic epidermal necrolysis. Arch. Dermatol. Res. 277:24, 1985.

170. Roujeau, J. C., et al: Involvement of macrophages in the pathology of toxic epidermal necrolysis. Brit. J. Dermatol. 113:425, 1985.

171. Safai, B., and Good, R. A.: Immunodermatology. Comprehensive Immunology. Vol. 7. Plenum Publishing Corp., New York, 1980.

172. Sanchez, N. P., et al: Clinical and histopathologic spectrum of necrotizing vasculitis. Report of findings in 101 cases. Arch. Dermatol. 121:220, 1985.

172a. Sauder, D. N.: Allergic contact dermatitis. In Thiers, B. H., and Dobson, R. L. (eds.): Pathogenesis of Skin Disease. Churchill Livingstone, New York, 1986, p. 3.

172b. Schemmer, K. R., and Halliwell, R. E.: Efficacy of alum-precipitated flea antigen for hyposensitization of flea-allergic dogs. Semin. Vet. Med. Surg. 2:195, 1987.

173. Schoeffer, M., and Sisk, L. C.: Allergenic extracts: A review of their safety and efficacy. Ann. Allergy 52:2, 1984.

174. Schick, R. O., and Fadok, V. A.: Responses of atopic dogs to regional allergens: 268 cases (1981–1984). J. Am. Vet. Med. Assoc. 189:1493, 1986.

175. Schindler, B. A.: Stress, affective disorders, and immune function. Med. Clin. North Am. 69:585, 1985.

176. Schmeitzel, L. P.: Focal cutaneous reactions at vaccination sites in a cat and four dogs. Proceedings, Ann. Meet. Am. Acad. Vet. Dermatol. and Am. Coll. Vet. Dermatol., 1986.

177. Schmeitzel, L. P.: The effects of multiple intradermal skin tests on skin reactivity. Vet. Allergist, Summer, 1986.

178. Schrader, L. E., and Hurvitz, A. I.: Cold agglutinin disease in a cat. J. Am. Vet. Med. Assoc. 183:121, 1983.

179. Schultz, K. T., and Maguire, H. C.: Chemically-induced delayed hypersensitivity in the cat. Vet. Immunol. Immunopathol. 3:585, 1982.

180. Schultz, R. D.: The effects of aging on the immune system. Compend. Cont. Ed. 6:1096, 1984.

181. Schultz, R. D., and Adams, L. S.: Immunologic methods for the detection of humoral and cellular immunity. Vet. Clin. North Am. 8:721, 1978.

182. Schultz, R. D.: ANA diseases. Calif. Vet. 38:23, 1984.

183. Schwartz, R. S., and Rose, N. R.: Autoimmunity: Experimental and Clinical Aspects. Ann. N.Y. Acad. Sci. 475, New York, 1986.

184. Schwartzman, R. M.: Immunologic studies of progeny of atopic dogs. Am. J. Vet. Res. 45:375, 1984.

185. Schwartzman, R. M.: Cutaneous amyloidosis associated with a monoclonal gammopathy in a dog. J. Am. Vet. Med. Assoc. 185:102, 1984.

186. Scott, D. W., et al: Staphylococcal hypersensitivity in the dog. J. Am. Anim. Hosp. Assoc. 14:666, 1978.

187. Scott, D. W.: Feline dermatology 1900–1978: A monograph. J. Am. Anim. Hosp. Assoc. 16:331, 1980.

187a. Scott, D. W.: Observations on canine atopy. J. Am. Anim. Hosp. Assoc. 17:91, 1981.

188. Scott, D. W.: Cutaneous eosinophilic granulomas with collagen degeneration in the dog. J. Am. Anim. Hosp. Assoc. 19:529, 1983.

189. Scott, D. W., et al: Canine lupus erythematosus. I. Systemic lupus erythematosus. J. Am. Anim. Hosp. Assoc. 19:461, 1983.

190. Scott, D. W., et al: Canine lupus erythematosus. II. Discoid lupus erythematosus. J. Am. Anim. Hosp. Assoc. 19:481, 1983.

191. Scott, D. W.: Pemphigus in domestic animals. Clin. Dermatol. 1:141, 1983.

192. Scott, D. W., et al: Unusual findings in canine pemphigus erythematosus and discoid lupus erythematosus. J. Am. Anim. Hosp. Assoc. 20:579, 1984.

193. Scott, D. W., et al: Pitfalls in immunofluorescence testing in canine dermatology. Cornell Vet. 73:131, 1983.

194. Scott, D. W., et al: Pitfalls in immunofluorescence testing in dermatology. II. Pemphigus-like antibodies in the cat, and direct immunofluorescence testing of normal dog nose and lip. Cornell Vet. 73:275, 1983.

195. Scott, D. W.: Sterile eosinophilic pustulosis in the dog. J. Am. Anim. Hosp. Assoc. 20:585, 1984.

196. Scott, D. W.: Feline dermatology 1979–1982: Introspective retrospections. J. Am. Anim. Hosp. Assoc. 20:537, 1984.

197. Scott, D. W.: Lichenoid reactions in the skin of dogs: Clinicopathologic correlations. J. Am. Anim. Hosp. Assoc. 20:305, 1984.

198. Scott, D. W.: Idiopathic lichenoid dermatitis in a dog. Canine Pract. 11:22, 1984.

199. Scott, D. W., et al: Hypereosinophilic syndrome in a cat. Feline Pract. 15:22, 1985.

200. Scott, D. W.: Localized scleroderma (morphea) in two dogs. J. Am. Anim. Hosp. Assoc. 22:207, 1986.

201. Scott, D. W., et al: Erythema multiforme and pemphigus-like antibodies associated with sulfamethoxazole-trimethoprim administration in a dog with polycystic kidneys. Canine Pract. 13:35, 1986.

202. Scott, D. W., et al: Miliary dermatitis. A feline cutaneous reaction pattern. Proceedings, Ann. Kal Kan Seminar 2:11, 1986.

203. Scott, D. W.: Granulomatous sebaceous adenitis in dogs. J. Am. Anim. Hosp. Asoc. 22:631, 1986.

204. Scott, D. W.: Pemphigoid in domestic animals. Clin. Dermatol. 5:155, 1987.

205. Scott, D. W., and Vaughan, T. C.: Papulonodular dermatitis in a dog with occult filariasis. Companion Anim. Pract. 1:31, 1987.

206. Scott, D. W., et al: Immune-mediated dermatoses in domestic animals: ten years after—Part I. Compend. Cont. Ed. 9:423, 1987.

207. Scott, D. W., et al: Immune-mediated dermatoses in domestic animals: ten years after—Part II. Compend. Cont. Ed. 9:539, 1987.

208. Scott, D. W.: Feline dermatology 1983–1985: "The Secret Sits." J. Am. Anim. Hosp. Assoc. 23:255, 1987.

209. Scott, D. W.: Sterile eosinophilic pustulosis in dog and man: Comparative aspects. J. Am. Acad. Dermatol. 16:1022, 1987.

210. Scott, D. W., and Buerger, R. G.: Nonsteroidal anti-inflammatory agents in the management of canine pruritus. J. Am. Anim. Hosp. Assoc. (in press).

211. Scott, D. W.: Unpublished observation.

211a. Scott, D. W.: Lichenoid dermatoses in dogs and cats. In Kirk, R. W. (ed.): Current Veterinary Therapy X. W. B. Saunders Company, Philadelphia (in press).

212. Sell, S.: Immunology, Immunopathology and Immunity III. Harper & Row, Hagerstown, 1980.

213. Shanley, K. J.: Lupus erythematosus in small animals. Clin. Dermatol. 3:131, 1985.

213a. Sheffy, B. E.: Nutrition, infection, and immunity. Compend. Cont. Ed. 7:990, 1985.

214. Shull, R. M., et al: Investigation of the nature and specificity of antinuclear antibody in dogs. Am. J. Vet. Res. 44:2004, 1983.

215. Skogh, M.: Atopic eczema unresponsive to evening primrose oil (linoleic and γ-linolenic acids). J. Am. Acad. Dermatol. 15:114, 1986.

216. Stanley, J. R., et al: Distinction between epidermal antigens binding pemphigus vulgaris and pemphigus foliaceus autoantibodies. J. Clin. Invest. 74:313, 1984.

217. Steinberg, A. D., et al: Systemic lupus erythematosus: insights from animal models. Ann. Intern. Med. 100:714, 1984.

217a. Stone, J.: Dermatologic Immunology and Allergy. C.V. Mosby Company, St. Louis, 1985.

217b. Stewart, L. J.: Isotretinoin in the treatment of sebaceous adenitis in two dogs. Ann. Meet. Am. Acad. Vet. Dermatol. and Am. Coll. Vet. Dermatol., 1988.

218. Storb, R., and Thomas, E. D.: Graft-versus-host disease in dog and man: The Seattle experience. Immunol. Rev. 88:215, 1985.

219. Susaneck, S. J.: Doxorubicin therapy in the dog. J. Am. Vet. Med. Assoc. 182:70, 1983.

220. Suarez-Chacon, R., et al: Clinical immunology: A reappraisal and new classification. Clin. Immunol. Immunopathol. 11:30, 1978.

221. Suter, M., et al: Pemphigus vulgaris und pemphigus foliaceus beim hund:9 falle. Schweiz. Arch. Tierheilkd. 126:249, 1984.

222. Suter, M. M., et al: Pemphigus in the dog: Comparison of immunofluorescence and immunoperoxidase method to demonstrate intercellular immunoglobulins in the epidermis. Am. J. Vet. Res. 45:367, 1984.

223. Talal, N.: New therapeutic approaches to autoimmune disease. Springer Sem. Immunopathol. 9:105, 1986.

224. Targowski, S.: Determination of immune complexes in sera from dogs with various diseases by mastocytoma cell assay. J. Clin. Micro. 15:64, 1982.

224a. Theilen, G. H., and Madewell, B. R.: Veterinary Cancer Medicine. Lea & Febiger, Philadelphia, 1987.

225. Theofilopoulos, A. N., and Dixon, F. J.: Immune complexes in human diseases: A review. Am. J. Pathol. 100:531, 1983.

225a. Thomsen, M. K., and Kristensen, F.: Contact dermatitis in the dog. A review and a clinical study. Nord. Vet. Med. 38:129, 1986.

226. Thornfeldt, C. R., and Menkes, A. U.: Bullous pemphigoid controlled by tetracycline. J. Am. Acad. Dermatol. 167:305, 1987.

227. Tizard, I. R.: An Introduction to Veterinary Immunology III. W. B. Saunders Company, Philadelphia, 1987.

228. Tizard, I.: Basic immunology—6: Histocompatibility antigens. Vet. Med. 81:574, 1986.

229. Tosti, A., et al: Therapies versus placebo in the treatment of patchy alopecia areata. J. Am. Acad. Dermatol. 15:209, 1986.

230. Van Hess, J., et al: Levamisole-induced drug eruptions in the dog. J. Am. Anim. Hosp. Assoc. 21:255, 1985.

231. Van Joost, T., et al: Oral lupus erythematosus: markers of immunologic injury. J. Cutan. Pathol. 12:500, 1985.

232. Van Joost, T., et al: Causative agents and pathogenicity in iatrogenic cutaneous autoimmunity. Int. J. Dermatol. 26:75, 1987.

233. Van Stee, E. W.: Risk factors in canine atopy. Calif. Vet. 37:8, 1983.

234. Vollset, I.: Atopic dermatitis in Norwegian dogs. Nord. Vet. Med. 37:97, 1985.

235. Vollset, I., et al: Immediate type hypersensitivity in dogs induced by storage mites. Res. Vet. Sci. 40:123, 1986.

236. Walton, G. S.: Allergic contact dermatitis. In Kirk, R. W., (ed): Current Veterinary Therapy VI. W. B. Saunders Company, Philadelphia, 1977, p. 571.

237. Weigand, D. A.: The lupus band test: A reevaluation. J. Am. Acad. Dermatol. 11:230, 1984.

238. Weigand, D. A.: Lupus band test: Anatomic regional variations in discoid lupus erythematosus. J. Am. Acad. Dermatol. 14:426, 1986.

239. Weisman, M. H., et al: Gold therapy in patients with systemic lupus erythematosus. Am. J. Med., 57(6A), 1983.

240. Werner, L. L., et al: Diagnoses of autoimmune skin disease in the dog: Correlation between histopathologic, direct immunofluorescent and clinical findings. Vet. Immunol. Immunopathol. 5:47, 1983.

241. Westly, E. D., and Wechsler, H. L.: Toxic epidermal necrolysis. Granulocyte leukopenia as a prognostic indicator. Arch. Dermatol. 120:721, 1984.

242. Whitbread, T. J., et al: Relative deficiency of serum IgA in the German Shepherd dog: A breed abnormality. Res. Vet. Sci. 37:350, 1984.

243. White, J. V.: Cyclosporine: prototype of a T-cell selective immunosuppressant. J. Am. Vet. Med. Assoc. 189:566, 1986.

244. White, S. D.: Bullous pemphigoid in a dog: Treatment with six-mercaptopurine. J. Am. Vet. Med. Assoc. 185:683, 1984.

245. White, S. D.: Food hypersensitivity in 30 dogs. J. Am. Vet. Med. Assoc. 188:695, 1986.

245a. White, S. D., et al: Corticosteroid (methylprednisolone sodium succinate) pulse therapy in five dogs with autoimmune skin disease. J.A.V.M.A. 191:1121, 1987.

246. Wilcock, B. P., and Yager, J. A.: Focal cutaneous vasculitis and alopecia at sites of rabies vaccination in dogs. J. Am. Vet. Med. Assoc. 188:1174, 1986.

247. Willemse, A., and Van Den Brom, W. E.: Evaluation of the intradermal allergy test in normal dogs. Res. Vet. Sci. 32:57, 1982.

248. Willemse, A.: Canine atopic disease: Investigations of eosinophils and the nasal mucosa. Am. J. Vet. Res. 45:1867, 1984.

249. Willemse, A., et al: Effect of hyposensitization on atopic dermatitis in dogs. J. Am. Vet. Med. Assoc. 184:1277, 1984.

249a. Willemse, A., and Van Den Brom, W. E.: Investigations of the symptomatology and the significance of immediate skin test reactivity in canine atopic dermatitis. Res. Vet. Sci. 34:261, 1983.

250. Willemse, A.: The allergologic tests. Proc. World Small Anim. Vet. Assoc. 11:A5, 1986.

251. Willemse, A., et al: Allergen specific IgGd antibodies in dogs with atopic dermatitis as determined by the enzyme linked immunosorbent assay (ELISA). Clin. Exp. Immunol. 59:359, 1985.

252. Willemse, A., et al: Induction of non-IgE anaphylactic antibodies in dogs. Clin. Exp. Immunol. 59:351, 1985.

252a. Willemse, T.: Canine atopic disease. Dermatol. Rep. 6:1, 1987.

252b. Willemse, T.: Atopic skin disease: a review and a reconsideration of diagnostic criteria. J. Small Anim. Pract. 27:771, 1986.

253. Winkelstein, J. A., et al: Genetically determined deficiency of the third component of complement in the dog. Science 212:1169, 1981.

254. Wintroub, B. U., and Stern, R.: Cutaneous drug reactions: Pathogenesis and clinical classification. J. Am. Acad. Dermatol. 13:167, 1985.

255. Wojnarowska, F., et al: The significance of an IgM band at the dermoepidermal junction. J. Cut. Pathol. 13:359, 1986.

256. Wright, S.: Atopic dermatitis and essential fatty acids: A biochemical basis for atopy? Acta Derm. Venereol. (Stockh.) Suppl. 114:143, 1985.

257. Yancy, K. B., and Lawley, T. J.: Circulating immune complexes and their immunochemistry, biology and detection in selected dermatologic and systemic diseases. J. Am. Acad. Dermatol. 10:711, 1984.

258. Yunginger, J. W.: Allergenic extracts: Characterization, standardization, and prospects for the future. Pediatr. Clin. North Am. 30:795, 1983.

10

Cutaneous Endocrinology

Many hormones affect the skin and adnexa. Although this chapter is limited to endocrine influences on skin, it must be remembered that hormones also have effects on the rest of the body. The specific actions of many proven and alleged hormonal imbalances on the skin are often poorly understood. Additionally, confusion is intensified by (1) species differences, (2) lack of adequate standardized or readily available diagnostic tests, (3) conflicting data in the literature, and (4) the complex physiologic and pathophysiologic inter-relationships between the endocrine glands and their hormonal products. The skin must also be regarded as having endocrine functions, as it is a major site for the metabolism and interconversion of many of the steroids.[107a]

Clinically bilaterally symmetric alopecia is often the first noticeable sign of a hormonal dermatosis. The hair coat is often dull, dry, and easily epilated, and it fails to regrow after clipping. Bilaterally symmetric pigmentary disturbances (usually *hyper*pigmentation) may accompany the alopecia. Endocrine dermatoses are classically nonpruritic.

However, exceptions to the above clinical rules are commonplace. The alopecia and pigmentary disturbances may be focal, multifocal, and asymmetric. Secondary seborrheic skin disease or pyoderma or both are frequent complications, resulting in varying degrees of dermatitis and pruritus.

Functional Anatomy of the Endocrine Hypothalamus and Hypophysis

Anatomically and functionally, the hypothalamus and hypophysis (pituitary gland) are most usefully thought of together as "the master gland" or "the endocrine brain."[9] The important portion of the hypophysis as it relates to dermatology is the adenohypophysis (anterior pituitary, pars distalis).

The hypothalamus contains a number of specialized cells that combine neural and secretory activity: the endocrine neurons. The endocrine hypothalamus produces hormones (adenohypophysiotropic releasing and inhibiting factors) that are transported as unstainable neurosecretions to the pituitary portal system and then to the adenohypophysis. Important hypothalamic releasing/inhibiting factors that control the adenohypophysis include:

Adrenocorticotropic hormone–releasing factor (ACTH–releasing factor); corticotropin-releasing factor (CRF)

Thyroid-stimulating hormone–releasing factor (TSH–releasing factor); thyrotropin-releasing factor (TRF); thyrotropin-releasing hormone (TRH)

Growth hormone–releasing factor (GHRF); somatotropin-releasing factor (SRF)

Growth hormone–inhibiting factor (GHIF); somatotropin-inhibiting factor (SIF), somatostatin

Follicle-stimulating hormone– and luteinizing hormone–releasing factor (FSH– and LH–releasing factor); gonadotropin-releasing hormone (GnRH)

Prolactin-releasing factor (PRF)

Prolactin-inhibiting factor (PIF)

These hypophysiotropic factors are presently thought to be regulated by higher brain centers, adenohypophyseal hormones ("short-loop" feedback system), and target endocrine gland hormones ("long-loop" system).

By means of light microscopy and acidic/basic dye staining characteristics, the adenohypophysis is seen to consist of three cell types: acidophils (producing GH and prolactin), basophils (producing FSH, LH, TSH, β-lipotropin, and ACTH), and chromophobes (producing ACTH and β-lipotropin).[9] When electron microscopy and immunohistochemical examination are used, the adenohypophysis is observed to consist of five cell types: thyrotropes (TSH), corticotropes (ACTH, β-lipotropin), gonadotropes (FSH, LH), somatotropes (GH), and mammotropes (prolactin).[9] The release of adenohypophyseal hormones is thought to be regulated by hypophysiotropic factors from the hypothalamus and negative feedback by target endocrine gland hormones.

In general, three factors determine the secretory rates of the endocrine glands: (1) humoral feedback loops, (2) neurologic stimulation or suppression, and (3) genetic influence. Effects of hormones depend on many factors, including chemical structure, concentration in the blood, method of transport in the blood, quantity of unbound target-cell receptors, integrity of target-cell post-receptor mechanism, and the rate of hormonal degradation and elimination.

Most peptide hormones (e.g., ACTH, TSH, FSH, LH, TRH) initiate their actions by activating the cell membrane enzyme adenyl cyclase and the cyclic AMP system. Steroid hormones (e.g., glucocorticoids, sex hormones) pass through target-cell membranes and bind to cytoplasmic receptors; the resultant steroid-receptor complex binds to nuclear chromatin to initiate activity. Thyroid hormones pass into target-cell cytoplasm to the nucleus, where they bind chromatin receptors and initiate activity.

The basic causes of endocrine disease include the following: (1) *primary hyperfunction* (e.g., hyperadrenocorticism due to functional pituitary and adrenal neoplasms; hyperestrogenism due to functional ovarian or testicular neoplasms), (2) *secondary hyperfunction* (e.g., hyperadrenocorticism due to bilateral adrenocortical hyperplasia), (3) *primary hypofunction* (e.g., congenital or acquired hypothyroidism; hypopituitarism due to cystic Rathke's cleft), (4) *secondary hypofunction* (e.g., secondary hypothyroidism due to hypopituitarism), (5) *ectopic hypersecretion* (e.g., ectopic ACTH syndrome), (6) *failure of target cell response*, (7) *abnormal degradation of hormone* (e.g., feminization due to chronic liver disease), and (8) *iatrogenic hormone excess* (glucocorticoids, progestogens, estrogens).[9]

Diagnosis of Endocrinopathies

The diagnosis of clinical endocrinopathies is usually based on finding an abnormal concentration of a hormone in the blood. The ideal endocrine assay does not exist. Although radioimmunoassay (RIA) and enzyme-linked immunosorbent assay (ELISA) are the most sensitive, specific, accurate, and precise available methodologies for measuring hormones,[9] these techniques are usually quite species specific and must be specially validated for dogs and cats. Any laboratory not willing to provide validation information on request is best avoided. The instructional staff at university veterinary teaching hospitals can usually direct practitioners to a laboratory that provides validated assays for the hormones desired.

Blood hormone levels are usually reported in *micrograms* (μg; 10^{-6} grams) *per deciliter* (dl) (e.g., cortisol, T_4, testosterone), *nanograms* (ng; 10^{-9} grams) *per dl* or *milliliter* (ml) (e.g., T_3, progesterone), or *picograms* (pg; 10^{-12} grams) *per ml* (e.g., estrogen). Because serum and plasma samples sent to a reference laboratory are subject to leaking in transit, being lost, and so forth, veterinarians should routinely freeze and store duplicate samples until laboratory results are obtained.

Basal (resting) levels of serum and plasma hormones frequently do not distinguish normal individuals from those with an endocrinopathy.[9] Basal blood hormone levels fluctuate in response to environmental, psychic, circadian, and drug-induced influences, and they vary with age, breed, sex, and so forth. Thus, various stimulation and suppression tests are routinely employed to overcome this unreliability of basal blood hormone levels.[9]

Thyroid Hormones

A deficiency of thyroid hormone action is the most common endocrine dermatosis of dogs but is rarely documented as a naturally occurring disorder in cats.[9, 66] The etiology of canine hypothyroidism is complex, with the most important cause being lymphocytic (autoimmune) thyroiditis.

THYROID PHYSIOLOGY

Canine thyroid physiology is a complex subject and has been exhaustively reviewed. It has been shown that dogs produce 3,5,3',5'-tetraiodothyronine (thyroxine, T_4), 3,5,3'-triiodothyronine (T_3), 3,3',5'-triiodothyronine (reverse T_3, rT_3), 3,3'-diiodothyronine (3,3'-T_2), and 3',5'-diiodothyronine (3',5'-T_2).[9, 29, 54, 66]

The thyroid gland secretes all the T_4, but up to 60 per cent of the daily T_3 requirement is formed via monodeiodination (thyroxine 5'-deiodinase) from T_4 in peripheral tissues. The preference of canine thyroid to secrete T_3, rather than T_4, is enhanced by TSH. T_3 is more potent and penetrates much faster into interstitial and intracellular spaces than does T_4. Iodine-deficient dogs show an 80 per cent reduction in their serum T_4 levels, but their serum T_3 levels remain normal, and the dogs remain eumetabolic. In addition, hypothyroid dogs being adequately maintained on only oral T_3 have *no* detectable serum T_4, whereas those maintained on only oral T_4 show normal levels of both serum T_3 and T_4. Thus, T_3 is the major metabolically active thyroid hormone in dogs, with T_4 serving mainly as a prohormone.

In dogs, rT_3, which is metabolically inactive, is formed via monodeiodination (thyroxine 5-deiodinase) from T_4. It is well known that in human beings and rodents a number of conditions—chronic illnesses, acute illnesses, surgical trauma, fasting, starvation, fever, glucocorticoid therapy—produce moderate-to-marked reduction of serum T_3 levels, mild-to-marked reduction of serum T_4 levels, and marked elevation of serum rT_3 levels.[4a, 20, 113] In these circumstances, the patients are euthyroid and in no need of thyroid medication. This situation is referred to as the "euthyroid sick syndrome" and is a common source of misdiagnosis concerning basal T_3 and T_4 serum levels. The "euthyroid sick syndrome" also occurs in dogs and cats (Table 10:1).[9, 28a, 29, 66, 84a] It is thought that this metabolic switch in the sick patient is (1) protective by counteracting the excessive calorigenic effects of T_3 in catabolic states, and (2) caused by an inhibition of one or more iodothyronine β-ring deiodinases, leading to both decreased production of T_3 from T_4 and decreased rT_3 degradation.

Studies in dogs have shown that T_2 is the major product of peripheral tissue deiodination of T_3 and rT_3. T_2 is metabolically inactive.

Information on thyroid physiology in cats is virtually nonexistent, and naturally occurring feline hypothyroidism has only rarely been documented as a congenital defect. It is known that cats produce both T_3 and T_4.[66, 93, 98]

THYROID HORMONES AND THE SKIN

Thyroid hormone plays a dominant role in controlling metabolism and is essential for normal growth and development.[9] The primary mechanisms of action of thyroid hormones are stimulation of cytoplasmic protein synthesis and increase of tissue oxygen consumption. These effects are thought to be initiated by the binding of thyroid hormone to nuclear chromatin and by augmentation of the transcription of genetic information. Available data suggest that thyroid hormone plays a pivotal role in differentiation and maturation of mammalian skin as well as in the maintenance of normal cutaneous function.

Hypothyroidism results in epidermal atrophy and abnormal keratinization because of decreased protein synthesis, mitotic activity, and oxygen consumption in dogs and humans.[9, 66] Thyroid hormone–deficient epidermis is characterized by both abnormal lipogenesis and decreased sterol synthesis by keratinocytes.[86] Epidermal melanosis may be seen in hypothyroid dogs and humans, but the pathomechanism is unclear.[66] Sebaceous gland atrophy occurs in hypothyroid dogs and humans, and sebum excretion rates are reduced in hypothyroid humans and rats.[66]

Table 10:1. RECOGNIZED CAUSES OF LOW T_3 AND T_4 LEVELS IN EUTHYROID DOGS: THE "EUTHYROID SICK SYNDROME"[29, 66]

Acute Illnesses	Chronic Illnesses	Related Drug
Bronchopneumonia, bacterial	Generalized demodicosis	Glucocorticoids
Distemper	Generalized furunculosis, bacterial	Phenylbutazone
Autoimmune hemolytic anemia	—	Phenobarbital
Systemic lupus erythematosus	Lymphosarcoma	Phenytoin
Intervertebral disc disease	Chronic renal failure	Salicylates
Polyradiculoneuritis	Diabetes mellitus	Diazepam
Starvation	Congestive heart failure	—
—	Hyperadrenocorticism	Primidone
—	Blastomycosis	—

Thyroid hormone is necessary for the initiation of the anagen phase of the hair follicle cycle.[66] Anagen is not initiated in hypothyroid dogs, resulting in the hair follicles being retained in telogen and leading to failure of hair growth and alopecia. It has been shown that the oral or topical administration of T_4 to normal dogs increases both the growth rate of hair and the numbers of anagen hair follicles, especially in the flanks.[34a]

In hypothyroid dogs, humans, and rats, hyaluronic acid accumulates in the dermis, leading to an increase in the interstitial ground substance and a thick, myxedematous dermis.[66] The exact cause of this tissue myxedema is unknown, although evidence has been presented to suggest that (1) elevated levels of TSH in primary hypothyroidism result in increased synthesis of ground substance and that (2) the transcapillary albumin escape rate is increased, while lymphatic drainage in myxedema is inadequate.[66, 116]

Thyroid hormone has been reported to heal the ulcers and to reduce the scarring associated with chronic radiodermatitis in humans and to improve the healing of deep dermal burns in rats.[66] These effects were thought to be due to thyroid hormone actions on the proliferation and metabolism of fibroblasts and collagen synthesis. In humans, hypothyroidism is associated with a 50 per cent reduction in plasma fibronectin levels.[103b] Not surprisingly, the skin of hypothyroid dogs and human beings exhibits poor wound healing and easy bruising.[66]

Pyoderma is a common complication of canine hypothyroidism.[66, 87] In various animal models it has been reported that (1) development of lymphoid tissue depends on the integrity of the thyroid gland, (2) thyroidectomy results in hypoplasia of lymphoid organs and thymus, and (3) depletion of thyroid hormones results in impaired neutrophil functions and B- and T-lymphocyte functions.[66]

Uncomplicated canine hypothyroidism is characterized by the absence of pruritus. It has been reported that tissue levels of histamine are decreased in experimental canine hypothyroidism.[66] Clinically, canine hypothyroidism is characterized by (1) bilaterally symmetric alopecia, (2) a dull, dry, easily epilated hair coat that fails to grow after clipping, (3) variable hyperpigmentation, (4) skin that is often dry, cool to the touch, thick, and puffy, (5) poor wound healing, (6) easy bruising, (7) frequent seborrheic skin disease or pyoderma, or both, and (8) variable changes of coat color. Histologically, the condition is characterized by orthokeratotic hyperkeratosis, follicular keratosis, follicular dilatation, follicular atrophy, telogenization of hair follicles, epidermal melanosis, sebaceous gland atrophy, thick dermis, and increased dermal mucin (myxedema).[95]

THYROID FUNCTION TESTS

No single area of veterinary diagnostics has become more misunderstood, confused, and abused than thyroid function testing. Most of this is referable to the failure to recognize (1) the significance of the euthyroid sick syndrome, (2) the unreliability of basal serum thyroid hormone levels, and (3) the unsatisfactory results obtained by sending samples to laboratories geared to testing human sera.

Thyroid function tests, such as basal metabolic rate, radioiodine uptake, protein-bound iodine, butanol extractable iodine, T_4 by competitive protein binding or column chromatography, T_3 resin uptake, and free thyroxine index (T_7 test) are either inaccurate, impractical, or inferior to modern techniques and will not be discussed here.

Serum Thyroid Hormones

Radioimmunoassay is the method of choice for determining serum levels of total T_3 and total T_4.[9, 29] However, radioimmunoassay techniques developed to measure thyroid hormone levels in human sera are unsatisfactory for dogs and cats. Serum samples may be held at room temperature for at least 1 week with no significant deterioration of T_3 and T_4 levels. Reported basal levels of serum total T_3 and total T_4 in the dog approximate 50 to 160 ng/dl and 1 to 4 µg/dl, respectively. However, even laboratories utilizing radioimmunoassay procedures adapted to dogs and cats may vary in their normal ranges of serum T_3 and T_4 levels, so one must exercise great caution when attempting to compare published data.

Other factors to consider when assessing basal serum T_3 and T_4 levels include the following: (1) low T_3 and T_4 levels occur in euthyroid patients with the "euthyroid sick syndrome" (discussed previously); (2) low T_3 and T_4 levels occur in euthyroid patients, associated with recent drug therapy (e.g., glucocorticoids, phenytoin, phenylbutazone)[9, 29, 66]; (3) normal T_3 and T_4 levels may be lower during warm weather[9, 66]; (4) normal T_3 and T_4 levels may be lower in certain breeds, such as the German shepherd, cocker spaniel, boxer, beagle, Labrador retriever, Alaskan malamute, Afghan, Saluki, and Siberian husky[9, 29, 66]; (5) normal T_3 and T_4 levels tend to be lower in large and giant breeds and old dogs, and higher in small breeds and very young dogs[9, 29, 66]; and (6) T_3 and T_4 levels may show sporadic daily fluctuations and a mild diurnal rhythm, with a peak around noon.[46, 66, 68] Additionally, in one study *low* basal serum T_3 and T_4 levels were found in 20 per cent of 100 normal dogs, and *normal* basal levels in 30 per cent of 250 hypothyroid dogs,[66] and in another study normal basal serum T_4 levels were found in over 50 per cent of 60 hypothyroid dogs.[9]

In humans, serum thyroid hormone–binding protein levels are known to markedly influence serum thyroid hormone levels (Table 10:2).[9, 29, 66] Thyroid hormone–binding proteins have been identified by electrophoresis in the albumin, inter-α-globulin, and two β-globulin regions of dog serum.[9, 29, 66] Alterations in thyroid hormone–binding protein levels and resultant changes in thyroid hormone levels have not been well studied in dogs. It has been reported that (1) glucocorticoids, phenylbutazone, salicylates, diazepam, primidone, phenytoin, androgens, and phenobarbital may decrease basal serum total T_3 and T_4 levels by interfering with protein binding, and (2) basal serum total T_3 and T_4 levels may be elevated in pregnancy, pseudopregnancy, and the feminization syndrome of male dogs with functional Sertoli cell testicular tumors, and in estrogen therapy, owing to increased protein binding capacity.[9, 29, 66, 84, 109]

Table 10:2. THYROID HORMONE–BINDING CAPACITY ABNORMALITIES

Factors Causing Increased Binding Capacity	Factors Causing Decreased Binding Capacity
Estrogens	Androgens
Oral contraceptives	Glucocorticoids
Pregnancy	Hypoproteinemia (malnutrition, protein-losing nephropathies and enteropathies)
Acute liver disease	Severe liver disease
Congenital increased thyroxine-binding globulin (TBG) levels	Congenital decreased TBG levels
	Drugs competing for binding sites (phenytoin, salicylates, phenylbutazone, penicillin, anticoagulants)

In summary, basal serum levels of T_3 and T_4 are significantly influenced by numerous conditions that have nothing to do with thyroidal disease and hypothyroidism. In the absence of classic, historical, clinical, and clinicopathologic evidence of thyroid hormone deficiency, low basal serum T_3 and T_4 levels are unreliable for a diagnosis of canine hypothyroidism. Basal serum T_3 levels are a particularly poor measure of thyroid dysfunction.[9, 29, 68] Because T_3 is predominantly an intracellular hormone and is preferentially produced in states of thyroid deficiency, T_4 levels drop before T_3 levels. In addition, T_3 levels are more severely affected by nonthyroidal illnesses and drugs and are inconsistently responsive to TSH and TRH stimulation.

Because the free concentration of T_4 (free T_4) appears to determine hormone availability to cells, and because total hormone concentrations may change with drugs, illness, and so forth without a change in free T_4, a direct or an indirect measurement of free T_4 provides a more consistent laboratory assessment of thyroid status than does the measurement of total T_4. The standard techniques for measurement of free T_4 are radioimmunoassay and equilibrium dialysis. These assays are technically difficult to perform and have not been widely available for dogs and cats. Free T_4 levels in normal dogs are reported to range from 0.7 to 2.1 ng/dl.[9, 28a, 29, 68] The diagnostic value of free T_4 determinations in dogs and cats has yet to be documented. In one study of 130 dogs,[28a] the simultaneous assessment of both total T_4 and free T_4 reduced the number of false-positive diagnoses by about 15 per cent. However, the assessment of free T_4 alone resulted in 10 per cent false-negative diagnoses. In addition, illness also produced reduced free T_4 levels in dogs, mimicking the effects of the euthyroid sick syndrome on total T_4 and total T_3.[28a]

In normal cats, basal serum T_3 and T_4 levels by radioimmunoassay are reported to range from 15 to 60 ng/dl and 1.5 to 5 μg/dl, respectively.[9, 66] T_4-binding serum globulins could not be found in the cat.[9, 66]

In dogs, basal serum rT_3 levels by radioimmunoassay are reported to approximate 100 ng/dl.[9, 29] Serum rT_3 levels would be expected to be elevated in the euthyroid sick syndrome. However, studies documenting the diagnostic value of rT_3 determinations in dogs and cats have not been reported.

Serum TSH

In humans, the determination of serum TSH levels by radioimmunoassay is the most sensitive and reliable indicator of hypothyroidism, often being abnormal for months before basal serum T_4 levels and TSH stimulation tests are abnormal.[9, 29, 66] Serum TSH levels should be elevated in primary hypothyroidism, and low to normal in secondary hypothyroidism. TSH is a species-specific protein, and attempts to utilize human TSH kits for analyzing canine TSH levels have been unsuccessful.[9, 28a, 29] A homologous radioimmunoassay for canine serum TSH was reported to accurately distinguish between normal dogs and dogs with experimental hypothyroidism.[81] Serum TSH levels in normal dogs were reported to range from 2.7 to 7.9 ng/ml.[41, 81] Evaluation of a commercially available, specific canine assay for serum TSH (Canine TSH Assay, Canadian Bioclinical Ltd) concluded that the test was no more predictive of hypothyroidism, normality, or response to thyroid supplementation than basal total T_4 alone.[81a] Another investigation of the same commercial assay found unexplained high levels of TSH in some normal dogs, and low levels in some *hypothyroid* dogs, also concluding that the assay could not be recommended for the diagnosis of canine hypothyroidism.[84b] Serum TSH assays would offer a major advancement in the area of thyroid diagnostics in dogs, and further progress in this area is eagerly awaited.

Provocative Thyroid Function Tests

To overcome the unreliability of basal blood T_4 and T_3 levels, various provocative tests of thyroid function have been developed.[9, 29, 66] There is controversy over the relative efficiency and accuracy of the various tests. Results are often difficult to compare because of variation in methodology (different products used at different doses; different time intervals of sampling; different laboratories performing and interpreting the tests).

TSH STIMULATION TEST

TSH is a species-specific glycoprotein, with a molecular weight of about 28,000 daltons, that is produced by the adenohypophysis.[1, 9] The secretion of TSH is stimulated by hypothalamic TRH and is inhibited by hypothalamic somatostatin, thyroid hormones, glucocorticoids, dopamine, and stress. Bovine TSH is biologically active in dogs and cats.

The TSH stimulation test has been widely evaluated in *dogs* and is vastly superior to the determination of basal blood T_4 and T_3 levels in the diagnosis of hypothyroidism.[9, 22, 28a, 29, 43, 66, 68, 71, 72, 117] A commonly used procedure for conducting the TSH stimulation test in dogs is as follows: Serum samples for T_4 determination are collected immediately before and 6 hours after the intravenous injection of 1 to 2.5 IU of bovine TSH (Dermathycin, Thytropar). Repeated intravenous injections of bovine TSH may produce anaphylaxis. Euthyroid dogs usually have pre-TSH serum T_4 levels within or below the normal pre-TSH range for the laboratory performing the assay, and post-TSH serum T_4 levels within the normal post-TSH range. The commonly espoused criterion, that euthyroid dogs double their basal serum T_4 levels after TSH stimulation, is unreliable. In general, measuring serum T_3 levels pre- and post-TSH is unreliable and not recommended.

The TSH stimulation test usually achieves normal post-stimulation serum T_4 levels in dogs with the euthyroid sick syndrome and drug-related low basal serum T_4 level.[9, 29, 66, 68] In some cases, especially in dogs with hyperadrenocorticism or dogs being treated with glucocorticoids, both the pre- and post-TSH serum T_4 levels will be below the expected normal ranges.[29, 48, 77] However, the slope of the response will parallel that seen in normal dogs. Glucocorticoids have been reported to suppress TRH secretion, suppress pituitary responsiveness to TRH, suppress TSH secretion, depress serum thyroid hormone–binding protein levels, supress basal serum T_4 and T_3 levels, inhibit the conversion of T_4 to T_3, and increase serum rT_3 levels.[9, 29, 48]

A single TSH stimulation test will *not* reliably distinguish between primary and secondary hypothyroidism in dogs.[9, 66] If secondary hypothyroidism is suspected, bovine TSH may be administered subcutaneously or intramuscularly for 3 to 5 consecutive days. After this period of time, the basal serum T_4 levels of dogs with secondary hypothyroidism should show a normal response to TSH.

If a clinician wishes to perform a TSH stimulation test on dogs receiving thyroid hormone treatment, the thyroid supplement should be stopped for at least 30 days.[9, 28a, 66, 68]

The TSH stimulation test can be conducted simultaneously with an ACTH stimulation test or a dexamethasone suppression test, with no compromise in the accuracy of either procedure.[65, 83]

In *cats*, the following two protocols have been reported to be accurate measurements of thyroid function: (1) serum T_4 determinations before and 6 hours after intravenous injection of 1 IU/kg bovine TSH,[37] or (2) serum T_4 determinations before and 10 hours after intramuscular injection of 2.5 IU bovine TSH.[47]

TRH STIMULATION TEST

Thyrotropin-releasing hormone (TRH) is a tripeptide produced by the hypothalamus.[1, 9] TRH stimulates the release of TSH and prolactin. TRH secretion is enhanced by norepinephrine, histamine, serotonin, and dopamine, and it is probably inhibited by thyroid hormones.

In humans, serum T_4 and TSH responses to exogenous TRH have been used to differentiate among primary, secondary, and tertiary hypothyroidism.[9, 29] Patients with primary hypothyroidism have low basal serum T_4 levels and high basal serum TSH levels, neither of which responds to TRH stimulation. Patients with secondary hypothyroidism have low basal serum T_4 and TSH levels, neither of which responds to TRH stimulation. Patients with tertiary hypothyroidism have low basal serum T_4 and TSH levels, both of which respond to TRH stimulation.

Detailed evaluation of the TRH stimulation test in the various forms of hypothyroidism in dogs and cats has not been conducted. In *dogs*, the TRH stimulation test has been reported to distinguish reliably between euthyroid and primary hypothyroid individuals.[22, 41, 43, 55, 58, 104] Serum T_4 levels are determined before and 6 hours after intravenous injection of 200 to 500 µg of TRH. Normal dogs at least double their basal serum T_4 levels. Serum T_3 determinations during this protocol are variable and nondiagnostic. TRH doses >900 µg or >0.1 mg/kg are reported to frequently cause various cholinergic side-effects, including hypersalivation, coughing, miosis, vomiting, diarrhea, urination, tachycardia and tachypnea.

In normal *cats*, serum T_4 levels were reported to show a reproducible doubling 6 hours after the intravenous injection of 0.1 mg/kg of TRH.[58] TRH doses in excess of 0.1 mg/kg often produced the cholinergic side-effects mentioned above for dogs.

Thyroid Biopsy

The distinction between primary and secondary canine hypothyroidism can be made rather easily by histologic examination of a biopsy of the thyroid.[9, 66] In primary hypothyroidism there is massive loss of follicular epithelium, usually associated with lymphocytic thyroiditis.[60] In secondary hypothyroidism the follicles are distended with colloid, the follicular epithelium is flattened, and there is no vacuolation of the colloid. Normal dogs treated with systemic glucocorticoid develop increased numbers of colloid droplets per thyroid follicular cell, suggesting inhibition of thyroid lysosomal hydrolysis of colloid.[43, 122] In these dogs, basal serum T_3 and T_4 levels were decreased, but TSH and TRH stimulation tests were normal.

Tests Used in Lymphocytic Thyroiditis

In dogs and human patients with lymphocytic (autoimmune) thyroiditis, a number of immunologic evaluations have been conducted, including serum levels of antithyroglobulin antibodies, serum levels of antimicrosomal and anticolloidal antibodies, in vitro lymphocyte blastogenesis to thyroid extract, delayed-type hypersensitivity skin test reactions to thyroid extract, and circulating immune complex levels.[9, 29, 31, 111] In dogs, antithyroglobulin antibodies are demonstrable in over 50 per cent of the cases of naturally occurring hypothyroidism by means of the enzyme-linked immunosorbent assay, hemagglutination, and indirect immunofluorescence techniques.[3a, 10a, 35, 36, 36a] Great Danes, Irish setters, borzois, Doberman pinschers, and old English sheepdogs may be predisposed. Interestingly, antithyroglobulin antibodies are also demonstrable in over 40 per cent of dogs with nonthyroid endocrine disorders and healthy relatives of antibody-positive patients, as well as in 13 per cent of hospital patients without endocrine disease. As these tests become more available, important applications may include (1) detecting family members that might develop hypothyroidism, and (2) helping to differentiate primary hypothyroidism (antibody positive) from secondary and tertiary hypothyroidism (antibody negative).

Glucocorticoids

Glucocorticoids are produced by the zona fasciculata of the adrenal cortex and are probably the most commonly used therapeutic agents in veterinary medicine.[9, 48, 94] Hyperglucocorticoidism may be produced by hypersecretion of ACTH or ACTH-like substances (ectopic, idiopathic, functional pituitary neoplasm); hypersecretion of endogenous glucocorticoids (functional adrenocortical neoplasm); and exogenous glucocorticoid administration (iatrogenic) (see pp. 205, 610).

GLUCOCORTICOIDS AND THE SKIN

The skin is a rather sensitive and specific indicator of hyperglucocorticoidism, reflecting both internal disease and inappropriate therapy.[9, 66, 94] The protein catabolic, antienzymatic, and antimitotic effects of glucocorticoids are manifested in numerous ways in canine, feline, and human skin: (1) The epidermis becomes thinned and hyperkeratotic (suppressed DNA synthesis, decreased mitoses, keratinization abnormalities); (2) the basement membrane zone becomes thinned and disrupted; (3) pilosebaceous atrophy becomes pronounced; (4) the dermis becomes thinned and dermal vasculature becomes fragile (inhibition of fibroblast proliferation, collagen and ground substance production); and (5) wound healing is delayed. Unique to the dog, presumably through changes in protein structure, collagen and elastin fibers become attractive sites for mineralization, resulting in dystrophic calcinosis cutis.[66] Additionally, due to the broad-spectrum anti-inflammatory and immunosuppressive effects of excessive glucocorticoids, patients have increased susceptibility to bacterial and fungal cutaneous infections.[9, 66]

Clinically, hyperglucocorticoidism in dogs and cats is characterized by (1) thin, hypotonic skin, (2) easy bruising (petechiae and ecchymoses), (3) poor wound healing, (4) seborrhea sicca, (5) phlebectasias, and (6) increased susceptibility to bacterial infection, demodicosis, and perhaps dermatophytosis. In dogs, calcinosis cutis, bilaterally symmetric alopecia, and variable hyperpigmentation are features of hyperglucocorticoidism, whereas these are not usually seen in cats and human beings. In human patients, but not in dogs and cats, hypertrichosis and cutaneous striae are common features of hyperglucocorticoidism.

Histologically, hyperglucocorticoidism in dogs and cats is characterized by orthokeratotic hyperkeratosis, follicular keratosis, telogenization of hair follicles, thin dermis, and telangiectasia.[95] The follicular dilatation, follicular atrophy, epidermal atrophy, epidermal melanosis, sebaceous gland atrophy, and dystrophic mineralization that are seen in dogs are very rare in cats.

ADRENAL FUNCTION TESTS

Adrenal function tests are basically of two types: those that are single measurements of basal glucocorticoid levels in blood or urine, and those that are provocative, dynamic response tests. Single measurements of basal glucocorticoid levels, while cheaper and easier to perform, are unreliable.[9, 28a, 66] Up to 90 per cent of the dogs with hyperadrenocorticism will have basal glucocorticoid levels in the normal range.

Urinary Glucocorticoids

In dogs, the major cortisol metabolites found in urine are cortol, 3-epiallocortol, cortolone, 3-epiallotetrahydrocortisol, and tetrahydrocortisol.[9, 66] These metabolites are excreted mainly as glucuronides, and a major portion of this fraction is represented by steroids reduced at C-20. Thus, the use of steroid assay procedures that measure only those steroids having a dihydroxyketotic side chain, such as the Porter-Silber reaction, would not measure these cortisol metabolites in dogs. In cats, virtually all glucocorticoid metabolites are excreted in bile (99 per cent), with only a small amount of Porter-Silber chromogens present as the free compounds in urine (1 per cent).[9, 93]

Urinary steroid assays (17-ketosteroids, 17-hydroxycorticosteroids) require 24-hour urine samples, metabolic cages, and collecting equipment; are easily contaminated; and must be measured before and after the administration of a provocative test agent. They are rarely used today.

Blood Cortisol

Blood cortisol levels in dogs and cats have been measured by three methods: fluorometric, competitive protein binding, and radioimmunoassay.[9] Radioimmunoassay (RIA) is the method of choice and the one in general use today. Basal blood cortisol levels by radioimmunoassay in normal dogs and cats approximate 0 to 8 μg/dl.[9, 28a, 66, 94]

It has been suggested that (1) plasma should be used to assay for cortisol, (2) plasma should be separated from the blood cellular elements within 15 minutes, and (3) plasma should be kept frozen; otherwise, cortisol levels may drop by as much as 50 per cent within 6 to 8 days.[66] However, researchers conducting other studies found no significant differences between serum and plasma cortisol levels and reported no significant decrease in serum or plasma cortisol levels that were stored in contact with erythrocytes for up to 8 days at 4 to 20°C.[66]

Important considerations to keep in mind when interpreting blood cortisol levels include the following: (1) different laboratories may differ in their normal and abnormal values, (2) stress can markedly elevate blood cortisol levels, (3) episodic cortisol secretion occurs in normal dogs and dogs with hyperadreno-corticism, and (4) single measurements of blood cortisol are of limited value in the diagnosis of hyperadrenocorticism.[9, 46, 66, 76] The clinical significance of diurnal cortisol rhythms in dogs and cats is unclear. In dogs, most investigators have found cortisol levels to be highest in the morning,[9, 66] while others have found no diurnal rhythm.[46, 66] Likewise, in cats, some investigators have found cortisol levels to be highest in the evening, while others have found no difference.[9, 66]

Cortisol Response Tests

To overcome the unreliability of basal blood cortisol levels, various provocative tests have been developed.[9, 18, 24-28, 66, 76, 79] There is controversy over the relative efficiency and accuracy of the various tests. Results are often difficult to compare, owing to differences in methodology (plasma versus serum samples; different products used at different doses; different time intervals of sampling; different laboratories performing and interpreting the tests). Cortisol response tests are traditionally begun at 8:00 to 10:00 AM.

ACTH STIMULATION TEST
(ACTH Response Test)

ACTH is a polypeptide with a molecular weight of about 4500 daltons secreted by the adenohypophysis as part of a large prohormone, pro-opiome-lanocortin, which also contains in its sequence β-lipotropin and the opioid peptides β-endorphin and enkephalins.[1, 9] Secretion of ACTH is controlled by circadian rhythm and stress mechanisms inherent in the central nervous system and by negative feedback from circulating glucocorticoids.

The ACTH stimulation test reliably documents a diagnosis of iatrogenic hyperadrenocorticism in dogs and cats.[9, 66] Basal blood cortisol levels are normal or low and show little or no response to ACTH. In addition, the ACTH stimulation test is very useful for monitoring therapeutic response to o,p'-DDD.[76, 79] The ACTH stimulation test is *not* as accurate as the low-dose dexamethasone suppression test for the diagnosis of spontaneous canine hyperadrenocorticism, as about 15 per cent of the cases of pituitary-dependent hyperadrenocorticism do not have an exaggerated response, and over 50 per cent of the cases of adrenocortical neoplasia are hyper-responsive.[9, 25, 28a, 26, 66, 75, 76, 79] In addition, dogs that are clinically stressed or that have various chronic illnesses frequently hyper-respond to ACTH.[8] Two commonly used protocols for ACTH stimulation are as follows: (1) plasma or serum cortisol samples collected before and 2 hours after the intramuscular injection or 2.2 IU/kg of ACTH gel (Acthar Gel), or (2) plasma or serum cortisol samples collected before and 1 hour after the intramuscular or intravenous injection of 0.25 mg synthetic ACTH (Cortrosyn). It has been shown that the ACTH stimulation test can be performed concurrently with the TSH stimulation test, while the accuracy of both tests is maintained.[83]

The ACTH stimulation test has been studied in normal cats and in a small number of cats with spontaneous hyperadrenocorticism.[9, 47, 66, 78, 80, 93, 124] Two protocols recommended for cats are as follows: (1) plasma or serum cortisol determinations before and 90 minutes after the intramuscular injection of 2.2 IU/kg ACTH gel, or (2) plasma or serum cortisol determinations before and 90 minutes after the intravenous injection of 0.125 mg synthetic ACTH. Other investigators reported no difference in the response of the healthy cats to 0.125 mg or 0.250 mg synthetic ACTH IM (peak cortisol responses at 30 minutes postinjection.[103c] It has been reported that cats with diabetes mellitus may hyper-respond to ACTH,[80] but another study failed to document this finding in diabetic and nondiabetic sick cats.[125]

LOW-DOSE DEXAMETHASONE SUPPRESSION TEST

The low-dose dexamethasone suppression test is presently the procedure of choice for confirming a diagnosis of spontaneous canine hyperadrenocorticism.[25, 27, 28a, 66, 76, 79] In normal dogs, the low dose of dexamethasone consistently suppresses blood cortisol levels to less than 1.0 μg/dl for the 8-hour test period. Inadequate suppression occurs in dogs with spontaneous hyperadrenocorticism (Fig. 10:1). However, dogs that are clinically stressed or that have various chronic illnesses may also fail to suppress with low-dose dexamethasone.[8] Thus, failure to suppress with low-dose dexamethasone is *not* pathognomonic for hyperadrenocorticism, and the diagnosis must be supported with other clinicopathologic data.[9] A commonly used protocol for the low-dose dexamethasone suppression test is to take plasma or serum cortisol samples before and 8 hours after the intravenous administration of 0.01 mg/kg dexamethasone. The dexamethasone suppression test has been performed concurrently with the TSH stimulation test, with the accuracy of both tests being preserved.[65]

The dexamethasone suppression test has been studied in a few normal cats and cats with spontaneous hyperadrenocorticism.[80, 124, 125] The methodologies have been quite variable, and specific recommendations cannot be made at present. One group of investigators reported that plasma cortisol responses of healthy cats to IV injections of dexamethasone at doses of 0.01 mg/kg, 0.1

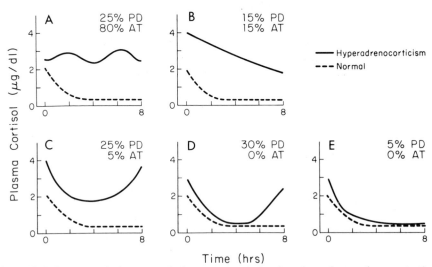

Figure 10:1. Patterns of plasma cortisol responses during low-dose dexamethasone testing in normal dogs and in dogs with hyperadrenocorticism. PD = pituitary-dependent hyperadrenocorticism, AT = adrenal tumor. (From Peterson, M. E.: Hyperadrenocorticism. Vet. Clin. North Am. [Small Anim. Pract.] *14*:731, 1984.)

mg/kg, and 1.0 mg/kg were similar (peak suppression at 6 to 10 hours postinjection).[103c] It was reported that the results of dexamethasone suppression testing were not different in normal, diabetic, and nondiabetic sick cats.[125]

HIGH-DOSE DEXAMETHASONE SUPPRESSION TEST

The high-dose dexamethasone suppression test is presently the procedure of choice for differentiating between pituitary-dependent hyperadrenocorticism and that caused by adrenocortical neoplasia in dogs.[26–28a, 66, 76, 79] Suppression of blood cortisol levels to below 1.5 μg/dl is diagnostic for pituitary-dependent hyperadrenocorticism (Fig. 10:2). Such suppression does not occur with adrenocortical neoplasia. However, about 15 per cent of the dogs with pituitary-dependent hyperadrenocorticism fail to adequately suppress with *any* dose of dexamethasone.[76, 79] This may be because these are neoplasms arising in the intermediate lobe of the pituitary gland.[9, 49, 76, 80a] The pars intermedia is avascular and innervated by dopaminergic and serotonergic fibers from the brain. Thus, this area is relatively unresponsive to blood-borne ACTH and dexamethasone. A commonly used protocol for the high-dose dexamethasone suppression test is to take plasma or serum cortisol samples before and 8 hours after the intravenous injection of 0.1 mg/kg dexamethasone. Some investigators have recommended a much higher dose, 1.0 mg/kg.[76, 79] While this larger dose markedly increases the expense of the test, it does *not* clearly enhance the diagnostic accuracy of the test.[9, 26, 28a, 49, 103] In fact, it has been suggested that the 1.0 mg/kg dose was less reliable than the 0.1 mg/kg dose.[26, 49]

Plasma ACTH

Plasma ACTH levels have been measured by RIA in normal dogs and in dogs with spontaneous hyperadrenocorticism.[9, 26, 28, 28a, 50, 76, 79] Endogenous plasma ACTH levels are extremely useful in determining the cause of spontaneous canine hyperadrenocorticism, especially when interpreted together with the results of dexamethasone suppression testing. Plasma ACTH levels range from normal to elevated (greater than 40 pg/ml) in dogs with pituitary-dependent

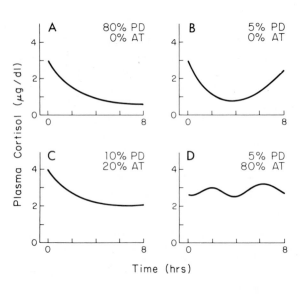

Figure 10:2. Patterns of plasma cortisol responses during high-dose dexamethasone suppression testing in dogs with hyperadrenocorticism. PD = pituitary-dependent hyperadrenocorticism, AT = adrenal tumor. (From Peterson, M. E.: Hyperadrenocorticism. Vet. Clin. North Am. [Small Anim. Pract.] *14*:731, 1984.)

hyperadrenocorticism, and from low to undetectable (less than 20 pg/ml) in dogs with functional adrenocortical neoplasms. As with plasma cortisol levels, plasma ACTH levels fluctuate episodically throughout the day, which results in some overlap of values between normal dogs and dogs with spontaneous hyperadrenocorticism.

Plasma ACTH levels have been measured by RIA in normal cats and are reported to approximate 20 to 100 pg/ml.[9, 28a, 80, 93] Plasma ACTH levels were markedly elevated in one cat with pituitary-dependent hyperadrenocorticism.

Accurate determination of plasma ACTH requires proper collection and handling of the specimen and a carefully performed, difficult RIA technique. Blood for ACTH assay must be collected in heparin- or EDTA-containing plastic tubes and spun immediately at 4°C. The plasma must be promptly separated into plastic or polypropylene tubes and kept frozen until assayed. At present, reliable plasma ACTH assays for dogs and cats are neither generally available nor economically feasible.

CRH Stimulation Test

Corticotropin-releasing hormone (CRH) is a peptide secreted in pulsatile fashion by the hypothalamus.[1, 9] CRH secretion is stimulated by epinephrine and serotonin, and it is inhibited by glucocorticoids and serotonin antagonists (e.g., cyproheptadine).

The recent isolation and synthesis of CRH makes possible an additional diagnostic test to differentiate the two causes of spontaneous hyperadrenocorticism.[9, 10] Synthetic ovine CRH was injected intravenously (0.1, 1.0, or 10.0 μ/kg) into normal dogs and produced peak plasma ACTH and cortisol levels within 30 to 60 minutes.[50] Preliminary information indicates that the CRH stimulation test is useful for distinguishing between canine pituitary-dependent hyperadrenocorticism (increased levels of ACTH and cortisol) and adrenocortical neoplasia (no response).[79]

However, until a relatively inexpensive, single-dose, sterilized CRH preparation becomes available, the CRH stimulation test will be of limited usefulness to most veterinarians.

Other Adrenal Function Tests

Recently, attempts have been made to devise more foolproof, inexpensive, and time-efficient adrenal function tests for the dog and cat. Tests evaluated include (1) the metyrapone response test, (2) the lysine-vasopressin test, (3) the insulin response test, (4) the glucagon response test, and (5) the combining of the ACTH response and dexamethasone suppression tests.[9, 18, 27, 28, 28a, 66] However, these tests are inferior to the standard dexamethasone suppression tests and cannot be recommended.

Growth Hormone

(Somatotropin)

Growth hormone (GH) is a polypeptide (molecular weight about 22,000 daltons) produced by the adenohypophysis.[1, 9] It has diametrically opposed intrinsic anabolic and catabolic activities. Its catabolic activity (enhanced lipolysis and restricted glucose transport caused by insulin resistance) is caused directly by the GH polypeptide, whereas its anabolic activity is mediated by somatomedins (insulin-like growth factors), which are primarily generated by the liver and controlled by GH.[15] The major function of GH is hormonal control of growth (in concert with thyroid hormones, insulin, cortisol, and sex steroids). GH is also important for the development of the thymus and T-cell function.[88, 89]

The secretion of GH is episodic and labile, and it is affected by the sleep-wake cycle, physical activity, nutritional state, physical and emotional stress, and pregnancy.[1, 9] Various neurotransmitters—norepinephrine, dopamine, and serotonin—as well as hypoglycemia, various amino acids, and progestogens stimulate GH secretion.

Excessive GH secretion produces acromegaly (see p. 619).[15, 97] The skin becomes thickened, myxedematous, and thrown into exaggerated folds. These changes are most obvious over the face and extremities. Hypertrichosis is common. Hyperpigmentation occurs in about 40 per cent of the human patients with acromegaly but has not been reported in dogs.[66] Histologically, acromegalic skin is characterized by increased dermal collagen and mucin and by hyperplasia of the epidermis and appendages.[97]

In dogs, juvenile GH deficiency results in retention of the puppy coat, followed by bilaterally symmetric alopecia and hyperpigmentation and by thin, hypotonic skin (see p. 611).[17, 66] Hyposomatotropism in the mature dog has similar cutaneous findings, but the retention of puppy coat is not seen (see p. 615).[101] Histologically, both entities are characterized by orthokeratotic hyperkeratosis, follicular keratosis, follicular dilatation, follicular atrophy, telogenization of hair follicles, epidermal melanosis, sebaceous gland atrophy, thin dermis, and decreased-to-absent elastin fibers.[95]

Specific radioimmunoassay techniques for measuring canine growth hormone have been developed.[15, 66, 101] Basal growth hormone levels in normal dogs and cats approximate 1.0 to 4.5 ng/ml.[9, 15, 66, 101] However, basal growth hormone levels in pituitary dwarfs and hypophysectomized dogs may approximate these values as well. Thus, basal growth hormone levels are inadequate for the documentation of growth hormone deficiency.

To document GH deficiency, clonidine or xylazine stimulation tests must be done.[9, 17, 66, 101] Clonidine (Catapres), an α-adrenergic/antihypertensive drug, has been used to stimulate GH release in dogs. Normal dogs showed a marked increase in plasma growth hormone levels within 15 to 30 minutes after the intravenous injection of 20 to 30 μg/kg of clonidine, whereas pituitary dwarfs and hypophysectomized dogs fail to respond. Clonidine may cause severe hypotension and shock.[103] Xylazine (Rompun), a sedative hypnotic drug, gives similar results when injected intravenously at 100 to 300 μg/kg. Proper interpretation of GH levels also requires the assessment of thyroid and adrenal gland function.[9, 17, 101] Both hyperglucocorticoidism and hypothyroidism impair GH secretion. In addition, pseudopregnancy, progestagen therapy, and sex hormone imbalances can cause elevation of basal plasma GH levels and poor responses to xylazine. The 300 μg/kg xylazine dose may cause severe hypotension and shock in toy and miniature breeds of dogs.[103]

In acromegaly, basal plasma growth hormone levels have been markedly elevated, ranging from 11 to 1476 ng/ml.[15, 16, 97] A hallmark of acromegaly is the nonsuppressibility of plasma GH levels during the administration of an intravenous glucose load. In canine acromegaly, plasma growth hormone levels were not suppressed by the intravenous administration of 1 gm glucose/kg.[9, 15, 16]

Somatomedins are polypeptides (molecular weight 5000 to 10,000 daltons) that can also be quantitated by radioimmunoassay to indirectly assess GH status.[9, 15–17] Somatomedin C (insulin-like growth factor 1) is most commonly assayed. Somatomedin C plasma levels parallel body size in dogs; normal values for cocker spaniels are 5 to 90 ng/ml, as opposed to 230 to 330 ng/ml for normal German shepherds. Somatomedin production is impaired by glucocorticoids and estrogens. Somatomedin C levels would be expected to be low or undetectable in GH-deficient states, and elevated in acromegaly.

Occasionally, assays for both GH and somatomedin C may be useful, as when (1) GH levels are normal (but the hormone is biologically inactive) and somatomedin C levels are low (Laron's type I dwarfism), or (2) GH levels are normal and somatomedin C levels are low (decreased hepatic GH receptors) (Laron's type II dwarfism).[9]

Sex Hormones

ESTROGENS

Estrogens are present in both males and females, and are produced by the ovarian follicles, the zona reticularis of the adrenal cortex, and Sertoli cells of the testicle.[9, 66] Pituitary FSH (follicle-stimulating hormone) stimulates ovarian follicular growth and estrogen production in females, and spermatogenesis in males.[1, 9] Hypothalamic GnRH (gonadotropin-releasing hormone) stimulates the pituitary to release FSH. In turn, estrogen inhibits GnRH release, and inhibin (produced by ovarian follicles and testicular Sertoli cells) inhibits FSH release.

Estrogens are reported to stimulate epidermal mitosis and to increase epidermal thickness in mice and humans, and also to reduce epidermal thickness in rats and humans. Epidermal atrophy was produced in dogs by daily intramuscular injections of 1 mg of diethylstilbestrol for 400 days.

Estrogens increase skin pigmentation in the guinea pig by increasing both free melanin and melanin within melanocytes, while ovariectomy has the opposite effect.[66] Cutaneous hyperpigmentation is a feature of clinical dermatoses associated with hyperestrogenism in dogs.

Estrogens reduce both sebaceous gland size and sebum production in rats and humans.[66] These effects appear to result from a local action on sebaceous glands, rather than from a feedback suppression of endogenous androgens. The daily intramuscular injection of 1 mg of diethylstilbestrol into dogs for 400 days produced marked sebaceous gland atrophy.

Estrogens suppress the initiation of anagen in rats, while ovariectomy has the opposite effect.[66] In addition, the rate of hair growth is greater in spayed female rats than in intact normal females, and estradiol implanted into spayed females or castrated males reduces the growth rate. In dogs, estrogens administered orally, subcutaneously, intramuscularly, and topically will produce alopecia. Bilaterally symmetric alopecia and easily epilated hair are striking features of clinical dermatoses associated with hyperestrogenism in dogs. There appears to be regional sensitivity of hair follicles to estrogenic abnormalities, as these dermatoses follow such a predictable pattern (see below). Evidence has also been presented that suggests that these estrogen-sensitive areas of skin may have increased numbers of estrogen receptors.[14]

Estrogens are reported to increase the amount of dermal ground substance in mice and humans.[66] The daily intramuscular injection of 1 mg of diethylstilbestrol in dogs for 400 days reduced the thickness of the subcutis.[41]

Estrogens are also known to affect thymic function, enhance antibody production, and inhibit suppressor T-cell function.[34]

Hyperestrogenism is thought to be the cause of two distinctive dermatoses in dogs: feminization of the male dog with a functional Sertoli cell tumor of the testicle (see p. 627) and hyperestrogenism (ovarian imbalance type I) of the intact female dog (see p. 622). Cutaneous changes in these syndromes include (1) bilaterally symmetric alopecia that begins in the perineal, genital, and ventral abdominal regions and spreads cranially and ventrally; (2) variable hyperpigmentation; (3) a dull, easily epilated hair coat that fails to regrow following clipping; (4) gynecomastia; (5) pendulous prepuce; (6) vulvar enlargement, and (7) variable seborrheic skin disease. In male dogs, linear prepucial dermatosis (see p. 628) appears to correlate with the presence of hyperestrogenism and testicular neoplasia. Histologically, both syndromes are characterized by orthokeratotic hyperkeratosis, follicular keratosis, follicular dilatation, follicular atrophy, telogenization of hair follicles, variable epidermal melanosis, and sebaceous gland atrophy.[95]

It has been stated that adrenalectomized and ovariectomized dogs maintained on only mineralocorticoids have normal skin and hair coats, indicating that estrogens or any other sex steroids are not necessary for normal skin and hair coat in dogs. However, hypoestrogenism has been hypothesized as an etiologic consideration in the estrogen-responsive dermatosis (ovarian imbalance type II) of spayed female dogs (see p. 625). Clinically, the dermatosis is characterized by (1) bilaterally symmetric alopecia that begins in the perineal, genital, and ventral abdominal areas and spreads cranially and ventrally and (2) an easily epilated hair coat that fails to regrow after clipping. Histologically, the dermatosis is characterized by follicular keratosis and follicular dilatation with telogenization of hair follicles.[95] In addition, spayed female cats with feline symmetric alopecia are known to respond to estrogen replacement therapy (see p. 701).

Assays (RIA) for plasma or serum estrogens are commercially available, but results are often difficult to interpret or are misleading.[9, 66] Most available assays measure ony *one* type of estrogen (e.g., estradiol, estrone), and as numerous estrogenic substances are produced in the body, such assays are often unsatisfactory. Thus, one can readily understand why only 40 per cent of the dogs with feminization due to functional Sertoli's cell neoplasms of the testicle could be shown to have hyperestrogenism (only estradiol is measured). Additionally, blood estrogen levels, along with the blood levels of the other sex steroids, fluctuate markedly during the day, necessitating multiple samples and unrealistic financial considerations. Evidence has been presented that suggests that dogs can have "cutaneous hyperestrogenism" (increased cutaneous estrogen receptors) in the *absence* of hyperestrogenemia.[14] Reported values for blood estradiol in the dog and cat approximate 0.5 to 5.0 pg/ml in males and 15 to 60 pg/ml in females.[9, 66, 98]

ANDROGENS

Androgens are present in both males and females, and they are produced by the interstitial cells of the testicle and by the zona reticularis of the adrenal cortex.[9, 66] Pituitary LH stimulates androgen secretion by testicular interstitial cells, and ovulation and corpus luteum formation/maintenance.[1, 9] Hypothalamic GnRH stimulates the pituitary release of LH. In turn, androgens and progestogens inhibit LH release, and estrogens and androgens (via hypothalamic aromatization to estrogens) inhibit GnRH release.

Androgens are reported to stimulate epidermal mitosis in mice and rats.[66] In humans, androgens are reported to increase epidermal mitotic activity and cell turnover time and thickness.

Androgens have no effect on pigmentation in the guinea pig but are reported to stimulate pigmentation in specialized areas of the skin, such as the subcostal region of the male golden hamster and the scrotum of the ground squirrel.[66] In humans, androgens increase cutaneous pigmentation, especially in sexual skin, apparently due to increased melanin synthesis. Men with an androgen deficiency develop hypopigmentation.

Androgens have been shown to enlarge the sebaceous glands in rats, rabbits, hamsters, mice, and human beings and to increase sebum production in humans and rats.[66] In humans, excessive androgens produce excessively oily skin, while androgen deficiency produces dry skin and hair. The action of androgens involves both an increase in rate of formation of new sebaceous cells and an increase in size of mature cells.

In rats, androgen administration retards the initiation of anagen, while gonadectomy enhances it.[66] However, neither castration nor treatment with testosterone has any effect on rate of hair growth in rats. In humans, an excess of androgens results in accelerated hair growth, whereas androgen deficiency in males results in the hair becoming sparse.

Androgens are reported to increase the relative and total amounts of hyaluronic acid and dermal ground substance in mice.[66] In humans, androgens cause thickening of the dermis with demonstrable increase in skin collagen content.

Androgens are also known to inhibit various T-cell functions.[34]

In the testosterone-responsive dermatosis of male dogs (see p. 633), hyponandrogenism is an etiologic hypothesis. The dermatosis is characterized by (1) bilaterally symmetric alopecia that begins in the perineal, genital, and ventral abdominal areas and spreads cranially and ventrally, (2) a dull, dry, easily epilated hair coat that fails to grow after clipping, (3) thin, hypotonic skin, and (4) seborrhea sicca. Histologically, the dermatosis is characterized by orthokeratotic hyperkeratosis, epidermal atrophy, follicular atrophy, telogenization of hair follicles, sebaceous gland atrophy, and thin dermis.[95] In addition, castrated male cats with feline symmetric alopecia are known to respond to testosterone replacement therapy (see p. 701). Conversely, hyperandrogenism is presumed to be the cause of seborrhea oleosa in "oversexed" intact male dogs, wherein the condition resolves with castration.[66] Hyperandrogenism has also been demonstrated in intact males with hyperplasia of the perianal glands and the tail gland.[100] Normal cats treated with mibolerone became virilized, showing thickening of the skin of the neck and clitoral hypertrophy.[9]

Assays (RIA) for plasma or serum androgens are commercially available and are accompanied by the same interpretational, financial, and practical considerations as previously mentioned for estrogens. Values for blood testosterone in normal male dogs and cats approximate 0.5 to 6 ng/ml, while those in normal female dogs and cats are usually less than 0.5 ng/ml.[9, 66, 98]

PROGESTERONE

Progesterone is present in both males and females, and it is produced by the corpus luteum of the ovary and by the zona reticularis of the adrenal cortex.[9, 66] The effects of progestational compounds on the skin have not been well studied. However, with the increased use of these compounds (e.g., megestrol acetate, medroxyprogesterone acetate) for the management of feline and canine skin disorders, the clinician must be alerted to some possible cutaneous side-effects.

Progesterone is known to have immunosuppressive action and various progesterone analogs are known to have glucocorticoid activity.[9, 66] Progestational compounds have also been shown to bind to the intracellular cytosol receptor for dihydrotestosterone and to inhibit the enzyme 5-α-reductase, which converts testosterone to dihydrotestosterone. By binding androgen receptors in multiple tissues, progestational compounds may be androgenic, synandrogenic, or antiandrogenic, depending on the compound and the dose.

In the skin, topically applied progesterone was shown to significantly suppress sebum excretion rate in women.[66] Medroxyprogesterone was reported to delay wound healing in rabbits. In the cat, subcutaneous injections of medroxyprogesterone acetate may produce local alopecia, atrophy, and pigmentary disturbances, and oral megestrol acetate can produce generalized cutaneous atrophy, alopecia, xanthomas, and poor wound healing (see p. 209). Bilateral flank alopecia was reported in a dog with hyperprogesteronemia and a testicular Sertoli's cell neoplasm.[23]

Assays (RIA) for plasma or serum progesterone are commercially available and are burdened by the same interpretational, financial, and practical considerations as previously mentioned for estrogens. Values for blood progesterone in female dogs and cats approximate <5 ng/ml (anestrus, estrus, proestrus) and 10 to 50 ng/ml (metestrus, pregnancy), and they approximate <1 ng/ml in male dogs and cats.[9, 66]

GONADOTROPINS AND PROLACTIN

The gonadotropins, FSH (follitropin, molecular weight about 32,000 daltons) and LH (lutropin, molecular weight about 30,000 daltons), are produced by the adenohypophysis.[1, 9] Gonadotropin secretion is stimulated by hypothalamic GnRH and inhibited by estrogens, glucocorticoids, and androgens (via aromatization to estrogens in the hypothalamus). FSH secretion is also inhibited by inhibin from the ovarian follicle and testicular Sertoli's cells. LH secretion is inhibited by progestogens and androgens. In normal dogs and cats, serum FSH levels by RIA are reported to approximate 40 to 70 ng/ml (higher in females in proestrus).[9] Serum LH levels by RIA in normal dogs and cats are reported as follows: 0 to 3 ng/ml in intact males, 6 to 10 ng/ml in females in estrus, and <2 ng/ml in females in metestrus or anestrus.[9] Gonadotropin deficiencies could be seen with hypothalamic or pituitary disorders.

Prolactin is a polypeptide (molecular weight about 22,500 daltons) produced by the adenohypophysis.[1, 9] Prolactin secretion is episodic and labile; stimulated by one or more hypothalamic releasing factors (including TRH), and inhibited by hypothalamic dopamine. In normal dogs and cats, serum prolactin levels by RIA are reported to approximate 1 to 10 ng/ml.[9] Hyperprolactinemia could be seen with hypothyroidism, pituitary neoplasms, and certain drug administrations (phenothiazines, cimetidine), resulting in galactorrhea, gynecomastia, and inhibition of FSH/LH secretion.

Clinical Aspects of Endocrine Skin Diseases

HYPERADRENOCORTICISM
(Cushing's Disease, Cushing's Syndrome)

Hyperadrenocorticism is a common disorder of the dog associated with excessive endogenous or exogenous glucocorticoids and characterized by polyuria and polydipsia, bilaterally symmetric alopecia, thin hypotonic skin, and skeletal muscle wasting. Hyperadrenocorticism is rare in cats.

CAUSE AND PATHOGENESIS

Canine hyperadrenocorticism may occur naturally or may be iatrogenic.[9, 28a, 66, 76, 92] The naturally occurring type may be associated with idiopathic bilateral adrenocortical hyperplasia, pituitary neoplasia, adrenocortical neoplasia, or the "ectopic" ACTH syndrome. Iatrogenic canine hyperadrenocorticism results from the misuse of exogenous glucocorticoids.

In about 90 per cent of the dogs with spontaneous hyperadrenocorticism, the disorder results from excessive pituitary ACTH secretion, which produces bilateral adrenocortical hyperplasia (pituitary-dependent hyperadrenocorticism). Controversy exists over the nature of the pituitary lesion in these dogs. Some reports indicate that most dogs with the syndrome have a functional (ACTH-producing) pituitary neoplasm,[28a, 66, 74, 76] while others indicate that most of these dogs have either histologically normal or hyperplastic pituitary glands.[9, 21, 66] In either condition, hypersecretion of ACTH results in bilateral adrenocortical hyperplasia that may be diffuse or nodular, or both. The zona glomerulosa is usually normal in width and histologic appearance, and enlargement is due to hyperplasia of the zona fasciculata and zona reticularis. In some cases, gross enlargement of the adrenals is not seen. The adrenal cortex may be grossly and histologically normal but functionally abnormal.

Idiopathic bilateral adrenocortical hyperplasia accounts for about 20 to 80 per cent of the cases of canine pituitary-dependent hyperadrenocorticism. It is currently thought that the underlying defect in idiopathic bilateral adrenocortical hyperplasia may be in hypothalamic regulation and the negative feedback mechanism. Serotonin appears to be an excitatory transmitter with regard to ACTH release. With increased serotonergic input there is no hippocampal inhibition of the release of corticotropin-releasing factor (CRF), resulting in increased CRF stimulation of pituitary ACTH release. Antiserotonergic agents, such as cyproheptadine, have been used successfully to treat human patients with hyperadrenocorticism resulting from idiopathic bilateral adrenocortical hyperplasia.

Bilateral adrenocortical hyperplasia secondary to a functional pituitary tumor accounts for about 20 to 80 per cent of the cases of canine pituitary-dependent hyperadrenocorticism. Chromophobe adenomas of the pars distalis are often large, compressive (hypothalamus, optic chiasm), and functional, especially in brachycephalic breeds. Adenomas arising from the pars intermedia are usually small, noncompressive, and nonfunctional and are found in non-brachycephalic breeds, but occasionally they may be functional. Canine pituitary-dependent hyperadrenocorticism has also been seen in association with pituitary adenocarcinomas. There appears to be no direct correlation between the size of the pituitary neoplasm, the degree of bilateral adrenocortical hyperplasia, and the severity of canine hyperadrenocorticism. Although the rate of growth of pituitary neoplasms is variable, it is usually slow. Great caution is in order in assessing the importance of pituitary neoplasms and "microadenomas" that occur in conjunction with hyperadrenocorticism. There is evidence to suggest that adenomatous changes in the adenohypophysis can be the *result* of hyperglucocorticoidism.

Functional (cortisol-producing) adrenocortical neoplasms account for about 10 per cent of the cases of naturally occurring canine hyperadrenocorticism. They may be adenocarcinomas or adenomas (which occur with about equal frequency) and usually appear in the right adrenal gland. These neoplasms are thought to function autonomously, producing excessive amounts of cortisol, which results in negative feedback suppression of CRF (hypothalamus) and ACTH (pituitary) and in atrophy of the contralateral adrenal gland. Adrenocortical adenocarcinomas tend to be large, often extending into the adrenal vein and caudal vena cava, and they usually metastasize to the liver, lung, kidney, and lymph nodes. Dogs with bilateral adrenocortical adenomas have been reported rarely.

The "ectopic" ACTH syndrome is a term used to describe conditions in which hyperadrenocorticism is associated with nonpituitary and nonadrenocortical neoplasia. In humans, the ectopic ACTH syndrome is most commonly seen with neoplasms of the lung and pancreas (thought to produce ACTH or an ACTH-like substance). In the dog, the ectopic ACTH syndrome appears to be very rare, and has been reported in association with lymphosarcoma and bronchial carcinoma.

By far, the most alarming cause of canine hyperadrenocorticism is the injudicious use of glucocorticoids for therapeutic purposes. Over 50 per cent of clinical hyperadrenocorticism in dogs is iatrogenic in origin.[92] Even the administration of topical glucocorticoids in ophthalmic,[30b, 85] otic,[65a] and skin[94, 123a] preparations can produce adrenocortical suppression, elevated hepatic enzymes, and iatrogenic hyperadrenocorticoidism in dogs.

Naturally occurring and iatrogenic hyperadrenocorticism are rare in the cat.[9, 66, 93] Naturally occurring feline hyperadrenocorticism has been reported in association with pituitary neoplasia and unilateral adrenocortical adenoma.[80, 93, 124] Iatrogenic hyperadrenocorticism can be produced only with great difficulty in the cat.[96]

CLINICAL FEATURES

Naturally occurring canine hyperadrenocorticism is a disease of middle-aged and older dogs (average 8 to 9 years), the range being 3 months to 18 years. Although there is no sex predilection for pituitary-dependent hyperadrenocorticism, females are affected by functional adrenocortical neoplasms three times as frequently as males. Boxers, Boston terriers, poodles, and dachshunds are predisposed to the disease; boxers and Boston terriers are predisposed to pituitary neoplasms, while dachshunds and poodles are predisposed to idiopathic adrenocortical hyperplasia. Dachshunds and large breeds of dogs are predisposed to adrenocortical neoplasms. Spontaneous hyperadrenocorticism has been reported in related Yorkshire terriers.[91] Iatrogenic canine hyperadrenocorticism knows no age, sex, or breed predilections. It most commonly occurs in dogs with chronic pruritus, since they are more likely to receive long-term systemic corticosteroids.

The clinical signs seen in canine hyperadrenocorticism are the result of excessive amounts of endogenous or exogenous glucocorticoids (see p. 204). In addition, some of the signs seen with naturally occurring canine hyperadrenocorticism may be caused by the compressive or invasive effects of a primary neoplasm or its metastases. The clinical signs can wax and wane. The frequency of various clinical signs in spontaneous canine hyperadrenocorticism are presented in Table 10:3.

The first signs recognized are usually polydipsia and polyuria (>100 ml/ kg/day water intake; >50 ml/kg/day urine output).[9, 66, 76] These may precede the more dramatic cutaneous changes by 6 to 12 months. Some owners do not recognize polydipsia and polyuria in dogs kept outdoors or in kennels. In addition, about 15 per cent of the cases do not manifest polydipsia and polyuria. Although polyphagia is also a common early sign, some dogs manifest varying degrees of anorexia.

The most spectacular signs are those related to the integument.[92] Cutaneous signs may include (1) bilaterally symmetric alopecia (which tends to spare the head and extremities and is less pronounced in short-coated dogs, in which the hair coat often appears patchy, thin, or moth eaten) (Fig. 10:3), (2) easily epilated hair, (3) variable pigmentary disturbances of the skin and hair coat (patchy or diffuse hyperpigmentation, hypopigmentation, or normal) (Fig. 10:4), (4) thin, hypotonic skin (mimics dehydrated skin, tends to wrinkle) (Figs. 10:4F and 10:5B), (5) easy bruising (petechiae; ecchymoses) (Figs. 10:4E, 10:5C), (6) comedones (Fig. 10:5D), (7) seborrhea sicca, (8) calcinosis cutis (Fig. 10:5E–H), (9) poor wound healing, (10) increased susceptibility to bacterial infection (Fig. 10:5H), and (11) phlebectasias (Fig. 10:4H). Cushingoid dogs may rarely present with only facial dermatoses.[118] Demodicosis may complicate hyperadrenocorticism in dogs and cats.[66, 124] Calcinosis cutis is seen in up to 40 per cent of the dogs with hyperadrenocorticism. It occurs most commonly over the dorsum

Table 10:3. CLINICAL SIGNS IN 300 DOGS WITH HYPERADRENOCORTICISM

Sign	Percentage of Dogs
Polyuria/polydipsia	82
Pendulous abdomen	67
Hepatomegaly	67
Hair loss	63
Lethargy	62
Polyphagia	57
Muscle weakness	57
Anestrus (69 females)	54
Obesity	47
Muscle atrophy	35
Comedones	34
Increased panting	31
Testicular atrophy (128 males)	29
Hyperpigmentation	23
Calcinosis cutis	8
Facial nerve palsy	7

From Peterson, M. E.: Hyperadrenocorticism. Vet. Clin. North Am. (Small Anim. Pract.) 14:731, 1984.

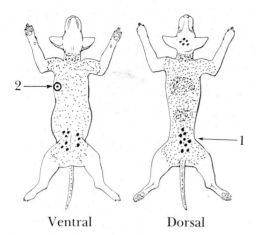

Ventral   Dorsal

Figure 10:3. Hyperadrenocorticism distribution pattern.

and in the inguinal and axillary regions, occasionally surrounded by an erythematous halo, and is frequently secondarily infected and pruritic. It may be mistaken for pyoderma. Cutaneous phlebectasias are seen in up to 40 per cent of the dogs with hyperadrenocorticism, especially over the ventrum and medial thighs.[99] These vascular lesions are macular to papular, erythematous, up to 6 mm in diameter, asymptomatic, and generally do not blanch with diascopy. These lesions do *not* regress following effective treatment. Pressure sores (decubital ulcers) are common in large dogs with hyperadrenocorticism.[28a]

Musculoskeletal abnormalities are common in canine hyperadrenocorticism.[9, 66, 76, 28a] Skeletal muscle atrophy and weakness are common, with atrophy being most pronounced over the head, shoulders, thighs, and pelvis. Abdominal enlargement ("potbelly") is frequent, with the abdomen being flaccid and the dog not being able to tense the abdomen normally (Fig. 10:4B). In addition, a cushingoid "myotonia" or "pseudomyotonia" may be seen, which is characterized by muscle stiffness and proximal appendicular muscle enlargement. Lameness associated with osteoporosis and osteomalacia, with or without pathologic fractures, is seen (Fig. 10:5A). Chronic hyperadrenocorticism can exaggerate common problems such as anterior cruciate ligament rupture and patellar luxation.[28a]

Persistent anestrus is frequently observed in intact bitches with hyperadrenocorticism.[9, 66, 76] In addition, clitoral enlargement is not uncommon (Fig. 10:4G) and presumably results from hypersecretion of adrenal androgens. Clitoral enlargement is *not* seen with iatrogenic hyperadrenocorticism. Testicular atrophy is often seen in intact males.

Lethargy and decreased exercise tolerance are commonly seen in dogs with hyperadrenocorticism.[9, 66, 76] Behavioral changes may also occur (aggressiveness, depression, psychoses, self-mutilation).

Respiratory complications reported to occur with canine hyperadrenocorticism include excessive panting, bronchopneumonia, dystrophic mineralization and fibrosis, and pulmonary thrombosis.[51]

Neurologic signs, including ataxia, blindness, head pressing, somnolence, Horner's syndrome, anisocoria, circling, hyperesthesias, and seizures, are occasionally seen in naturally occurring canine hyperadrenocorticism and are caused by pituitary neoplasia or metastatic adrenocortical neoplasia (Fig. 10:4B).[9, 66, 76] Exophthalmos and indolent corneal ulcers have also been reported in association with canine hyperadrenocorticism.

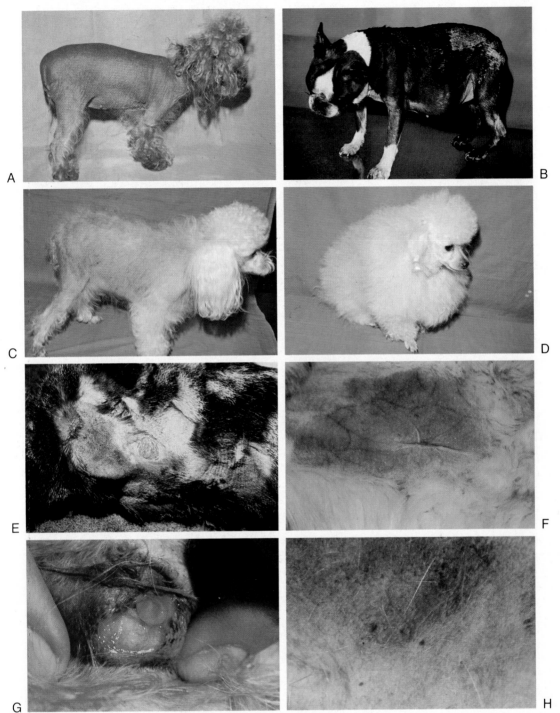

Figure 10:4. Hyperadrenocorticism. *A*, Toy poodle showing typical advanced alopecic pattern and hyperpigmented skin. This dog regrew a good hair coat with o,p'-DDD treatment. *B*, Boston terrier with muscle wasting, pendulous abdomen, and patchy alopecia. *C*, Poodle growing diffuse, fuzzing hair coat during early treatment with o,p'-DDD. *D*, Same poodle as in *C* after 4 months of treatment with o,p'-DDD. Hair is growing luxuriantly, and the animal made complete recovery but is maintained on once weekly therapy. *E*, Bruising and ulceration (torn skin) on the back of a cat with iatrogenic hyperglucocorticoidism. The area has been clipped. (From Scott, D. W.: Feline dermatology 1900—1978: A monograph. J.A.A.H.A. *16*:331, 1980.) *F*, Thin, hypotonic skin with a central wrinkle, prominent vasculature, and a few petechiae in a cat with iatrogenic hyperglucocorticoidism. *G*, Clitoral hypertrophy in a female dog with hyperadrenocorticism. *H*, Multiple red telangiectases on the abdomen of a dog with hyperadrenocorticism.

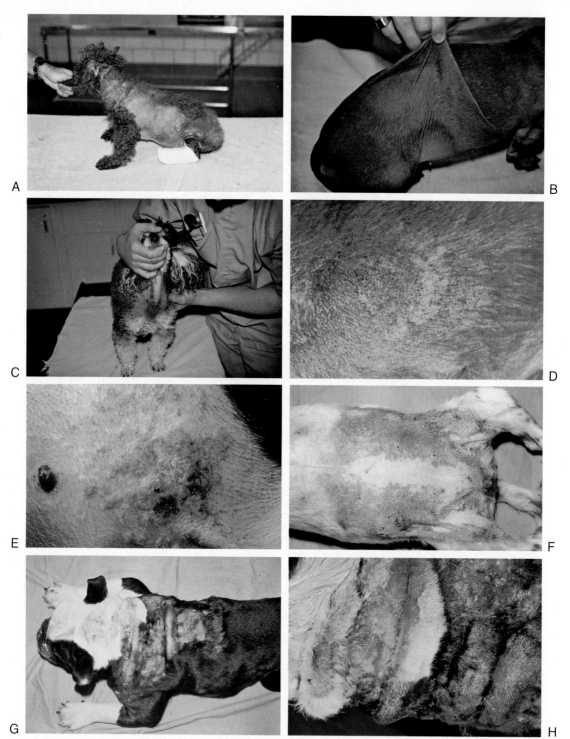

Figure 10:5. Hyperadrenocorticism. *A*, Poodle demonstrates the spectacular alopecic pattern typically seen in long-coated breeds. There was a metatarsal fracture due to osteoporosis. This patient had an adrenal tumor. (Courtesy M. D. Lorenz.) *B*, Hypotonia of skin in a dachshund with hyperadrenocorticism. *C*, Patients bruise easily, and hematomas commonly occur at sites of venipuncture. Note bruising evident in jugular region. *D*, Dark keratin plugs ("comedones"), which are inactive hair follicles filled with keratin and debris. They appear as "pepper" or "pinfeathers." *E*, Whitish nodules of calcinosis cutis, some with inflammatory reaction. *F*, Dog with iatrogenic Cushing's disease has extensive calcinosis cutis with severe erythema on the ventral surface. *G*, English bulldog with large areas of ulceration due to foreign-body reaction in mineralized skin (calcinosis cutis). *H*, Same patient as in *G* with closer view of secondary pyoderma in folds and regions involved with cutaneous mineralization.

600

Palpable hepatomegaly is a common feature of canine hyperadrenocorticism.[9, 66, 76] As many as 10 to 15 per cent of the dogs with naturally occurring hyperadrenocorticism may have concurrent diabetes mellitus and elevated blood insulin levels. Dogs with chronic hyperadrenocorticism appear to be predisposed to pancreatitis.[28a]

Clinical signs reported in association with feline hyperadrenocorticism are similar to those described for the dog. However, the cat appears to be more resistant to the development of alopecia, tends to develop fragile, easily torn skin (Fig. 10:4E), and has not been reported to develop calcinosis cutis.[66, 80, 93, 124] In one series of 9 cats with naturally occurring hyperadrenocorticism,[28a] the age ranged from 7 to 15 years; seven of nine cats were female; eight of nine had concurrent diabetes mellitus; six of nine had abnormal, unkempt haircoats; and less than 50 per cent of the cats had alopecia, muscle wasting, easy bruising, and cutaneous abscesses. Interestingly, cats with iatrogenic hyperadrenocorticism developed medial curling of the tips of the pinnae.[96]

DIAGNOSIS

Before the onset of the cutaneous signs the differential diagnosis of hyperadrenocorticism is basically that of polyuria-polydipsia: chronic renal disease, chronic hepatic disease, diabetes mellitus, diabetes insipidus (pituitary or renal), psychogenic polydipsia, hyperthyroidism, hypercalcemia, hypernatremia, hypokalemia, hypoadrenocorticism, polycythemia vera, and pyrexia.[9, 66] After the endocrine alopecia develops, the differential includes hypothyroidism, hyposomatotropism, and sex hormone "imbalances." Definitive diagnosis is based on history, physical examination, hemogram, urinalysis, serum chemistries, radiography, skin biopsy, and adrenal function tests.

Hemograms classically reveal leukocytosis (25 to 60 per cent of cases; 17,000 to 68,000/μl), neutrophilia (25 to 60 per cent; 11,500 to 65,000/μl), lymphopenia (33 to 70 per cent; 0 to 1000/μl), and eosinopenia (76 to 95 per cent; 0 to 100/μl).[9, 66, 76] Erythrocytosis (polycythemia), thrombocytosis, and hypersegmentation of neutrophil nuclei may also be seen.

Urinalysis usually reveals a low specific gravity (85 per cent; average 1.012).[9, 66, 76] In addition, 50 per cent of the dogs have urinary tract infection, usually manifested only by bacteriuria. Proteinuria is commonly seen. About 10 to 15 per cent of the dogs have glucosuria in association with concurrent diabetes mellitus.

Serum chemistry panel abnormalities may include mild-to-marked elevations in levels of cholesterol (56 to 88 per cent of cases), serum alanine transaminase (ALT) (52 to 90 per cent), serum aspartate transaminase (AST) (30 to 50 per cent), and glucose (10 to 50 per cent) and a decreased blood urea nitrogen (BUN) (10 to 50 per cent) level. Hypophosphatemia is seen in about 33 per cent of dogs with spontaneous hyperadrenocorticism. Abnormal glucose tolerance tests and elevated serum insulin levels are common.

The serum alkaline phosphatase level is usually elevated in canine hyperadrenocorticism (80 to 95 per cent) and is mainly due to a steroid-induced isoenzyme that is hepatic in origin.[9, 66, 76] Cellulose acetate electrophoretic separation of serum alkaline phosphatase isoenzymes may be helpful in the diagnosis of canine hyperadrenocorticism. Unlike the situation in dogs, serum alkaline phosphatase levels are *not* usually elevated in feline hyperadrenocorticism.

Basal thyroid hormone levels (T_4 and T_3) are usually low in canine hyperadrenocorticism.[9, 28a, 66,77] These spuriously low thyroid hormone levels are caused by glucocorticoids (see p. 578) and do *not* usually indicate concurrent hypothyroidism. The results of TSH stimulation tests are usually normal, but pre- and post-TSH levels may be below the normal ranges (however, the slope of the charted response parallels that of normal dogs). When the hyperadrenocorticism is corrected, thyroid hormone levels return to normal. Occasionally, a dog truly has concurrent hypothyroidism and requires thyroid maintenance therapy.

Dogs with hyperadrenocorticism may also have elevated systolic (180 to 280 mmHg; normal $\leqq170$) and diastolic (110 to 180 mmHg; normal $\leqq100$) blood pressures, which may predispose to congestive heart failure.[9, 28a, 66] In dogs with cushingoid myopathies, electromyographic studies have revealed bizarre high-frequency discharges in association with histopathologic findings in skeletal muscle (atrophy, degeneration, necrosis) and peripheral nerves (segmental demyelination).

Dogs with hyperglucocorticoidism have decreased blood GH levels, which respond poorly or not at all to xylazine or clonidine.[9, 66, 76] Glucocorticoids can also suppress serum gonadotropin (LH, FSH) levels, prolactin levels, and testosterone and estrogen levels.[28a, 43, 48, 104] Serum testosterone responses to exogenous LH or hCG (human chorionic gonadotropin) injections are normal in this situation.

Radiography may reveal (1) hepatomegaly, (2) osteoporosis and osteomalacia (especially of vertebrae, ribs, and flat bones), with or without pathologic fractures, (3) dystrophic mineralization of soft tissues (especially of the lung, kidney, and skin), and (4) adrenocortical neoplasms.[9, 28a, 66, 76] An important finding is unilateral mineralization in the area of an adrenal gland, which can be seen in about 25 per cent of dogs with adrenocortical neoplasms. Gamma camera imaging of adrenal glands in normal dogs and in dogs with naturally occurring hyperadrenocorticism has been reported.[9, 66] This technique requires sophisticated equipment and several days, and it is expensive. In addition, it must be remembered that adrenal glands can be grossly normal, yet hyperfunctional.

Dogs with hyperadrenocorticism may have significant elevations of coagulation factors I (fibrinogen), V, VII, IX, and X, as well as elevated levels of antithrombin III and plasminogen.[9, 51, 66] These abnormalities may predispose the patient to hypercoagulability and thromboembolism.

In cats, hemograms, serum chemistry panels, and urine specific gravities are usually unremarkable.[28a] The most consistent abnormalities are hyperglycemia, hypercholesterolemia, and glucosurine.

Histopathology. Skin biopsy in canine hyperadrenocorticism may reveal many nondiagnostic changes consistent with endocrinopathy (orthokeratotic hyperkeratosis, epidermal atrophy, epidermal melanosis, follicular keratosis, follicular dilatation, follicular atrophy, telogenization of hair follicles, sebaceous gland atrophy).[95] Histopathologic findings highly suggestive of hyperadrenocorticism include dystrophic mineralization (collagen fibers, basement membrane zone of epidermis and hair follicles), thin dermis, and absence of arrector pili muscles (Figs. 10:6 to 10:9). Histopathologic findings consistent with secondary pyoderma and foreign body granuloma (associated with dystrophic mineralization) may be seen. Histopathologic characteristics of cutaneous phlebectasias range from marked dilatation and congestion of superficial dermal

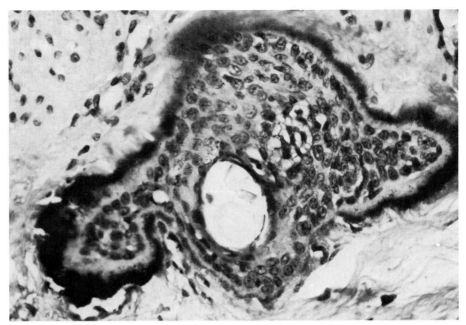

Figure 10:6. Canine hyperadrenocorticism. Dystrophic mineralization of glassy membrane of hair follicle.

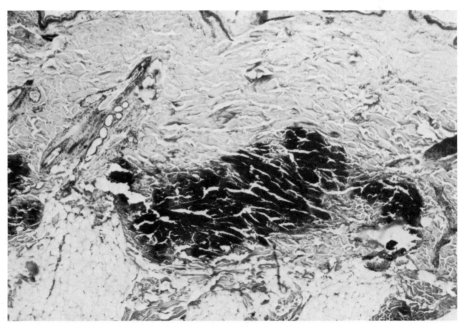

Figure 10:7. Dystrophic mineralization of dermal collagen.

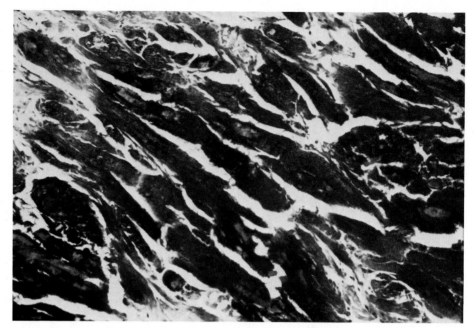

Figure 10:8. Close-up of Figure 10:7. Mineralization tracks collagen bundles.

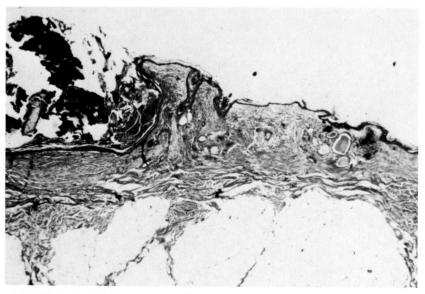

Figure 10:9. Canine hyperadrenocorticism. Note follicular keratosis and atrophy. Absence of hair shafts, sebaceous gland atrophy, thin dermis, and dystrophic mineralization of dermis (right) and surface (left).

blood capillaries (macular stage) to a lobular proliferation of normal appearing superficial dermal blood vessels, which may be encased by an epidermal collarette (papular stage).[99]

Adrenal Function Tests. Once spontaneous hyperadrenocorticism is suspected (based on clinical signs and routine laboratory findings), the diagnosis is substantiated and further defined by a two-stage protocol.[9, 76, 79] The objective of the first or "screening" stage is to confirm or rule out the diagnosis of hyperadrenocorticism. Once the diagnosis is confirmed, the purpose of the second stage is to differentiate pituitary-dependent hyperadrenocorticism from that caused by adrenal neoplasia. Figure 10:10 is a flow sheet of diagnostic tests that are useful for evaluating dogs with suspected hyperadrenocorticism.

Adrenal function tests are basically of two types: those that are single measurements of basal glucocorticoid levels in urine or blood and those that are provocative, dynamic response tests of the glucocorticoid levels in urine or blood (see p. 585). Single measurements of basal glucocorticoid levels are unreliable, with up to 50 per cent of the dogs with naturally occurring hyperadrenocorticism having levels within the normal range. Urinary steroid assays are cumbersome and rarely used. Presently, the most commonly used adrenal function tests are the ACTH response test, the dexamethasone suppression test, or some combination thereof.

Tests to Diagnose Hyperadrenocorticism. The *ACTH stimulation test* reliably documents a diagnosis of iatrogenic hyperadrenocorticism in dogs and cats.[9, 66] Basal blood cortisol levels are low or normal and show little or no response to ACTH. The ACTH stimulation test is *not* as accurate as the low-dose dexamethasone suppression test in diagnosing spontaneous canine hyperadrenocorticism, as about 15 per cent of the cases of pituitary-dependent hyperadrenocorticism do not have an exaggerated response, and over 50 per cent of the cases of adrenocortical neoplasia are hyper-responsive (see p. 586).[9, 25, 66, 76, 79] In addition, dogs that are clinically stressed or that have various chronic

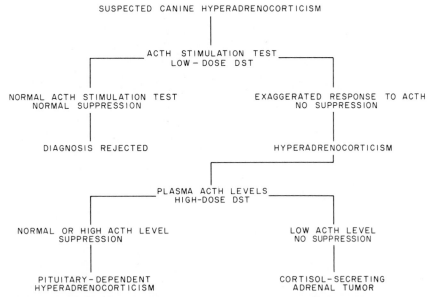

Figure 10:10. Flowchart for evaluation of dogs with suspected hyperadrenocorticism. (From Peterson, M. E.: Hyperadrenocorticism. Vet. Clin. North Am. [Small Anim. Pract.] *14*:731, 1984.)

illnesses frequently hyper-respond to ACTH stimulation (see p. 586).[8] It has been reported that cats with uncomplicated diabetes mellitus may also hyper-respond to ACTH stimulation.[80]

Two commonly used ACTH stimulation test protocols for dogs are as follows: (1) plasma or serum cortisol determinations are collected before and 2 hours after the intramuscular injection of 2.2 IU/kg ACTH gel, and (2) plasma or serum cortisol determinations are collected before and one hour after the intramuscular or intravenous injection of 0.25 mg synthetic ACTH (see p. 586). The ACTH stimulation test has been utilized in a limited number of normal cats and cats with naturally occurring and iatrogenic hyperadrenocorticism (see p. 586).[66, 78, 93, 98] Two recommended ACTH stimulation test protocols for cats are as follows: (1) plasma or serum cortisol determinations before and 90 minutes after the intramuscular injection of 2.2 IU/kg ACTH gel, and (2) plasma or serum cortisol determinations before and 90 minutes after the intramuscular injection of 0.125 mg synthetic ACTH (see p. 586).

The *low-dose dexamethasone suppression test* is presently the procedure of choice for diagnosing spontaneous hyperadrenocorticism in dogs (see p. 587).[9, 25, 66, 76, 79] In normal dogs, the low dose of dexamethasone consistently suppresses cortisol levels to less than 1.0 μg/dl for the 8-hour test period. Inadequate suppression occurs in dogs with spontaneous hyperadrenocorticism. However, dogs that are clinically stressed or that have various chronic illnesses may also fail to suppress.[8] Plasma or serum cortisol levels are determined before and 8 hours after an intravenous injection of 0.01 mg/kg of dexamethasone. *In cats,* there is little information available on the diagnostic benefit of dexamethasone suppression tests.

Tests to Differentiate the Cause of Hyperadrenocorticism. The *high-dose dexamethasone suppression test* is presently the procedure of choice for differentiating between pituitary-dependent hyperadrenocorticism and that caused by adrenocortical neoplasia in dogs (see p. 588).[9, 26, 28, 66, 76, 79] Suppression of blood cortisol levels to below 1.5 μg/dl is diagnostic for pituitary-dependent hyperadrenocorticism. Such suppression does not occur with adrenocortical neoplasia. However, about 15 per cent of the dogs with pituitary-dependent hyperadrenocorticism fail to adequately suppress with *any* dose of dexamethasone.[9, 49, 66, 76, 79] Plasma or serum cortisol levels are determined before and 8 hours after the intravenous injection of 0.1 mg/kg dexamethasone. Some investigators have recommended a dexamethasone dosage of 1.0 mg/kg.[76, 79] However, this dosage does not clearly increase the accuracy of the test, and greatly increases the cost of the procedure.[9, 26, 49, 103]

Recently, attempts have been made to streamline adrenal function testing in the dog by combining the ACTH stimulation test and the dexamethasone suppression test (see p. 589).[9, 18, 27, 28, 66] Such combination tests appear to be less reliable than single tests of adrenal function, and cannot be recommended at present. Other tests that have been evaluated in spontaneous canine hyperadrenocorticism include the metyrapone response test, the lysine-vasopressin test, and the insulin response test.[9, 66] These tests cannot be recommended.

Endogenous plasma ACTH levels are extremely useful in determining the cause of spontaneous canine hyperadrenocorticism, especially when interpreted together with the results of dexamethasone suppression tests (see p. 588).[9, 26–28, 76, 79] Plasma ACTH levels are normal to elevated (>40 pg/ml) in dogs with pituitary-dependent hyperadrenocorticism, and low to undetectable (<20 pg/

ml) in dogs with functional adrenal neoplasms. Unfortunately, accurate determination of plasma ACTH levels requires proper collection and handling of specimens and technically difficult radioimmunoassay procedures. Many commercial laboratories may be unable to provide dependable results (see p. 589).[9, 76, 79]

The recent isolation and synthesis of CRH offers an additional diagnostic test to differentiate the two causes of spontaneous canine hyperadrenocorticism (see p. 589).[9, 50, 76, 79] Preliminary information indicates that the *CRH stimulation test* (plasma ACTH or cortisol levels measured before and 30 to 60 minutes after the intravenous injection of 1.0 µg/kg CRH) is useful for distinguishing between pituitary-dependent hyperadrenocorticism (increased levels of ACTH or cortisol) and adrenocortical neoplasia (no response) in dogs. However, until a relatively inexpensive, single-dose, sterilized CRH preparation becomes available, the CRH stimulation test appears to be of limited usefulness for most veterinarians.

Ultrasonography (adrenal glands), *gamma camera imaging* (adrenal glands), and *computed tomography* (pituitary gland, adrenal glands) are also useful techniques for differentiating between pituitary-dependent hyperadrenocorticism and adrenocortical neoplasia but are generally unavailable to most veterinarians.[19, 28, 28a, 40, 80b, 108, 110a]

CLINICAL MANAGEMENT

The prognosis for untreated naturally occurring canine hyperadrenocorticism is poor, with death often occurring within 2 years (septicemia, diabetes mellitus, heart failure, pancreatitis, pyelonephritis thromboembolism, and so on).[9, 28a, 66, 92] Although the prognosis is much better with therapy, it is still unpredictable. Death may occur in association with either adrenalectomy, hypophysectomy, o,p'-DDD, or concurrent diseases. In addition, death may occur at any time during or after therapy in association with growth of a pituitary neoplasm or metastasis of an adrenocortical adenocarcinoma. Since hyperadrenocorticism is a disease of older dogs, most will die or be euthanized within 2 years of diagnosis, as a result of any of the aforementioned conditions. Spontaneous remission of pituitary-dependent canine hyperadrenocorticism rarely has been reported. The average life expectancy of 256 treated cases of canine hyperadrenocorticism was 2 years (18 days to over 7 years).

The cause of hyperadrenocorticism determines therapy.[28a, 76, 79] Pituitary-dependent hyperadrenocorticism can be treated surgically with bilateral adrenalectomy or hypophysectomy, or it can be managed medically with the adrenocorticolytic agent o,p'-DDD. Unilateral adrenocortical neoplasms should be surgically removed. Regardless of the treatment method chosen, hyperadrenocorticism cannot be treated easily, inexpensively, or without close monitoring and follow-up. Some dogs with pituitary-dependent hyperadrenocorticism have relatively mild, slowly progressive disease, and observation alone may be best for these dogs and owners.

Pituitary-Dependent Hyperadrenocorticism. This disorder can be treated with either *bilateral adrenalectomy or hypophysectomy.*[9, 66, 76] Both procedures require a skilled surgeon, intensive intraoperative and postoperative monitoring and supportive care, lifelong hormone replacement therapy, and considerable expense. Surgical techniques and management protocols have been described.[19a, 28a, 59]

Pituitary-dependent hyperadrenocorticism has also been treated with drugs that act on the central nervous system, adenohypophysis, and adrenal gland.[9, 66, 76] *Cyproheptadine* (Periactin) is an antiserotonin agent that blocks serotonin-mediated CRH and ACTH release. The drug has been used to treat spontaneous canine hyperadrenocorticism (0.3 to 3.0 mg/kg/day orally), but most dogs were not helped.[76, 105] *Bromocriptine* (Parlodel) is a potent dopamine receptor agonist that inhibits ACTH secretion. This drug has also been used to treat dogs with spontaneous hyperadrenocorticism (up to 0.1 mg/kg/day) with rare benefit.[9, 66, 76] Side-effects seen with these drugs include vomiting, depression, behavioral changes, and changes in appetite. Because of their frequent side-effects and infrequent benefit, these drugs appear to have limited usefulness in the management of hyperadrenocorticism.[28a]

Ketoconazole is an antifungal imidazole drug that also inhibits adrenocortical steroidogenesis in dogs and humans (see p. 180).[28a] Normal dogs treated with 10 to 30 mg/kg/day ketoconazole orally developed significant decrease in basal plasma cortisol levels, and 45 to 90 per cent reductions of plasma cortisol responses to exogenous ACTH.[120] Ketoconazole has been helpful for the treatment of some humans and dogs with pituitary-dependent hyperadrenocorticism.[120] Fifteen cushingoid dogs, including four with adrenal tumors, were treated with ketoconazole orally, 15 mg/kg BID, and all showed rapid improvement.[28a] It has been ineffective in a small number of cushingoid dogs.[103] Ketoconazole failed to suppress basal plasma cortisol levels in normal cats given 30 mg/kg/day orally for 30 days.[121]

The drug of choice for pituitary-dependent hyperadrenocorticism in dogs is o,p'-DDD (mitotane, Lysodren).[9, 28a, 57, 66, 76, 79] o,p'-DDD is a chlorinated hydrocarbon derivative that causes selective necrosis and atrophy of the zona fasciculata and zona reticularis of the adrenal cortex, while the zona glomerulosa (mineralocorticoid-producing zone) is relatively resistant. Initial dosage of o,p'-DDD is 25 to 50 mg/kg/day for 7 to 10 days. The daily dose may be divided in half and administered BID. Small doses of glucocorticoid (oral prednisone or prednisolone at 0.2 mg/kg/day; or oral hydrocortisone at 1.0 mg/kg/day) are often given during the initial 7 to 10 days of o,p'-DDD therapy to minimize the side-effects associated with acute glucocorticoid withdrawal. Some authors advise against using glucocorticoids because (1) it makes evaluation of early responses very difficult, and (2) it is necessary in only about 5 per cent of the cases.[28a] In dogs with concurrent diabetes mellitus, treatment with o,p'-DDD reduces the daily insulin requirement, and can predispose to insulin overdosage and hypoglycemia. A low initial dose of o,p'-DDD (25 mg/kg/day) and a higher daily maintenance dose of prednisone or prednisolone (0.4 mg/kg) or hydrocortisone (20 mg/kg) prevent the rapid reductions in circulating glucocorticoid levels and daily insulin requirements and allow for easier regulation of the diabetes.

The most common side-effects observed during initial o,p'-DDD therapy include lethargy, vomiting, diarrhea, anorexia, and weakness. Less common side-effects include disorientation, ataxia, and head pressing. About 25 per cent of dogs develop one or more side-effects during initial therapy, but the effects are relatively mild in most dogs. Side-effects develop when plasma cortisol levels either fall below normal basal range (>1.0 µg/dl) or drop too rapidly into normal range (glucocorticoid withdrawal syndrome), and resolve promptly with increased glucocorticoid supplementation. If adverse signs occur during initial o,p'-DDD therapy, the drug should be stopped and the glucocorticoid dose doubled until the dog can be evaluated. If clinical signs persist longer than 3 hours after increasing the glucocorticoid dose, other medical problems should be considered.

There are many ways to assess the effectiveness of initial o,p'-DDD therapy.[9, 28a, 66, 76, 79] Measurement of daily water consumption and eosinophil counts can be used, but may be misleading, as they only indirectly reflect circulating cortisol levels. In addition, up to 15 per cent of cushingoid dogs do not manifest polydipsia or eosinopenia. Some dogs with hyperadrenocorticism may *not* consume large quantities of water in a foreign environment. Thus, water consumption and urine specific gravity are best determined in the dog's normal surroundings. A more direct approach is to perform an ACTH stimulation test. Since prednisone, prednisolone, and hydrocortisone all cross-react in most cortisol assays, glucocorticoid supplementation should not be given on the morning of ACTH stimulation testing. To insure adequate control of hyperadrenocorticism with o,p'-DDD, both basal and post-ACTH cortisol levels should remain within normal range. Following o,p'-DDD induction therapy and ACTH stimulation testing, o,p'-DDD should be discontinued and glucocorticoid supplementation should be continued until cortisol results are available.

About 15 per cent of dogs still have exaggerated ACTH stimulation tests after initial o,p'-DDD therapy. In these dogs, daily o,p'-DDD therapy should be continued and ACTH stimulation tests repeated at 5- to 10-day intervals until basal and post-ACTH cortisol levels are in the normal range. This may require as long as 30 to 60 days in some dogs. In contrast, about 33 per cent of dogs will have basal and post-ACTH cortisol levels *below* normal range following initial o,p'-DDD therapy. In these dogs, o,p'-DDD should be stopped and glucocorticoid supplementation continued as needed, until basal cortisol levels normalize. This usually takes about 2 to 6 weeks.

Once normal cortisol levels are documented by ACTH stimulation testing, o,p'-DDD is continued at a weekly maintenance dosage of 50 mg/kg. The weekly maintenance dosage may be divided in half and given twice weekly. During maintenance therapy with o,p'-DDD, glucocorticoid supplementation is rarely required. In the rare dog that manifests poor appetite, depression, weakness, and mild weight loss in spite of normal cortisol levels, alternate-morning doses of prednisone or prednisolone (0.4 mg/kg) are very beneficial. One author (G. H. M.) prefers to skip the induction period of 7 to 10 days and immediately starts the patient on the weekly maintenance dose. Although response time is prolonged, he reports no adverse effects.

About 5 per cent of the dogs treated with maintenance o,p'-DDD therapy develop iatrogenic hypoadrenocorticism characterized by low basal and post-ACTH cortisol levels and hyperkalemia/hyponatremia. Adverse clinical signs resolve after stopping o,p'-DDD and supplementing with appropriate doses of glucocorticoid and mineralocorticoid. Iatrogenic hypoadrenocorticism may be temporary or permanent, and further o,p'-DDD therapy is not indicated unless the hypoadrenocorticism resolves and basal and post-ACTH cortisol levels increase above normal range.

About 50 per cent of dogs treated with initial loading and maintenance doses of o,p'-DDD relapse within 12 months of treatment as evidenced by recurrence of clinical signs and elevated basal and post-ACTH cortisol levels. To ensure continued control and prevent serious relapse during o,p'-DDD therapy, ACTH stimulation testing should be repeated every 6 months during maintenance therapy. If basal and post-ACTH cortisol levels rise above normal range, the o,p'-DDD dosage should be increased to 25 to 50 mg/kg/day for 5 days, and the weekly maintenance dose should be increased by 50 per cent. Because of multiple relapses, some dogs eventually require maintenance o,p'-DDD doses as high as 100 to 300 mg/kg/week.

Medical management of spontaneous feline hyperadrenocorticism has not been reported. Because cats are quite sensitive to chlorinated hydrocarbon toxicosis, o,p'-DDD may be inappropriate therapy.[66, 93] Recently o,p'-DDD was administered orally (12.5 to 25 mg/kg BID) to four normal cats.[124] Each dose was administered for 7 days, and adrenal responses were monitored by ACTH stimulation testing. Two cats had progressive suppression of cortisol levels (one of these developed vomiting, diarrhea, and anorexia), and two cats appeared to be unaffected. One cat with naturally occurring hyperadrenocorticism was treated for 45 days with o,p'-DDD with no response (either clinically or with ACTH stimulation tests).[28a] Further evaluation of o,p'-DDD in cats is required before its usage can be recommended.

Adrenocortical Neoplasia. The therapy of choice for adrenocortical neoplasia is unilateral adrenalectomy.[9, 66, 76, 79, 90] Because the contralateral adrenal gland is severely atrophied, these dogs have to be supported as glucocorticoid-deficient patients with maintenance and stress doses of glucocorticoids for 2 to 12 months. ACTH stimulation testing can be performed every 2 to 3 months so as to determine when the remaining adrenal gland has returned to normal function.

If the adrenal neoplasm is malignant, if the owner refuses surgery for the dog, or if the dog is considered to be an unsuitable surgical candidate, medical adrenalectomy with o,p'-DDD can be attempted.[76, 79] However, only limited success has been achieved in the treatment of canine adrenocortical neoplasms with o,p'-DDD. In general, the drug is administered at a daily dose of 50 to 150 mg/kg, and ACTH stimulation testing is repeated every 2 weeks. If remission does occur, maintenance glucocorticoid supplementation is recommended. Subsequent dosage adjustments are based on the results of periodic ACTH stimulation tests.

Iatrogenic Hyperadrenocorticism. Therapy of canine iatrogenic hyperadrenocorticism requires ceasing excessive exogenous glucocorticoids, while continuing maintenance and stress therapy for the concomitant secondary adrenocortical (glucocorticoid) deficiency.[9, 66, 76, 92] When glucocorticoid therapy is withdrawn, patients may be susceptible to hypothalamic-pituitary-adrenal insufficiency for 3 to 12 months. Hydrocortisone is the glucocorticoid of choice for replacement therapy and is given at 0.2 to 0.5 mg/kg every morning. Recovery usually occurs within 3 to 4 months. Exogenous ACTH should *not* be used in iatrogenic hyperadrenocorticism. This is because the block after prolonged glucocorticoid therapy is not at the level of the adrenocortical response to ACTH, but at the level of the ability of the hypothalamic-pituitary unit to resume release of CRH-ACTH. Therefore, ACTH may actually aggravate the problem.

Whichever method of therapy is employed, the skin may initially show increasing scaling and pigmentation, and new hair regrowth may be of different color from normal (for example, gray hair grows in black, black grows in red). With successful therapy, the cutaneous signs of hyperadrenocorticism including calcinosis cutis usually regress within 3 to 4 months.

HYPOPITUITARISM

Hypopituitarism can be caused by failure or loss of one or more of the pituitary hormones.[1, 9, 11] The endocrine manifestations of hypopituitarism are related to the type and degree of hormonal deficiency and the stage in life during which the deficiency occurs.

Hypopituitarism may be caused by pituitary or hypothalamic deficiencies. Pituitary deficiencies may be caused by congenital hypoplasia, destructive lesions (infections, lymphocytic hypophysitis, infiltrative diseases, trauma, neoplasms), vascular lesions, and the inherited disorder of German shepherds and carnelian bear dogs (see following discussion). Hypothalamic deficiencies may be caused by trauma, encephalitis, aberrant parasite migration, hamartoma, neoplasia, and neurosecretory dysfunction.

Hypopituitarism is diagnosed on the basis of various clinical signs, responses of various target organs and pituitary hormones to challenges with pituitary and hypothalamic hormones and releasing factors, and various sophisticated radiographic techniques.[1, 9]

PITUITARY DWARFISM

Canine pituitary dwarfism is usually a hereditary hypopituitarism associated with proportionate dwarfism, bilaterally symmetric alopecia and hyperpigmentation, and variable thyroidal, adrenocortical, and gonadal abnormalities.

CAUSE AND PATHOGENESIS

In the German shepherd and carnelian bear dog, pituitary dwarfism is thought to be inherited as a simple autosomal recessive condition.[9, 17, 66] Most affected dogs appear to have a variably sized cyst (Rathke's cleft cyst) in the pituitary gland resulting in varying degrees of anterior pituitary insufficiency (Fig. 10:11E,F). However, a few dogs have had either hypoplastic or normal anterior pituitary glands.[61, 66] The clinical signs are related to growth hormone deficiency, with or without concurrent thyroidal, adrenocortical, and gonadal abormalities (see p. 589).

Immunodeficient dwarfism has been reported in an inbred colony of Weimaraners with growth hormone deficiency and congenital absence of thymic cortex.[88, 89]

CLINICAL FEATURES

Canine pituitary dwarfism has been reported in many breeds, but predominantly in the German shepherd and carnelian bear dog.[9, 10b, 66] No sex predilection is evident.

For the first 2 to 3 months of life, the dog may appear normal and indistinguishable from normal litter mates. After this time, the dog fails to grow, the hair coat is notably shorter, and no primary hairs develop. The puppy coat of secondary hairs is retained. This hair is soft, woolly, and easily epilated. Primary hairs are often present only on the face and distal extremities (Fig. 10:11A,B). Bilaterally symmetric alopecia then develops, especially in the wear areas of the neck and caudolateral aspects of the thighs. The alopecic skin

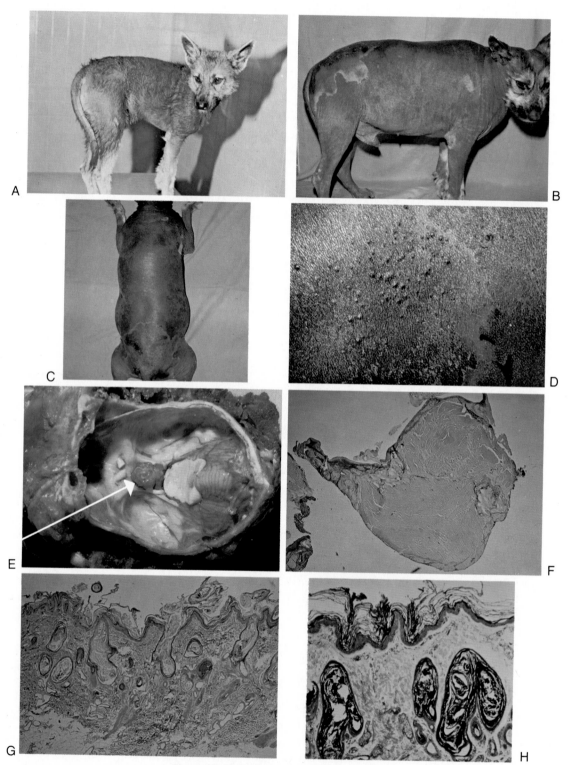

Figure 10:11 *See legend on opposite page*

is at first normally pigmented, then progresses through increasing degrees of hyperpigmentation. The skin becomes thin, hypotonic, and scaly. Comedones may be numerous (Fig. 10:11C,D). These dogs may have behavioral abnormalities such as fear biting and aggressiveness. Gonadal status may vary from atrophic testicles or absence of estrus to normal. If there are concurrent deficiencies of TSH and/or ACTH, the dogs may manifest signs of hypothyroidism and adrenocortical insufficiency. As dwarfs grow older, they often become progressively more listless, dull, and inactive, and most die between 3 and 8 years of age due to infections, degenerative diseases, or neurologic dysfunction.[28a]

Immunodeficient dwarfism in Weimaraners is characterized by puppies, which appear normal at birth, developing a wasting syndrome at a few weeks of age.[88, 89] Clinical signs include unthriftiness, emaciation, lethargy, and persistent infections, usually resulting in death.

DIAGNOSIS

The differential diagnosis includes congenital hypothyroidism, juvenile diabetes mellitus, gonadal dysgenesis, malnutrition, severe metabolic diseases (portal caval shunts, congenital renal disease, congenital heart defects), and skeletal dysplasias (chondrodysplasia in Alaskan malamutes, pseudoachondroplastic dysplasia in miniature poodles, mucopolysaccharidosis).[9] Definitive diagnosis is based on history, physical examination, laboratory tests, skin biopsy, radiography, insulin-induced hypoglycemia, and growth hormone stimulation tests. Depending on the degree of anterior pituitary insufficiency, affected dogs may have laboratory findings consistent with hypothyroidism and secondary adrenocortical insufficiency. Immunodeficient dwarf Weimaraners have deficient lymphocyte blastogenic responses to phytomitogens, as well as thymic cortical hypoplasia.[88, 89]

Histopathology of the skin reveals changes consistent with endocrinopathy (orthokeratotic hyperkeratosis, follicular keratosis, follicular dilatation, follicular atrophy, telogenization of hair follicles, sebaceous gland atrophy, epidermal melanosis, thin dermis) (Fig. 10:11G,H).[95] A highly suggestive finding is the decreased amount and size of dermal elastin fibers. In cases with concurrent hypothyroidism, histopathologic findings may include vacuolated and/or hypertrophied arrector pili muscles.

Radiography may reveal delayed closure of growth plates of long bones, delayed eruption of permanent teeth, failure of the os penis to completely

Figure 10:11. Pituitary dwarfism. *A,* Dwarf German shepherd at nine months of age showing puppy coat of secondary hair on body, primary hairs on face and distal portions of legs, and alopecia on posterolateral aspect of thigh. Dog has a "coyote-like" appearance. *B,* Dwarf German shepherd at nearly four years of age. Note hyperpigmentation, peeled epidermis over hips, flaccid penile sheath, and chunky conformation. This is the same dog shown in *A. C,* Dorsal view of dwarf German shepherd immediately after euthanasia. Note obesity, hyperpigmentation, and areas of epidermal peeling and scarring. *D,* Close-up of skin showing alopecia, hyperpigmentation, and papules (cystic follicles). (*A, B, C,* and *D* from Muller, G. H., and Jones, S.: Pituitary dwarfism associated with cystic Rathke's cleft in a dog. J.A.A.H.A. 7:567, 1973.) *E,* Multinodular pituitary gland (arrow) in the pituitary fossa at necropsy. *F,* Histologic section of pituitary gland showing almost complete replacement of cystic Rathke's cleft, which was filled with eosinophilic mucinous substance (× 11, H & E stain). *G,* Hyperkeratosis and follicular keratosis of skin of dwarf German shepherd (× 22, H & E stain). *H,* Skin from back of dwarf German shepherd. Note absence of black elastic fibers in dermis around keratotic follicles (× 80). (Figures *F, G,* and *H* courtesy Armed Forces Institute of Pathology, Washington, D.C.)

mineralize by 1 year of age, open fontanelles of the skull and smaller-than-normal heart, liver, and kidney (Fig. 10:12).[9, 10b, 66]

A characteristic metabolic abnormality of growth hormone–deficient dogs is hypersensitivity to the hypoglycemic effect of injected insulin.[9, 17, 66] The intravenous injection of 0.025 units/kg of regular insulin into growth hormone–deficient dogs produces severe, prolonged hypoglycemia.

Basal plasma growth hormone levels (by radioimmunoassay) in normal dogs approximate 1.0 to 4.5 ng/ml in most reports.[9, 66] However, basal growth hormone levels in pituitary dwarfs and hypophysectomized dogs may approximate these values. Thus, basal growth hormone levels are inadequate for the documentation of growth hormone deficiency. Clonidine (an α-adrenergic antihypertensive drug) and xylazine have been used to stimulate growth hormone release in the dog and to document the existence of growth hormone deficiency.[9, 17, 66] Normal dogs show a marked increase in plasma growth hormone levels within 15 to 30 minutes after the intravenous injection of 10 to 30 μg/kg of clonidine or 100 to 300 μg/kg xylazine, whereas pituitary dwarfs and hypophysectomized dogs fail to respond (see p. 590). Hypothyroidism, hyperadrenocorticism, and sex hormone abnormalities must *always* be ruled out, as they can impair growth hormone secretion.

The measurement of plasma somatomedin C levels could also be diagnostic (<5 ng/ml), but test results must be evaluated in light of the size of the dog (see p. 591).[9, 17] It has been shown that heterozygous carriers of the pituitary dwarfism trait have intermediate levels of plasma somatomedin C, as compared with dwarfs and normal dogs. In some instances, it may be of value to assess both growth hormone and somatomedin C levels, such as when (1) growth hormone levels are normal (and the hormone is biologically inactive), but somatomedin C levels are low (Laron's type I dwarfism), or (2) growth hormone levels are normal, but somatomedin C levels are low (decreased hepatic GH receptors) (Laron's type II dwarfism).[9]

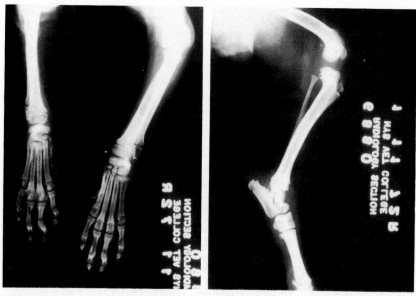

Figure 10:12. Radiographs of extremities of 18-month-old standard poodle with pituitary dwarfism. Note the open epiphyseal lines, especially the distal radius and ulna.

Recently, human GHRH has been used to evaluate GH responses in the dog.[28a] When administered to normal dogs at a dose of 1 μg/kg, GHRH produced a twofold-to-fourfold increase in GH levels, whereas there was no response in dogs with hyposomatotropism.

CLINICAL MANAGEMENT

The owner should be made aware of the chronic nature of the disease and the general unavailability of growth hormone for treatment, and of the shortened life expectancy. If the owner is willing to accept these possibilities, the dwarf dog can be kept as a pet.

Bovine growth hormone (10 IU subcutaneously, every other day for 30 days) and porcine growth hormone (2 IU subcutaneously, every other day or 0.1 IU/kg subcutaneously three times weekly for 4 to 6 weeks) have been used experimentally to treat canine pituitary dwarfism.[9, 10b, 28a, 66, 82] A beneficial response in the skin and hair coat is seen within 6 to 8 weeks. However, growth plates close rapidly, and no appreciable increase in stature is achieved. Although not reported during the treatment of canine pituitary dwarfism, repeated injections of bovine and porcine growth hormone could result in hypersensitivity reactions or diabetes mellitus. Concurrent hypothyroidism or secondary adrenocortical insufficiency would require additional specific therapy with L-thyroxine or glucocorticoids, respectively. If secondary adrenocortical insufficiency is present, this should always be treated first.

HYPOSOMATOTROPISM IN THE MATURE DOG
(Pseudo-Cushing's Syndrome, Growth Hormone–Responsive Dermatosis)

Hyposomatotropism is a rare, bilaterally symmetric alopecia occurring in mature dogs.

CAUSE AND PATHOGENESIS

The cause and pathogenesis of this disorder are unknown.[17, 28a, 101] Clonidine and xylazine stimulation tests have shown that affected dogs have inadequate or absent ability to secrete growth hormone. Necropsy examination of two dogs has revealed pituitary atrophy in one, and a normal pituitary in the other. The preponderance of cases occurring in certain breeds and familial occurrence of the condition suggest that the etiology has a genetic component. It is likely that these dogs have a GH neurosecretory dysfunction, such as deficient hypothalamic GHRH activity.[4]

CLINICAL FEATURES

Hyposomatotropism has been reported predominantly in male dogs of the chow chow, keeshond, Pomeranian, and miniature poodle breeds.[101] Age of onset is between 9 months and 11 years of age, with about 50 per cent of the dogs beginning at less than 2 years of age. The disorder is characterized by (1) bilaterally symmetric alopecia and hyperpigmentation, which occurs mainly on the trunk, neck, pinnae, tail, and caudomedial thighs (Fig. 10:13A–D), (2) bilaterally symmetric trunk alopecia without hyperpigmentation, or (3) bilater-

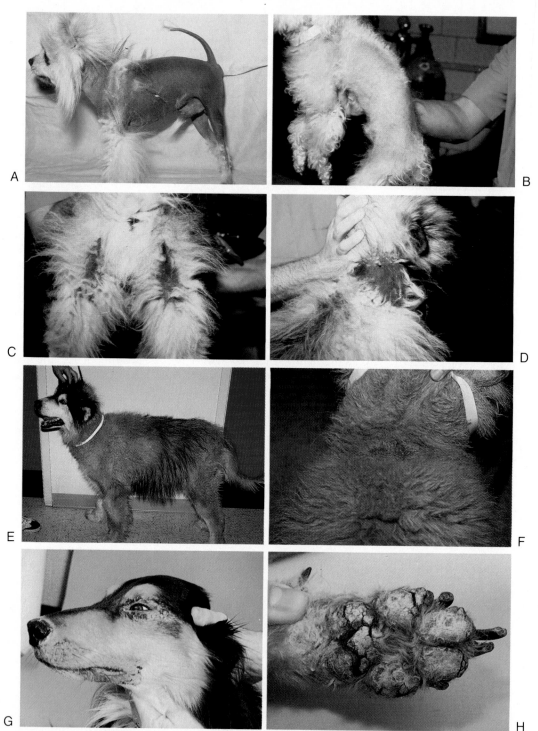

Figure 10:13. Hyposomatotropism (growth hormone–responsive dermatosis). *A*, Pomeranian with hyposomatotropism. Note the distribution pattern of the alopecia and hyperpigmentation. *B*, Alopecia and brownish-tinged hyperpigmentation of the trunk in a poodle with hyposomatotropism. (From Parker, W. M., and Scott, D. W.: Growth hormone–responsive alopecia in the mature dog: a discussion of 13 cases. J.A.A.H.A. *16*:824, 1980.) *C*, Alopecia and hyperpigmentation of the caudal thighs in a dog with hyposomatotropism. *D*, Alopecia and hyperpigmentation in the neck of a dog with hyposomatotropism. *E*, Castration-responsive dermatosis in a "woolly" malamute. (Courtesy of W. H. Miller, Jr.) *F*, Close-up of dog in *E*. Frictional alopecia under neck collar. (Courtesy of W. H. Miller, Jr.) *G*, Canine hepatocutaneous syndrome (diabetic dermatosis). Erythema, crusting, and alopecia around nose, mouth, and eye. *H*, Canine hepatocutaneous syndrome (diabetic dermatosis). Hyperkeratosis and fissuring of footpads.

ally symmetric flank alopecia, with or without hyperpigmentation (Fig. 10:14). Hairs in affected areas are often easily epilated. In chronic cases, the skin may be thin and hypotonic. In cases in which previous skin biopsies had been performed, the hair grew back over the biopsy sites. The dogs are normal, except for the dermatologic signs. In Airedales, boxers, and English bulldogs, a seasonal growth hormone deficiency is seen, wherein dogs develop flank alopecia and hyperpigmentation in winter.[103, 103a]

DIAGNOSIS

The differential diagnosis includes hypothyroidism, hyperadrenocorticism, and sex hormone "imbalances." Definitive diagnosis is based on history, physical examination, laboratory rule-outs, skin biopsy, and response to therapy. Skin biopsy reveals changes consistent with endocrinopathy (orthokeratotic hyperkeratosis, follicular keratosis, follicular dilatation, telogenization of hair follicles, epidermal melanosis, sebaceous gland atrophy, thin dermis).[95] A highly suggestive histopathologic finding is decreased amounts and small size of dermal elastin fibers (Figs. 10:15 and 10:16), but this finding may be present only in dogs that have been clinically affected for 2 years or more.[101] Measurements of plasma growth hormone levels before and after the intravenous injection of clonidine or xylazine documents growth hormone deficiency (see p. 590).[101] In dogs with seasonal (winter) growth hormone deficiency (Airedales, boxers, English bulldogs), xylazine responses are suppressed in winter and become normal in summer.[103] Hypothyroidism, hyperadrenocorticism and sex hormone abnormalities must always be ruled out before interpreting growth hormone test results, as these conditions will impair growth hormone secretion.[9, 17, 101, 103] Recently human GHRH has been used to evaluate GH responses in the dog (see pituitary dwarfism).

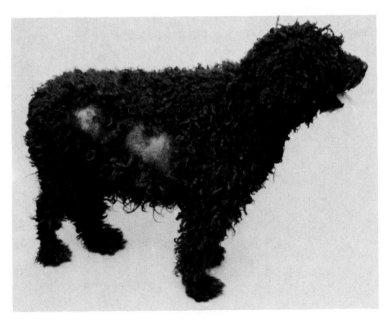

Figure 10:14. Hyposomatotropism. Symmetric flank alopecia.

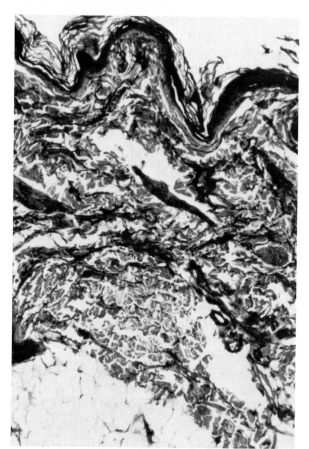

Figure 10:15. Normal canine skin. Numerous thick, long elastin bundles and fibers are present in the dermis (Verhoeff's stain). (From Parker, W. M., and Scott, D. W.: Growth hormone–responsive alopecia in the mature dog: a discussion of 13 cases J.A.A.H.A. *16*:824, 1980.)

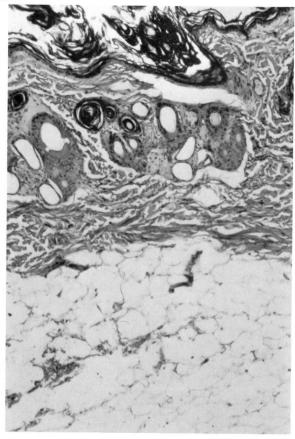

Figure 10:16. Hyposomatotropism (growth hormone–responsive dermatosis) in a dog. Marked absence of dermal elastin (Verhoeff's stain). (From Parker, W. M., and Scott, D. W.: Growth hormone–responsive alopecia in the mature dog: a discussion of 13 cases. J.A.A.H.A. *16*:824, 1980.)

CLINICAL MANAGEMENT

Therapy with bovine or porcine GH has been reported to be effective.[17, 101] Doses of 2.5 IU (dogs weighing less than 14 kg) or 5.0 IU (dogs weighing over 14 kg) are given subcutaneously every other day for 10 treatments. A good response is seen within 3 months. Remission may last from 6 months to over 3 years. Possible side-effects include diabetes mellitus, acromegaly, and hypersensitivity reactions. Ovine growth hormone has been reported to be ineffective for treating dogs.[101] Recently human GH (0.15 IU/kg subcutaneously twice weekly for 6 weeks) was reported to be effective for the treatment of Pomeranians.[90a] At present, no commercial source of GH is available for use in dogs. Fortunately, dogs with adult-onset hyposomatotropism are usually otherwise healthy, and their disease is primarily an aesthetic problem.

Until the genetics of adult-onset hyposomatotropism are more carefully analyzed, the use of affected dogs for breeding should be discouraged.

ACROMEGALY

Acromegaly in the dog is characterized by inspiratory stridor, thick skin, hypertrichosis, abdominal enlargement, polyuria-polydipsia, and fatigue associated with hypersecretion of growth hormone in the mature animal. It is a rare disease.

CAUSE AND PATHOGENESIS

Acromegaly is caused by hypersecretion of growth hormone in the mature animal (after epiphyseal closure). Hypersecretion of growth hormone results in an overgrowth of connective tissue, bone, and viscera (see p. 590). In the dog, acromegaly has been reported in association with injections of anterior pituitary gland extracts, acidophilic hyperplasia or adenoma of the anterior pituitary gland, diestrus in the intact cycling bitch, and administration of progestational compounds.[9, 15, 16, 28a, 97] In the cat, acromegaly has been associated with pituitary tumors.[9, 13]

CLINICAL FEATURES

No breed or age predilections are evident for canine acromegaly. Most cases have occurred in intact female dogs that are in diestrus or are being treated with progestational compounds. The most common signs noted in acromegaly include inspiratory stridor (due to soft-tissue increases in the orolingual-oropharyngeal regions), increased body size (especially paws and skull) (Fig. 10:17), abdominal enlargement, polyuria, polydipsia, polyphagia, fatigue, frequent panting, prognathism, widening of the interdental spaces, and galactorrhea. Cutaneous changes include thickened, myxedematous skin thrown into excessive folds, hypertrichosis, and thick hard nails (Fig. 10:18).

DIAGNOSIS

The definitive diagnosis of acromegaly is based on history, physical examination, serum chemistries, skin biopsy, persistent elevation of plasma growth hormone levels, and the nonsuppressibility of plasma growth hormone

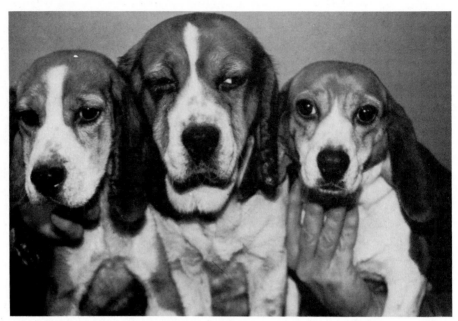

Figure 10:17. Acromegaly. Acromegalic beagle (center) and two normal littermates.

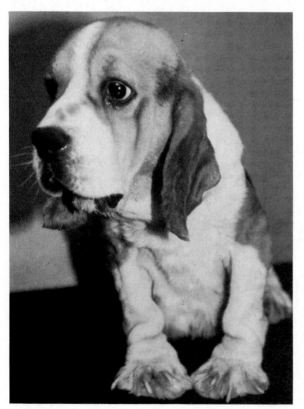

Figure 10:18. Acromegaly. Note large head and paws.

levels after intravenous glucose administration.[9, 15, 16, 97] Many acromegalic dogs have mild-to-moderate hyperglycemia and mild-to-severe elevations of serum alkaline phosphatase levels. Basal plasma growth hormone levels have ranged from 11 to 1476 ng/ml and could not be suppressed by an intravenous glucose load (1 gm glucose/kg). Nonsuppressibility of plasma growth hormone levels during an intravenous glucose load is considered to be a hallmark of acromegaly. The levels of plasma growth hormone do not always correlate with the degree of acromegaly. GH levels may also be elevated in response to stress, acute illness, chronic renal and liver disease, diabetes mellitus, and starvation.[28a] The measurement of plasma somatomedin C levels (mean 679 ± 116 ng/ml in acromegalic dogs, mean 280 ± 23 ng/ml in normal German shepherds) could also be diagnostic, but must be evaluated in light of the size of the dog (see p. 591).[9, 15, 16] Acromegalic patients also manifest insulin resistance.

In dogs and human beings, histologic examination of acromegalic skin reveals collagenous hyperplasia, myxedema, and hyperplasia of the epidermis and appendages (Figs. 10:19 and 10:20).[97]

CLINICAL MANAGEMENT

Dogs with acromegaly associated with diestrus or with progestational compound treatment have responded well to ovariohysterectomy and to stopping progestogen therapy, respectively.[9, 15, 16, 97]

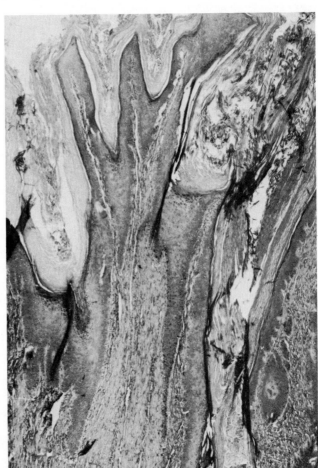

Figure 10:19. Acromegaly. Papillated hyperplasia and orthokeratotic hyperkeratosis.

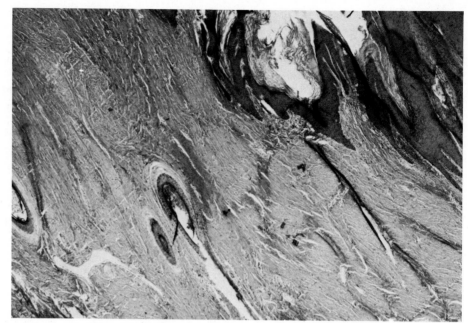

Figure 10:20. Acromegaly. Collagenous hyperplasia.

HYPERESTROGENISM IN THE FEMALE DOG
(Ovarian Imbalance Type I)

Hyperestrogenism in the female dog is a rare disorder characterized by bilaterally symmetric alopecia, gynecomastia, vulvar enlargement, and estrus cycle abnormalities. It is associated with cystic ovaries or functional ovarian tumors.

CAUSE AND PATHOGENESIS

This disorder is usually associated with cystic ovaries and rarely with functional ovarian tumors.[9, 66] Most estrogen-producing ovarian neoplasms are granulosa-theca cell in origin, and 10 to 20 per cent are malignant. Estrogenic substances have been administered to dogs by a number of investigators (see p. 592), resulting in cutaneous syndromes identical with the naturally occurring disease. An identical syndrome may also be seen with overdoses of estrogens used to treat mismating and urinary incontinence after an ovariohysterectomy.[3, 66, 114] Recent evidence suggests that some dogs have "cutaneous hyperestrogenism" (blood estrogen levels normal), owing to increased numbers of cutaneous estrogen receptors.[14]

CLINICAL FEATURES

Hyperestrogenism associated with polycystic ovaries is usually seen in the middle-aged intact female dog. English bulldogs may be predisposed to the disorder.[9] Hyperestrogenism associated with functional ovarian neoplasia is usually seen in older intact females, and no breed predilections are reported. The disorder is characterized by bilaterally symmetric alopecia beginning in the perineal and genital regions (Figs. 10:21 and 10:22A–C). Diffuse alopecia appears

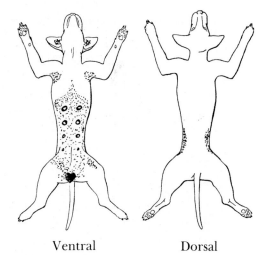

Figure 10:21. Hyperestrogenism distribution pattern.

Ventral   Dorsal

and may eventually affect (1) the caudomedial thighs, ventral abdomen, thorax, and neck, (2) the flanks, and (3) the feet. Hairs in affected areas are easily epilated. Some dogs present with symmetric alopecia that is confined to the flank areas, and the alopecia may fluctuate with the estral cycle. The nipples and vulva are enlarged. Secondary seborrheic skin disease, pruritus, and ceruminous otitis externa are common features of this disorder. In addition, estrus cycle abnormalities (irregular cycles, prolonged estrus) often occur, and endometritis/pyometra may be seen. Nymphomania and estrogen-induced bone marrow depression are rare.

DIAGNOSIS

The differential diagnosis includes hypothyroidism, hyperadrenocorticism, hormonal hypersensitivity, and seborrheic skin disease complex. Definitive diagnosis is based on history, physical examination, laboratory rule-outs, and response to therapy. Skin biopsy is nondiagnostic, revealing changes consistent with endocrinopathy (orthokeratotic hyperkeratosis, follicular keratosis, follicular dilatation, follicular atrophy, telogenization of hair follicles, sebaceous gland atrophy) or inflammatory skin disease (superficial perivascular dermatitis, either spongiotic or hyperplastic) or both disorders (Fig. 10:23).[95] Elevated blood estrogen levels may support the diagnosis (see p. 592). Ultrasonography and laparoscopy are useful for delineating ovarian neoplasms.[9]

CLINICAL MANAGEMENT

Therapy of hyperestrogenism in the female dog consists of ovariohysterectomy. A good response is usually evident within 3 months but occasionally may not be seen for 6 months. Symptomatic therapy with topical antiseborrheic agents may be indicated. If an ovarian neoplasm is suspected, chest radiographs should be taken prior to surgery, as 10 to 20 per cent of these are malignant.[9]

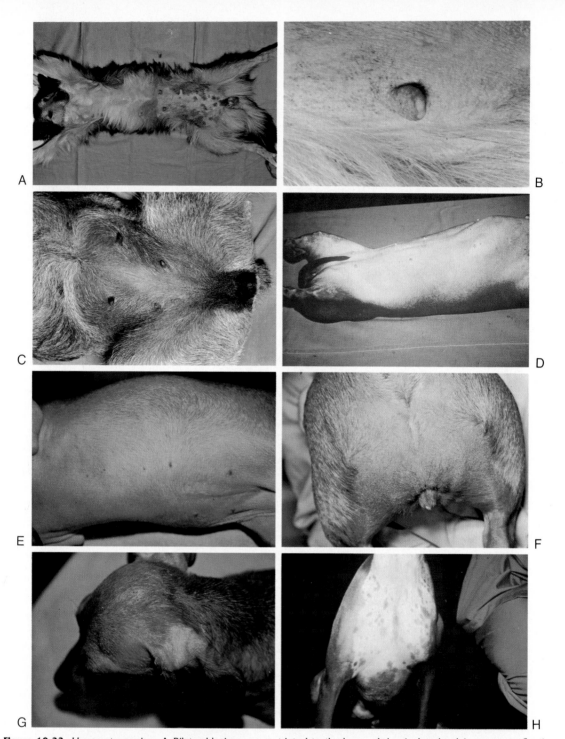

Figure 10:22. *Hyperestrogenism: A,* Bilateral lesions are restricted to the lower abdominal and pelvic areas, a reflection of the internally caused gonadal disturbance. *B,* Close-up of an enlarged nipple with comedones. The nipples are as large as those of a lactating female, although this bitch has never whelped. *C,* Note the hypertrophied, hyperpigmented vulva. *Estrogen-responsive dermatosis: D,* Mature dachshund bitch with typical alopecia of ventral chest and abdomen. The skin is pale, thin, and soft. *E,* Closer view of a similar case rolled over on the side. Note the fine soft hair that is apparent on the sides of the chest. *F,* Perineal region of a typical early case. Alopecia is complete, and the vulva is small. *G,* Alopecia starting on the temporal regions. It is complete at the base of the ears. (Poodles may lose all the hair on both ears with a syndrome resembling "alopecia areata" in man. This is *not* the syndrome pictured here.) *H,* Mature boxer bitch shows affected hair coat on brisket and ventral neck. The skin is pale, soft, and alopecic.

624

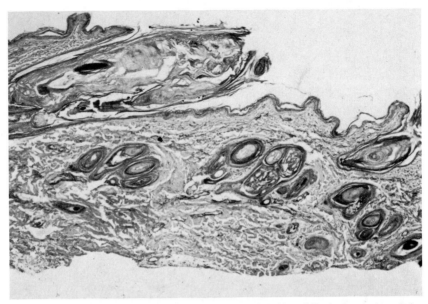

Figure 10:23. Hyperestrogenism (ovarian imbalance I) in a dog. Note follicular keratosis and plugging, absence of hair shafts, and sebaceous gland atrophy.

ESTROGEN-RESPONSIVE DERMATOSIS OF THE FEMALE DOG
(Ovarian Imbalance Type II, "Hypoestrogenism")

Estrogen-responsive dermatosis is a rare, bilaterally symmetric alopecia of unknown etiology seen in spayed female dogs.

CAUSE AND PATHOGENESIS

The cause and pathogenesis of estrogen-responsive dermatosis in female dogs are unknown.[9, 66, 109] Hypoestrogenism has been suggested as the cause of this endocrine-like dermatosis seen in prematurely ovariohysterectomized female dogs. Estrogen-responsive dermatoses have also been described in female dogs before their first estrus, during pseudopregnancy, and in association with estrus cycle abnormalities. Although some investigators have reported abnormally low urinary or blood estrogens in association with these dermatoses, hypoestrogenism has *not* been documented in the vast majority of cases.

CLINICAL FEATURES

Estrogen-responsive dermatosis is usually seen in female dogs that have been prematurely ovariohysterectomized. No age or breed predilections are documented, but most reported cases involve dachshunds and boxers. The dermatosis is characterized by bilaterally symmetric alopecia that begins in the perineal and genital regions. Diffuse alopecia is observed, which may eventually affect the caudomedial thighs, the ventral abdomen, thorax, neck, and pinnae (Fig. 10:24). Hairs in affected areas are easily epilated. The nipples and vulva are infantile. Some dogs present with only bilateral flank alopecia. Although pruritus and skin lesions are usually absent, some dogs may manifest pruritus, dermatitis, and secondary seborrheic skin disease. Aside from the dermatologic

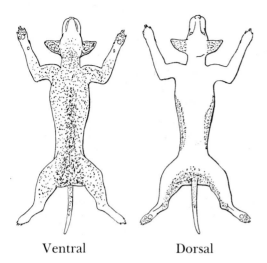

Ventral   Dorsal

Figure 10:24. Estrogen-responsive dermatosis (ovarian imbalance type II) distribution pattern.

signs, dogs with estrogen-responsive dermatosis are usually normal (see Fig. 10:22D–H). Concurrent estrogen-responsive urinary incontinence is occasionally seen.

DIAGNOSIS

The differential diagnosis includes hypothyroidism, hyperadrenocorticism, hyposomatotropism, and pattern baldness. Definitive diagnosis is based on history, physical examination, laboratory rule-outs, and response to therapy. Skin biopsy is nondiagnostic, revealing orthokeratotic hyperkeratosis, follicular keratosis, follicular atrophy, follicular dilatation, and telogenization of hair follicles (Fig. 10:25).[95]

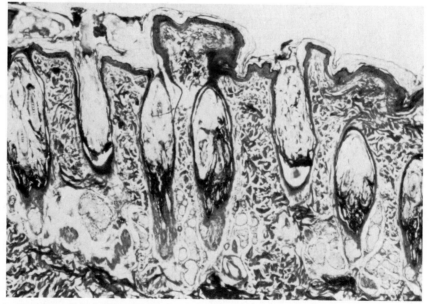

Figure 10:25. Estrogen-responsive dermatosis (ovarian imbalance type II). Note follicular keratosis and plugging and absence of hair shafts.

CLINICAL MANAGEMENT

Therapy consists of 0.1 to 1 mg of diethylstilbestrol, given orally once daily. Therapy is continued on the basis of 3 weeks "on" and 1 week "off," until hair growth is evident. If a satisfactory response is not seen within 3 months, the diagnosis must be questioned. When a good response is seen, a maintenance dose of 0.1 to 1 mg given once or twice weekly is established. If signs of estrus occur, the dose should be lowered. Great caution is warranted when prolonged estrogen therapy is administered to dogs, as they are susceptible to severe estrogen-induced bone marrow depression (thrombocytopenia, leukopenia, anemia).

Recently, a dog that was suspected of having estrogen-responsive dermatosis and that had hypoestrogenemia was successfully treated with FSH (0.75 mg/kg/day intramuscularly until signs of proestrus appeared).[6] It was theorized that the FSH stimulated "sluggish" ovaries to produce adequate amounts of estrogen.

SERTOLI'S CELL TUMOR
(Alopecia and Feminization with Functional Sertoli's Cell Tumor)

Hyperestrogenism due to a functional Sertoli's cell testicular tumor is an uncommon disorder, causing bilaterally symmetric alopecia and feminization in male dogs.

CAUSE AND PATHOGENESIS

A syndrome of endocrine alopecia and feminization occurs in about one-third of the dogs with a testicular Sertoli's cell tumor.[9, 66] An identical clinical syndrome has been reported rarely in association with testicular interstitial cell tumors and seminomas. One should remember, however, that more than one type of tumor may be present in the testis simultaneously, and that bilateral testicular neoplasia is not uncommon. In addition, a hereditary syndrome of male pseudohermaphroditism, cryptorchidism, Sertoli's cell neoplasia, and feminization has been reported in miniature schnauzers.[5, 9] Many investigators have demonstrated increased levels of estrogens in the peripheral blood and the neoplastic tissue of dogs with Sertoli's cell testicular neoplasia and feminization. Hyperestrogenism results in the cutaneous, prostatic, behavioral, and hematologic abnormalities associated with these functional Sertoli's cell neoplasms (see p. 592). Bilateral flank alopecia has been reported in a male dog with hyperprogesteronemia and a testicular Sertoli's cell tumor.[23]

CLINICAL FEATURES

Functional Sertoli's cell tumors are most commonly found in cryptorchid testicles. The incidence of feminization increases from about 15 per cent with scrotally located tumors to 50 per cent in cases of inguinal and 70 per cent in cases of abdominal localization. Feminization is more likely to occur with larger tumors and tends to be increasingly severe as tumor size increases. Although any breed of dog may be affected, boxers, Shetland sheepdogs, Weimaraners, Cairn terriers, Pekingese, and collies are predisposed.[9, 66, 115] The disease usually affects middle-aged to older dogs.

The functional Sertoli's cell tumor feminizing syndrome is characterized by varying combinations of bilaterally symmetric alopecia, gynecomastia, pendulous prepuce, and attraction of other male dogs (Fig. 10:26). It is important to emphasize that affected dogs may present with alopecia or feminization, or both. The alopecia begins in the perineal and genital regions and may eventually involve the ventral abdomen and chest, flanks, and neck (Figs. 10:27A–C). Hairs in affected areas are easily epilated. The skin may be thin or of normal thickness. Pruritus, dermatitis, and hyperpigmentation are uncommon. Linear prepucial dermatosis (Fig. 10:28) appears to be very suggestive of hyperestrogenism and testicular neoplasia (Sertoli's cell tumor, interstitial cell tumor) in dogs.[33, 103] A well-demarcated linear area of macular erythema and/or melanosis is present along the ventral aspect of the prepuce.

In addition to gynecomastia and attraction of other males, signs of feminization may include decreased libido, aspermatogenesis, and galactorrhea. The tumor may be palpated in a retained or scrotal testicle (Fig. 10:29). The non-neoplastic testicle is usually atrophied. Caution is warranted here, as functional Sertoli's cell tumors may occur in palpably normal scrotal testicles. The prostate is often enlarged (estrogen-induced squamous metaplasia) and infected, and there may be clinical signs referable to prostatomegaly or prostatitis, or both. Rarely, spermatic cord torsion with an intra-abdominal testicular Sertoli's cell tumor occurs, resulting in an acute abdomen.[52] Estrogen-induced bone marrow depression (thrombocytopenia, neutropenia, anemia) is a life-threatening complication in dogs with functional Sertoli's cell tumors.[64, 66] Pseudohermaphroditism in miniature schnauzers consists of unilateral or bilateral cryptorchidism, small penis and prepuce, feminization, and endocrine alopecia.[5, 9] These dogs may also have anorexia, depression, and pyrexia with concurrent pyometra.

DIAGNOSIS

The differential diagnosis includes hypothyroidism, hyperadrenocorticism, adult-onset hyposomatotropism, idiopathic feminizing syndrome of male dogs, and castration-responsive dermatosis of male dogs. Definitive diagnosis is based on history, physical examination, laboratory rule-outs, and response to therapy. Skin biopsy is nondiagnostic, revealing orthokeratotic hyperkeratosis, follicular keratosis, follicular dilatation, follicular atrophy, telogenization of hair

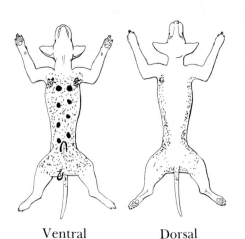

Figure 10:26. Sertoli's cell tumor distribution pattern.

Ventral   Dorsal

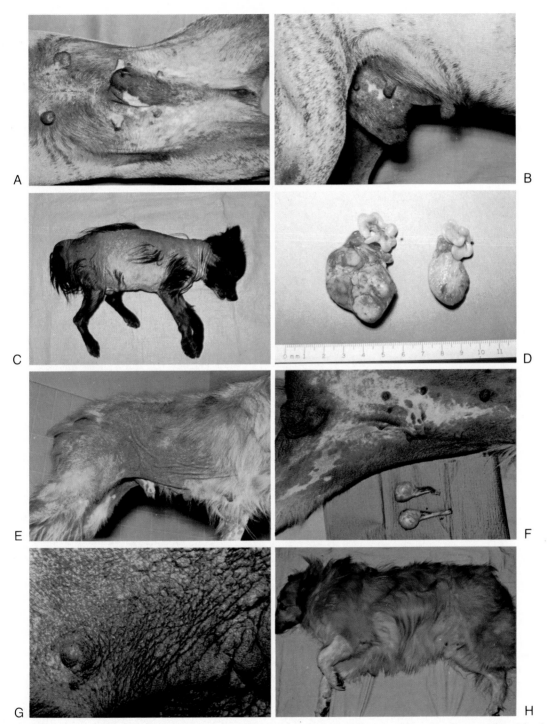

Figure 10:27. *Sertoli's cell tumor:* A, Genital area of boxer with a Sertoli's cell tumor. Note the absence of testicles in the scrotum, the gynecomastia, and the blotchy hyperpigmentation. *B,* Lateral view of *A. C,* Pomeranian whose death was caused by a Sertoli's cell tumor 8 cm in diameter. Note the distribution pattern of the alopecia in this extremely advanced case. *D,* Cryptorchid testes removed surgically from dog in *A.* The left testis is neoplastic, whereas the right testis is atrophied. *Male feminizing syndrome:* E, Alopecia with hyperpigmented, hyperkeratotic, lichenified skin in the flanks and thighs. The entire area is greasy and scaly. *F,* At the time of castration two small, soft testes were removed. Enlarged nipples and typical lesions of the flank and scrotum are also evident. *G,* Close-up of skin showing gynecomastia, hyperpigmentation, hyperkeratosis, and lichenification. *H,* Same patient as in *E* and *F* 8 months after castration.

629

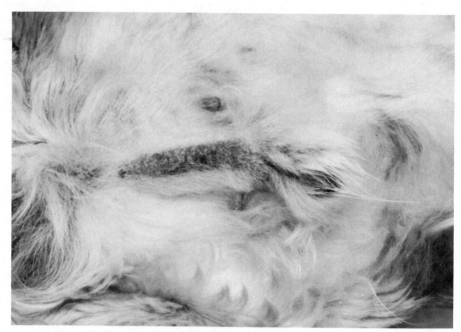

Figure 10:28. Linear preputial dermatosis in a dog with a Sertoli's cell tumor.

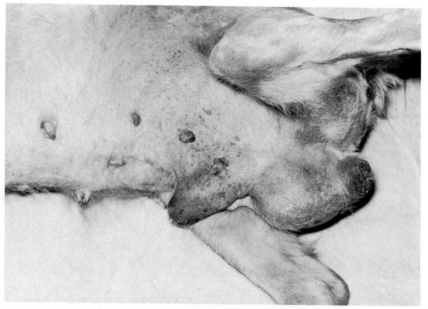

Figure 10:29. Intrascrotal testis with Sertoli's cell tumor constituting most of the scrotal mass. The small node at the posterior edge of the scrotum is the uninvolved but atrophied testis. Note enlarged nipples.

follicular keratosis, follicular dilatation, follicular atrophy, telogenization of hair follicles, and sebaceous gland atrophy (Fig. 10:30).[95] Elevated blood estrogen levels may support the diagnosis (see p. 592). Diagnosis is confirmed by histopathology of the neoplastic testicle.

CLINICAL MANAGEMENT

Therapy consists of castration. Careful abdominal palpation and thoracic radiographs are indicated prior to surgery, as about 10 per cent of Sertoli's cell tumors are malignant. A good clinical response is usually seen within 3 months. Remission followed by relapse indicates functional metastases. Concurrent prostatic or bone marrow disease must also be treated. Aplastic anemia secondary to hyperestrogenism warrants a guarded prognosis.

Therapy of pseudohermaphroditism in miniature schnauzers may require simultaneous castration and hysterectomy.

IDIOPATHIC MALE FEMINIZING SYNDROME

Male feminizing syndrome is a very rare, idiopathic disorder characterized by bilaterally symmetric alopecia, severe seborrheic skin disease and hyperpigmentation, gynecomastia, and normal testicles.

CAUSE AND PATHOGENESIS

The cause and pathogenesis of idiopathic feminizing syndrome of male dogs are unknown.[9, 66] The disorder is not associated with gross or histologic testicular abnormalities. In addition, studies on the plasma concentrations and concentration ratios of estradiol and testosterone in peripheral and spermatic cord venous blood failed to document any differences between dogs with

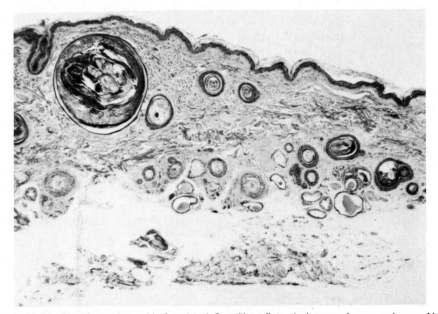

Figure 10:30. Skin from dog with functional Sertoli's cell testicular neoplasm syndrome. Note follicular keratosis and dilatation, absence of hair shafts, and sebaceous gland atrophy.

idiopathic feminizing syndrome and normal dogs. Skin biopsy reveals no evidence of endocrinopathy.[95]

CLINICAL FEATURES

Idiopathic feminizing syndrome usually affects middle-aged male dogs. No breed predilections are reported. The disorder is characterized by bilaterally symmetric alopecia, seborrheic skin disease, and severe hyperpigmentation that begins in the perineal and genital regions (Fig. 10:31). These dermatologic changes may eventually involve the ventral abdomen and chest, flanks, neck, and face. The secondary seborrheic skin disease is usually inflammatory and greasy, and pruritus may be severe (Fig. 10:27E–G). Ceruminous otitis externa is common. Gynecomastia is a constant finding, but the testicles are usually normal. Attraction of other male dogs, decreased libido, and aspermatogenesis may or may not be noted.

DIAGNOSIS

The differential diagnosis includes the functional Sertoli's cell tumor syndrome, hypothyroidism, the seborrheic skin disease complex, hormonal hypersensitivity, and food hypersensitivity. Definitive diagnosis is based on history, physical examination, laboratory rule-outs, and response to therapy. Skin biopsy is nondiagnostic, revealing hyperplastic or spongiotic superficial perivascular dermatitis wherein mononuclear cells or neutrophils may predominate.[95]

CLINICAL MANAGEMENT

The therapy of idiopathic feminizing syndrome is as mysterious as the disease itself.[66] Some investigators have reported that bilateral castration is very effective. Others have reported that testosterone is quite efficacious. Methyl testosterone may be given orally at 1 mg/kg up to a maximum of 30 mg total dose, every other day. Maintenance doses may then be given once or twice weekly. Repositol testosterone 2.2 mg/kg intramuscularly every 6 months has also been reported to be effective. Regardless of the method of therapy employed, a good response should be evident within 3 months.

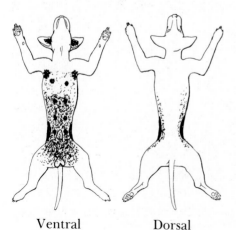

Figure 10:31. Feminizing syndrome of male dogs (hypoandrogenism) distribution pattern.

Ventral   Dorsal

TESTOSTERONE-RESPONSIVE DERMATOSIS OF THE MALE DOG

("Hypoandrogenism")

Testosterone-responsive dermatosis is a very rare, bilaterally symmetric alopecia of unknown etiology seen in male dogs.

CAUSE AND PATHOGENESIS

The cause and pathogenesis of testosterone-responsive dermatosis in male dogs are unknown.[66, 95] Hypoandrogenism has been suggested, but not documented as the cause of this endocrine-like dermatosis.

CLINICAL FINDINGS

Testosterone-responsive dermatosis is usually seen in older male dogs with normal, atrophied, cryptorchid, or neoplastic testicles or in dogs that were prematurely castrated. No breed predilections are reported. The dermatosis is characterized by bilaterally symmetric alopecia that begins in the perineal and genital regions (Fig. 10:32). There is diffuse-to-patchy alopecia that may eventually affect the caudomedial thighs, ventral abdomen, and flanks. Hairs in

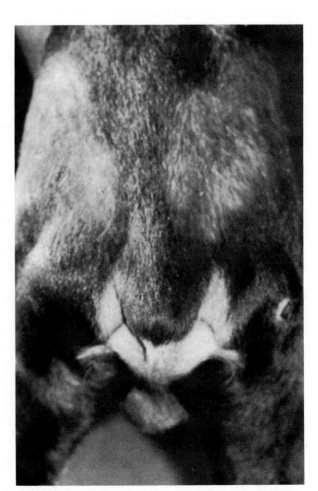

Figure 10:32. Testosterone-responsive dermatosis. Alopecia and scaling over rump.

affected areas are easily epilated. The skin is usually thin and hypotonic, the hair coat is dry and dull, and seborrhea sicca is present (Fig. 10:33).

DIAGNOSIS

The differential diagnosis includes hypothyroidism, hyperadrenocorticism, hyposomatotropism, castration-responsive dermatosis, and functional Sertoli's cell tumor syndrome. Definitive diagnosis is made by history, physical examination, laboratory rule-outs, and response to therapy. Skin biopsy is nondiagnostic, revealing orthokeratotic hyperkeratosis, epidermal atrophy, follicular keratosis, follicular atrophy, follicular dilatation, telogenization of hair follicles, thin dermis, and sebaceous gland atrophy.[95]

CLINICAL MANAGEMENT

Therapy consists of methyl testosterone given orally at 1 mg/kg, up to a maximum total dose of 30 mg, every other day. A good response should be evident within 3 months. At this point, a maintenance dose may be established (once or twice weekly). Large doses of testosterone may result in seborrhea oleosa, cholestatic liver disease, and behavioral changes (aggression).

HYPERANDROGENISM

Hyperandrogenism is a cause of perianal gland hyperplasia and tail gland hyperplasia, with or without seborrhea oleosa, in male dogs with testicular neoplasia.[100, 103] Hyperandrogenism is a *suspected* cause of seborrhea oleosa in "oversexed" intact male dogs.[66]

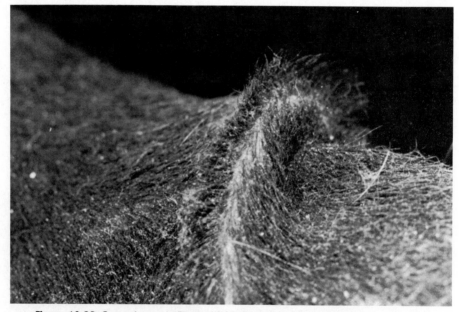

Figure 10:33. Same dog as in Figure 10:32. Note thinning, hypotonicity, and scaling.

CAUSE AND PATHOGENESIS

The circumanal glands and the tail gland of the dog are composed of the same perianal (hepatoid) gland tissue (Fig. 10:34). This tissue is androgen responsive. Hypertestosteronemia, usually in association with testicular neoplasia (especially interstitial cell tumors), results in glandular hyperplasia at both sites. Hyperandrogenism is a suspected, but not documented, cause of hypersexuality and seborrhea oleosa in intact male dogs (testicles usually normal).

CLINICAL FEATURES

Hyperandrogenism with testicular neoplasia produces diffuse perianal gland hyperplasia circumanally and hyperplasia of the tail gland (Figs. 10:35 to 10:37). The circumanal hyperplasia results in a donut-like appearance around the anus. The tail gland hyperplasia appears as an oval enlargement of the dorsal surface of the proximal tail. The tail gland area may become alopecic, greasy, and crusted. The skin in the area of the tail gland, perianal area, scrotum, ventral tail, and ventral abdomen often develops macular hyperpigmentation. A testicular mass can usually be palpated. In some instances, the testicular mass is palpated several months before or after the development of the cutaneous abnormalities.

DIAGNOSIS

Diagnosis is based on history, physical examination, determination of blood testosterone levels (see p. 593), and response to castration. Histopathologic examination of the testicular tumor usually reveals an interstitial cell neoplasm.

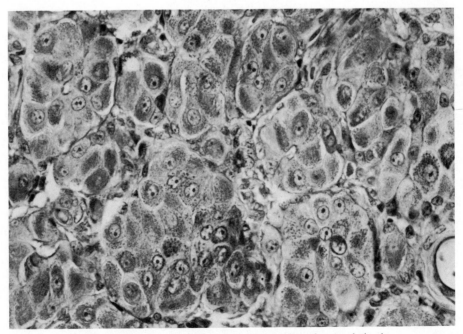

Figure 10:34. Tail gland hyperplasia. Hyperplasia of perianal glands.

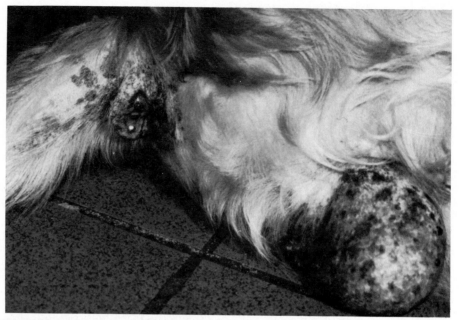

Figure 10:35. Dog with interstitial cell tumor of testicle and hypertestosteronemia. Note enlarged scrotum and macular melanosis of scrotum and perianal area.

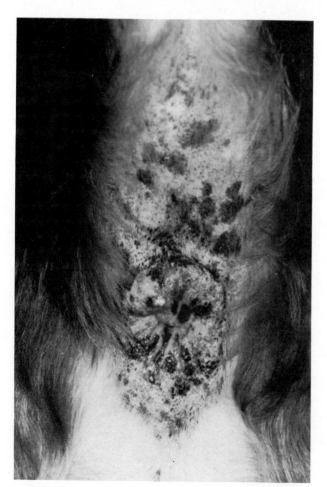

Figure 10:36. Same dog as in Figure 10:35. Perianal gland hyperplasia and macular melanosis.

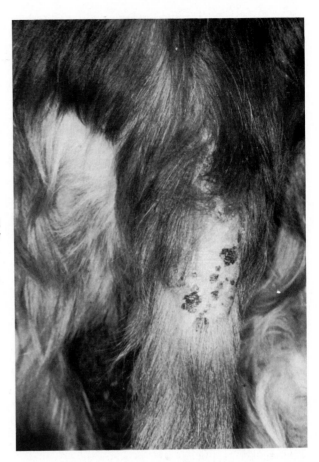

Figure 10:37. Same dog as in Figures 10:35 and 10:36. Alopecia, macular melanosis, and hypertrophy of tail gland.

CLINICAL MANAGEMENT

In general, a beneficial cutaneous response to therapy is seen within 2 to 3 months following castration.

TESTICULAR NEOPLASIA AND THE SKIN

Functional testicular neoplasia is associated with numerous cutaneous abnormalities in dogs.[9, 66] The cryptorchid testicle is about 13 times more likely to develop a Sertoli's cell tumor or seminoma than is a scrotal testicle. In addition, the signs referable to Sertoli's cell tumors usually begin at an earlier age when a cryptorchid testicle is involved. Cryptorchidism and, therefore, Sertoli's cell tumors and seminomas more commonly involve the right testicle. Boxers are predisposed to all three of the common canine testicular neoplasms. Bilateral castration should always be performed, as bilateral testicular involvement (either palpable or nonpalpable!) is not uncommon.

Sertoli's cell tumors are the most commonly associated with dermatologic disease (see p. 627). Boxers, Shetland sheepdogs, Weimaraners, Cairn terriers, Pekingese, and collies are predisposed. The average age of dogs at the time of diagnosis is 9 to 10 years. About 10 per cent of the dogs with Sertoli's cell tumors have one in both testicles, and about 20 per cent have another tumor type. About 10 per cent of the Sertoli's cell tumors are malignant. Blood estrogen levels are not always elevated (see p. 592). In addition, the hyperestrogenism could be a local (tissue-level) effect with the peripheral aromatization of androgens to estrogens. Bilateral flank alopecia has been reported in a dog with hyperprogesteronemia and Sertoli's cell tumor.

Seminomas have rarely been associated with feminization and alopecia. Whether this situation truly reflects a hormonally active seminoma or the failure to detect another coexisting tumor type is unknown. Boxers and German shepherds are predisposed. The average age of dogs at the time of diagnosis is 10 years. Seminomas can occur concurrently with other tumor types. About 10 per cent of seminomas are malignant.

Interstitial (Leydig) cell tumors have rarely been associated with feminization and alopecia, but more commonly with perianal gland hyperplasia and adenoma, tail gland hyperplasia, and seborrhea oleosa. About 30 per cent of dogs with this tumor have prostatic disease, and about 15 per cent have perineal hernias. About 90 per cent of these tumors occur in scrotal testicles, and right and left testicles are affected with equal frequency. About 30 per cent of the dogs have bilateral interstitial cell tumors. Boxers are predisposed. The average age of dogs at the time of diagnosis is 10 years. These tumors frequently occur in conjunction with other tumor types.

CASTRATION-RESPONSIVE DERMATOSIS OF MALE DOGS
("Woolly" Syndrome)

This is a poorly understood and uncommon dermatosis of intact male dogs.

CAUSE AND PATHOGENESIS

The etiology of this syndrome is unknown but is clearly testicle dependent.[63, 103] The testicles are usually palpably and histologically normal. Sex hormone values are variable, and occasionally normal (see later discussion). It would appear that this "syndrome" may represent a number of testicular-origin deficiencies, excesses, or imbalances in sex hormones.

CLINICAL FEATURES

Adult intact male dogs are affected, and Siberian huskies, malamutes and keeshonds may be predisposed. The initial clinical sign is often an abnormality of hair coat texture and/or color. The hair coat usually becomes fluffy and crimped (woolly) (Fig. 10:13E,F, p. 616), and occasionally dull and brittle. Darker hair coats often fade or develop a reddish or bronze hue. Symmetric alopecia develops over rump, perineum, caudomedial thighs, ventral abdomen and thorax, and around the neck (collar). Hyperpigmentation is variable and, when present, is diffuse. The testicles are usually normal on palpation. The dogs are usually otherwise normal.

DIAGNOSIS

Differential diagnosis includes hypothyroidism, hyperadrenocorticism, and adult-onset hyposomatotropism. Diagnosis is based on history, physical examination, sex hormone blood levels, and response to castration. Blood sex hormone levels are variable and occasionally normal.[30a, 63, 103] However, if testosterone, estradiol, and progesterone are all measured simultaneously, an abnormality (too high, too low) is usually found in one of the hormones. Animals with high testosterone or low estradiol levels may have low basal total serum T_4 levels (decreased thyroid hormone–binding proteins?) but normal response to TSH. Conversely, animals with low testosterone or high estradiol levels may have elevated basal total serum T_4 levels (increased thyroid hormone–binding proteins?), but normal responses to TSH. Dermatohistopathologic findings are typically endocrinopathy-like and nondiagnostic.

CLINICAL MANAGEMENT

The therapy of choice is bilateral castration. Clinical improvement should be obvious within 2 to 3 months.

DIABETES MELLITUS

In human beings, diabetes mellitus is associated with a number of dermatologic disorders, including vascular complications (microangiopathy, atherosclerosis), diabetic dermopathy, necrobiosis lipoidica, granuloma annulare, scleredema, fibrovascular papillomas, yellow nails, rubeosis, bacterial and fungal infections, diabetic neuropathy, pruritus, idiopathic bullae, alopecia, xanthomatosis, and poor wound healing.[38] Up to 30 per cent of humans with diabetes mellitus develop a skin disorder that is either an early indicator of undiagnosed diabetes or a complication of known diabetes. In dogs and cats, skin lesions have been reported to occur rarely or in as many as one-third of the cases.[28a, 66, 98, 119]

The most common dermatologic manifestations of diabetes in dogs and cats appear to be pyoderma, seborrheic skin disease, thin and hypotonic skin, and varying degrees of alopecia. The thin, hypotonic skin, with or without alopecia, probably results from protein catabolism. The seborrheic skin disease (usually generalized seborrhea sicca) is probably due to protein catabolism and abnormal lipid metabolism.

Diabetics are predisposed to infections, particularly those caused by coagulase-positive *Staphylococci* and *Candida* spp.[38, 53, 66] This susceptibility appears to be due to abnormalities in neutrophil chemotaxis, phagocytosis, intracellular killing, and cell-mediated (T-cell) immune responses. These abnormalities may or may not be totally corrected by restoring normoglycemia with insulin therapy.

The *hepatocutaneous syndrome* ("diabetic dermatosis") is a rare condition in dogs.[103, 112] Most affected dogs have been older females. The cutaneous lesions, which include erythema, crusting, oozing, and alopecia of the face, genitals, and distal extremities as well as hyperkeratosis and ulceration of the footpads, usually precede the onset of the typical signs of diabetes mellitus and hepatic disease by weeks or months (occasionally 2 years) (Fig. 10:13G,H, p. 616). Affected dogs may be predisposed to dermatophyte infections. Histopathologic findings are diagnostic and include superficial perivascular-to-lichenoid dermatitis with marked diffuse parakeratotic hyperkeratosis and striking inter- and intracellular edema limited to the upper half of the epidermis (Figs. 10:38 and 10:39). Canine hepatocutaneous syndrome is remarkably similar to the gluca-

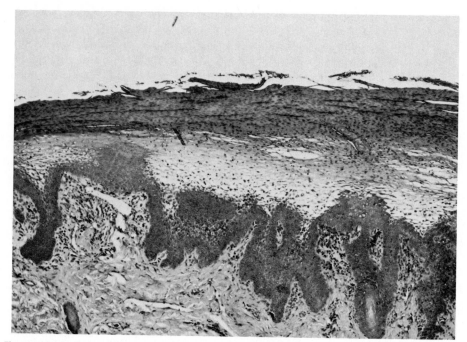

Figure 10:38. Canine hepatocutaneous syndrome (diabetic dermatosis). Marked edema of upper one-half of epidermis with diffuse parakeratotic hyperkeratosis.

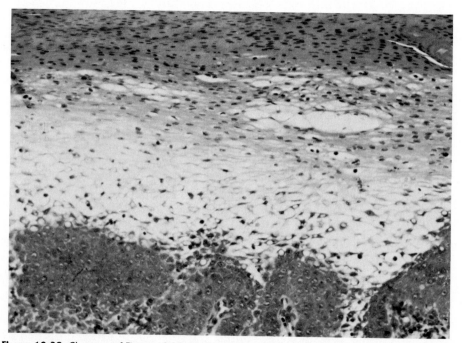

Figure 10:39. Close-up of Figure 10:38. Marked intercellular and intracellular edema with parakeratotic hyperkeratosis.

gonoma syndrome (necrolytic migratory erythema) of humans, which is usually associated with hyperglucagonemia and a glucagon-secreting alpha-cell neoplasm of the pancreas. Hyperglucagonemia has also been documented in dogs with hepatocutaneous syndrome, but pancreatic tumors have not been found. Eight of nine dogs studied developed diabetes mellitus, which was very difficult to control with insulin.[103] The consistent necropsy finding in dogs has been hepatic cirrhosis. In dogs, therapy (including glucocorticoids, aspirin, and eicosapentaenoic acid) is unrewarding, and the prognosis is grave.

Rarely, pruritus vulvae, xanthomatosis, and necrobiosis lipoidica have been reported to occur in association with diabetes mellitus in dogs.[9, 70, 119] Xanthomatosis has been reported in cats with naturally occurring and megestrol acetate–induced diabetes mellitus (see p. 945).[98]

HYPOTHYROIDISM

Hypothyroidism is the most common endocrine disorder of the dog and is characterized by a plethora of cutaneous and noncutaneous clinical signs associated with a deficiency of thyroid hormone activity.[9]

CAUSE AND PATHOGENESIS

Canine hypothyroidism may be naturally occurring or iatrogenic in origin (Table 10:4).[9, 28a, 29, 66] Naturally occurring, acquired primary hypothyroidism accounts for over 90 per cent of all canine hypothyroidism. The two main causes of acquired primary hypothyroidism are lymphocytic thyroiditis and idiopathic thyroid necrosis and atrophy.

Table 10:4. POSSIBLE CAUSES OF CANINE HYPOTHYROIDISM

Inadequate mass of functioning thyroid tissue (primary hypothyroidism)
  Congenital
    Thyroid agenesis (athyreosis)
  Acquired
    Lymphocytic thyroiditis
    Idiopathic necrosis and atrophy
    Thyroid neoplasia
    Iatrogenic surgical thyroidectomy and radiation therapy

Lack of thyroid stimulation by TSH
  Secondary (pituitary) hypothyroidism
    Hypopituitarism (pituitary dwarfism)
    Pituitary neoplasia
  Tertiary (hypothalamic) hypothyroidism

Deficiency of precursors for synthesis of thyroid hormone
  Iodine deficiency

Intrinsic defect in synthesis of thyroid hormone
  Dyshormonogenesis

Peripheral abnormalities
  Inadequate conversion of T_4 to T_3
  Antithyroid hormone antibodies
  Thyroid hormone–binding protein abnormalities
  Target organ resistance

Antithyroid drugs
  Thiouracil, thiourea

Lymphocytic (Hashimoto's) thyroiditis is the most common cause of hypothyroidism in dogs.[9, 28a, 60, 66] Lymphocytic thyroiditis has long been recognized as a familial disorder of colony-raised beagles, with polygenic inheritance. Lymphocytic thyroiditis is thought to be an autoimmune disorder in which humoral autoimmunity and cell-mediated autoimmunity are involved in the pathogenesis. Antithyroglobulin antibodies are demonstrable in the sera of over 50 per cent of dogs with naturally occurring hypothyroidism, and Great Danes, Irish setters, borzois, and old English sheepdogs appear to be predisposed (see p. 584). However, antithyroglobulin antibodies have also been found in about 40 per cent of dogs that have other nonthyroid endocrine diseases and healthy dogs that are closely related to antibody-positive hospital patients, as well as in 13 per cent of canine hospital patients that do not have endocrine disorders. Interestingly, dogs with various dermatoses also had an increased prevalence of antithyroglobulin antibodies. Twenty per cent of the dogs with naturally occurring hypothyroidism also have circulating immune complexes. Lymphocytic thyroiditis has been produced in normal dogs by injections of thyroglobulin or thyroid antigens with adjuvants, intrathyroidal injections of antithyroglobulin antibodies, and intrathyroidal injections of allogenic lymphocytes.[31, 36a] Thyroid lesions in dogs with naturally occurring lymphocytic thyroiditis are characterized by multifocal-to-diffuse interstitial infiltration of lymphocytes, plasma cells, and macrophages associated with destruction of thyroid follicles and by the presence of electron-dense deposits in the follicular basement membrane that resemble antigen-antibody complexes. Because lymphocytic thyroiditis is a focal disease and because inflammation is minimal in the late stages, it has been suggested that so-called idiopathic thyroid necrosis and atrophy may, in fact, be an end stage of lymphocytic thyroiditis.

Naturally occurring secondary hypothyroidism accounts for less than 10 per cent of all canine hypothyroidism and has been reported in association with pituitary dwarfism and pituitary neoplasia.[9, 66, 67] Other causes of canine hypothyroidism are rare.

Other than congenital disease,[2] naturally occurring hypothyroidism has *not* been documented in the cat.[93] Experimentally, iodine deficiency in cats resulted in bilaterally symmetric alopecia, commonly involving the lateral neck, thorax, and abdomen.[93] The hair coat became dry and easily epilated, and the skin was dry, scaly, and thickened. Radiothyroidectomized cats develop marked, nonpruritic seborrhea sicca, matting of the hair coat due to failure to groom, and alopecia and crusting of the distal half of the pinna.[107]

CLINICAL FEATURES

Although hypothyroidism may affect any breed of dog, certain breeds are predisposed. In a study of 250 hypothyroid dogs, breeds that were at risk included the chow chow (RR* 11.0), Great Dane (RR 4.1), Irish wolfhound (RR 4.1), boxer (RR 3.8), English bulldog (RR 3.2), dachshund (RR 2.8), Afghan hound (RR 2.7), Newfoundland (RR 2.6), malamute (RR 2.5), Doberman pinscher (RR 2.2), Brittany spaniel (RR 2.0), poodle (RR 2.0), golden retriever (RR 2.0), and miniature schnauzer (RR 2.0).[66] Others report the Irish setter to

---

*RR = Relative Risk. For instance, the chow chow was seen for hypothyroidism 11 times more frequently than it should have been, based on general hospital population.

be at risk.[28a] Interestingly, the following breeds were found to have a *reduced* risk for hypothyroidism: beagle, cocker spaniel, English springer spaniel, German shepherd, and mongrel. However, clinicians do commonly diagnose hypothyroidism in dogs of these breeds. Familial hypothyroidism has been suspected in Great Danes, Doberman pinschers, and German shorthaired pointers.[12, 35, 103]

There is no sex predilection for canine hypothyroidism. Although a dog of any age may be affected, the RR is great (2.0) for dogs between the ages of 6 and 10 years. The onset of hypothyroidism tends to occur at an earlier age (2 to 3 years old) in large and giant breeds.

Clinical signs seen in association with canine hypothyroidism are truly legion (Table 10:5).[9, 28a, 66, 68] It must be emphasized that a dog may exhibit any one or a combination of these signs. Thus, canine hypothyroidism could definitely be labeled "the great impersonator."

Although lethargy, mental depression, obesity, and thermophilia are classic manifestations of hypothyroidism, many hypothyroid dogs are active, alert, well-fleshed or thin, and non–heat-seeking. In general, if a dog is obviously obese, it probably is *not* hypothyroid. The rectal temperature of most hypothyroid dogs is in the normal range.

The classic cutaneous signs of canine hypothyroidism include:
1. Bilaterally symmetric alopecia, which tends to spare the extremities (Figs. 10:40 to 10:42).

Table 10:5. CLINICAL SIGNS ASSOCIATED WITH CANINE HYPOTHYROIDISM

General
Lethargy
Increased sleeping
Mental depression
Personality changes
"Tragic" facies
Obesity or weight loss
Thermophilia
Hypothermia
Lack of endurance

Cutaneous
Alopecia
Hyperpigmentation
Thick, cool, puffy skin
Poor wound healing
Easy bruising
Dry, dull, brittle, and easily epilated hair coat
Seborrhea
Pyoderma
Pruritus
Staphylococcal hypersensitivity
Otitis externa
Hypertrichosis
"Rat tail"
Puppy coat
Coat color change

Neuromusculoskeletal
Myopathy, myalgia
Arthropathy, arthralgia
Neuropathy
Hoarseness
Central nervous system disorders (stupor, coma, ataxia, seizures)

Gastrointestinal
Vomiting
Diarrhea or constipation
Decreased or increased appetite

Cardiovascular
Bradycardia
Weak apex beat
Cardiac arrhythmias
Vascular insufficiency (atherosclerosis, thrombosis)

Reproductive
Infertility (male or female)
Decreased libido
Decreased spermatogenesis
Anestrus
Prolonged postestral bleeding
Testicular atrophy
Galactorrhea
Gynecomastia

Ocular
Blepharoptosis
Corneal lipidosis
Corneal ulceration
Uveitis
Retinopathy

Hematologic
Pale mucous membranes (anemia)
Purpura (coagulopathy)

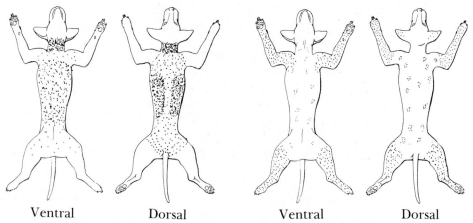

| Ventral | Dorsal | Ventral | Dorsal |

Figure 10:40. Hypothyroidism (left) and hypothyroidism, giant breeds (right), distribution patterns.

2. A dull, dry, brittle, easily epilated hair coat that fails to regrow following clipping.
3. Thick, puffy, nonpitting skin (myxedema) that is cool to the touch (Fig. 10:41C).
4. Variable hyperpigmentation (Fig. 10:42C).
5. Lack of pruritus.

However, the clinical variations from this classic picture are enormous and frequent. Alopecia may be focal, multifocal, generalized, symmetric, or asymmetric (Fig. 10:43). Seborrhea may be dry (sicca), greasy (oleosa), or dermatitic, and may be focal, multifocal, generalized, symmetric or asymmetric (Figs. 10:41 and 10:42).[66, 87]

> **Dogs with unexplained pyodermas should be checked for hypothyroidism.**

Pyoderma frequently occurs secondarily to hypothyroidism in dogs.[66, 87] The pyoderma may be localized (e.g., pododermatitis), multifocal, or generalized and may be superficial (folliculitis) or deep (furunculosis). The pathomechanism of this increased susceptibility to pyoderma is unclear. However, in various laboratory animals it has been reported that depletion of thyroid hormone results in impaired B-lymphocyte and T-lymphocyte functions.[66] In addition, it has been found that some dogs with pyoderma secondary to hypothyroidism have depressed neutrophil or T-lymphocyte function as assessed by bactericidal assay or in vitro lymphocyte blastogenesis to phytomi-

Figure 10:41. Hypothyroidism. *A*, The rear quarters of the St. Bernard illustrate the typical hair loss on the extremities seen with hypothyroidism in giant breeds. *B*, Alopecia of foreleg of same dog as in *A*. *C*, Hypothyroidism. "Tragic facies" associated with facial myxedema. *D*, Severely hypothyroid black cocker spaniel. He also has an advanced case of secondary seborrhea. Note sleepy look, secondary conjunctivitis, and scaly seborrhea. *E*, Same dog as in *D*, showing poor skin tone and excess skin folds with intertriginous seborrhea. *F*, Same dog as *D*, showing severe chronic otitis. *G*, Hypothyroidism, "rat tail." *H*, Purpura at the margin of the pinna of a dog with hypothyroidism.

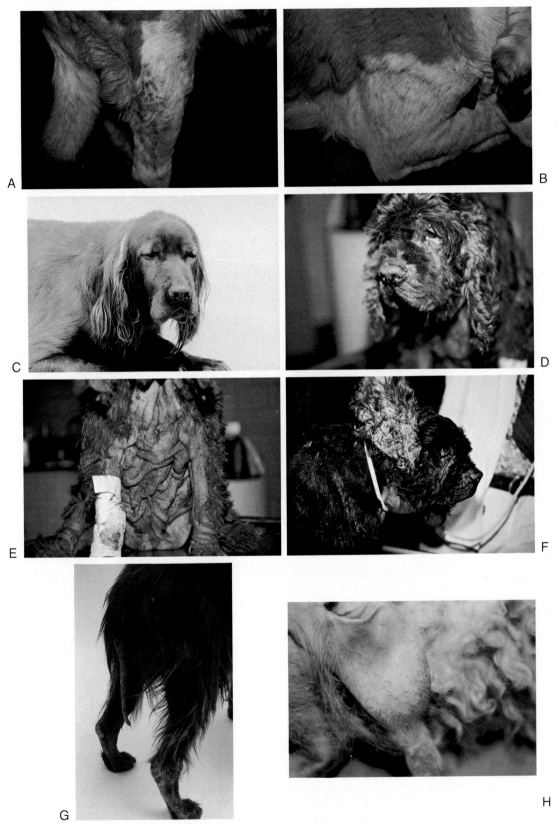

Figure 10:41 *See legend on opposite page*

togens, respectively.[66] These laboratory abnormalities returned to normal with T_4 therapy, whether or not systemic antibiotics were used concurrently. If seborrheic skin disease is also present, pyoderma could be secondary to the seborrhea.[66]

When seborrhea or pyoderma or both are present secondary to canine hypothyroidism, pruritus may be considerable. Poor wound healing is probably referable to defects in fibroblast function and collagen metabolism (see p. 578). Easy bruising is a common feature of canine hypothyroidism. Easy bruising may be associated with the collagen metabolism defects mentioned previously or with thrombasthenia and clotting factor defects that respond to thyroid hormone therapy.[9, 66] An unusual cutaneous manifestation of canine hypothyroidism is hypertrichosis (Fig. 10:44), in which the retarded turnover of hair coat leads to a very thick coat that resembles a carpet (especially boxers and Irish setters). This hypertrichosis may also occur in female dogs (especially Irish setters) that respond to ovariohysterectomy or estrogen therapy. Coat color changes may be seen in hypothyroid dogs.

Peripheral neuropathies are occasionally recognized in association with canine hypothyroidism.[9, 39, 66] Affected dogs may show facial palsy, laryngeal paralysis, vestibular dysfunction, paraparesis, or tetraparesis (Fig. 10:42D). If diagnosed and treated early, these neuropathies appear to respond to thyroid hormone. Dogs with hypothyroidism due to a pituitary neoplasm may show associated central nervous system signs. Myopathy is also seen in conjunction with canine hypothyroidism.[9, 66] In dogs, muscle wasting and weakness are most pronounced in the temporal, masseter, shoulder, pelvic, thigh, and lumbar regions. A stiff gait, "cramps," and rarely myalgia may be seen. Muscle biopsy reveals atrophy of type II fibers or lymphoplasmacytic myositis.

The most common gastrointestinal sign of hypothyroidism in humans, but not in dogs, is constipation. In dogs, the most common gastrointestinal signs of hypothyroidism are diarrhea or vomiting, or both[66]; these are occasional. Cardiovascular complications of hypothyroidism in dogs include bradycardia, weak apex beat, atherosclerosis, thrombosis, and cardiac arrhythmias associated with cardiomyopathy.[28a, 66, 68] Cerebrovascular atherosclerosis may produce a myriad of neurologic dysfunctions, including ataxia, vestibular disease, and seizures.[56, 79]

In addition to the classically described reproductive abnormalities seen with canine hypothyroidism, galactorrhea and gynecomastia may occasionally be seen.[9, 66] It is thought that the increased secretion of thyrotropin-releasing hormone (TRH) in dogs with primary hypothyroidism stimulates increased prolactin release, which in turn produces galactorrhea and gynecomastia.

Ocular abnormalities that may be associated with canine hypothyroidism include corneal lipidosis, corneal ulceration, keratoconjunctivitis sicca, uveitis, and retinopathy.[9, 28a, 66, 68]

Figure 10:42. Hypothyroidism. *A*, Hypothyroid patient showing obesity and patchy alopecia. *B*, Pekingese with advanced hypothyroidism showing alopecia, change in hair color, dry skin, and scaliness. Skin and hair coat returned to normal after 4 months' treatment with levothyroxine *C*, Close-up of affected area showing dry skin, ridges, hyperpigmentation, and alopecia. *D*, Beagle showing blepharoptosis. *E*, Photomicrograph shows thick dermis and periadnexal myxedema (blue). *F*, Photomicrograph shows orthokeratotic hyperkeratosis, follicular keratosis, and marked hypertrophy of arrector pili muscles. *G*, Photomicrograph shows myxedema. *H*, Photomicrograph shows vacuolated arrector pili muscle. (*E, F, G,* and *H* from Scott, D. W.: Histopathologic findings in the endocrine skin disorders of the dog. J.A.A.H.A. *18*:173, 1982.)

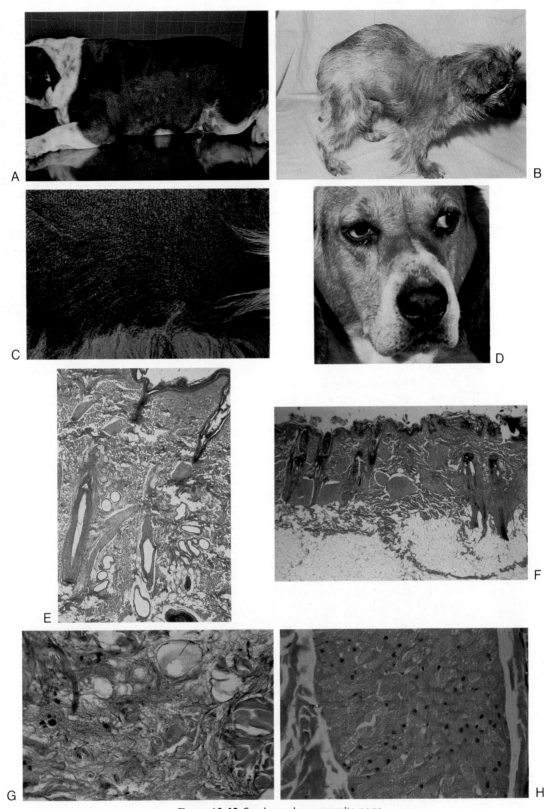

Figure 10:42 *See legend on opposite page*

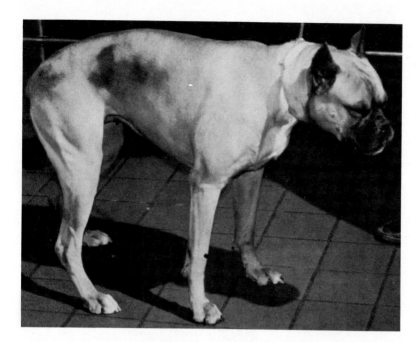

Figure 10:43. Hypothyroidism. Symmetric flank alopecia and hyperpigmentation.

Myxedema coma is a dangerous possible sequela of severe canine hypothyroidism, and most recognized cases have occurred in Doberman pinschers.[9, 42] Suggestive clinical signs include hypothermia without shivering, stupor progressing to coma, hypoventilation, hypotension, and bradycardia.

Renal lesions have been recognized in human beings and laboratory animals with hypothyroidism.[66] Renal lesions and renal failure have also been recognized in association with canine hypothyroidism, especially in dogs with lymphocytic thyroiditis. In addition, an association between primary hypothy-

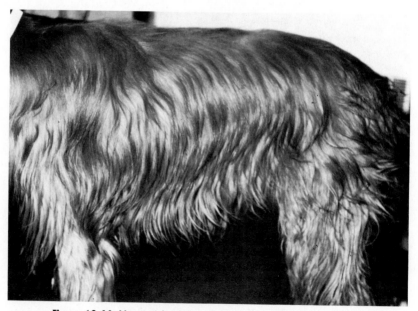

Figure 10:44. Hypertrichosis in an Irish setter with hypothyroidism.

roidism and diabetes mellitus has been proposed in dogs and humans.[9, 66] Such an association could represent an autoimmune disorder affecting multiple endocrine glands, with lymphocytic thyroiditis and "insulitis" (lymphocytic infiltration of the pancreatic islets).

Congenital hypothyroidism has been reported in dogs[7, 9, 32, 62] and cats.[2] Affected animals present with disproportionate dwarfism, mental retardation (cretinism), and variable hair coat abnormalities. Congenital hypothyroidism may be goitrous or nongoitrous.

DIAGNOSIS

Because of the plethora of clinical signs that are possible in canine hypothyroidism, the differential diagnosis is quite exhaustive, as would be expected from a "great impersonator" such as this disease. Definitive diagnosis is based on history, physical examination, hematology, serum chemistry, urinalysis, skin biopsy, thyroid function tests, and thyroid biopsy.

The hemogram classically reveals a normocytic, normochromic, nonregenerative anemia (PCV 25 to 36).[9, 28a, 66, 68] However, this is found in only 25 per cent of the cases. In addition, macrocytic and microcytic-hypochromic anemias may be seen in canine hypothyroidism, possibly reflecting defects in vitamin B_{12} folic acid metabolism or iron metabolism, respectively. Leptocytosis may be prominent in the anemic hypothyroid dog.

Another classic laboratory finding in hypothyroidism is hypercholesterolemia (260 to 1000 mg/dl).[9, 66, 68] However, serum cholesterol levels are greatly influenced by diet and after a 24-hour fast are significantly elevated in only about 33 per cent of the cases. They tend to be elevated with severe degrees of thyroid failure. Analysis of serum lipids in lipemic hypothyroid dogs may reveal hypercholesterolemia, hypertriglyceridemia, and intense electrophoretic bands at the origin, β_1-lipoprotein and α_2-lipoprotein positions.

Serum creatine phosphokinase (CPK) is mildly to markedly elevated in about 50 per cent of the dogs with hypothyroidism with or without concurrent myopathy.[9, 66] Other serum enzyme levels that may be mildly to markedly elevated in hypothyroidism include lactate dehydrogenase (LDH), aspartate transaminase (AST), alanine transaminase (ALT), and alkaline phosphatase. These elevations presumably result from the aforementioned hypothyroid myopathy and from the degenerative hepatopathies (fatty infiltration, cirrhosis) that may accompany canine hypothyroidism.

Urinalysis is usually normal in canine hypothyroidism. A few dogs with lymphocytic thyroiditis have had proteinuria and immune complex glomerulonephritis.

Electrocardiographic examination of hypothyroid dogs may reveal bradycardia, low voltage in all leads, flat T waves, and arrhythmias.[9, 66, 68] Radiographic examination of animals with congenital hypothyroidism reveals epiphyseal dysgenesis.[9]

Skin biopsy in canine hypothyroidism may reveal many nondiagnostic changes consistent with endocrinopathy (orthokeratotic hyperkeratosis, epidermal atrophy, epidermal melanosis, follicular keratosis, follicular dilatation, follicular atrophy, telogenization of hair follicles, sebaceous gland atrophy (see Fig. 10:42E,F).[95] Histopathologic findings highly suggestive of hypothyroidism include vacuolated, hypertrophied arrector pili muscles, increased dermal mucin (myxedema), and a thick dermis (see Fig. 10:42G,H). About 50 per cent of the biopsies from hypothyroid dog skin reveal variable degrees of inflammation, reflecting the common occurrence of secondary seborrhea or pyoderma, or both.

Basal serum levels of T_3 and T_4 are unreliable for diagnosing hypothyroidism (see p. 581). Common causes of low basal T_3 and T_4 levels in euthyroid dogs include concurrent drug therapy (especially glucocorticoids) and any number of acute or chronic illnesses (the "euthyroid sick syndrome"). In addition, one study found *low* basal T_3 and T_4 levels (as low as 0.0 μg/dl) in 20 per cent of 100 normal dogs, and *normal* basal T_3 and T_4 levels in 30 per cent of 250 hypothyroid dogs.[66] In another study, *normal* basal serum T_4 levels were found in over 50 per cent of 60 hypothyroid dogs.[9]

The *TSH stimulation test* is vastly superior to the determination of basal serum T_3 and T_4 levels for the diagnosis of hypothyroidism (see p. 582). A commonly used procedure for the TSH stimulation test in dogs is as follows: serum samples for determinations are collected before and 6 hours after the intravenous injection of 1 to 2.5 IU of bovine TSH. Euthyroid dogs should have basal serum T_4 levels and post-TSH serum T_4 levels within the normal pre- and post-TSH ranges for the laboratory that is assaying the samples. Dogs with the euthyroid sick syndrome or hyperglucocorticoidism usually have normal TSH stimulation tests, but occasionally have pre- and post-TSH serum T_4 levels below the expected normal ranges. However, the slope of the charted response parallels that seen in normal dogs. The determination of serum T_3 levels pre- and post-TSH is unreliable and not recommended.

A single TSH stimulation test does *not* reliably distinguish between primary and secondary hypothyroidism. If secondary hypothyroidism is suspected, TSH may be administered daily for 3 to 5 days. After this period of time, serum T_3 and T_4 levels should show a brisk response to TSH in secondary hypothyroidism. If repeated injections of TSH are given, the intravenous route must be avoided (see p. 582).

Occasionally, the clinician would like to do a TSH stimulation test on a dog that is receiving thyroid hormone therapy. It is recommended that thyroid hormone therapy be stopped for at least 30 days prior to doing a TSH stimulation response test.

The *TRH stimulation test* has recently been used to distinguish between euthyroid dogs and dogs with primary hypothyroidism (see p. 583). Serum T_4 levels are determined before and 6 hours after intravenous injection of 200 to 500 μg of TRH. Normal dogs at least double their basal serum T_4 levels. Serum T_3 determinations during this protocol are variable and nondiagnostic. TRH doses >900 μg or >0.1 mg/kg may cause severe cholinergic side-effects (see p. 583).

Antithyroglobulin antibodies are demonstrable in over 50 per cent of the cases of naturally occurring canine hypothyroidism (see p. 584). Important applications of such findings may include (1) detecting family members that could develop hypothyroidism and (2) helping to differentiate primary hypothyroidism (antibody positive) from secondary and tertiary hypothyroidism (antibody negative).

In humans, the determination of *serum TSH levels* and TSH responses to TRH injections have been successfully used to distinguish between primary, secondary, and tertiary hypothyroidism (see p. 581). These tests are presently unreliable in dogs.

The diagnosis of hypothyroidism, as well as the distinction between primary and secondary hypothyroidism, can be made rather easily by *thyroid biopsy* (see p. 583).

In cats, the following two TSH stimulation test protocols have been reported to be accurate measurements of thyroid function: (1) serum T_4 levels before and 6 hours after intravenous injection of 1 IU/kg bovine TSH or (2) serum T_4 levels before and 10 hours after intramuscular injection of 2.5 IU bovine TSH (see p. 583). Normal cats were also reported to double their basal serum T_4 levels 6 hours after the intravenous injection of 0.1 mg/kg of TRH (see p. 583).

Although the response to thyroid hormone therapy is often listed as a diagnostic feature of hypothyroidism, it is unreliable.[9, 28a, 66] The metabolic effects of thyroid hormones may produce varying degrees of improvement in such symptoms as lethargy, depression, and obesity, regardless of their etiology. By the same token, it is well known that thyroid hormone administration may produce varying degrees of hair regrowth in normal dogs, and in dogs and cats having numerous dermatoses that are unrelated to hypothyroidism (see p. 206).[34a, 103]

Recently a complicated equation for the diagnosis of canine hypothyroidism has been proposed.[52a] This needs further evaluation.

CLINICAL MANAGEMENT

Once treatment for primary hypothyroidism has been started, it is continued for the remainder of the patient's life.[9, 66, 69] Early regimens of thyroid hormone replacement therapy for dogs were hindered by a lack of knowledge about canine thyroid physiology and by attempts to anthropomorphize the dog. Confusion and controversy remain in regard to the dosage and the frequency of administration of thyroid hormones for canine hypothyroidism today.

In most cases, the drug of choice for treating canine hypothyroidism is L-thyroxine (T_4).[9, 30, 66, 69] An effective, commonly used regimen for canine hypothyroidism is to give L-thyroxine orally at 0.02 mg/kg BID. Side-effects are *rare* and include anxiety, panting, polydipsia, polyuria, polyphagia, diarrhea, tachycardia, heat intolerance, pruritus, and pyrexia (signs of hyperthyroidism). In dogs, it is difficult to cause an overdose with thyroid hormone because of their rapid metabolic turnover rate for T_3 and T_4 (serum half-life of T_3 and T_4 in dogs approximating 5 hours and 12 to 24 hours, respectively, as compared with 24 hours and 7 days, respectively, in humans), pronounced fecal excretion of T_3 and T_4, and incomplete absorption from the gut. Dogs with attitudinal abnormalities (lethargy, depression, and so on) usually respond very rapidly (within 2 to 4 weeks) to L-thyroxine therapy, but up to 5 months may pass before those with skin and hair coat abnormalities show a good response. Therapy should *always* be given for a *minimum* of 3 months before any judgment about its effectiveness is rendered. Most dogs will ultimately progress well on 0.02 mg/kg L-thyroxine SID. A reasonable approach to therapy would be first to establish that the condition being treated is responsive to thyroid hormone (L-thyroxine given BID for 3 months) and then to reduce the frequency of administration to SID. If the patient continues to do well, this would certainly make therapy easier and less expensive. There is no indication that proprietary L-thyroxine is any more efficacious than the less expensive L-thyroxine.

Dogs with cardiac disease, regardless of whether it is related to their hypothyroidism, should be started on *lower* doses of L-thyroxine, or heart failure may be precipitated.[9, 66] The following protocol for L-thyroxine is recommended: 0.005 mg/kg BID for 2 weeks, then 0.01 mg/kg BID for 2 weeks, then 0.015 mg/kg BID for 2 weeks, then up to routine maintenance dosage. In addition, patients with concurrent hypoadrenocorticism should not be treated for hypothyroidism until their adrenal insufficiency is corrected and stabilized with medication. Thyroid hormone therapy may also necessitate increased doses of insulin and certain anticonvulsants (phenytoin, phenobarbital) in patients being managed with those agents.

L-Triiodothyronine (T_3) may also be used to treat canine hypothyroidism but is rarely indicated.[9, 30, 66, 69] It should be given orally at 4 to 6 μg/kg TID, thus requiring more frequent administration and greater expense. It is usually reserved for dogs that are not satisfactorily able to absorb T_4 or to convert T_4 to T_3 peripherally.

Desiccated thyroid may be unsatisfactory for the treatment of hypothyroidism, due to variable potency, variable absorption from the gut, variable shelf life, production of unphysiologic serum T_3 and T_4 levels, and other idiopathic reasons for treatment failure.[9, 30, 66] After noting the unreliability of desiccated thyroid and the basic parity of expense between generic L-thyroxine and desiccated thyroid, one is forced to echo the sentiments of other investigators: "Why does anyone still use desiccated thyroid USP?"

Treatment of myxedema coma is a medical emergency.[9, 42] It consists of intravenous levothyroxine sodium (Synthroid for injection) or oral liothyronine sodium by gastric tube, mechanical respiratory support, intravenous glucocorticoids, broad-spectrum antibiotics, and passive rewarming.

Reasons for therapeutic failure with thyroid hormones are numerous (Table 10:6). Those most commonly encountered are incorrect diagnoses (usually as a result of measuring only *basal* serum T_3 and T_4 levels), wrong dose, wrong frequency of administration of T_3 and T_4 (usually due to using the earlier, *lower* doses SID), and use of desiccated thyroid. Rare individuals fail to absorb T_3 or T_4 from the gut. Such dogs are reported to respond to injectable L-thyroxine, but such therapy is impractical. Other rare dogs will fail to respond due to development of autoantibodies against T_3 and T_4.[66, 103, 123] In these cases, T_4 and/or T_3 levels are abnormally high in the face of clinical hypothyroidism. Such dogs may respond to concurrent L-thyroxine and glucocorticoid therapy.

Therapeutic monitoring of the serum T_3 and T_4 levels in hypothyroid dogs is rarely necessary.[9, 30, 66, 69] Physical examination usually suffices. If the response to therapy is inadequate, the clinician may wish to check "post-pill" serum T_3 and T_4 levels. It is recommended that the dog undergo the therapy for at least

---

Table 10:6. POTENTIAL REASONS FOR THERAPEUTIC FAILURE WITH THYROID HORMONES

1. Wrong diagnosis
2. Wrong dose
3. Wrong frequency of administration
4. Wrong product (desiccated thyroid)
5. Inadequate peripheral conversion of T_4 to T_3
6. Rapid metabolism/excretion
7. Poor absorption from gut
8. Autoantibodies to T_3 and T_4
9. Failure to ingest medication
10. Irregular administration
11. Target organ resistance

30 days before post-pill testing. If T_4 is being used for therapy BID, serum samples may be taken 2 to 3 hours post-pill for T_3 determination, and 4 to 8 hours post-pill for T_4 determination. The T_3 and T_4 levels should be within or slightly above the normal basal range. Dogs being treated with T_4 SID should also be sampled *before* the medication is normally given. If T_3 is being used for therapy, a serum sample is taken for T_3 determination 2 to 3 hours post-pill, and T_4 should be undectectable.

Treatment for secondary hypothyroidism would essentially be as that described for primary hypothyroidism. Dogs with concurrent secondary adrenocortical insufficiency would also require glucocorticoid therapy.

Dietary iodine deficiency is corrected by supplementing dogs with dietary iodine at 34 µg/kg/day, and cats with 100 µg/day.[9, 30, 69]

Appropriate doses of thyroid hormones for cats have not been determined. Data from cats that were bilaterally thyroidectomized and anecdotal clinical recommendations indicate that 0.05 to 0.1 mg L-thyroxine, once daily, or 30 µg L-triiodothyronine TID is sufficient.[9, 66, 98, 107]

FELINE HYPERTHYROIDISM

Hyperthyroidism is the second most common endocrinopathy of cats (diabetes mellitus being the first).[9] The etiology of feline hyperthyroidism is usually a solitary thyroid adenoma (feline Plummer's disease) or multinodular adenomatous hyperplasia of the thyroid (feline Marine-Lenhart syndrome). Thyroid carcinomas are seen rarely. Clinical signs are due to an accelerated basal metabolic rate and increased sensitivity to catecholamines.

Feline hyperthyroidism is seen in older cats, 6 to 20 years of age, with no apparent breed or sex predilections. Common clinical signs include polyphagia, polydipsia, polyuria, weight loss, hyperactivity, and tachycardia. Cutaneous abnormalities that may be seen with feline hyperthyroidism include excessive shedding and matting of the hair coat, focal or symmetric alopecia associated with excessive grooming, increased rate of nail growth, seborrhea sicca, and peripheral arteriovenous fistula.[28a, 102]

Diagnosis is based on history, physical examination, and elevated basal T_4 and T_3 levels. Common biochemical abnormalities in hyperthyroid cats include elevated levels of serum alkaline phosphatase, serum lactate dehydrogenase, and serum aspartate transaminase.

Therapy includes surgical excision, radioactive iodine treatment, or administration of antithyroid drugs (propylthiouracil, methimazole).

References

1. Abboud, C. F.: Laboratory diagnosis of hypopituitarism. Mayo Clin. Proc. *61*:35, 1986.
2. Arnold, U., et al.: Goitrous hypothyroidism and dwarfism in a kitten. J.A.A.H.A. *20*:735, 1984.
3. Barsanti, J. A., et al.: Diethylstilbestrol-induced alopecia in a dog. J.A.V.M.A. *182*:63, 1983.
3a. Beale, K. M.: Hypothyroidism and thyroglobulin autoantibodies in the Doberman Pinscher dog: incidence and significance. Ann. Meet. Am. Acad. Vet. Dermatol. and Am. Coll. Vet. Dermatol., 1988.
4. Bercu, B. B., and Diamond, F. B.: Growth hormone neurosecretory dysfunction. Clin. Endocrinol. Metab. *15*:537, 1986.
4a. Brent, B. A., and Hershman, J. M.: Thyroxine therapy in patients with severe nonthyroidal illnesses and low thyroxine concentration. J. Clin. Endocrinol. Metab. *63*:1, 1986.
5. Bruinsma, D. L., and Ackerman, L. A.: Male pseudohermaphroditism in a miniature schnauzer. Vet. Med. Small Anim. Clin. *78*:1568, 1983.
6. Carlson, R. A.: Endocrine alopecia in a dog show-

ing response to FSH administration. J.A.A.H.A. 21:735, 1985.

7. Chastain, C. B., et al.: Congenital hypothyroidism in a dog due to an iodide organification defect. Am. J. Vet. Res. 44:1257, 1983.

8. Chastain, C. B., et al.: Evaluation of the hypothalamic-pituitary-adrenal axis in clinically stressed dogs. J.A.A.H.A. 22:435, 1986.

9. Chastain, C. B., and Ganjam, V. K.: Clinical Endocrinology of Companion Animals. Lea & Febiger, Philadelphia, 1986.

10. Chrousos, G. P., et al.: Clinical applications of corticotropin-releasing factor. Ann. Int. Med. 102:344, 1985.

10a. Conaway, D. H., et al.: Clinical and histological features of primary progressive, familial thyroiditis in a colony of Borzoi dogs. Vet. Pathol. 22:439, 1985.

10b. DeBowes, L. J.: Pituitary dwarfism in a German Shepherd puppy. Compend. Cont. Ed. 9:931, 1987.

11. Eigenmann, J. E., et al.: Panhypopituitarism caused by a suprasellar tumor in a dog. J.A.A.H.A. 19:377, 1983.

12. Eigenmann, J. E., et al.: Polyendocrinopathy in two canine littermates: simultaneous occurrence of carbohydrate intolerance and hypothyroidism. J.A.A.H.A. 20:143, 1984.

13. Eigenmann, J. E., et al.: Elevated growth hormone levels and diabetes mellitus in a cat with acromegalic features. J.A.A.H.A. 20:747, 1984.

14. Eigenmann, J. E.: Estrogen-induced flank alopecia in the female dog: evidence for local rather than systemic hyperestrogenism. J.A.A.H.A. 20:621, 1984.

15. Eigenmann, J. E.: Acromegaly in the dog. Vet. Clin. North Am. (Small Anim. Pract.) 145:827, 1984.

16. Eigenmann, J. E.: Disorders associated with growth hormone oversecretion: diabetes mellitus and acromegaly. In Kirk, R. W.: Current Veterinary Therapy IX. W. B. Saunders Company, Philadelphia, 1986, p. 1006.

17. Eigenmann, J. E.: Growth hormone–deficient disorders associated with alopecia in the dog. In Kirk, R. W.: Current Veterinary Therapy IX. W. B. Saunders Company, Philadelphia, 1986, p. 1015.

18. Eiler, H., et al.: Stages of hyperadrenocorticism: response of hyperadrenocorticoid dogs to the combined dexamethasone suppression/ACTH stimulation test. J.A.V.M.A. 185:289, 1984.

19. Emms, S. G., et al.: Evaluation of canine hyperadrenocorticism, using computed tomography. J.A.V.M.A. 189:432, 1986.

19a. Emms, S. G., et al.: Adrenalectomy in the management of canine hyperadrenocorticism. J.A.V.M.A. 23:557, 1987.

20. Engler, D., and Burger, A. G.: The deiodination of the iodothyronines and of their derivatives in man. Endocr. Rev. 5:151, 1984.

21. Etreby, M. F. E., et al.: Functional morphology of spontaneous hyperplastic and neoplastic lesions in the canine pituitary gland. Vet. Pathol. 17:109, 1980.

22. Evinger, J. V., et al.: Thyrotropin-releasing hormone stimulation testing in healthy dogs. Am. J. Vet. Res. 46:1323, 1985.

23. Fadok, V. A., et al.: Hyperprogesteronemia associated with Sertoli cell tumor and alopecia in a dog. J.A.V.M.A. 188:1058, 1986.

24. Feldman, E. C., et al.: Comparison of aqueous porcine ACTH with synthetic ACTH in adrenal stimulation tests of the female dog. Am. J. Vet. Res. 43:522, 1982.

25. Feldman, E. C.: Comparison of ACTH response and dexamethasone suppression as screening tests in canine hyperadrenocorticism. J.A.V.M.A. 182:506, 1983.

26. Feldman, E. C.: Distinguishing dogs with functioning adrenocortical tumors from dogs with pituitary-dependent hyperadrenocorticism. J.A.V.M.A. 183:195, 1983.

27. Feldman, E. C.: Evaluation of a combined dexamethasone suppression/ACTH stimulation test in dogs with hyperadrenocorticism. J.A.V.M.A. 187:49, 1985.

28. Feldman, E. C.: Evaluation of a six-hour combined dexamethasone suppression/ACTH stimulation test in dogs with hyperadrenocorticism. J.A.V.M.A. 189:1562, 1986.

28a. Feldman, E. C., and Nelson, R. W.: Canine and Feline Endocrinology and Reproduction. W. B. Saunders Company, Philadelphia, 1987.

29. Ferguson, D. V.: Thyroid function tests in the dog. Recent concepts. Vet. Clin. North Am. (Small Anim. Pract.) 14:783, 1984.

30. Ferguson, D. V.: Thyroid hormone replacement therapy. Current Veterinary Therapy IX. W. B. Saunders Company, Philadelphia, 1986, p. 1018.

30a. Fourrier, P., and Lepesant, V.: Dysendocrinie sexuelle chez un caniche male age de 5 ans. Prat. Med. Chirurg. Anim. Comp. 22:395, 1987.

30b. Glaze, M. R., et al: Ophthalmic corticosteroid therapy: systemic effects in the dog. J.A.V.M.A. 192:73, 1988.

31. Gosselin, S. J., et al.: Autoimmune lymphocytic thyroiditis in dogs. Vet. Immunol. Immunopathol. 3:185, 1982.

32. Greco, D. S., et al.: Juvenile-onset hypothyroidism in a dog. J.A.V.M.A. 187:948, 1985.

33. Griffin, C.: Linear prepucial erythema. Proceedings, Am. Acad. Vet. Dermatol. and Am. Coll. Vet. Dermatol. New Orleans, 1986, p. 35.

34. Grossman, C. J.: Regulation of the immune system by sex steroids. Endocr. Rev. 5:435, 1984.

34a. Gunaratnam, P.: The effect of thyroxine on hair growth in the dog. J. Small Anim. Pract. 27:17, 1986.

35. Haines, D. M., et al.: Survey of thyroglobulin autoantibodies in dogs. Am. J. Vet. Res. 45:1493, 1984.

36. Haines, D. M., et al.: The detection of canine autoantibodies to thyroid antigens by enzyme-linked immunosorbent assay, hemagglutination, and indirect immunofluorescence. Can. J. Comp. Med. 48:262, 1984.

36a. Haines, D. M., and Penhale, W. J.: Experimental thyroid autoimmunity in the dog. Vet. Immunol. Immunopathol. 9:221, 1985.

37. Hoenig, M., and Ferguson, D. C.: Assessment of thyroid functional reserve in the cat by the thyrotropin-stimulation test. Am. J. Vet. Res. 44:1229, 1983.

38. Huntley, A. C.: The cutaneous manifestations of diabetes mellitus. J. Am. Acad. Dermatol. 7:427, 1982.

39. Indrieri, R. J., et al.: Neuromuscular abnormalities associated with hypothyroidism and lymphocytic thyroiditis in three dogs. J.A.V.M.A. 190:544, 1987.

40. Kantrowitz, B. M., et al.: Adrenal ultrasonography in the dog: detection of tumors and hyperplasia in hyperadrenocorticism. Vet. Radiol. 27:91, 1986.

41. Kaufman, J., et al.: Serum concentrations of thyroxine, 3,5,3'-triiodothyronine, thyrotropin, and prolactin in dogs before and after thyrotropin-releasing hormone administration. Am. J. Vet. Res. 46:486, 1985.

42. Kelly, M. J., and Hill, J. R.: Canine myxedema stupor and coma. Comp. Cont. Ed. 6:1049, 1984.

43. Kemppainen, R. J., et al.: Effects of prednisone on thyroid and gonadal endocrine function in dogs. J. Endocrinol. 96:293, 1983.

44. Kemppainen, R. J., et al.: Use of a low dose synthetic ACTH challenge test in normal and prednisone-treated dogs. Res. Vet. Sci. 35:240, 1983.

45. Kemppainen, R. J., and Sartin, J. L.: Effects of single intravenous doses of dexamethasone on baseline plasma cortisol concentrations and responses to synthetic ACTH in healthy dogs. Am. J. Vet. Res. 45:742, 1984.

46. Kemppainen, R. J., and Sartin, J. L.: Evidence for episodic but not circadian activity in plasma concentrations of adrenocorticotrophin, cortisol, and thyroxine in dogs. J. Endocrinol. 103:219, 1984.

47. Kemppainen, R. J., et al.: Endocrine responses of normal cats to TSH and synthetic ACTH administration. J.A.A.H.A. 20:737, 1984.

48. Kemppainen, R. J.: Effects of glucocorticoids on endocrine function in the dog. Vet. Clin. North Am. (Small Anim. Pract.) 14:721, 1984.

49. Kemppainen, R. J., and Zenoble, R. D.: Non–dexamethasone-suppressible, pituitary-dependent hyperadrenocorticism in a dog. J.A.V.M.A. 187:276, 1985.

50. Kemppainen, R. J., et al.: Ovine corticotrophin-releasing factor in dogs: dose-response relationships and effects of dexamethasone. Acta Endocrinol. 112:12, 1986.

51. King, R. R., et al.: Pulmonary function studies in a dog with pulmonary thromboembolism associated with Cushing's disease. J.A.A.H.A. 21:555, 1985.

52. Laing, E. J., et al.: Spermatic cord torsion and Sertoli cell tumor in a dog. J.A.V.M.A. 183:879, 1983.

52a. Larsson, M. G.: Determination of free thyroxine and cholesterol as a new screening test for canine hypothyroidism. J.A.A.H.A. 24:209, 1988.

53. Latimer, K. S., and Mahaffey, E. A.: Neutrophil adherence and movement in poorly and well-controlled diabetic dogs. Am. J. Vet. Res. 45:1498, 1984.

54. Laurberg, P.: Iodothyronine deiodination in the canine thyroid. Dom. Anim. Endocrinol. 1:1, 1984.

55. Li, W. I., et al.: Effects of thyrotropin-releasing hormone on serum concentrations of thyroxine and triiodothyronine in healthy, thyroidectomized, thyroxine-treated, and propylthiouracil-treated dogs. Am. J. Vet. Res. 47:163, 1986.

56. Liu, S. K., et al.: Clinical and pathologic findings in dogs with atherosclerosis: 21 cases (1970–1983). J.A.V.M.A. 189:227, 1986.

57. Lorenz, M.D.: Canine hyperadrenocorticism: diagnosis and treatment. Compend. Cont. Ed. 1:315, 1979.

58. Lothrop, C. D., et al.: Canine and feline thyroid function assessment with the thyrotropin-releasing hormone response test. Am. J. Vet. Res. 45:2310, 1984.

59. Lubberink, A. A. M. E.: Therapy for spontaneous hyperadrenocorticism. Current Veterinary Therapy VII. W. B. Saunders Company, Philadelphia, 1980, p. 979.

60. Lucke, V. M., et al.: Thyroid pathology in canine hypothyroidism. J. Comp. Pathol. 93:415, 1983.

61. Lund-Larsen, T. R., and Grondalen, J.: Ateliotic dwarfism in the German shepherd dog. Low somatomedin activity associated with apparently normal pituitary function (2 cases) and with pan-adenopituitary dysfunction (1 case). Acta Vet. Scand. 17:298, 1976.

62. Medleau, L., et al.: Congenital hypothyroidism in a dog. J.A.A.H.A. 21:341, 1985.

63. Miller, W. H.: Gonadal aberration in a Keeshond. Dermatol. Rep. 1:1, 1982.

64. Morris, B. J.: Fatal bone marrow suppression as a result of Sertoli cell tumor. Vet. Med. Small Anim. Clin. 78:1070, 1983.

65. Moriello, K. A., et al.: Determination of thyroxine, triiodothyronine, and cortisol changes during simultaneous adrenal and thyroid function tests in healthy dogs. Am. J. Vet. Res. 48:458, 1987.

65a. Moriello, K. A., et al.: The effect of otic glucocorticoids on adrenal and hepatic function. Proceedings, Am. Acad. Vet. Derm. and Am. Coll. Vet. Derm., Phoenix, 1987, p. 4.

66. Muller, G. H., et al.: Small Animal Dermatology III. W. B. Saunders Company, Philadelphia, 1983.

67. Neer, T. M., et al.: Craniopharyngioma and associated central diabetes insipidus and hypothyroidism in a dog. J.A.V.M.A. 182:519, 1983.

68. Nelson, R. W., and Ihle, S. L.: Hypothyroidism in dogs and cats: a difficult deficiency to diagnose. Vet. Med. 82:60, 1987.

69. Nelson, R. W., and Ihle, S. L.: Treating hypothyroidism through hormone supplementation. Vet. Med. 82:153, 1987.

70. Niemand, H. G.: Bildbericht. Kleintier-Praxis 16:193, 1971.

71. Oliver, J. W., and Waldrop, V.: Sampling protocol for thyrotropin stimulation test in the dog. J.A.V.M.A. 182:486, 1983.

72. Oliver, J. W., and Held, J. P.: Thyrotropin stimulation test—new perspective on value of monitoring triiodothyronine. J.A.V.M.A. 187:931, 1985.

73. Patterson, J. S., et al.: Neurologic manifestations of cerebrovascular atherosclerosis associated with primary hypothyroidism in a dog. J.A.V.M.A. 186:499, 1985.

74. Peterson, M. E., et al.: Immunocytochemical study of the hypophysis in 25 dogs with pituitary-dependent hyperadrenocorticism. Acta Endocrinol. 101:15, 1982.

75. Peterson, M. E., et al.: Plasma cortisol response to exogenous ACTH in 22 dogs with hyperadrenocorticism caused by adrenocortical neoplasia. J.A.V.M.A. 180:542, 1982.

76. Peterson, M. E.: Hyperadrenocorticism. Vet. Clin. North Am. (Small Anim. Pract.) 14:731, 1984.

77. Peterson, M. E., et al.: Effects of spontaneous hyperadrenocorticism on serum thyroid hormone concentrations in the dog. Am. J. Vet. Res. 45:2034, 1984.

78. Peterson, M. E., et al.: Adrenal function in the cat: comparison of the effects of cosyntropin (synthetic ACTH) and corticotropin gel stimulation. Res. Vet. Sci. 37:331, 1984.

79. Peterson, M. E.: Canine hyperadrenocorticism. Current Veterinary Therapy IX. W. B. Saunders Company, Philadelphia, 1986, p. 963.

80. Peterson, M. E., and Steele, P.: Pituitary-dependent hyperadrenocorticism in a cat. J.A.V.M.A. 189:680, 1986.

80a. Peterson, M. E., et al.: Plasma immunoreactive and cortisol in normal dogs and dogs with Addison's disease and Cushing's syndrome: Basal concentrations. Endocrinol. 119:720, 1986.

80b. Poffenbarger, E. M., et al: Gray-scale ultrasonography in the diagnosis of adrenal neoplasia in dogs: six cases (1981–1986). J.A.V.M.A. 192:228, 1988.

81. Quinlan, W. J., and Michaelson, S.: Homologous radioimmunoassay for canine thyrotropin: response of normal and x-irradiated dogs to propylthiouracil. Endocrinol. 108:937, 1981.

81a. Rachofsky, M. A.: Clinical relevance of results

from the new canine specific endogenous TSH assay: a review of 79 cases. Ann. Meet. Am. Acad. Vet. Dermatol. and Am. Coll. Vet. Dermatol., 1988.

82. Ranke, M. B., and Bierich, J. R.: Treatment of growth hormone deficiency. Clin. Endocrinol. Metab. 15:495, 1986.

83. Reimers, T. J., et al.: Changes in serum thyroxine and cortisol in dogs after simultaneous injection of TSH and ACTH. J.A.A.H.A. 18:923, 1982.

84. Reimers, T. J., et al.: Effects of reproductive state on concentrations of thyroxine, 3,5,3'-triiodothyronine and cortisol in serum of dogs. Biol. Reprod. 31:148, 1984.

84a. Reimers, T. J., et al.: Effect of fasting on thyroxine 3,5,3'-triiodothyronine, and cortisol concentrations in serum of dogs. Am J. Vet. Res. 47:2485, 1986.

84b. Richardson, H. W.: Evaluation of endogenous cTSH assay RIA test kit in clinically normal and suspect hypothyroid dogs. Ann. Meet. Am. Acad. Vet. Dermatol. and Am. Coll. Vet. Dermatol., 1988.

85. Roberts, S. M., et al.: Effect of ophthalmic prednisolone acetate on the canine adrenal gland and hepatic function. Am. J. Vet. Res. 45:1711, 1984.

86. Rosenberg, R. M., et al.: Abnormal lipogenesis in thyroid hormone-deficient epidermis. J. Invest. Dermatol. 86:244, 1986.

87. Rosenkrantz, W., et al.: Alopecia in dogs and cats. Dermatol. Rep. 3 (3), 1, 1984.

88. Roth, J. A., et al.: Thymic abnormalities and growth hormone deficiency in dogs. Am. J. Vet. Res. 41:1256, 1980.

89. Roth, J. A., et al.: Improvement in clinical condition and thymus morphologic features associated with growth hormone treatment of immunodeficient dwarf dogs. Am. J. Vet. Res. 45:1151, 1984.

90. Scavelli, T. D., et al.: Results of surgical treatment for hyperadrenocorticism caused by adrenocortical neoplasia in the dog: 25 cases (1980–1984). J.A.V.M.A. 189:1360, 1986.

90a. Schmeitzel, L. P., and Lothrop, C. D.: Evaluation of hormonal abnormalities in normal coated Pomeranians and Pomeranians with growth hormone responsive dermatosis. Ann. Meet. Am. Acad. Vet. Dermatol. and Am. Coll. Vet. Dermatol., 1988.

91. Schulman, J., and Johnston, S. D.: Hyperadrenocorticism in two related Yorkshire Terriers. J.A.V.M.A. 182:524, 1983.

92. Scott, D. W.: Hyperadrenocorticism (hyperadrenocorticoidism, hyperadrenocorticalism, Cushing's disease, Cushing's syndrome). Vet. Clin. North Am. 9:3, 1979.

93. Scott, D. W.: Feline dermatology 1900–1978: a monograph. J.A.A.H.A. 16:331, 1980.

94. Scott, D. W.: Dermatologic use of glucocorticoids: systemic and topical. Vet. Clin. North Am. 12:19, 1982.

95. Scott, D. W.: Histopathologic findings in the endocrine skin disorders of the dog. J.A.A.H.A. 18:73, 1982.

96. Scott, D. W., et al.: Iatrogenic Cushing's syndrome in the cat. Feline Pract. 12:30, 1982.

97. Scott, D. W., and Concannon, P. W.: Gross and microscopic changes in the skin of dogs with progestagen-induced acromegaly and elevated growth hormone levels. J.A.A.H.A. 19:523, 1983.

98. Scott, D. W.: Feline dermatology 1979–1982: introspective retrospections. J.A.A.H.A. 20:537, 1984.

99. Scott, D. W.: Cutaneous phlebectasias in Cushingoid dogs. J.A.A.H.A. 21:351, 1985.

100. Scott, D. W., and Reimers, T. J.: Tail gland and perianal gland hyperplasia associated with testicular neoplasia and hypertestosteronemia in a dog. Canine Pract. 13:15, 1986.

101. Scott, D. W., and Walton, D. K.: Hyposomatotropism in the mature dog: a discussion of 22 cases. J.A.A.H.A. 22:467, 1986.

102. Scott, D. W.: Feline dermatology 1983–1985: "The Secret Sits." J.A.A.H.A. 23:255, 1987.

103. Scott, D. W.: Unpublished observations.

103a. Shanley, K. J., and Miller, W. H.: Adult-onset growth hormone deficiency in sibling Airedale terriers. Compend. Cont. Ed. 9:1076, 1987.

103b. Shirakami, A., et al.: Changes in plasma fibronectin levels in thyroid diseases. Horm. Metab. Res. 18:345, 1986.

103c. Smith, M. C., and Feldman, E. C.: Plasma endogenous ACTH concentrations and plasma cortisol responses to synthetic ACTH and dexamethasone sodium phosphate in healthy cats. Am. J. Vet. Res. 48:1719, 1987.

104. Stolp, R., et al.: Plasma cortisol response to thyrotropin releasing hormone and luteinizing hormone releasing hormone in healthy kennel dogs and in dogs with pituitary-dependent hyperadrenocorticism. J. Endocrinol. 93:365, 1982.

105. Stolp, R., et al.: Results of cyproheptadine treatment in dogs with pituitary-dependent hyperadrenocorticism. J. Endocrinol. 101:311, 1984.

106. Thoday, K. L., et al.: Radioimmunoassay of serum total thyroxine and triiodothyronine in cats: assay methodology and effects of age, sex, breed, heredity, and environment. J. Small Anim. Pract. 25:457, 1984.

107. Thoday, K. L.: Differential diagnosis of symmetric alopecia in the cat. Current Veterinary Therapy IX. W. B. Saunders Company, Philadelphia, 1986, p. 545.

107a. Thoday, A. J., and Friedmann, P. S.: Scientific Basis of Dermatology. A Physiological Approach. Churchill Livingstone, New York, 1986.

108. Turrell, J. M., et al.: Computed tomographic characteristics of primary brain tumors in 50 dogs. J.A.V.M.A. 188:851, 1986.

109. Van Der Walt, J. A., et al.: Functional endocrine modification of the thyroid following ovariectomy in the canine. J. So. Afr. Vet. Assoc. 54:225, 1983.

110. Vollset, I., and Jakobsen, G.: Feline endocrine alopecia-like disease probably induced by medroxyprogesterone acetate. Feline Pract. 16:16, 1986.

110a. Voorhout, G., et al.: Computed tomography in the diagnosis of canine hyperadrenocorticism not suppressible by dexamethasone. J.A.V.M.A. 192:641, 1988.

111. Wall, J. R., and Kuroki, T.: Immunologic factors in thyroid disease. Med. Clin. North Am. 69:913, 1985.

112. Walton, D. K., et al.: Ulcerative dermatosis associated with diabetes mellitus in the dog: a report of four cases. J.A.A.H.A. 22:79, 1986.

113. Wartofsky, L., and Burman, K. D.: Alterations in thyroid function in patients with systemic illness: the "euthyroid sick syndrome." Endocr. Rev. 3:164, 1982.

114. Watson, A. D. J.: Oestrogen-induced alopecia in a bitch. J. Small Anim. Pract. 26:17, 1985.

115. Weaver, A. D.: Survey with follow-up of 67 dogs with testicular Sertoli cell tumours. Vet. Rec. 113:105, 1983.

116. Wheatley, T., and Edwards, O. M.: Mild hypothyroidism and oedema: evidence for increased capillary permeability to protein. Clin. Endocrinol. 18:627, 1983.

117. Wheeler, S. L., et al.: Serum concentrations of thyroxine and 3,5,3'-triiodothyronine before and after intravenous or intramuscular thyrotropin administration in dogs. A.J.V.R. 46:2605, 1985.

118. White, S. D.: Facial dermatosis in four dogs with hyperadrenocorticism. J.A.V.M.A. *188*:1441, 1986.
119. Wilkinson, J. S.: Spontaneous diabetes mellitus. Vet. Rec. *72*:548, 1960.
120. Willard, M. D., et al.: Ketoconazole-induced changes in selected canine hormone concentrations. Am. J. Vet. Res. *47*:2504, 1986.
121. Willard, M. D., et al.: Effects of long-term administration of ketoconazole in cats. Am. J. Vet. Res. *47*:2510, 1986.
122. Woltz, H. H., et al.: Effect of prednisone on thyroid gland morphology and plasma thyroxine and triiodothyronine concentrations in the dog. Am. J. Vet. Res. *44*:2000, 1983.
123. Young, D. W., et al.: Abnormal canine triiodothyronine-binding factor characterized as a possible triiodothyronine autoantibody. Am. J. Vet. Res. *46*:1346, 1985.
123a. Zenoble, R. D., and Kemppainen, R. J.: Adrenocortical suppression by topically applied corticosteroids in healthy dogs. J.A.V.M.A. *191*:685, 1987.
124. Zerbe, C. A., et al.: Hyperadrenocorticism in a cat. J.A.V.M.A. *190*:559, 1987.
125. Zerbe, C. A., et al.: Effect of nonadrenal illness on adrenal function in the cat. Am. J. Vet. Res. *48*:451, 1987.

11

Congenital and Hereditary Defects

Cutaneous Asthenia
(Ehlers-Danlos Syndrome, Rubber Puppy Disease,
Dermal Fragility Syndrome, Dominant Collagen Dysplasia, Dermatosparaxis)

Cutaneous asthenia is a group of inherited, congenital connective tissue diseases characterized by loose, hyperextensible, and abnormally fragile skin that is easily torn by minor trauma.

CAUSE AND PATHOGENESIS

This disease complex resembles the Ehlers-Danlos syndrome of humans, which consists of at least eleven different disorders that are distinguishable clinically, biochemically, and genetically.[14a, 15] Dermatosparaxis means "torn skin"; because of the collagen defects the skin of affected animals often tears easily, which results in large gaping "fish mouth" wounds (Fig. 11:1*A,B*). These lacerations heal readily but leave thin, highly visible "cigarette paper" scars (Figs. 11:1*C,D*). The tensile strength of the skin of affected dogs is reduced 40-fold, while that from affected cats is reduced 9-fold.[15b, 24] Cutaneous asthenia has been reported in sheep, cattle, mink, dogs, and cats as well as in human beings.[15a, 15b, 22, 24] Cases include Himalayan and domestic shorthair cats and beagle, dachshund, boxer, St. Bernard, German shepherd, English springer spaniel, greyhound, and mixed breed dogs. The genetic background of the syndrome is complex.[23]

Recessive cutaneous asthenia has only recently been described in cats,[9, 11, 26] but it was the first collagen defect to be reported in any animal (initially sheep and cattle).[22] In animals, the disease only occasionally has the hyperextensibility and laxity of joints commonly seen in human patients with the syndrome. The morphology of collagen fibrils from affected human beings is different from that of fibrils from animals.[24, 41] Holbrook[26] has shown that the affected dermal collagen forms twisted ribbons rather than cylindrical fibrils and fibers (Figs. 11:2 and 11:3). Biochemical studies show a deficiency of procollagen peptidase and an accumulation of pN-collagen in the skin of some affected cats.[11]

Dominant cutaneous asthenia is a simple autosomal trait found in mink, cats, and dogs. The abnormal physical properties of the skin result from a defect in the packing of collagen into fibrils and fibers. A mixture of abnormal and normal fibers are found in heterozygous animals. In normal fibers all the fibrils are cylindrical, of uniform diameter, and packed in uniform parallel arrays. Abnormal fibers are recognized by the severe disorganization in the packing of the fibrils and by the presence of many abnormally large fibrils. Abnormal

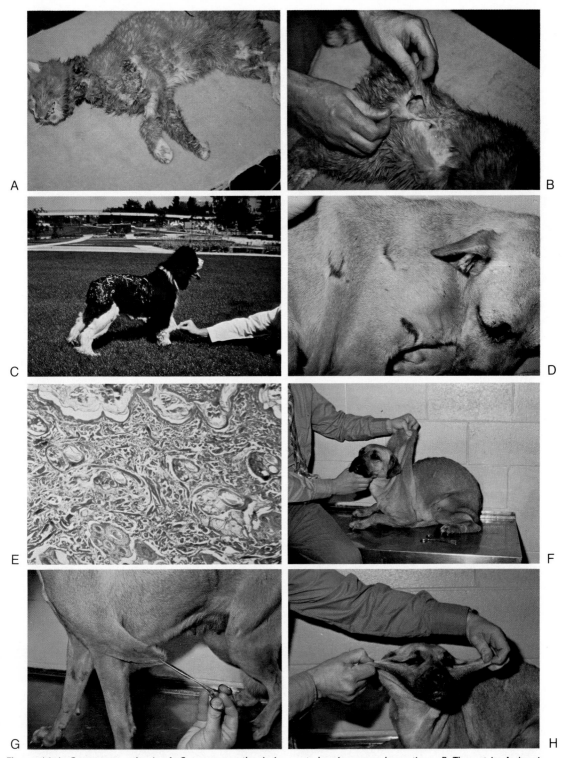

Figure 11:1. Cutaneous asthenia. *A,* Cutaneous asthenia in a cat showing many lacerations. *B,* The cat in *A* showing a laceration at the lower back. The skin will tear easily. *C,* Typical appearance of springer spaniel with cutaneous asthenia. Note the numerous scars on the back. (Courtesy G. A. Hegreberg.) *D,* Young boxer showing pigmented scars on shoulder. (Courtesy G. Ackland.) *E,* Photomicrograph of the skin of a springer spaniel with cutaneous asthenia. Dermal changes consist of fragmentation, disorientation, and sparsity of mature collagen bundles. (Courtesy G. A. Hegreberg.) *F,* Boxer in *D* showing extremely loose skin of the neck. (Courtesy G. Ackland.) *G,* Boxer in *D* with elbow skin stretched. (Courtesy G. Ackland.) *H,* Boxer in *D* with stretched cheeks. (Courtesy G. Ackland.)

659

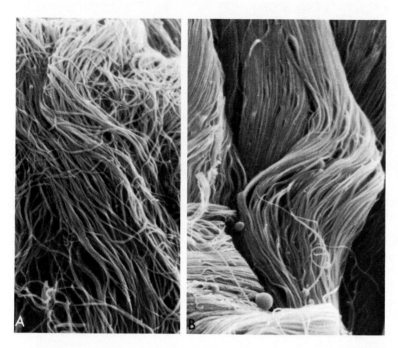

Figure 11:2. Scanning electron microscopic views (SEMs) of collagen fibrils in a fiber bundle from the dermis of A, the dermatosparactic cat, and B, the normal cat (× 6000). (From Holbrook, K. A., Byers, P.H., Counts, D. F., and Hegreberg, G. A.: Dermatosparaxis in a Himalayan cat: II. Ultrastructural studies of dermal collagen. J. Invest. Dermatol. 74:100, 1980.)

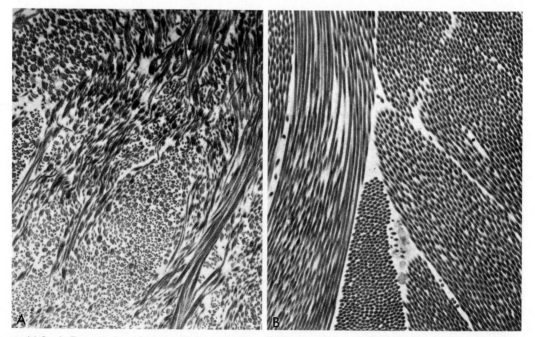

Figure 11:3. A, Transmission electron microscopic view (TEM) of a collagen fiber bundle from the dermis of the dermatosparactic cat showing fibers and fibrils in various planes of section within the bundle (× 10,000). B, TEM of a dermal collagen fiber bundle from the normal control cat. All fibrils within a fiber are organized in the same plane (× 6200). (From Holbrook, K. A., Byers, P. H., Counts, D. F., and Hegreberg, G. A.: Dermatosparaxis in a Himalayan cat: II. Ultrastructural studies of dermal collagen. J. Invest. Dermatol. 74:100, 1980.)

fibers are scattered among normal fibers (Fig. 11:1E). These collagen defects are seen at all ages, including in the midterm fetus. If the trait is present in a homozygous state, it is probably lethal.[41, 54]

Electron microscopic studies of cases of this disorder have shown a variety of morphologic abnormalities in the dermal collagen in unrelated animals. Thus, it appears that these diseases may be due to different sporadic dominant mutations involving structural proteins.

CLINICAL FEATURES

The skin is soft, pliable, thin, very loosely attached to underlying tissues, and hyperextensible. It has decreased elasticity and a moist, blanched appearance. The skin can be stretched to extreme lengths (Fig. 11:1F–H) and may hang loosely in folds, especially on the legs and throat. Minimal trauma from traction or scratching may produce skin tears, but there is little or no bleeding. Healing is rapid, but irregular thin white scars are prominent disfiguring features (Fig. 11:1C). Widening of the bridge of the nose and subcutaneous hematomas, which may develop at trauma sites, elbow hygromas, and epicanthal folds, are minor signs in some affected animals. Some animals manifest only cutaneous hyperextensibility *or* only fragility, while others exhibit both features.

DIAGNOSIS

Histopathologic changes, electron microscopic examination, or sophisticated biochemical studies (such as procollagen peptidase activity) may be needed for accurate diagnosis. The clinical syndrome of easily torn, hyperextensible skin with multiple scars is usually highly suggestive of the proper diagnosis. Breed incidence may also be useful. In affected dogs the dermis is thinner than normal (1.21 mm affected versus 1.71 mm normal), but the epidermis is normal.[15b] In cats no signifcant abnormalities were found in dermal or epidermal thickness between normal and diseased animals.[15b] The skin extensibility index devised by Patterson and Minor[47] is helpful. Extensibility is quantified by manually extending a fold of dorsolumbar skin to the maximum distance above the spine that can be attained without pain. This distance is measured, as is the body length from the base of the tail to the occipital crest. Extensibility is calculated as follows:

$$\text{Extensibility index} = \frac{\text{vertical height of skin fold}}{\text{body length}} \times 100$$

In affected dogs the skin extensibility index is greater than 14.5 per cent, while in affected cats it is greater than 19 per cent.[15b]

Histopathology. Skin biopsy may reveal striking dermal abnormalities or normal skin. Collagen fibers may be fragmented, shortened, and disoriented (Fig. 11:4). Additionally, collagen fibers may form irregular sized bundles, may demonstrate improper interweaving, and may be surrounded by mucinous degeneration.[24] Alternately, the collagen may appear normal on light microscopic examination.[47]

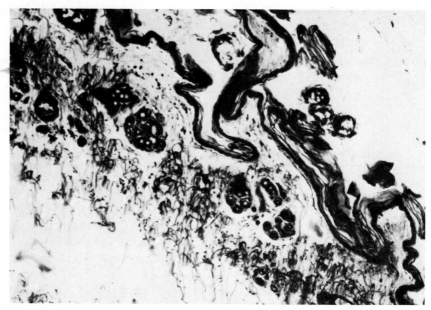

Figure 11:4. Cutaneous asthenia histopathology showing fragmented collagen fibrils that are shortened and disoriented.

CLINICAL MANAGEMENT

The clinician should inform the owner of the nature, heritability, and chronic incurable course of the disease. The animal should not be used for breeding.

Every precaution must be taken to prevent injury to the patient. Not only must fights and automobile accidents be avoided, but also special protection is necessary during simple daily activities. Declawing the hind feet of affected cats may be helpful in reducing self-mutilation from scratching. Any laceration must be promptly sutured, preferably using retention (mattress) sutures, and care must be taken to prevent disruption of the sutures before healing is complete.

Aplasia Cutis

(Epitheliogenesis Imperfecta)

Aplasia cutis is a congenital inherited discontinuity of squamous epithelium.[19, 25, 44] It is considered to be an autosomal recessive trait in cattle, horses, sheep, and pigs, but little is known of its inheritance in dogs and cats. The condition is characterized by areas of abrupt absence of epithelium, with resultant ulcers. Histologically, the ulcerated areas are distinguished by the complete absence of epidermis, hair follicles, and glands. The lesions of aplasia cutis in the newborn rapidly become infected, and septicemia soon results in death. Small lesions may, with supportive therapy, heal by scar formation. Skin grafting techniques may be beneficial.

Acanthosis Nigricans

Canine acanthosis nigricans is an uncommon cutaneous reaction pattern characterized by axillary hyperpigmentation, lichenification, and alopecia in association with various known and unknown causes.

CAUSE AND PATHOGENESIS

Canine acanthosis nigricans is best thought of as a cutaneous reaction pattern with multiple causes.[1a, 29, 58] The pathogenesis of the reaction pattern is poorly understood. Canine acanthosis nigricans may be divided into primary (idiopathic) and secondary types.

Primary (idiopathic) canine acanthosis nigricans is almost exclusively a disease of dachshunds. The striking breed predilection and early age of onset strongly suggest that this type of canine acanthosis nigricans is a genodermatosis. Indeed, one form of acanthosis nigricans in humans is known to be inherited.[50]

Secondary canine acanthosis nigricans is associated with underlying disorders, including (1) friction or intertrigo (conformational abnormalities or obesity, or both, resulting in excessive axillary friction and dermatitis), (2) endocrinopathy (underlying hypothyroidism, hyperadrenocorticism, sex hormone "imbalances" and so on), and (3) hypersensitivity (chronic axillary pruritus and dermatitis associated with canine atopy, food hypersensitivity, or contact dermatitis). In humans, about 20 per cent of the cases of acanthosis nigricans are associated with malignant neoplasms.[50] Only two cases of canine acanthosis nigricans have been reported to occur in association with malignant neoplasms (hepatic carcinoma, thyroid adenocarcinoma), and a true cause-and-effect relationship was not established.[51] In humans, acanthosis nigricans can also occur as a disorder that is secondary to drugs (e.g., nicotinic acid, diethylstilbestrol, glucocorticoids), regressing when the offending drugs are stopped.[50] Drug-induced acanthosis nigricans has not been reported in dogs.

CLINICAL FEATURES

Although primary canine acanthosis nigricans has been reported in several breeds, dachshunds are overwhelmingly the breed at risk. Secondary canine acanthosis nigricans may also occur in any breed and is more commonly recognized in those predisposed to the various underlying diseases. Primary canine acanthosis nigricans occurs in either sex and begins in dogs less than 1 year of age. Secondary canine acanthosis nigricans generally mimics any sex or age predilection inherent in the underlying diseases.

The earliest sign of primary canine acanthosis nigricans is usually bilateral axillary hyperpigmentation (Figs. 11:5A and 11:6). With time, lichenification and alopecia develop (Fig. 11:7). In severe cases, the dermatosis may spread to involve the forelimbs, ventral neck, chest, abdomen, groin, perineum, hocks, periocular area, and pinnae (Fig. 11:5B,C). Seborrheic skin disease (greasy, with rancid odor) and secondary pyoderma are common complicating factors. Pruritus is variable and is usually most severe when seborrheic skin disease or pyoderma, or both, are present.

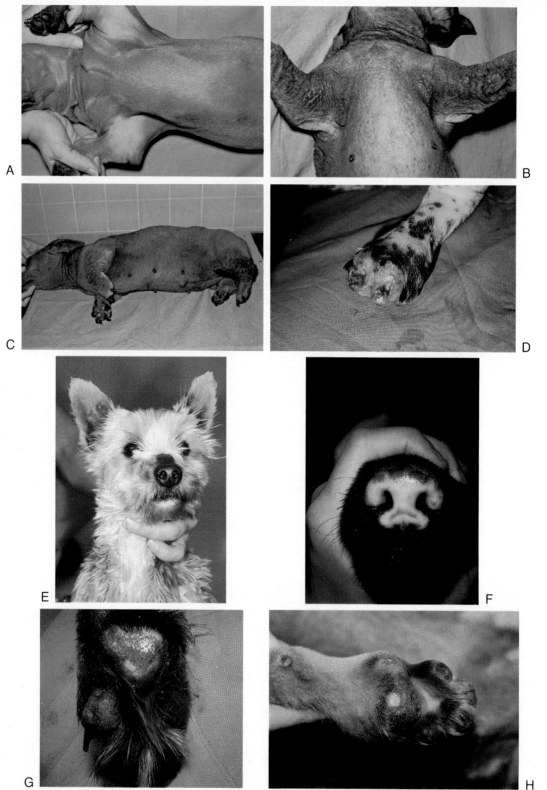

Figure 11:5. *A,* Acanthosis nigricans, juvenile stage. Note the small hyperpigmented patches in the axillae of this 6-month-old dachshund. *B,* Acanthosis nigricans, severe hyperpigmentation and lichenification in a 5-year-old dachshund. *C,* Acanthosis nigricans, chronic, advanced stage, in a 13-year-old dachshund. *D,* Acral mutilation in an English pointer. *E,* Facial and pinnal hyperpigmentation and alopecia in a Yorkshire terrier. *F,* Canine tyrosinemia. Depigmentation and ulceration of nose. (Courtesy G. A. Kunkle.) *G,* Canine tyrosinemia. Ulceration of footpads. (Courtesy G. A. Kunkle.) *H,* Collagen disorder of footpads of German shepherd. (Courtesy W. H. Miller, Jr.)

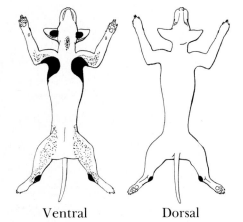

Figure 11:6. Acanthosis nigricans distribution pattern.

Ventral   Dorsal

DIAGNOSIS

The *differential diagnosis* of canine acanthosis nigricans includes the previously mentioned causes of primary and secondary disease. *Definitive diagnosis* is based on history, physical examination, laboratory rule-outs, skin biopsy, and response to therapy. Juvenile-onset acanthosis nigricans in a dachshund is most likely to be primary and genetic. Thyroid function is usually normal in dachshunds with acanthosis nigricans. Histopathology is nondiagnostic, revealing hyperplastic superficial perivascular dermatitis with focal parakeratosis, epidermal melanosis, pigmentary incontinence, and follicular keratosis (Fig. 11:8). The perivascular inflammatory infiltrate is usually mixed mononuclear cells and neutrophils. A similar histopathologic pattern may be seen with many chronic inflammatory dermatoses.

CLINICAL MANAGEMENT

The prognosis for cure in canine acanthosis nigricans varies with the underlying cause. Primary canine acanthosis nigricans in the dachshund is a controllable, but not a curable, disease. The disparity in responses to various recommended treatments undoubtedly reflects the multifactorial etiology of canine acanthosis nigricans.

Early therapeutic regimens for canine acanthosis nigricans focused on the thyroid gland. Thus, thyroid hormones, antithyroid drugs (propylthiouracil), thyroidectomy, thyroid-stimulating hormone (TSH), and synthetic thyrotropin-releasing factor, were all tried and recommended. Propylthiouracil may produce reversible or irreversible thyroid atrophy and fibrosis and has *no* place in the treatment of canine acanthosis nigricans. It is recommended that any type of thyroid hormone therapy be reserved for those rare cases of canine acanthosis nigricans that are documented to be associated with hypothyroidism (see p. 641).

Melatonin, a pineal gland hormone, has been effective in the treatment of canine acanthosis nigricans.[1, 29, 48] It has been postulated that melatonin may be a physiologic antagonist to melanocyte-stimulating hormone (MSH) and that the acanthosis nigricans may represent an imbalance between metabolism and

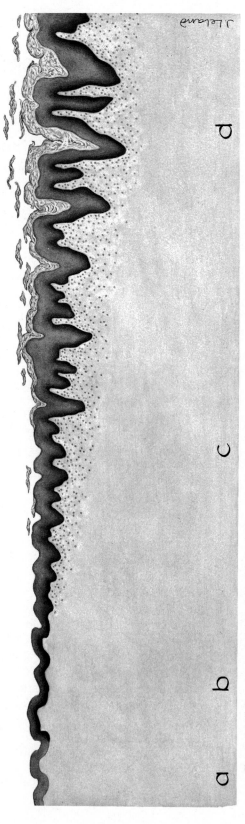

Figure 11:7. Acanthosis nigricans dermogram. *A*, Normal skin. *B*, In the early stage, hyperpigmented patches appear in the axillae. *C*, Elongated rete pegs, acanthosis, hyperpigmentation, hyperkeratosis, and mild dermal infiltration account for the thickened, gray, lichenified skin of more advanced cases. Scales and a greasy film form on the surface. *D*, In the chronic stage, the skin in many ventral areas of the body becomes thickened and the changes shown in *C* are even more pronounced.

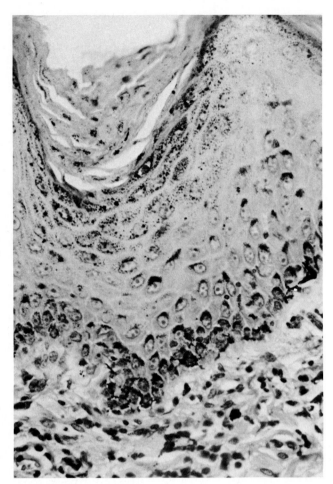

Figure 11:8. Canine acanthosis nigricans. Epidermal hyperplasia and full-thickness hypermelanosis.

MSH. Melatonin* is given subcutaneously at 2 mg per dog, daily for 3 to 5 days, then weekly or monthly, as needed.

Systemic glucocorticoids are effective in the treatment of canine acanthosis nigricans,[1] presumably via their anti-inflammatory, antiseborrheic, and anti–MSH effects. Prednisolone or prednisone is given orally at 1.0 mg/kg BID for 7 to 10 days, and then on an alternate-morning regimen (see p. 203). In mild cases, topical glucocorticoid therapy alone may suffice (see p. 168).

Vitamin E (dl-α-tocopherol acetate), 200 IU given orally BID as the only treatment, produced improvement within 30 to 60 days in eight cases of primary acanthosis nigricans.[58] Hyperpigmentation was not reduced, but inflammation, lichenification, pruritus, greasiness, and objectionable odor all subsided. There were no side-effects, and improvement was maintained while treatment continued.

Several ancillary therapeutic procedures may be indicated, including weight reduction, systemic and/or topical antibiotics, and topical antiseborrheic agents.

---

*Rickards Research Foundation, 18235 Euclid Avenue, Cleveland, Ohio, 44112.

Familial Canine Dermatomyositis

Familial canine dermatomyositis is a hereditary, idiopathic inflammation of the skin and muscles of young collies and Shetland sheepdogs.

CAUSE AND PATHOGENESIS

The cause is not well understood in dogs or in humans. The suggestion of an immune-mediated pathogenesis is favored for humans, in whom viral, bacterial, and parasitic agents as well as neoplasia, immunization and trauma have all been purported causes.[7, 20a–d, 33] A family history of the syndrome almost never occurs in humans, but it is a common finding in dogs. Test breedings in collies support an autosomal dominant mode of inheritance with variable expressivity. It has been described in the collie, Shetland sheepdog, and in cross-bred dogs involving one of those breeds. The disease has been reported from many geographic regions. Early skin lesions appear to favor locations over bony prominences that are especially exposed to mechanical trauma.

CLINICAL FEATURES

Dermatomyositis has no sex predilection and is found in all color phases of the breeds and in both individuals with smooth coats and those with rough coats. Signs may appear as early as 7 to 11 weeks of age, most cases being recognized by 3 to 6 months of age. Early lesions vary markedly in intensity. Some regress spontaneously, and indeed it is characteristic of the disease for lesions to wax and wane. In some instances, the early lesions heal and do not reappear. Almost all individuals with skin lesions have some degree of muscle involvement. Muscle abnormalities may be hard to demonstrate, and some older dogs with myositis and atrophy have a negative history of skin lesions. (Perhaps the cutaneous aspects were minor and transitory or not observed.)

Initial lesions are small pustules, papules, vesicles, or plaques with erosions, ulcers and crusts. There are alopecia, pigmentation disturbances and scarring. Lesions first appear around the face, lips and nose, the tips of the ears; later, they are seen on the tip of the tail, sides of the paws, and the stifle (Figs. 11:9A–H and 11:10). Mucocutaneous junctions may be involved early but rarely persist until the pups mature. Lesions are nonpainful and nonpruritic and may last 3 to 21 days in the early stages. Some regress, but many become worse and persist for 6 to 8 months. Permanent scarring and alopecia may result. Relapse of quiescent cases may be triggered by trauma, estrus, or exposure to sunlight.

Individuals with minor skin lesions often have minimal evidence of myositis, while more severe cases often show clinical, electromyographic and histologic evidence of polymyositis.[20] There may be evidence of temporal and masseter muscle atrophy by 1 year of age, and some individuals have difficulty lapping water or chewing and swallowing. Patients with severe cases may show stunted growth, extensive muscle atrophy, megaesophagus, and poor fertility.

DIAGNOSIS

Diagnosis is made by history, physical examination, biopsy of affected skin and muscle, electromyographs, and laboratory rule-outs.

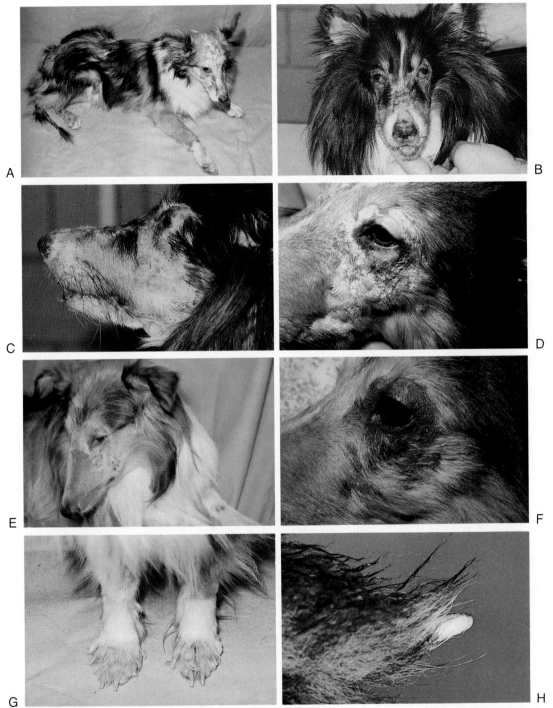

Figure 11:9. Dermatomyositis. *A,* Shetland sheepdog with typical lesions on face, legs, and tail. *B,* Shetland sheepdog with dermatomyositis. Severe facial scarring and drop-jaw. *C,* Close-up of dog in *B. D,* Shetland sheepdog with severe, typical lesions on cheek and eyelids. *E,* Shetland sheepdog with crusting, alopecia, and scarring. Note the lesions on the radial area of the leg. *F,* Same Shetland sheepdog as in *E* after six weeks of treatment with topical and systemic corticosteroids. Hyperpigmentation and hair replaced the inflammatory lesions. *G,* Shetland sheepdog with dermatomyositis. Alopecia, erythema, and scarring of feet. *H,* Collie with dermatomyositis. Alopecia of tip of tail.

669

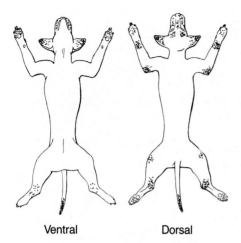

Ventral   Dorsal

Figure 11:10. Dermatomyositis distribution pattern.

Biopsy of affected skin shows follicular atrophy (Fig. 11:11), moderate perifolliculitis and perifollicular fibrosis (Fig. 11:12), and superficial perivascular dermatitis. Less commonly, hydropic degeneration of basal epidermal cells, and colloid (Civatte) bodies are associated with intrabasal or subepidermal clefts and vesicles (Fig. 11:13).[18] Muscle biopsy may show mixed inflammatory

Figure 11:11. Canine dermatomyositis. Fibrosing dermatitis, with orphaned apocrine glands and pigmentary incontinence.

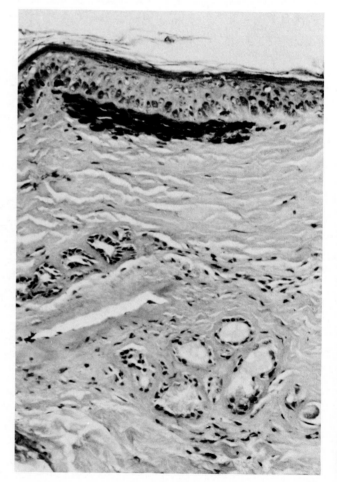

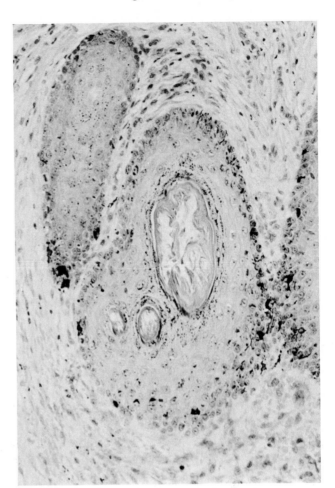

Figure 11:12. Canine dermatomyositis. Perifollicular fibrosis.

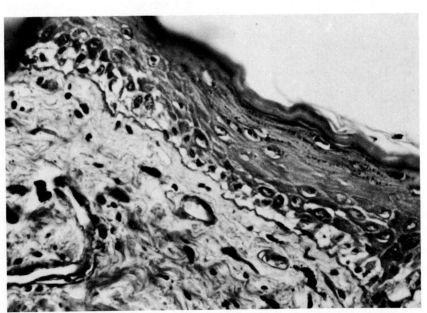

Figure 11:13. Dermatomyositis (epidermolysis bullosa simplex) in a collie. Marked hydropic degeneration of epidermal basal cells without inflammation. (From Scott, D. W., and Schultz, R. D.: Epidermolysis bullosa simplex in the collie dog. J.A.V.M.A. *171:*721, 1977.)

exudates, accompanied by muscle fiber necrosis and atrophy. In some cases a vasculitis may be found. Needle electromyographic abnormalities include positive sharp waves and fibrillation potentials in muscles of the head and of distal extremities.

Hemograms and serum chemistry profiles are usually unremarkable. Neurologic examination and nerve conduction studies are usually normal. Elevated concentrations of circulating immune complexes may be found in active disease.

The differential diagnosis should include demodicosis, staphylococcal folliculitis, dermatophytosis, discoid lupus erythematosus, and epidermolysis bullosa. The latter might be considered if there are no muscle signs or lesions and if vesicles are present (Fig. 11:14). In active cases, vesicles or erythematous plaques can often be induced by frictional trauma applied to a warmed area of the skin. Biopsy of the induced lesion should be typical.

CLINICAL MANAGEMENT

Therapy is difficult to assess because the disease waxes and wanes and often spontaneously regresses naturally. Treatment with large doses of systemic corticosteroids is suggested during periods of exacerbation, but results are often inconclusive.[33] Patients should be protected from sunlight and from trauma (this is especially difficult with pups). Oral doses of vitamin E (100 to 400 IU/day) may be useful.[4]

It is most important that affected animals and siblings be excluded from a breeding program.

Because the outcome is so variable, the prognosis for individual pups is difficult to determine.[33] The prognosis for life is usually good. Mild cases may have long periods of remission, while severe cases may have such chronic, poorly responsive problems that euthanasia is administered.

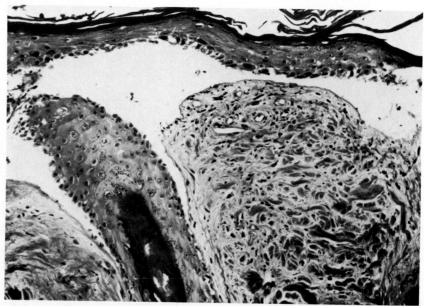

Figure 11:14. Dermatomyositis (epidermolysis bullosa simplex) in a collie. Subepidermal vesicle due to hydropic degeneration of epidermal basal cells. (From Scott, D. W., and Schultz, R. D.: Epidermolysis bullosa simplex in the collie dog. J.A.V.M.A. *171:721*, 1977.)

Epidermolysis Bullosa

(Mechanobullous Diseases)

This syndrome has been reported as a group of hereditary mechanobullous diseases of unknown cause that are characterized by cutaneous blisters in response to trauma.[39, 43, 57] Subsequent work in collies and Shetland sheepdogs suggests that the condition actually is a mild form of canine familial dermatomyositis in which the muscle lesions are not recognized (see p. 668).[33] The myositis in the latter disease may vary in time of onset and intensity and may be difficult to demonstrate by clinical signs, biopsy, or laboratory tests. Therefore, it is possible that epidermolysis bullosa simplex may exist as a separate entity in collies, Shetland sheepdogs, and cross-bred dogs involving one of those breeds.[21]

A single male toy poodle delivered by cesarean section developed multiple vesicles and bullae on the footpads, the oral cavity, and the tongue within 24 hours of birth.[14] Vesicles were produced on haired skin subjected to friction and pressure. Owing to the severity of the lesions, the pup was euthanized at 3 days of age. Histologic examination of the skin lesions showed subepidermal vesicles without inflammation. Ultrastructural evaluation showed cleavage of the basement membrane through the lamina lucida, leaving the lamina densa attached to the dermis. The findings were similar to those described for junctional epidermolysis bullosa in humans.

Acral Mutilation Syndrome

Acral mutilation and analgesia is an unusual hereditary sensory neuropathy of dogs that results in progressive mutilation of the distal extremities.

CAUSE AND PATHOGENESIS

The disorder has been reported in German shorthaired pointers[12] and English pointer dogs. It probably is an inherited autosomal recessive condition.[27] Pathologic lesions are identified at the level of the primary sensory neuron. Necropsy changes are seen grossly as a decrease in prominence of the spinal ganglia and dorsal roots. The nerve cell bodies of the subcapsular mantle zone are decreased in number (22 to 50 per cent) and the neuron mantle is decreased in thickness. The numbers of small neurons (20 µm or less) in the affected ganglia are disproportionately increased in affected dogs. The only spinal cord changes occur in the dorsolateral fasciculus, where reduced fiber density correlates well with the loss of pain perception that is seen clinically. Light and electron-microscopic examinations of spinal roots, ganglia, and peripheral nerves show myelinated and unmyelinated fiber degeneration. Neuronal degeneration does not account for the deficiency of sensory cell bodies. This mutilating acropathy is a manifestation of a sensory neuropathy in which the neuronal deficiency results from insufficient development and slowly progressive postnatal degeneration.[12]

CLINICAL FEATURES

The syndrome first appears in affected pups at 3 to 5 months of age. Both sexes and more than one pup per litter may be affected. The pups may be smaller than littermates. They begin to bite and lick their paws. There is total loss of temperature and pain sensation in the toes and in some cases in the proximal legs and trunk. Usually, the hind legs are most severely involved, and occasionally only the toes of the rear legs are affected.

The toes and feet become swollen and the skin of the footpads, the plantar surface, and the area over the tuber calcis may be ulcerated (Figs. 11:5D, p. 664, and 11:15). Paronychia is present and, possibly, autoamputation of the toes. The puppies walk unflinchingly on the mutilated feet. Proprioception is normal, tendon reflexes are intact, and no motor or autonomic impairment is present. Electromyographic studies reveal no denervation potentials.

DIAGNOSIS

History and a thorough clinical examination of puppies of predisposed breeds should provide a presumptive diagnosis. Histopathologic examination of nerve tissues at necropsy provide a definitive diagnosis.

CLINICAL MANAGEMENT

Attempts to prevent further mutilation by means of bandages, restraint collars, or sedation are of little benefit, and euthanasia is usually requested by the owners.

The hereditary aspects of this syndrome are important, as it has been seen in several strains of English pointers.[37] Parents of affected pups should not be used as breeders. Siblings should not be used either, although further breeding trials are necessary to more firmly establish the genetic mechanism of the disorder before this recommendation can be made with certainty.

Acrodermatitis

Acrodermatitis has been reported as an inherited, autosomal recessive trait that produces a lethal syndrome in bull terriers.[28]

The clinical, pathologic, and genetic features of the syndrome resemble acrodermatitis enteropathica in humans, lethal trait A46 in Black Pied Danish cattle, and experimental zinc deficiency in dogs. Although affected bull terriers

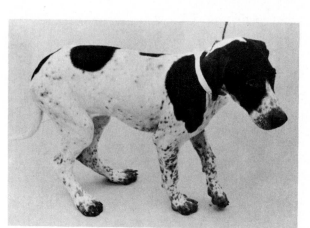

Figure 11:15. Pointer pup with acral mutilation of four feet. (Courtesy J. MacDonald.)

had significantly lowered serum zinc levels, they did not respond to high-dose zinc replacement therapy. Recent studies have demonstrated a zinc absorption defect in affected dogs.[44a] In addition, metallothionein levels—the major zinc-binding protein in tissues—were found to be similar between affected and normal dogs.[44a]

CLINICAL FEATURES

At birth, affected pups have skin pigmentation that is lighter than normal, and they are physically weaker. They cannot chew or swallow well, and their growth is retarded. By 6 weeks of age their feet are splayed, the footpads are cracked, and crusted skin lesions appear between the toes. Ulcerated, exudative crusted lesions are also found on the ears and muzzle; and papular or pustular dermatitis may be found around all body orifices, but most notably around those of the head. The foot lesions progress rapidly to severe interdigital pyoderma and paronychia. Later, there is nail dystrophy and a frondlike keratinization of the noncontact areas of the footpads. A generalized folliculitis may develop, being most severe in areas prone to frictional trauma, such as the elbows and hocks. They may have diarrhea and respiratory infections with chronic nasal discharges. At weaning time they appear especially aggressive, but by 14 to 16 weeks they become less active and spend a lot of time sleeping. Many have ocular abnormalities. The average survival time is 7 months, but almost all die before 15 months of age.

Laboratory evaluation of hemogram, serum chemistry findings, and enzyme and immunologic tests produced minor abnormalities, but no highly significant diagnostic results. Serum zinc levels are low. Pathologic findings in affected skin included parakeratotic hyperkeratosis and ulceration with superficial bacterial skin infection. There is a severe reduction in lymphocytes in the T lymphocyte areas of lymphoid tissue. Most pups have mild to severe dilation of the cerebral ventricles. Severe bronchopneumonia is the usual cause of death.

CLINICAL MANAGEMENT

No treatment exists. The prognosis is hopeless.

In this mode of inheritance, the parents of affected dogs are heterozygous carriers, and two-thirds of clinically normal siblings of affected dogs can be carriers. None of the family should be used for breeding. There is no laboratory test for recognition of carriers.[28]

Dermoid Sinus

(Dermoid Cyst)

A dermoid sinus is a neural tube defect resulting from incomplete separation of the skin and neural tube during embryonic development. The sinus is a tubular indentation of skin extending from the dorsal midline as a blind sac ending in the subcutaneous tissue or extending through the spinal canal to the dura mater. The lumen becomes filled with sebum, keratin debris, and hair. It may become cystic and is often inflamed. If infected, it may produce meningomyelitis and neurologic clinical abnormalities.

Dermoid sinus has been reported in the Rhodesian ridgeback dog and in a Shih Tzu and a boxer.[2, 15c, 38, 45, 59] The dermoid sinus of Rhodesian ridgeback dogs may be caused by a gene complex; if so, most individuals of this breed carry some of the factors. The only available data concerning inheritance of the dermoid sinus suggested that the factor may be inherited as a simple recessive gene.[38] If this is so, complete eradication of the problem can be achieved only by a program of progeny testing. However, by not breeding from affected individuals the incidence can be rapidly reduced (as is now done). When additional cases occur, breeders should extend that policy by not using either parent or any sibling of an infected pup for breeding. The problem is complicated further because dermoid sinus is not always easy to detect in a young pup.

CLINICAL FEATURES

Lesions are often noted in young dogs. Whorled hair may be seen along the topline (normal in the Rhodesian ridgeback), or isolated whorls may appear at the dorsal midline at the cervicothoracic junction. A tuft of hair may protrude from single or multiple small openings in the skin and a cord of tissue may be palpated, descending from the skin toward the spine (Fig. 11:16).

Diagnosis can be suspected on the basis of the anamnesis and the clinical appearance, but it is confirmed by a metrizamide fistulagram. A tract may be delineated from the skin to the dorsal processes of the thoracic vertebrae. Lumbar myelograms may demonstrate attenuation of the subarachnoid space near the termination of the fistula.

CLINICAL MANAGEMENT

If the lesion is quiescent, observation without treatment may be suitable. On the other hand, if drainage or neurologic signs are present, surgical

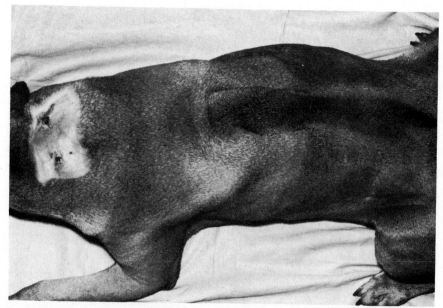

Figure 11:16. Dual fistulas opening on either side of the midline in the cervical region of the Rhodesian ridgeback dog are typical lesions of a dermoid sinus. (Neck has been clipped.) Notice whorled ridge of hair on the lower back form which the breed derived its name.

dissection is the treatment of choice. However, because of the deep attachments of the dermoid sinus, complete removal is not always possible. The tissue at the base is often fibrous, and careful blunt dissection is needed. Meningitis often complicates these cases; therefore, extreme care should be taken to ensure an aseptic technique during surgery. Successful surgery often results in complete recovery. Affected individuals should not be bred.

Chédiak-Higashi Syndrome

Chédiak-Higashi syndrome is an inherited disease of Persian cats (smoke color), white tigers, Hereford cattle, Aleutian mink, and humans. It is an immune disorder associated with a defect in cell structure that results in the production of abnormally large granules in leukocytes and enlarged melanin granules. It can be diagnosed by the examination of a stained blood smear for the presence of grossly enlarged granules in leukocytes or by examining hair shafts for enlarged melanin granules.[63]

The abnormal melanin granules give rise to a very pale coat color and light-colored irises (pseudoalbinism). Cats also have red fundic light reflection instead of yellow-green. Because of the immunologic deficiency, affected cats may be especially susceptible to bacterial, viral, and fungal infections or lymphoid tumors.

There is no treatment. Affected animals should not be bred.

Congenital and Hereditary Alopecias

Alopecia is defined as absence of hair from areas of skin where it normally is present. The loss can be complete or partial and diffuse or circumscribed. Animals normally are covered with a hair coat typical of their breed, and the coat creates a major impression about the animal. Any deviation from normal is readily apparent. Almost all the disease states listed in this text have some influence on the hair. Accordingly, in this section we will emphasize disorders that are primarily congenital and hereditary abnormalities of hair.

COLOR MUTANT ALOPECIA
(Blue Doberman Syndrome, Fawn Irish Setter Syndrome, Blue Dog Disease)

Color mutant alopecia is a hereditary ectodermal defect of color mutants of certain breeds, which is characterized by partial alopecia, a dry, lusterless hair coat, scaliness, and papules.

CAUSE AND PATHOGENESIS

The disease is most commonly found and is most characteristic in blue Doberman pinschers (Fig. 11:17A). It was formerly called the "blue Doberman syndrome" until it also appeared in other colors and other breeds. The condition occurs in most fawn Irish setters (Fig. 11:17E,F), some red and fawn Doberman pinschers, blue dachshunds, blue chow chows, blue standard poodles, blue

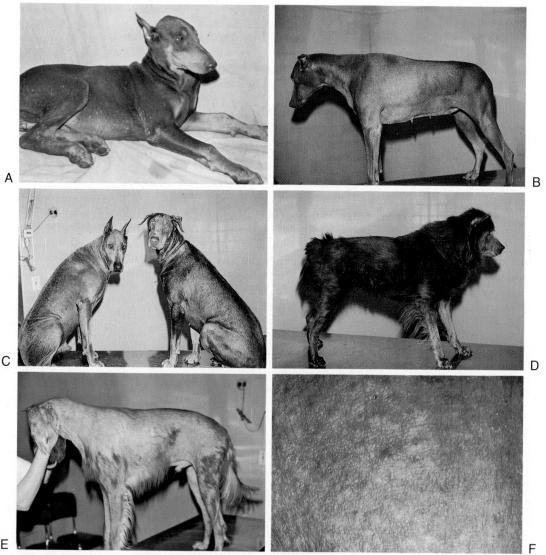

Figure 11:17. Color mutant alopecia. *A,* Four-month-old blue Doberman pinscher showing diffuse, alopecic, scaly patches. *B,* Fawn Doberman pinscher. *C,* Fawn and blue Doberman pinschers. Note poor hair coats. *D,* Blue chow chow dog. *E,* Fawn Irish setter, several years old, who has lost most of the hair of the trunk. *F,* Close-up of the skin of the Irish setter in Figure 11:17*E,* showing papulopustules and alopecia.

Great Danes, blue Italian greyhounds, and blue whippets (Figs. 11:17B–D).[3, 6, 15a, 45] The genetic factors are not known at this time, but observation has shown the color mutation to be heritable and the skin defects to be associated with the coat color. Defects in melanization and cortical structure of affected hairs have recently been described.[6a]

CLINICAL FEATURES

Most color mutant patients have a normally textured coat at birth and while they are very young. Soon, however, a "moth-eaten" alopecia appears and the skin becomes scaly. The hair coat is more brittle and drier than in normally colored littermates. The alopecia usually affects only the blue areas of the coats; the tan points remain normal. The blue Doberman female in Fig. 11:17A was 4 months old when photographed. She had normal littermates. Some blue Dobermans do not begin to show the defect until 3 years of age, at which time they have often won championships and have been used for breeding.

In many, but not all, cases there is papule formation. The papules are cystic hair follicles that are devoid of hair. Some papules develop into pustules (Fig. 11:17F). Secondary pyodermas may develop. After several years, almost all hair on the trunk of the body is lost and the alopecic areas are very scaly. The head, legs, and tail are least affected and sometimes almost normal.

The disease is incurable, although the condition of the skin can be improved slightly with treatment. Except for the dermatologic lesions, color-mutant dogs seem to be in good general health.

DIAGNOSIS

The first diagnostic hint is the occurrence of a scaly, "moth-eaten" alopecia in a dog whose color is different from the standard for that breed. Examples are fawn or blue Doberman pinschers and some red Doberman pinschers who are color mutants. The normal color for Doberman pinschers is black, tan, or red.

Differential diagnoses include seborrhea (with all its causes), bacterial folliculitis, dermatophytosis, demodicosis, zinc-responsive dermatosis, and hypothyroidism.

While some dogs with color mutant alopecia have "low-normal" thyroxine (T_4) levels, they do not usually have primary hypothyroidism. In addition, they do not grow a normal hair coat with thyroid supplementation. Thyroid, given empirically to some of these dogs, may slightly improve the hair coat (although this may only be the wishful clinical impression).

As in many skin disorders, fungal tests should be performed to check for dermatophytosis. Skin scrapings for ectoparasites (especially demodectic mites) should be done. One author (R. W. K.), in evaluating three blue Doberman pinschers, has analyzed the hair coat for zinc levels (normal), examined skin biopsies, and used high levels of zinc supplements for 3 months without benefit.

Histopathologic findings are characteristic. Cystic hair follicles predominate; they are often devoid of hairs and filled with keratin. Many hairs are dystrophic, and clumps of melanin (melanotic mush) are found within hair follicles. Examination of affected hairs reveals large aggregates of melanin within the cortex and medulla, which are associated with deformation and fracture of the hair cortex.[6a] A dense cellular infiltrate often forms around some cystic follicles to produce the perifolliculitis, folliculitis, and furunculosis that are seen clinically as papulopustules. Variable degrees of hyperplastic superficial perivascular dermatitis are usually present, reflecting the seborrheic skin disease seen clinically.

CLINICAL MANAGEMENT

The chronic nature and poor response to any treatment should be carefully explained to the owner. Frequent submerged baths or wet dressings hydrate the skin. Antiseborrheic shampoos help to remove scales. Benzoyl peroxide shampoos (OxyDex shampoo), given once or twice a week, help to remove papulopustules. Alpha-Keri spray applied daily makes the coat look shinier and helps to lubricate the dry, brittle hairs.

If thyroid function tests reveal a low or low-normal value, thyroid supplementation in some cases is justified. Affected dogs should not be used for breeding.

One of the authors (D.W.S.) has tried an oral eicosapentaenoic acid-containing product (Derm Caps) on two blue Doberman pinschers with color mutant alopecia. The appearance of the skin improved markedly, but there was no hair regrowth after 3 months.

FELINE ALOPECIA UNIVERSALIS
(Sphinx Cat, Canadian Hairless Cat)

The cat pictured in Figure 11:18A,B and 11:19A has a rare case of naturally occurring feline generalized alopecia. A male cat was born to a normal mother that had several normal kittens in the litter.

The cat resembled a Chihuahua at first glance, since it was almost hairless. Its smooth, hairless skin had a greasy feel. This resulted from the cat's reluctance to lick itself. The rough, barbed tongue is equipped for combing hair but causes pain when glabrous skin is groomed. The cat instinctively attempted to clean itself but stopped when the tongue touched the naked skin. Sebaceous glands were active, however, and a surface lipid film contributed to the oiliness of the skin and the greasy odor. It was necessary for the owner to wash the cat with soap and water twice a week. Grayish black deposits of grease that formed under the nail folds had to be removed regularly. The claws were slightly deformed. Cats with alopecia universalis are being bred and are called "sphinx cats" by some breeders. Anyone who plans to own such a cat should be aware of the difficulties in grooming just described.

Microscopically, the skin shows a complete absence of primary hairs (Fig. 11:19B). Secondary hair follicles are found only in certain areas. The epidermis is eight to ten cells thick, which is much thicker than normal feline skin. Sebaceous and apocrine glands are both present, but they open directly onto the surface of the skin. The dermis appears to be normal.

Figure 11:18. Ectodermal defects. *A,* Alopecia universalis (sphinx cat). *B,* Alopecia universalis (sphinx cat). Same cat as in *A.* Except for a few lanugo hairs, this cat has complete alopecia. *C,* Hypotrichosis in a Devon rex cat. *D,* Hypotrichosis in a Lhasa apso. (Courtesy of W. H. Miller, Jr.) *E,* Ventral neck and chest of an Irish water spaniel with hereditary hypotrichosis. *F,* Hindquarters of an Irish water spaniel with hereditary hypotrichosis. *G,* Head and face of toy poodle with hypotrichosis and partial alopecia present since birth. *H,* Body and extremities of poodle shown in *G.*

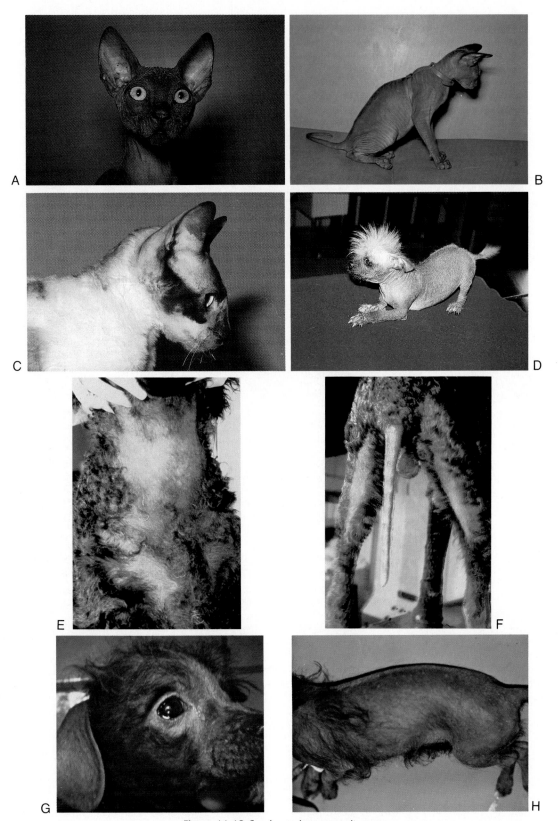

Figure 11:18 *See legend on opposite page*

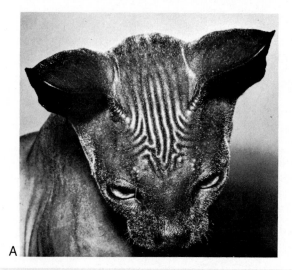

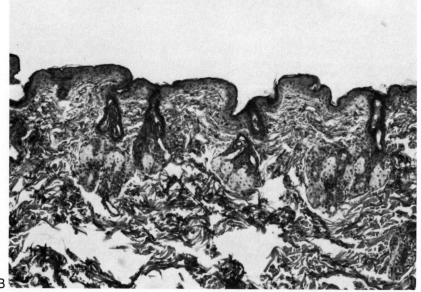

Figure 11:19. *A*, Feline alopecia universalis. *B*, Hereditary hypotrichosis in a Siamese cat. Poorly developed hair follicles devoid of hair shafts. (From Scott, D. W.: Feline Dermatology 1900–1978: A Monograph. J.A.A.H.A. *16*:331, 1980.)

The hairs are grossly abnormal. Only two types, secondary hairs (down or awn hairs) and other shorter hairs, can be found; the long, straight guard hairs are absent. The length of the hair increases from anterior to posterior regions of the body, but it is not normal anywhere. All hairs lack a well-formed bulb and can therefore be easily epilated.[49]

These cats are being bred and sold. Certain breed standards have been established.

1. Forehead is wrinkled.
2. Face is covered with a fine plush pile.
3. Eye color is golden.
4. Whisker pores, but no whiskers, are present.

5. Skin is taut in adults, freeing the body of wrinkles except on the head.
6. Paws are covered with fine down that is longer than facial hair.
7. Scrotum is covered with fine, long hair (longest on the body).
8. Tail is free of hair, except at the tip.
9. Back is covered with fine secondary hairs.

FELINE HYPOTRICHOSIS

Hereditary hypotrichosis has been reported in the Siamese cat.[53] The condition is an autosomal recessive trait. Affected cats have thin, downy hair at birth and develop alopecia by 10 to 14 days of age. Some hair regrowth is seen by 8 to 10 weeks of age, but total alopecia returns by about 6 months of age. Histopathologic examination of affected skin reveals small, poorly developed primary hair follicles, most of which are in telogen and devoid of hair (see Fig. 11:19B).

Recently, hereditary hypotrichosis was reported in the Devon rex cat (Fig. 11:18C).[64]

CANINE ALOPECIC BREEDS

At least two breeds have been established by selection for partial alopecia as part of the breed standard. The Chinese crested dog, which is illustrated in Figure 11:20, has hair on the top of the head and feet, but the rest of the body is almost glabrous. The Mexican hairless breed and the Chihuahua have varying degrees of hypotrichia with much individual variation. Other alopecic breeds include the Abyssinian dog, African sand dog, Turkish naked dog, Peruvian hairless dog, and Xoloitzcuintl.

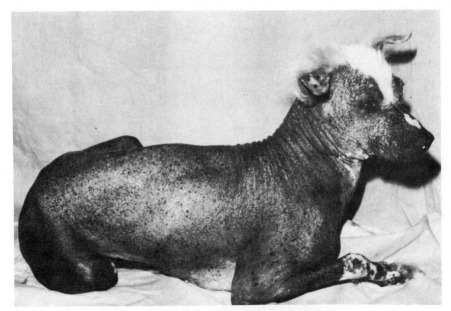

Figure 11:20. Chinese crested dog, a recognized breed.

Color mutant alopecia is seen in a hereditary partial alopecia that is associated with unusual coat color in blue Dobermans, fawn Irish setters, blue dachshunds, and blue whippets (see p. 677). Breeding of these color mutants should be discouraged.

CONGENITAL ALOPECIA AND ECTODERMAL DEFECTS

Congenital alopecia and other ectodermal defects have been reported in several breeds (Figs. 11:18D–F). Two dermatologists described a cocker spaniel with bilaterally symmetric alopecia of the entire ventral surface, noted from birth.[30] One author (R.W.K.) has observed a Belgian shepherd puppy with cranial alopecia and absence of ectodermal appendages since birth (Fig. 11:21). He also observed two male littermate toy poodles that had partial alopecia and a short hair coat affecting the face, ears, and dorsal trunk regions (Figs. 11:18G,H). The puppies appeared to be healthy and active. Unfortunately, no further information is available.

A congenitally hypotrichotic male whippet with partial absence of the hair coat in a bilaterally symmetric pattern similar to that shown by Selmanowitz's alopecic poodles was described.[65]

Similar cases have been reported in a male beagle,[31] a male bichon frise,[16] and in four male basset hound littermates.[8]

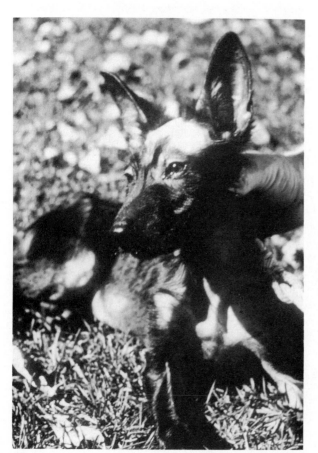

Figure 11:21. Four-month-old Belgian shepherd with congenital alopecia of head.

The basset hounds were born of normal parents, and two female littermates were normal. The affected males were mahogany in color and had identical patterns of focal alopecia involving the temporal regions, ear pinnae, dorsal pelvic region, and the proximal dorsal tail. The normal females were predominantly black. Kunkle,[31] however, reported a congenital lack of hair in a female black Labrador retriever. Six littermates (both yellow and black and both sexes of each) were normal. The affected pup had well-delineated symmetric alopecia over the temporal regions, the dorsum of the ears, the sacrum, and the entire ventral abdomen. At 9 months of age she lacked two incisors and several premolars and had marginal lacrimal secretion. Numbers of hair follicles and adnexa were markedly decreased. Her nails were normal.

Extensive information has been reported about a litter of five "miniature" (toy) poodles.[60] The dam, sire, and three female puppies were normal, but the two male puppies had bilaterally symmetric alopecia affecting about two-thirds of their body surface. These puppies are shown in Figures 11:22 and 11:23. Figure 11:24 illustrates histologic sections of affected skin and a transitional area between normal and affected skin. Affected skin was characterized histologically by a complete absence of hair follicles, sebaceous glands, and apocrine glands. There was absence of hair on the head, ears, ventral body, sacral region, and the posterior and medial surfaces of the legs. Early in life the alopecic skin was pinkish gray; but as the puppies matured, they developed slate-gray hyperpigmentation and scaliness of both alopecic and normal-haired skin. In alopecic areas, there was complete absence of cutaneous appendages (hair follicles, arrector pili muscles, sebaceous and sweat glands). Subsequently, abnormalities in dentition have been found. Extensive laboratory and clinical

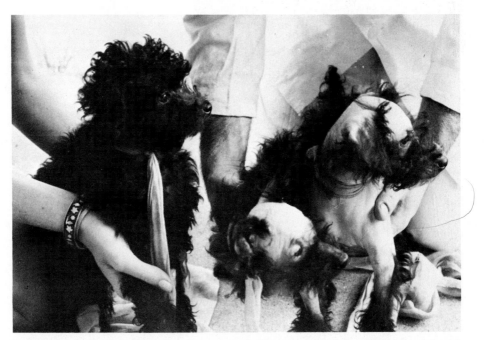

Figure 11:22. The partially alopecic males compared with a full-coated sister. The pattern of alopecia, which is bilaterally symmetric and includes about two-thirds of the body surface, is the same in both males. (From Selmanowitz, V. J., Kramer, K. M., and Orentreich, N.: Congenital ectodermal defect in miniature poodles. J. Hered. 61:196, 1970.)

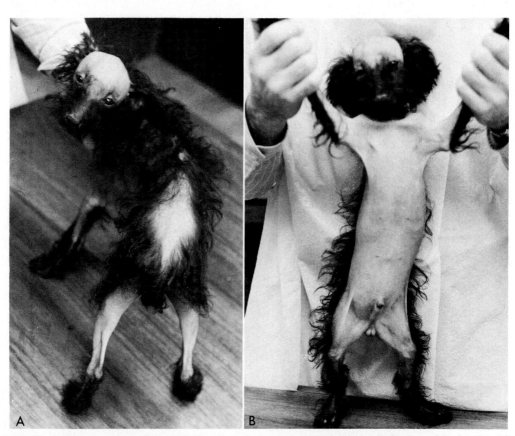

Figure 11:23. *A* shows the diamond-shaped alopecic region over the dorsal pelvis and alopecia of the head and limbs. *B,* Ventral view of affected male, showing the pattern of alopecia on the trunk and legs. (From Selmanowitz, V. J., Kramer, K. M., and Orentreich, N.: Congenital ectodermal defect in miniature poodles. J. Hered. *61*:196, 1970.)

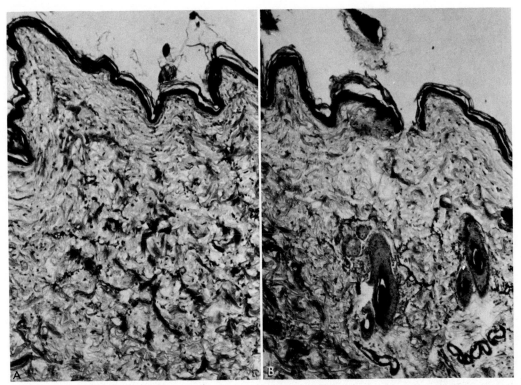

Figure 11:24. *A,* Appendage-free skin from the head; hair follicles, sebaceous glands and sweat glands are absent. (Acid orcein elastica stain × 70.) *B,* Transition zone of appendage-free and appendage-containing skin. Hair follicles, sweat glands, and sebaceous gland cells (seen near the upper portion of the section of the follicle in the center of the photograph) appear normal. The portion of dermis lacking appendages marks the beginning of a large area of alopecia. There is no overt difference in the appearance of the epidermis and connective tissue on either side of the transition. (From Selmanowitz, V. J., Kramer, K. M., and Orentreich, N.: Congenital ectodermal defect in miniature poodles. J. Hered. *61*:196, 1970.)

investigation did not reveal other abnormalities. Although the numbers are few, one might suspect a sex-linked mechanism of inheritance.

Another study was made on a similar litter of miniature poodles. In the study, progressive hypotrichosis was detected in two silver male miniature poodle siblings at 5 weeks of age. A male and two female siblings had normal black coats. The sire (a 3-year-old black miniature poodle) and the dam (a 2-year-old silver miniature poodle) also had normal coats. Histologically, the hypotrichotic skin had accumulations of keratotic debris in and around inactive and dystrophic hair bulbs (Fig. 11:25). Sex-linked or sex-limited inheritance may have been involved, inasmuch as both affected dogs were males. This result was also found by other investigators.[10]

Canine hereditary black hair follicular dysplasia has been reported in two black and white mongrel siblings, a male and a female. Defective hair coats were found only in the black hair coat regions and included these features: hypotrichosis; fractured, stubby hairs lacking a normal sheen; and periodic scaliness of the skin (Fig. 11:26). These abnormalities were found diffusely in the black hair coat regions, with the exception of parts of the margins and the sides of the necks of both animals. The white portions of the coat were normally full and lustrous. Observation of subsequent litters has shown that, although some black and white mongrels appeared normal at birth, all eventually (by 4 weeks) showed the black hair follicular dysplasia.[61] Of 15 offspring from two matings

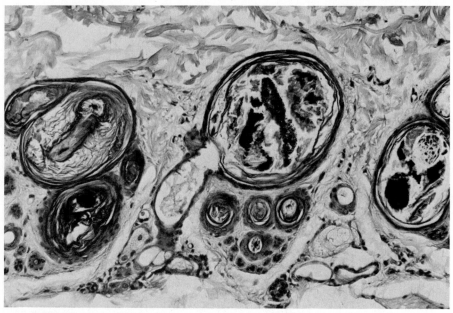

Figure 11:25. Canine hypotrichosis. Dystrophic hair follicles and abortive hair shafts.

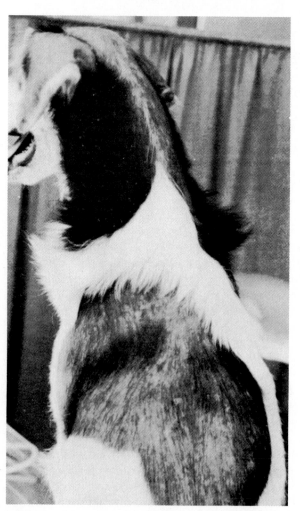

Figure 11:26. Hypotrichosis of black haircoat on body, head, and dorsal midline of neck, excepting sides of neck. (From Selmanowitz, V. J., Kramer, K.M., and Orentreich, N.: Canine hereditary black hair follicular dysplasia. J. Hered. *63*:43, 1972.)

of an affected pair of dogs, 12 spotted pups developed the disorder in the black regions; the remaining 3 were all white and appeared normal.

Histologic examination showed the white hairs to be of the normal multiple-hair-follicle composite type with hairs egressing through a common infundibulum and orifice. Affected black hair coat regions had irregular distortions and bulges of hair follicle walls and keratinous blockage of the hair canals.

When the two affected animals were interbred, six puppies were produced. Two had the same condition as that seen in their parents, two were normal (although spotted), one was all white (normal), and one had uniformly wavy black hair. Selmanowitz[61] and associates were intrigued by the disorder "because melanocytes are of neural crest derivation and neural factors have been implicated in the morphogenetic induction of cutaneous appendages."

In human beings, certain disorders inherited in an autosomal dominant mode manifest multiple derangements of neural crest derivatives (multiple lentigines syndrome). We suspect a similar modus operandi in this canine disorder in which only pigmented skin displays abnormalities of hair. The population of melanocytes that is operative in hair pigmentation is clearly associated with the follicular dysplasia.

Black hair follicular dysplasia has also been recognized in bearded collies, a dachshund, a schipperke, a bassett hound, and a Papillon.[15a, 43, 45]

PATTERN BALDNESS

This is an inherited condition seen especially in the dachshund breed. Alopecia begins at less than 1 year of age, and different forms appear in males and females. Males develop bilateral pinnal alopecia that progresses to completely bald ears by 8 to 9 years of age. In females, a ventral thinning of hair progresses to complete alopecia of the ventrum (Fig. 11:27). The female baldness must be differentiated from hypoestrogenism, which usually also involves loss of hair on the perineum and an infantile vulva. Alopecia due to hypoestrogenism responds to estrogen replacement, while pattern baldness is unresponsive to any therapy.

MELANODERMA AND ALOPECIA OF YORKSHIRE TERRIERS

This syndrome is well recognized, but poorly studied and reported.[1, 55] It is probably a genetic dermatosis, but the mode of inheritance is unknown. Typically, the syndrome affects Yorkshire terriers, of either sex, beginning at 6 months to 3 years of age.

The dogs develop a symmetric alopecia and marked hyperpigmentation over the bridge of the nose, the pinnae, and occasionally the tail and feet (Fig. 11:5E, p. 664). Affected skin is smooth and shiny. There is no pruritus or pain, and affected dogs are otherwise healthy.

Skin biopsies are reported to show orthokeratotic hyperkeratosis of the epidermal surface and of the hair follicles.

Some dogs with mild lesions appear to spontaneously recover. Most dogs remain affected throughout their lifetime.

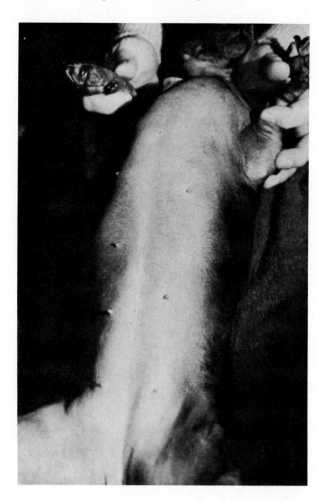

Figure 11:27. Pattern baldness in a dachshund.

Miscellaneous Congenital and Hereditary Defects

LYMPHEDEMA

Lymphedema is swelling of some part of the body due to a lymph system disorder.

CAUSE AND PATHOGENESIS

Lymphedema can be primary or secondary.[13, 17, 35] Primary lymphedema is caused by developmental defects in lymphatics and lymph nodes. Secondary lymphedema occurs as a result of the obstruction of lymphatic flow by inflammatory or neoplastic disease or by interruption of lymphatics resulting from surgery or trauma. In some dogs, primary lymphedema has been shown to be inherited as an autosomal dominant trait with variable expressivity.[36, 46] Canine primary lymphedema has been classified by lymphangiography and histopathology into two basic structural defects: (1) lymphatic hypoplasia, with or without hypoplasia or absence of the regional lymph nodes, and (2) lymphatic hyperplasia and dilatation.[13, 17, 35, 36]

CLINICAL FEATURES

Primary lymphedema has been recognized in several breeds of dogs, including the English bulldog, German shepherd, borzoi, Belgian Tervuren, Labrador retriever, Great Dane, and poodle. There appears to be no sex predilection. The onset of disease is usually within the first 12 weeks of life.

The hind limbs are the most commonly affected, although the front limbs, ventrum, tail, and pinnae may be involved. Affected skin is usually normal in surface appearance but is thickened and spongy, and it pits with digital pressure. Regional lymph nodes may not be palpable, and the dogs are usually healthy otherwise. However, lymphedema predisposes affected tissues to secondary bacterial infection and delayed healing, and these complications may be clinically apparent.

DIAGNOSIS

Differential diagnosis includes other causes of obstructive, inflammatory, and hypoproteinemic edema. Definitive diagnosis is based on history, physical examination, laboratory rule-outs, skin biopsy, and lymphangiography. Skin biopsy reveals variable degrees of subcutaneous and dermal edema.[62] Lymphatics may be dilated and hyperplastic or may be hypoplastic. Chronic cases may show variable degrees of fibrosis and epidermal hyperplasia. Inflammatory cells are usually few in number to absent, unless secondary infection is present.

CLINICAL MANAGEMENT

The prognosis and indicated therapy vary with the severity of the lymphedema. Mild cases may wax and wane, spontaneously regress, or persist indefinitely with no adverse consequences to the patient. More severe cases may require (1) frequent bandaging (e.g., modified Robert Jones splint) to reduce the lymphedema,[62] (2) surgical extirpation of the edematous tissues, or (3) amputation of the affected part. Dogs with severe primary lymphedema often die shortly after birth, owing to pleural and abdominal effusions.[34]

TYROSINEMIA

A single case of congenital tyrosinemia in a young dog was reported.[32] It appeared to be similar to tyrosinemia type II in humans or pseudodistemper in mink. Tyrosinemia, inherited as an autosomal recessive trait, is a group of distinct metabolic diseases with five phenotypes in humans. The case reported in the dog is characterized by a very early age onset of characteristic eye and skin lesions with varying degrees of mental retardation.

CAUSE AND PATHOGENESIS

It is apparently hereditary (both parents of this dog had elevated serum tyrosinase levels), the serum tyrosinase levels being elevated because of a deficiency of cytosolic hepatic tyrosine aminotransferase. The pathophysiology is considered to be an inflammatory response to tyrosine crystals deposited in tissues. This appears to be the case with the corneal lesions, but many skin lesions have no crystals. Instead there may be increased numbers of highly condensed tonofibrils and increased numbers of keratohyalin granules in the granular layer. Tyrosine is known to influence the number of microtubules in the tonofibrils.

CLINICAL FEATURES

The 7-week-old German shepherd puppy was small for its age when it first developed conjunctivitis and cloudy corneas. The globes were small, and cataracts and corneal granulation were present, but no ulceration. There was ulceration of the nose, tongue, and central portions of the footpads (Fig. 11:5F,G, p. 664). As the disease progressed, ulcers involved the metatarsal pads and the nail folds, and nails were broken. Erythematous bullae were found on the abdomen. The planum nasale developed erythema, focal ulceration with marginal crusting, and hypopigmentation.

DIAGNOSIS

Diagnosis was based on suspicion of a metabolic defect found on physical examination and from the history. High levels of tyrosine in the serum and urine were identified.

Histopathology of ulcerated skin lesions revealed large granules of tyrosine surrounded by an eosinophilic, amorphous material, which resembled the Splendore-Hoeppli reaction.

CLINICAL MANAGEMENT

The prognosis for a cure is not good. In humans, dramatic reduction of plasma tyrosine levels and dramatic clearing of skin and eye lesions occur in patients placed on diets of low tyrosine and low phenylalanine. Symptoms recur when a regular diet is resumed.[119] This might be tried in canine cases, but it is probably not practical.

COLLAGEN DISORDER OF THE FOOTPADS OF GERMAN SHEPHERD

This disorder is probably a genetic dermatosis, but the mode of inheritance has not been established.[40] It first appears in German shepherds, of either sex, at a few weeks to a few months of age. Usually multiple dogs of a litter are affected.

In general, all footpads become softer than normal and are often tender. Discrete ulcers develop on one or more pads (Fig. 11:5H, p. 664), especially the carpal and tarsal pads. Initially, the dogs are otherwise healthy.

Histopathologic findings include multifocal areas of collagenolysis and a predominantly neutrophilic inflammation (Figs. 11:28 and 11:29).

Therapy with antibiotics, glucocorticoids, and topicals has been unsuccessful. The condition usually regresses spontaneously by 1 year of age. However, the dogs usually develop renal amyloidosis and die at 2 to 3 years of age.

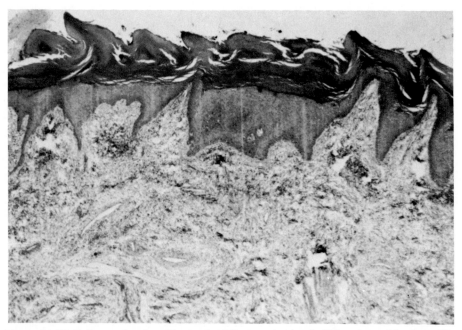

Figure 11:28. Collagen disorder of footpads of German shepherds. Diffuse-to-nodular dermatitis.

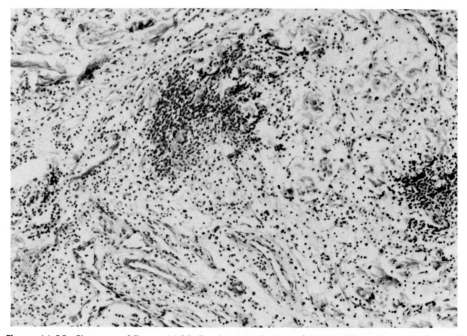

Figure 11:29. Close-up of Figure 11:28. Focal accumulations of neutrophils and mononuclear cells around degenerate collagen.

DIGITAL HYPERKERATOSIS OF IRISH TERRIERS

This disorder is widely recognized in western and eastern Europe, but has apparently not been well studied and reported.[30] It is apparently a genetic dermatosis, but the mode of inheritance has not been established.

Irish terriers of either sex develop hyperkeratosis of the footpads of all four paws at a very early age. The condition becomes more severe with age, and the affected pads tend to fissure, become secondarily infected, and painful. Affected dogs are usually otherwise healthy.

Histopathologic findings include mild-to-moderate epidermal hyperplasia with marked papillated orthokeratotic hyperkeratosis (Fig. 11:30). Therapy is for symptoms (see p. 718) and is rather unrewarding.

ICHTHYOSIS

Ichthyosis is a congenital syndrome of abnormal keratinization that is discussed on page 741.

EPIDERMAL DYSPLASIA OF WEST HIGHLAND WHITE TERRIERS

Epidermal dysplasia of West Highland white terriers is probably a genetic syndrome involving defects in keratinization. It is discussed on page 730.

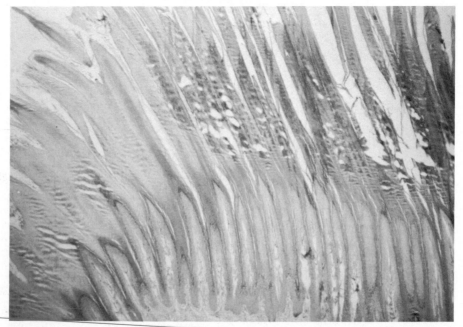

Figure 11:30. Digital hyperkeratosis of Irish terrier. Marked papillated hyperplasia and orthokeratotic hyperkeratosis.

CYCLIC HEMATOPOIESIS
(Gray Collie Syndrome)

Cyclic hematopoiesis is an hereditary disorder of gray collies. It is discussed on page 710.

LICHENOID-PSORIASIFORM DERMATOSIS OF SPRINGER SPANIELS

Lichenoid-psoriasiform dermatosis of springer spaniels is probably a hereditary syndrome involving defects in keratinization. It is discussed on page 728.

PITUITARY DWARFISM

Pituitary dwarfism is a hereditary disorder most commonly reported in the German shepherd dog. It is discussed on page 611.

VITILIGO

Vitiligo is probably a hereditary pigmentary disorder of Doberman pinschers and Rottweilers. It is discussed on page 711.

NEVI

Nevi are often congenital hyperplastic disorders in the skin. A syndrome of multiple collagenous nevi is hereditary in the German shepherd dog. Nevi are discussed on page 937.

GRANULOMATOUS SEBACEOUS ADENITIS

Sebaceous adenitis appears to be a hereditary disorder in black and apricot standard poodles. It is discussed on page 555.

References

1. Allen, L. S. S.: Skin condition in Yorkshire terriers. Canine Pract. *12*:29, 1985.
1a. Anderson, R. K.: Canine acanthosis nigricans. Compend. Cont. Ed. *1*:466, 1979.
2. Antin, I. P.: Dermoid sinus in a Rhodesian ridgeback dog. J.A.V.M.A. *157*:961, 1970.
3. Austin, V.: Blue dog disease. Mod. Vet. Pract. *36*:31, 1975.
4. Ayres, S., Jr., and Mihan, R.: Epidermolysis bullosa: vitamin E as an effective treatment. Arch. Dermatol. *4*:482, 1981.
5. Bornfors, S.: Acanthosis nigricans in dogs. Acta Endocrinol. (Suppl.)*28*:1, 1958.
6. Briggs, O. M., and Botha, W. S.: Color mutant alopecia in a blue Italian greyhound. J.A.A.H.A. *22*:611, 1986.

6a. Brigrac, M. M., et al.: Microscopy of color mutant alopecia. Ann. Meet. Am. Acad. Vet. Dermatol. and Am. Coll. Vet. Dermatol., 1988.
7. Callen, J. P.: Dermatomyositis. Dermatol. Clin. *1*:461, 1983.
8. Chastain, C. B., and Sawyer, D. E.: Congenital hypotrichosis in male bassett hound littermates. J.A.V.M.A. *187*:845, 1985.
9. Collier, L. A., Leathers, C. W., et al.: A clinical description of dermatosparaxis in a Himalayan cat. Feline Pract. *10*:25, 1980.
10. Conroy, J. D.: Hypotrichosis in miniature poodle siblings. J.A.V.M.A. *166*:697, 1975.
11. Counts, D. F., Byers, B. F., et al.: Dermatosparaxis in a Himalayan cat. 1. Biochemical studies of dermal collagen. J. Invest. Dermatol. *74*:96, 1980.

12. Cummings, J. F., deLahunta, A., et al.: Acral mutilation and nociceptive loss in English pointer dogs. Acta Neuropathol. (Bul.)53:119, 1981.

13. Davies, A. P., et al.: Primary lymphedema in 3 dogs. J.A.V.M.A. 174:1316, 1979.

14. Dunstan, R. W., Sills, R. C., et al.: A mechano-bullous disease (junctional epidermolysis bullosa) in a toy poodle. Proceedings, Am. Acad. Vet. Derm. annual meeting. Phoenix, March, 1987.

14a. Duvic, M., and Pinnell, S. R.: Ehlers-Danlos syndrome. In Thiers, B. H., and Dobson, R. L. (eds.): Pathogenesis of Skin Disease. Churchill Livingstone, New York, 1988, p. 565.

15. Fitzpatrick, T. B., et al.: Dermatology in General Medicine. 2nd ed. McGraw-Hill Book Company, New York, 1981.

15a. Foil, C. S.: Comparative genodermatoses. Clin. Dermatol. 3:175, 1985.

15b. Freeman, L. J., et al.: Ehlers-Danlos syndrome in dogs and cats. Semin. Vet. Med. Surg. 2:221, 1987.

15c. Gammie, J. S.: Dermoid sinus removal in a Rhodesian ridgeback dog. Can. Vet. J. 27:250, 1986.

16. Grieshaber, T. L., Blakemore, J. C., et al.: Congenital alopecia in a bichon frise. J.A.V.M.A. 188:1053, 1986.

17. Griffin, C. E., and MacCoy, D. M.: Primary lymphedema: a case report and discussion. J.A.A.H.A. 14:373, 1978.

18. Gross, T. L., and Kunkle, G. A.: The cutaneous histology of dermatomyositis in collie dogs. Vet. Pathol. 24:11, 1987.

19. Gupta, B. N.: Epitheliogenesis imperfecta in a dog. Am. J. Res. 34:443, 1973.

20. Hargis, A. M., Haupt, K. H., et al.: A skin disorder in three Shetland sheepdogs: Comparison with familial canine dermatomyositis of collies. Compend. Cont. Ed. 7:306, 1985.

20a. Hargis, A. M., et al.: Familial canine dermatomyositis. Initial characterization of the cutaneous and muscular lesions. Am. J. Pathol. 116:234, 1984.

20b. Hargis, A. M., et al.: Familial canine dermatomyositis. Am. J. Pathol. 120:323, 1985.

20c. Hargis, A. M., et al.: Post mortem findings in four litters of dogs with familial canine dermatomyositis. Am. J. Pathol. 123:480, 1986.

20d. Hargis, A. M., et al.: Post-mortem findings in a Shetland sheepdog with dermatomyositis. Vet. Pathol. 23:509, 1986.

21. Haupt, K. H., Prieur, J. D., et al.: Familial canine dermatomyositis. Am. J. Vet. Res. 46:1861, 1985.

22. Hegreberg, G. A., and Padgett, G. A.: Ehlers-Danlos syndrome in animals. Bull. Pathol. 8:247, 1967.

23. Hegreberg, G. A., Padgett, G. A., et al.: A heritable connective tissue disease of dogs and mink resembling the Ehlers-Danlos syndrome of man. II. Mode of inheritance. J. Hered. 60:249, 1969.

24. Hegreberg, G. A., Padgett, G. A., et al.: A heritable connective tissue disease of dogs and mink resembling the Ehlers-Danlos syndrome of man. III. Histopathologic changes of the skin. Arch. Pathol. 90:159, 1970.

25. Hewitt, M. P., Mills, J. H., et al.: Epitheliogenesis imperfecta in a black Labrador puppy. Can. Vet. J. 16:371, 1975.

26. Holbrook, K. A., Byers, B. F., et al.: Dermatosparaxis in the Himalayan cat. II. Ultrastructural studies of dermal collagen. J. Invest. Dermatol. 74:100, 1980.

27. Hutt, F. B.: Necrosis of the toes. In: Genetics for Dog Breeders. W. H. Freeman, San Francisco, 1979.

28. Jezyk, P. F., Haskins, M. E., et al.: Lethal acrodermatitis in bull terriers. J.A.V.M.A. 188:833, 1986.

29. Kirk, R. W.: Acanthosis nigricans. Vet. Clin. North Am. 9:49, 1979.

30. Kral, F., and Schwartzman, R. M.: Veterinary and Comparative Dermatology. J. B. Lippincott Company, Philadelphia, 1964.

31. Kunkle, G. A.: Congenital hypotrichosis in two dogs. J.A.V.M.A. 185:84, 1984.

32. Kunkle, G. A., Jezyk, P. F., et al.: Tyrosinemia in a dog. J.A.A.H.A. 20:615, 1984.

33. Kunkle, G. A., Gross, T. L., et al.: Dermatomyositis in collie dogs. Compend. Cont. Ed. 7:185, 1985.

34. Ladds, P. W., Dennis, S. M., et al.: Lethal congenital edema in bulldog pups. J.A.V.M.A. 155:81, 1971.

35. Leighton, R. L., and Suter, P. F.: Primary lymphedema of the hind limb in a dog. J.A.V.M.A. 174:369, 1979.

36. Luginbuhl, H., et al.: Congenital hereditary lymphedema in the dog, part II. Pathological studies. J. Med. Genet. 4:153, 1967.

37. MacDonald, J. M.: Personal communication, 1982.

38. Mann, G. E., and Stratton, J.: Dermoid sinus in the Rhodesian ridgeback. J. Small Anim. Pract. 7:631, 1966.

39. Miller, W. H., Jr.: Canine facial dermatoses. Compend. Cont. Ed. 1:640, 1979.

40. Miller, W. H., Jr.: Personal communication, 1987.

41. Minor, R. R.: Animal models of heritable diseases of the skin. In Goldsmith, E. L. (ed.): Biochemistry and Physiology of Skin. Oxford University Press, New York, 1982.

42. Minor, R. R., et al.: Defects in collagen fibrillogenesis causing hyperextensible fragile skin in dogs. J.A.V.M.A. 182:142, 1983.

43. Muller, G. H., Kirk, R. W., and Scott, D. W.: Small Animal Dermatology. 3rd ed. W. B. Saunders Company, Philadelphia, 1983.

44. Munday, B. L.: Epitheliogenesis imperfecta in lambs and kittens. Br. Vet. J. 126:xlvii, 1970.

44a. Mundell, A. C.: Mineral analysis in Bull Terriers with lethal acrodermatitis. Ann. Meet. Am. Acad. Vet. Dermatol. and Am. Coll. Vet. Dermatol., 1988.

45. O'Neill, C. S.: Hereditary skin disease in the dog and the cat. Compend. Cont. Ed. 3:791, 1981.

46. Patterson, D. F., et al.: Congenital hereditary lymphedema in the dog, part I. Clinical and genetic studies. J. Med. Genet. 4:145, 1967.

47. Patterson, D. F., Minor, R. R.: Hereditary fragility and hyperextensibility of the skin of cats. Lab. Invest. 37:170, 1977.

48. Rickards, R. A.: A new treatment for canine melanosis. Mod. Vet. Pract. 47:38, 1966.

49. Robinson, R.: The Canadian hairless or sphinx cat. J. Hered. 64:47, 1973.

50. Rook, A., Wilkinson, D. S., et al.: Textbook of Dermatology. 3rd ed. Blackwell Scientific Publications, Oxford, 1979, pp. 1307–1310.

51. Schwartzman, R. M., and Orkin, M.: A Comparative Study of Skin Diseases of Dog and Man. Charles C. Thomas, Springfield, Illinois, 1962, pp. 313–318.

52. Scott, D. W.: Cutaneous asthenia in a cat. Vet. Med. (S.A.C.) 69:1256, 1974.

53. Scott, D. W.: Feline dermatology 1900–1978: a monograph. J.A.A.H.A. 16:313, 1980.

54. Scott, D. W.: Feline dermatology. Introspective retrospections. J.A.A.H.A. 20:537, 1984.

55. Scott, D. W.: Unpublished data, 1987.

56. Scott, D. W., and McGrath, C. J.: Acanthosis nigricans in a Lhasa apso. Vet. Med. (S.A.C.), 68:676, 1973.

57. Scott, D. W., and Schultz, R. D.: Epidermolysis bullosa simplex in a collie dog. J.A.V.M.A. 171:721, 1977.

58. Scott, D. W., and Walton, D. K.: Clinical evaluation of oral vitamin E for the treatment of primary acanthosis nigricans. J.A.A.H.A. *21*:345, 1985.

59. Selcer, E. A., Helman, R. G., et al.: Dermoid sinus in a Shih Tzu and a boxer. J.A.A.H.A. *20*:634, 1984.

60. Selmanowitz, V. J., Kramer, K. M., et al.: Congenital ectodermal defect in poodles. J. Hered. *61*:196, 1970.

61. Selmanowitz, V. J., Markotsky, J., et al.: Black hair follicular dysplasia in dogs. J.A.V.M.A. *171*:1079, 1977.

62. Takahashi, J. L., Farrow, C. S., et al.: Primary lymphedema in a dog: A case report. J.A.A.H.A. *20*:849, 1984.

63. Tizard, I.: Veterinary Immunology. 3rd ed. W. B. Saunders Company, Philadelphia, 1987.

64. Thoday, K.: Skin diseases of the cat. In Pract. *3*:21, 1981.

65. Thomsett, L. R.: Congenital hypotrichia in the dog. Vet. Rec. *73*:915, 1961.

CHAPTER
12

Acquired Alopecias

An acquired alopecia is a hair loss that develops sometime during the life of an animal. Not included in this chapter are the hereditary alopecias (Chapter 11) and hair losses that develop as a result of specific disease processes, such as dermatophytosis, endocrine abnormalities, immunologic diseases, or self-inflicted hair loss from hypersensitivity or parasitism.

The remaining assorted conditions include canine and feline pinnal alopecia, pattern baldness, feline symmetric alopecia, short-hair syndrome of silky breeds, preauricular alopecia of cats, excessive shedding, and anagen and telogen defluxion. The knowledge about the cause of most of these alopecias is sparse, although the clinical features are well recognized.

Canine and Feline Pinnal Alopecia

Pinnal alopecia is most common in dachshunds but has also been observed in other breeds such as Chihuahuas, Boston terriers, whippets, and Italian greyhounds.[3] The pinnal alopecia is seldom noticed in animals less than 1 year of age. At first, the hair coat is thinner than normal on the pinnae and can progress into total alopecia as the dog reaches 8 to 9 years of age. In general, no treatment is available, but if the dog's owner is very concerned about this hair loss, hormones can be tried empirically. If a trial period of thyroid supplementation does not produce new hair in 3 months, it should be discontinued. In males, testosterone therapy can be tried for about 3 months. If either of the above hormones causes hair to regrow, a low maintenance dose can be used.

It is important to differentiate such spontaneous alopecias from dermatoses that cause hair loss on the pinnae. A vasculitis can occur on the pinna that causes alopecia with severe erythema, scaling, crusting, and eventually ulceration and tissue loss at the pinna margin. Pinnal vasculitis may respond to systemic corticosteroids. Unfortunately, the damaged pinnal margin is often left with irregular "scalloped" edges. After healing, surgical trimming can restore the natural appearance.

Estrogen-responsive dermatosis of the female dog (ovarian imbalance II) may cause pinnal alopecia, in addition to causing hair loss of the neck, chest, ventral abdomen, and caudomedial thighs (see p. 625). Ventral alopecia of female dogs (especially dachshunds) must also be differentiated from hypoestrogenism (ovarian imbalance II).

Some Siamese cats develop a spontaneous, periodic alopecia of the ears

698

(Fig. 12:1A). After several months the hair regrows without treatment. The cause is unknown.[5]

Seborrhea of the margin of the pinnae (seen in dachshunds and some other breeds, especially cocker spaniels) is often accompanied by alopecia. In these cases the seborrheic pinna is scaly and greasy, with the alopecia being only a secondary manifestation (see discussion of ear margin dermatoses, p. 737).

Periodic alopecia of the ears of miniature poodles is of unknown cause. It has many similarities to alopecia areata in humans. Mature poodles suddenly lose large tufts of hair from their pinnae. The loss continues over a period of several months until both pinnae are alopecic in a bilaterally symmetric pattern. In almost every case, the hair regrows spontaneously within 3 to 4 months.

Pattern Baldness

Pattern baldness is most commonly seen in dachshunds but may be seen in breeds such as the Manchester terrier, miniature Doberman pinscher, and the Chihuahua.[3] The cause is unknown but is probably genetically determined (see also p. 689).

Preauricular Feline Alopecia

On an area of the temporal region between the ear and eye of cats, the hair is sparser than on other parts of the head (Fig. 12:1B). This is a physiologic, not a pathologic, condition.[5] In long-haired or densely coated cats, this area is not noticeable; however, in cats with short or less dense hair coats it mimics an alopecia. When cat owners ask their veterinarians about the condition, it can be explained as a normal condition that, of course, neither requires nor would respond to treatment. Certainly, skin scrapings, fungal cultures, or biopsies are totally unnecessary.

Anagen and Telogen Defluxion

In *anagen defluxion*, a special circumstance (antimitotic drugs, infectious diseases, endocrine disorders, or metabolic diseases) interferes with anagen, resulting in abnormalities of the hair follicle and hair shaft. Hair loss occurs suddenly within days of the insult, as the growth phase continues (Fig. 12:1C).[1, 5]

In *telogen defluxion*, a stressful circumstance (high fever, pregnancy, shock, severe illness, surgery, or anesthesia) causes the abrupt, premature cessation of growth in anagen hair follicles and the sudden synchronization of many hair follicles in catagen, then in telogen. Two to three months later, a large number of telogen hairs are shed as a new wave of hair follicle cyclic activity begins (Fig. 12:1D).

Diagnosis is based on history, physical examination, and microscopic examination of affected hairs. Telogen hairs are characterized by a uniform shaft diameter and a slightly clubbed, nonpigmented root end that lacks root sheaths. Anagen defluxion hairs are characterized by irregularities and dysplastic changes. The diameter of the shaft may be irregularly narrowed and

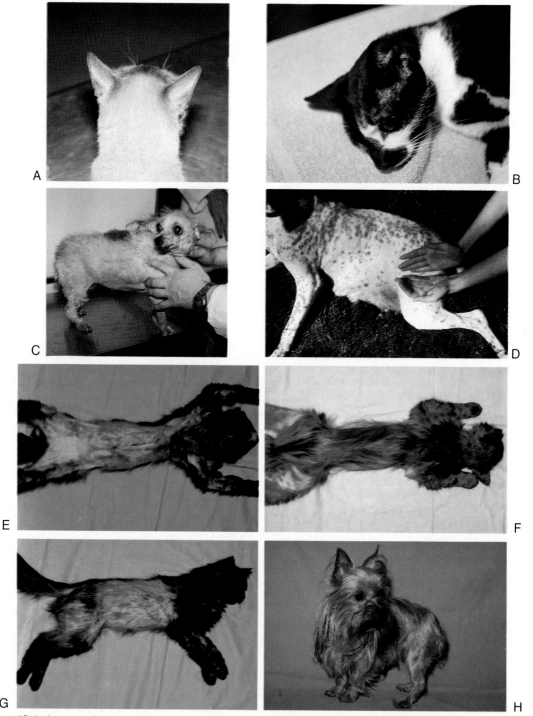

Figure 12:1. *Acquired alopecias. A,* Periodic alopecia of ears of a Siamese cat. Hair will regrow spontaneously. The cause is unknown. (Courtesy W. H. Miller, Jr.) *B,* Preauricular feline alopecia. Note normal sparseness of hair between eye and ear. *C,* Anagen defluxion. Diffuse alopecia due to arrest of hair cycle by cytoxan. (Courtesy W. H. Miller, Jr.) *D,* Telogen defluxion. Postpartum shedding resulting from physiologic stress of gestation and lactation. *Feline symmetric alopecia.* *E,* Ventral view showing characteristic bilateral alopecia without skin reaction or lesions. *F,* Bilateral alopecia showing normal hair along the dorsal midline. *G,* Characteristic alopecia from the sternum posteriorly, sparing hair on the lower legs. *H,* Yorkshire terrier with short hair syndrome. This dog previously had long, silky hair that reached the floor.

deformed, and breaking often occurs at such structurally weakened sites, resulting in ragged points.

Both anagen and telogen defluxion spontaneously resolve when the constitutional stress is relieved.

Excessive Shedding

Owners often ask "Why does my dog (or cat) shed so much?" They are naturally concerned about large amounts of hair getting on their rugs, furniture, and clothing. If excessively shed hairs are quickly replaced and no alopecia results, the condition may cause inconvenience to the owner but causes no problem for the animal. Since the hair growth cycle is controlled by a number of factors (see p. 4), the questions about shedding are difficult to answer. Very little information about it is available in the literature. In the absence of obvious clinical disease, modification of diet, or adjustment of light and temperature can be considered as treatment. If no abnormal conditions can be discovered, the only treatment is to remove the dead telogen hairs from the animal by combing, brushing, or in some cases vacuuming.

Feline Symmetric Alopecia

(Feline Endocrine Alopecia)

Feline symmetric alopecia is a rare acquired bilaterally symmetric hypotrichosis of unknown etiology.[4-6]

CAUSE AND PATHOGENESIS

The exact cause and pathogenesis of feline symmetric alopecia is unknown. The former name, feline endocrine alopecia, is changed in this edition because a true endocrine cause could not be proved.[3] Also, it has been observed that an identical pattern of alopecia can be self-inflicted by the cat. Since cats are sometimes "secret groomers," the owners are not aware that the cat is licking or pulling excessively at the hairs. The success of therapy with gonadal or thyroid hormones to cause regrowth of hair may be due to a more rapid replacement of the pulled hair, rather than to an endocrine deficiency. It has been established that affected cats have normal thyroid function. Some clinicians have placed Elizabethan collars or buckets on the cat's head for several weeks in order to document whether or not the alopecia is self-inflicted. When the device is removed, if the alopecia has been self-induced, the alopecia will recur in the same pattern. Such devices are inhumane and eventually ineffective. Their long-term use is discouraged.

CLINICAL FEATURES

Feline symmetric alopecia is seen mostly in neutered male and female cats. No breed predilection has been reported, but purebred cats are rarely affected. Ages of affected cats range from 2 to 12 years (average is 6 years).

Feline symmetric alopecia is characterized by bilaterally symmetric hypotrichosis, which begins in the genital and perineal regions (Figs. 12:1*E* to *G* and

12:2). There is diffuse thinning of the hair, rather than complete baldness, affecting the anogenital region, proximal tail, caudomedial thighs, and ventral abdomen. Long-standing cases may have hypotrichosis of the lateral thorax, flanks, and caudomedial front limbs, but the dorsum is spared. Hairs in the affected areas are easily epilated. Pruritus and skin lesions are usually absent.

DIAGNOSIS

The first diagnostic question is whether the cat has bitten or licked the hairs and caused the alopecia by self-trauma or whether the hairs fell out by themselves. A trichogram can provide the answer. Twenty or more hairs are plucked and the distal ends are examined. If the hair tips are intact and pointed, the hairs are falling out. If, however, the distal end of the hair shows a broken or "chewed off" edge, the cat is doing damage to itself. For anyone not experienced in reading trichograms, practicing on normal cat hairs is helpful.

The differential diagnosis includes psychogenic alopecia, dermatophytosis, feline demodicosis (rare), flea bite hypersensitivity, atopy, food hypersensitivity, hypothyroidism (extremely rare), hyperadrenocorticism (extremely rare), excessive shedding, and telogen and anagen defluxion. Definitive diagnosis is based on history, physical examination, laboratory rule-outs, and response to therapy. Hemogram, serum chemistries, urinalysis, and tests of thyroid and adrenal function are normal. Skin biopsy reveals telogenization of hair follicles.

CLINICAL MANAGEMENT

If the hair loss is induced by the cat, the cause must be found and treated. Systemic corticosteroids can be tried, and after about 1 month the patient can be evaluated for new hair growth. Mechanical devices, such as Elizabethan collars, may prevent further hair loss, but their long-term use is not recommended.

If the cat has definitely not caused the hair loss by licking or biting, the treatment becomes more difficult and empirical. The owner should be informed of the likely chronic course of the condition. Treatment is then the same as

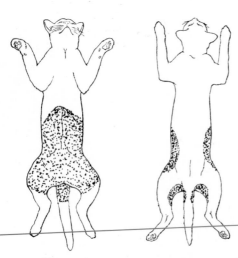

Figure 12:2. Feline symmetric alopecia distribution pattern.

Ventral   Dorsal

that recommended when the condition was thought to have been caused by an endocrine abnormality.[2] Therapy consists of (1) combined androgen-estrogen injections, (2) progestational compounds, or (3) thyroid hormone. Combined androgen-estrogen therapy appears to be more effective than either sex hormone alone. Excellent results have been obtained with repositol testosterone (12.5 mg/cat); and repositol diethylstilbestrol (0.625 mg/cat) or estradiol (0.5 mg/cat), given intramuscularly. The cats are re-examined in 6 weeks, and if new hair growth is not evident, a second injection is given. Relapse occurs after a variable period of time (6 months to 2 years) in about 50 per cent of the cats so treated. Retreatment is effective.

The occasional transient side-effects that are seen with androgen-estrogen therapy are signs of estrus in females and aggressiveness or urine spraying, or both, in males. These signs are seen during the first week of therapy. Overdose of either testosterone or estrogen can result in severe hepatobiliary disease and death. Repositol testosterone, repositol diethylstilbestrol, and repositol estradiol are not licensed for use in cats in the United States.

Progestational compounds are also effective for the treatment of feline symmetric alopecia. Repositol progesterone (2.2 to 22 mg/kg) or medroxyprogesterone acetate (50 to 175 mg/cat) may be given intramuscularly or subcutaneously. The cats are re-examined in 6 weeks, and a second injection is given if hair regrowth is not evident. Relapse rate and retreatment success are described above for androgen-estrogens. Megestrol acetate may be given orally (2.5 to 5 mg/cat), once every other day, until hair growth is evident. A maintenance dose of 2.5 to 5 mg/cat, once every 1 to 2 weeks, is usually required. Because potential side-effects of progestational compounds in the cat are numerous and occasionally severe, other alternative treatments are recommended (see p. 210). These compounds are not licensed for use in cats in the United States. Interestingly, progestational compounds can *produce* feline symmetric alopecia–like hair loss.

In spite of the fact that cats with feline symmetric alopecia are not hypothyroid, thyroid hormones have been recommended for therapy. Sodium levothyroxine (0.05 to 0.1 mg orally BID) is reported to be effective. Sodium liothyroxine (50 μg orally BID) was reported to produce complete hair regrowth in 73 per cent of the cats treated.[3] With either thyroid hormone, hair regrowth was good within 3 months of beginning treatment. Side-effects are apparently rare. It must be emphasized here, that thyroid hormone therapy can force varying degrees of hair growth in many nonthyroidal illnesses, and such responses must not be misinterpreted as being indicative of hypothyroidism.

Short-Hair Syndrome of Silky Breeds

Yorkshire terriers and silky terriers normally have long, silky hair coats. The luxurious coat was achieved by many generations of selective breeding. The coat is a source of great pride to the pet's owner. Occasionally, an apparently normal-coated mature dog loses its coat, and it is replaced with hairs that never grow to their former full length (Fig. 12:1H). The owner is distressed by this and seeks help, often after unsuccessfully trying vitamin and mineral supplements or coat conditioners containing fatty acids. The affected dogs have no itching, erythema, or scaling of the skin. Onset occurs from 1 to 5 years of age. There are no broken or bitten hairs. Because the long silky hairs are gone, the remaining hair coat would be most adequate for a mixed-breed dog or a more short-haired purebred dog.

It can only be theorized that the hair cycle has been shortened by some unknown factor, so that the hairs are shed before they reach their normal full length. The most important differential diagnosis is to rule out endocrine (especially hypothyroidism) and congenital disorders, psychogenic alopecia, and other more obvious dermatoses. There is no known treatment.

This condition also occurs in younger dogs. In such cases the puppy coat is normal, but it is replaced with a permanent, shorter coat. The abnormal new coat is apparent at 5 months of age. The hair on the head is normal length. However, the posterior abdominal area, hind legs, and chest have hairs that are shorter than normal. There is no scaliness or inflammation of the skin.

References

1. Fadok, V. A.: The dynamics of hair growth and development. Dermatology reports. Vol. 4, No. 1, 1985.
2. Kral, F., and Schwartzman, R. M.: Veterinary and Comparative Dermatology. J. B. Lippincott Company, Philadelphia, 1964.
3. Muller, G. H., Kirk, R. W., and Scott, D. W. (eds.): Small Animal Dermatology. 3rd ed. W. B. Saunders Company, Philadelphia, 1983.
4. Scott, D. W.: Thyroid function in feline endocrine alopecia. J.A.A.H.A. *11*:798, 1975.
5. Scott, D. W.: Feline Dermatology 1900–1978; a monograph. J.A.A.H.A. *16*:331, 1980.
6. Thoday, K. L.: Differential diagnosis of symmetrical alopecia in the cat. *In* Kirk, R. W. (ed.): Current Veterinary Therapy IX. W. B. Saunders Company, Philadelphia, 1986.

13

Pigmentary Abnormalities

The Normal Process of Skin Pigmentation

The color of normal skin depends primarily on the amount of melanin, carotene, and oxyhemoglobin or reduced hemoglobin that it contains. Skin pigmentation, which depends largely on the melanin content of the keratinocytes, is not visible unless melanosomes have entered the keratinocytes. Pigmentation occurs according to the following sequence:

1. Formation of melanosomes in the melanocyte
2. Melanization of the melanosomes in the melanocyte
3. Secretion of the melanosomes into the keratinocytes
4. Transport of the melanosomes by the keratinocytes, with degradation of the melanosomes in white skin or without degradation in dark skin

The basic unit of the melanin pigment system is the melanocyte. This cell contains specialized pigment organelles called melanosomes, which constitute the site of melanin synthesis and are rich in the enzyme tyrosinase. When fully melanized, melanosomes lose their tyrosinase activity and become melanin granules. Melanin is a polymer of 5,6-indole quinone, and the initial step in its formation is the oxidation of tyrosine to 3,4-dihydroxyphenylalanine (dopa) in the presence of tyrosinase.

All normal skin, within a particular species or subspecies, has the same proportion of melanocytes. Differences in skin color are attributable to genetically determined or acquired differences in the production of melanosomes within the melanocytes and to the rate at which the melanin granules are transferred to the keratinocytes.

Melanin-stimulating hormone (MSH or melanotropin) increases melanin pigmentation, presumably by means of an effect on cyclic adenosine monophosphate (cAMP) in the melanocyte and the consequent activation of the enzyme tyrosinase. Therefore, a blockade against MSH could cause a lightening of pigmented skin. Many hormonal and inflammatory influences tend to produce secondary changes in pigmentation.

Disorders of melanin pigmentation are very common in many canine and feline dermatoses.[5, 6] Their etiologic diagnosis often requires a very methodical clinicopathologic approach. A careful history and a physical examination permit the clinician to establish an inclusive differential diagnosis, which determines the laboratory tests used.

Hyperpigmentation

(Hypermelanosis, Melanoderma)

Hyperpigmentation means that the pigmentation (usually melanin) is greater than normal for the area of skin in question. This is a result of the increased amount of melanin in either the dermis or epidermis, or both. Excess melanin in the superficial dermis can be caused by inflammation, trauma, or endocrine changes. Excess pigment in the hair is called melanotrichia.

Hyperpigmentation in animals may be genetic or acquired and may result from endocrine abnormalities, reactions to chronic inflammations or irritations, or pigmented neoplasms. Examples of such hyperpigmentation are seen in pigmented healing lesions of generalized demodicosis, chronic canine scabies, the center of healing circular dermatophytoses and staphylococcal folliculitides, acanthosis nigricans, male feminizing syndrome, ovarian dysfunction, hypothyroidism, and Sertoli cell tumors. These disorders are discussed in other chapters.

CANINE LENTIGO

Lentigo (pl., lentigines) in dogs is a common macular melanosis that is benign and intensely black, and that usually occurs as multiple lesions. Lentigines appear in mature dogs, often increasing in number and size over a period of several months, subsequently becoming static and remaining unchanged for the life of the dog. These sharply circumscribed macules do not itch and are of no consequence to the patient. The lesions are usually not raised and resemble "tar spots" *in* the skin (Fig. 13:1). The lesions are sometimes grouped in clusters or may be spread rather diffusely over the ventral surface of the body. Occasionally the lesions have a hyperkeratotic surface.

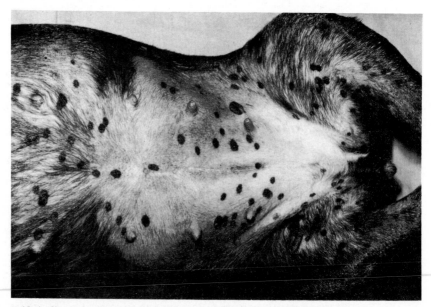

Figure 13:1. Close-up view of 7-year-old French bulldog with multiple lentigines. Note the intensity of the pigmentation and the sharply demarcated borders.

A hereditary form of lentigo called "lentiginosis profusa" has been reported in pugs.[1] The mating of two unrelated dogs that were affected with the disorder produced one with the same condition. This was thought to be an autosomal dominant mode of inheritance as is found in humans.[1]

Histologically, early lentigines are characterized by a sharply localized increase in melanocytes and basal cell melanin.[17] Usually, no structural change occurs in the epidermis. As the lesion develops, the epidermis may thicken, hyperkeratosis may occur, and a slight rete ridge may form. The epidermal pigmentation is greatly increased, as almost every keratinocyte is stuffed with melanin granules.

The significance of lentigo mainly concerns the differential diagnosis of pigmented tumors (melanomas). In humans lentigines may become malignant, but to our knowledge no malignancy in dogs has been reported.

Clinical management of these lesions entails early recognition and biopsy to establish a definitive diagnosis. Lentigo does not respond to treatment (except excision) and none is necessary. Lesions should be observed carefully for possible indications of malignant change.

LENTIGO SIMPLEX IN ORANGE CATS

Lentigo simplex in orange cats is analogous to human lentigo simplex.[3, 7, 14] The condition in cats is characterized by asymptomatic macular melanosis, usually beginning in those less than 1 year of age, and typically affecting the lips, gums, eyelids, and nose. Affected cats are at no risk of developing melanoma.

The lesions start on the lips and begin as tiny, black, asymptomatic spots that gradually enlarge and become more numerous with time.[14] In addition to

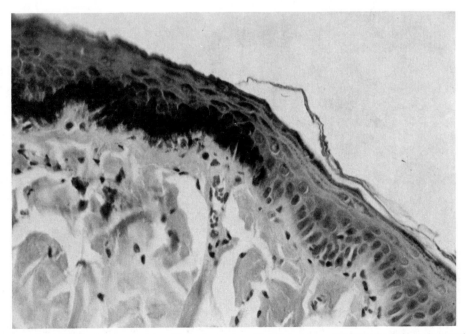

Figure 13:2. Feline lentigo simplex. Note abrupt transition between melanotic area (left) and normal epithelium (right).

the lip there can be lesions on the nose, gingiva, and eyelids. Well circumscribed, generally circular areas of intense, uniform macular melanosis, ranging from one to nine mm in diameter, occasionally coalescent, are present in variable numbers (Figs. 13:3A,B). Surrounding tissue is normal. The lesions are not pruritic, painful, crusted, or eroded, nor does any dermatosis, injury, drug administration, or illness precede the development of the lesions. The lesions do not vary in intensity of hyperpigmentation with time of year.

Histopathologic findings included marked hypermelanosis of predominantly the basal cell layer of the epithelium, owing to increased numbers of melanocytes and hypermelanosis of neighboring basal keratinocytes (Figs. 13:2 and 13:4). Occasionally melanophages have been seen in the superficial dermis.

There is no known treatment to remove these pigmented spots. Nor is one necessary since the condition causes no pain or discomfort. It is only a noticeable cosmetic defect. Whether or not lentigo simplex occurs in all orange cats or in other cats and how often, is not known. With increased awareness of this condition, larger and more complete studies may provide this information.

ACROMELANISM

Siamese, Himalayan, Balinese, and Burmese kittens are born white and develop "points" as adults, owing to the influence of external temperature.[11, 13] In addition to being influenced by external temperature (high temperatures producing light hairs, low temperatures producing dark hairs), coat color also appears to be affected by physiologic factors determining heat production and loss (inflammation, alopecia). These phenomena appear to be associated with a temperature-dependent enzyme involved in melanin synthesis. These changes in coat color are usually temporary, and the normal color returns with the next hair cycle, if the temperature influences are remedied.

Hypopigmentation

(Hypomelanosis, Leukoderma)

Hypopigmentation refers to a lack of pigment in the skin or hair coat in areas that normally should be pigmented. The disorder may be congenital or acquired. Lack of melanin pigment in hair is called leukotrichia.

CONGENITAL HYPOPIGMENTATION

Albinism is a hereditary lack of pigmentation that is transmitted as a recessive trait.[3a, 5] Albino individuals have a normal complement of melanocytes, but they lack tyrosinase for melanin synthesis and therefore have a biochemical inability to produce melanin. Albino animals have unpigmented (pink) irides, as well as skin, and are extremely rare. They should not be used as breeders.

Nasal solar dermatitis is a condition that almost always starts from a small patch of depigmented skin on the planum nasale or on the area slightly posterior to it. Unless the skin is exposed to excess sunlight, it is possible that no disease process will occur.

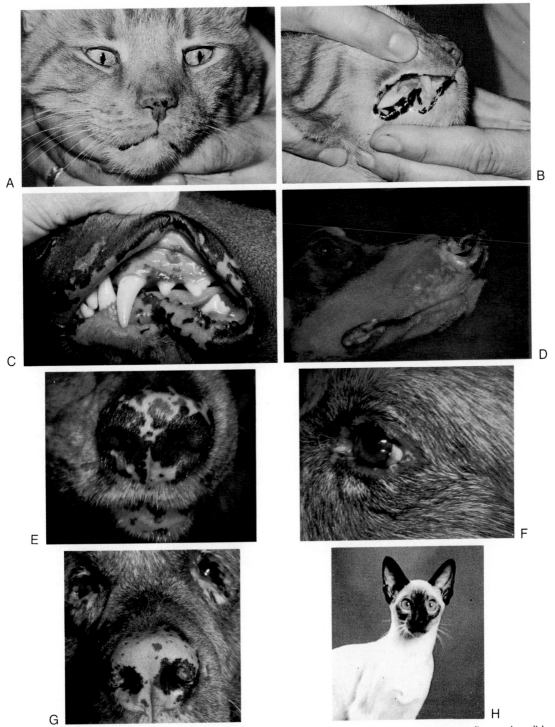

Figure 13:3. Pigment abnormalities. *A,* Lentigo simplex in an orange cat. Melanotic macules on nose, lips, and eyelids. *B,* Same cat as in *A.* Marked macular melanosis of lips. *C,* Patchy, hypopigmentation present from birth on the lips of a mature Doberman pinscher. *D,* Face and nose of Doberman with progressive hypopigmentation. The dog was normal at birth, but hypopigmentation started on the sides of the nostrils and slowly spread to the lips. Treatment was not effective. *E,* Two-year-old Newfoundland that had a normal black color at birth but gradually developed patchy hypopigmentation evident in skin and hairs. *F,* Face and eye of dog illustrated in *C. G,* Front view of dog in *C,* showing progressive nature of the hypopigmentation. *H,* Periocular leukotrichia ("goggles") in a Siamese cat postestrus.

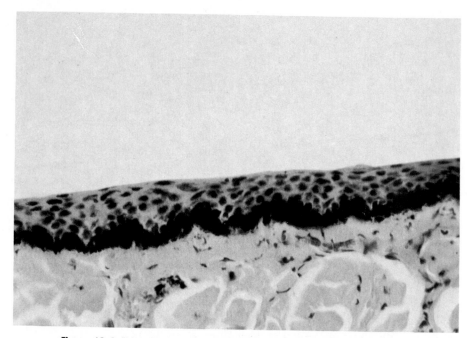

Figure 13:4. Feline lentigo simplex. Marked melanosis of basilar epithelium.

Nasal solar dermatitis must be differentiated from several other diseases in which nasal depigmentation is one of the secondary manifestations. Dorsal nasal lesions occur with discoid lupus erythematosus, systemic lupus erythematosus, pemphigus, Vogt-Koyanagi-Harada syndrome, and bullous pemphigoid. Cases of nasal solar dermatitis and mild, early cases of the above autoimmune diseases are sometimes difficult to differentiate clinically. Histopathology and immunofluorescent testing usually establish the correct diagnosis.

Hypopigmentation of the lips and nose occurs as a congenital condition in Doberman pinschers and other breeds (Figs. 13:3C,D).[4] The cause is unknown, and, in fact, it is not a pathologic process. Although many owners object to the cosmetic appearance, it is best not to attempt treatment, which is ineffective.

Canine Cyclic Hematopoiesis (Gray Collie Syndrome, Canine Cyclic Neutropenia). This is a lethal autosomal recessive syndrome wherein collie puppies are born with a silver-gray hair coat that differs from the normal sable or tricolor coat.[5, 8, 16] In some of these puppies a slight yellow pigmentation may be present, which produces a mixture of light beige and light gray hair. The light-colored nose is a characteristic and diagnostic lesion.

In addition to the hair color change, gray collie puppies are usually smaller and weaker than their littermates, a difference observable by 1 week of age. By 8 to 12 weeks of age, signs of clinical illness appear, including fever, diarrhea, lymphadenopathy, infections, conjunctivitis, and arthralgia. The term *cyclic neutropenia* reflects the appearance of neutropenia alternating with rebounding neutrophilia. This cycle continues at 10- to 12-day intervals until death. Other hematologic abnormalities include nonregenerative anemia as well as cyclical reticulocytosis, monocytosis, and thrombocytosis.[16] Other clinicopathologic abnormalities include hyperglobulinemia, depressed mitogenic responses of lymphocytes, and cyclic hormonogenesis (cortisol, adrenocorticotropic hormone [ACTH], thyroxine [T_4], and triiodothyronine [T_3]).[8, 16]

There is no effective treatment, and parents and littermates should not be used for breeding. Lithium carbonate (20 to 25 mg/kg/day) stabilizes the level of neutrophils, but it is toxic. Affected animals usually die before 6 months of age without supportive care. Even with optimal care, most die before 2 years of age owing to hepatic and/or renal failure associated with amyloidosis. Bone marrow transplantation is effective but impractical. In differential diagnosis, this syndrome must not be mistaken for the dominant or Maltese gray collie and a transient dilution called powder puff.

Chédiak-Higashi Syndrome. An autosomal recessive disorder, this syndrome is reported in Persian cats with yellow eyes and "blue smoke" hair color.[7] It is characterized by a partial oculocutaneous albinism, a bleeding disorder, an increased susceptibility to infection, photophobia, and enlarged granules in many cell types, including melanocytes and leukocytes. Examination of unstained hairs from affected cats reveals large, elongated, irregular clumps of melanin. Histopathologic findings in affected skin include melanin granules that are much larger than normal, but they are markedly decreased in number when compared with normal cat skin. There is no effective treatment, and affected cats should not be used for breeding (see also p. 677).

Tyrosinase Deficiency in the Chow Chow. Puppies with this condition exhibit a dramatic color change. The normally bluish black tongue turns pink, and portions of the hair shafts turn white. The buccal mucosa also may become rapidly depigmented.

The change in color is the result of a deficiency of tyrosinase, the enzyme necessary in the chemical reactions that produce melanin. This can be confirmed by skin biopsy. After tyrosine is added, the specimen is incubated, and the melanin is measured after tissue staining.[2]

There is no effective treatment. However, melanin reappears spontaneously in 2 to 4 months. Chow chow breeders have claimed success with the use of vitamins, unsaturated oils, and dietary changes, but probably the improvement was spontaneous.

Color Mutant Alopecia. This is a hereditary hypotrichosis associated with coat color dilution (see p. 677).

ACQUIRED HYPOPIGMENTATION

Loss of skin pigment is called *leukoderma*, and loss of hair pigment is called *leukotrichia*. Each can be present alone or in combination with the other. *Vitiligo* is a specific, often idiopathic leukoderma of human beings, which may have a hereditary, autoimmune, or neurogenic pathogenesis. A presumptive hereditary vitiligo has been described in Belgian Tervurens, German shepherds, and Siamese cats.[7, 9, 10] In the United States, Rottweilers and Doberman pinschers ("Dudley nose") are commonly affected.[13] The animals develop more-or-less symmetric macular depigmentation, especially of the nose, lips, buccal mucosa, and the facial skin. The footpads and nails, as well as the hair coat, may be affected. The onset usually occurs in young adulthood. In some cases, pigment returns to affected areas, whereas in others, the depigmentation is permanent. Recently vitiligo was reported in two Old English sheepdog littermates and in a dachshund with juvenile-onset diabetes mellitus.[14a] Histologically, the condition is characterized by an absence of epidermal melanocytes and melanin (Figs. 13:5 and 13:6). Recently antimelanocyte antibodies were demonstrated in the serum of all 17 Belgian Tervuren dogs with vitiligo, and in none of 11 normal Belgian Tervuren dogs tested.[9a] There is no effective therapy.

Acquired depigmentation of previously normal skin and hair can result from many factors that destroy or depress melanocytes. Consequently, trauma, burns, infections, and ionizing irradiation may have potent local effects. These are often most dramatic when they affect the hair color. We have seen a red Irish setter puppy that had severe pustular dermatitis and developed white bands around the hair shafts—presumably, as a result of effects on pigment production in the hair bulb during the infection. Deficiencies of nutrients such as zinc, pyridoxine, pantothenic acid, and lysine have produced graying of the hair. Copper deficiency is said to cause black hair to develop a reddish brown hue.

Normal black Newfoundlands, at 18 months of age, may develop patches of depigmentation on the nose, lips, and eyelids (Figs. 13:3 *E* to *G*). The lesions steadily progress and also affect the hair follicles in a diffuse manner. The animals become "gray roans." Supplementation with trace minerals, vitamins, and zinc produces no improvement.

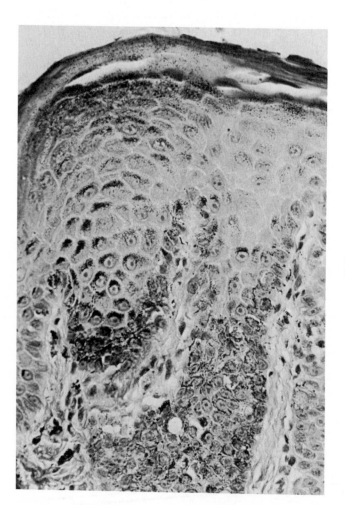

Figure 13:5. Canine vitiligo. Normal skin adjacent to vitiliginous macule.

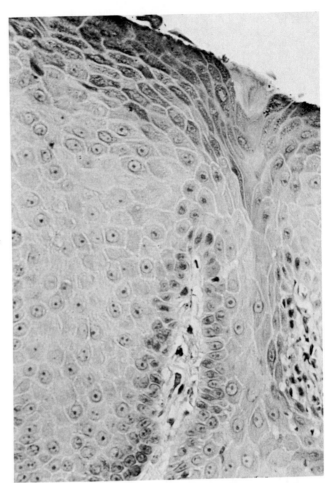

Figure 13:6. Canine vitiligo. Complete absence of melanin in vitiliginous area.

Acquired depigmentation of the nose and lips can result from contact dermatitis from plastic or rubber food dishes (see p. 464). It may also be idiopathic (Fig. 13:3D).

Nasal depigmentation is a syndrome of unknown etiology. It has been reported in Afghan hounds, Samoyeds, Siberian huskies, white German shepherds, golden retrievers, poodles, Doberman pinschers, Irish setters, and pointers.[4] The dogs are normal at birth, but gradually the black of the planum nasale fades into a chocolate brown or whitish color. The cause is unknown and to date no treatment has worked effectively. A few patients recover spontaneously, and in others the degree of pigmentation waxes and wanes, sometimes seasonally. Since this discoloration is a show ring fault, breeders of show animals are understandably concerned.

PERIOCULAR LEUKOTRICHIA

Bilateral periocular leukotrichia ("goggles") was described in Siamese cats.[13] There is no apparent age predilection, but the condition is seen more commonly in females. Commonly recognized precipitating factors include pregnancy, dietary deficiency, and systemic illnesses. The condition is characterized by patchy or complete lightening of the hairs of the mask in a halo-like appearance around both eyes (Fig. 13:3H). The condition is transient and usually resolves within the next two hair cycles.

A syndrome of unilateral periocular depigmentation (Aguirre syndrome) has been described in Siamese cats associated with Horner's syndrome, or corneal necrosis with uveitis and upper respiratory tract infections.[5, 15]

References

1. Briggs, O. M.: Lentiginosis profusa in the pug: three case reports. J. Small Anim. Pract. 26:675, 1985.
2. Engstrom, D.: Tyrosinase deficiency in the chow chow. In Kirk, R. W., (ed.): Current Veterinary Therapy II. W. B. Saunders Company, Philadelphia, 1966.
3. Fitzpatrick, T. B., et al.: Dermatology In General Medicine, 3rd ed. McGraw-Hill Book Company, New York, 1987.
3a. Foil, C. S.: Comparative genodermatoses. Clin. Dermatol. 3:175, 1985.
4. Griffin, C. E.: Nasal dermatitis. Dermatol. Rep. 2:1, 1983.
5. Guaguere, E., et al.: Troubles de la pigmentation melanique en dermatologie des carnivores: 2. hypomelanoses et amelanoses. Point Vet. 18:5, 1986.
6. Guaguere, E., et al.: Troubles de la pigmentation melanique en dermatologie des carnivores: 3. hypermelanoses. Point Vet. 18:699, 1986–1987.
7. Holzworth, J.: Diseases of the Cat. Medicine & Surgery, Vol. I. W. B. Saunders Company, Philadelphia, 1987.
8. Lothrop, C. D., et al.: Cyclic hormonogenesis in gray collie dogs: interactions of hematopoietic and endocrine systems. Endocrinology 120:1027, 1987.
9. Mahaffey, M. B., Yarbrough, K. M., et al.: Focal loss of pigment in the Belgian Tervuren dog. J.A.V.M.A. 173:390, 1978.

9a. Naughton, G. K., et al: Antibodies to surface antigens of pigmented cells in animals with vitiligo. Proc. Soc. Exp. Biol. Med. 181:423, 1986.
10. Nordlund, J. J.: Vitiligo. In: Thiers, B. H., Dobson, R. L., (eds.): Pathogenesis of Skin Disease. Churchill Livingstone, New York, 1986, p. 99.
11. Scott, D. W.: Feline dermatology 1900–1978: a monograph. J.A.A.H.A. 16:331, 1980.
12. Scott, D. W.: Unpublished observations, 1987.
13. Scott, D. W.: Feline dermatology 1983–1985: the secret sits. J.A.A.H.A. 23:255, 1987.
14. Scott, D. W.: Lentigo simplex in orange cats. Companion Anim. Pract. 1:23, 1987.
14a. Scott, D. W., and Randolph, J. F.: Vitiligo in two old English Sheepdog littermates and a dachshund with juvenile-onset diabetes mellitus. Companion Anim. Pract. (in press).
15. Simon, M.: Observation clinique. Depigmentation perioculaire chez deux chats siamois. Prat. Med. Chirurg. Anim. Comp. 20:49, 1985.
16. Trail, P. A., and Yang, T. J.: Canine cyclic hematopoiesis: alterations in T lymphocyte populations in peripheral blood, lymph nodes, and thymus of gray collie dogs. Clin. Immunol. Immunopathol. 41:216, 1986.
17. VanRensburg, I. B. J., Briggs, O. M.: Pathology of canine lentiginosis profusa. J. So. Afr. Vet. Assoc. 57:159, 1986.

14

Keratinization Defects

Keratinization defects are among the most visible and annoying skin diseases because they involve the outermost layer of the skin, the epidermis. Seborrhea, nasodigital hyperkeratosis, and callus formation are examples of such defects. Seborrhea is included in this chapter because it refers to excess scales that are shed from the horny layer of the skin (the stratum corneum); this process is usually secondary to some underlying cause. Although seborrhea in dogs is a scaly condition, human seborrhea is more oily or greasy. Therefore, the word seborrhea, which literally means "flow of sebum," is more accurately applied to humans than to dogs.

The keratinization defects consist of hyperkeratosis, hypokeratosis, and dyskeratosis. Hyperkeratosis is common in chronic dermatoses. It is further divided histopathologically into parakeratotic (nucleated) and orthokeratotic (anuclear) types. Hypokeratosis is not as common, but it is seen histologically in some seborrheas, presumably as a result of very rapid exfoliation. Another fault in epidermopoiesis is dyskeratosis, which is seen in neoplastic skin diseases (such as squamous cell carcinoma), pemphigus, lichenoid reactions, and some types of seborrhea.

Ichthyosis is also included in this chapter. Although it is usually congenital, it is clearly a keratinization defect with its laminated orthokeratotic hyperkeratosis.

Nasodigital Hyperkeratosis

Nasodigital hyperkeratosis is characterized by increased amounts of horny tissue originating from and tightly adherent to the epidermis of the footpads or planum nasale.

CAUSE AND PATHOGENESIS

Nasal hyperkeratosis occurring without digital changes is a specific entity. Figure 14:1*A* shows such a case: A standard poodle suddenly developed nasal hyperkeratosis at the age of 5 years, and his nose remained dry and horny until the end of his life at 15 years. The numerous topical medications that were applied did not alter the hyperkeratosis. Fissures that developed in the dry nose were treated, and they responded favorably to the application of corticosteroid-antibiotic ointment.

Cases of nasal hyperkeratosis may occur in the absence of diseases such as distemper, pemphigus foliaceus, or discoid lupus erythematosus. The cause

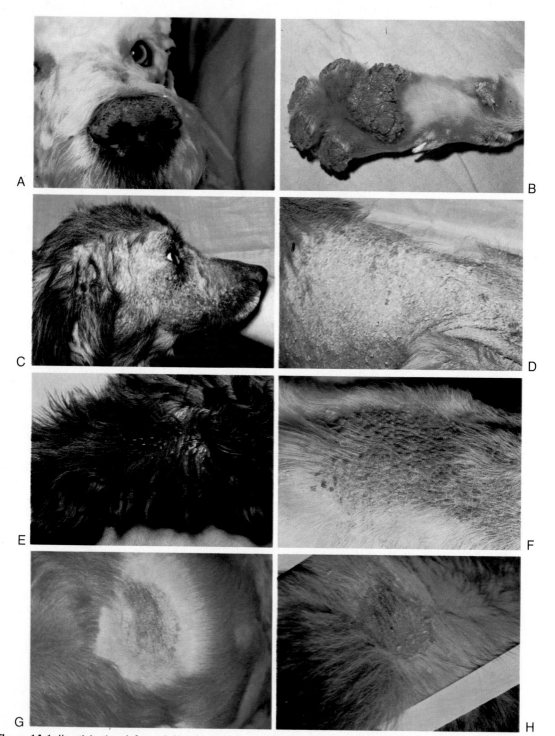

Figure 14:1. Keratinization defects. *A,* Nasal hyperkeratosis. Horny growths of keratin adhere tightly to the epidermis of the dry planum nasale. *B,* Hyperkeratotic laminations on the digital pads of a German shepherd. This is suggestive of pemphigus foliaceus. *C,* Head of a dog with seborrheic dermatitis of the face. Notice the severe "dandruff" among the hairs. *D,* Generalized seborrhea in a dog, showing extreme scaling, flaking, and alopecia. *E,* Seborrhea oleosa on the back of a cocker spaniel. Note that clusters of fatty particles adhere to the hairs and resemble louse nits. *F,* Seborrhea. Skin from the leg of a blond cocker spaniel showing tightly adhering, greasy particles on a patch of alopecia. *G,* Alopecia patch with seborrhea from a brown cocker spaniel. Notice the pigmented center and the halo of erythema. Lesion was clipped. *H,* Localized seborrheic patch showing scaly alopecia on an erythematous base. Hair is not clipped but flattened on each side to expose the lesion better.

716

is unknown. Idiopathic nasal hyperkeratosis tends to occur in older dogs and tends to be an abnormality more focal than that seen on the nose secondary to such disorders as canine distemper and immunologic disorders.

Digital hyperkeratosis occurs spontaneously in some adult dogs. The cause is unknown when it is not associated with "hard pad" distemper, pemphigus foliaceus, discoid or systemic lupus erythematosus, zinc-responsive dermatosis, ichthyosis, or the hepatocutaneous syndrome. Severe digital hyperkeratosis also occurs as a hereditary disorder of Irish terriers (see p. 694). Idiopathic digital hyperkeratosis tends to occur in older dogs and tends to be a more focal abnormality, affecting only the periphery (junction of pad with haired skin) of the pads. A similar change is seen at the periphery of pads in dogs that have chronic pododermatitis of numerous causes.

Hyperkeratosis of the footpads and nasal tip does occur in some cases of distemper. In fact, some clinicians feel that "hard pad disease" is a rare special form of distemper, characterized by hyperkeratotic changes.

CLINICAL FEATURES

The hyperplastic keratin that develops in this disease grows in a variety of shapes, depending on its location, its stage of development, and the variation among individual animals. At times, small verrucous keratin growths appear in a regular pattern. At other times, the keratin is ridged, grooved, or feathered. Dryness is the common characteristic of all lesions. The planum nasale, which is moist, black, soft, and shiny in normal dogs, becomes hard, dry, and rough. Fissures, erosions, and ulcers develop in the dry epidermal tissue.

The hard, cracked pads of large breeds of dogs contain excess keratin tissue, which makes walking painful for heavy dogs. Fissures and erosions add significantly to the discomfort. "Corns" form in the feet of some individuals, as excess keratin develops into deep, circular plaques. These press into the surrounding footpad and cause pain when pressure is applied as the animal walks. The condition appears to be hereditary, as several related Kerry blue terriers were affected.

DIAGNOSIS

A *definitive diagnosis* of simple nasal or digital hyperkeratosis is easily made, provided it is not secondary to other keratinizing diseases. The *differential diagnosis* includes "hard pad distemper," ichthyosis, pemphigus foliaceus and erythematosus, discoid and systemic lupus erythematosus, zinc-responsive dermatosis, and the hepatocutaneous syndrome (diabetic dermatosis).

It is necessary to distinguish between the nasodigital hyperkeratosis that accompanies certain cases of distemper (or a distemper-like disease) and those cases pictured here that arise spontaneously and of unknown cause. When distemper patients recover, those with "hard pad" changes often lose their cutaneous lesions after several months, whereas the spontaneous hyperkeratoses are chronic and often present for life.

Simple nasodigital hyperkeratosis must be differentiated from canine ichthyosis, which is congenital and involves large areas of the dog's skin.

Pemphigus foliaceus may show digital hyperkeratosis (see p. 502). Some cases of pemphigus foliaceus involve only the pads and are characterized by extreme, chronic thickening of the pads with "feathering" of keratin deposits

(Fig. 14:1*B*). A biopsy of the affected digital area may show the characteristic histopathologic features and positive results of direct immunofluorescence test for pemphigus foliaceus. This cause of digital hyperkeratosis is more common than was formerly suspected.

Discoid lupus erythematosus (DLE) usually has no digital involvement, but nasal changes must be differentiated from simple nasal hyperkeratosis. In DLE the primary clinical lesion shows erythema, erosions, and ulceration of the planum nasale and all or part of the dorsal nasal surface. Such inflammatory and ulcerative changes are not found in nasal hyperkeratosis. In DLE, histologic examination and direct immunofluorescence testing of skin of the lesion will establish the diagnosis.

Systemic lupus erythematosus may produce hyperkeratosis of the nose and/or footpads. However, other systemic disorders are usually present (see p. 519). Diagnosis is based on the antinuclear antibody (ANA) test, biopsy (interface dermatitis, hydropic and/or lichenoid), direct immunofluorescence testing, and fulfilling the American Rheumatism Association criteria.

Zinc-responsive dermatoses may be associated with nasodigital hyperkeratosis (see p. 801). Onset at less than 1 year of age, breed predilection for Siberian huskies and Alaskan malamutes, crusting of other cutaneous sites, and skin biopsy (marked, diffuse parakeratosis) help to establish the diagnosis.

The hepatocutaneous syndrome is characterized by severe hyperkeratosis of the footpads and mucocutaneous crusting and ulceration (see p. 639). Skin biopsy is diagnostic.

Histopathologic findings in idiopathic nasodigital hyperkeratosis include irregular-to-papillated epidermal hyperplasia and marked orthokeratotic-to-parakeratotic hyperkeratosis.

CLINICAL MANAGEMENT

Since the formation of excess keratin cannot usually be stopped, treatment is directed toward relieving discomfort. Excess keratin can be trimmed away with scissors when it overlaps the margins of the digital pads, and corns can be carefully pared or shaved. Care must be taken to cut only into keratin and not into the deeper, living tissue. Wet dressings or water soaks are useful to hydrate the keratin (which easily absorbs water). Petroleum jelly, applied immediately after the wet dressings or soaks, helps to hold moisture in the pad or nasal tissues. For erosions, fissures, and ulcers, ointments containing antibiotics and corticosteroids are helpful. The hyperkeratotic feet can be bandaged for short periods of time (2 to 5 days) to protect them and to allow healing of the erosions and fissures. Nitrofurazone (Furacin) or chlorhexidine (Nolvasan) dressing under the bandage combats or prevents secondary bacterial infection. Ichthammol (fortified—Maurry Biologics) ointment used once a day for 2 weeks exerts a beneficial keratolytic and healing effect on digital hyperkeratinized pads. Kerasolv Gel (DVM Corp.) can be used twice a day on the affected areas.

Canine Seborrhea

Seborrhea is a chronic skin disease of dogs that is characterized by a defect in keratinization with increased scale formation, occasionally by excessive greasiness of the skin and hair coat, and sometimes by secondary inflammation.

Clinically, the disorder is divided into the following categories:

1. *Seborrhea sicca* is characterized by dry skin with focal or diffuse scaling and accumulations of white to gray nonadherent scales. The coat is dry and dull, and Irish setters, German shepherds, dachshunds, and Doberman pinschers are typically affected.

2. *Seborrhea oleosa* is characterized by focal or diffuse scaling associated with excessive lipid production that produces brownish yellow clumped material that adheres to the skin and hair. "Nitlike" flakes are present on the hairs, and the coat is odoriferous and greasy to the touch. Cocker spaniels, springer spaniels, and Chinese Shar Pei are typically affected.

3. *Seborrheic dermatitis* is characterized by scaling and greasiness with gross evidence of local or diffuse inflammation. It is often associated with folliculitis. Classic *localized* seborrheic dermatitis has circular bull's-eye lesions with alopecia, erythema, marginal epidermal scaling with central clearing, and, later, hyperpigmentation. This must be differentiated from other disorders causing target lesions. There may be breed predilection for cocker and springer spaniels, West Highland white terriers, and Basset hounds.

It should be noted that this morphologic classification is not three distinct diseases but is a complex in which each type may have certain characteristics of the others.

An etiologic classification of seborrhea into primary and secondary types is useful in considering therapy, and thus it is most important to distinguish between the two types. Primary seborrhea is idiopathic. Primary idiopathic seborrhea in cocker and springer spaniels, West Highland white terriers, and basset hounds often occurs in young animals and may have a genetic component. Seborrhea is called "secondary" if the signs occur in association with a number of unrelated disease processes (Table 14:1).[9–12]

Reserve the term seborrhea for primary idiopathic seborrhea; secondary seborrhea accompanies other skin diseases.

Table 14:1. CLASSIFICATION OF SEBORRHEA*

Primary Seborrhea
  Idiopathic seborrhea

Secondary Seborrhea
  Metabolic seborrhea
    Endocrine-related
      Hypothyroidism, hyperadrenocorticism, gonadal aberrations, hyposomatotropism, diabetes
        mellitus
    Nutrition-related (especially fat)
      Dietary deficiency (fat, protein, vitamin A, zinc), malabsorption/maldigestion (intestinal,
        hepatic, pancreatic), defects in fat metabolism ("fat responsive")
  Ectoparasites (cheyletiellosis, pediculosis, demodicosis, scabies)
  Endoparasites (intestinal, dirofilariasis)
  Pyoderma and bacterial hypersensitivity
  Dermatophytosis
  Hypersensitivity and drug eruption
  Local trauma or irritants
  Autoimmune disease
  Subcorneal pustular dermatosis
  Neoplasia
  Any chronic catabolic state
  Environmental (dry heat)

---

*Modified from Ihrke, P. J.: Canine seborrheic disease complex. Vet. Clin. North Am. *9*:93, 1979.

CAUSE AND PATHOGENESIS

The *epidermal turnover* has been shown to be more rapid in seborrheic dogs than in normal dogs. By using radioactive thymidine to label epidermal cells, it has been found that the epidermal turnover of seborrheic dogs is 3 to 4 days, while in normal dogs it is 3 weeks.[1a]

Research on human epidermal keratinocytes from psoriatic skin revealed that the growth fraction of the cells is more significant than the epidermal turnover time.[7] This growth fraction may also be a factor in primary canine seborrhea.

Cutaneous bacteria on normal skin are low in number and consist mainly of aerobic micrococci (see p. 247). Seborrheic skin has tremendous numbers of bacteria, predominantly *Staphylococcus* spp., coagulase positive. These large numbers in addition to the associated pruritus and self-trauma may account for the high incidence of secondary pyoderma.

Surface lipids provide a normal protective film composed of sterol, wax esters, and free cholesterol and triglycerides with very few fatty acids (see p. 17). In both dry and oily seborrhea the surface film contains a smaller percentage of diester waxes but a large increase in free fatty acids.[9, 10] It has also been shown that cutaneous bacteria counts increased with both larger amounts and smaller amounts of surface lipid on seborrheic skin, as compared with such bacteria counts on normal skin.[9, 10] Reedy compared lipid films from normal and from seborrheic cocker spaniels (in quantitative titers) as to their ability to inhibit the growth of standard cultures of coagulase-positive staphylococci and found no difference between them.[20] Thus, canine surface lipids from seborrheic dogs do not appear to enhance bacterial growth.

Endocrine factors have a profound effect on sebum production and general skin health (see Chapter 10). Sebum production tends to be increased by thyroxine and androgens and tends to be decreased by estrogens and corticosteroids. However, although changes in the delicate balance of production and utilization of these hormones may contribute to seborrhea, the other clinical signs of gross hormonal abnormality are not always evident. In addition, replacement therapy with medication or reduction of hormones by castration, spaying, or withdrawing medication cannot be counted on to produce dramatic dermatologic effects. Individual cases may respond satisfactorily, but each case must be considered on its own merits, and these principles should be used only as guidelines. Hypothyroidism is undoubtedly the most common endocrine cause of seborrhea, but the patients sometimes do not show other typical clinical signs of an endocrine disorder. Careful laboratory work-ups are necessary for diagnosis. Gonadal abnormalities may cause cyclical seborrhea in intact bitches—especially those with estrus cycle abnormalities. Seborrheic male dogs that are especially aggressive or show signs of virilism should be suspected of having endocrine-caused seborrhea. Unfortunately, there are few laboratory tests or endocrine assays that help define the diagnosis in such cases.

Dietary factors may influence the onset of seborrhea. While deficiencies of protein, zinc, and vitamin A should be considered, dietary fat deficiency is the only common nutrition-related cause of seborrhea. Strangely, this may appear clinically as either a dry or a greasy skin and coat. These problems may develop as a result of a low fat intake, malabsorption or maldigestion, or a defect in fat metabolism. Dogs with diabetes mellitus may develop a dry secondary seborrhea. The specific mechanism is unclear.

CLINICAL FEATURES

Primary seborrhea is typified by oiliness and scaliness that are often accumulated in patches that adhere to the skin or clusters of fatty particles that attach to the hair (Fig. 14:1C,D,F). The latter resemble louse nits (Fig. 14:1E). The yellow-brown masses on the skin have a typical rancid and unpleasant odor. Lesions may be especially severe on ears, elbows, and hocks. Pruritus is variable in primary seborrhea; if it is present, the clinician should first suspect secondary seborrhea, perhaps resulting from an ectoparasite, a hypersensitivity skin disease, or primary seborrhea complicated by a bacterial infection. A local seborrheic lesion characteristically appears as an alopecic, scaly macule or patch, with a pigmented center surrounded by an erythematous halo and a flaking keratin rim (Fig. 14:1G,H). These lesions are especially typical on the trunk and chest (Fig. 14:2), and they mimic dermatophytosis. They also vaguely resemble human psoriasis lesions.

Secondary seborrhea is typically dry and scaly, yet in some cases an oily film will remain on one's hand after handling the coat. The dry scales may be localized or generalized. When localized, they may be associated with crusts or may appear quite thick (scabies, demodicosis, dermatophytosis, zinc deficiency, pemphigus foliaceus, and so on).

Seborrheic Breeds. Certain breeds have interesting and almost specific breed syndromes of seborrhea.[10, 12]

Primary, idiopathic seborrhea is a most stubborn, commonly familial disease found in cocker and springer spaniels and sometimes in West Highland white terriers and basset hounds. It is typified by tightly adherent, scaly patches on the back and chest. The entire hair coat is scaly and greasy.

Doberman pinschers are even more prone to a dry seborrhea and folliculitis than are other short-coated breeds. In black and tan Dobermans the white scales have high visibility—much to the owner's distress. Mild scratching or combing will immediately accentuate the flaking. Red, fawn, and blue Dobermans often have color mutant alopecia with seborrhea as a complication. They have diffuse alopecia, papules, and scales. This syndrome does not respond to treatment, and a lifelong problem can be expected (see p. 677).

Irish setters commonly have dry seborrhea as a complication of hypersensitivity skin disease. Although atopy and flea bite hypersensitivity may be

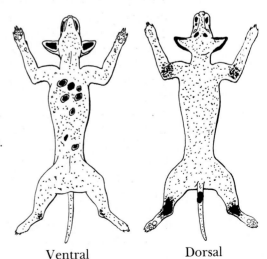

Figure 14:2. Seborrhea distribution pattern.

Ventral   Dorsal

common causes, folliculitis, hypothyroidism, and color mutant alopecia (in fawn Irish setters) may also be underlying factors in the disease.

The Chinese Shar Pei has a very high incidence of oily seborrhea that is made more troublesome by the accumulation of sebum and apocrine sweat in the ample body skin folds. The intertriginous irritation produces fold dermatitis with unpleasant odors.

Certain black Labrador retrievers have a severe idiopathic dermatitis ("waterline disease") that defies specific diagnosis and treatment (see pg. 842). These individuals have a chronic secondary seborrhea.

Dachshunds and other breeds with pendulous ears may develop seborrhea of the ear margins. It may appear as a local disorder or as part of a generalized seborrhea (see p. 737).

DIAGNOSIS

Diagnosis is suggested by the history, a careful physical examination, and a systematic elimination of possible secondary causes. The diagnosis of idiopathic primary seborrhea is usually made by exclusion of other possible diagnoses. Laboratory and clinical tests to consider include skin scraping, fecal flotation, analysis of fecal fat or estimation of protein-fat-starch digestion, thyroid function tests, Wood's light examination, fungal and bacterial cultures, skin biopsy, and possibly a chemistry panel and hemogram.

Histopathology. Histopathologic evaluation of a skin biopsy may be suggestive of seborrhea, but the pathologic lesions are not specifically diagnostic. Seborrhea appears microscopically as a spongiotic and/or hyperplastic superficial perivascular dermatitis. There is usually a marked keratinization defect, characterized by orthokeratotic and/or parakeratotic hyperkeratosis, follicular keratosis, and variable dyskeratosis. The perivascular cellular infiltrate consists of variable numbers of mononuclear cells, neutrophils, and plasma cells. The classic appearance of primary (idiopathic) seborrhea in cocker and springer spaniels includes a mildly hyperplastic superficial perivascular dermatitis with papillomatous and focal areas of parakeratotic hyperkeratosis (parakeratotic "caps") overlying edematous dermal papillae (papillary "squirting") (Figs. 14:3 and 14:4). Evidence of secondary bacterial infection is commonly seen as intraepidermal pustular dermatitis and perifolliculitis or folliculitis. Likewise, evidence of an underlying endocrinopathy may be present (see p. 641).

Differential Diagnosis. Differential diagnosis of seborrhea is one of the most challenging in dermatology. If the diagnosis of primary seborrhea is made, endocrine and metabolic causes must be carefully ruled out before considering the case as idiopathic seborrhea. The following comments allude to some of the common differential diagnoses.

Idiopathic seborrhea is a diagnosis made by exclusion of other diagnoses. Breeds commonly affected—especially early in life—include cocker and springer spaniels, poodles, dachshunds, West Highland white terriers, bassett hounds, and German shepherds.

Endocrine-related seborrheas are often caused by hypothyroidism. Thyroid function should always be evaluated even if the seborrheic dog has few other signs suggestive of hypothyroidism. Thyroid function tests are diagnostic, but dry seborrhea with secondary inflammation in Irish setters, Doberman pinschers, and Afghan hounds is highly suggestive. Response to thyroid replacement in these cases can be dramatic (see p. 651).

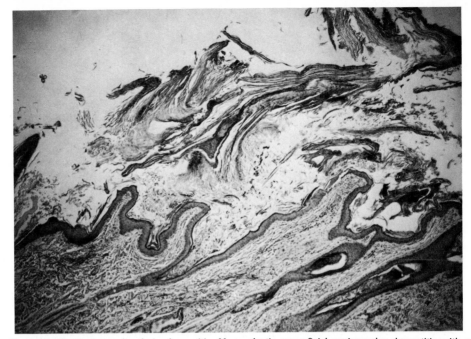

Figure 14:3. Canine seborrheic dermatitis. Hyperplastic superficial perivascular dermatitis with a marked keratinization defect and parakeratotic cuffing.

Figure 14:4. Close-up of Figure 14:3. Papillary squirting.

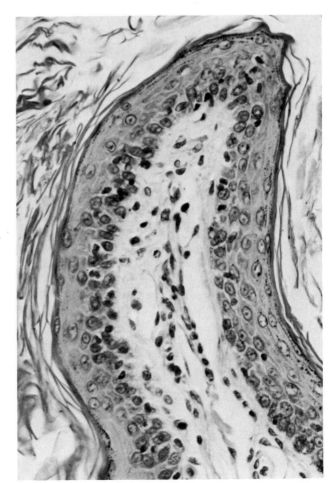

Male feminizing syndrome and ovarian imbalance type I are accompanied by ceruminous otitis and a severe oily seborrhea at points of intertriginous wear. There may be a mild, diffuse seborrhea, too. Diagnosis must be made by history and physical examination and response to treatment, since gonadal hormone assays in dogs and cats are unreliable. Although acanthosis nigricans is not a hormonal problem, it does present a somewhat similar clinical seborrhea syndrome.

Lipid-related seborrhea may affect any breed. Some clues that a problem exists may include diarrhea or pancreatic or other digestive disturbances. A history of dry, semimoist, or unbalanced commercial diets or poorly supplemented home diets may also be suggestive. Many of these patients are diagnosed only by placing them on special high-fat diets and noting the response. Zinc-responsive dermatosis causes a thick focal hyperkeratosis resembling dry seborrhea that affects the face and pressure points.

Vitamin A–responsive dermatosis presents as severe, medically refractory localized or generalized seborrheic dermatitis, especially in cocker spaniels.

Granulomatous sebaceous adenitis may present as a medically refractory seborrhea sicca or follicular seborrhea.

Ectoparasites produce dramatic but easily diagnosed and treated seborrheic problems. Scabies produces severe scaling and crusting of the lower body, especially the ears, elbows, and legs. There is severe pruritus. Demodicosis, especially in its localized form, mimics several other disorders. The fine white scales and alopecia may be complicated by focal pyoderma. Cheyletiellosis is characterized by an especially heavy dorsal concentration of diffuse or localized white scales—the so-called walking dandruff. Lice, especially biting lice, produce an irritation that causes epidermal scaling.

Hypersensitivity disorders produce a secondary scaling due to the erythema, papules, and associated local trauma from excoriations. Dogs with atopy, food and flea allergies, and contact dermatitis are prone to develop secondary seborrhea as part of the disease. Diagnosis by skin tests, diet exclusion, and other methods of identifying allergens will pinpoint the problem. Local irritation from a dry environment, too-frequent wetting and shampooing, and contact with local irritants such as soaps, organic solvents, and propylene glycol may produce scaling.

Dermatophytosis causes focal scaly, hairless patches. Although in some cases the alopecia and keratin scales are diffuse and mild, in others the scales are mixed with crusts to form thick, tightly adherent lesions in single or multiple locations. Fungal cultures and skin biopsy are diagnostic.

Autoimmune diseases such as pemphigus foliaceus and systemic lupus erythematosus may produce seborrhea-like lesions of the face, head, and body. In pemphigus foliaceus, the scales are epidermal collarettes secondary to vesicles and pustules.

Neoplasms that produce severe inflammation and alopecia may develop focal seborrheic plaques. Cutaneous lymphoreticular neoplasms, including mycosis fungoides, are examples.

Secondary seborrhea can also be produced by staphylococcal folliculitis, subcorneal pustular dermatosis, bacterial hypersensitivity (the target lesions produced look much like local seborrhea), and dermatomyositis.

CLINICAL MANAGEMENT

Management of primary seborrhea in dogs involves a good understanding of the chronic nature of the disease. The veterinarian's common sense and sympathetic and enthusiastic attitude will help the client bear the burden of a disease that can be controlled but seldom cured.

Primary idiopathic seborrhea is a chronic disease that can be ameliorated but not cured.

The objectives of treatment are to remove scales and crusts, reduce oiliness, control the seborrheic odor, relieve itching, and decrease inflammation.

Management of secondary seborrhea involves the elimination of the primary etiologic agent. Then symptomatic care of the skin will enhance its natural recovery. The following suggestions provide guidelines for symptomatic care of seborrheic skin.

Antiseborrheic shampoos applied at intervals of 3 to 14 days are extremely helpful. Shampoo intervals can be determined by instructing the client to repeat the dog's bath when the scaling or odor returns. As the treatment becomes effective, the need for shampoos decreases and the interval can be expanded. In severe idiopathic seborrhea, the best that usually can be expected is shampooing every week for the life of the animal. Common ingredients of medicated shampoos are salicylic acid, sulfur, tar, and antiseptics.

Ointments containing tar, salicylic acid, and sulfur are useful to reduce focal crusting and scaling. Sulfur reduces oiliness. In general, oily seborrheas are best managed with sulfur-containing or benzoyl peroxide–containing products, and dry seborrheas are most effectively managed with emollient-type shampoo (Allergroom, HY-LYT efa) and rinses (Humilac, HY-LYT efa) (see p. 154).

Corticosteroids may be given systemically to relieve erythema and pruritus, but continuous long-term therapy should not be used. These drugs tend to aggravate dry seborrhea, and may lead to bacterial infection. Topical corticosteroid creams and lotions can be used for local lesions.

Sebaceous gland suppression can be tried in severe cases. Pochi and Strauss found that in human females the administration of ethinyl estradiol and diethylstilbestrol depressed sebum production up to 35 per cent.[19] It is questionable whether this hormonal therapy is useful or even indicated in dogs, as it could be harmful. In human males, systemic corticosteroids reduced sebum production by 19 per cent, whereas castration followed by corticosteroid therapy reduced it by 40 per cent.

If there is secondary bacterial infection, antibiotics should be used to control it.

The ceruminous otitis present in many cases needs special attention (see p. 811).

Therapy for some types of lipid-related seborrheas entails dietary fat supplements. This is most effective if *equal parts* of saturated (lard or animal fat) and unsaturated (vegetable oil) fats are used. The treatment is as follows: Start the patient with a small amount of the mixture (1 to 3 tsp) in the food per day, depending on the animal's size. Slowly increase the quantity daily, until soft stools result. Then reduce the amount to a nonreacting level and continue daily for at least 8 weeks. Fat supplementation may be difficult in patients with chronic pancreatitis.

Other commercial dietary supplements containing multiple vitamins, minerals, amino acids, and essential fatty acids are rarely needed if the diet is complete and balanced. The supplements may be useful in cases of multiple deficiencies. A relative zinc deficiency may be produced by excess calcium in the diet. See p. 801 for other information.

The prognosis for complete recovery varies from excellent for secondary seborrhea, or for endocrine-related or metabolic conditions in which the cause can be removed or modified, to hopeless for primary idiopathic seborrhea. In all cases, special attention to coat care and hygiene will be necessary for a long time. In longer-coated dogs, regular clipping of the hair to a length of ½ to 1 inch is often a helpful adjunct to therapy. Experimentation with various topical medications is necessary to provide the best result for an individual. This approach must be carefully discussed with the owner for complete understanding and cooperation. A large number of topical medications are available commercially. A few should be selected from each category in Table 14:2 and their use and effects should be thoroughly understood. More specific details are available in the discussion of topical treatment in Chapter 4.

Oral retinoids have been used in the management of many keratinization disorders in humans.[6, 23] In dogs with primary seborrhea, despite anecdotal reports of success,[2] larger studies of the effect of oral retinoids (isotretinoin, 1 to 3 mg/kg orally BID) have produced disappointing results.[5, 23]

One of the authors (D.W.S.) has had encouraging results recently in treating primary seborrhea of cocker and springer spaniels with an eicosapentaenoic acid–containing product (Derm Caps).

Vitamin A–Responsive Dermatosis

A vitamin A–responsive dermatosis in cocker spaniels has been described.[8a, 11, 23] The condition is characterized by a medically refractory seborrheic skin disease, wherein marked follicular plugging and hyperkeratotic plaques with surface "fronds" typically are seen (Fig. 14:5A–E). The follicular plugging and hyperkeratotic plaques are especially prominent on the ventral and lateral chest and abdomen. Skin biopsy reveals disproportionately marked follicular orthokera-

Table 14:2. SEBORRHEIC MEDICATIONS

Antiseborrheic Shampoos	**Non-oily Spray Rinse (Humectant)**
Sebbafon	Humilac
Seba-Lyt	**Emollients**
Mycodex Tar and Sulfur	V.F. Soothing Lotion
Lytar	Nivea Lotion
V.F. Tar Shampoo	Johnson's Baby Oil
Allergroom	**Keratolytics**
OxyDex, Pyoben	OxyDex Gel, Pyoben Gel
Selsun	KeraSolv Gel
Thiomar	Lime-sulfur solution
Allerseb T	Vitamin A acid
Adams Sulfur	**Antiseborrheic Creams**
Pragmatar shampoo	Diprosone Creme
Topical Bath Oils/Sprays	Aristocort Creme (0.1%)
Alpha Keri	Pragmatar ointment
Lubath	
HY-LYT efa	
V.F. Oil Rinse	
Groom Aid Spray	

totic hyperkeratosis (Fig. 14:5F). Other lesions include varying degrees of focal crusting, scaling, alopecia, and follicular papules. A ceruminous otitis externa is usually present. A generally dry, dull, disheveled, easily epilated hair coat is present, as well as a rancid skin odor and mild to moderate pruritus. Except for the skin disease, the dogs are generally healthy.

Treatment consists of 10,000 U vitamin A (retinol) given orally, once daily, with a fatty meal. Improvement can be expected in 3 weeks with complete clinical remission within 8 to 10 weeks. Treatment should be continued for life. When treatment is discontinued, the lesions and symptoms reappear. Cocker spaniels have long been recognized as a breed with a predisposition to an idiopathic, possibly hereditary form of seborrheic skin disease. Although it would be inappropriate (if not inaccurate) to equate all "Cocker Spaniel Seborrhea" with the vitamin A–responsive dermatosis, the breed predilection inherent in each syndrome suggests a genetic basis for both. At present, the final diagnosis of vitamin A–responsive dermatosis can be confirmed only by response to therapy.

Lichenoid-Psoriasiform Dermatosis of Springer Spaniel Dogs

This dermatosis has been recently described.[8, 14] The dermatosis began in young dogs (4 to 18 months of age) of both sexes. Asymptomatic, generally symmetric, erythematous, lichenoid papules and plaques were initially noted on the pinnae, in the external ear canal, and in the inguinal region. With time, lesions became increasingly hyperkeratotic (some, almost papillomatous), and spread to involve the face, ventral trunk, and perineal area. Chronic cases resembled "severe seborrhea." The exclusive occurrence, to date, of this dermatosis in springer spaniels could suggest a genetic predilection.

Skin biopsy revealed a lichenoid dermatitis with areas of psoriasiform epidermal hyperplasia, intraepidermal microabscesses (containing eosinophils and neutrophils), and Munro's microabscesses (Fig. 14:6). Chronic hyperkeratotic lesions frequently show papillated epidermal hyperplasia and papillomatosis.

This dermatosis was characterized by a waxing and waning course for periods of 1 to 3 years. Neither spontaneous nor therapeutic remissions were reported. Various medicaments—including antibiotics, anti-inflammatory doses of glucocorticoids, oral vitamin A, levamisole, dapsone, autogenous vaccine, and antiseborrheic shampoos—were of little or no benefit. Repeated courses of erythromycin were of partial benefit to one dog, and large doses of prednisolone (2.2 mg/kg/day) benefited another.

Feline Seborrhea

Cats only occasionally develop signs that suggest seborrhea.[21] Perhaps this is partially a result of their fastidious cleaning habits, which remove scales quickly. When cats do become seborrheic they usually have secondary seborrhea sicca (dry) with fine white or gray flakes and scales ("dandruff") in the coat. If it is

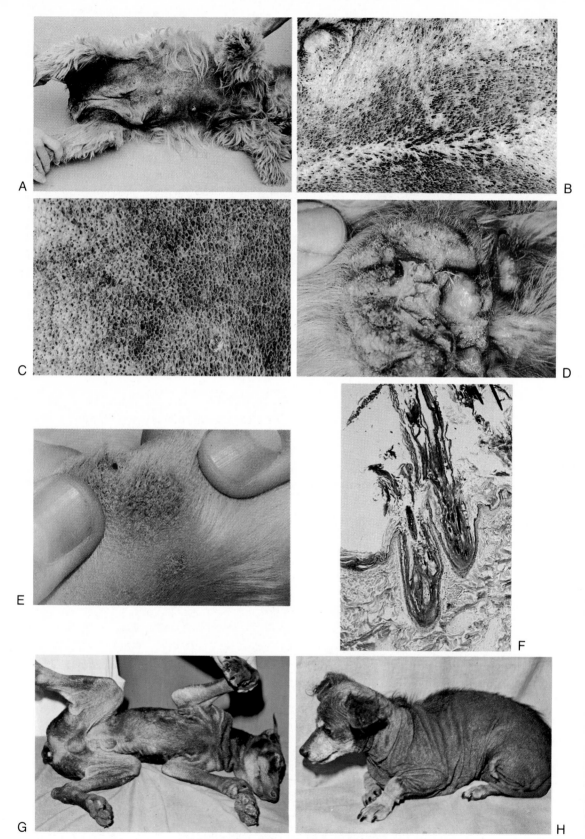

Figure 14:5 *See legend on opposite page*

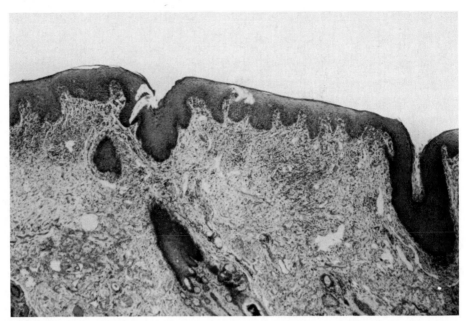

Figure 14:6. Lichenoid psoriasiform dermatosis of English springer spaniel. Lichenoid dermatitis with overlying psoriasiform hyperplasia.

fairly generalized, the following should be suspected: a systemic illness, intestinal parasites, a too-dry environment, too-frequent shampooing or powdering, contact with irritating chemicals, diabetes mellitus, chronic liver disease, hyperthyroidism, a low-fat diet, or ectoparasites such as cheyletiella or lice. More localized lesions suggest dermatophytosis.

If oily or inflammatory processes are present, suspect liver disease, systemic lupus erythematosus, feline leukemia virus infection, drug eruption, or toxic reactions. Therapy for any of these conditions should be directed at the underlying cause, with topical medications used selectively from the principles described for dogs. In general, emollient shampoos (Allergroom, HY-LYT efa, Nolvasan) or sulfur or benzoyl peroxide–containing shampoos should be used. Emollient rinses (Humilac, HY-LYT efa) may be especially useful in cats with severe seborrhea sicca, although the subject of skin moisturizers is presently being re-evaluated. (See Chapter 4.)

> *Because of their potentially toxic effects,* do not use tar, selenium, quaternary ammonium compounds, or phenol-containing preparations on cats.

Some cats may benefit from the oral administration of linoleic acid and arachidonic acid.

Figure 14:5. *A,* Vitamin A–responsive dermatosis in a cocker spaniel. Alopecia and hyperpigmentation. *B,* Same dog as in Figure 14:5*A.* Marked comedo formation on abdomen. *C,* Same dog as in *A* and *B.* Close-up of comedones. *D,* Same dog as in *A, B,* and *C.* Ceruminous otitis externa. *E,* Hyperkeratotic plaque with surface fronds. *F,* Disproportionate orthokeratotic hyperkeratosis of hair follicles. *G,* Five-month-old Doberman pinscher with congenital canine ichthyosis. Most of the dog's ventral surface is hyperkeratotic. Note how the extreme digital hyperkeratosis has caused enlargement of the paws. *H,* Canine ichthyosis in a terrier-cross with generalized dry, hyperkeratotic, alopecic skin. The dog has appeared this way since birth.

Epidermal Dysplasia of West Highland White Terriers

This disorder is probably a genetic dermatosis, but the mode of inheritance is unknown. It typically appears in West Highland white terriers, of either sex, at a few weeks to a few months of age.

Initially, the dermatosis begins with erythema and pruritus, especially on the feet, legs, and ventrum. As the disease intensifies, erythema becomes widespread, and alopecia and other chronic inflammatory changes develop (Fig. 14:7A). Peripheral lymphadenopathy becomes moderate to marked. With the passage of time, the dogs become hyperpigmented, lichenified, greasy, and malodorous, a situation that has led to the popular description, "The Armadillo Westie Syndrome" (Fig. 14:7B,C). Pruritus is generalized and severe.

The differential diagnosis includes atopy, food hypersensitivity, ectoparasitisms (especially canine scabies), ichthyosis, and seborrheic skin disease. Typically, the condition does not improve significantly with glucocorticoid therapy or hypoallergenic diets. Intradermal skin testing is negative. The breed, early age of onset, and progressive, medically refractory dermatosis should suggest epidermal dysplasia. Histopathologic findings include variable degrees of hyperplastic perivascular dermatitis with epidermal dysplasia (Figs. 14:8 and 14:9). The epidermis shows varying degrees of hyperchromasia, excessive keratinocyte mitoses, crowding of basilar keratinocytes, epidermal "buds," and loss of polarity. Parakeratosis is prominent, and inflammatory infiltrates consist of varying numbers of neutrophils and mononuclear cells.

The prognosis for improvement is very poor. The condition responds poorly to antibiotics, systemic glucocorticoids (even immunosuppressive doses), azathioprine, megadoses of vitamin E, oral zinc, and oral vitamin A. One of the authors (D.W.S.) has used isotretinoin (Accutane 1 mg/kg BID orally) and eicosapentaenoic acid–containing oral product (Derm Caps) with no benefit.

This condition is frustrating for the breeder, owner of a new puppy, and the veterinarian who treats the dogs. Owners usually request euthanasia. However, there seem to be two forms of the disease. In one, all treatment fails and the young dog is still extremely seborrheic at 6 months of age or older. In the other form, recovery is possible and permanent. These latter cases respond favorably to the administration of systemic corticosteroids (high doses for a short time) much like the response seen in juvenile cellulitis (see p. 840). Therefore euthanasia should not be performed without attempting therapy and allowing a reasonable time for possible recovery. As a rule, the dog's general health otherwise is good.

Figure 14:7. Epidermal dysplasia of West Highland white terriers and schnauzer comedo syndrome. A, Epidermal dysplasia in a West Highland white terrier. Early erythroderma. B, Epidermal dysplasia. Chronic alopecia, hyperpigmentation, and lichenification. C, Pinna and periocular region of the dog in B. D, Individual papulopustules on back of miniature schnauzer (close-up of F, below). E, Comedones, papules, and scaliness that also form on backs of affected individuals (close-up of G, below). F, Miniature schnauzer whose back has been clipped to expose the area affected with lesions. G, Clipping allows visualization of affected areas on the back of this miniature schnauzer. Note the distribution of lesions extending from the shoulder to the tail. There are visible erythematous patches. H, Prominent, soft comedones on the skin of another schnauzer.

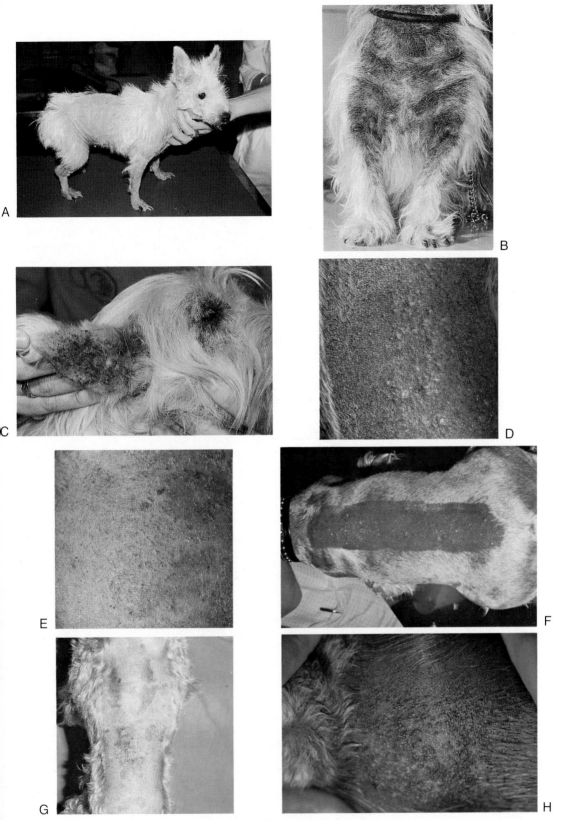

Figure 14:7 *See legend on opposite page*

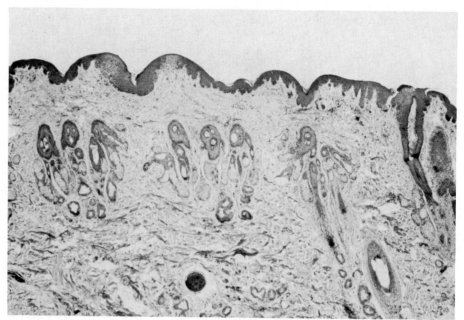

Figure 14:8. Epidermal dysplasia of West Highland white terriers. Hyperplastic superficial perivascular dermatitis with epidermal "budding."

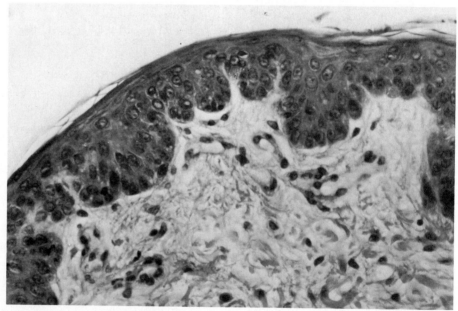

Figure 14:9. Close-up of Figure 14:8. Epidermal buds, composed of crowded, often hyperchromatic basal cells, and resultant dysplasia.

Schnauzer Comedo Syndrome

The schnauzer comedo syndrome affects the backs of miniature schnauzer dogs and is typified by multiple comedones that may become crusted, nonpainful papules.

CAUSE AND PATHOGENESIS

This condition has been observed exclusively in miniature schnauzers. It seems to be a seborrheic disorder and occurs only in certain predisposed individuals. The exclusive occurrence in schnauzers and the clinicopathologic similarity to nevus comedonicus in humans[6, 13] suggest that this syndrome may be a developmental dysplasia of hair follicles with an inherited basis. Once recognized, schnauzer comedo syndrome usually can be treated and easily controlled, but recurrences are common. However, there is much variability, with some cases responding to therapy more favorably than others.

CLINICAL FEATURES

Certain predisposed individual schnauzers tend to form comedones (blackheads) on their backs (Fig. 14:7D,E). These can be felt as sharp, crusted, papular projections above the surface of the skin. Some comedones are soft and waxy (Fig. 14:7E).

The lesions are most numerous at the midspinal area of the back, fanning out laterally and extending from the neck to the sacrum (Figs. 14:7F,G and 14:10).[9] Schnauzer comedo syndrome is seldom noted in the early stage before the comedo extrudes from the follicular orifice. At that stage there is no pain or discomfort. In some individuals, the comedo changes into a soft small acne-like pustule and causes slight irritation (Fig. 14:7H). Dogs seldom display visible pain or itching, unless secondary bacterial infection results in folliculitis.

DIAGNOSIS

Clipping a small spot on the back with a shaving blade exposes the affected skin so the individual comedones and papules can be seen.

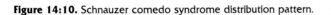

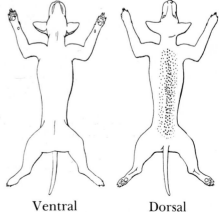

Figure 14:10. Schnauzer comedo syndrome distribution pattern.

Ventral   Dorsal

Histopathology. A section through one of the comedones reveals a keratinous plug blocking the hair follicle and sebaceous gland. A small cystic cavity is formed, lined by thin, stretched follicular epithelium and filled with keratin and sebum (Fig. 14:11). Sebum secretion accumulates behind the plug, which further dilates the cyst. If the follicle ruptures into the dermis, and its irritating contents escape, perifollicular inflammatory infiltrate appears. Eventually there is communication with the epidermal surface, and the spilled keratosebaceous material forms a crust.

Differential Diagnosis. Seborrhea is similar to schnauzer comedo syndrome but is not restricted to the back. Calcinosis cutis, another possible diagnosis, is accompanied by other symptoms of hyperadrenocorticism. Lesions are often on the abdomen or flanks and may be white or other colors. Flea bite hypersensitivity is pruritic, whereas schnauzer comedo syndrome is not.

CLINICAL MANAGEMENT

The pathogenesis is explained to the owner. The affected area should be clipped if severe crust formation exists, and the back should be shampooed twice a week with a benzoyl peroxide shampoo (OxyDex, Pyoben). Daily alcohol rubs to the back are beneficial. Benzoyl peroxide gel applied to loosen comedones is very useful if applied once or twice a day. For follow-up treatment or prophylaxis, the owner should give an alcohol rub at least twice a week to discourage further comedo formation. Periodic antiseborrheic or follicular flushing shampoos (OxyDex, Pyoben) are also necessary.

Recently, isotretinoin (Accutane), 1 mg/kg, orally BID, has been used to manage schnauzer comedo syndrome that is refractory to topical therapy.[15a]

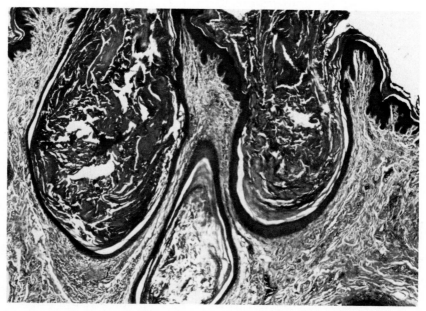

Figure 14:11. Comedones (acne) are dilated follicles with keratin plugs blocking the follicular opening.

Canine Tail Gland Hyperplasia

All dogs have an oval spot on the dorsal surface of the tail, about 1 to 2 inches distal to the anus, that is different from other skin. The area has single, instead of multiple, hair follicles and has numerous large sebaceous and perianal glands (see p. 38).

In some dogs, especially in individuals with testicular neoplasms or elevated blood androgen levels, or in those inclined toward seborrhea, there is sebaceous and/or perianal gland hyperplasia in the tail gland, and the area is enlarged grossly (see p. 634). As the dog sits on its tail, friction causes hair loss on the now-prominent oval spot, and an alopecic, tumor-like area appears clinically. The size of the enlargement differs greatly with individual dogs. When the spot is only slightly enlarged and occurs in long-haired dogs, it may not be noticeable. However, gross enlargement with frictional alopecia, especially in a short-haired dog, is an obvious cosmetic defect (Fig. 14:12A). In such cases, the owner may seek veterinary advice and treatment. The overlying skin may be scaly, greasy, or hyperpigmented, or some combination of these.

There seem to be two syndromes: one in seborrheic dogs and another in dogs with testicular disorders and perianal hyperplasia.

The area of tail gland hyperplasia has been observed to become infected, although this is not common. Grouped or single pustules may develop (Fig. 14:12B). Each pustule represents an acne-like sebaceous or perianal gland infection. Puncturing these pustules, expressing the contents, and administering systemic antibiotics usually provide relief. In some cases the infection may recur.

Surgical treatment of tail gland hyperplasia may be necessary. An elliptic piece of skin is removed from the dorsal area of the tail over the enlargement. Blunt dissection and curettage are then used to remove the excess glandular material that is under and lateral to the incision. Before suturing, more loose skin can usually be removed to provide a normal conformation of skin around the tail. The area should be bandaged to prevent self-damage or suture removal by the dog. Usually, excellent cosmetic correction results, with only a small scar visible. Recurrence often occurs in 1 to 3 years.

Castration or progestational compounds are often helpful, and a beneficial response is usually seen within 2 months.

Feline Tail Gland Hyperplasia

(Stud Tail)

Cats have the same tail gland area as dogs, but it is located in a line along the dorsal aspect of the tail and commonly called the "supracaudal organ" (see p. 39). As in dogs, this area is rich in sebaceous and apocrine glands (Fig. 14:13), and a waxy secretion accumulates on the surface.

In some cats, especially those kept in catteries or small enclosures, unusually large amounts of excess secretions accumulate and cause matting of the hair and the formation of scales and crusts (Fig. 14:12C,D). In some cases, the overlying hair coat is thinned and the skin may be hyperpigmented. Rarely, secondary bacterial folliculitis and furunculosis may complicate the condition. This condition is of great concern to owners of uncastrated male show cats,

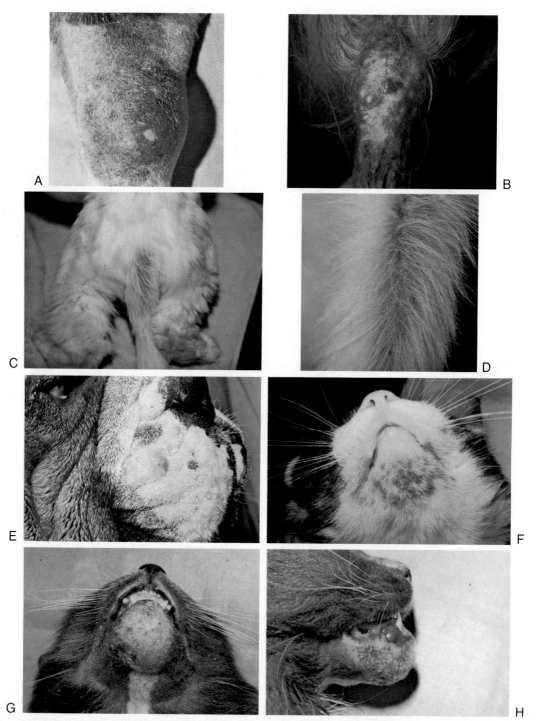

Figure 14:12. Tail gland hyperplasia and acne. *A,* Tail gland hyperplasia in an 8-year-old male beagle. Note the tumor-like swelling on the dorsal surface of the tail. *B,* Infected tail gland hyperplasia in a dog. Notice the multiple acne-like pustules. (Courtesy T. McKenna.) *C,* Hind quarters of an uncastrated male cat with "stud tail." Even from this distance, a dirty-appearing patch can be seen at the proximal dorsal surface of the tail. *D,* Close-up of tail in *C* showing a greasy, reddish brown streak on the dorsal tail surface. *E,* Canine acne. Pustules on the lip of an English bulldog. *F,* Early case with erythematous folliculitis. *G,* Advanced case with edema of the chin, alopecia, and pustule formation. Hair has been removed from periphery of lesion for better visualization. *H,* Side view of *G* clearly shows grayish black comedones and edema of the entire chin.

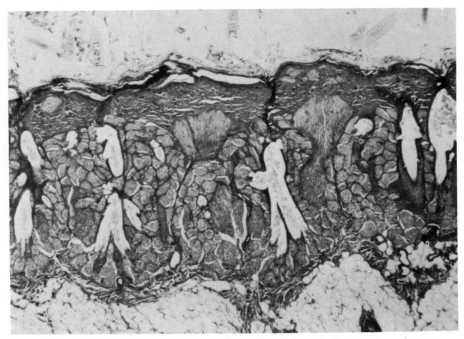

Figure 14:13. Feline stud tail. Marked sebaceous gland hyperplasia.

which accounts for the popular name "stud tail."[21] However, it has also been observed in females and in altered males. Castration does not help the condition.

Treatment consists of clipping the affected area and washing it with soap and water. Benzoyl peroxide shampoo can be very useful. This can be followed by daily cleansing with alcohol. It is advisable to provide affected cats with as much freedom and as little confinement as possible. The outdoors with fresh air and sunshine may help prevent recurrence. The unconfined cat usually resumes cleaning itself (and the tail gland area) with the customary fastidiousness characteristic of healthy, well-adjusted cats. Progestational compounds may be helpful, but because of their common side-effects, their use in treating a benign, asymptomatic disease is of questionable wisdom.

If the cat fails to care for the problem, the owner must carefully and frequently comb and groom the area to prevent recurrence.

Canine Ear Margin Dermatosis

Marginal seborrhea affecting the pinna of the ear is characterized by numerous small, greasy plugs adhering to the skin and hairs of the medial and lateral margins. It is most common in dachshunds but also occurs in other breeds with pendulous ears (Fig. 14:14). The small particles can be removed easily with the thumb nail or a flat instrument for diagnosis. Occasionally, these particles resemble the nits of lice, but they are softer, more irregular, and greasy. The condition can be accompanied by partial alopecia of the pinna. In severe cases, inflammation, necrosis, ulceration, and permanent deformities may occur. In some cases, thrombosis of one or more vessels supplying blood

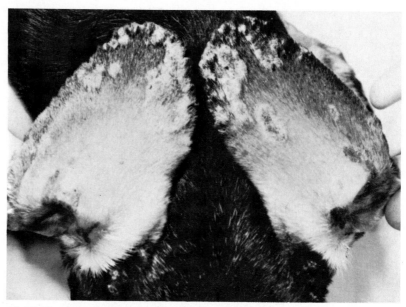

Figure 14:14. Ear margin dermatosis in a dachshund, showing flat waxy crusts at margins of pinnae.

to the pinna is the cause. Pruritus is rare. In severe cases, the entire ear margin of both pinnae is encased in a thick keratosebaceous material.

Histopathology shows marked orthokeratotic and/or parakeratotic hyperkeratosis (Fig. 14:15).

Treatment consists of removing the accumulated material and treating the underlying dermatitis. A sebolytic or ceruminolytic agent, such as benzoyl peroxide or sulfur, is useful in softening and partially dissolving the cutaneous debris. After the keratosebaceous debris is removed, inflammation can be

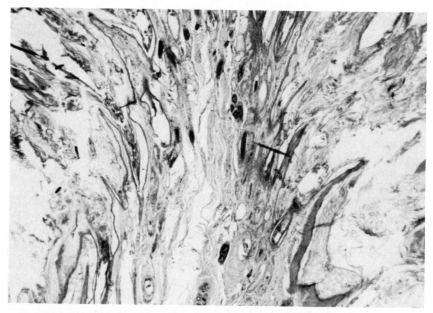

Figure 14:15. Histopathologic section of ear margin dermatosis. Tangential section shows a papillary epidermis with orthokeratotic hyperkeratosis.

controlled with topical glucocorticosteroids, such as 1 per cent hydrocortisone cream or ointment. In most patients the treatment should be repeated periodically on a permanent basis.

Acne

Acne is characterized by comedones and pustules in localized areas of the chin and lips of dogs and cats. It is a disorder of follicular keratinization that may become secondarily infected (folliculitis). Canine acne differs clinically from feline acne; therefore, the two conditions will be discussed as separate entities.

CANINE ACNE

CAUSE AND PATHOGENESIS

Canine acne is common in short-coated breeds, especially English bulldogs (Fig. 14:12E), boxers, Great Danes, and Doberman pinschers.[16] Canine acne resembles acne vulgaris of humans in many ways, but it is of only minor clinical importance. It begins during the dog's adolescence, which lasts only a few months compared with several years in humans. Canine acne occurs between 3 and 12 months, the time of sexual maturity. Sometimes acne persists into adult life in the susceptible breeds mentioned previously. The pathogenesis may be similar to that in humans,[3] involving increased circulatory androgens leading to greater androgen turnover and greater production of dihydrotestosterone in "acne-prone" skin. This, in turn, causes hypertrophy and hyperplasia of the sebaceous glands, and more sebum is released into the hair follicle. Theoretically, this is followed by the reaction and formation of fatty acids through the action of bacterial lipases from *Staphylococcus* sp. in the dog, with altered keratinization of follicular epithelium and comedo formation (blackheads).

CLINICAL FEATURES

The lesions of canine acne are the typical papulopustules that usually develop from comedones. The areas of the skin that are rich in sebaceous glands around the chin and lips are common sites. The disease is mild—often inapparent to the owner—and usually heals spontaneously at sexual maturity. In the predisposed breeds referred to previously, acne may persist into adulthood, usually for the life of the dog. The chin is studded with firm-to-fluctuant furuncles, often with draining tracts.

DIAGNOSIS

Diagnosis can easily be made by history, age, breed, and clinical appearance. The differential diagnoses to be considered are demodicosis, dermatophytosis, staphylococcal folliculitis and juvenile cellulitis. Histopathology of a follicular papule reveals marked follicular keratosis, plugging and dilatation (comedo), and perifolliculitis (see Fig. 14:11). Eventually the papule becomes a pustule and the histopathologic findings include suppurative folliculitis and, if follicular rupture ensues, furunculosis.

CLINICAL MANAGEMENT

Mild cases of acne need no treatment. Only occasionally will the lesions of a severely affected dog warrant therapy and prophylaxis. The drug of choice is benzoyl peroxide, first as a 5 per cent gel (OxyDex gel) used once daily and then as a 2.5 per cent shampoo (OxyDex shampoo). Shampoos are usually given twice a week until improvement occurs and then once a week as a preventative measure.

In chronic cases, treatment of an acute flare-up usually requires systemic antibiotics (antistaphylococcal) for 3 to 4 weeks, topical wet soaks, and benzoyl peroxide. Foreign body granulomatous dermatitis (hair, keratin) tends to be chronic and persistent in these cases and may require short courses of systemic glucocorticoids (prednisolone 1.1 mg/kg orally SID) or maintenance therapy with a potent, penetrating topical glucocorticoid such as fluocinolone acetonide in DMSO (Synotic). Surgical excision of affected tissue has not been satisfactory. Owners must be aware of the chronic, waxing and waning course of these cases.

FELINE ACNE

Feline acne is a somewhat different syndrome.[21] One major difference of feline acne from the canine and human form is that it is not confined to adolescence and also occurs in mature cats.

CAUSE AND PATHOGENESIS

Cats clean their bodies meticulously by licking. However, they use their saliva-moistened front paws to cleanse the face. Some cats have difficulty washing their chin in that manner, so surface lipids and dirt accumulate and predispose the skin to comedo formation. Perhaps cats with feline acne are seborrheic individuals. As in canine and human acne, comedones of the feline disease may progress into papules and finally pustules. An explanation for the periodic occurrence of feline acne may be associated with the cat's shedding cycle. Acne starts when hairs are in the telogen (resting) phase, and the comedo forms because the telogen hair is unable to push out the keratin plug and keep the follicle open. Both etiologic theories are unproven, and the real cause may still be undiscovered.

CLINICAL FEATURES

The lesions consist of comedones, papules, and pustules on the chin and sometimes the lips (Fig. 14:12F–H). Severe cases may develop suppurative folliculitis, furunculosis, or cellulitis (*Pasteurella multocida*, β-hemolytic streptococci, coagulase-positive *Staphylococcus* spp.). There can also be edema of the chin with spongy thickening of the lower lip; this has been referred to as "fat chin" by cat breeders. However, the most common cause of fat chin is eosinophilic granuloma (see p. 564).

DIAGNOSIS

Abscesses and dermatophytosis must be differentiated from feline acne, and this can usually be done by history and fungal and bacterial cultures.

Feline demodicosis is rare, but there have been cases that resemble feline acne. Demodicosis will be more alopecic, scaly, and hyperpigmented rather than pustular.

The histopathology of feline acne is similar to human and canine acne. The dermogram (Fig. 14:16) shows the histopathologic features as they relate to the clinical appearance. There is a progression of comedo → papule → pustule → rupture of follicle wall and dermal infiltrate. Thus, after the initial follicular keratosis, plugging, and dilatation (comedo), the histopathologic findings may include perifolliculitis, folliculitis, and furunculosis (Fig. 14:17).

CLINICAL MANAGEMENT

Treatment consists primarily of cleansing the cat's chin to remove sebum, debris, and bacteria. Daily gentle washing with soap, detergent, or alcohol is effective. Benzoyl peroxide shampoo 2.5 per cent (OxyDex Shampoo) is occasionally useful. Benzoyl peroxide gel is not recommended because it can be irritating to cats. Prior to treatment, the hair should be clipped with a shaving blade (No. 40 clipper). Cleansers for human acne may be effective but are usually too irritating. Alcohol and other defatting agents may be needed periodically. If an occasional case appears to progress into a pyoderma-like condition, penicillin or tetracycline is usually effective. Other useful antibiotics are ampicillin and cephalexin. Acne lesions often involve an influx of neutrophils into the hair follicle. In humans, it has been shown that *low levels* of certain antibiotics (tetracycline, erythromycin) inhibit leukocyte chemotaxis—resulting in a certain anti-inflammatory effect.[4]

About half the cases of feline acne recur. The owners are then instructed to become regular "chin washers," cleaning the cat's chin one to three times weekly for the life of the cat. However, if the condition causes no pain to the cat (and it usually does not) and is not cosmetically objectionable to the owner, no treatment is required. Given a choice, most cats prefer just to be left alone.

The short-term use of systemic glucocorticosteroids has been recommended.[2b] However, great caution should be used in prescribing such potent drugs for such an innocuous dermatosis.

Canine Ichthyosis

(Fish Scale Disease)

Canine ichthyosis is a very rare congenital skin disease of dogs, characterized by extreme hyperkeratosis on all or part of the skin and by exaggerated thickening of the digital, carpal, and tarsal pads.

CAUSE AND PATHOGENESIS

Canine ichthyosis resembles human ichthyosis, although not enough cases have been studied to reveal whether different forms of the disease occur.[1, 6a, 17, 18, 22] In humans, there are at least eleven major and rare forms of ichthyosiform dermatoses.[6, 25] The major forms of human ichthyosis are presently classified genetically into four types:

1. Ichthyosis vulgaris (autosomal dominant)
2. X-linked ichthyosis (sex-linked to males)

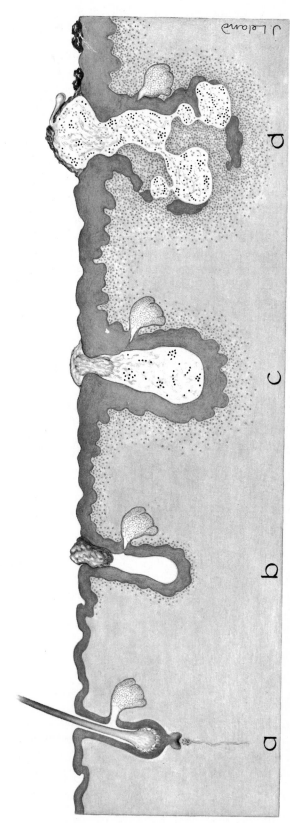

Figure 14:16. Feline acne dermogram. *A*, Hair follicle in telogen. *B*, The hair has been shed and a comedo plugs the follicular orifice. The epidermis is slightly acanthotic, and a mild perifollicular infiltrate forms. *C*, As bacteria (black dots) invade the follicle, acanthosis and inflammation increase. The follicle dilates, and a pustule begins to form. At the same time, the comedo disintegrates. *D*, Pustule formation is complete. The thin crust at the former follicular opening is breaking away as the first drop of pus oozes out. The former follicle is now a small intradermal abscess surrounded by a dense inflammatory infiltrate. This represents the severe form of feline acne on the chin.

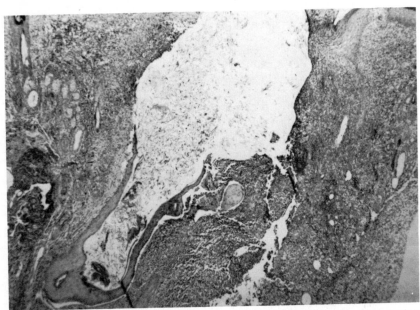

Figure 14:17. Feline acne. Ruptured comedo (follicular plug) with surrounding pyogranulomatous dermatitis.

3. Lamellar ichthyosis (autosomal recessive)

4. Epidermolytic hyperkeratosis (autosomal dominant)

Ichthyosis in humans, a disorder of keratinization, shows various clinical and histologic characteristics. In ichthyosis vulgaris, mild scaling and a diminished granular layer are observed. In X-linked ichthyosis, there is moderately severe scaling and a normal granular layer. In lamellar ichthyosis, severe scaling and a thickened granular layer are seen. In epidermolytic hyperkeratosis, severe verrucous thickening and a coarse, thick, degenerate granular layer appear.

The gene responsible for lamellar ichthyosis is autosomal and recessive; thus, the parents are usually not affected. Canine ichthyosis is probably also an autosomal recessive trait, inasmuch as the dogs with the cases reported so far had normal parents.[17, 18] The possibility of different types in dogs remains to be determined, but the lamellar form is the most likely form. An ichthyotic mouse has been described, with an appearance that closely resembles human lamellar ichthyosis (nonbullous, congenital ichthyosiform erythroderma).[24] A congenital scaly dermatosis of young West Highland white terriers may be lamellar ichthyosis.[15]

CLINICAL FEATURES

Much of the body is covered with tightly adhering, verrucous, tannish gray scales (Fig. 14:5H) and feathered keratinous projections, which give a rough texture to the skin (Fig. 14:18). While some of these adhere to the skin, others constantly flake off, producing large quantities of scaly, seborrheic-smelling debris. Scaly, dry patches are particularly prominent in the flexural creases and intertriginous areas. Marked thickening of the horny layer of the digital pads is observed (Fig. 14:19). Masses of hard keratin accumulate at the margins of the pads and often extend upward from the margin in winglike projections. The entire paw of some individuals appears grossly enlarged, and

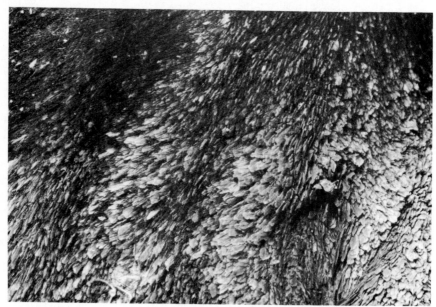

Figure 14:18. Close-up of skin from chest of a 5-month-old Doberman pinscher with canine ichthyosis, showing the laminated, tightly adhering scales.

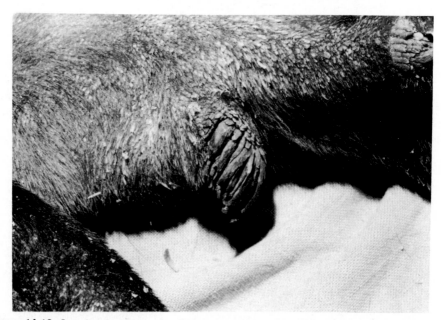

Figure 14:19. Carpal pad of dog in Figure 14:18. Note the "feathered" hyperkeratosis of the carpal pad.

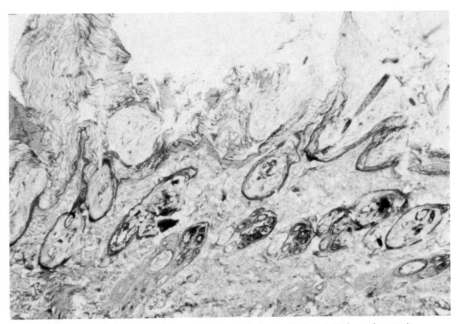

Figure 14:20. Acquired canine ichthyosis. Marked orthokeratotic hyperkeratosis.

the whole foot seems "heavier" than normal (Fig. 14:5G, p. 727). There is pain and discomfort of the feet. Hyperkeratosis may surround the eye if the skin of the periorbital area is affected. Some dogs may have severe erythroderma.[22]

DIAGNOSIS

Histopathology. Skin biopsy usually reveals characteristic histopathologic changes, especially the prominent granular layer and the presence of many mitotic figures in keratinocytes. Marked orthokeratotic hyperkeratosis (Figs. 14:20 and 14:21) and focal digitate projections of hyperkeratosis may be seen.

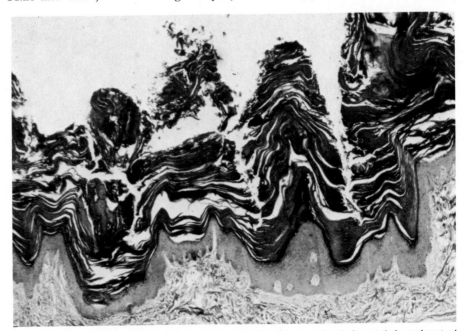

Figure 14:21. Congenital canine lamellar ichthyosis. Marked laminated orthokeratotic hyperkeratosis.

Follicular keratosis and plugging are common. The epidermis may or may not be hyperplastic. One of the most characteristic histopathologic changes is marked hypergranulosis (Fig. 14:22). Mitotic figures may be numerous. Although canine ichthyosis is usually characterized by hypergranulosis, some cases will have hypogranulosis similar to that seen in human ichthyosis vulgaris.[22]

The superficial epidermis may contain numerous vacuolated keratinocytes, which may rupture and result in reticular degeneration. Severe reticular degeneration may lead to microvesicle formation.

Differential Diagnosis

1. Nasodigital hyperkeratosis is not present at birth and is not accompanied by hyperkeratosis in other parts of the body.

2. Seborrhea differs by developing after several months of age instead of at birth. The skin is usually oily and greasy, instead of dry and rough as in ichthyosis.

3. Zinc-responsive dermatosis is not congenital, is a *crusting* dermatosis, and can be treated with zinc sulfate so that complete recovery results in 1 to 5 months. There is a breed predisposition in Siberian huskies and Alaskan malamutes.

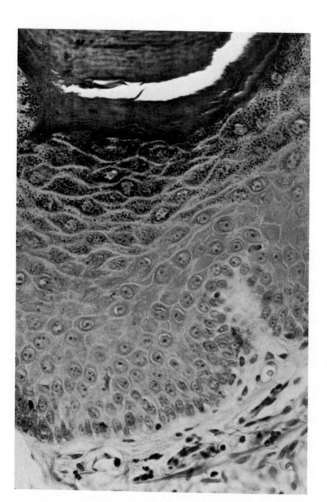

Figure 14:22. Close-up of Figure 14:21. Epidermal hyperplasia and hypergranulosis.

CLINICAL MANAGEMENT

The owner should understand the chronic nature, incurability, and difficult treatment of ichthyosis. Although the afflicted dog's general health seems to be good, the skin changes are so severe and their management so difficult that the patients are troublesome house pets. Still, a devoted owner may be capable of tolerating the burden of caring for these dogs.

Warm water baths and soaks soften the dry skin and horny projections so that they can be washed away more easily. Antiseborrheic and keratolytic shampoos (Sebutone, Sebbafon, Thiomar, Pragmatar) are useful. KeraSolv (DVM) (6 per cent salicylic acid gel) or Retin-A ointment is applied once or twice daily as a keratolytic agent. Alpha-Keri spray can be applied daily to lubricate the dry skin and help to mask the seborrheic odor.

Spectacular results have been obtained in human ichthyosis using alpha-hydroxy acids topically. The most practical treatment appears to be 5 per cent lactic acid in either hydrophilic ointment or petrolatum or as a spray or rinse (Humilac, HY-LYT efa). A thin film is applied twice daily to affected skin. Results are dramatic in 2 weeks. The treatment seems to affect the keratinization process itself and is not a keratolytic. It may be useful in various ichthyosiform dermatoses.[6] Propylene glycol may be useful as a topical medication, since it acts as a hygroscopic lipid solvent that penetrates the horny layer to increase its water content and makes the skin less taut. It works even more effectively when applied with polyethylene films under occlusion.[6, 22] In environments with low humidity, it may cause dehydration by taking moisture from the skin, rather than the air.

One American pit bull terrier with lamellar ichthyosis and one Boston terrier with acquired ichthyosis were described.[22] Oral isotretinoin (40 mg BID, approximately 1.5 mg/kg/day) produced remarkable remission in the American pit bull terrier. Oral retinoids have produced dramatic improvement in many human patients with various forms of ichthyosis.[6] The Boston terrier received daily topical application of 50 per cent propylene glycol, which also produced dramatic improvement.

Exfoliative Dermatoses

Exfoliative dermatoses are characterized by more-or-less generalized severe desquamation, with or without generalized erythema (erythroderma).[23a] These dermatoses are uncommon in dogs and cats and may be caused by immunologic disorders (pemphigus foliaceus, systemic lupus erythematosus, drug eruptions, severe atopy, or food hypersensitivity), contact dermatitis, scabies, dermatophytosis, ichthyosis, or lymphosarcoma. Recently, exfoliative dermatoses in a dog and a cat resembling large plaque parapsoriasis in humans were reported.[23a] The dermatoses were characterized by widespread erythematous, scaly plaques that spared the head, pinnae, and distal limbs. Histopathologic study revealed a focally parakeratotic, regularly hyperplastic, superficial perivascular-to-lichenoid dermatitis with diffuse exocytosis of normal lymphocytes. These cells were often arranged in a row within the stratum basale. Both cases were well controlled with long-term systemic glucocorticosteroid therapy.

References

1. August, J. R., et al.: Congenital ichthyosis in a dog: Comparison with the human ichthyosiform dermatoses. Comp. Cont. Ed. *10*:40, 1988.
1a. Baker, B. B., and Maibach, H. I.: Epidermal cell renewal in seborrheic skin of dogs. Am. J. Vet. Res. *48*:726, 1987.
2. Bates, J. R.: Treatment of idiopathic seborrhea in a dog. Mod. Vet. Pract. *65*:725, 1984.
2a. Carlotti, D.: Seborrhee canine. Point. Vet. *17*:355, 1985.
2b. Chastain, C. B., and Ganjam, V. K., Clinical Endocrinology of Companion Animals. Lea & Febiger, Philadelphia, 1986.
3. Dobson, R. L.: Acne. *In*: Thiers, B. H., Dobson, R. L., (eds.): Pathogenesis of Skin Disease. Churchill Livingstone, New York, 1986. p. 35.
4. Easterly, N. B., Furey, N. L., et al.: The effect of antimicrobial agents on leukocyte chemotaxis. J. Invest. Dermatol. *70*:51, 1978.
5. Fadok, V. A.: Treatment of canine idiopathic seborrhea with isotretinoin. Am. J. Vet. Res. *47*:1730, 1986.
6. Fitzpatrick, T. B., et al.: Dermatology in General Medicine. 3rd ed. McGraw-Hill Book Company. New York, 1987.
6a. Foil, C. S.: Comparative genodermatoses. Clin. Dermatol. *3*:75, 1985.
7. Gelfant, S.: The epidermal cell cycle and its significance in psoriasis. *In* Farber, E. M., and Cox, A. J.: Psoriasis. Grune & Stratton, New York, 1982.
8. Gross, T. L., et al.: Psoriasiform lichenoid dermatitis in the springer spaniel. Vet. Pathol. *23*:76, 1986.
8a. Guaguere, E.: Cas clinique: Seborrhee primaire repondant a l'administration de vitamine. A. Point. Vet. *16*:689, 1984.
9. Halliwell, R. E. W.: Seborrhea in the dog. Compend. Cont. Ed. *1*:227, 1979.
10. Ihrke, P. J.: Canine seborrheic disease complex. Vet. Clin. North Am. *9*:93, 1979.
11. Ihrke, P. J., and Goldschmidt, M. H.: Vitamin A–responsive dermatosis in the dog. J.A.V.M.A. *182*:687, 1983.
12. Kunkle, G. A.: Managing canine seborrhea. *In* Kirk, R. W. (ed.): Current Veterinary Therapy VIII. W. B. Saunders Company. Philadelphia, 1983.
13. Lever, W. F., and Lever, G. S.: Histopathology of the Skin. 6th ed. J. B. Lippincott Company, Philadelphia, 1983.
14. Mason, K. V., et al.: Characterization of lichenoid-psoriasiform dermatosis of springer spaniels. J.A.V.M.A. *189*:897, 1986.
15. McDonald, J.: Dermatosis of terriers. A.A.H.A. seminar, March, 1983.
15a. Miller, W. H., Jr.: Personal communication, 1987.
16. Muller, G. H.: Acne vulgaris. *In* Andrews, E. J., et al. (eds.): Spontaneous Animal Models of Human Disease. Vol. 2. Academic Press, Inc., New York, 1979.
17. Muller, G. H.: Ichthyosis in two dogs. J.A.V.M.A. *169*:1313, 1976.
18. O'Neill, C. S.: Hereditary skin diseases in the dog and cat. Compend. Cont. Ed. *3*:791, 1981.
19. Pochi, P. E., and Strauss, J. S.: Sebaceous gland suppression with ethinyl estradiol and diethylstilbestrol. Arch. Dermatol. *108*:210, 1973.
20. Reedy, L.: Presentation. A.A.H.A. Annual Meeting, Las Vegas, 1982.
21. Scott, D. W.: Feline dermatology 1900–1978: a monograph. J.A.A.H.A. *16*:331, 1980.
22. Scott, D. W., and Rosychuck, R. A. W.: Ichthyosis in two dogs: congenital and acquired forms. Companion Anim. Pract. (Submitted), 1988.
23. Scott, D. W.: Vitamin A–responsive dermatosis in the cocker spaniel. J.A.A.H.A. *22*:125, 1986.
23a. Scott, D. W.: Exfoliative dermatoses in a dog and a cat resembling large plaque parapsoriasis in humans. Companion Anim. Pract. (in press, 1988).
24. Selmanowitz, F. J.: Ichthyosis. *In* Andrews, E. J., et al.: Spontaneous Animal Models of Human Diseases. Vol. 2. Academic Press, New York, 1979.
25. Williams, M. L., and Elias, P. M.: The ichthyoses. *In* Thiers, B. H., and Dobson, R. L. (eds.): Pathogenesis of Skin Disease. Churchill Livingstone, New York, 1986. p. 519.

15

Psychogenic Dermatoses

Psychodermatology (psychocutaneous medicine, dermatopsychosomatics) is a growing field of interest to those involved in clinical work and research in human medicine.[2] Workers in this field believe that the body (soma) and the mind (psyche), which have been treated separately for too long, constitute a single unit. In fact, it is believed that the role of emotional factors in diseases of the skin is of such significance that if it is ignored, the effective management of at least 40 per cent of the patients attending departments of dermatology is impossible. Research in laboratory animals and humans indicates that the central nervous system, through the effects of neurohormones, can significantly modulate immune responses and pruritus. The relationship between the hypothalamus and the immune system seems to involve (1) neurohormones secreted by the hypothalamus itself—thyrotropin-releasing hormone, growth hormone–releasing factor, corticotropin-releasing factor, prolactin-releasing factor, gonadotropin-releasing hormone, (2) the neurotransmitters—norepinephrine, serotonin, dopamine, acetylcholine, γ-aminobutyric acid, and (3) the polypeptide neuroregulators—somatostatin, vasoactive intestinal peptide, substance P, neurotensin, enkephalins, and endorphins.[2]

This exciting field of psychodermatology promises to improve our understanding of the pathomechanisms involved in many skin disorders and to improve our ability to successfully and specifically treat these conditions. Applications of such information and technology to small animal dermatology are anxiously awaited.

Most lesions of psychogenic dermatoses are the result of self-induced damage. There is good clinical evidence that psychologic disturbances are the cause. Three general factors are involved in the etiopathogenesis:

1. Breed predisposition. The more emotional and nervous breeds develop more psychogenic dermatoses. Abyssinian and Siamese cats are especially at risk. Among dogs, the predisposed breeds include Doberman pinschers, Great Danes, Irish setters, and German shepherds.

2. The "lifestyle" of the animal can be the cause. Individuals of nonpredisposed breeds, when they are forced into stressful, isolated or boring situations, without human or canine companionship, may develop psychogenic dermatoses. Long confinement in crates, continual chain restraint, small pen housing, or domination by a forceful or inconsiderate owner may precipitate problems. A rival animal in the same home or an aggressive neighborhood animal can trigger a psychogenic disturbance.

3. The individual animal, regardless of breed or lifestyle, can be particularly nervous, hyperesthetic, fearful, or shy.

Physical causes must always be eliminated before a diagnosis of psychogenic dermatosis is made. This process includes such causative factors as trauma, pruritus, local pain, parasites, and bacteria or fungal infections, as well as internal diseases.

Psychogenic dermatoses include the following syndromes: acral lick dermatitis (lick granuloma), feline psychogenic alopecia, feline psychogenic dermatitis (feline neurodermatitis), and miscellaneous psychogenic manifestations such as tail sucking (feline), tail biting (canine), flank sucking, foot licking, self-nursing, and anal licking. There are also some nondermatologic manifestations of psychomotor epilepsy or psychosis, such as tail chasing and "imaginary fly catching."

Acral Lick Dermatitis

Acral lick dermatitis (lick granuloma) results from an urge to lick the lower anterior portion of a leg, producing a thickened, firm, oval plaque. The condition may be organic or psychogenic in origin.[5, 6]

CAUSE AND PATHOGENESIS

Boredom is often the major cause of the dog's habit of licking its leg. A carefully taken history will often reveal that the dog is alone much of the day while the owners are away. The classic patient is a large, active dog; the owners work and there are no children. Either there is no companion dog or the other dog provides no particular play activity.

Boredom may be a major cause.

Unusual restrictions on the dog's freedom can be a causative factor. Dogs kept in crates for long periods each day or dogs that are chained become bored and relieve their frustrations by constantly licking a leg. In other dogs, a pre-existing focal dermatosis (infection, neoplasm, wound, etc.) precipitates the vicious cycle.[5, 6]

A definite breed predilection exists, with a tendency toward large, active, vigorous or affectionate dogs—the Doberman pinscher, Great Dane, Labrador retriever, Irish setter, golden retriever, and German shepherd. Other similar breeds or smaller dogs can also develop acral lick dermatitis. It can occur at any age, although most of the dogs are over 5 years when presented clinically. Males with the disorder outnumber females, two to one. The pathogenesis is explained as a constant licking that produces an eroded area on the skin, which itches exquisitely. An itch–lick cycle is established until a firm, ulcerated lesion results.

The most common organic causes of acral lick dermatitis are staphylococcal furunculosis, pre-existing wounds, and hypersensitivity disorders (atopy, food hypersensitivity, flea bite hypersensitivity).

CLINICAL FEATURES

At first, constant licking causes alopecia. Next, the epidermis erodes and, with sensory nerve exposure, the licking reaches deeper skin layers. Finally, ulceration develops and the licking keeps the ulcer from healing. Epidermal hyperplasia and dermal fibrosis account for the nodular plaque that is characteristic of the disease. Formerly, the lesion at this stage was mistakenly called a granuloma or tumor. It is neither neoplastic nor granulomatous.

In almost all cases, the lesion is single and unilateral (Fig. 15:1A). However, in some cases multiple legs may be affected, and these cases usually respond poorly to treatment. The most common site is the anterior carpal or metacarpal area (Figs. 15:1 and 15:2). The next most usual sites are the anterior radial, metatarsal, or tibial regions. In rare cases, the dog picks the tail or back as a site for licking. Chronic lesions become hard, thickened plaques or nodules that have an ulcerated surface and a hyperpigmented halo (Fig. 15:1B,C). Extremely large lesions on the joints that have been present for years may be associated with arthritis or ankylosis of the underlying joint (Fig. 15:1D).

Secondary bacterial infection seldom occurs on the surface of the lesion, because licking keeps it clean. Purulence develops only in fistulas below the surface or under the crusts on the skin.

DIAGNOSIS

A definitive diagnosis can usually be made from the clinical examination and history.

Differential diagnoses include neoplasia, pressure point granulomas, calcinosis circumscripta, bacterial furunculosis, dermatophytosis, mycotic or mycobacterial granulomas, and underlying hypersensitivity disorders. A fungal culture shows mycotic infections. Histiocytomas and mastocytomas may be mistaken for acral lick dermatitis, if they occur on the anterior surface of the leg. Exfoliative cytologic findings and biopsy provide the basis for diagnosis.

Histopathologically, the lesions usually show features that are characteristic of the disorder, but that are not diagnostic by themselves.[5] An ulcerated surface is bordered by irregular epidermal hyperplasia, which may be papillated or pseudocarcinomatous. A mild perivascular accumulation of neutrophils and mononuclear cells is usually present. The dermis shows varying degrees of fibroplasia, and dermal papillae often show "vertical streaking" of fibroblasts and collagen fibrils (Figs. 15:3 and 15:4). Common findings are moderate-to-marked numbers of plasma cells around the apocrine sweat glands and inferior segments of hair follicles, and sebaceous gland hyperplasia (Fig. 15:5). It should always be determined whether there is a coexisting folliculitis or secondary pyoderma.

Radiographs usually reveal secondary periosteal reaction of bones that underlie large chronic acral lick dermatitis lesions.

CLINICAL MANAGEMENT

"Psychologic counseling" with the client should be the first step in the management of acral lick dermatitis of psychogenic origin. The client needs to understand that the dog's problem is "in his head" and not on the leg. Together, the clinician and client must become psychologic detectives to find

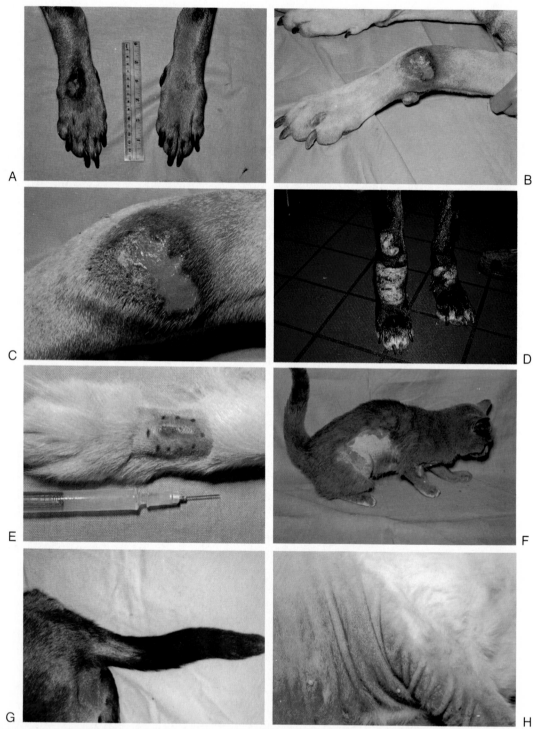

Figure 15:1. Acral lick dermatitis and psychogenic alopecia and dermatitis. *A,* Unilateral appearance on anterior metacarpal region. *B,* The carpal area is commonly affected. *C,* Close up of *B* shows the thickened nodule with the characteristic ulcerated epidermis surrounded by a hyperpigmented halo. *D,* Bilateral acral lick dermatitis in a Great Dane. *E,* Blue dots mark the needle entrance of area to be infiltrated with intralesional corticosteroid. *F,* Licking removes the hair and causes a chronic inflammation of skin in the favored area. *G,* Unilateral alopecia of the tail and rump may be initiated by anogenital pain or inflammation of anal sacs. *H,* Lichenification. Thickened skin in the axilla, a response to the irritation of constant licking.

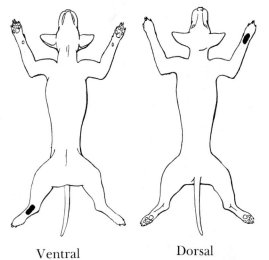

Figure 15:2. Acral lick dermatitis distribution pattern.

Ventral   Dorsal

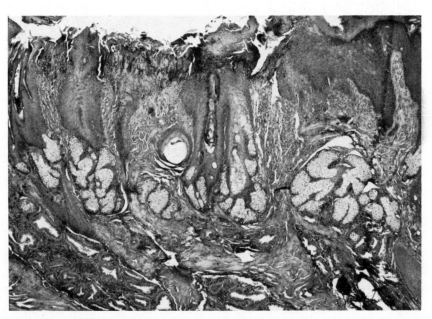

Figure 15:3. Acral lick dermatitis in a dog. Ulcerative, hyperplastic perivascular dermatitis with sebaceous gland hyperplasia.

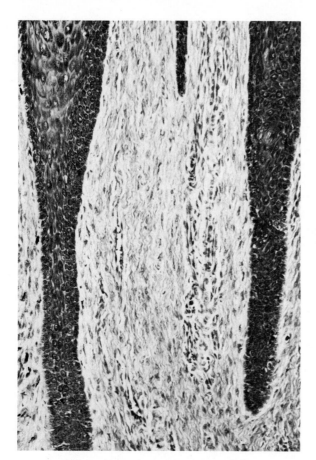

Figure 15:4. Vertical "streaking" of collagen fibrils between rete ridges.

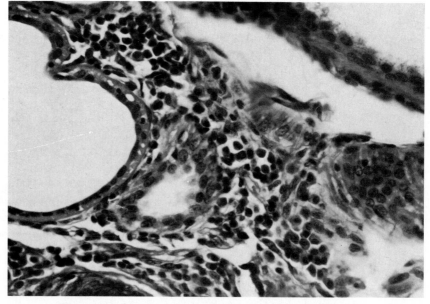

Figure 15:5. Canine acral lick dermatitis. Periapocrine plasma cells.

what caused the dog to lick its leg. The search must be for a "displacement phenomenon" and to single out events or situations that triggered the dog's psychosis. Examples of causes are:

1. Dog left alone all day.
2. Lengthy confinement to crate, kennel, cage, or run.
3. New pet in the home.
4. New baby in the home.
5. Female dog "in heat," close but not accessible to male dog.
6. New dog in the neighborhood.
7. Death in the family.
8. Death of long-time companion dog.

The first step in treatment is to recognize the cause and eliminate it, if possible. Sometimes a change in the dog's "lifestyle" is the answer. Each situation differs, but the following are examples of successful corrective measures that have worked.

1. More walks and human companionship are very helpful. Some owners can take their dog to work if they own a small shop or business.

2. For a kennel dog, such as a breeding dog, avoidance of confinement to cages, kennels, or runs can be beneficial. The owner can make a house pet of the afflicted dog. Even nightly confinement to a cage may cause enough frustration to trigger acral lick dermatitis.

3. A new puppy as a companion can act as a diversion that may discourage further licking. The success of this method depends on the extent to which a friendship develops between the two dogs. For a male dog, a spayed female is very suitable. The owner should be aware that the companion dog is not a guarantee of cure.

4. Freedom to leave the house and premises enables the dog to develop a "life of his own" in the neighborhood. This suggestion is suitable for some rural areas but is usually impossible in suburban or urban areas where leash laws are in effect.

If the psychogenic cause cannot be found and corrected, the acral lick dermatitis may never be cured.

When presented with acral lick dermatitis, one should always rule out organic causes such as initial wounds or trauma; subcutaneous injections of drugs intended for intravenous use; foreign body; furunculosis; and underlying joint, muscle, or bone disease. Bilateral lesions should prompt a consideration of food or flea bite hypersensitivity.

Systemic, topical, and surgical treatment are used simultaneously with psychologic therapy. One or more of the following may be useful.

Treating the Mind. *Phenobarbital* is given orally in doses of 2.2 to 6.6 mg/kg BID. This has a sedative effect and can be used for short or long periods of time. Other "antianxiety" drugs that have occasionally been useful include diazepam and primidone.

Tranquilizers, given orally, have not been particularly successful but may be used during especially stressful periods (during fireworks, when neighboring female dogs are in estrus, and so on). They must be given before the onset of the stress.

Progestagens have a calming effect, especially on male dogs. An injection of repositol progesterone (Depo-Provera) 20 mg/kg every 3 weeks has been successful in selected cases. Megestrol acetate (Megace, Ovaban) has been used orally at 1 mg/kg SID, then tapered to minimal maintenance doses and frequencies. These have to be continued for several months and, of course, should not be used in intact female dogs.

Recently, *naltrexone* (Trexan, an endorphin blocker used in various self-mutilation syndromes in humans) has been used in dogs with severe, chronic acral lick dermatitis.[7] Dogs were treated with 2.2 mg/kg orally SID. Seven of ten dogs responded well, but four dogs relapsed when the drug was discontinued. Long-term control may be accomplished with reduced dosages or increased intervals between doses. Significant side-effects have not been seen.

Treating the Lesion. In the past, treatment has been restricted to attacking the lesion with surgery or drugs. This has yielded disappointing results. Attempts have also been made to protect the lesion by the use of Elizabethan collars, muzzles, bandages, casts, and wire-cloth devices. None of these has been routinely successful, and they often further frustrate the psychotic dog. Repellent liquids and creams have shown only limited success. However, in many cases, it is necessary to radically treat the lesion itself. Some of these methods follow, along with comments on their value.

1. Topical corticosteroids. One commercially available product contains fluocinolone acetonide 0.01 per cent in 60 per cent dimethyl sulfoxide (DMSO [Synotic]). This is applied twice a day.

Dissolved in DMSO, corticosteroids can penetrate the lesion. A formula devised by a California veterinarian is useful, especially in cases with secondary bacterial fistulas. Use in equal parts: 90 per cent DMSO solution; H-B 101 solution (1 per cent hydrocortisone acetate and 2 per cent Burow's solution in propylene glycol). Paint or rub the lotion on the lesion twice a day for several weeks. Use rubber gloves when handling this product.

2. A combination of fluocinolone and DMSO (Synotic) with flunixin (Banamine R). This has been reported to be effective in many cases.[5] Three ml of Banamine are added to one 8-ml vial of Synotic. The solution is applied twice a day with rubber or plastic gloves until the lesion has healed. The treatment time varies from 3 to 8 weeks.

3. Intralesional injections of triamcinolone acetonide (Vetalog) or methyl-prednisolone (Depo-Medrol) (Fig. 15:1E). These are helpful in early lesions smaller than 3 cm in diameter. They are useless in larger, chronic cases.

Intralesional injections of diluted modified cobra venom have been used extensively in the past. The method is described in detail in the previous edition of this text. Although the mechanism of action is unknown, people bitten by cobras often have prolonged hypalgesia in the bitten area, and it is possible that this treatment does have a potent local effect. Cobroxin is no longer marketed, but processed cobra venom, although expensive, is available from the Miami Serpentarium in Miami, Florida.

4. Surgical removal. In some cases, surgical excision of the entire lesion is the treatment of choice. It is easily and quickly accomplished if the lesion is small enough to allow surgical repair without undue skin tension. The clinician should always close the incision with mattress sutures and use bandages or protective devices to prevent removal of the sutures or trauma by the dog before healing is complete (requires at least 2 to 3 weeks).

In extreme cases, excision of the lesion and replacement with a full-thickness skin graft can be performed.

5. Radiation therapy is occasionally effective.

6. Cryosurgery may be used as a last resort for lesions that are so large that they cannot be removed surgically, cannot be grafted with a full-thickness skin flap, and have not responded to other treatment. Properly used, the hardened mass of tissue is frozen and sloughs over a period of several weeks. New, healthy skin begins to grow from the wound margins. Freezing destroys nerve endings, thereby blocking the itch–lick cycle. The procedure usually must be repeated two or three times. It should be attempted only by those familiar with cryosurgery (see Skin Surgery p. 213).

7. Acupuncture has been reported to be effective, but its usefulness must be further documented.

8. If bacterial infection is present, several weeks of antibiotic therapy is useful. The bacterial component can be revealed by biopsy or stained smears.

In chronic acral lick dermatitis, one must *treat both the skin lesion* and the mind

---

In summary, a guarded prognosis should be given before beginning any treatment. This is one of the most obstinate skin disorders, but at least it is not life threatening.

Feline Psychogenic Alopecia and Dermatitis

Psychogenic alopecia or dermatitis is an alopecia or a chronic skin inflammation produced by constant licking and scratching of local skin areas.[1, 4] The dermatitic form may be considered the feline equivalent of acral lick dermatitis in dogs.

CAUSE AND PATHOGENESIS

The primary or initiating cause may be a dermatitis with pruritus, infected ears or anal sacs, or excessive nervousness of the cat. It frequently is an anxiety neurosis caused by psychologic factors such as displacement phenomena (new pet or baby in the household, move to new surroundings, boarding, hospitalization, loss of favorite bed or companion). There is a breed predilection for the more emotional breeds, such as Siamese and Abyssinian cats.

Feline psychogenic alopecia and dermatitis may be expressed in many ways. Some cats lick vigorously at a particular area until the sharp barbs on the tongue produce alopecia, abrasion, ulceration, and secondary infection. Other cats lick and chew more gently or over a more widespread area, so alopecia is the predominant lesion.

CLINICAL FEATURES

Areas that the cat can lick conveniently are the most common sites: the inside of the thigh, the lower abdomen, the center of the back (Figs. 15:1F,G

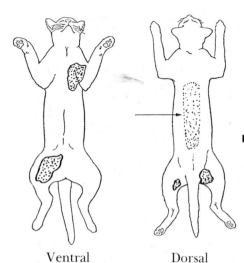

Figure 15:6. Psychogenic alopecia and dermatitis distribution pattern.

Ventral   Dorsal

and 15:6), the limbs, and the tail. A symmetric alopecia may also involve the caudomedial thighs and ventrum. The characteristic lesion of the dermatitic form is a bright red oval plaque or red streak. Animals with chronic cases develop lichenification and hyperpigmentation (Fig. 15:1*H*). The course is long and progresses slowly, sometimes remaining static for months. Siamese or Siamese-cross cats often lick out the hair in a localized area of the back, the ventral abdomen, or a leg, without causing skin reaction (Fig. 15:7). Because

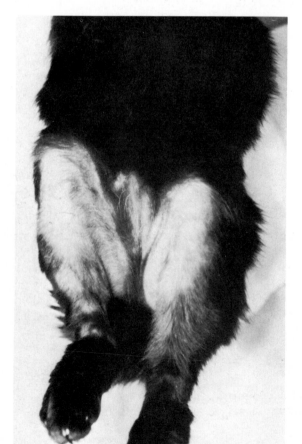

Figure 15:7. Feline psychogenic alopecia. Hair has been removed from the inguinal area by the cat's licking and biting.

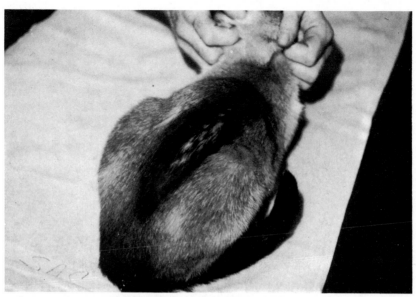

Figure 15:8. Constant licking removed hair from the back, thus reducing the skin temperature and causing the hair to grow in dark in color.

the temperature-labile enzymes that convert melanin precursors into melanin are active (high temperatures produce white hair, low temperatures produce pigmented hair, and the hairless area is cool), the hair becomes dark (Fig. 15:8). After the next shedding, the hair is usually replaced by normal-colored hair (see p. 8).

> *Affected cats have an uncontrollable urge to lick their lesions.*

DIAGNOSIS

Lesions of the dermatitic form may be confused with or possibly develop into indolent ulcers, eosinophilic plaques, or eosinophilic granulomas (see pp. 561–564). The alopecic forms may be confused with dermatophytosis, demodicosis, atopy, food or flea bite hypersensitivity, and feline symmetric alopecia. Because cats are often reclusive groomers, owners may not know that the cat is licking or chewing excessively (see p. 701). A helpful technique for differentiating between self-induced hair loss and spontaneous alopecia is the epilation and microscopic examination of hairs from the affected areas, or the application of an Elizabethan collar (see p. 129). In psychogenic alopecia, hairs do *not* epilate easily, they appear broken off when examined microscopically, and the hair regrows while the cat is wearing an Elizabethan collar.

CLINICAL MANAGEMENT

Response to treatment may be poor, and the condition requires much patience on the part of the owner and the veterinarian. If licking can be stopped, the lesions heal promptly.

Because of the potential side-effects of many of the commonly used treatments, cats with the alopecic form of the disease may best be served by *no* treatment.

Much has been written about acral lick dermatitis of dogs. Its psychologic cause and treatment apply also to feline psychogenic alopecia and dermatitis. In cats, boredom is a less significant factor than are disturbing influences. Cats are such territorial creatures that a change in the pecking order of animals in the territory has tremendous "anxiety potential." One needs to look for a new cat that entered the household or a neighborhood tomcat invading the cat's territory. Other factors are barking dogs, a new baby, moving to a new home, or major changes in the present home.

Topical medications are of little value, since the cat immediately licks them off.

The first systemic treatment for the dermatitic form should be corticosteroids. After an initial injection, oral medication can be used in gradually reduced dosages. Because of the severity of some cases, corticosteroids are necessary for 3- to 4-week periods. Tranquilizers and sedatives can be tried alone or in combination with corticosteroids. Valium, 1.0 to 2.0 mg twice daily with or without 8.0 to 15.0 mg phenobarbital, or phenobarbital alone has been effective in many cases. Some authors have reported occasional success with 12.5 to 25 mg of primidone given orally SID, BID, or TID.[1]

Mechanical devices (such as Elizabethan collars) are resented by cats and should be replaced by sedation, if possible. In either case, reduction of medication or removal of the collar often allows a relapse to take place. Once the areas are healed, recurrence can be triggered by emotional upsets. Susceptible cats with tendencies toward anxiety begin licking themselves as soon as they are boarded or psychologically stressed in other ways, and the cycle begins again.

The alopecic form may be successfully managed with phenobarbital (2.2 to 6.6 mg/kg BID orally), diazepam (Valium) (total dose of 1 to 2 mg, orally SID to BID), or progestational compounds (total dose of 2.5 to 5.0 mg megestrol acetate [Ovaban], orally every other day, then weekly; or 100 mg medroxyprogesterone acetate [Depo-Provera] subcutaneously, as needed). Again, the side-effects of these drugs can be striking, and one must weigh the gravity of the disease against the possible drug toxicities. (See p. 210.)

Miscellaneous Psychogenic Manifestations

A group of six psychogenic manifestations involve sucking or licking a specifically selected anatomic area. The animal concentrates on one area to which it habitually returns. The treatment regimens that can be tried are those discussed for canine acral lick dermatitis and feline psychogenic alopecia and dermatitis.

Tail sucking occurs mostly in cats, specifically Siamese cats. It is easily recognized by a wetness of the distal 2 to 3 cm of the tail. Close examination of the skin reveals normal skin without inflammation or scaling. Whenever the cat ceases to lick the tail and the hair dries, the condition can no longer be detected. This drying occurs during times when the cat's attention is focused on interesting activities. When bored, the cat resumes licking its tail. Treatment is not successful until the cat's boredom is relieved, possibly by changing its lifestyle.

Tail biting is occasionally seen in young, long-tailed, mostly long-haired dogs. These dogs chase their tail (*tail chasers*) and then bite the tip. Many of the afflicted dogs stop this habit when they get older.

Flank sucking in dogs is similar, in most respects, to tail sucking in cats, but it is more common and is especially prevalent in Doberman pinschers. At one time trichuriasis was thought to be a cause of the disorder, but this has not been documented. It has been suggested that tail biters and flank suckers may have a form of psychomotor epilepsy. Therapy with phenobarbital or primidone may be helpful. One investigator suggested one intramuscular injection of medroxyprogesterone acetate (20 mg/kg) for possible therapy.[3]

Self-nursing is restricted, of course, to female dogs and cats. Usually the self-nursing is confined to one nipple, and the animal repeatedly suckles that nipple. Spaying the animal seems to be helpful in correcting this annoying habit. Sedation and psychologic training to break the habit may also be useful.

Anal licking occurs only in dogs, and a breed predilection exists for poodles. It is almost impossible to break the habit. Although it is tempting to blame anal sac irritation for this condition, removal of the anal sac usually does not solve the problem. Anorectal disease and food hypersensitivity should be ruled out. Neurotic poodles that lick the anal area cause their owners much anguish. The perianal skin of chronic anal-licking dogs becomes thickened, hyperpigmented, verrucous, and lichenified.

One radical treatment is to overfeed the dog to such an extent that its obesity makes it physically impossible for it to reach the anal area. Then the owner can try to identify and remove the psychogenic cause.

Foot licking is rare when it is not associated with atopy or other hypersensitivities. It is a difficult habit to break.

References

1. Holzworth, J.: Diseases of the Cat: Medicine and Surgery. Vol. I. W. B. Saunders Company, Philadelphia, 1987.
2. Panconesi, E.: Stress and skin diseases: Psychosomatic dermatology. Clin. Dermatol. 2:4, 1984.
3. Pemberton, P. L.: Canine and feline behavior control: progestin therapy. *In* Kirk, R. W., (ed.): Current Veterinary Therapy VIII. W. B. Saunders Company, Philadelphia, 1983.
4. Scott, D. W.: Feline dermatology 1900–1978: a monograph. J.A.A.H.A. 16:331, 1980.
5. Scott, D. W., and Walton, D. K.: Clinical evaluation of a topical treatment for canine acral lick dermatitis. J.A.A.H.A. 20:562, 1984.
6. Walton, D. K.: Psychodermatoses. *In* Kirk, R. W., (ed.): Current Veterinary Therapy IX. W. B. Saunders Company, Philadelphia, 1986, p. 557.
7. White, S. D.: Treatment of acral-lick dermatitis with the endorphin-blocker naltrexone. Ann. Meet. Am. Acad. Vet. Dermatol. Am. Coll. Vet. Dermatol., 1988.

16

Environmental Diseases

Photodermatitis

Electromagnetic radiation comprises a continuous spectrum of wavelengths varying from fractions of angströms (Å) to thousands of meters (m). A useful wavelength is the nanometer (nm) (1 nm equals 10 μ or 10 Å). The ultraviolet (UV) spectrum is of particular importance in dermatology.[6] UV-B (290 to 320 nm) is often referred to as the sunburn, or erythema, spectrum and is about 1000 times more erythemogenic than UV-A. UV-A (320 to 400 nm) is the spectrum associated with photosensitivity reactions.

Photodermatitis is defined as ultraviolet light–induced (UVL–induced) inflammation of the skin. *Phototoxicity* is a dose-related response of all animals to light exposure (e.g., sunburn). *Photosensitivity* implies that the skin has been rendered increasingly susceptible to the damaging effects of UVL. *Photoallergy* is a reaction to a chemical (systemic or topical) and UVL, in which an immune mechanism can be demonstrated. *Photocontact dermatitis* occurs when contactants cause photosensitivity or photoallergy.

The pathogenesis of UVL–induced dermatitis is complex and incompletely understood.[6] Two main mechanisms have been proposed to account for the dermal vascular changes that follow UVL exposure. The diffusion mechanism theory postulates the diffusion of mediators released by UVL–damaged keratinocytes into the dermis. The direct-hit mechanism theory suggests a direct action of UVL on dermal blood vessels. Numerous mediator substances have been studied, including histamine, serotonin, free radicals, and especially prostaglandins and leukotrienes.

SOLAR DERMATITIS

Solar dermatitis occurs from an actinic reaction upon white skin, depigmented skin, or light skin that is not sufficiently covered by hair. The condition develops when such skin is exposed to direct sunshine in the middle of the day (from 10:00 AM to 4:00 PM) in sunny climates. The dermatitis is purely a phototoxic reaction ("sunburn") and has no apparent relationship to a hypersensitivity state. For the sake of discussion, the subject is divided into canine nasal solar dermatitis, feline solar dermatitis, and canine solar dermatitis of the trunk and extremities. The nasal and feline forms are common disease entities and therefore are discussed in the greatest detail.

Canine Nasal Solar Dermatitis

Nasal solar dermatitis is an actinic reaction upon poorly pigmented nasal skin of dogs.[12, 23]

CAUSE AND PATHOGENESIS

This is a phototoxic reaction occurring in poorly pigmented skin. Affected dogs may be born without pigment, or the nose may undergo spontaneous noninflammatory depigmentation (see p. 708).

CLINICAL FEATURES

The lesions are found principally at the junction of the haired and hairless skin of the nose (Figs. 16:1*A,C* and 16:2*A*). Initially, the area that was devoid of pigment becomes erythematous, and alopecia develops. Exudation and crusting are common, and ulceration may appear later (Fig. 16:1*C*). Progress and enlargement of the lesions are evident with the passage of each year but are especially rapid during periods of prolonged exposure to intense sunlight. This may occur in the summer months or during the winter as a result of reflection from snow. If the patient is housed to eliminate exposure to sun, the lesions may heal by regeneration of a thin, fragile epithelium that is devoid of hair, pigment, or glandular structures. Neglect allows these irritative reactions to develop (rarely) into squamous cell carcinomas. Deep ulcers form, and extensive tissues of the nares and nasal tip disappear, exposing unsightly nasal tissues that bleed easily. Sometimes, vertical fissures occur at the nasal tip, dorsal to and involving the nares. Once established, these fissures are often permanent.

DIAGNOSIS

The clinical appearance is typical, and both history and improvement upon removal from sunlight provide circumstantial support for the diagnosis.

In the past, discoid and systemic lupus erythematosus, pemphigus erythematosus, and pemphigus foliaceus with nasal lesions were mistakenly called nasal solar dermatitis. When identification of these autoimmune diseases became possible, some veterinarians began to doubt the existence of nasal solar dermatitis. The disorder does exist, although it is more common in very sunny climates; even there, differentiation must be made accurately. A definitive diagnosis depends on a substantial case history, early age of onset, lesions confined to the nose, histopathologic examination, and negative direct immunofluorescence testing. Skin biopsy should be performed in advanced cases to allow pathologic examination for squamous cell carcinoma.

Histopathology. The early depigmented areas of the nose show fewer melanocytes and less melanin pigment than are seen in normal skin. Following solar radiation, epidermal hyperplasia with intraepidermal edema is observed. Perivascular accumulations of inflammatory cells are seen in the upper dermis, and vascular dilatation is noted in the lower dermis. Ulceration can cause disappearance of the epidermis and even of the dermis and underlying cartilages. In rare advanced cases, activity in the cells of the basal layer is increased, and large, polyhedral tumor cells that invade the dermis and

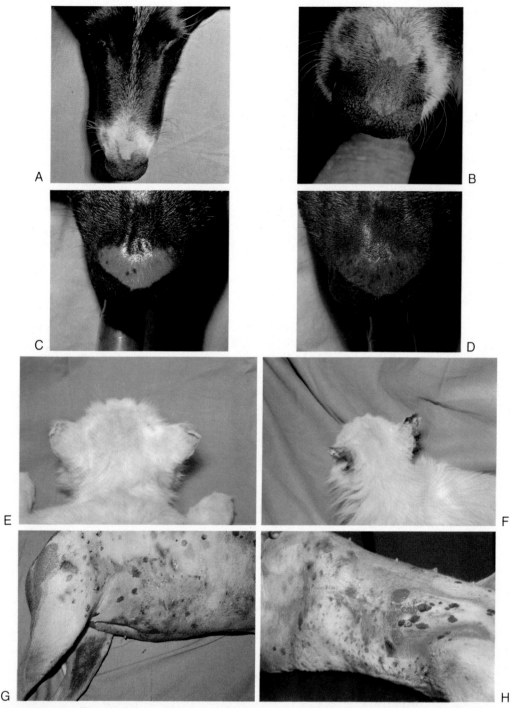

Figure 16:1. Nasal solar dermatitis. *A*, Nose of dog predisposed to nasal solar dermatitis. Tattoo applied at this stage is excellent prophylaxis. *B*, Same nose as in *A*, one year after tattoo. *C*, Hypopigmented nose with erythema from solar radiation. *D*, Same nose as in *C*, immediately after tattooing. Note cosmetic improvement. *E*, Sunburned erythematous margins of the pinnas precede the more serious stage of the disease. Note the characteristic curling of the tips. *F*, This 14-year-old cat had the disease for several years until a squamous cell carcinoma developed on both ears. *G*, Truncal solar dermatitis. Squamous cell carcinoma has developed on posterior abdomen of "sun-loving" brown and white Staffordshire terrier. *H*, Close-up of same dog as in *E*.

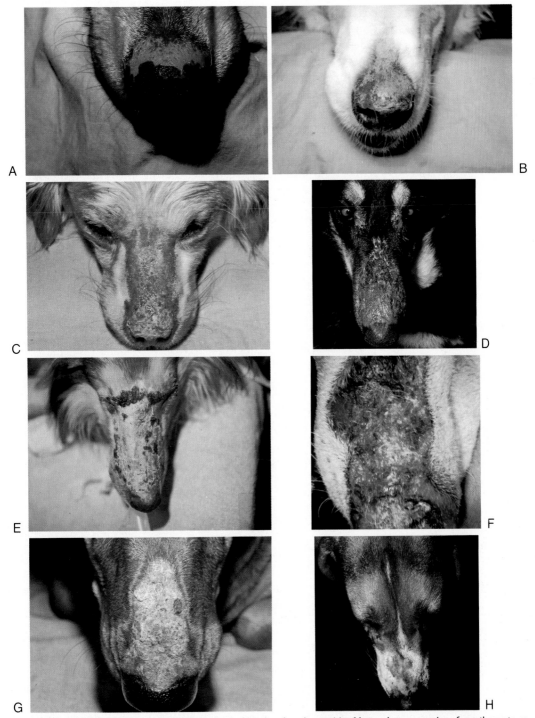

Figure 16:2. Differential diagnosis of nasal lesions. *A,* Nasal solar dermatitis. Note sharp margin of erythematous, sunburned depigmented area. Negative direct immunofluorescent test. *B,* Discoid lupus erythematosus. *C,* Systemic lupus erythematosus. Note "butterfly pattern." *D,* Nasal folliculitis and furunculosis has sudden onset and rapid response to proper therapy. *E,* Nasal dermatitis as result of neomycin sensitivity. Cessation of topical neomycin ointment treatment, which had been used for 18 months, and daily soaks with Burow's solution resulted in prompt healing. *F,* Nasal abrasion resulting from automobile trauma. Sudden onset and sharp margins are differential features. Complete, prompt healing follows conservative treatment. *G,* Typical case of *Microsporum gypseum* dermatophytosis probably resulting from "rooting" in ground is suggestive of nasal solar dermatitis. *H, Trichophyton mentagrophytes* infection in a coonhound following a racoon bite wound.

subcutaneous tissue are formed. A squamous cell carcinoma forms, and cords of neoplastic cells invade the tissue to the level of the nasal cartilage.

Differential Diagnosis. A knowledge of the numerous causes of nasal lesions is required before a definitive diagnosis of nasal solar dermatitis can be made.[8] There are many causes of the condition other than the nasal dermatoses pictured in Figures 16:1 and 16:2. The following are the main conditions that must be differentiated.

Discoid lupus erythematosus is an autoimmune disease that is more severe and may involve an area larger than nasal solar dermatitis (Fig. 16:2B) (see p. 526). It occurs in all climates, although sunshine exacerbates the lesions. Histopathologic findings are typical, and the direct immunofluorescence test will be positive with fluorescence at the dermoepidermal junction. Discoid lupus erythematosus is *the* most common cause of nasal dermatitis in dogs.

Systemic lupus erythematosus may have nasal lesions but may also have other severe dermatologic and systemic lesions; therefore, it should not be mistaken for nasal solar dermatitis. The skin lesions of systemic lupus erythematosus may involve the face, forming a so-called butterfly pattern (Fig. 16:2C).

Dermatomyositis is a disease of Shetland sheepdogs and collies, accompanied by nasal, facial, and extremity lesions that can resemble nasal solar dermatitis (see p. 668). The histopathology shows hydropic degeneration of basilar cells and subepidermal clefts and vesicles, with a negative direct immunofluorescence test.

Pemphigus erythematosus and foliaceus may have vesicular or pustular, erosive and crusted lesions of the face and nose, which may have been diagnosed as nasal solar dermatitis. However, histopathologic findings, direct immunofluorescence testing, and the presence of other lesions on haired portions of the body should differentiate these disorders.

Plastic dish dermatitis can cause hypopigmentation and severe erythema of the nose. However, there is no ulceration of the planum nasale.

Nasal folliculitis and furunculosis due to bacterial infection or dermatophytosis has a sudden, acute onset and rarely affects the planum nasale (Fig. 16:2D). With folliculitis and furunculosis, skin lesions *begin* in the haired skin and may progress to involve the planum nasale.

Tumors. Basal cell tumors, squamous cell carcinomas, mycosis fungoides, and fibrosarcomas (see Fig. 20:27G) can occur in the nasal regions of dogs in the absence of solar dermatitis. History, clinical course, and biopsy are means of differentiation.

Topical hypersensitivity to drugs (Fig. 16:2E), *fixed drug eruption, trauma* (Fig. 16:2F), *candidiasis, dermatophytosis* (Fig. 16:2G,H), *aspergillosis, other mycoses,* and *leishmaniasis* must also be considered in the differential diagnosis.

CLINICAL MANAGEMENT

Avoidance of sun exposure is the most important prophylactic therapeutic factor. During the period from 10:00 AM to 4:00 PM, the dog should be kept indoors or in the shade as much as possible. Systemic topical corticosteroids during the early treatment period help to heal eroded surface lesions. Systemic antibiotic therapy may be needed if secondary bacterial infection occurs.

Sunscreen agents (containing para-aminobenzoic acid [PABA]) can be used but must be massaged into the tissue. This may be especially helpful if the dog must be exposed to the sun on special occasions, such as hunting or walking during the day. A black felt marking pen may be used to mark the nasal tip and help to shield the skin from the sun. Its effectiveness has never been confirmed.

Tattooing with black ink is the treatment of choice. It has two uses. First, the tattooed skin seems to be less susceptible to solar irritation. Although, admittedly, the ink is in the upper dermis and not in the epidermis, clinical experience shows that the actinic reaction is reduced. Second, the cosmetic improvement is enthusiastically welcomed by the dog's owner (Fig. 16:1B,D).

The tattoo ink can be applied with a tattoo vibrating machine, a hypodermic needle, or a Mizzi jet.[12] If a hypodermic needle is used, the ink is carefully injected with a 25-gauge, five-eighths-inch needle and a tuberculin syringe. Naturally, general anesthesia should be used, and the ulcers must first be healed. It may be necessary to repeat the tattoo procedure in 30 to 60 days to cover any remaining hypopigmented spots. Annual "touch-up" tattoos are needed if the depigmented area enlarges. Ideally, the tattoo procedure should be applied to young dogs *before* the disease progresses.

Allergic reactions to tattoo ink are rare but have occurred as severe local edema, which responds well to systemic corticosteroids. Contaminated tattoo ink or a severe allergic reaction can cause mild-to-extensive sloughs of nasal tissue.

Neglected patients that have developed squamous cell carcinoma have a poor prognosis.

Feline Solar Dermatitis

Feline solar dermatitis is a chronic actinic dermatitis of the white ears and, occasionally, the eyelids, nose, and lips of cats, which is caused by repeated sun exposure.[10, 28] It can develop into a squamous cell carcinoma.

CAUSE AND PATHOGENESIS

The disease occurs in white cats or in colored cats with white ears. Blue-eyed white cats are most susceptible. Actinic damage to the ear tip occurs from repeated sunburn and exposure to solar UV waves of the 290 to 320 nm unit band. This erythema-producing band of sunlight is not filtered by thin clouds. The disease occurs mostly in warm, sunny climates such as those of California, Florida, Hawaii, Australia, and South Africa. Sixteen cats with solar dermatitis were examined for heme biosynthesis abnormalities, but none were demonstrated.[13]

CLINICAL FEATURES

The earliest sign is erythema of the margin of the pinna (Fig. 16:1E). The hair is lost in this area, making it even more accessible to solar radiation. There is almost no discomfort to the cat at this stage. In susceptible cats the first lesions can occur as early as 3 months of age. Lesions become progressively more severe each summer. The advancing lesions consist of severe erythema of the pinna, peeling of the skin, and formation of marginal crusts (Fig. 16:3). At this stage cats show pain and will further damage their ears by scratching. The margins of the pinnae may be curled. The margins of the lower eyelids, nostrils, and lips may be affected, especially in white, blue-eyed cats. A

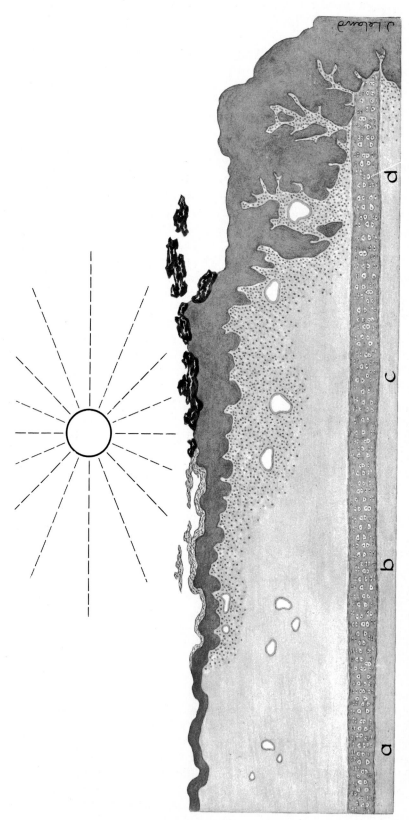

Figure 16:3. Feline solar dermatitis dermogram. *A,* Normal skin and cartilage of the ear's pinna. *B,* Sunburned skin showing mild acanthosis, scaling, and vascular dilatation. *C,* With increasing solar radiation, the skin responds with more acanthosis, inflammation, hyperemia, and crusting. *D,* Squamous cell carcinoma formation results from continued actinic effects of susceptible skin. Masses of neoplastic epidermal cells invade the dermis to the level of the cartilage. Skin and cartilage are eventually replaced by the squamous cell carcinoma.

squamous cell carcinoma develops in some cases on the ears, and in rare cases there has been metastasis to the regional lymph nodes. Carcinomatous change may occur, usually after 6 years of age, but sometimes as early as 3 years. The squamous cell carcinoma appears as an ulcerating, hemorrhagic, and locally invasive lesion. It is partially crusted and in advanced cases destroys the pinna (Fig. 16:1F).

DIAGNOSIS

A definitive diagnosis of feline solar dermatitis can be made from the clinical appearance, the color of the cat, and the history. Biopsy of the lesion is valuable in order to determine whether the disease is in the inflammatory phase or whether it has developed into a squamous cell carcinoma. However, by the time significant ulceration has occurred, carcinoma is almost always present.

Histopathology. A biopsy can be performed to determine if the lesion is premalignant or has already developed into a squamous cell carcinoma. Histopathologic study shows that in the early stages superficial perivascular dermatitis (spongiotic, hyperplastic) is present. Basophilic degeneration ("solar elastosis") of the superficial dermal connective tissue may be seen. With the formation of squamous cell carcinoma, the epidermal surface is ulcerated and the dermis is invaded by nests of polyhedral epithelial tumor cells. In a disorganized manner, these cells resemble the stratum spinosum. Their nuclei vary moderately in size, and mitotic figures are frequent. In advanced cases the masses of tumor tissue extend to the level of the cartilage.

Differential Diagnosis. Severe ear mite infestation or feline scabies will sometimes cause an erythema similar to that of early solar dermatitis; however, mite eradication allows the lesion to heal. Fight wounds on the ear, especially those with crusting and granulation, resemble solar dermatitis. They heal nicely, however, with antibiotic therapy. Frostbite and cold agglutinin disease result in marginal ear dermatitis and curling, in which case the history of occurrence in cold weather is diagnostic.

Pemphigus and systemic lupus erythematosus often severely affect the ears and nose. However, other body lesions and illness differentiate these conditions easily from feline solar dermatitis.

CLINICAL MANAGEMENT

Affected cats should be kept out of the sunshine from 10:00 AM to 4:00 PM when the ultraviolet rays are most damaging. During the summer, the ears should be protected with topical sunscreen lotions or a solution containing PABA. Once early lesions develop, serious consideration should be given to a cosmetic amputation of the ear tips. This merely "rounds off" the ears, removes the thinly haired tips, and allows hair to cover and protect the pinna. Results are usually excellent, cosmetically and prophylactically.

Once a carcinoma has developed, surgical excision of the affected portion of the pinna is necessary. Radical amputation of the pinna is necessary for advanced cases, but the cosmetic result is surprisingly satisfactory after the hair has regrown. In amputation it is important to achieve good skin-to-skin apposition over the cartilage so that hair will cover the margin.

Beta-carotene and canthaxanthin (25-mg doses of active carotenoids) were administered orally to treat feline solar dermatitis.[13] Only the most severely affected cats failed to respond. Carotenoids have been used to treat the photosensitivity associated with erythropoietic protoporphyria in human beings.[6] Carotenoids are thought to quench the triplet state of singlet oxygen and free radicals and possibly to form a lipid-carotene complex in skin that absorbs the damaging solar radiation.

> *Early amputation of the pinna saves further trouble, is usually curative, and provides surprisingly good cosmetic results.*

Canine Solar Dermatitis of the Trunk and Extremities

While the nose and ears are the areas most exposed and are therefore most susceptible to actinic damage, other regions of the body can also be affected. A combination of factors are necessary for sun damage to occur. First, the skin must be unpigmented or poorly pigmented. Second, only a sparse hair coat covers the skin, allowing the ultraviolet rays of the sun to reach the epidermis. Third, the areas so predisposed must be regularly and frequently exposed to the sun. This occurs in dogs that like to "sunbathe" or that are confined to areas where no sun shelter is available during the middle of the day, especially if the ground cover is highly reflective. As is true of the other types of solar dermatitis, the chance of actinic disease is increased in sunny climates.

Breeds predisposed to truncal solar dermatitis include the dalmatian and white bull terriers.[19, 23] The flank and abdomen are the areas most severely affected (Fig. 16:1G,H). At first, regular sunburning occurs and the affected areas are erythematous and scaly. Running a hand over affected areas of skin may produce a bumpy feeling, as the white areas of skin are thickened, while the black areas are normal. At this stage, biopsy reveals variable degrees of superficial perivascular dermatitis with necrotic keratinocytes. Superficial dermal fibrosis may be prominent. Solar elastosis may be seen. After two or more summers, the sunburned areas become thicker and develop erosion, ulceration, crusting, and comedones, and they occasionally develop necrosis, fistulae, and scarring. At this stage, a skin biopsy may reveal follicular cysts, pyogranulomatous inflammation, and premalignant actinic keratosis. Finally, a squamous cell carcinoma can develop, especially if the dog continues to be exposed to direct sunlight. Such squamous cell carcinomas should be removed surgically, and the procedure should be repeated if necessary. There is always a danger of metastasis, to the regional lymph nodes and internally. Solar dermatitis of the distal portions of the legs and the paws and of the bridge of the nose is less common. The tip of the tail, especially in dalmatians, can be affected if it has lost most or all of its hair. In such cases, amputation of several inches of the tail is always a good alternative treatment.

Therapy involves photoprotection by keeping the animal out of the sun and by using topical sunscreens where practical. It has been reported that β-carotene (30 mg orally BID for 30 days, then SID for life) in combination with anti-inflammatory doses of prednisone or prednisolone, is effective in early cases.[19]

Actinic Keratosis

Actinic keratoses may be seen in dogs and cats, and are premalignant epithelial dysplasias (see p. 941).

Irritant Contact Dermatitis

Contact dermatitis is an inflammatory skin reaction caused by direct contact with an offending substance.[6, 21, 23]

CAUSE AND PATHOGENESIS

The disease is divided into two types, primary irritant contact dermatitis and contact hypersensitivity (see p. 464).

Primary irritant contact dermatitis causes cutaneous inflammation in most exposed dogs and cats, without requiring an allergic response. A number of primary irritants such as soaps, detergents, weed and insecticidal sprays, fertilizers, strong acids and alkalies, and flea collars are potential causative agents. Although most primary irritants are chemicals, similar skin lesions can be produced by thermal injuries, solar overexposure, and contact with living organisms.

Primary irritants are often divided into absolute and relative types. Absolute primary irritants are corrosive substances such as strong acids and alkalies, which injure the skin immediately following the first contact. Relative primary irritants are less toxic, commonly used substances such as soaps, detergents, and solvents, which require repeated contact to cause injury.

CLINICAL FEATURES

Irritating substances come in contact with and may produce dermatitis in areas where the hair coat is thin or missing. The abdomen, chest, axillae, flanks, interdigital spaces, legs, perianal area, ventral surface of the tail, and eyelids are the most susceptible areas (Fig. 16:4A–D). Only when the offending agent is liquid or aerosol are hairy regions involved. The distribution pattern of flea collar dermatitis is illustrated in Figure 16:5.

Patches of erythema and papules represent primary lesions (Fig. 16:4A,B). Vesicles are rarely present in dogs and cats. As the disease progresses, crusts, excoriations, hyperpigmentation, and lichenification occur. Intense pruritus may promote severe self-trauma in the form of scratching and biting. Pyotraumatic dermatitis and eventual ulceration may obliterate primary lesions.

Single episodes are common in primary irritant contact dermatitis, as in scrotal involvement from soap that is not rinsed off (Fig. 16:4D). Seasonal recurrence results from exposure to plants, lawn fertilizer, herbicides, and salted roads (Fig. 16:4A).

DIAGNOSIS

Diagnosis is made on the basis of patch testing, an accurate history, and elimination and provocative exposure testing.

In most clinical cases, the histopathologic changes of primary irritant contact dermatitis consist of nondiagnostic superficial perivascular dermatitis (spongiotic, hyperplastic). The exact appearance depends on the stage of contact dermatitis and the effects of secondary infection and excoriation. Neutrophils or mononuclear cells may predominate in a given case.

Differential diagnosis should include a number of disorders. One of these, atopy, includes many features of contact dermatitis but is differentiated by evidence of paw licking, face rubbing, or generalized pruritus, and by the use

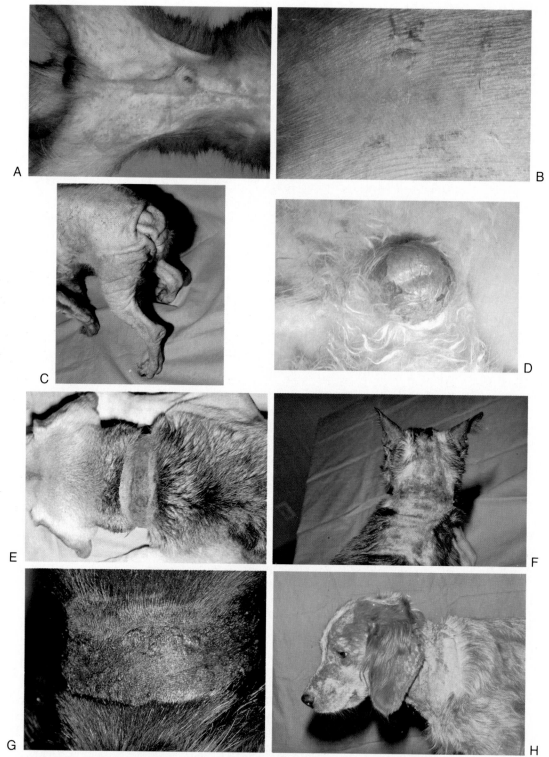

Figure 16:4. Irritant contact dermatitis. *A*, Pruritic papules on glabrous abdomen of keeshond from contact with irritant plant materials in field. *B*, Local erythema and superficial exfoliation on abdomen from contact irritant. *C*, Overtreatment dermatitis (repeated irritating topical medication). *D*, Irritant contact dermatitis affecting the delicate scrotal skin. *E*, Acute erythema, erosion due to flea collar dermatitis. *F*, Erythema, papules, and erosions spreading on head and neck on cat with flea collar dermatitis. *G*, Chronic scaling and crusts. Seven months after onset of flea collar dermatitis. *H*, Severe generalized lesions of flea collar dermatitis. Head and shoulders are covered with papules, crusts, and scales.

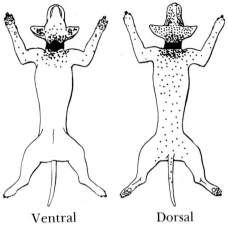

Ventral   Dorsal

Figure 16:5. Flea collar dermatitis distribution pattern. The skin around the neck is always the most severely affected and the last to heal. This is the diagnostic clue. In generalized cases, other parts of the body can be affected and are shown in the diagram by dots. The more dense the number of dots, the more intense is the irritation. (From Muller, G. H.: Flea collar dermatitis in animals. J.A.V.M.A. *157*:1616, 1970.)

of intradermal skin testing. Food hypersensitivity may produce similar clinical signs and can only be documented with a hypoallergenic diet and a rechallenge with the normal diet. Canine scabies may produce a ventrally distributed, severely pruritic papular dermatitis. In scabies cases, peripheral lymph nodes are enlarged, skin scrapings may be positive, and the response to therapy is diagnostic. Staphylococcal folliculitis may also produce a ventrally oriented, pruritic, papulocrustous dermatitis. Cytologic examination suggests the diagnosis, and appropriate antibiotic therapy is curative. Dermatophytosis has more circumscribed, circular lesions and fewer diffuse patches. Pruritus usually is minimal. Culture or microscopic examination reveal fungal elements. Seborrheic dermatitis is usually chronic, with more scaling and variable pruritus. Solar dermatitis characteristically affects hairless, exposed anatomic areas, such as the nose and ears, in actinically predisposed individuals. Suspected drug eruptions can often be documented by finding a history of drug administration. Insect bites are accompanied by the sudden appearance of localized edema or urticarial wheals. The "id" reaction to dermatophytes, especially *Trichophyton mentagrophytes,* may mimic contact dermatitis and is a very common reaction in humans.

CLINICAL MANAGEMENT

Find the offending substance and remove it.

The difficult task of discovering and eliminating offending substances depends on the correlation of a detailed history and a careful examination of the environment of the dog. Soap, flea collars, grasses, pollens, insecticides, petrolatum, paint, wool, carpets, rubber, and wood preservatives are examples of contact irritants. If the location of the initial inflammation can be correlated with an agent that came in contact with that area, the cause can sometimes be found.

When the contactant cannot be found, relief depends on systemic and topical therapy. Corticosteroids can be administered systemically for 1 to several weeks. They must often be repeated during recurrences. Topical treatment may include wet dressings (Burow's solution), baths, or emollients (Nivea Creme or lotion), and corticosteroid ointments, creams, or aerosols, depending on the stage of the eruption (see Chapter 4).

FLEA COLLAR DERMATITIS

Flea collar dermatitis is an especially obvious contact dermatitis that occurs in some dogs and cats wearing a polyvinyl chloride plastic collar that is impregnated with an insecticidal chemical.[22, 23, 28]

Skin lesions start in areas of the skin in close contact with the collar. Circular erythematous patches develop. There may be edema, erosions, ulceration, and even a purulent discharge (Fig. 16:4E,F). In some cases, the lesions spread to the head and neck and become generalized over much of the body (Fig. 16:4H). Later in the course of the condition, the skin becomes thickened and crusted, and exfoliation of the superficial epidermis may occur (Fig. 16:4G).

> *Advanced flea collar dermatitis often takes months to heal, even after the collar is removed.*

CLINICAL MANAGEMENT

The flea collar is removed, and affected areas should be clipped. Wet dressings should be applied to all crusted lesions every 4 to 6 hours, using lukewarm water or Burow's solution. Topical corticosteroid ointment is applied twice a day. In cases complicated by pyoderma, a bacterial culture and antibiotic sensitivity test should be performed; treatment with the appropriate systemic antibiotics should follow. The clinician must always examine the external ear canals and must treat for otitis. When severe systemic signs occur, one should hospitalize and treat for toxicosis with supportive therapy (intravenous fluids and systemic corticosteroids in large doses).

PREVENTION

The flea collar is applied loosely enough to permit two to three fingers to be inserted easily under the collar. Tightness is a major cause of flea collar dermatitis. Owners should inspect the throat and neck of all dogs and cats wearing flea collars every few days. One should avoid using similar insecticides in other forms (powders, dips, vermifuges, etc.) in animals wearing flea collars.

Burns

Superficial and deep burns are often complicated by bacterial infections and sepsis, and they present a dermatologic healing problem.

CAUSE AND PATHOGENESIS

Most severe burns seen in small animal practice are caused by heat. The causative agents are varied and can be boiling water, electric hot pads, dog driers, the underside of car motors, or fire. The full thickness of the skin is often burned.

Burns of dogs and cats have been categorized into two types: *partial-thickness burns* and *full-thickness burns*.[20] In *partial-thickness burns*, only incomplete destruction of the skin occurs, so the chance of re-epithelialization is greater. In *full-thickness burns*, there is complete destruction of all parts of the skin (including the adnexa and nerves), and re-epithelialization depends on migration of epidermal cells from the edges of the burns. The human classification of first, second, and third degree burns depends on the extent of blistering, which is not seen in dogs and cats.

The pathophysiologic events observable in the burned patient result from three proximate causes: the effects of thermal injury on the skin, the effects of heat injury on the blood vessels and the blood elements, and the general metabolic disturbances.[6, 7, 20] Loss of the skin as a protective barrier opens the underlying tissue to invasive infection. While microcirculation is restored within 48 hours to areas of partial-thickness injury, the full-thickness burn is characterized by complete occlusion of the local vascular supply. The avascular, necrotic tissue of the full-thickness burn, with impaired delivery of humoral and cellular defense mechanisms, provides an excellent medium for bacterial proliferation, with the ever-present potential for life-threatening sepsis. Initial colonization of the burn wound surface by gram-positive organisms shift by the third to fifth day after the burn to an invasive gram-negative flora (especially *Pseudomonas aeruginosa*).

CLINICAL FEATURES

Immediately after the burn, the hair coat may hide the trauma and the owner may only be aware of the animal's apparent pain and its accompanying behavioral changes. When the animal is presented to the veterinarian for treatment, the skin is often hard and dry. Infection causes a purulent discharge and sometimes an unpleasant odor. Large areas of necrotic skin may slough and reveal a deep, suppurating wound (Fig. 16:6A). If the skin is débrided and sutured, temporary closure may be achieved (Fig. 16:6B). However, the sutured area almost always sloughs, leaving a large, raw surface (Fig. 16:6C).

If 25 per cent of the body is involved in the burn, there are usually systemic manifestations. These can be septicemia, shock, renal failure, anemia, and respiratory difficulty.

DIAGNOSIS

The diagnosis is easy if the client has observed the accidental burning. However, if the animal was not observed during the occurrence of the burn, the resulting wound and slough can present a diagnostic puzzle. In the case of a dog drier burn, the condition may not be discovered for several days.

CLINICAL MANAGEMENT

For minor and major burns, the initial wound management, following evaluation and stabilization as needed, is the same.[6, 7, 20, 23] Regardless of the location or the depth of the wound, removal of all debris and loose skin and stripping of the necrotic epidermis are imperative. The wound is thoroughly cleansed with povidone-iodine and débrided as needed. Daily hydrotherapy is

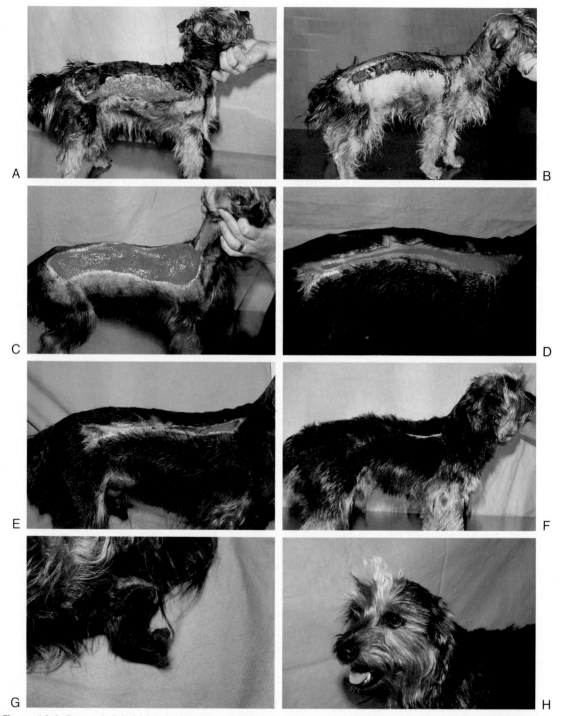

Figure 16:6. Burns. *A,* Full-thickness thermal burn in a silky terrier, with sloughing and infection. *B,* Appearance after debridement and suturing. *C,* After slough of sutured area and silver sulfadiazine cream dressings. *D,* Healing wound after bacterial infection was treated with nitrofurazone (Furacin Soluble Dressing) and, later, silver sulfadiazine cream under occlusive dressing. *E,* Two months after *A. F,* Complete closure three months after *A.* Later, hair coat covered most of the scar. *G,* Full-thickness burn and slough of pinna of the same dog. *H,* Left ear after pinna slough surgery and healing.

utilized for complete cleansing of all burn wounds and sharp débridement of loose, necrotic eschar. Once all burn wounds have been adequately cleansed and débrided, local care consists of the application of topical antibiotics. Occlusive burn wound dressings are avoided because of their tendency to produce a closed wound with bacterial proliferation and to delay healing. Nonocclusive dressings, changed frequently, can be useful in certain cases. The wound should be cleaned two or three times daily and the topical antibiotic should be reapplied.

The most acceptable topical antibiotic found to date is silver sulfadiazine (Silvadene). It is a broad-spectrum antibacterial agent with satisfactory eschar penetration, and it is painless and nonstaining. The often-used nitrofurazone (Furacin) has no place in the treatment of major burns. It has a narrow range of antibacterial activity and does *not* penetrate eschar in sufficient quantity. Systemic antibiotics are *not* effective for preventing local burn wound infections and may permit the growth of resistant organisms.

Suturing, as shown in Figure 16:6B, is seldom necessary, since the sutured area almost always sloughs. Cleansing and débriding (preferably under sedation or general anesthesia) is the initial treatment of choice.

Burns heal slowly, so the owner must be informed that many weeks may be required to allow the wound to close by granulation (Fig. 16:6D–F). If *full-thickness burns* occur on the ear (Fig. 16:6G), amputation of the pinna is usually needed. However, the results in long-haired dogs can be very satisfactory (Fig. 16:6H).

In deep burns, anticipate sepsis and a lengthy, costly healing process.

Frostbite

CAUSE AND PATHOGENESIS

Frostbite affects the tips of the ears of cats and dogs or the tip of the tail, the digits, or the scrotum of dogs—places where the hair covering is sparse and where peripheral circulation may be poor.[23, 28] Affected animals have usually been left outdoors (accidentally?) for many hours in subzero (°F) weather or have recently moved from a warm climate to a cold one and have not had a chance to become acclimated.

CLINICAL FEATURES

While frozen, the skin appears pale and is hypoesthetic and cool to the touch. After thawing, there may be mild erythema, pain, and eventual scaliness of the skin. In mild cases the hair of affected areas may turn white (see Fig. 16:11H). Later, the tips and margins of the pinnae may curl. In severe cases, the skin becomes necrotic and sloughs (Fig. 16:7). Healing proceeds slowly; but if the tips of the ears are lost, the remaining pinna of the ear has a rounded contour that usually is so cosmetically acceptable as to be unnoticed. Often the lesions look similar to burns.

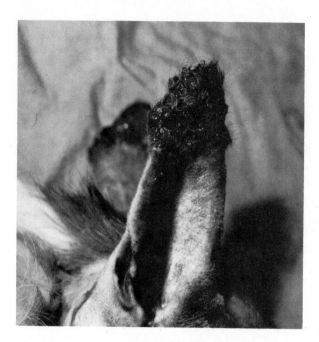

Figure 16:7. Necrosis, ulceration, and crusting on the ear tip of a dog with frostbite.

CLINICAL MANAGEMENT

One should rapidly thaw frozen tissues by the *gentle* application of warm water. *Tissues must be handled gently.* With mild frostbite resulting in erythema and scaliness, a bland protective ointment such as petroleum jelly (Vaseline) or cod-liver-oil ointment is applied. Healing is rapid. In severe cases with necrosis, affected tissue should be amputated, but not too early, since more tissue may actually be viable than is initially suspected (Fig. 16:7). Once frozen, tissues may be more susceptible to subsequent damage by the cold. Ear tips that are permanently scarred and alopecic could be treated beneficially by plastic surgery. This should remove the hairless portion and leave the remaining pinna well covered with hair for protection from the cold. Every effort should be made to keep these patients in protected quarters during cold weather.

Miscellaneous Causes of Necrosis and Sloughing of the Extremities

There are many well-documented causes of peripheral cutaneous necrosis in small animals, including solar dermatitis, frostbite, severe burns, caustic contactants, cold agglutinin disease, systemic lupus erythematosus, vasculitis, snakebite, septicemia, and various forms of vascular insufficiency.[5] There are also some rare, often poorly documented or poorly understood associations.

It has been reported that dogs may rarely develop peripheral necrosis with *ergotism* and *leptospirosis*.[16] Dry gangrene of the pinnae was reported in cats fed decomposed scallops.[10] Peripheral necrosis and sloughing has been reported in dogs and cats with disseminated intravascular coagulation.[10, 30] Necrosis and sloughing of the digits have been reported as sequelae of hepatitis in dogs.[18] Necrosis and sloughing of the digits has also been seen in puppies fed highly concentrated formulas containing evaporated milk.[14, 29]

Snake Bite

Two subfamilies of venomous snakes are indigenous to the United States: Crotalidae and Elapidae. Crotalidae, commonly called pit vipers, include the copperhead, cottonmouth moccasin, and rattlesnake. One or more species of this subfamily are found in virtually all of the 48 contiguous states. Elapidae are represented in this country by two genera of coral snakes, which are found only in the southeastern and southwestern United States.

Snake venoms contain many toxic polypeptides, low molecular weight proteins, and enzymes.[17, 26, 32] In general, venoms produce alterations in the resistance and integrity of blood vessels, changes in blood cells and blood coagulation mechanisms, direct or indirect changes in cardiac dynamics, alterations of nervous system function, depression of respiration, and necrosis at the site of envenomation. The severity of a poisonous snake bite depends on the type and size of the snake, the amount of venom injected in relation to the victim's weight, the site of venom injection, and the time interval between the venom injection and the onset of medical therapy.

Most snake bites occur during spring and summer. The face and legs are most commonly involved. Bites around the face are potentially serious because of rapid swelling and respiratory embarrassment. Cutaneous manifestations of snake bites include rapid, progressive edema, which usually obliterates the fang marks, pain, and occasionally local hemorrhage. This area may progress to necrosis and sloughing.

The treatment of snake bite remains one of the most controversial areas in medical practice.[17, 26, 32] In general, treatment should be directed toward the: (1) prevention or retardation of local venom absorption, (2) removal of local venom, (3) neutralization of venom locally and systemically, and (4) prevention of the onset of local and systemic complications. Techniques such as tourniquets, incision and suction, cryotherapy, corticosteroid therapy, and antivenin therapy are shrouded in controversy. The reader is referred to recent references for specifics.[17, 26]

Foreign Bodies

Foreign bodies occasionally cause skin lesions in dogs and cats. Most commonly, the foreign material is of plant origin (seeds and awns, wood slivers). One of the most notorious plants in the United States in this regard is the foxtail (*Hordeum jubatum*).[2]

In a retrospective study of 182 cases of grass awn migration in dogs and cats in California, younger dogs (increased activity) and hunting and working breeds (increased exposure) were at greater risk.[2] The most common site of grass awn localization was the external ear canal (51 per cent of the cases), with the other common cutaneous sites being the interdigital webs. Lesions consist of nodules, abscesses, and draining tracts. Secondary bacterial infection is exceedingly common.

The only effective treatment is surgical removal of the foreign body.

Arteriovenous Fistula

An arteriovenous fistula is a vascular abnormality, defined as a direct communication between an adjacent artery and vein that bypasses the capillary circulation.[1] Arteriovenous fistulae may be congenital or acquired, and are rarely reported in dogs and cats.[1, 3, 9, 15, 31] Most clinically relevant cutaneous arteriovenous fistulae are acquired, and most of these result from penetrating wounds or blunt trauma, although they may also be secondary to infection, neoplasia, and iatrogenic factors (surgical dewclaw procedures, injections of irritating substances). Recurrent peripheral arteriovenous fistula has been reported in a cat with hyperthyroidism.[9]

Acquired arteriovenous fistulae most commonly involve the paws (following dewclaw procedures, following injury) and the neck (secondary to neoplasms), but they have involved the legs, the flank, and the pinnae. Affected areas show persistent or recurrent edema, pain, and, occasionally, secondary infection and hemorrhage. Superficial blood vessels may be distinct and tortuous. Arteriovenous fistulae are generally characterized by pulsating vessels, palpable thrills, and continuous machinery murmurs.

Diagnosis is based on the history, physical examination, and demonstration of the arteriovenous fistula by contrast radiography. Therapy includes surgical extirpation of the fistula or, in some instances, amputation of the affected part.

Myospherulosis

Myospherulosis is a rare granulomatous reaction thought to be due to the interaction of ointments, antibiotics, or endogenous fat with erythrocytes.[11] It is associated with small saclike structures (parent bodies) filled with endobodies (spherules) and has been reported in humans and dogs. The condition has been induced experimentally in laboratory animals. Myospherulosis is most commonly reported following injections of oil medicaments or after the topical application of oily products in open wounds.

Patients are usually presented for solitary subcutaneous or dermal nodules, which may or may not be discharging.[11, 29] Histologic examination reveals several solid and cystic masses. The walls of the cystic area and most solid areas are composed of histiocytes with abundant vacuolated cytoplasm. Histiocytes surround parent bodies (30 to 350 μm) composed of thin eosinophilic walls and filled with homogeneous eosinophilic, 3- to 7-μm spherules (Fig. 16:8). Parent bodies and spherules do not stain with periodic acid-Schiff (PAS), Gomori's methenamine silver (GMS), or Ziehl-Neelsen stains but are positive for endogenous peroxidase (diaminobenzidine reaction) and hemoglobin, indicating that the spherules are erythrocytes.

The only effective treatment is surgical excision.

Thallium Toxicosis

(Thallium Poisoning)

Thallium is a cumulative, general cell poison that may produce skin lesions or systemic toxicity.[10, 23, 28]

CAUSE AND PATHOGENESIS

The common use of thallium as a rodenticide and roach poison in the United States has been terminated because of its toxicity. *Thallium toxicosis is*

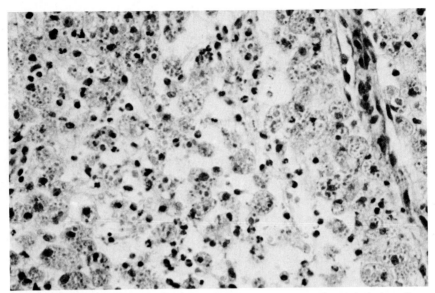

Figure 16:8. Myospherulosis. Macrophages containing many intracytoplasmic inclusions (fragments of erythrocytes).

probably of historic interest only, although cases are still occasionally recognized in the United States.[25] With doses over 20 to 40 mg/lb of body weight, the fatality rate is 100 per cent and the clinical signs are those of damage to the central nervous system and circulatory system. Nervousness, convulsions, tremors, salivation, weakness, and paralysis, together with a rapid weak pulse, are seen. Reliable early signs of less acute toxicity include vomiting, hemorrhagic gastroenteritis, polydipsia, pyrexia, and "brick-red" mucous membranes. Colic and dyspnea are often apparent. Smaller doses of thallium may be cumulative and may produce the subacute or chronic syndrome described. Even with the best of care, the mortality rate is extremely high (70 per cent); therefore, the prognosis is poor. Thallium is rapidly absorbed through the oral and intestinal mucosa and through the skin. It is mainly excreted in the urine but may persist in various tissues for up to 3 months. Thallium and potassium move together through cell walls and are excreted together in the urine. Therefore, increased turnover of one substance increases the secretion of the other. Cystine and methionine seem to protect against the alopecic and toxic effects of thallium (in rats).

Researchers emphasize that thallium poisoning may be commonly unrecognized in cats that do not show cutaneous involvement.[10] Although the syndrome with skin lesions is classic and highly suggestive, cases of poisoning without skin lesions exhibit multisystemic problems that require a detailed case work-up and laboratory support for accurate diagnosis. Even with intensive supportive care, only 19 per cent of the feline patients in one study recovered; thus, a poor prognosis must be given.[10] Many of the antidotal drugs suggested for other species are highly toxic to cats, and consequently the clinician is further handicapped in treating this species.

CLINICAL FEATURES

Thallium poisoning is divided into two syndromes. In acute toxicity, the onset of signs is delayed 24 to 36 hours after ingestion, but the length of the course until death is only 4 to 5 days. In the chronic syndrome, 7 to 21 days may pass before signs appear, and the course may extend to 3 weeks. Treatment should last 7 to 21 days, depending on the severity of the case. Lesions of the chronic form show ulceration and hyperemia of mucous membranes, and there is occasional vomiting, diarrhea, and depression. Often the first sign (12 to 21 days after ingestion) is alopecia accompanied by erythema and necrosis of the skin. Feline cutaneous lesions are illustrated in Figure 16:9A–G. These lesions are located on the axillae, the ears, the posterior abdomen and genitalia, and the interdigital frictional areas and at mucocutaneous junctions (Fig. 16:9H,I). The lesions are slowly reversible in some cases. Other lesions include nephrosis, polyneuritis, and necrosis of skeletal and myocardial muscle fibers. In addition, there may be inflammation and necrosis of the liver, tongue, pancreas, and other organs.

DIAGNOSIS

Thallium toxicosis mimics many diseases.

Diagnosis is based on (1) a history showing that thallium baits were available, (2) a positive urine test for thallium—Gabriel's test with rhodamine B is a simple procedure that accurately detects thallium in the dog but may produce false positives in cats, (3) biopsy of skin lesions.

Histopathology. Thallium exerts a local toxic effect on epidermal cells in the process of differentiation leading to keratin formation. Degenerative changes are evident in the hair follicle and in the surface epidermis.[27] The direct insult to the hair follicle is especially noteworthy in anagen hairs; the hair shaft is converted to an amorphous mass, the bulb degenerates, and the hair is lost. Follicular plugging and parakeratosis are prominent.

The surface epidermis shows massive parakeratotic hyperkeratosis and dyskeratosis with vacuolar degeneration of keratinocytes (Fig. 16:10A). Multiple spongiform microabscesses are present in the superficial epidermis and hair follicle outer root sheath (Fig. 16:10B).

The superficial dermis shows edema, vascular dilatation, and extravasation of erythrocytes.

Differential Diagnosis. Differential diagnosis includes arsenic poisoning, organophosphate poisoning, encephalitis, leptospirosis, distemper, gastroenteritis, pancreatitis, bacterial pyoderma, candidiasis, autoimmune dermatoses (pemphigus, pemphigoid, lupus erythematosus), lymphoreticular neoplasia

---

Figure 16:9. Thallium toxicosis. *A*, Early inflammation and crusting of the eyelids and lips of cat with thallium poisoning. *B*, Closer view of the lips, illustrating cracking of the superficial epidermis. *C*, Inflammation and ulceration of the footpads. *D*, The skin of the entire head is affected; the superficial epidermis is loosened and peeling over extensive areas. *E*, After three weeks, the face, ears, and top of the head are bald, but all inflammation has subsided. In this cat and another that recovered, the hair eventually grew in completely. *F*, Ultimately the skin becomes red, ulcerated, and covered with purulent exudate. *G*, In cats that live long enough, the skin anywhere on the body may eventually become affected. The first change is focal cracking and peeling of the thin dry superficial layer of epithelium, with loosening of the hair. *H*, Erythema, alopecia, and erosion of the digits and interdigital spaces. *I*, Severe ulceration and crusting of skin of the nasal region. A purulent exudate is present. (Figures *A* through *G* from Zook, B. C., Holzworth, J., and Thornton, G. W.: Thallium poisoning in cats. J.A.V.M.A. *153*:285, 1968.)

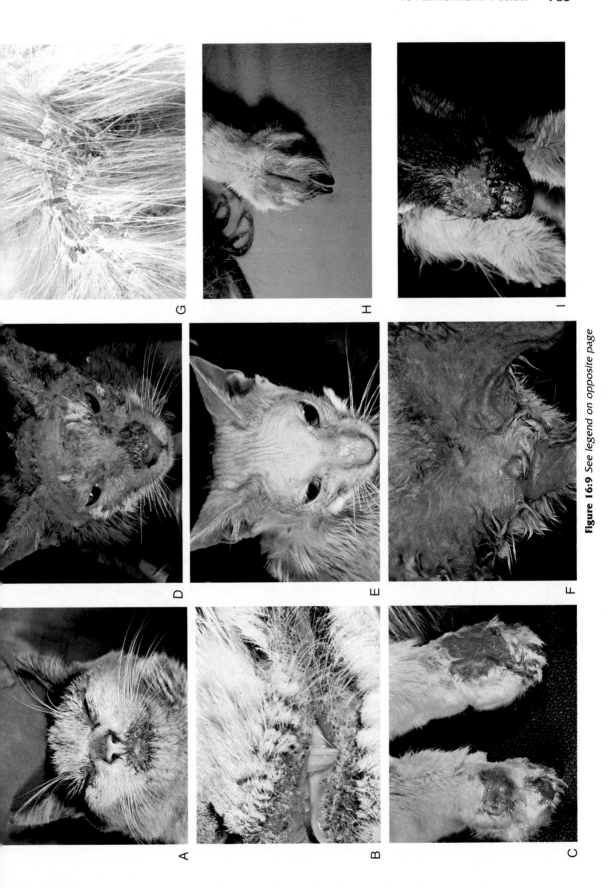

Figure 16:9 *See legend on opposite page*

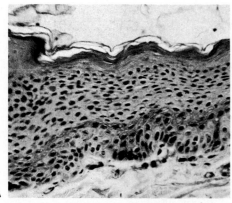

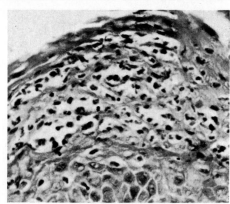

Figure 16:10. Histologic sections of skin from canine axilla. *A,* Note hyperkeratosis and parakeratotic scale, constituting approximately 65 per cent of epidermis. Epidermal cells are vacuolated. (× 195, H & E stain.) *B,* Higher magnification of spongiform abscesses, showing multilocular spaces containing neutrophils (× 360, H & E stain.) (From Schwartzman, R. M., and Kirschbaum, J. O.: The cutaneous histopathology of thallium poisoning. J. Invest. Dermatol. *39:*169, 1962.)

(especially mycosis fungoides), toxic epidermal necrolysis, erythema multiforme, and drug eruption.

CLINICAL MANAGEMENT

The primary objective is to remove thallium from the body.[10, 23] Emetics can be used early in the course. Once absorbed, thallium excretion can be promoted by oral administration of diphenylthiocarbazone (70 mg/kg of body weight TID) or diethyldithiocarbamate (30 mg/kg of body weight TID). Potassium chloride (orally, 2 to 6 gm per day) may help, too. Peritoneal dialysis may be used in early cases. Prussian blue (ferric hexacyanoferrate) may be an effective antidote. It prevents absorption and cyclic reabsorption from the intestinal tract. The substance is said to be relatively nontoxic, and a dosage of 100 mg/kg orally TID has been suggested for dogs and cats.[25] Further research is needed, but this may prove to be the most effective antidote.

Later, the affected skin should be protected with antibiotic ointments and padded bandages. Other supportive treatment may be vitally needed. Fluid injections to encourage renal function (5 per cent dextrose and water), B-complex vitamins, and sodium bicarbonate to combat the acidosis may all be useful.

Arsenic Toxicosis

Arsenic is a general tissue poison that combines with and inactivates sulfhydryl groups in tissue enzymes.[34] Sources of arsenic include herbicides, rodenticides, pesticides, and arsenical medicaments. Signs of arsenic toxicosis vary according to the dose, physical form, route of administration, and composition (organic or inorganic).

Arsenic toxicosis was reported in a mature dog presented for listlessness, anorexia, weight loss, rough coat, swollen muzzle, and necrosis and ulceration of the pinnae, feet, lips, and prepuce.[4] A container of liquid insecticide (44 per cent sodium arsenite) was found to be leaking into the dog's house. Arsenic concentrations were found at toxic levels in the urine, blood, feces, and hair. Bathing the dog and cleaning up its environment resulted in complete remission within 1 month.

Callus and Hygroma

A *callus* is a round or oval hyperkeratotic plaque that develops on the skin or over bony pressure points. In dogs, the elbow and hock are the most common sites. Large breeds are especially susceptible if the dog sleeps on cement, brick, or wood. However, many adult dogs develop varying degrees of callus. Callosities are a normal, protective response to pressure-induced ischemia and inflammation.[23] The callus is hairless and gray and has a wrinkled surface (Figs. 16:11A–D, 16:12, and 16:13). Histologically there is irregular-to-papillated epidermal hyperplasia and orthokeratotic-to-parakeratotic hyperkeratosis. Small follicular cysts are seen in the dermis.

Dog owners are often alarmed when they discover a callus, and they mistake it for ringworm, mange, or some other skin disorder. Actually, most calluses are harmless and require no treatment. Only when they become extremely hyperplastic, ulcerated (Fig. 16:11E), or infected, need therapy be considered. Foam rubber pads, air mattresses, straw beds, carpets, or blankets can make the bed or doghouse a softer place. The breeches illustrated in Figure 16:12 may be useful in reducing excess pressure. In extreme cases, the callus can be removed surgically. This has to be performed carefully because there can be much hemorrhage and, owing to constant movement, the sutures often do not hold. Wound dehiscence is a possible complication of surgery.

Hygroma is a false or acquired bursa that develops subcutaneously over bony prominences.[23] Hygromas develop following repeated trauma-induced necrosis and inflammation over pressure points. They are initially soft to fluctuant (fluid filled) but may become abscesses or may become granulomatous or fistulous, especially if secondarily infected.

Histologically, hygromas are characterized by cystic spaces surrounded by dense walls of granulation tissue, the inner layer of which is a flattened layer of fibroblasts. Early lesions usually respond well to loose, padded bandages applied for 2 to 3 weeks, and corrective housing. More severe lesions may require extensive drainage, extirpation, or skin grafting procedures.

Pressure point granuloma[23] may develop in regions subject to repeated trauma (Fig. 16:11F).

CALLUS DERMATITIS AND PYODERMA

This is a secondary infection of a callus subjected to repeated trauma between a bony prominence and a hard surface of the environment.

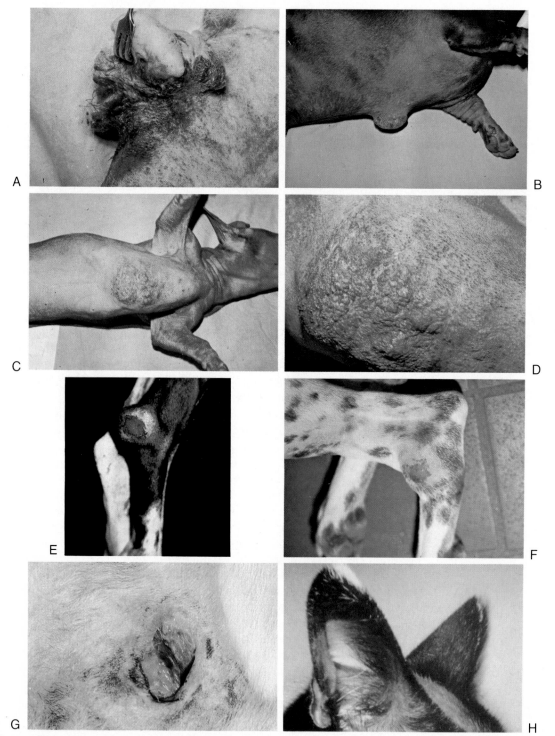

Figure 16:11. Callus syndrome. *A*, Very large elbow callus in an Alaskan malamute with extreme epithelial proliferation. This callus was excised surgically. *B*, Dachshund with a well-circumscribed sternal callus that responded to surgical excision. *C*, Sternal callus in a dachshund. *D*, Close-up of callus in *C* showing hyperkeratosis, hyperpigmentation, papules, and comedones. *E*, Ulcerated callus on wear area of hock. *F*, Pressure point granuloma of hock region, Dalmatian dog. Notice the erythema and ulcerated surface from licking (acral lick dermatitis). *G*, Pressure sore on rump over trochanter major. Hair has been clipped. *H*, Mild frostbite in this Siamese cat caused the hair on the ear tips to turn white.

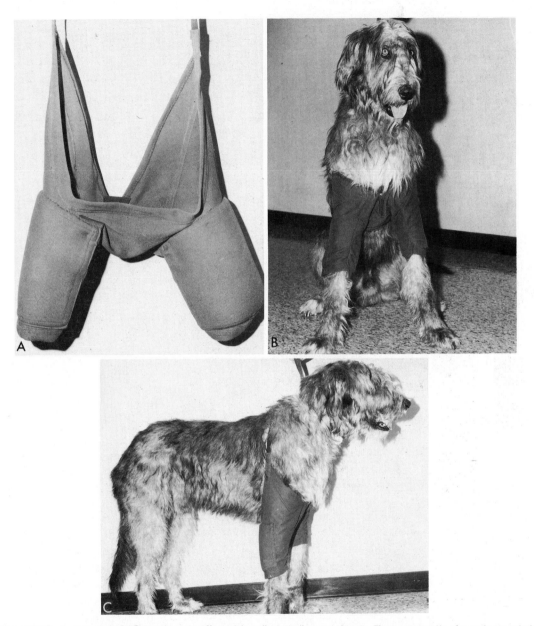

Figure 16:12. *A,* Breeches for giant breeds affected by elbow callus pyoderma. They are made of tough stretchable jersey material with foam rubber pad inserts in the region of the elbow. A strap and buckle (suspenders) attach over the back to hold them up. They are comfortable and worn constantly until the lesions heal, and then "nighttime only" usually suffices. These breeches are also useful for hygromas. *B,* Irish wolfhound with his breeches in place. *C,* Side view shows strap over the shoulders. (In *B* and *C,* E. M. Farber's Irish wolfhound "Finnegan.")

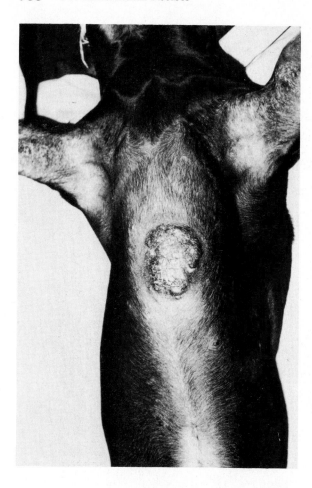

Figure 16:13. Sternal callus. Ventral view of dachshund in Figure 16:11*B*.

CAUSE AND CLINICAL FEATURES

The callus is the initial response to trauma. Continued trauma and the proliferative skin reaction that follows produce crevices in the callus and intertriginous areas, which results in a fold dermatitis. Additional trauma causes epidermal breakdown, ulceration of pressure points, and fistulas. The lesions are most common over the hock and elbow joints of giant breeds such as Great Danes, St. Bernards, Newfoundlands, and Irish wolfhounds (Fig. 16:14*A*). Sternal calluses on the chest of dachshunds, setters, pointers, boxers, and Doberman pinschers may also become secondarily ulcerated and infected (Figs. 16:13 and 16:15). Often there is no specific bacterial flora involved in this infection, although staphylococci commonly are isolated. Doberman pinschers, especially, are "callus formers." Pressure point granulomas, which often contain free hair shafts, may develop (Fig. 16:16) (see also Fig. 16:11*F*).

CLINICAL MANAGEMENT

Primary attention must be given to relieving the trauma so the tissue can heal. This can be accomplished through water beds, special bedding, padded breeches, or a combination of those measures (Fig. 16:12). In severe cases surgical excision of the callus or hygroma may be indicated. This is major surgery with a difficult postoperative course, and the reader is referred to texts on soft-tissue surgery for details of treatment.

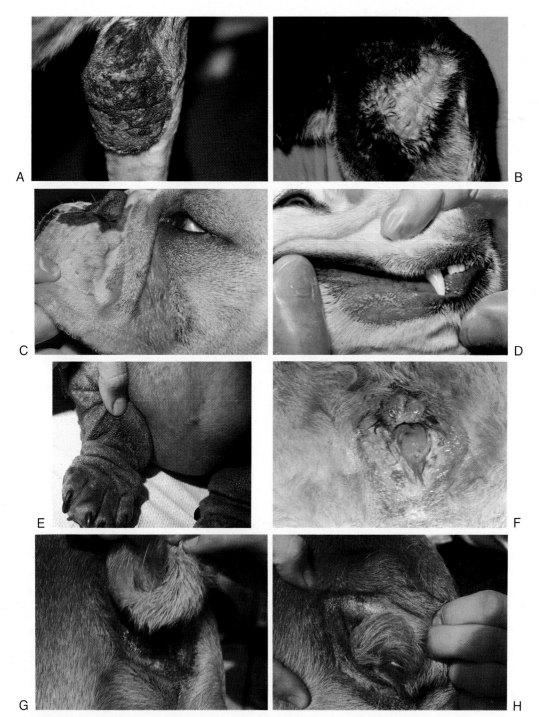

Figure 16:14. Pyotraumatic and fold dermatitis. *A,* Callus dermatitis. Note intertriginous folds in thick, rugose callus. (Courtesy W. H. Miller, Jr.) *B,* Acute moist dermatitis typically develops rapidly into a glistening, suppurative, hairless lesion bordered by a band of erythematous skin. *C,* Facial fold dermatitis. The thumb is pulling the lip forward to expose the erythematous, infected crevice hidden in the fold. *D,* Lipfold dermatitis characterized by erythema, exudation, and fetid odor. *E,* Body fold dermatitis. Finger is lifting the skin fold on foreleg of obese dachshund. (Courtesy W. H. Miller, Jr.) *F,* Vulvar fold dermatitis showing chronic purulent exudate. *G,* Tail fold dermatitis in a dog with "screw tail" conformation. Same dog as seen in Figure 16:19. (Courtesy P. J. Ihrke.) *H,* Close-up of same dog as in Figures 16:14 and 16:19. (Courtesy P. J. Ihrke.)

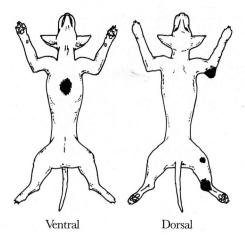

Ventral   Dorsal

Figure 16:15. Distribution pattern of callus dermatitis.

Medical management of minor fold dermatitis and fistulas is possible in many cases. Relief from pressure in these cases is also important. Wet soaks applied three times a day or warm whirlpool baths (p. 151) given daily, to cleanse the folds and stimulate circulation and healing, are beneficial.

Topical medication with antibacterial creams and bandaging, if necessary, may help control infection. One of the better medications for topical stimulation of wound healing is an ointment with live yeast cell extract and shark liver oil (Preparation H). This can be applied twice daily or used under a bandage, if it is changed daily.

Decubital ulcers produced by constant pressure on normal skin in paralyzed animals can be managed by the methods just described. Daily whirlpool baths, bedding on water beds with frequent turning, and careful attention to nutrition often prevent the development of decubital sores. Specific details on their management is contained in textbooks of surgery.

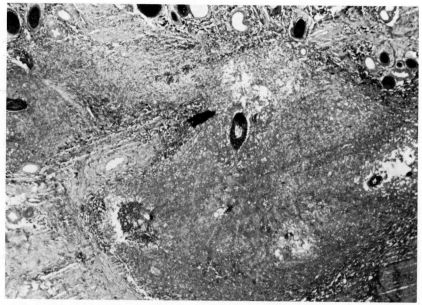

Figure 16:16. Pressure point granuloma in a dog. Deep dermal/subcutaneous pyogranuloma containing naked hair shafts.

Pressure Sores

(Decubitus Ulcers)

Pressure sores usually occur as a result of prolonged application of pressure concentrated over a bony prominence in a relatively small area of the body and sufficient to compress the capillary circulation, causing tissue damage or frank necrosis.[33] Tissue anoxia and full-thickness skin loss rapidly progress from a small localized area to produce ulceration, which almost invariably becomes infected with a variety of pathogenic bacteria. Within 24 to 48 hours the edges of the ulcerated area are undermined. The ulceration may extend to the underlying bone. Because of the area of capillary and venous congestion in the base of the ulcer and at the tissue margins, systemic antibiotics do not penetrate, and their use in therapy, therefore, is virtually useless.

Animals that are emaciated or recumbent are at an increased risk of pressure sores. Lesions are initially characterized by an erythematous to reddish purple discoloration. This progresses to oozing, necrosis, and ulceration. The resultant ulcers tend to be deep, undermined at the edges, secondarily infected, and very slow to heal (Fig. 16:11G).

The most important aspect of treatment is to identify and correct the cause. Routine wound care includes daily cleansing and drying agents, and topical or systemic antibiotics, if indicated. Surgical débridement, surgical excision, or skin grafting may be necessary in certain instances. Prevention is vastly more important than any kind of therapy.

Pyotraumatic Dermatitis

(Acute Moist Dermatitis "Hot Spots")

This disorder is produced by self-induced trauma as the patient bites, rubs, or scratches at a part of its body in an attempt to alleviate some pain or itch.[23] The majority of cases are complications of flea bite hypersensitivity, but allergic skin diseases, other ectoparasites, anal sac problems, inflammations such as otitis externa, foreign bodies in the coat, irritant substances, dirty unkempt coats, psychoses, and painful musculoskeletal disorders may be underlying causes. Owners usually believe that some factor producing a diet that is too rich may create the problem, but only a severe, essential fatty acid *deficiency* has been shown to be a cause (see p. 797). These factors initiate the itch–scratch cycle, which varies in intensity with individuals. The intense trauma produces severe large lesions in a few hours. Animals particularly disposed to this problem are those with a heavy pelage that has a dense undercoat, such as golden and Labrador retrievers, collies, German shepherds, and St. Bernards. The problem is much more common in hot, humid weather and may have something to do with lack of ventilation in the coat. A typical lesion is red, moist, and exudative. There is a coagulum of proteinaceous exudate in the center of the area surrounded by a red halo of erythematous skin. The hair is lost from the area, but the margins are sharply defined from the surrounding normal skin and hair (Fig. 16:14B). The lesion progresses rapidly if appropriate therapy is not started at once. Much pain is associated with the local area, and this may eventually deter the animal from further trauma. Lesions are often located in close proximity to the primary painful process, i.e., near infected ears, anal sacs, and flea bites on the rump.

A study of the type of bacteria found in lesions of pyotraumatic dermatitis revealed multiple organisms, with *Staphylococcus intermedius* being the most common. It also showed that St. Bernard and golden retriever dogs tended to have deeper pyogenic infections (see p. 261).[24]

Diagnosis is made by the history of acute onset, the physical appearance, and the association with a more or less primary cause. If the condition is persistent or recurrent, consider bacterial folliculitis, dermatophytosis, demodicosis, candidiasis, dermatophilosis, or neoplasia (lymphosarcoma, apocrine sweat gland carcinoma) as differential diagnoses. True pyotraumatitis dermatitis is a relatively flat, eroded-to-ulcerated lesion. Lesions that are thickened, plaquelike, and bordered by papules and/or pustules (satellite lesions) should always suggest a primary eruptive process, especially a staphylococcal infection.

Therapy is effective if applied promptly and vigorously. Sedation or anesthesia is usually needed to allow thorough cleansing of the area. Cleansing is the first and most important step in local therapy. The hair is clipped away from the lesion and the skin is thoroughly cleaned with a mild antiseptic solution or scrub such as povidone-iodine. A single application of 5 per cent tannic acid and 5 per cent salicylic acid in 70 per cent alcohol is used as an astringent. This can be followed by wet soaks with 5 per cent aluminum acetate (Domeboro solution) applied three to four times daily for 10 minutes each time. This action is drying, astringent, and antiseptic. Topical application of antibiotic corticosteroid cream three times daily is useful. Five days of systemic corticosteroids in anti-inflammatory doses (prednisolone 1.1 mg/kg SID) is useful in alleviating the pruritus, pain, and local inflammation. As the lesion becomes dry and crusted, topical medication should be changed to softening creams and emollients.

At the time of the initial treatment, it is most important to find the predisposing factor and eliminate or modify it to stop the patient's reflex self-trauma. The treatment to accomplish this varies, depending on the primary cause.

Clients always clamor for ways to prevent future lesions, since some unfortunate dogs may have repeated problems. There is no simple prophylaxis. However, constant attention to grooming, hygiene, baths, and parasite control and periodic cleaning of the ears and anal sacs will help. Owners should be particularly vigilant during periods of hot, humid weather. Although diet is often suggested as a cause, except for severe fatty acid deficiency or food hypersensitivity, this has never been proven.

Intertrigo

(Skin Fold Dermatitis)

Intertrigo is produced by friction and minor trauma to skin caused by anatomic defects in certain breeds (Figs. 16:17 and 16:18).[23] Skin rubbing against skin is irritating, and the areas where this occurs have poor air circulation. In combination with moisture, glandular secretions, and excretions such as tears, saliva, and urine these areas provide an environment that favors skin maceration and bacterial growth. These conditions cause the bacterial infection to be a problem greater than that seen in pyotraumatic dermatitis. Inflammations are rarely deep, however, and even here the bacterial colonization of the skin does not constitute a severe infection. The bacteria acting on the skin secretions do

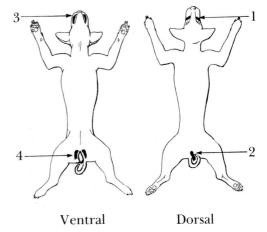

Figure 16:17. Fold dermatitis. *1*, Facial fold; *2*, tail fold; *3*, lip fold; *4*, vulvar fold.

Ventral   Dorsal

produce breakdown products that have an unpleasant odor, however, and this may be a major client concern. Moisture and maceration are critical factors. Obesity can be a contributing cause, especially in vulvar fold dermatitis.

Medical treatment of fold dermatitis may palliate some lesions, but surgical correction of the anatomic defect and elimination of the fold is the only permanent treatment. However, in cases where obesity causes body fold dermatitis, fasting to reduce weight, and hence the folds, may be curative. Brief comments will be made about each of the skin fold syndromes.

Facial fold dermatitis is seen in brachycephalic breeds, especially Pekingese, English bulldogs, and pugs (Fig. 16:14C).[23] The fold may rub on the cornea and cause severe keratitis and ulceration. The breed standards in some cases require a facial fold, so even though its presence may damage the eye, one should be careful to explain the ramifications of surgical correction to owners and should obtain their approval before ablating the folds. Daily or twice-weekly cleansing of intertriginous folds with 2.5 per cent benzoyl peroxide, thorough rinsing, and application of ointment to the hairs to keep them from irritating the cornea may be temporarily palliative. Surgical removal of the fold is the only definitive treatment.

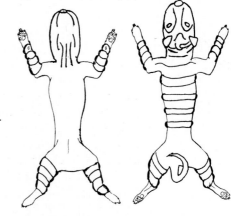

Figure 16:18. Body fold dermatitis—Chinese Shar Pei.

Ventral   Dorsal

Lip fold dermatitis is primarily an esthetic problem to owners, since it produces severe halitosis.[23] Owners may need to be convinced that the small lip fold can produce all that odor. They often feel certain that it is coming from the dog's throat. To convince them, make swabs of fluid from the throat and from the lip fold and have the owner compare odors. This problem is prevalent in dogs with a large lip flap, such as spaniels and St. Bernards (Fig. 16:14D). Again, benzoyl peroxide washes may be palliative, but surgical correction (cheiloplasty) is curative.

Body fold dermatitis, primarily found in obese individuals (Fig. 16:14E), is now seen in certain Chinese Shar Pei dogs (Fig. 16:18).[23] It is most common in puppies of that breed, which have an increased number of folds, and in those with a tendency to seborrhea. As the puppies mature, they do "grow out" of their folds on parts of the body, and therefore fold dermatitis in the adult Shar Pei is more concentrated on the head and face, where the folds persist. It may also be seen on the ventral midline of female dogs and cats with intertrigo between pendulous mammary glands or with rolls of body fat.[10, 23] There is no real therapy except frequent antiseborrheic shampoos with medications that are also antibacterial, such as OxyDex and Sebbafon shampoos. In obese dogs, body weight reduction is, of course, indicated. As with many breed standards, undesirable features unfortunately are often associated with anatomic features that the breed standard prescribes.

Vulvar fold dermatitis is common in obese older females that have infantile vulvas as a result of spaying at a young age (Fig. 16:14F).[23] The vulva is recessed, and vaginal secretions and drops of urine may accumulate in the folds of the perivulvar region. This is a special stimulus to ulceration and bacterial growth, and the odors produced are especially unpleasant. Ascending bacterial urinary tract infections are not an uncommon sequela to vulvar fold dermatitis. Several methods of management may help. Since obesity is usually present, weight reduction is indicated. Modest doses of oral diethylstilbestrol or estrogenic hormone injections will cause vulvar enlargement and may reduce the folds. The potential danger of such endocrine therapy must be considered.

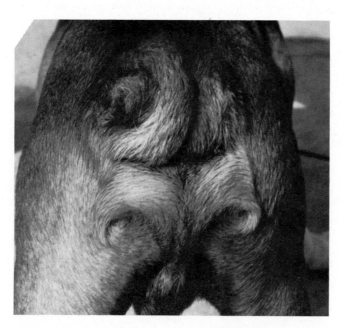

Figure 16:19. "Screw tail" conformation in a dog. (Courtesy P. J. Ihrke, University of California, Davis.)

Daily hygienic cleansing would be useful, but because there is so much pain from the ulcers, the bitch usually will not permit it. Surgical vulvoplasty (episioplasty), with fixation of the dorsal vulvar commissure to elevate the vulva out of the crevice, is curative. Squamous cell carcinoma has been reported to arise from chronic vulvar fold dermatitis.[23]

Tail fold dermatitis results from pressure of "corkscrew tails" on the skin of the perineum (Figs. 16:14G,H and 16:19). It is seen in English bulldogs, pugs, Boston terriers, and other breeds with that type of tail.[23] In addition, a rump fold dermatitis may be seen in certain Manx cats.[10] In some cases, the tail may partially obstruct the anus, so that feces, anal sac secretions, and other skin gland products enhance the skin maceration from the intertrigo. Do not hesitate to amputate the tail. Amputation resolves the problem, but the surgery is not as simple as one might expect.[33] Hemorrhage can be persistent and the surgical site is inconvenient.

References

1. Bouayad, H., et al.: Peripheral acquired arteriovenous fistula: A report of four cases and literature review. J. Am. Anim. Hosp. Assoc. *23*:205, 1987.
2. Brennan, K. E., and Ihrke, P. J.: Grass awn migration in dogs and cats: A retrospective study of 182 cases. J. Am. Vet. Med. Assoc. *182*:1201, 1983.
3. Butterfield, A. B., et al.: Acquired peripheral arteriovenous fistula in a dog. J. Am. Vet. Med. Assoc. *176*:445, 1980.
4. Evinger, J. V., and Blakemore, J. C.: Dermatitis in a dog associated with exposure to an arsenic compound. J. Am. Vet. Med. Assoc. *184*:1281, 1984.
5. Fadok, V. W.: Necrotizing skin diseases. In Kirk, R. W., (ed.): Current Veterinary Therapy VIII. Philadelphia, W. B. Saunders Company, 1983, p. 473.
6. Fitzpatrick, T. B., et al.: Dermatology in General Medicine III. New York, McGraw-Hill Book Company, 1987.
7. Fox, S. M.: Management of thermal burns—part I. Compend. Cont. Ed. *7*:631, 1985.
8. Griffin, C. E.: Nasal dermatitis. Dermatol. Rep. *2*:1, 1983.
9. Harari, J., et al.: Recurrent peripheral arteriovenous fistula and hyperthyroidism in a cat. J. Am. Anim. Hosp. Assoc. *20*:759, 1984.
10. Holzworth, J.: Diseases of the Cat: Medicine and Surgery. Philadelphia, W. B. Saunders Company, 1987.
11. Hargis, A. M., et al.: Myospherulosis in the subcutis of a dog. Vet. Pathol. *21*:248, 1984.
12. Ihrke, P.: Nasal solar dermatitis. In Kirk, R. W., (ed.): Current Veterinary Therapy VII. Philadelphia, W. B. Saunders Company, 1981, p. 440.
13. Irving, R. A., et al.: Porphyrin values and treatment of feline solar dermatitis. Am. J. Vet. Res. *43*:2067, 1982.
14. Israel, E., et al.: Microangiopathic hemolytic anemia in a puppy: Grand Rounds Conference. J. Am. Anim. Hosp. Assoc. *14*:521, 1978.
15. Jones, D. G. C., et al.: Arteriovenous fistula in the metatarsal pad of a dog: A case report. J. Small Anim. Pract. *22*:635, 1981.
16. Kral, F., and Schwartzman, R. M.: Veterinary and Comparative Dermatology. Philadelphia, J. B. Lippincott Company, 1964.
17. Mansfield, P. D.: The management of snake venom poisoning in dogs. Compend. Cont. Ed. *6*:988, 1984.
18. Mason, B. J. E.: Necrosis of a dog's toes following hepatitis. Vet. Rec. *101*:286, 1977.
19. Mason, K. V.: The pathogenesis of solar induced skin lesions in bull terriers. Proceedings, Am. Memb. Meeting. Am. Acad. Vet. Dermatol. and Am. Coll. Vet. Dermatol., 1987, p. 12.
20. McKeever, P. J.: Thermal injuries. In Kirk, R. W., (ed.): Current Veterinary Therapy VII. Philadelphia, W. B. Saunders Company, 1980, p. 191.
21. Muller, G. H.: Contact dermatitis in animals. Arch. Dermatol. *96*:423, 1967.
22. Muller, G. H.: Flea collar dermatitis in animals. J. Am. Vet. Med. Assoc. *157*:1616, 1970.
23. Muller, G. H., Kirk, R. W., and Scott, D. W.: Small Animal Dermatology III. Philadelphia, W. B. Saunders Company, 1983.
24. Reinke, S. I., Stannard, A. A., et al.: Histopathologic features of pyotraumatic dermatitis. J. Am. Vet. Med. Assoc. *190*:57, 1987.
25. Ruhr, L. P., and Andries, J. K.: Thallium intoxication in a dog. J. Am. Vet. Med. Assoc. *186*:498, 1985.
26. Schaer, M.: Eastern diamondback rattlesnake envenomation of 20 dogs. Compend. Cont. Ed. *6*:997, 1984.
27. Schwartzman, R. M., and Kirschbaum, J. O.: The cutaneous histopathology of thallium poisoning. J. Invest. Dermatol. *39*:169, 1962.
28. Scott, D. W.: Feline dermatology, 1900–1978: A monograph. J. Am. Anim. Hosp. Assoc. *16*:331, 1980.
29. Scott, D. W.: Unpublished observations, 1987.
30. Shakespeare, A. C., et al.: Infarction of the digits and tail secondary to disseminated intravascular coagulation and metastatic hemangiosarcoma in a dog. J. Am. Anim. Hosp. Assoc. (in press).
31. Slocum, B., et al.: Acquired arteriovenous fistula in two cats. J. Am. Vet. Med. Assoc. *162*:271, 1973.
32. Springer, T. R., and Bailey, W. J.: Snake bite treatment in the United States. Int. J. Dermatol. *25*:479, 1986.
33. Swain, S. F.: Surgery of Traumatized Skin: Management and Reconstruction in the Dog and Cat. Philadelphia, W. B. Saunders Company, 1980.
34. Van Gelder, G. A., (ed.): Clinical and Diagnostic Veterinary Toxicology II. Dubuque, Kendall/Hunt Publishing Company, 1976.

17

Nutritional Skin Diseases

A dermatosis may result from numerous nutritional deficiencies, excesses, or imbalances, but the skin responds with only a few types of clinical reactions and lesions. These include scaling, crusting, alopecia, and a dry, dull hair coat. Consequently, with physical examinations alone the specific nutritional cause can seldom be found.

Nutritional dermatoses have multiple causes, but often similar clinical signs.

As we enter the 1990s we need to take a new look at the relationship between nutrition and skin disease. It is important to re-evaluate old ideas that have been quoted and requoted during the past 50 years. Does a fatty acid deficiency that was experimentally produced in 1943[4] have any bearing on dogs of today that are fed well-balanced, nutritionally complete commercial dog foods?

It is useful to know the nutritional requirements of dogs and cats[1, 10] but it is difficult to prove that a specific deficiency causes a specific skin disease. During the last decade a few new skin diseases were described that were definitely connected to nutritional factors. It became fashionable to name these dermatoses in terms of being responsive to a nutrient, rather than in terms of a deficiency. Notable examples of these are the zinc-responsive dermatosis and the vitamin A-responsive dermatosis (rather than zinc deficiency and vitamin A deficiency). In many instances these entities may represent genetically related inabilities to absorb or metabolize the nutrients rather than true nutritional deficiencies. In others the response obtained may be the result of presently unknown effects of supraphysiologic doses of the nutrients.

As we evaluate what is new in nutrition as it is related to dermatology, we must be very cautious. Are certain diets, supplements, and pharmaceuticals really intended to cure skin diseases?

Major nutritional problems of concern are deficiencies of essential fatty acids, protein, zinc, copper, vitamins A, B, and E, and excessive levels of vitamin A. See also Systemic Therapy, page 195. Food hypersensitivity may also produce dermatoses (see p. 470).

Fatty Acid Deficiency

Fatty acid deficiency is uncommon and only seen in animals fed dry rations, commercial diets that have been poorly preserved (storage, temperature, preservative problems), or homemade diets.[1, 5, 10, 16] A deficiency may occur because fat is expensive and was left out of the food, because it leaked from the bag during storage, or because it became rancid. It also may occur with diets containing fat, but with inadequate antioxidants such as vitamin E.

Dog food should have a minimum of 3 per cent fat in a canned diet and 7 to 8 per cent in a dry diet. Cats usually have 35 to 40 per cent of their calories provided by fat—a much higher intake, because they need a dense caloric formula. The oxidation of fat during storage is a great concern, since it becomes rancid and destroys not only the essential fatty acids but vitamins D, E, and biotin. This may occur in canned food after 1 year or in dry food after 6 months, especially if they are stored at high temperatures. Animals may also develop fatty acid deficiency in association with intestinal malabsorption, pancreatic disease, and chronic hepatic disease.

Animals must be on a diet deficient in essential fatty acids for several months before skin problems become evident.[3, 4, 5, 10, 11, 17, 18] Fatty acid deficiency causes dry and lusterless hair, fine scaling, thickened skin, and alopecia and later causes pruritus, pyotraumatic dermatitis, and greasy skin and hair from excess sebaceous activity. At first there is a decrease in sebum production, but later it increases markedly, especially in the ear canals and between the toes. Initially, the hair coat is dry and lusterless, and a fine desquamation of keratin scales and alopecia appear. Erythema, edema, and pruritus are variable. When the sebaceous glands become more active later in the course of the dermatosis, the hair and skin become greasy. The skin thickens and is predisposed to secondary bacterial pyoderma. The fatty acid deficiency causes a change in the lipid film on the skin surface, which allows a change in the bacterial flora.

Fatty acid deficiency in a number of species produces abnormal keratinization, resulting in epidermal hyperplasia, hypergranulosis, and orthokeratotic and/or parakeratotic hyperkeratosis. This abnormal keratinization is thought to result from arachidonic acid deficiency with resultant prostaglandin E deficiency, which causes aberrations in ratios of epidermal cyclic adenosine monophosphate (cyclic AMP) to cyclic guanosine monophosphate (cyclic GMP) and in DNA synthesis.

The polyunsaturated fatty acid linoleic acid is essential in the diet of all animals. Arachidonic and linolenic acids are also required, but with the exception of arachidonic acid in the cat, they can be synthesized from linoleic acid. The cat seems to lack an active Δ-6-desaturase to initiate the conversion of linoleic acid to arachidonic acid and thus is an obligate carnivore.[1, 5, 11] Therapy produces visible responses after 3 to 8 weeks of fatty acid supplementation *if* the dermatosis is indeed an essential fatty acid deficiency. In such cases the coats may in fact develop more luster. If supplementation is needed, equal parts of vegetable and animal fats are recommended, because even though dogs (not cats) can convert linoleic acid to arachidonic acid, if it is provided in the diet, the conversion is not necessary. Animal fats contain arachidonic acid; vegetable fats do not. The concentration of unsaturated essential fatty acids in various fats is as follows:

Safflower oil	70%
Pork fat	29%
Soybean oil	50%
Poultry fat	24%
Corn oil	59%
Beef and butter fat	3%

Palm, olive, and coconut oil are low in linoleic acid and should not be used.[11]

Although fat is needed in the diet for energy as a source of essential fatty acids and fat-soluble vitamins, excess supplementation should be avoided because it causes obesity and unbalances the diet. Do not supplement with more than 2 tsp (10 ml) of oil per cup or can of food, as this amount increases the caloric intake by 25 per cent. Usually one-half this amount (1 tsp) of equal parts animal and vegetable fat per cup or can of food is a reasonable and effective supplement. The fatty acid deficiency responds within 1 to 3 months. Because the clinical syndrome can be caused by several deficiencies, supplements of fatty acids, vitamin A, and zinc and riboflavin assure that the skin condition is being adequately treated.[10, 11]

We know of no controlled data to support claims that the addition of extra fatty acids above minimum requirements promotes a glossy coat. Be cautious about supplementing fats in diets of dogs with pancreatitis or with maldigestion or malabsorption syndromes.

Protein Deficiency

Protein deficiency may be produced by inanition, starvation, feeding kittens commercial dog food, or feeding dogs "special" or very low-protein diets. Many commercial pet foods are actually extremely high in protein; therefore, the problem is rare.

Hair is 95 per cent protein with a high percentage of sulfur-containing amino acids. The normal growth of hair (the sum of growth in all follicles being 100 feet per day) and the keratinization of skin require 25 to 30 per cent of the animal's daily protein requirement.[5, 10, 11] Animals with protein deficiency have hyperkeratosis, epidermal hyperpigmentation, and loss of hair pigment. There is patchy alopecia with hairs that become thinner, rough, dry, dull, and brittle, so that they are easily broken and grow slowly. Shedding is prolonged. These lesions, together with scales and crusts, may appear symmetrically on the head, back, thorax, abdomen, and feet and legs. Lesions are more prominent in young, growing dogs, whose protein needs are higher. In humans, a mean hair root diameter of less than 0.06 mm suggests protein deficiency. Similar data are not available for animals. An analysis of the diet and the provision of protein on a dry matter basis, 25 per cent for the dog and 33 per cent for the cat, should be therapeutic. High quality protein from eggs, meat, or milk is important in supplementation.

Vitamin Deficiencies

Vitamin A. This vitamin has a function to maintain healthy skin and epithelial cells, and therefore deficiency or toxicity signs (which are similar) are manifested cutaneously.[5, 10, 11, 16] There is hyperkeratinization of the epithelial surfaces. Hyperkeratosis occurs in the sebaceous glands, occluding their ducts and blocking secretion. Firm papular eruptions with a firm center are formed, and they may be local or general. A poor coat, alopecia, scaling of the skin, and an increased susceptibility to bacterial infection are also observed. A single injection of 6000 IU aqueous vitamin A solution/kg body weight is adequate therapy for 2 months for a serious deficiency. Overtreatment can produce vitamin A toxicity.

Because vitamin A is stored so well, toxicity may be of more concern than deficiency. There is real danger from oversupplementation or from excess liver in the diet. A level 30 times the requirement for 2 to 3 months will produce toxicity. Do not give high daily doses orally. Maximum dosage for dogs and cats should not exceed 400 IU/kg/day vitamin A orally for 10 days.

Vitamin A–Responsive Dermatosis. Some cases of severe seborrhea in cocker spaniels have responded to vitamin A supplementation and are discussed in detail in Chapter 14.

Vitamin E. Vitamin E, selenium, and fatty acids have a balanced relationship. Experimental vitamin E deficiency in dogs also results in severe suppression of in vitro lymphocyte blastogenesis.[9] In cats, a similar imbalance produces pansteatitis.[5, 16] This syndrome results when high-fat diets such as canned red tuna are fed almost exclusively. If food processing or fat oxidation has inactivated vitamin E, the imbalance results. Cats show pain on gentle palpation and are anorectic, lethargic, and excitable. They may die in several weeks. There are large firm "lumps" in the subcutaneous tissues and abdominal cavity. Diagnosis can be made at biopsy or autopsy by finding yellow fat and steatitis. Biopsy reveals lobular panniculitis with "ceroid" within lipocytes, macrophages, and giant cells. Ceroid is a pink-to-yellow homogenous material on H & E stain and deep crimson on acid-fast stain.

Naturally-occurring vitamin E deficiency has not been reported in dogs. However, experimentally induced vitamin E deficiency has been studied in dogs.[19] Researchers showed that skin lesions can be produced. They consisted of an early keratinization defect (seborrhea sicca), a later inflammatory stage (erythroderma), and a tendency to develop secondary pyoderma. The dermatohistopathologic findings in dogs with experimentally produced vitamin E deficiency are nondiagnostic. Morphologically, the findings are characterized by hyperplastic superficial perivascular dermatitis. This is a common reaction pattern in canine skin, most commonly seen with hypersensitivity reactions, ectoparasitisms, and seborrheic disorders. When experimental dogs fed a vitamin E–deficient diet were provided a vitamin E supplement equal to or twice the National Research Council recommendations, the dermatosis responded dramatically. The erythema and greasiness subsided within 3 to 6 weeks, and the scaling was absent by 8 to 10 weeks.

A number of dermatoses in dogs and humans have been treated successfully with oral vitamin E, including discoid lupus erythematosus, acanthosis nigricans, and epidermolysis bullosa. It is unlikely that vitamin E deficiency would occur in dogs on commercial diets. It would enter into the differential diagnosis of the dog with seborrhea or erythroderma. Diagnosis would be based on dietary history, physical examination, ruling out other more common canine dermatoses, compatible skin biopsy results, and response to vitamin E therapy.

Vitamin E is used in doses of 10 mg (13.5 IU)/kg daily as an antioxidant and for therapy of pansteatitis in cats (resulting from excess tuna or fat in the diet). In severe cases it is mandatory to use systemic corticosteroids during the painful period of treatment (2 to 3 weeks).

Vitamin E in doses of 400 to 800 IU BID has been used successfully in discoid lupus erythematosus, systemic lupus erythematosus, and in disorders involving the basement membrane zone.

Vitamin B. B-complex vitamins are considered as a group. Single deficiencies of these vitamins are very rare, and even the clinical syndromes are quite similar.[5, 10, 11] They are synthesized by intestinal bacteria, but because they are water soluble and not stored, a constant supply is needed. On the other hand, toxicities do not occur. It is possible for biotin, riboflavin, niacin, and pyridoxine deficiencies to have clinical ramifications.

Biotin can be inactivated by feeding a diet high in uncooked eggs.[5, 10, 11] The whites contain avidin, which binds biotin so it cannot be absorbed. Biotin deficiency also results from prolonged oral antibiotic therapy. The most striking sign is a "spectacle eye" of alopecia around the face and eyes. This should be differentiated from demodicosis, dermatophytosis, and other facial dermatoses (discoid lupus erythematosus, pemphigus, dermatomyositis, epidermolysis bullosa). In severe cases, crusted lesions of the face, neck, body, and legs are present. There may also be lethargy, emaciation, and diarrhea. Biotin deficiency has been shown to cause a widespread papulocrustous dermatitis in cats.[4]

Riboflavin deficiency may produce a dry, flaky dermatitis (seborrhea) especially around the eyes and ventrum, but the outstanding sign is cheilosis.[10, 11] It also produces alopecia on the head of cats.[5] Deficiencies are all but impossible if *any* meat or dairy products are present in the diet.

Niacin deficiency is manifested as pellagra and is characterized by ulcerated mucous membranes, diarrhea, and emaciation. It may produce a pruritic dermatitis of the rear legs and abdomen.[10, 11] To produce a deficiency, diets must be low in animal protein and high in corn, which is low in tryptophan. All cereals are low in tryptophan. All animals, except the cat, convert tryptophan to niacin. Commercial pet diets contain more than enough niacin, and therefore supplementation is not needed.

Pyridoxine deficiency, produced experimentally in cats, causes a dull, waxy, unkept hair coat with generalized fine, white scales.[12] In some experimental cats it also caused multiple areas of alopecia in the temporal and periauricular area, on the dorsum of the muzzle, periorally, and on the extremities. When these experimental cats, after being on a pyridoxine-deficient diet, were fed a balanced diet, all skin lesions resolved. This condition has not been clinically observed and remains a laboratory phenomenon.

The most common signs of B-complex deficiencies are a dry, flaky seborrhea with alopecia, anorexia, and weight loss. These can be effectively treated with brewer's yeast or B-complex injections, or both. These may only be needed if animals are anorectic and having problems that cause excess water turnover.

Mineral Imbalances

Zinc, copper, and calcium are three minerals that influence iodine metabolism and each other, and abnormal levels of any one may be reflected in the skin. Because of the great variation among individuals, only one or several of a group of animals may show lesions, even though all are fed and managed alike.

Copper deficiency should only appear as a balance problem if excess zinc is added to the diet.[10, 11] Copper is needed by enzymes that convert L-tyrosine to melanin and by the follicular cells in the conversion of prekeratin to keratin. A deficiency is manifested by hypopigmentation and faulty keratinization of the skin and hair follicles, with the hair becoming dull and rough. Because commercial pet foods have adequate copper levels, supplements are not needed.

ZINC-RESPONSIVE DERMATOSIS

Zinc is an important cofactor and modulator of many critical biologic functions.[11a, 13a] Two dermatologic syndromes that respond to zinc supplementation occur in dogs.[2, 8, 13]

Syndrome I is a condition that occurs primarily in Siberian huskies and Alaskan malamutes but has also been recognized in Doberman pinschers and Great Danes. Lesions first develop before puberty in some puppies, but adult dogs may also develop them. There is early erythema followed by alopecia, crusting, scaling, and underlying suppuration around the mouth, chin, eyes, and ears (see Fig. 17:1A–G). Other body openings and the scrotum, prepuce, and vulva may be affected. Although the coat is dull, there is excess sebum production. Thick crusts may appear on the elbows and other joints, too. The skin may be inelastic and the legs stiff, as a result of hardened crusts. The footpads may become hyperkeratotic (Fig. 17:1H). In chronic cases, hyperpigmentation occurs in the area of the lesions. There may be a decreased sense of smell (hyposmia) and taste (hypogeusia). Clinical signs may be precipitated or intensified by stress, estrus, and so forth.

It has been shown that malamutes have a genetic defect of decreased capability for zinc absorption from the intestines.[8, 11] In some huskies, hypothyroidism and decreased serum zinc levels have been reported, but the significance of this is unknown.[8] Dogs on high-calcium or high-cereal diets (which have high levels of phytate) show poor zinc absorption, owing to binding of the zinc. Prolonged enteritis or diarrhea also prevents normal absorption. A severe deficiency may cause poor growth and weight loss in young pups and poor wound healing in any animal.[14, 15]

Syndrome II occurs in rapidly growing puppies that are on zinc-deficient diets or are oversupplemented with mineral and vitamins. Many breeds may be affected, but Great Danes, Doberman pinschers, beagles, German shepherds, German shorthaired pointers, Labrador retrievers, Rhodesian ridgebacks, and standard poodles have been reported.[8, 13, 22] Severity of lesions can vary greatly within a litter. Some animals may be normal, while others are stunted, depressed, and anorectic. The skin lesions are hyperkeratotic plaques over areas of repeated trauma or where calluses might normally occur (Fig. 17:2). The footpads and planum nasale may be affected and any thickened area may have deep fissures. There may be secondary infection of the crusts and an associated lymphadenopathy.

In both syndromes, serum or hair zinc levels may be decreased, but proper analysis for zinc is difficult and may be unreliable, as a result of contamination of samples by zinc in glassware, rubber stoppers, and influences of various environmental, physiologic, and disease-related factors.[22, 24]

Diagnosis may be made by the history, physical examination, and skin biopsy. Hyperplastic superficial perivascular dermatitis, with marked diffuse and follicular parakeratotic hyperkeratosis, is suggestive of zinc deficiency (Figs. 17:3 and 17:4). Eosinophils are often prominent in the perivascular cellular infiltrate. Papillomatosis and/or diffuse spongiosis, intraepidermal pustular dermatitis, and suppurative folliculitis reflect secondary bacterial infection.

Therapy is usually successful, especially in syndrome II, in which response is rapid. Zinc sulfate ($ZnSO_4$) in a dose of 10 mg/kg/day is adequate in most cases. Excess amounts block copper and iron absorption.[8, 11] Large dogs are usually given 100 to 200 mg $ZnSO_4$, twice daily, and syndrome I dogs may

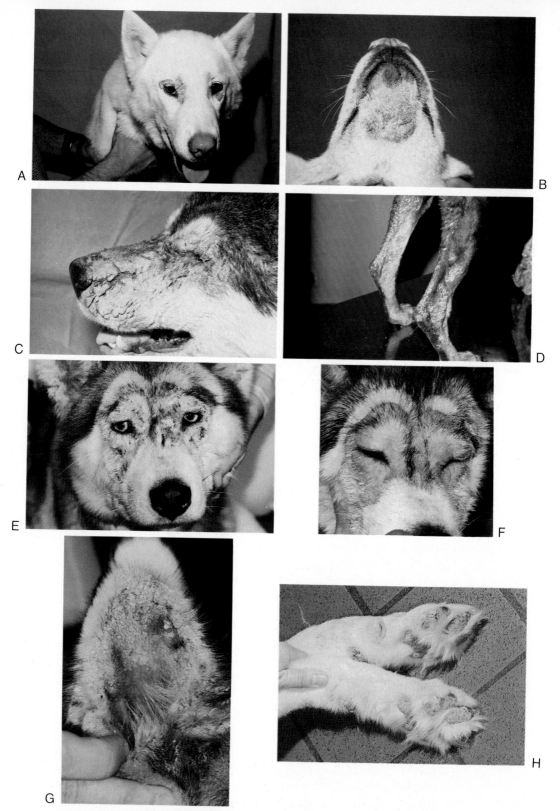

Figure 17:1. Zinc-responsive dermatosis. *A*, Siberian husky with alopecia and crusting around eyes. *B*, Same dog as in *A*, with lesions on the chin. *C*, Alaskan malamute with severe crusting and alopecia of face, eyelids, and lips. *D*, Doberman pinscher with erythema, scaling, crusts, and alopecia of legs. Previously called "dry juvenile pyoderma." *E*, Zinc-responsive dermatosis. Facial crusting. *F*, Same dog as in *E*. Severe erythema underlying crusts. *G*, Same dog as in *E* and *F*. Erythematous, crusted pinna. *H*, Same dog as in *E*, *F*, and *G*. Hyperkeratosis of foot pads.

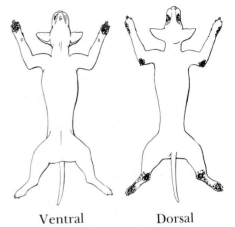

Figure 17:2. Zinc-responsive dermatosis distribution pattern.

Ventral   Dorsal

need to be kept on therapy indefinitely. Zinc sulfate tablets should be crushed and mixed with a little food. Zinc methionine (Zinpro) may be given orally at 1.7 mg/kg SID. The medication can usually be withdrawn from puppies when they are mature. If obvious dietary imbalances are present, they should be corrected. It has been noted that high-protein diets and increased vitamin D may enhance absorption of zinc. Local therapy may help to soften the dry crusts. This can include wet dressings, 10 minutes twice a day, and the use of antiseborrheic shampoos.

In kittens, dietary zinc deficiency was reported to cause thinning of the hair coat, slow hair growth, scaly skin, and ulceration of the buccal margins.[7] The cat's requirement for dietary zinc was estimated at between 15 and 50 ppm.

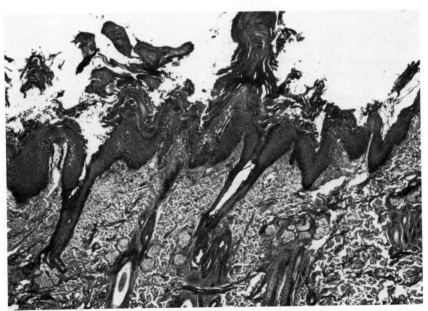

Figure 17:3. Zinc-responsive dermatosis in a Siberian husky. Hyperplastic perivascular dermatitis with marked diffuse parakeratotic hyperkeratosis.

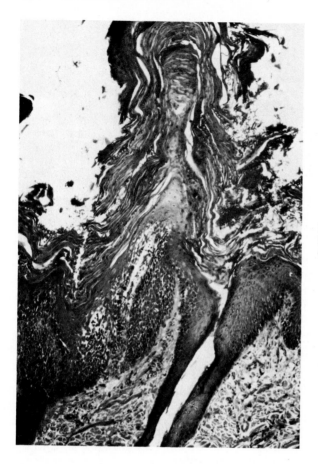

Figure 17:4. Zinc-responsive dermatosis in a Siberian husky. Marked parakeratotic hyperkeratosis. Close-up of Figure 17:3.

GENERIC DOG FOOD SKIN DISEASE
(Zinc Deficiency?)

Dogs fed only generic dog foods for 2 to 4 weeks developed bilateral symmetric scaling and crusting dermatoses.[20, 21] The lesions involved the bridge of the nose, mucocutaneous junctions, pressure points, and distal extremities. Well-demarcated older lesions had erythematous borders with scales, crusts, and variable hyperpigmentation and lichenification. A few cases had alopecia, focal erosions, papules, and pustules. Most dogs had fever, depression, lymphadenopathy, and pitting edema of dependent areas.

Skin biopsies showed hyperplastic superficial perivascular dermatitis with diffuse parakeratotic hyperkeratosis and focal epidermal dyskeratosis and a mixed dermal cellular infiltrate (Fig. 17:5). The dietary history, physical, and histopathologic findings suggest that, in all likelihood, this syndrome is due to a zinc deficiency.

The differential diagnosis should include relative or absolute zinc deficiency, immune-mediated skin diseases (especially pemphigus foliaceus and systemic lupus erythematosus), demodicosis, dermatophytosis, staphylococcal folliculitis, and other exfoliative skin diseases.

Treatment with antibiotics or corticosteroids was unsuccessful, but rapid

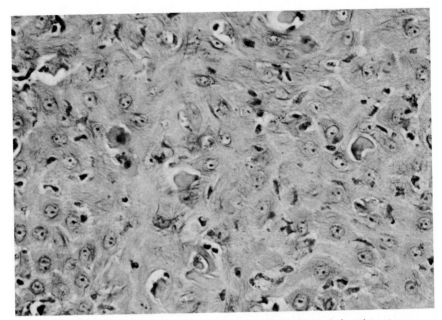

Figure 17:5. Zinc-responsive dermatosis. Multiple dyskeratotic keratinocytes.

response occurred 1 week after simply changing the diet to a national brand of dog food meeting NRC requirements.

Further work is needed to precisely define the problem, but since it mimics more serious dermatoses, clinicians should recognize the syndrome and be aware of its simple resolution by dietary measures.

Supplement Formula

Lewis[10, 11] has suggested feeding the supplements in the formula below to correct most skin conditions caused by nutritional deficiencies. If the condition persists in spite of the supplementation, it undoubtedly does not have a nutritional origin.

SUPPLEMENT FORMULA

1 tsp vegetable cooking oil
2 to 3 oz cooked liver
100 mg zinc sulfate
1 drop tincture of iodine

Add the supplement to the diet daily for a 20- to 30-pound dog. It provides fat, protein, vitamins A and E, biotin, riboflavin, niacin, and iodine and zinc.

It would be better yet to change from the generic diet to a superior brand of dog food.

References

1. Anderson, R. W., (ed.): Nutrition of the Dog and Cat: Proceedings of an International Symposium. Elmsford, New York, Pergamon Press, 1980, p. 67.
2. Fadok, V. A.: Nutritional therapy in veterinary dermatology. *In* Kirk, R. W., (ed.): Current Veterinary Therapy IX. Philadelphia, W. B. Saunders Company, 1986.
3. Hansen, A. E., and Weise, H. F.: Fat in the diet in relation to nutrition of the dog. I. Characteristic appearance and gross changes of animals fed diets with and without fat. Tex. Rep. Biol. Med. *52*:205, 1951.
4. Hansen, A. E., and Weise, H. F.: Studies with dogs maintained on diets low in fat. Proc. Soc. Exp. Biol. Med. *52*:205, 1943.
5. Holzworth, J.: Diseases of the Cat: Medicine and Surgery. Philadelphia, W. B. Saunders Company, 1987.
6. Ihrke, P. J., and Goldschmidt, H. H.: Vitamin A–responsive dermatosis in the dog. J. Am. Vet. Med. Assoc. *182*:687, 1983.
7. Kane, E., et al.: Zinc deficiency in the cat. J. Nutr. *111*:488, 1981.
8. Kunkle, G. A.: Zinc-responsive dermatoses in dogs. *In* Kirk, R. W. (ed.): Current Veterinary Therapy VII. Philadelphia, W. B. Saunders Company, 1980.
9. Langweiler, M., Schulz, R. D., and Sheffy, B. E.: Effect of vitamin E deficiency on the proliferative response of canine lymphocytes. Am. J. Vet. Res. *42*:1681, 1981.
10. Lewis, L. D.: Cutaneous manifestations of nutritional imbalances. Proceedings, Am. Anim. Hosp. Assoc. *48*:263, 1981.
11. Lewis, L. D., and Morris, M. L., Jr.: Small Animal Clinical Nutrition. 2nd ed. Topeka, Mark Morris Associates, 1984.
11a. Norris, D.: Zinc and cutaneous inflammation. Arch. Dermatol. *121*:985, 1985.
12. Norton, A.: Skin lesions seen in cats with vitamin B (pyroxidine) deficiency. Proceedings, Am. Acad. Vet. Dermatol. and Am. Coll. Vet. Dermatol. Phoenix, 1987.
13. Ohlen, B., and Scott, D. W.: Zinc responsive dermatitis in puppies. Canine Pract. *13*:2, 1986.
13a. Russell, R. M., et al: Zinc and the special senses. Ann. Int. Med. *99*:227, 1983.
14. Sanecki, R. K., et al.: Tissue changes in dogs fed a zinc-deficient ration. Am. J. Vet. Res. *43*:1642, 1982.
15. Sanecki, R. K., Corbin, J. E., and Forbes, R. M.: Extracutaneous histologic changes accompanying zinc deficiency in pups. Am. J. Vet. Res. *46*:2119, 1985.
16. Scott, D. W.: Feline dermatology 1900–1978: A monograph. J. Am. Anim. Hosp. Assoc. *16*:331, 1980.
17. Scott, D. W.: Feline dermatology 1979–1982: Introspective retrospections. J. Am. Anim. Hosp. Assoc. *20*:537, 1984.
18. Scott, D. W.: Feline dermatology 1983–1985: "The secret sits." J. Am. Anim. Hosp. Assoc. *23*:255, 1987.
19. Scott, D. W., and Sheffy, B. E.: Dermatosis in dogs caused by vitamin E deficiency. Comp. Anim. Pract. *1*:42, 1987.
20. Sousa, C. A., et al.: Dermatosis associated with feeding generic dog food: 13 cases (1981–1982). J.A.V.M.A. *192*:676, 1988.
21. Sousa, C. A.: Nutritional dermatoses. *In* Nesbit, G. H., (ed.): Dermatology Contemporary Issues in Small Animal Practice. New York, Churchill Livingstone, Inc., 1987.
22. van den Broek, A. H. M., and Thoday, K. L.: Skin disease in dogs associated with zinc deficiency: A report of 5 cases. J. Small Anim. Pract. *27*:313, 1986.
23. Wolf, A. M.: Zinc-responsive dermatosis in a Rhodesian Ridgeback. Vet. Med. *82*:908, 1987.
24. Wright, R. P.: Identification of zinc-responsive dermatoses. Vet. Med. *80*:37, 1985.

18

Diseases of Ears, Eyelids, Nails, and Anal Sacs

Ear Diseases

OTITIS EXTERNA

Otitis externa is an acute or chronic inflammation of the epithelium of the external ear canal but may also involve parts of the pinna. It is a complicated multifactorial disease.

Glands of the external auditory canal. The skin lining of the external ear canal is stratified squamous epithelium with sebaceous and apocrine glands and hair follicles. Just under the epithelium, the sebaceous glands are abundant. The tubular apocrine glands are located deeper in the dermis. Normal ear wax is thought to be a mixture of the secretions of both types of glands. In inflammation, the apocrine glands become cystic and their secretion increases markedly.

CAUSE AND PATHOGENESIS

Otitis externa is exceedingly common. Studies[8] covering many years and many thousands of clinic patients report the incidence to be 5 to 8 per cent of total admissions, but 18 to 20 per cent of patients admitted for other conditions. The incidence is highest at 5 to 8 years of age. There is no sex or seasonal predisposition. However, seasonal growth of plant awns or good weather for swimming may influence the types of causes of the disorder. In addition, seasonal otitis externa may be seen with atopy, chiggers, and ticks. Approximately 80 per cent of cases involve long-eared dogs, especially spaniels, poodles, Kerry blue terriers, Labrador retrievers, and breeds with abundant hair growth in the ear canal. The pinna folding down over the entrance to the ear canal restricts air circulation and promotes infection. This anatomic feature is of primary concern in otitis externa (Fig. 18:1). Of the erect-eared breeds, the German shepherd is especially prone to ear infections. Feline otitis is less common, perhaps because of the erect pinna.[15]

Water dogs may develop yeast infections (*Candida albicans* and *Malassezia pachydermatis*) if the ear canals remain wet after swimming. These organisms are increasingly common in association with otitis externa. Plant awns (foxtails) and foreign objects may cause otitis in dogs that frequent the fields. Parasites, especially *Otodectes cynotis*, but also *Sarcoptes scabiei* (var. *canis*), *Notoedres cati*,

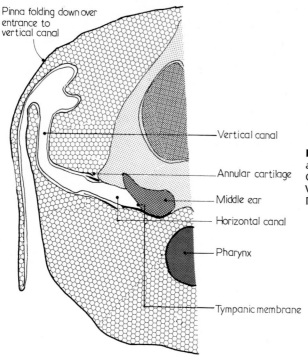

Pinna folding down over entrance to vertical canal

Vertical canal

Annular cartilage

Middle ear

Horizontal canal

Pharynx

Tympanic membrane

Figure 18:1. Section of the head of a lop-eared dog at the level of the external auditory meatus. (From Grono, L. R.: Otitis externa. *In* Kirk, R. W. (ed): Current Veterinary Therapy VII. W. B. Saunders Company, Philadelphia, 1980.)

chiggers and demodectic mites, may be irritating factors. Ear mites are the most common cause of otitis in cats. Tumors and polyps are found especially in cats, and extension of middle ear infections and external skin diseases may be primary causes in both dogs and cats. Atopy and seborrhea are of special concern in that regard. Primary bacterial otitis externa is a rare entity, but the anatomy and ecology of the ear canal make it so ideal an incubator that once inflammation starts, secondary infections perpetuate themselves.

Common organisms of the normal canine ear canal have been reported as *Staphylococcus intermedius* (coagulase positive) and *M. pachydermatis* (Table 18:1). Organisms isolated from ears with otitis externa included those mentioned plus

Table 18:1. ORGANISMS ISOLATED FROM NORMAL EAR CANALS AND FROM EARS AFFECTED WITH OTITIS EXTERNA*

Organism	Clinically Normal Ear Canals			Ears with Otitis Externa			
	Grono, Frost (1969) %	Sampson et al. (1973) %	Marshall et al. (1974) %	Grono, Frost (1969) %	Boyle, Grono (data to be published) %	Sampson et al. (1973) %	Marshall et al. (1974) %
Coagulase-positive Staphylococcus	47.6	15	1.7	30.9	30.4	35.0	38.0
Pityrosporum spp.	37.9	6	28.3	35.9	44.3	23.0	86.2
Pseudomonas spp.	2.4	4	0.0	34.6	16.5	5.0	16.4
Proteus spp.	1.6	0	0.0	20.8	9.9	5.0	3.4
Streptococcus spp.	0.0	2	0.0	7.4	4.3	6.0	8.6
Aspergillus spp.	0.0	—	—	0.8	1.1	—	—

*From Grono, L. R.: Otitis externa. *In* Kirk, R. W. (ed.): Current Veterinary Therapy VII. W. B. Saunders Company, Philadelphia, 1980.

Proteus spp. and *Pseudomonas* spp., especially in chronic infections. Other reports have indicated that β-hemolytic streptococci, *E. coli*, and *Bacillus* spp. are frequently isolated from infected ears.[5] In about 30 per cent of otitis cases, more than one organism is cultured. In cats, the most commonly reported organisms from otitic ears are coagulase-positive staphylococci and *M. pachydermatis*.[15]

Poor air circulation in the ear canal favors infection.

Comparison of antibiotic sensitivity of bacteria from recent otitis externa cases with those of many years ago suggests the emergence of strains that are resistant to antibacterial agents used for routine treatment. Table 18:2 provides data on sensitivity tests of 467 cultures of otitis externa.[8]

August[3] proposes three categories of factors causing otitis externa in dogs and cats: (1) primary causes—parasites, foreign bodies, hypersensitivity diseases, disorders of keratinization, autoimmune diseases, systemic diseases; (2) predisposing causes—conformational predisposition, ear canal maceration (moisture), treatment errors, obstructive ear disease, pyrexia; (3) perpetuating causes—bacteria, yeasts, water, otitis media, progressive pathologic changes.

Table 18:2. RESULTS OF SENSITIVITY TESTS OF 467 SWABS FROM CANINE EARS AFFECTED WITH OTITIS EXTERNA*

Agent		Pseudomonas	Proteus	Staph. Aureus†	Coliforms	Streptococci	Diphtheroids	Micrococci
Penicillin	S‡	0.0	11.8	60.9	0.0	100.0	75.0	50.0
	R	100.0	88.2	39.1	100.0	0.0	25.0	50.0
Streptomycin	S	46.2	52.9	95.4	66.7	60.0	50.0	100.0
	R	53.8	47.1	4.6	33.3	40.0	50.0	0.0
Chloramphenicol	S	3.8	58.8	97.7	55.6	100.0	100.0	100.0
	R	96.2	41.2	2.3	44.4	0.0	0.0	0.0
Tetracycline	S	25.0	17.6	92.0	44.4	100.0	100.0	100.0
	R	75.0	82.4	8.0	55.6	0.0	0.0	0.0
Ampicillin	S	0.0	11.8	69.0	0.0	100.0	75.0	100.0
	R	100.0	88.2	31.0	100.0	0.0	25.0	0.0
Trimethoprim-Sulfadiazine	S	3.8	29.4	66.7	33.3	20.0	50.0	100.0
	R	96.2	70.6	33.3	66.7	80.0	50.0	0.0
Neomycin	S	86.5	76.5	97.7	77.8	80.0	50.0	100.0
	R	13.5	23.5	2.3	22.2	20.0	50.0	0.0
Polymyxin B	S	86.5	0.0	97.7	77.8	80.0	75.0	100.0
	R	13.5	100.0	2.3	22.2	20.0	25.0	0.0
Gentamycin	S	100.0	88.2		100.0			
	R	0.0	11.8		0.0			
Carbenicillin	S	64.7	82.4		100.0			
	R	35.3	17.6		0.0			

*From Grono, L. R.: Otitis externa. *In* Kirk, R. W. (ed.): Current Veterinary Therapy VII. W. B. Saunders Company, Philadelphia, 1980.

†This organism, a coagulase-positive *Staphylococcus*, would probably be identified today as *Staphylococcus intermedius*.

‡S = susceptible; R = resistant.

The following list summarizes the causes of otitis externa.

1. Foreign bodies (foxtails)
2. Bacterial otitis
3. Yeast otitis (*Malassezia, Candida*)
4. Mycotic otitis of pinna (secondary to generalized dermatophytosis)
5. Otodectic otitis
6. Seborrheic otitis
7. Demodectic otitis (otodemodicosis)
8. Pemphigus and other autoimmune diseases causing pinnal lesions with secondary otitis
9. Hairs in ears acting as foreign bodies (in poodles, etc.)
10. Overtreatment of otitis (primary irritant or allergic contact dermatitis, etc.)
11. Hypersensitivity reactions (atopy, food), scratching of inflamed, pruritic ears
12. Pendulous pinnae
13. Ticks (*Otobius megnini*)
14. Chiggers
15. Water
16. Fly bites (*Stomoxys calcitrans*)
17. Polychondritis

CLINICAL FEATURES

Otitis externa is a single clinical syndrome with many stages. Grono[8] has divided otitis into two broad categories: infective and reactive. The infective group includes inflammations that are acute purulent, chronic purulent, chronic ulcerative, parasitic, and fungal. The reactive group includes acute erythematous, chronic proliferative, and verrucous disorders. Early inflammations are characterized by erythema and swelling of the lining of the epithelium. This may be a hypersensitivity or irritant reaction. The fragile skin may easily become traumatized or ulcerated and secondarily infected. A purulent or bloody exudate develops. If infection persists for long periods, the skin that lines the canal becomes thick and hyperplastic, and a cauliflower-like growth or ossification of the cartilage may result. If ear mites are a cause, the exudate is typically tan or reddish brown and waxy or of the consistency of coffee grounds. The white mites are easily seen moving against that background. As infection progresses, the discharge becomes more purulent. Foreign bodies, water, tumors, and parasites all have a marked effect in prolonging the otitis, and they often incite the disease. Fungal infection produces a moist, caseous, gray exudate with a musty odor. Seborrheic otitis may be misdiagnosed as purulent otitis. Its appearance can vary from an oily yellow film or flakes to dry adherent flakes and scales. There may be a characteristic rancid, sweet odor, and the ear lesions may be associated with generalized seborrhea.

Pain, head shaking, and scratching are common in otitis externa, especially when foreign objects, parasites, or acute otitis are present. Spots of acute moist dermatitis can develop on or near the ear. Rubbing or cleaning the ear may cause the animal to lean into the side being handled while involuntarily scratching with the hind leg on that side and groaning with pleasure.

DIAGNOSIS

The history and physical examination makes the diagnosis of otitis externa obvious in most cases. The problem is to define the type of reaction and to determine the cause. Significant bilateral pinnal involvement suggests systemic disease. This must be searched for diligently using an otoscope and good lighting. Careful inspection of the canal for awns, foxtails, mites, and foreign objects is essential. It is important to examine the tympanum. The most common cause of chronic recurrent otitis externa in dogs is an undiagnosed otitis media resulting from tympanic rupture. Removal of accumulated hair and irrigation of the ear canal with water and antiseptic solutions will often expose foreign objects that were not visible previously. Because of pain the patient may resent examination. It is imperative to use deep tranquilization or light anesthesia to properly examine and treat the ears.

Biopsy of the ear canal is rarely performed, unless a tumor is suspected. The histopathology in otitis shows a spongiotic and/or hyperplastic perivascular dermatitis. Epidermal hyperplasia, rete ridge formation, and epithelial ulceration are present. The dermis is fibroplastic and the sebaceous glands are small and displaced by dilated ducts of the prominent ceruminous glands that may be filled with an eosinophilic, colloidal material.

CLINICAL MANAGEMENT

Treatment depends on the immediate cause, which must be removed or modified. Next, the predisposing causes must also be eliminated or modified.[7] In general, Grono[8] advocates these principles:

1. Sedate or anesthetize the patient.

2. Take swab/cultures for a Gram's or Diff Quik stain and culture.

3. Examine ear with otoscope and 6.0 cm speculum of the largest convenient diameter.

4. Pluck any hair and remove debris by gently irrigating the ear canal with warm antiseptic solution (0.5 per cent chlorhexidine, 10 per cent solution of povidone-iodine), or ceruminolytic agents (Cerumene, Panoprep, propylene glycol, or Surfak), if wax and sebum from seborrhea are a problem. A small catheter, polyethylene tubing, or a Water-Pik (Fig. 18:2) may help to irrigate effectively. Do not use pressure against the tympanum or in the canal. Do not use cotton swabs except to wipe *out* the canal and cleanse the pinna and outer part of the canal.

5. Gently dry the canal with suction and re-examine the ear with the otoscope. Otic Domeboro, Oti-Clens, or Epi Otic are effective drying and cleansing agents.

Establishing good drainage is the key to successful ear treatment.

---

6. If the ears are pendulous, tape them over the head to improve air circulation in the ear canal. Leave them taped over the head for 7 to 10 days, as needed.

7. Apply specific medication in a thin film to the entire lining of the clean canal.

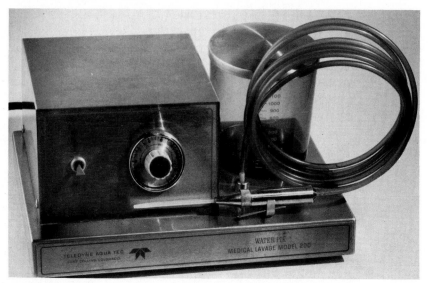

Figure 18:2. Water-Pik uses warm solutions of chlorhexidine povidone iodine at low pressures to thoroughly irrigate and cleanse the external auditory canal of exudates, secretions, and debris.

8. Change and repeat treatment as needed or as indicated by laboratory reports.

Specific treatment depends on clinical and laboratory findings.

Infective Types of Otitis

Acute Otitis. Early erythematous stages are swollen, red, and easily traumatized. Gentle handling and daily applications of a few drops of bland antibiotic-steroid preparations, such as Liquichlor, Gentocin Otic, or Panalog, are indicated.

Acute Purulent. After thorough initial cleansing, control infection by daily application of ear drops containing either gentamicin or chloramphenicol. When culture and sensitivity results are known, change medication as needed. Occasionally, stubborn cases respond to daily irrigation with a 10 per cent solution of povidone-iodine, white vinegar (diluted 1:1 with water), or 70 per cent isopropyl alcohol. In each case, it is important to be sure the tympanum is intact and to dry the canal after irrigation. Venker-van Haagen has emphasized that thorough cleansing is only possible with a fine, forceful stream of water.[17] She uses the Elpa otologic flusher (Stümer, Haugerring 5, 8700 Würtzburg, West Germany) designed for flushing the human ear. It delivers thermostatically controlled water with variable force through specially designed cannulas and efficiently and safely cleans the ear canal.

Chronic Purulent. These may involve middle ear infections; therefore, systemic therapy with laboratory test guidance may be necessary. The irrigation procedure described above is helpful, and the schedule illustrated in Fig. 18:3 is advocated by Venker-van Haagen for management of these cases.[17] The Water-Pik (Teledyne Water-Pik, Fort Collins, Colorado, 80525) oral hygiene appliance works well if low pressure is used.

Chronic Ulcerative. Treat as for purulent otitis. However, topical therapy should include chemical cauterization of frank ulcers with 5 per cent silver nitrate or 5 per cent tannic or salicylic acid in 70 per cent alcohol.

Fungal or Yeast. Treat daily with 0.5 per cent chlorhexidine in propylene glycol (a good general-purpose ear drop), miconazole (Conofite), povidone-iodine in water 1:10, or thiabendazole solution (Tresaderm). Nystatin ointment is effective against *Candida albicans* infections.

Parasitic. Apply a topical parasiticide to the ear canal. After the animal shakes its head, wipe medication away from external surfaces. Venker-van Haagen recommends 2 per cent lindane, but rotenone (Canex) and mineral oil 1:3 and thiabendazole solution are also excellent. Treat affected animals all over with flea sprays or powders, and treat all other dogs and cats on the premises weekly for 3 weeks. When treating outdoor cats on which only a single treatment is possible, Pellitol ointment and mineral oil are effective. Ivermectin injected subcutaneously at 300 μg/kg and repeated in 3 weeks is very effective against ear mites in dogs and cats (see p. 182).

Reactive. Reactive otitis is treated differently, since the inflammation is proliferative and may be more refractory to treatment.

Acute reactive. Try to control the reaction with systemic and topical corticosteroids, and prevent secondary bacterial infection.

Chronic reactive. Control the reaction with corticosteroids or antiseborrheic creams, or both. Treating the seborrheic ear canal requires the same measures as treating the rest of the body of a seborrheic patient (see p. 724). If some response is not seen in 4 to 6 weeks, surgical measures should be considered to establish drainage and ventilation.

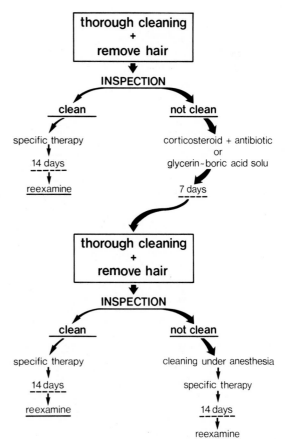

Figure 18:3. A schedule for cleaning ears is important for successful management of chronic otitis. (From Venker-van Haagen, A. J.: Managing diseases of the external ear. *In* Kirk, R. W. (ed): Current Veterinary Therapy VIII. W. B. Saunders Company, Philadelphia, 1983.)

Table 18:3. RESULTS OF MEDICAL TREATMENT OF 100 CANINE OTITIS EXTERNA CASES*

Type of Otitis Externa	Cured (%)	Temporary Response (%)	No Response (%)	No Record (%)
Acute (eczematous; purulent)	86.5	0	4.5	9.0
Chronic (purulent; ulcerative)	48.4	25.6	12.0	14.0
Otomycosis	77.0	14.0	5.0	4.0
Parasitic	96.1	0	0	3.9
Proliferative	0	0	100	0

*From Grono, L. R.: Otitis externa. *In* Kirk, R. W. (ed.): Current Veterinary Therapy VII. W. B. Saunders Company, Philadelphia, 1980.

In general, ear problems can be handled successfully if they are properly diagnosed and treated diligently and thoroughly the first time. Small amounts of correct medication, applied in a thin film to a clean canal, often produce a good response in 7 to 10 days. Treatment should continue for an additional 2 weeks if the condition is improving. Grono reported results of therapy of 100 unselected cases of otitis externa (Table 18:3). Failure to respond suggests consideration of surgical treatment. This step should not be delayed too long. Surgery is designed either to resect the lateral wall of the canal to improve ventilation and drainage or to completely ablate the ear canal. These measures are discussed in veterinary surgery texts and articles.[7, 10]

EAR FISSURE

Ear fissures develop on the distal edge of the pinna from scratching or "flapping" the ears. They start as small marginal wounds but constantly enlarge with further trauma, because the natural healing process of the skin is constantly interrupted. Fissures vary in size from 2 to 3 mm to deep triangular tears of up to 3 cm. Hemorrhage accompanies further ear flapping, and the dog's surroundings often are splattered with blood.

Treatment is difficult. The cause should be found and eliminated. Ear mites, otitis, foreign objects, and generalized pruritus are common etiologic factors. Topical antibiotics and corticosteroids can be used, but they are usually not effective and radical treatment is needed. The following three surgical procedures can be used:

1. The edges of the fissures can be trimmed and the new wounds sutured so that the fissure is obliterated. Cosmetic results are excellent, but the dog usually succeeds in removing or loosening the sutures before healing is complete, and a new, larger fissure results. Immobilizing the ear flap in a protective bandage over the top of the head for 3 weeks may ensure primary healing.

2. Trimming the edges of the fissures and suturing the skin of the medial edge to that of the lateral edge over the exposed cartilage allows healing but leaves a punched-out notch in the ear flap. This is cosmetically disfiguring and does not always prevent further deepening of the triangle. However, this simple method will often successfully stop the bleeding and allow the wound to heal.

3. The most successful repair method is the surgical removal of the distal segment of the pinna. Serrated scissors are used to make a rounded incision that resects the distal pinna to a point just above the proximal edge of the

fissure. It is advisable to mark the line of incision with a sterile marking pen. The more carefully this cut is made, the more pleasing are the results. During healing, the ear should be bandaged across the head to prevent trauma caused by shaking. The shortened pinna seldom attracts attention after healing is complete and the hair has regrown.

EAR MARGIN NECROSIS

Ear margin necrosis may be produced by vasculitis, cold agglutinin disease, frostbite, solar dermatitis, and ear margin seborrhea. They are discussed elsewhere in the text. Holzworth[10a] reported necrosis of the pinna of cats that had eaten decomposed scallops from a seafood processing plant, and in cats with various severe systemic diseases and hematologic disorders (disseminated intravascular coagulation).

CANINE STERILE EOSINOPHILIC PINNAL FOLLICULITIS

Sterile eosinophilic pinnal folliculitis is an idiopathic, nonseasonal, bilaterally symmetric dermatosis of dogs.[15a] It is characterized by restriction of lesions to the pinnae, tissue eosinophilia, negative cultures, and a good response to topical or systemic glucocorticosteroids. Affected dogs are otherwise healthy, and the disorder is chronic in nature, requiring long-term maintenance therapy.

Eyelid Diseases

The eyelids are complex folds of skin susceptible to many structural and functional disorders that can, in turn, affect the eyeball (globe) itself (Fig. 18:4A).

ANATOMY

Canine and feline eyelids consist of an upper eyelid, a lower eyelid, a third eyelid (membrana nictitans), a row of cilia in the upper lid only, the orbicularis oculi muscles, nerves, blood vessels, lymphatics, and a number of glands. Meibomian glands (tarsal glands) are modified, large sebaceous gland units that produce a viscous, oily secretion. Zeis's glands are sebaceous glands associated with cilia. Moll's glands are modified apocrine sweat glands associated with cilia. Glands of the third eyelid (nictitans glands, Harder's glands) are masses of lymphoid tissue located on the inner surface of the membrana nictitans. In addition, there are accessory lacrimal glands in the eyelids that discharge tears into the conjuctival sac and contribute to the precorneal film. The largest of these in the dog is the superficial gland of the membrana nictitans, also known (erroneously) as the Harder's gland (or harderian gland).

DISEASES

Many dermatoses may appear first on the eyelids or are limited to the lids (Table 18:4).[2, 5a] Others are known for their periocular distribution, although they are not limited to that area (Table 18:5).[2]

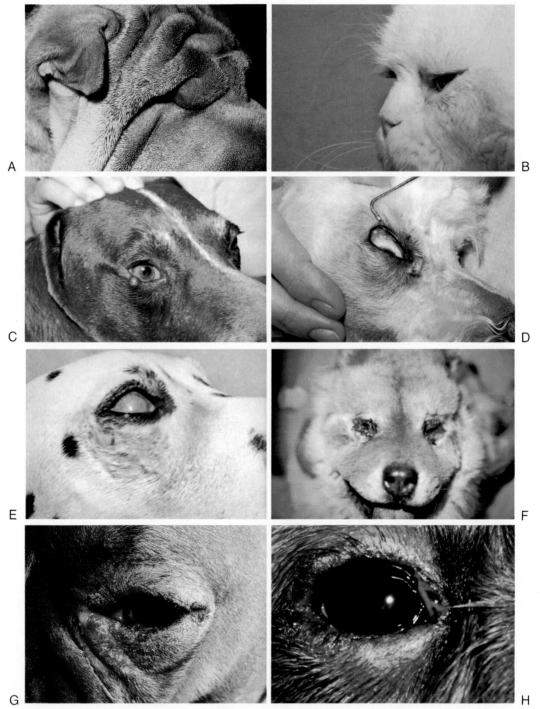

Figure 18:4. Eyelid diseases. *A,* This Shar Pei dog cannot see because the facial and eye folds cover the orbit. *B,* Entropion in a Persian cat. Note the narrowed palpebral fissure (squint), the wet hair from continual epiphora, and the conjunctival irritation. Surgical correction is curative. *C,* Chalazion, chronic inflammation of a meibomian gland—external appearance. *D,* Chalazion, internal view of the early stage. A cystic meibomian gland has a similar appearance. *E,* Mycotic blepharitis *(M. canis)* affecting the lower lid. The keratitis is secondary. *F,* Chronic blepharitis due to *Aspergillus niger.* Gentle cleansing and topical application of nystatin ointment produced an excellent response. (Courtesy S. Bistner and R. Riis.) *G,* Marked focal alopecia due to demodectic blepharitis. *H,* Small papules and pustules at the lid edges from staphylococcal infection produced this marginal blepharitis. (Courtesy S. Bistner.)

Table 18:4. DISEASES LIMITED TO OR THAT MAY FIRST PRESENT AS EYELID OR PERIOCULAR DERMATOSES

Demodicosis
Dermatophytosis
Bacterial folliculitis
Facial fold dermatitis
Atopy (allergic inhalant dermatitis)
Food hypersensitivity
Zinc-responsive dermatosis
Juvenile cellulitis
Facial keratosis
Idiopathic periocular alopecia
Self-trauma secondary to ocular disease

Entropion and Ectropion. Entropion (inversion or turning in) (Fig. 18:4*B*) and ectropion (eversion or turning out) of the lid margins are best corrected by surgery. Chronic conjunctivitis or other diseases of the eye that may result in distortion of the lids should also receive attention.

Hordeolum (Sty). This is an acute, painful pyogenic infection of a sebaceous gland of the eyelid. Two types are recognized: The external hordeolum (zeisian sty) involves the glands of Zeis and the cilia on the outer eyelid. The internal hordeolum (meibomian sty) involves the meibomian gland in the inner surface of the eyelid. The internal type is the most common hordeolum in dogs. Treatment consists of incising the abscess and applying an antibiotic ointment. Appropriate systemic antibiotics are useful when the hordeolum is caused by staphylococci.

Chalazion. A chronic inflammation of a meibomian gland (Fig. 18:4*C,D*), the chalazion appears externally on the skin surface of the lid as a painless nodule, and internally on the palpebral conjunctiva as a yellow, smaller nodule. The irritation from the inner swelling causes conjunctivitis. Treatment consists of incision and curettage of accumulated sebaceous material. Large chalazia should be excised completely to prevent recurrence.

Blepharitis. This erythematous, crusted inflammation of eyelid *margins* is often accompanied by a mucous discharge. Many generalized skin diseases extend to the lids, producing an inflammation that can be named after its cause.

Seborrheic Blepharitis. This is characterized by greasy scales and flakes on the lids. Corticosteroid ointments are a valuable symptomatic treatment.

Mycotic Blepharitis. When a dermatophytosis extends to the lids and cilia (Fig. 18:4*E*), this condition can occur. It is usually caused by *Microsporum canis*, *Microsporum gypseum*, or *Trichophyton mentagrophytes*. Systemic griseofulvin is

Table 18:5. DISEASES THAT AFFECT THE EYELID OR PERIOCULAR AREA IN ADDITION TO OTHER SITES

Pemphigus foliaceus (PF)
Pemphigus erythematosus (PE)
Systemic lupus erythematosus (SLE)
Discoid lupus erythematosus (DLE)
Vogt-Koyanagi-Harada syndrome
Canine familial dermatomyositis
Canine hepatocutaneous syndrome
Erythema multiforme

effective treatment. Figure 18:4F illustrates a case attributable to *Aspergillus niger* that responded to topical nystatin.

Demodectic Blepharitis. This disorder is very common in young dogs (Fig 18:4G). An alopecic, frequently erythematous patch on the upper or lower lid usually yields demodectic mites when skin scrapings are made. As long as the condition remains localized and free of staphylococcus infection, it is not serious. *Canine scabies* can also affect the eyelids. For treatment, a mild rotenone (Goodwinol) ointment, applied once a day, is sufficient. The cornea should be protected with ophthalmic ointment when irritating medication is used on the eyelids.

Distemper Blepharitis. Accompanying most cases of canine distemper, this condition is closely related to the conjunctivitis that is common in distemper, and copious mucous eye discharge is seen. The eyes should be cleansed frequently and an antibiotic ointment (such as chloramphenicol ointment) should be used three times a day. A similar blepharitis accompanies some other acute infectious diseases of dogs and cats.

Staphylococcal Marginal Blepharitis. This condition (Fig. 18:4H) may affect skin of the eyelids, just as it may involve other parts of the body.

Juvenile Cellulitis. This disorder usually involves much of the face and is often accompanied by swelling of the eyelids, blepharitis, and a purulent ocular discharge.

Autoimmune Diseases. These diseases, especially pemphigus vulgaris and bullous pemphigoid, often involve the mucocutaneous junction of the eyelids.

Atopy and Food Hypersensitivity. Dogs with these conditions often rub their eyes and have conjunctivitis with accompanying blepharitis.

Trichiasis. This disorder is an abnormal position or direction of the cilia resulting in epiphora, mucous eye discharge, and sometimes corneal vascularization and even corneal ulceration. Treatment consists of meticulous electro-epilation in the involved cilia.

Distichiasis. Animals with distichiasis (Fig. 18:5A) display aberrant cilia on the lid. They may emerge from the openings of the meibomian glands or the inner-lid margin. Electroepilation is the treatment of choice. Distichiasis has been reported in poodles, boxers, Pekingese, Alsatians, cocker spaniels, Shetland sheepdogs, and Bedlington and Yorkshire terriers, as well as in the Shih Tzu, pug, and St. Bernard.[12, 13]

Nictitans gland hypertrophy ("Cherry eye"). A bright red nodule protrudes into the medial canthus from under the third eyelid, in animals with this disorder. It is most common in Boston terriers and cocker spaniels. Although the condition may be unilateral, the opposite eye frequently becomes involved later. Surgical removal of the protruding nictitans gland is a simple operation

---

Figure 18:5. Eyelid diseases (continued) and feline nail diseases. *A,* Distichiasis. Note carefully the aberrant cilia projecting onto the bulbar conjunctiva. They will cause constant irritation and chronic lacrimation and conjunctivitis and should be removed by electroepilation or by the surgical lid-splitting operation. (Courtesy S. Bistner.) *B,* Epiphora. The chronic discharge of tears is common in poodles and results in brown staining of the wet hair. (This phenomenon is seen anywhere that white hair is constantly wet.) If nasolacrimal blockage is not the cause, careful removal of the gland of the membrana nictitans is often helpful, as it reestablishes the lacrimal "lake." *C,* Nasolacrimal blockage and severe chronic epiphora produced this severe secondary blepharitis. Treatment should attempt to reestablish the normal lacrimal drainage. (Courtesy S. Bistner.) *D,* Mastocytomas involving this boxer's eyelids produce a most serious and painful disease process. Prognosis is poor. *E,* Sebaceous adenoma, upper eyelid. *F,* Paronychia in a cat with pemphigus foliaceus. *G,* Feline paronychia associated with FeLV infection. *H,* Close-up of cat foot in *G.*

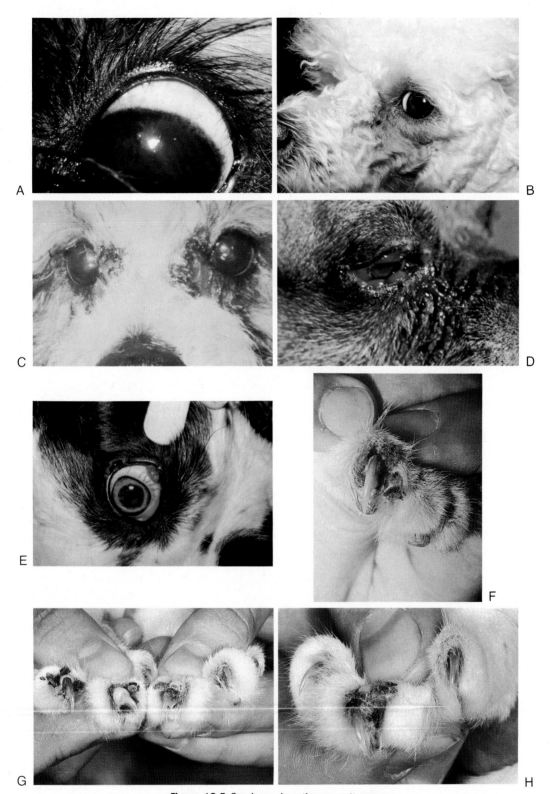

Figure 18:5 *See legend on the opposite page*

Table 18:6. NEOPLASTIC CONDITIONS THAT MAY AFFECT THE EYELID OR PERIOCULAR AREA

Squamous cell carcinoma
Actinic keratosis
Melanoma
Sebaceous gland tumors
Fibrous histiocytoma
Dermoid
Lymphosarcoma
Mycosis fungoides
Papilloma
Mastocytoma
Histiocytoma

that provides excellent results. It is most important to avoid damage to the third eyelid itself during this surgery.

Epiphora. This disorder is common in poodles (Fig. 18:5B,C). The cause may be atresia, blockage of the nasal lacrimal system, or lid or membrana nictitans deformities.[4] Surgical correction of the lid problem or deepening of the "lacrimal lake" frequently permits improved function of the lower puncta. Correction of possible causes of chronic lacrimation from ocular irritation should also be implemented.

Tumors of the eyelids. These tumors are difficult to manage because of the problems with plastic repair following surgery or with protection to the globe, if radiation therapy is contemplated. Papilloma, sebaceous gland tumor and melanomas, basal cell tumor and mastocytoma (Fig. 18:5D) are often found. A histiocytoma of the eyelid of a 10-month-old Afghan that regressed spontaneously has been reported.[6]

In older dogs, eyelid tumors are very common (Table 18:6).[2] These can be adenomas and adenocarcinomas of Zeis's and Moll's glands as well as meibomian gland tumors (Fig.18:5E). For *treatment*, surgical removal is indicated when the tumor is on the palpebral junction and touches the cornea. This can be accomplished by surgical excision, electrosurgery, or cryosurgery. Tumors that touch the conjunctiva and cause irritation (and sometimes ulceration) must be removed. It is important to remove the entire tumor; otherwise, it will regrow. The surgery can be performed with a sedative (tranquilizer) plus local anesthesia. A small V-shaped incision exposes the entire tumor for removal and can be closed with one or two sutures. Massive eyelid tumors that require removal of a large section of lid should be referred to an ophthalmologist, as correct plastic repair is necessary for proper lid function.

Nail (Claw) Diseases

ANATOMY

The nail (claw) is a specialized structure that is a direct continuation of the dermis and epidermis (Fig. 18:6). The distal phalanx of each toe has a crescent-shaped dorsal process called the ungual crest. The dermis of adjacent skin is continuous with, and extends distally from, this bony process as the periosteum of the phalanx. It has a rich blood supply and is the source of the profuse

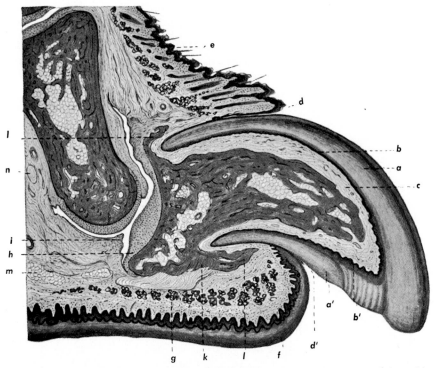

Figure 18:6. Midsagittal section through the claw of the dog: *a*, stratum corneum of the epidermis of the claw; *a'*, stratum corneum of the epidermis of the sole; *b,b'*, deep, noncornified epidermal layers of the dorsum and sole of the claw; *c*, corium (papillated in the area of the sole); *d*, claw fold; *d'*, limiting furrow separating the sole from the digital pad; *e*, skin with hair and glands; *f*, epidermis of the digital pad with stratum granulosum and lucidum; *g*, tubular glands in the digital pad; *h*, articular cartilage of the third phalanx; *i*, meniscus; *k*, Sharpey's fibers from a tendon insertion; *l*, ungual crest; *m*, fat cushion within the digital pad; *n*, lamellar corpuscle. (From Trautmann, A., and Fiebiger, J.: Fundamentals of the Histology of Domestic Animals. Copyright 1952 by Cornell University. Reprinted by permission of Cornell University Press.)

hemorrhage if the claw is trimmed too short. The structures constituting the claw are compressed laterally, and the dermis can thus be divided into the sole (ventral), the dorsal ridge of the coronary band, and the lateral and medial walls. Most of the claw is formed from the coronary band and the dorsal ridge. In many areas the dermis has fine papillae that project distally and interdigitate with soft epidermal lamellae.

The epidermis of adjacent skin is also continuous with that of the claw. The basal layer of the epidermis, supported by the dermis, is most active in the coronary and dorsal ridge areas and causes growth in a circular fashion, producing a curved claw. This is why the claw may grow around into the volar surface of the footpad. The horny walls grow over the sole of the claw for the same reason. During the first 2 years of life, the claws of beagles grow an average of 1.9 mm/week, but this rate declines with age. The epidermis of the claw sole has distinct granular and clear layers, as well as the usual structures. However, the epidermis of the rest of the claw is largely composed of a thick horny layer that consists of flat cornified epidermal cells fused into a horny plate, with an absent stratum granulosum. On the ventral surface the claw is separated from the footpad by a distinct furrow. A fold of modified skin hides the dorsal junction of hairy skin and claw. This claw fold is free of hair on its inner surface and produces the thin stratum tectorium that is the outer layer of the proximal claw.

The nails of animals have important functions as prehensile and locomotor organs. Cats use their nails to fight and to climb trees. Cats may cause anguish to their owners when they pick furniture as they keep their nails sharp. A dog's nails should be kept properly trimmed for good foot health, and normal locomotion. Abnormal nails predispose the feet to trauma, strains and podo-dermatitis. Because of the long growth cycle, the correction of abnormalities may require 6 to 8 months.

Many systemic diseases and drugs are reflected in human nail deformities. A single disease can present widely differing lesions and, conversely, a particular nail malformation can be the expression of a number of diseases of varying etiology.[1] Some human diseases that commonly involve nails are psoriasis, epidermolysis bullosa, lichen planus, alopecia areata, various forms of dermatitis, phototoxicity, contact dermatitis, trauma, drugs, and bacterial and mycotic infections. Only a few of these have been implicated in animal nail dystrophies. Veterinarians should be alert to recognition of the effects of disease on nails (claws). Veterinary problems associated with nail diseases include trauma, demodicosis, infection, pemphigus (Fig. 18:5F), feline leukemia virus infection (Fig. 18:5G,H), systemic lupus erythematosus, pemphigoid, acromegaly, feline hyperthyroidism, vascular insufficiency, seborrheic derma-titis, and senility.

DISEASES

The nails and nail folds are subject to injury, bacterial infection (paronychia), and fungal infection (onychomycosis). Defects in keratinization of the nail plate also occur. In general, true nail diseases are relatively uncommon in dogs and cats.

Paronychia. This is an inflammatory condition of the soft tissue around the nail. It is most commonly caused by bacteria, but dermatophytes or yeasts can also produce it. A single nail or several may be involved. When many or all nails are affected, one should suspect that it is secondary to a systemic disease such as pemphigus, bullous pemphigoid, systemic lupus erythemato-sus, feline leukemia, lymphosarcoma, generalized demodicosis, or diabetes mellitus. Diagnosis can be established by the case history, physical examination, stained smears of exudate, skin scrapings, fungal and bacterial cultures, and biopsy (especially utilizing a direct immunofluorescent test).

Bacterial paronychia. This disorder (Fig. 18:7A) may be acute or chronic, the latter being more common. Since the seat of the infection is at the base of the nail under the fold, surgical removal of the nail plate (shell) provides satisfactory drainage and is the treatment of choice. In most cases, the nail grows back. With the animal under general anesthesia, the nail plate is grasped firmly with a strong hemostat and stripped from its attachment in one steady downward motion. Because the diseased nail usually is loose, the procedure is easily accomplished and there is little or no hemorrhage (see Figs.18:7B–E and 18:8). Systemic antibiotics and antimicrobial soaks are indicated. In cats, primary bacterial paronychia is very rare. The clinician should always consider under-lying causes, such as pemphigus foliaceus, feline leukemia virus infection, arteriovenous fistulae, and metastatic bronchial carcinoma.

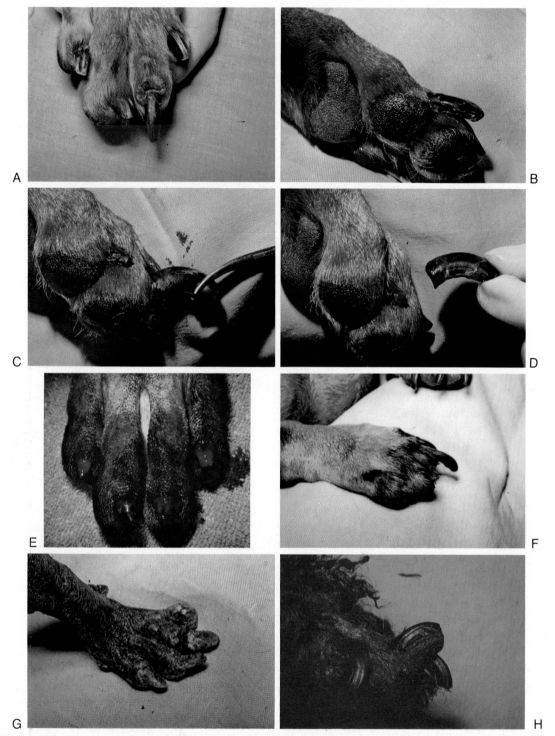

Figure 18:7. Canine nail diseases. *A,* Bacterial paronychia with ulceration of the nail fold. Note the purulent exudate at the base of the nail. *B,* Paronychia in a Doberman pinscher showing one infected nail before removal. *C,* The nail plate is grasped with a hemostat or needle holder and twisted along its curvature, while dog is under general anesthesia. *D,* The nail plate has been removed exposing the subungual nail bed. *E,* The paw after removal of all nail plates. Nitrofurazone (Furacin Soluble Dressing) should be applied and a well-padded bandage placed on the paw to protect the sensitive nail beds. *F,* Paronychia from which *Candida albicans* was isolated. The nails fell out and the nail folds were painful. *G,* Onychomycosis in a dog caused by *Trichophyton mentagrophytes*. Nails are grossly deformed, and there is secondary paronychia in the central toe. *H,* Deformed nail following an injury. Note the split and exposed matrix.

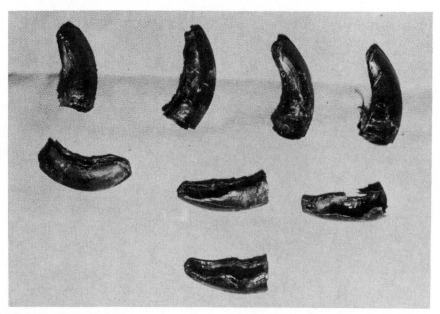

Figure 18:8. The nail plates of dog in Figure 18:7*B* after removal. Notice the rough edges and deteriorated state of the keratin.

Candidal paronychia. This condition is rare (Fig. 18:7*F*). When a candida infection is established in the nail fold, pain is considerable, and the affected nails may fall out. Other involved nails usually are painful and loosely attached. Topical nystatin or miconazole or oral ketoconazole (10 mg/kg BID) can be used for treatment. The latter has shown excellent results recently. Animals with candidiasis always should be checked for diabetes mellitus and various types of endogenous or exogenous immunosuppression.

Onychomycosis. Found in dogs, onychomycosis is usually caused by *Trichophyton mentagrophytes*. It frequently accompanies generalized dermatophytosis. The nail shown in Fig. 18:7*G* came from a dog with a *T. mentagrophytes* infection involving over half of its skin surface. In cats, *Microsporum canis* is the most common cause of onychomycosis. Treatment consists of permanent surgical excision of the affected nails (the entire third phalanx), followed by griseofulvin or ketoconazole orally for several months. To prevent relapses, griseofulvin or ketoconazole must be continued until mycotic cultures fail to grow dermatophytes.

Onychorrhexis (Brittle Nails). This is a tendency of the nail to break from the free edge. It occurs spontaneously in some dogs. There is a breed predilection for dachshunds. Some or all nails may be involved, and the condition is usually chronic. When only one nail is involved, the cause may be an injury (Fig. 18:7*H*). However, when several nails on more than one foot are involved, the cause is unknown and there is no response to treatment. Warm water soaks and removal of splintered pieces provide temporary relief. If the condition persists for 1 year, permanent amputation of the nail (declawing) is the treatment of choice. Although the surgery is more difficult than the declawing of cats, it provides complete relief to the affected dog, who gets along well without nails.

Onychomadesis. This separation of the hard keratin "shell" results in loss (slough) of the nail. It can be caused by trauma, infection, vascular insufficiency, pemphigus, or systemic lupus erythematosus. Treatment depends on the cause and usually involves treatment of a systemic disorder, as well as topical medication.

Miscellaneous. Nails may grow very rapidly and be abnormally thick and hard in canine acromegaly, feline hyperthyroidism, and zinc-responsive/deficient conditions (see appropriate sections of this text). Congenital nail disorders such as *arthronychia* (abnormal curvature) and *anonychia* (absence) are rarely reported.[18]

Anal Sac Diseases

There are three anal sac abnormalities discussed here: impaction, chronic infection, and acute infection (abscessation).

CAUSE AND PATHOGENESIS

Anal sacs are paired invaginations of the skin located between the internal and external sphincters of the anus. Each is connected to the surface by a single duct that opens at the mucocutaneous junction of the anus of the dog but that opens on a pyramid prominence 0.25 cm lateral to the anus of the cat. Most of each sac is lined with abundant large sebaceous glands, but the fundic portion of the canine sac has numerous apocrine glands (Fig. 18:9). The total secretion of these glands is a brownish, oily fluid that develops a characteristic disagreeable odor with infection or impaction or both (Table 18:7). The odor of the fluid may have a function in social recognition among dogs. Normally, defecation causes compression of the sacs and expression of some of their contents. However, change in character of the secretion, oversecretion, or

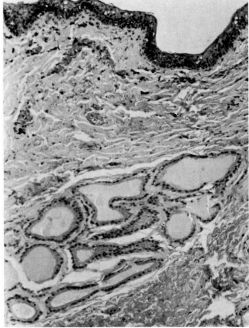

Figure 18:9. Section through wall of the anal sac showing apocrine-type glands in the dermis.

Table 18:7. ANAL SAC SECRETIONS

Color	Consistency	Odor	Disease Process
Straw	Thin liquid with small brownish flecks, or thick liquid pus	Pungent	None
Greenish yellow	Medium-thick liquid	Fetid	Infection
Red	Oily thick paste	Fetid	Infection
Clay	Dry paste	Very little	Impaction
Black	Dry or thick liquid	Very little	Chronic impaction

change in the muscle tone or fecal form may cause overfilling of the sacs, plugging of the ducts with resulting fermentation, inflammation, and infection.

Abnormalities of the anal sacs cause "scooting," licking, biting, or rubbing the anus, and acute moist dermatitis from self-trauma may result in the surrounding region. Infected anal sacs are a focus of infection that has the potential for several untoward results. Some veterinarians are convinced that dogs licking the anal region in such cases transfer infection to the mouth with resultant pharyngitis, gagging, and so on. Treatment of both areas (anal sacs and pharynx) has produced good results.

Anal sacs are probably vestigial structures that the ancestors of dogs and cats used as a spraying defense mechanism similar to that used by the skunk. Anal sac problems occur more commonly in smaller breeds (under 15 kg), especially poodles (miniature and toy), Chihuahuas, and seborrheic spaniels. They are less common in German shepherds and giant breeds. There is no sex or age predisposition. The overall incidence was 2 per cent among the animals examined in a nonreferral hospital.[9] The anal sac is sometimes called the "anal gland," which is an erroneous term that should not be used. There are, however, multiple perianal glands in the cutaneous border of the anus and modified sebaceous and apocrine cells in the lining and ducts of the anal sacs.

CLINICAL FEATURES

The distended sacs can often be palpated just lateral to and below the midpoint of the anus (at "4 o'clock" and "8 o'clock"). Localized erythema, swelling, pain, and subsequent rupture and draining of an acutely infected sac may occur 1 to 2 cm lateral to the anus. The abscess is usually unilateral, and the course is short (7 to 10 days). Impaction and chronic infection may have a prolonged course (months) with many periods of quiescence and exacerbation.

CLINICAL MANAGEMENT

Feline impactions usually occur without infection, and manual expression (by lateral external compression) usually relieves clinical signs for a relatively long time.[9, 16]

Canine impactions tend to recur. They should be gently but thoroughly expressed. This may have to be repeated several times at weekly intervals by gently placing a gloved finger in the posterior rectum and compressing the sac between the finger and the thumb (positioned lateral to the distended sac). A fetid brownish yellow or black discharge is expressed. If recurrence is frequent, the following irrigation should be performed.

Chronically infected anal sacs should be treated as any infection—by drainage. This need not be surgical. Frequent expression of the purulent or bloody exudate followed by instillation of an antibiotic solution may be curative.

Inferior results are often obtained with this method because the tenderness of the region precludes thorough treatment. It is preferable to lightly anesthetize the patient and thoroughly lavage *both* sacs with lactated Ringer's solution, using a blunt needle or cannula attached to a syringe. Ceruminolytic agents such as hexamethyltetracosane (Ceruminex) may also be useful as lavage fluids. After the sac is thoroughly flushed, it is important to instill an antibiotic cream (chloramphenicol), nitrofurazone solution, or a lotion containing chloramphenicol and a topical corticosteroid in a ceruminolytic base. This may be repeated in 5 to 7 days. If recurrence develops after initial response, surgical removal of the sacs is indicated.

An acutely infected anal sac (abscess) must be treated by liberal incision at the point of localization and by curettage and application of 5 per cent Lugol's solution. Healing occurs by granulation. If the anal sac abscess does not heal with the above treatments or if it recurs repeatedly, surgical excision of the anal sacs is indicated. (Their function is unknown, and they are unnecessary for good health.)

References

1. Achten, G., and Parent, D.: The normal and pathologic nail. Int. J. Dermatol. *22*:556, 1983.
2. Angarano, D. W.: Dermatologic disorders of the eyelid and periocular region. *In* Kirk, R. W., (ed.): Current Veterinary Therapy X, W. B. Saunders Company, Philadelphia, 1986.
3. August, J. R.: Diseases of the ear canal. Complete Manual of Ear Care, Veterinary Learning Systems, Princeton Junction, New Jersey, 1986.
4. Bistner, S. I.: Diseases of the nasolacrimal system. *In* Kirk, R. W., (ed.): Current Veterinary Therapy V. W. B. Saunders Company, Philadelphia, 1974.
5. Blue, J. L., and Wooley, R. E.: Antibacterial sensitivity patterns of bacteria isolated from dogs with otitis externa. J.A.V.M.A. *177*:362, 1977.
5a. Charbonne, L., and Clerc, B.: Les blepharites des carnivores domestiques. Point. Vet. *20*:33, 1988.
6. Gelatt, K. N.: Histiocytoma of the eyelid of a dog. Vet. Med. (S.A.C.) *70*:305, 1975.
7. Griffin, C.: Principles for treatment of the diseased ear canal. Complete Manual of Ear Care. Veterinary Learning Systems. Princeton Junction, New Jersey, 1986.
8. Grono, L. R.: Otitis externa. *In* Kirk, R. W., (ed.): Current Veterinary Therapy VII. W. B. Saunders Company, Philadelphia, 1980.
9. Harvey, C. E.: Incidence and distribution of anal sac disease in the dog. J.A.A.H.A. *10*:573, 1974.
10. Harvey, C. E.: Ear canal disease in the dog. Medical and surgical management. J.A.V.M.A. *177*:136, 1980.
10a. Holzworth, J.: Diseases of the Cat. W. B. Saunders Company, Philadelphia, 1987.
11. Joshua, J. O.: Anal sac lesions in the cat. Mod. Vet. Pract. *52*:53, 1971.
12. Ketring, K. L.: Diseases of the eyelids. *In* Kirk, R. W. ed.: Current Veterinary Therapy VII. W. B. Saunders Company, Philadelphia, 1980.
13. Lawson, D. D.: Canine distichiasis. J. Small Anim. Pract. *14*:469, 1973.
14. Nesbitt, G. H., and Schmitz, J. A.: Chronic bacterial dermatitis and otitis; a review of 195 cases. J.A.A.H.A. *13*:442, 1977.
15. Scott, D. W.: Feline dermatology 1900–1978: A monograph. J.A.A.H.A. *16*:331, 1980.
15a. Scott, D. W.: Canine sterile eosinophilic pinnal folliculitis. Companion Anim. Pract. (in press, 1988).
16. Seim, H. B.: Diseases of the anus and rectum. *In* Kirk, R. W., (ed.): Current Veterinary Therapy IX, W. B. Saunders Company, Philadelphia, 1986.
17. Venker-van Haagen, A. J.: Managing diseases of the external ear. *In* Kirk, R. W., (ed.): Current Veterinary Therapy VIII, W. B. Saunders Company, Philadelphia, 1983.
18. Wallace, L. J., et al.: Arthronychia and anonychia in greyhound dogs. J.A.V.M.A. *160*:421, 1972.

19

Miscellaneous Diseases

Subcorneal Pustular Dermatosis

Subcorneal pustular dermatosis is a very rare, idiopathic, sterile, superficial pustular dermatosis of dogs.[8, 10, 15]

CAUSE AND PATHOGENESIS

The cause of subcorneal pustular dermatosis is unknown. It has been postulated that a product of the stratum corneum or stratum granulosum (antigen-antibody complexes?) of skin may act as a chemotactic factor for neutrophils.[10]

CLINICAL FEATURES

In 24 cases of subcorneal pustular dermatosis reported in the literature,[8, 10, 15] no apparent age (6 months to 14 years old) or sex predilection exists. Although many breeds have been affected, miniature schnauzers have accounted for 38 per cent of the cases.

Affected dogs usually have a multifocal-to-generalized pustular-to-seborrhea–like dermatitis. The head and trunk are particularly affected. Intact pustules are usually nonfollicular, commonly greenish yellow, and often very transient in nature (persisting for only 2 to 4 hours at a time) (Fig. 19:1A,B). Thus, the affected dogs often have only circular areas of alopecia, erosion, scaling, crusting, and epidermal collarettes. Rarely the footpads may be affected and show a superficial peeling. Pruritus varies from extreme to nonexistent. The course of the dermatosis often erupts and regresses. Usually, the dogs are otherwise healthy.

DIAGNOSIS

Since this dermatosis is diagnosed by exclusion of other conditions, improved diagnostic techniques should make it an *extremely rare* entity.

Figure 19:1. *A,* Multiple nonfollicular pustules on the abdomen of a dog with subcorneal pustular dermatosis. *B,* Close-up view of Figure 19:1*A. C,* Sterile panniculitis in a dachshund. Two subcutaneous nodules on trunk. *D,* Sterile panniculitis in a cat. Ulcerated nodule in groin. *E,* Lupus erythematosus panniculitis in a dog. Multiple ulcers over hindquarters. *F,* Close-up of dog in Figure 19:1*E. G,* Perianal fistulas, anus. (Courtesy R. E. Hoffer.) *H,* Face of dachshund pup with juvenile cellulitis.

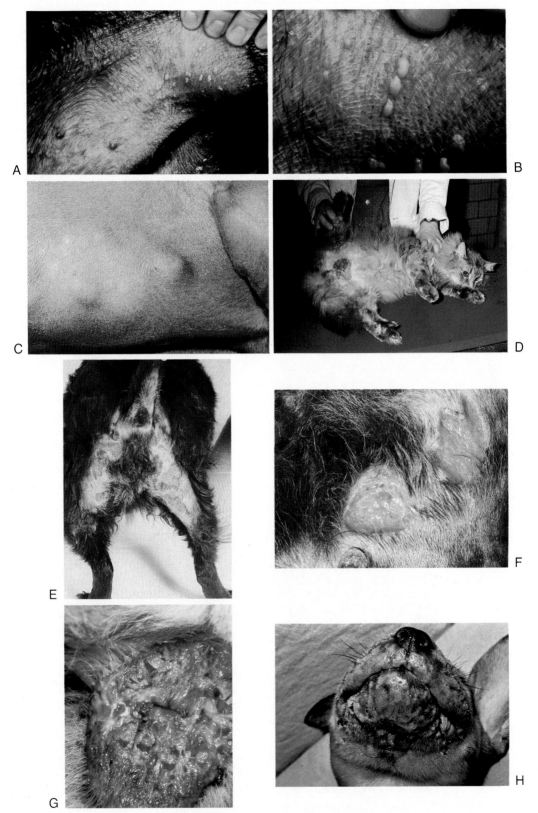

Figure 19:1 *See legend on opposite page*

Differential diagnosis includes bacterial folliculitis, dermatophytosis, demodicosis, pemphigus foliaceus, systemic lupus erythematosus, sterile eosinophilic pustulosis, seborrheic skin disease, atopy, and food hypersensitivity. Definitive diagnosis is based on history, physical examination, laboratory ruleouts, and response to therapy. Subcorneal pustular dermatosis is poorly responsive to systemic antibiotics, systemic glucocorticoids, and topical agents. Direct smears from intact pustules usually reveal numerous neutrophils, occasional acantholytic keratinocytes, and no microorganisms. Carefully performed cultures from intact pustules are usually negative, but a few colonies of coagulase-negative staphylococci are occasionally isolated. Immunofluorescence testing is negative. Skin biopsy reveals intraepidermal (subcorneal) pustular dermatitis.[15] Acantholysis is usually minimal, occasionally marked. Hair follicles are rarely involved (Figs. 19:2 and 19:3).

CLINICAL MANAGEMENT

The drug of choice in subcorneal pustular dermatosis is dapsone (see p. 194), which is given orally at 1 mg/kg TID. A beneficial response is usually seen within 1 to 4 weeks. The therapy can be either stopped with long-term remission resulting (in the minority of cases) or tapered to maintenance levels (variable from dog to dog: from 1 mg/kg SID to twice a week).

In humans, the side-effects of dapsone are numerous (see p. 194). In dogs, the major side-effects to date have been hematologic and hepatic. Many dogs develop mild nonregenerative anemia and leukopenia, and mild-to-moderate elevations of serum alanine aminotransferase (ALT) during induction therapy. If these laboratory abnormalities are not associated with clinical signs, it is not necessary to stop therapy, and the levels will return to normal when maintenance doses are achieved. Dapsone has also caused fatal thrombocytopenia in one dog,[9] profound leukopenia in one dog, occasional vomiting and diarrhea,

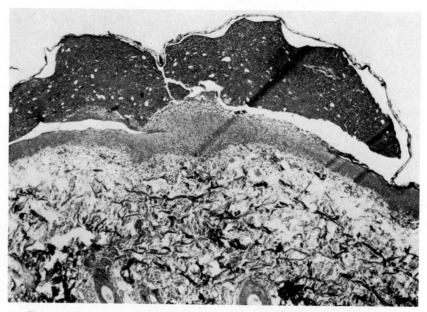

Figure 19:2. Canine subcorneal pustular dermatosis. A large subcorneal pustule.

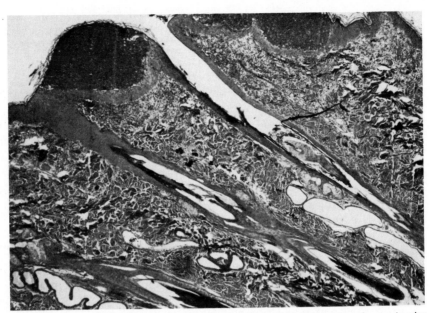

Figure 19:3. Canine subcorneal pustular dermatosis. Subcorneal pustules that do not involve hair follicles.

and generalized, pruritic erythematous maculopapular skin eruptions in two dogs.[15, 16] Dapsone is *not* licensed for use in dogs.

Very rarely, dogs have apparently become "resistant" to dapsone. These dogs may benefit from the administration of sulfasalazine (Azulfidine), orally at 10 to 20 mg/kg TID until the dermatosis is controlled, then as needed. Chronic administration of sulfasalazine may be associated with keratoconjunctivitis sicca.

Panniculitis

Panniculitis is a multifactorial inflammatory condition of the subcutaneous fat, characterized by deep-seated cutaneous nodules that often become cystic and ulcerated and develop draining tracts. The disorder is more common than the literature may suggest.

CAUSE AND PATHOGENESIS

The lipocyte (fat cell, adipocyte) is particularly vulnerable to trauma, ischemia, and neighboring inflammatory disease.[6, 17] In addition, damage to lipocytes results in the liberation of lipid, which undergoes hydrolysis into glycerol and fatty acids. Fatty acids are potent inflammatory agents, and they incite further inflammatory and/or granulomatous tissue reactions.

Multiple etiologic factors are involved in the genesis of panniculitis in human beings (Table 19:1). Many of these factors have yet to be recognized in dogs and cats, but this may only reflect lack of awareness. Infectious and nutritional causes of canine and feline panniculitis are discussed elsewhere (see pp. 270, 799) and therefore are not to be addressed here. This section concentrates on sterile forms of panniculitis.

Table 19:1. DIFFERENTIAL DIAGNOSIS OF HUMAN PANNICULITIS

Infectious
  Bacterial,* mycobacterial,* actinomycetic,* fungal,* chlamydial, viral
Immunologic
  Lupus erythematosus,* rheumatoid arthritis, drug eruption, erythema nodosum*
Physicochemical (factitial)
  Trauma, pressure, cold, foreign body* (e.g., post-subcutaneous injection of bulky, oily, or
    insoluble liquids)
Pancreatic disease
  Inflammation, neoplasia
Postglucocorticoid therapy
Vasculitis
  Leukocytoclastic, periarteritis nodosa, thrombophlebitis, embolism*
Nutritional
  Vitamin E deficiency*
Enteropathies
*Idiopathic**

*Recognized in dogs and cats.

"Nodular panniculitis" refers to sterile subcutaneous inflammatory nodules and is *not* a specific disease. It is purely a descriptive term, clinically representing the end result of several known and unknown etiologic factors.[5, 17] "Weber-Christian panniculitis" has been a frequently misused term and does *not* exist as a specific disease. In dogs and cats, the majority of cases of sterile nodular panniculitis are solitary lesions of idiopathic origin. A few cases of lupus erythematosus panniculitis and erythema nodosum have been recognized in dogs.[11, 17]

CLINICAL FEATURES

Panniculitis is manifested clinically as deep-seated cutaneous nodules. The lesions may occur singly or in crops, either localized to specific areas or generalized, and they vary from a few mm to several cm in diameter (Fig. 19:1C–F). Nodules may be firm and well circumscribed, or soft and ill defined (Fig. 19:4). They are initially subcutaneous, but may fix the overlying skin as they progress. The lesions may become cystic, may ulcerate, and may develop draining tracts that discharge an oily, yellowish brown to bloody substance (Fig. 19:5). The lesions may or may not be painful and often heal with depressed scars.

In a study of 22 dogs (14 reported in the literature; 8 seen by D.W.S.), idiopathic sterile nodular panniculitis was found to occur most commonly in the dachshund (13 cases).[11] Other breeds that were represented included the miniature poodle, wire-haired fox terrier, Manchester terrier, boxer, collie, German shepherd, old English sheepdog, and Weimaraner. There was no sex predilection. Ages of affected dogs varied from 10 weeks to 11 years, with 13 of the 22 dogs first developing lesions at less than 6 months of age.

In a later study of 57 canine cases, multiple breeds were involved and no age, sex, or breed predilection existed.[17] Eighty per cent had solitary, firm-to-fluctuant subcutaneous lesions of 2 to 9 cm in diameter. Lesions were most commonly present in the ventrolateral chest, neck, and abdomen. In 35 per cent of the dogs, lesions were associated with ulceration or fistula formation.

In a report of 21 cats, 17 were domestic short hair and the ages ranged from 10 weeks to 13 years, but 70 per cent were less than 4 years old. There was no sex or neutering factor in these cases. Ninety-five per cent of the cats

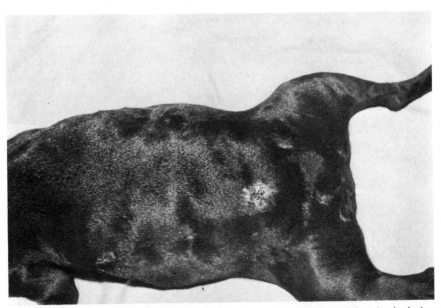

Figure 19:4. Panniculitis. Dorsal view of Boston terrier showing multiple nodular, circular lesions. A large draining fistula can be seen in the sacral lesion. Note the "lumpy" appearance of the lower back.

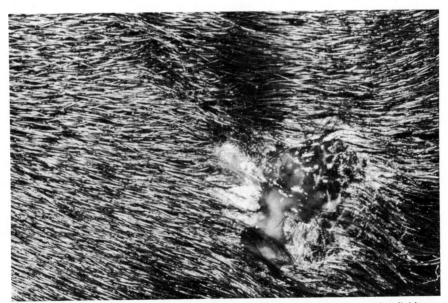

Figure 19:5. Close-up of the draining nodule seen in Figure 19:4. Note the oozing lipid pus and superficial crusts.

displayed solitary lesions, while 24 per cent developed ulceration and fistula formation associated with the lesion.[17] Lesions were most commonly present in the ventral abdomen and ventrolateral thorax.

A few cases of canine and feline idiopathic sterile nodular panniculitis are associated with constitutional signs, including poor appetite, depression, lethargy, and pyrexia.[17, 18] These signs are usually intermittent and often herald a new crop of skin lesions. If the panniculitis is associated with lupus erythematosus (lupus erythematosus panniculitis, lupus panniculitis, lupus profundus), concurrent signs of this disease may also be present. If erythema nodosum is present, concurrent signs may include pyrexia, depression, and arthralgia.

DIAGNOSIS

Sterile nodular panniculitis is most commonly misdiagnosed as deep pyoderma, cutaneous cysts, or cutaneous neoplasms. Aspirates from intact lesions usually reveal numerous neutrophils, "foamy" macrophages, and no microorganisms. Sudan stains may reveal extracellular and intracellular lipid droplets.

The diagnosis of panniculitis can only be made by biopsy. Excision biopsy is the *only* biopsy technique that is satisfactory for subcutaneous nodules.[6, 11, 12] Punch biopsies fail to deliver tissue sufficient to be of diagnostic value in about 75 per cent of the cases. Panniculitis may be lobular, septal, diffuse, or a combination of these characteristics.[17] In addition, panniculitis may be granulomatous, pyogranulomatous, suppurative, eosinophilic, necrotizing, or fibrosing. Thrombosis of subcuticular blood vessels, lymphoid nodules, and radial fat crystals may be seen. In a recent study of canine and feline panniculitis,[17] the histopathologic pattern and cytomorphology of the reactions had *little* diagnostic, therapeutic, or prognostic significance (Figs. 19:6 to 19:8). It is imperative to realize that most panniculitides, regardless of cause, look histo-

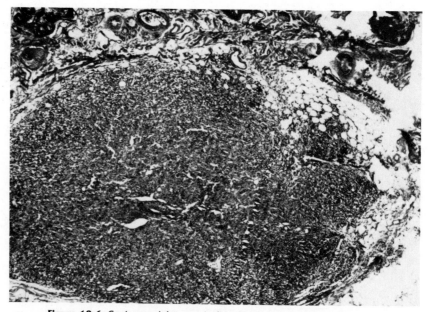

Figure 19:6. Canine nodular panniculitis. Pyogranulomatous panniculitis.

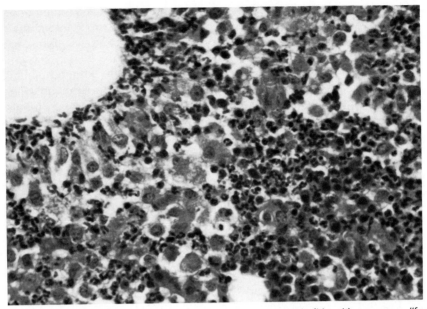

Figure 19:7. Canine nodular panniculitis. Pyogranulomatous panniculitis with numerous "foamy" macrophages (lipophages).

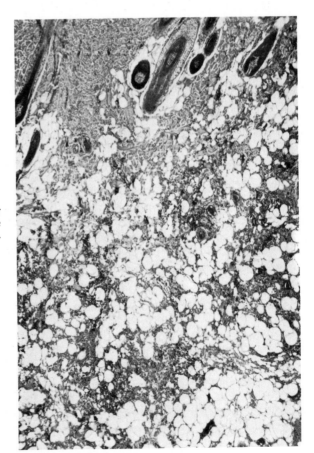

Figure 19:8. Feline nodular panniculitis. Marked lobular panniculitis and fat necrosis. (From Scott, D. W.: Feline dermatology 1900–1978: a monograph. J.A.A.H.A. *16*:331, 1980.)

logically identical. Thus, one cannot diagnose sterile nodular panniculitis from a biopsy specimen. Special stains and cultures are *always* indicated to rule out infectious agents, and polarized light examination is indicated to rule out foreign bodies.

If the panniculitis is predominantly lymphohistioplasmacytic, with or without concurrent neutrophilic vasculitis, or if other clinical signs suggest lupus erythematosus, other diagnostic tests may include antinuclear antibody (ANA), lupus erythematosus (LE) cell test, and direct immunofluorescence testing of lesional skin. If a vasculitis is present, diagnostic tests indicated may reflect the differential diagnosis of vasculitis (Figs. 19:9 and 19:10) (see p. 533). If the panniculitis is persistent and refractory or if the patient shows concurrent signs of gastrointestinal disease, pancreatic disease should be ruled out.

Erythema nodosum is characterized histologically by a *septal* panniculitis and is thought to represent a hypersensitivity reaction (Fig. 19:11).[6, 12] Thus, diagnostic considerations should include concurrent infections (bacterial endocarditis, coccidioidomycosis) and drug reactions.[6, 11, 12]

CLINICAL MANAGEMENT

Careful surgical excision of solitary lesions is usually curative.[17] Dogs and cats with multiple sterile panniculitis lesions usually respond well to systemic glucocorticoids.[7b, 17, 18] Prednisolone or prednisone may be administered orally

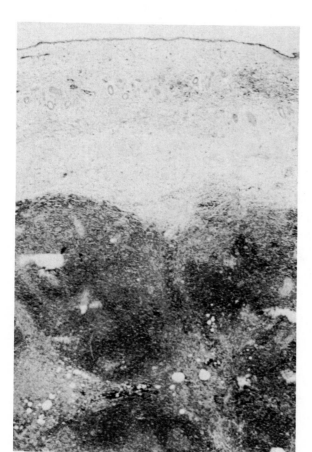

Figure 19:9. Lupus erythematosus panniculitis in a dog. Lobular to diffuse panniculitis with marked lymphoid nodule formation.

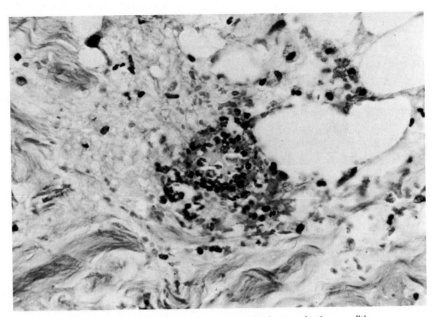

Figure 19:10. Close-up of Figure 19:9. Leukocytoclastic vasculitis.

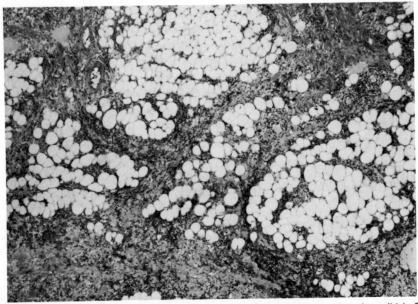

Figure 19:11. Canine erythema nodosum (associated with staphylococcal endocarditis). Septal panniculitis.

at 2 mg/kg SID (dog) or 4 mg/kg SID (cat) until the lesions have regressed (3 to 8 weeks). Therapy should be stopped at that point, since many dogs, especially young dogs, enter long-term or permanent remission. In recurrent cases, alternate-day steroid therapy may be required for prolonged periods.

In a few canine and feline cases, good results have been obtained with oral vitamin E (dl-α-tocopherol acetate), 400 IU BID.[11] The vitamin E must be given at least 2 hours before or after a meal for maximum effectiveness. In humans, oral potassium iodide has been used successfully in cases of sterile nodular panniculitis.[6]

Subcutaneous Fat Sclerosis

A single case of subcutaneous fat sclerosis has been described in a 1-year-old male domestic short hair cat.[4] An inguinal abscess had been treated by surgical drainage and antibiotics 5 weeks prior to the time a rapidly growing abdominal subcutaneous mass appeared. It was a firm, nonpainful subcutaneous plaque that extended from the xiphoid to the pelvic inlet and laterally to the lumbar processes. The borders were raised and distinct, and the normal overlying skin was cool, indurated, and adherent. The mass was large enough to restrict movement of the legs.

Differential diagnosis included neoplasia, panniculitis, and nutritional steatitis. A hemogram, extensive serum chemistry findings, and a feline leukemia test (ELISA) were normal. Bacteria and fungal cultures were negative.

Oral treatment with prednisolone was not effective. Later, small subcutaneous satellite nodules could be palpated on the chest wall, cranial to the mass.

On necropsy the abdominal subcutaneous tissues were thickened and fibrous, and were adhered to the dermis. Histopathologic findings revealed extensive subcutaneous fibrosis with minimal fat necrosis and inflammation. Within the subcutaneous fat, or within the fat-rich interstitial tissues of abdominal muscles, were bands of septal fibrosis, fat cells of increased size (fat micropseudocyst formation), and lipocytes containing needle-shaped fat clefts (fat crystals) (Figs. 19:12 and 19:13). Although a few scattered lymphocytes, histiocytes, and multinucleated histiocytic giant cells were found, and although there were isolated foci of neutrophils, the process was largely noninflammatory.

These findings are similar to two rare human disorders, sclerema neonatorum and subcutaneous fat necrosis of the newborn. The latter is indistinguishable from poststeroid panniculitis, but this cat had no history of being administered corticosteroids.

Perianal Fistulas

Multiple perianal fistulas (perianal pyoderma, anal furunculosis) is a deep infection involving the perianal skin and mucocutaneous junction with ulceration, sinuses, and deep fistulous tracts.

It affects German shepherds or crossbreed shepherds almost exclusively. However, isolated cases have been reported in Irish and English setters, English springer spaniels, Great Danes, Labrador and Chesapeake retrievers, Dandi Dinmont terriers, and crossbreeds. Either sex may be involved; the age range is about 3 to 8 years.

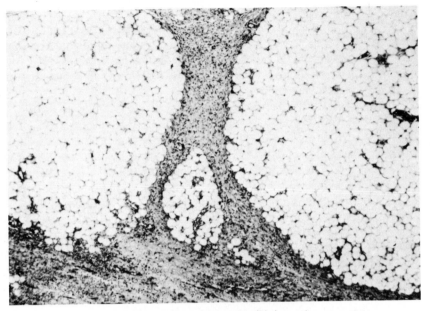

Figure 19:12. Septal panniculitis in a cat.

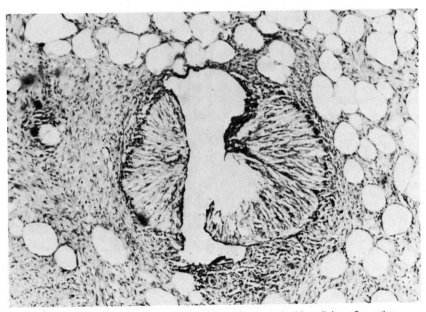

Figure 19:13. Sclerosing panniculitis in a cat. Fat crystal with radial configuration.

In a series of 54 cases, 36 per cent previously had anal sacculitis, 56 per cent had hind leg weakness (hip dysplasia?), and 67 per cent had a history of diarrhea.[1]

It has been suggested that the disease may result from fecal impaction of the crypts of Morgagni or from contamination of anal sacs, hair follicles, and apocrine and sebaceous glands of the perianal region by a fecal film spread by the broad tail of the German shepherd. Poor ventilation of the area may accentuate the problem.

Clinical signs include tenesmus, pain, constipation or diarrhea, rectal bleeding, constant licking or biting at the lesions, dyschezia, and weight loss. In chronic cases, the constant pain can produce personality changes and an unstable disposition.

The lesions consist of epidermal necrosis, perianal ulceration, multiple fistulas and sinuses lined with granulation tissue or stratified squamous epithelium, dilated perianal gland ducts, and dense fibrosis. (Fig. 19:1G).

Medical treatment is ineffective. It may offer temporary control but may delay more definitive measures and jeopardize long-term results.

Sharp surgical excision of the crypts of Morgagni, the anal pillars, the perianal gland tissue, and the anal sacs has been advocated, but up to 35 per cent of cases so treated result in fecal incontinence.[3] Electrosurgical deroofing and fulguration of fistulas and allowing the lesions to heal by granulation have also been advocated.[1] Cryosurgery repeated two or more times has resulted in 48 to 87 per cent satisfactory results, with only minor problems of stenosis or incontinence, or both.[1, 3, 20]

Because of problems with stenosis or fecal incontinence in other methods, the treatment of choice now appears to be tail amputation.[19] Minor local débridement or fistulectomy may be necessary for the most severe lesions.[7] Surgery must be accomplished carefully to eliminate folds or problems with skin tension and the anal opening. Secondary treatment with fulguration or deroofing of persisting fistulas, or more regular clipping of hair in the region, may be necessary in 10 per cent of cases that do not heal completely in 4 to 6 weeks.

Postoperative care with whirlpool baths or antiseptic irrigations and the use of stool softeners, systemic corticosteroids, and antibiotics have all been indicated. This disorder is a major problem that requires careful surgical management. It should be referred to those who have experience and expertise in these procedures. (See also References and textbooks on soft-tissue surgery.)

Juvenile Cellulitis

Juvenile cellulitis (juvenile pyoderma, puppy strangles) is a vesiculopustular disease of puppies that are less than 4 months but more than 3 weeks of age. It usually affects short-coated breeds, especially dachshunds, golden retrievers, and pointers. A single pup, several pups, or a whole litter may be involved. There may be positive cultures of *Staphylococcus* spp., but with careful technique and unbroken lesions the cultures usually fail to grow bacteria. A hypersensitivity reaction has been suggested as a cause. Although the etiology is unknown, one author (D.W.S.) has shown that the pups have suppressed in vitro lymphocyte blastogenesis, secondary to a serum factor. Total globulins, serum protein electrophoresis, immunoelectrophoresis, and bactericidal assays are

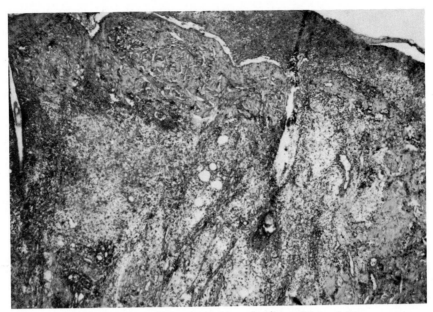

Figure 19:14. Juvenile cellulitis in a dog. Note diffuse cellulitis.

normal, however. Skin biopsy reveals diffuse dermatitis (cellulitis), with neutrophils and mononuclear cells predominating.

The lesions are concentrated around the face and head, especially the mucocutaneous junction, but the ears, anus, and prepuce may be involved. Although regional lymphadenopathy is present, many puppies are alert and afebrile; others have fevers. Some have whole body infection with fever, anorexia, and depression. The skin may be red, glistening, and alopecic, and serum or pus may ooze from the surface and may form tan crusts (Fig. 19:1*H*). The epidermis is fragile, and even mild trauma causes erosions. Because the inflammation is deep and fulminating, hair follicles are destroyed and permanent scarring results (Fig. 19:14).

Therapy should include systemic pediatric antibiotics, and the cephalosporins are suggested for most cases. Corticosteroids are the most important part of the treatment. Prednisolone or prednisone (2 mg/kg SID per os), triamcinolone, or dexamethasone should be administered, in all cases. This should be started after the antibiotics, and both should be continued for at least 2 weeks. Topical therapy is also important and entails wet soaks, especially Burow's solution (Domeboro), three to four times daily for 5 to 10 minutes each time. Be gentle to avoid more extensive scarring.

Because the puppies may be stressed by parasites, poor diet, and hygienic problems, these aspects of their management should receive close attention. The prognosis is favorable after 4 to 5 days of therapy. Once healing starts, the response is dramatic.

Infantile Pustular Dermatosis

Infantile pustular dermatosis is an acutely developing pustular skin reaction occurring in young puppies from 3 days to 3 weeks of age. It has been observed in Chinese Shar Pei, pointers, and Labrador retrievers. By the time puppies are examined, the pustules have progressed to tiny yellow, reddish, or brown crusts that are present mostly on the head and body. They may be incorporated into mats of hair. The pups are afebrile but depressed and anorectic. It is not unusual for some pups in a litter to be unaffected, some to have a mild disease, and others to be so severely affected that they die unless treated promptly.

Although it is not believed to be a bacterial disease, it may be wise to use a pediatric formulation of systemic antibiotic such as cephalosporin as a "cover." The most effective therapy is the administration of systemic corticosteroids, either prednisolone orally SID or triamcinolone acetonide (Vetalog), 0.1 mg intramuscularly or subcutaneously once daily for 5 days, with appropriate nursing and supportive care. Without such treatment, severely affected pups may die; with it, the prognosis is favorable. Complete recovery can be expected in 1 to 2 weeks. Systemic corticosteroids should be given only for the shortest possible time—seldom longer than 5 days.

Idiopathic Acquired Cutaneous Laxity

An unusual dermal collagen disorder was reported in a 9-year-old male English setter.[11a] The dog recently developed large folds of pendulous skin on each side of the head and under the neck. The folds were composed of thin skin with a jelly-like subcutis. Other areas of the dog's body were covered with normal skin. On necropsy, the dermis in the affected areas was found to be only two-thirds of the normal thickness, and the dermal collagen bundles were of smaller-than-normal diameter, fragmented, and widely separated by ground substance. The elastin was normal. The affected tissues contained areas of necrotic subcutaneous fat and vessels with endothelial swelling and a decreased lumen. No inflammation was observed. A vascular insufficiency was proposed as the cause.

Idiopathic Mucinosis of Chinese Shar Pei

This poorly understood condition is usually seen in young Shar Pei of either sex.[7a, 12a] Affected dogs present with generalized pitting "edema," variable pruritus, and often severe puffiness and wrinkling of the head and extremities. Vesicles may be present which, when ruptured, drain a clear, viscous, stringy substance. Biopsies reveal severe diffuse, full-thickness dermal mucinosis. Some cases may spontaneously resolve ("deflate") as the dogs mature, and others appear to benefit from glucocorticosteroid therapy.

"Waterline Disease" of Black Labrador Retrievers

This is a poorly understood condition of black Labrador retrievers of either sex.[4a] Affected dogs present with severe pruritus, secondary seborrhea and alopecia of the legs and ventrum, and occasionally the head. Scrapings and cultures are negative, as are responses to intradermal skin testing and hypoallergenic diets. The disorder is poorly responsive to systemic glucocorticosteroids.

References

1. Bloomsburg, M. S.: The clinical management of perianal fistulas in the dog. Compend. Cont. Ed. 2:615, 1980.

2. Buck, G. E., Stewart, D.D., et al.: Isolation of a corynebacterium from a beagle dog affected with alopecia. Am. J. Vet. Res. 35:297, 1974.

3. Budsbery, S. C., Robinette, J. D., et al.: Cryosurgery performed on perianal fistulas in dogs. Vet. Med. (S.A.C.) 76:667, 1981.

4. Buerger, R. G., Walton, D. K., et al.: Subcutaneous fat sclerosis in a cat. Compend. Cont. Ed. 9:1198, 1987.

4a. DeBoer, D. J.: Common skin diseases of retrievers and setters. Ann. Meet. Am. Acad. Vet. Dermatol. and Am. Coll. Vet. Dermatol. Washington, D. C., April 20, 1988.

5. Edgar, T. P., and Furrow, R. D.: Idiopathic nodular panniculitis in a German shepherd. J.A.A.H.A. 20:603, 1984.

6. Fitzpatrick, T. B., et al.: Dermatology in General Medicine. 2nd ed. McGraw-Hill Book Company, New York, 1979.

7. Flanders, J.: Personal communication, 1987.

7a. Griffin, C. E.: Common dermatoses of the Akita, Shar Pei and Chow Chow. Ann. Meet. Am. Acad. Vet. Dermatol. and Am. Coll. Vet. Dermatol. Washington, D.C., April 20, 1988.

7b. Guaguere, E., et al.: Panniculite nodulaire sterile. A propos d'un cas. Prat. Med. Chirurg. Anim. Comp. 23:27, 1988.

8. Halliwell, R. E. W., et al.: Dapsone for treatment of pruritic dermatitis (dermatitis herpetiformis and subcorneal pustular dermatosis) in dogs. J.A.V.M.A. 170:697, 1977.

9. Lees, G. E., McKeever, P. J., et al.: Fatal thrombocytopenic hemorrhagic diathesis associated with dapsone administration to a dog. J.A.V.M.A. 174:49, 1979.

10. McKeever, P. J., and Dahl, M. V.: A disease in dogs resembling human subcorneal pustular dermatosis. J.A.V.M.A. 170:704, 1977.

11. Muller, G. H., Kirk, R. W., and Scott, D. W.: Small Animal Dermatology. 3rd ed. W. B. Saunders Company, Philadelphia, 1983.

11a. Pieraggi, M. T., et al.: An unusual dermal collagen disorder in a dog. J. Comp. Pathol. 96:289, 1986.

12. Rook, A., Wilkinson, D. S., et al.: Textbook of Dermatology. 3rd ed. Blackwell Scientific Publications, Oxford, England, 1979.

12a. Rosenkrantz, W. S., et al.: Idiopathic mucinosis in a dog. Comp. Anim. Pract. 1:39, 1987.

13. Scott, D. W.: Immunologic skin disorders in the dog and cat. Vet. Clin. North Am. 8:641, 1978.

14. Scott, D. W.: Feline dermatology 1900–1978: A monograph. J.A.A.H.A. 16:331, 1980.

15. Scott, D. W., et al.: Comparative pathology of nonviral bullous skin diseases in domestic animals. Vet. Pathol. 17:257, 1980.

16. Scott, D. W.: Unpublished data. New York State College of Veterinary Medicine, Cornell University, Ithaca, 1987.

17. Scott, D. W., Anderson, W. I.: Nodular panniculitis in dogs and cats: A retrospective analysis of 78 cases. J.A.A.H.A. In press, 1987.

17a. Seim, H. B.: Diseases of the anus and rectum. In Kirk, R. W., (ed.): Current Veterinary Therapy IX. W. B. Saunders Company, Philadelphia, 1986.

18. Shanley, K. J., and Miller, W. H., Jr.: Panniculitis in a dog: A report of five cases. J.A.A.H.A. 21:545, 1985.

19. van Ee, R. T., Palminteri, A.: Tail amputation for treatment of perianal fistulas in dogs. J.A.A.H.A. 23:95, 1987.

20. Vasseur, P. B.: Perianal fistulas in dogs, a retrospective analysis of surgical techniques. J.A.A.H.A. 17:177, 1981.

20

Neoplastic Diseases

Cutaneous Oncology

Veterinary oncology has come into its own as a specialty. Detailed information on the various aspects of the etiopathogenesis and immunology of neoplasia is available in other publications[114, 144, 199, 207a, 223] and is therefore not presented here. This chapter serves as an overview of canine and feline cutaneous neoplasia as well as of non-neoplastic tumors (Table 20:1).

The combined *incidence rates* (the number of new cases of a disease diagnosed in 1 year divided by the population at risk and expressed as cases per 100,000 of the population at risk) for benign and malignant neoplasms in dogs and cats were reported to be about 1077 and 188, respectively.[144, 199] Thus, dogs have about six times as many tumors as do cats. The incidence rates for canine and feline skin neoplasms are about 728 and 84, respectively.[144, 199]

The *peak age period* of neoplasm occurrence in dogs and cats is 6 to 14 years.[144, 199] The *median ages* of cutaneous neoplasm occurrence in dogs and cats are 10.5 years and 12 years, respectively.[144, 199] Among dogs breeds differ in their predilection for various skin neoplasms (Table 20:2). Canine breeds that have the highest neoplasm incidence are the boxer, Scottish terrier, bull mastiff, basset hound, Weimaraner, Kerry blue terrier, and Norwegian elkhound.[144, 145, 199] Canine breeds having the lowest neoplasm incidence are the Brittany spaniel, Chihuahua, Pekingese, Pomeranian, and poodle. There appears to be no breed predilection for neoplasia in the cat.[144, 172, 199] The overall incidence of neoplasia is greater in female dogs than in males (56 per cent versus 44 per cent); in cats, however, males predominate (56 per cent versus 44 per cent).[144, 172, 199]

There are no completely satisfactory criteria for distinguishing benign neoplasms from certain proliferative inflammatory lesions and hyperplastic processes and for distinguishing benign from malignant neoplasms.[144] In general, malignant neoplasms are usually characterized by sudden onset, rapid growth, infiltration, recurrence, and metastasis (Table 20:3). The most important criterion of malignancy is metastasis. In dogs, the number of malignant neoplasms is only about half the number of benign neoplasms.[144, 199] However, in cats, there are about three times as many malignant neoplasms as benign neoplasms.[144, 172]

The skin is the most common site of occurrence of neoplasms in the dog (about 30 per cent of the total), and the second most common site in the cat (about 20 per cent of the total.)[24, 144, 172, 199] The most common skin neoplasms in dogs and cats vary somewhat from one report to another. In general, canine

Table 20:1. SKIN TUMORS

Epithelial Neoplasms
Cutaneous papilloma
  Canine viral papillomatosis
Intracutaneous cornifying epithelioma
Squamous cell carcinoma
Basal cell tumor
Hair follicle tumors
  Trichoepithelioma
  Tricholemmoma
  Trichofolliculoma
  Dilated pore of Winer
  Warty dyskeratoma
  Pilomatrixoma
Sebaceous gland tumors
  Nodular sebaceous hyperplasia
  Sebaceous adenoma
  Sebaceous epithelioma
  Sebaceous adenocarcinoma
Sweat gland tumors
  Apocrine sweat gland tumors
    Apocrine cysts
    Apocrine adenoma
    Apocrine adenocarcinoma
  Eccrine sweat gland tumors
    Eccrine adenoma
    Eccrine adenocarcinoma
Perianal gland tumors
  Nodular perianal gland hyperplasia
  Perianal adenoma
  Perianal adenocarcinoma
  Apocrine anal gland tumor
  Apocrine tumors of anal sac origin
Epithelioid sarcoma

Mesenchymal Neoplasms
Fibroma
Fibrovascular papilloma
Fibrosarcoma
Myxoma and myxosarcoma
Undifferentiated sarcoma
Nodular fasciitis
Leiomyoma and leiomyosarcoma
Tumors of neural origin
  Schwannoma
  Neurothekeoma
  Granular cell tumor
Lipoma
  Infiltrative lipoma
  Angiolipoma
Liposarcoma
Tumors of vascular origin
  Hemangioma
  Hemangiosarcoma
  Hemangiopericytoma
  Angiokeratoma
  Lymphangioma
  Lymphangiosarcoma
Mast cell tumor
Osteoma and osteosarcoma

Lymphohistiocytic Neoplasms
Histiocytoma
Malignant histiocytosis
Systemic histiocytosis
Cutaneous histiocytosis
Transmissible venereal tumor
Fibrous histiocytoma
Malignant fibrous histiocytoma
Cutaneous lymphosarcoma
Epitheliotropic lymphosarcoma
  Mycosis fungoides
  Alopecia mucinosa
  Pagetoid reticulosis
  Sézary syndrome
Leukemia cutis
Pseudolymphoma
Cutaneous plasmacytoma
Primary cutaneous neuroendocrine tumor

Melanocytic Neoplasms
Melanomas
  Benign melanoma
  Malignant melanoma

Secondary Skin Neoplasm

Non-Neoplastic Tumors
Cutaneous cysts
  Epidermoid cyst
  Dermoid cyst
  Follicular cyst
  Trichilemmal cyst
Nevi
  Collagenous nevus
  Organoid nevus
  Vascular nevus
  Sebaceous gland nevus
  Epidermal nevus
  Melanocytic nevus
Keratoses
  Seborrheic keratosis
  Actinic keratosis
  Lichenoid keratosis
  Cutaneous horn
Keloids
Xanthomas
Calcinosis cutis
Cutaneous mucinosis

Table 20:2. BREED PREDILECTIONS FOR CUTANEOUS NEOPLASMS
IN THE DOG

Papilloma	Cocker spaniel, Kerry blue terrier
Intracutaneous cornifying epithelioma	Norwegian elkhound, collie, German shepherd, keeshond
Squamous cell carcinoma	Scottish terrier, Pekingese, boxer, poodle, Norwegian elkhound
Squamous cell carcinoma, ventral trunk (actinic)	Dalmatian, bull terrier
Squamous cell carcinoma, digit	Black Labrador retriever, black standard poodle
Basal cell tumor	Cocker spaniel, poodle
Trichoepithelioma	Cocker spaniel
Pilomatrixoma	Kerry blue terrier, poodle
Sebaceous gland tumors	Cocker spaniel, Boston terrrier, poodle, Kerry blue terrier, beagle, dachshund, basset hound, Norwegian elkhound
Sweat gland tumors	Cocker spaniel
Perianal gland tumors	Cocker spaniel, English bulldog, Samoyed, beagle
Fibroma	Boxer, Boston terrier, fox terrier, Afghan, dachshund
Fibrosarcoma	Cocker spaniel
Schwannoma	Fox terrier
Lipoma	Cocker spaniel, dachshund, Labrador retriever, Weimaraner
Liposarcoma	Dachshund, Brittany spaniel
Hemangioma	Boxer
Hemangiosarcoma	Boxer, German shepherd, Bernese Mountain dog
Hemangiopericytoma	Boxer, cocker spaniel, fox terrier, German shepherd, springer spaniel
Mast cell tumor	Boxer, Boston terrier, bull terrier, Staffordshire terrier, English bulldog, Weimaraner, Labrador retriever, fox terrier, dachshund
Histiocytoma	Boxer, dachshund, cocker spaniel, Great Dane, Shetland sheepdog
Systemic histiocytosis	Bernese Mountain dog
Malignant histiocytosis	Bernese Mountain dog
Fibrous histiocytoma	Collie
Lymphosarcoma	Boxer, cocker spaniel, Scottish terrier, beagle, German shepherd, golden retriever, basset hound, St. Bernard
Melanoma	Scottish terrier, Boston terrier, boxer, chow chow, Airedale terrier, cocker spaniel, springer spaniel, Irish setter, Irish terrier, Chihuahua, Doberman pinscher
Collagenous nevi	German shepherd
Calcinosis circumscripta	German shepherd, boxer, Boston terrier

Table 20:3. CRITERIA FOR DISTINGUISHING BETWEEN BENIGN AND
MALIGNANT NEOPLASMS

Criterion	Benign	Malignant
Growth rate	Slow	Rapid
Growth limits	Limited, circumscribed, encapsulated	Unrestricted
Mode of growth	Expansion, pedunculation	Expansion, infiltration
Metastasis	None	Frequent
Recurrence after removal	Rare	Frequent
Anaplasia	No	Yes
Tissue structure	Near normal	Abnormal
Stroma	Usually abundant	Usually scanty
Mitotic figures	Few	Usually numerous
Invasion of vessels and other structures	Rare	Frequent
Tissue destruction	Minimal	Frequent
Cell size	Uniform	Pleomorphic
Nuclear chromatin	Nearly normal amount	Hyperchromatic
Nucleoli	Normal	Large, may be multiple

Table 20:4. CYTOMORPHOLOGIC CHARACTERISTICS SUGGESTIVE OF MALIGNANCY

General Findings
Pleomorphism (variable cell forms)
Variable nucleus: cytoplasm ratios
Variable staining intensity

Nuclear Findings
Marked variation in size
Coarsely clumped, sometimes jagged chromatin
Nuclear molding
Peripheral displacement by cytoplasmic secretions or vacuoles
Prominent, occasionally giant, or angular nucleoli

Cytoplasmic Findings
Variable staining intensity, sometimes dark blue
Discrete, punctate vacuoles
Variable amounts

skin neoplasms may be broadly categorized as about 55 per cent mesenchymal and 45 per cent epithelial in origin.[12, 24, 125, 172, 195] In the dog, the most common skin neoplasms, in approximate descending order, are lipoma, mast cell tumor, sebaceous gland hyperplasia and adenoma, and papilloma (squamous and fibropapilloma). In the cat, the approximate order is basal cell tumor, squamous cell carcinoma, fibrosarcoma, and mast cell tumor.

The key to appropriate management and accurate prognosis of cutaneous neoplasm is *specific diagnosis*. This can only be achieved by biopsy and histologic evaluation. Exfoliative cytologic techniques (aspiration, impression smear) are easy and rapid, and often provide valuable information about neoplastic cell type and differentiation. The techniques, methodologies, and interpretation used in cytologic studies have been beautifully described and illustrated (see Chap. 3).[4, 10, 136, 137, 199] Cytomorphologic characteristics suggestive of malignancy are presented in Table 20:4. However, exfoliative cytologic evaluation is inferior to and no substitute for biopsy and histopathologic examination. Historical and clinical considerations often allow the experienced clinician to formulate an inclusive differential diagnosis on a cutaneous neoplasm, but variability renders such "odds playing" unreliable. In short, "a lump is a lump" until it is evaluated histologically.

The detailed histopathologic description of canine and feline cutaneous neoplasms is beyond the scope of this chapter. Only the histopathologic "essence" of individual neoplasms is presented here. For in-depth information and photomicrographic illustrations, the reader is referred to other texts on cutaneous neoplasia[120, 144, 199] and the individual references cited for each neoplasm.

Recently, the use of "markers"—enzyme histochemical and immunohistochemical methods for identifying specific cell types—have been increasingly employed and touted for the diagnosis of neoplastic conditions in humans.[32, 120, 133, 139, 162] Examples of these markers are presented in Table 20:5. Although it is presently employed in few veterinary research facilities,[169a] the development of marker technology in veterinary medicine could greatly enhance the understanding of neoplasia in dogs and cats.

Clinical management of cutaneous neoplasms may include surgery, cryosurgery, electrosurgery, radiotherapy, chemotherapy, immunotherapy, hyperthermia, phototherapy, and combinations of these. Detailed information on the

Table 20:5. EXAMPLES OF MARKERS FOR THE IDENTIFICATION OF CELL TYPES

Marker	Cell Type
Enzyme Histochemical	
Alpha naphthyl acetate esterase	Monocyte, histiocyte, Langerhans' cell, plasma cell
Chloracetate esterase	Neutrophil, mast cell
Acid phosphatase	Monocyte, histiocyte, plasma cell
Alkaline phosphatase	Neutrophil, endothelial cell
Beta-glucuronidase	Histiocyte, T lymphocyte, plasma cell
Adenosine triphosphatase	Histiocyte, plasma cell, B lymphocyte, endothelial cell
5' nucleotidase	Endothelial cell
Nonspecific esterase	Monocyte, histiocyte
Lysozyme	Monocyte, histiocyte
Alpha-1-antitrypsin	Monocyte, histiocyte
Immunohistochemical	
Cytokeratin	Squamous and glandular epithelium
Vimentin	Fibroblast, Schwann cell, endothelial cell, lymphocyte, monocyte, histiocyte, melanocyte, Langerhans' cell
Desmin	Skeletal muscle, smooth muscle
Neurofilament	Axon cell bodies, dendrites
S100 protein	Melanocyte, Schwann cell, Langerhans' cell, myoepithelial cell, sweat gland acini and ducts, lipocyte
Myoglobin	Skeletal muscle
Factor VIII–related antigen	Endothelial cell
Ulex europaeus agglutinin I	Endothelial cell
Leukocyte common antigen	Leukocyte
Peanut agglutinin	Histiocyte
Myelin basic protein	Schwann cell
Laminin	Basement membrane
Leu and OKT (various numerical designations)	Lymphocytes (various developmental and functional types)

various treatment modalities is available in a number of excellent references.[49, 60, 81, 152, 155, 156, 167, 169, 199, 201, 220] Brief comments on treatment are included under clinical management sections of each tumor. Table 20:6 converts body weight to surface area, which is necessary for chemotherapy.

Epithelial Neoplasms

CUTANEOUS PAPILLOMA
(Wart, Verruca)

Cutaneous papillomas are common (in dogs) to rare (in cats) benign neoplasms arising from squamous epithelial cells.[12, 125, 144, 145, 172] The cause of cutaneous papillomas is unclear, although viral infection appears to be involved in some cases among dogs.

Canine viral papillomatosis is common and caused by a DNA papovavirus.[144, 199] A retrospective study of selected canine papillomas, using a peroxidase-antiperoxidase technique, demonstrated papilloma structural antigens in the lesions.[193] It affects young dogs, with no breed or sex predilection. It has *not* been described in cats. The disease is contagious and has an incubation period of about 30 days. Canine viral papillomatosis almost always occurs as

Table 20:6. CONVERSION OF BODY WEIGHT TO SURFACE AREA*

Body Weight		Surface Area	
Kilograms	Pounds	Sq. Meters	Sq. Centimeters
2	4.4	0.16	1600
4	8.8	0.25	2500
6	13.2	0.33	3300
8	17.6	0.40	4000
10	22.0	0.46	4600
12	26.5	0.52	5200
14	30.9	0.58	5800
16	35.3	0.64	6400
18	39.7	0.69	6900
20	44.1	0.74	7400
22	48.5	0.79	7900
24	52.9	0.83	8300
26	57.3	0.88	8800
28	61.7	0.92	9200
30	66.1	0.97	9700
32	70.6	1.01	10,100
34	75.0	1.05	10,500
36	79.4	1.09	10,900
38	83.8	1.13	11,300
40	88.2	1.17	11,700
42	92.6	1.21	12,100
44	97.0	1.25	12,500
46	101.4	1.28	12,800

*From Davis, L. E.: Treatment and management of burns. Veterinary Scope, 8:7–11, April, 1963.

multiple lesions. The papillomas vary from white, flat, smooth papules and plaques of a few mm in diameter to whitish gray, pedunculated or cauliflower-like masses of up to 2 cm in diameter (Fig. 20:1A). Viral papillomas affect the buccal mucosa, tongue, palate, pharynx, epiglottis, lip, skin (Fig. 20:1B), eyelids, conjunctiva, and cornea.[144, 199]

Cutaneous papillomas occur in older dogs and cats (Figs. 20:2 and 20:3). Cats show no breed or sex predilection, but among dogs papillomas are more common in males, cocker spaniels, Kerry blue terriers.[145] In both species, cutaneous papillomas may be single or multiple, occurring mainly on the head, eyelids, and feet. They are usually pedunculated or cauliflower-like, firm to soft, well circumscribed, alopecic, smooth to keratinous, and usually less than 0.5 cm in diameter.

Recently, *cutaneous inverted papillomas* were reported in dogs.[36a] Affected dogs were 8 months to 3 years of age, and lesions appeared on the ventral abdomen. The lesions were raised and firm, and they contained a central pore opening to the surface of the skin. Skin biopsies revealed inverted papillomas with central keratin-filled crypts, ballooning degeneration (koilocytosis) of cells in the stratum granulosum, and eosinophilic intranuclear inclusion bodies. Papillomavirus group-specific antigens were detected in the lesions, and electron microscopy revealed papillomavirus-like inclusion bodies.

Although both cutaneous and viral papillomas are usually benign, apparent transformation into squamous cell carcinoma has been recognized in a few canine cases.[145] Some dogs treated with a live-virus vaccine that was made from papillomavirus isolated from naturally occurring oral papillomas developed squamous cell carcinomas at the sites of vaccine inoculation.[194, 256] Rare cases of viral papillomatosis have been completely unresponsive to treatment, perhaps owing to immunologic defects.

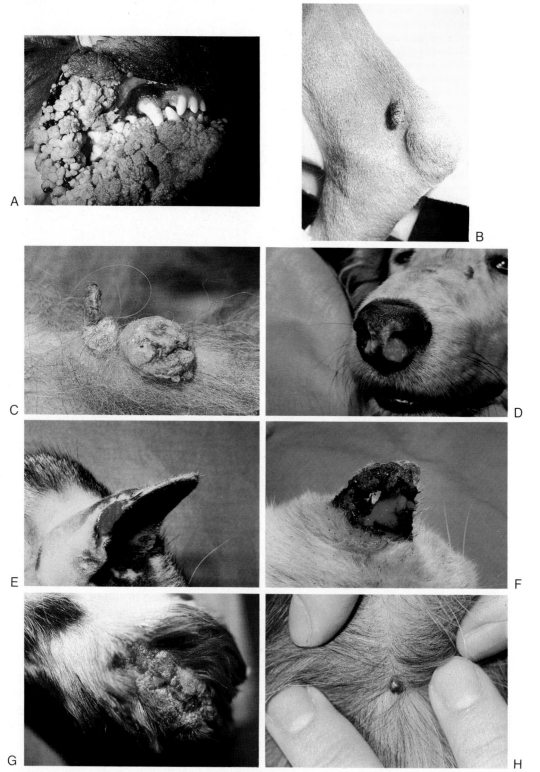

Figure 20:1. *A,* Severe case of oral papillomatosis. *B,* Squamous papilloma in the hock of a dog. *C,* Canine intracutaneous cornifying epithelioma. One of the neoplasms has an overlying cutaneous horn. *D,* Squamous cell carcinoma inside the left nostril of a collie, with area of depigmentation of the nasal tip. Surgical removal resulted in complete recovery. *E,* Early squamous cell carcinoma on margin of cat pinna. Photo was taken after removal of crust. There was a complete response to surgical excision and to avoidance of sunlight. *F,* Advanced squamous cell carcinoma involving entire cat pinna, which required radical amputation of pinna. *G,* Digital squamous cell carcinoma in a dog. *H,* Pigmented basal cell tumor on the rump of a cat.

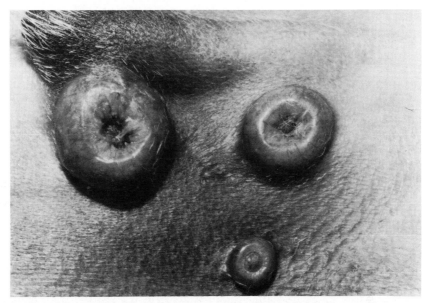

Figure 20:2. Viral papillomas on the flank of a dog. The neoplasm developed rapidly over several months. Surgical excision was successful.

Histologically, papillomas are usually divided into two types: (1) *Squamous papilloma* (the most common type) (Figs. 20:4 and 20:5) is characterized by papillated epidermal hyperplasia and papillomatosis, with ballooning degeneration (koilocytosis) and basophilic intranuclear inclusion bodies as variable findings. (2) *Fibropapilloma* (fibrous polyp) (Fig. 20:6) is characterized by a fibroma-like proliferation of collagen with a hyperplastic epidermis.[144, 145]

Clinical management of cutaneous papillomas may include surgical excision, cryosurgery, electrosurgery, or observation without treatment. Canine viral papillomatosis *usually* undergoes spontaneous regression within about 3 months, and solid immunity follows experimental or natural infection. Autogenous or commercially produced wart vaccines and immunomodulating drugs (e.g., levamisole and thiabendazole) are without documented value. In certain

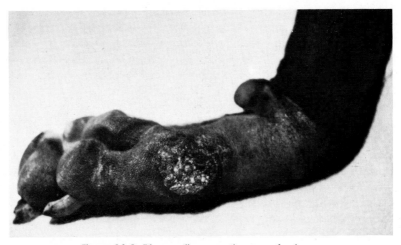

Figure 20:3. Fibropapilloma on the paw of a dog.

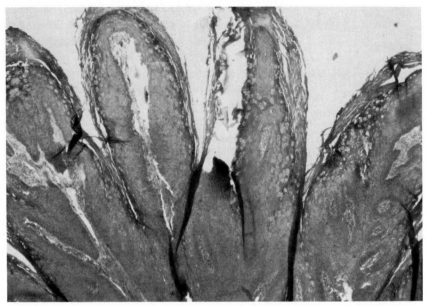

Figure 20:4. Canine squamous papilloma. Note papillomatosis and vacuolated epidermal cells.

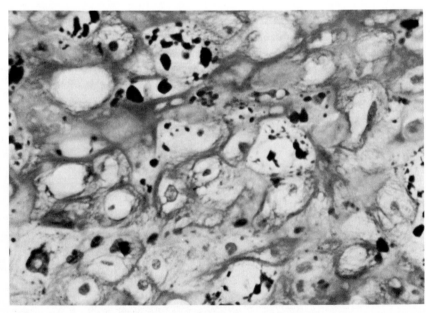

Figure 20:5. Canine viral papillomatosis. Note ballooning degeneration and clumping of keratohyalin granules.

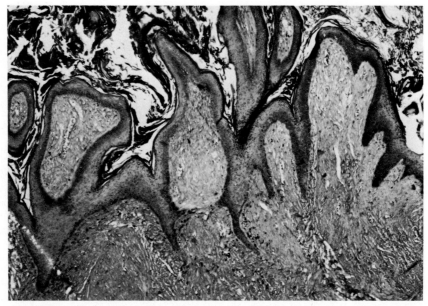

Figure 20:6. Canine fibropapilloma. Papillomatous proliferation of epidermis and fibroblasts.

cases with large masses of proliferating tissue, eating and oral hygiene may be facilitated by surgically removing some of the larger papillomas, which is usually performed by cryosurgery or electrosurgery. Reports have indicated that intralesional injections of bleomycin or α interferon are beneficial to humans with recalcitrant papillomas.[7, 183]

INTRACUTANEOUS CORNIFYING EPITHELIOMA
(Keratoacanthoma)

Intracutaneous cornifying epitheliomas are common benign neoplasms of the dog and are thought to arise from the epidermis between hair follicles.[144, 145, 199] There are unsubstantiated references to the occurrence of intracutaneous cornifying epitheliomas in the cat.[8] The cause of intracutaneous cornifying epitheliomas is unknown, although the generalized forms may have a hereditary basis in dogs and humans.

Usually, these epitheliomas occur in dogs 5 years of age or less. Males are more commonly affected than females.[144, 199] The incidence is higher in purebred dogs and particularly in the Norwegian elkhound and keeshond, which are predisposed to the generalized form.[144, 199] However, the generalized form has also been recognized in the German shepherd and Old English sheepdog.[145, 199] Collies are also reported to be breeds at risk.[145]

Although intracutaneous cornifying epitheliomas are usually solitary, they may be multiple in the Norwegian elkhound, keeshond, German shepherd, and Old English sheepdog (Fig. 20:1C). Most tumors occur on the back, neck, thorax, and shoulders. There is considerable variation in the gross appearance of intracutaneous cornifying epitheliomas. Most of the tumors appear as firm-to-fluctuant, well-circumscribed dermal or subcutaneous masses varying from 0.5 to 4 cm in diameter, with a pore opening onto the skin surface that ranges

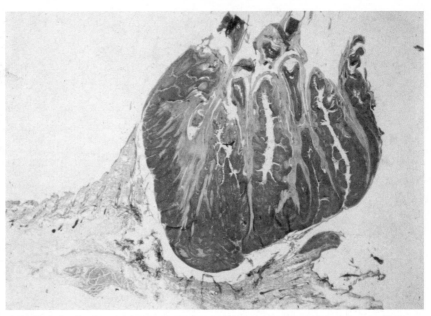

Figure 20:7. Section of entire intracutaneous cornifying epithelioma. It is a keratin-filled crypt of folded stratified squamous epithelium that opens to the skin surface.

from less than 1 mm to several mm in diameter. The opening usually contains a hard keratinized plug, varying from small and inconspicuous to large and hornlike. Very superficial lesions with large keratinous plugs are easily mistaken for cutaneous horns. Some of the tumors are entirely dermal or subcutaneous, do not communicate with the surface of the skin, and are easily confused with "cysts." Intracutaneous cornifying epitheliomas are not invasive or metastatic. However, in the generalized form (up to 50 lesions) a recurrent problem should be anticipated, because affected dogs tend to develop new tumors at other sites throughout their lives.

Histopathologically, intracutaneous cornifying epitheliomas are characterized by a keratin-filled crypt in the dermis that opens to the skin surface (Fig. 20:7).[144] The wall of the crypt is composed of a thick, complex, folded layer of well-differentiated stratified squamous epithelium, with columns of squamoid cells projecting peripherally from the basal surface of the wall and forming small epithelial "nests" (Fig. 20:8).

Clinical management of intracutaneous cornifying epitheliomas may include surgical excision, cryotherapy, electrotherapy, or observation without treatment.[51, 199] Chemotherapy with cyclophosphamide and prednisone and immunotherapy with autogenous vaccine or levamisole have been ineffective in dogs.[51] Recently, the oral administration of retinoids or intralesional injections of 5-fluorouracil have provided good results in the treatment of keratoacanthomas in humans.[15, 50, 150]

SQUAMOUS CELL CARCINOMA
(Epidermoid Carcinoma)

Squamous cell carcinomas are common malignant neoplasms of the dog and cat, arising from squamous epithelial cells.[12, 13, 144, 172, 199] The etiology of squamous cell carcinoma is not clear in all cases. White cats and humans show a strong

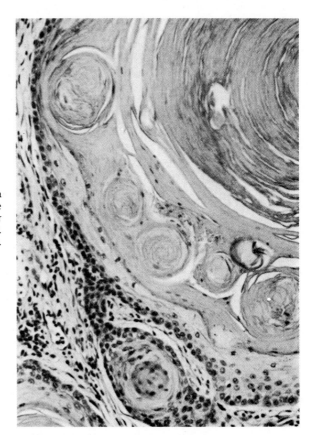

Figure 20:8. Intracutaneous cornifying epithelioma of a dog showing the concentric lamellae of keratin. Note the complex wall structure and the lack of a granular cell layer in the stratified squamous cell epithelial lining. (From Weiss, E., and Frese, K.: VII Tumors of the skin. Bull. WHO *50*:79, 1974.)

correlation existing between the development of squamous cell carcinomas and exposure to ultraviolet light. This does *not* appear to be the case in dogs,[13, 20, 123] except in individuals with nasal depigmentation associated with conditions such as discoid lupus erythematosus, pemphigus erythematosus, and vitiligo (see p. 526) or in individuals with unnatural, enhanced exposure to sunlight.[85, 199] These tumors may occur multifocally in sparsely haired areas of white-coated dogs (Dalmatians and pit bull terriers) who habitually sleep in the sun and sustain excessive actinic skin damage. Rarely, squamous cell carcinoma has been reported to arise from burn scars.[7, 199] In humans squamous cell carcinomas are known to occasionally arise from burn and frostbite scars, radiation burns, stasis dermatitis, and various chronic infectious processes.[105a] In a retrospective study,[193] papillomavirus structural antigens were demonstrated in five of nine canine cutaneous squamous cell carcinomas, suggesting that papillomaviruses have an etiologic role in this neoplasm. Squamous cell carcinomas occurred at the site of injection of a live canine oral papillomavirus vaccine in some dogs.[23a]

In dogs and cats squamous cell carcinomas occur at an average of 9 years of age. No sex predilection exists. There is no breed predilection in cats, although white cats develop cutaneous squamous cell carcinoma about 13 times more frequently than do other cats.[172] Among dogs, squamous cell carcinoma has been reported to occur more frequently in Scottish terriers, Pekingese, boxers, poodles, and Norwegian elkhounds.[145] The reported increased incidence in Norwegian elkhounds may be misleading, because this breed is known to be predisposed to intracutaneous cornifying epithelioma, a neoplasm that may be misdiagnosed as squamous cell carcinoma on histologic grounds.[120, 144]

Squamous cell carcinomas are usually solitary. In dogs, the most common sites of occurrence are the trunk, limbs, digits, scrotum, lips, nose, and oral cavity (Fig. 20:1*D*). In cats, the most common sites are the pinnae, lips, nose, and eyelids (Fig. 20:1*E,F*). Squamous cell carcinomas may be *proliferative* or *ulcerative*. The proliferative types are papillary masses of varying size, many of which have a cauliflower-like appearance. The surface tends to be ulcerated and bleeds easily. Cutaneous horns may develop on the surface of such lesions. The ulcerative types initially appear as shallow, crusted ulcers that become deep and crateriform. Squamous cell carcinomas are generally locally invasive but are slow to metastasize. In dogs and cats, squamous cell carcinomas arising from the digits (Fig. 20:1*G*) appear to be much more aggressive and may be misdiagnosed as paronychia or some form of pyoderma.[145, 157, 199] In dogs, black-skinned breeds (Labrador retriever, black standard poodle) appear predisposed to multiple subungual (nail bed) squamous cell carcinomas.[126, 148] These dogs usually present with a single affected digit, which is swollen and painful with a misshapen or absent nail and paronychial discharge, and they develop multiple lesions in other digits over a period of 2 to 4 years. In light-skinned, lightly haired dogs such as bull terriers and Dalmatians, multiple squamous cell carcinomas may arise on the ventral chest and abdomen following chronic sunburn and actinic keratoses (see p. 941).[165a, 199] Pseudohyperparathyroidism has been reported in association with a squamous cell carcinoma.[78]

Histologically, squamous cell carcinomas are characterized by irregular masses or cords of epidermal cells that proliferate downward and invade the dermis.[144] Frequent findings include keratin formation, "horn pearls," "intercellular bridges" (desmosomes), mitoses, and atypia (Figs. 20:9 and 20:10). Squamous cell carcinomas may rarely have confusing "clear cell" or "spindle cell" histologic variants.[86, 205] In cats with cutaneous squamous cell carcinoma, it was reported that prognosis correlated with the degree of histopathologic differentiation, but not with anatomic sites.[19] Fifty per cent of the cats with poorly differentiated neoplasms were destroyed within 12 weeks, and the longest survival time was 20 weeks.

Clinical management of squamous cell carcinomas may include surgical excision, cryosurgery, electrosurgery, hyperthermia, or radiotherapy.[81, 105, 199] Hyperthermia is often effective for the treatment of superficial cutaneous squamous cell carcinomas in cats and dogs.[63] Chemotherapy with bleomycin, cisplatin, benzaldehyde, thioproline, and oral retinoids has been ineffective.[64, 82, 91, 124, 159a, 199]

BASAL CELL TUMOR
(Basal Cell Carcinoma, Basal Cell Epithelioma, Basalioma,
"Rodent Ulcer")

These tumors are common benign neoplasms of the dog and cat that are thought to arise from the basal cells of the epidermis, hair follicle, sebaceous gland, and sweat gland.[12, 56, 144, 145, 172, 199] The cause of basal cell tumors in dogs and cats is unknown. In humans, there is a strong correlation between exposure to ultraviolet light and the development of basal cell tumors.[67]

Basal cell tumors occur in dogs and cats at an average of 7 and 9 years of age, respectively. There is no sex predilection. Basal cell tumors are the most

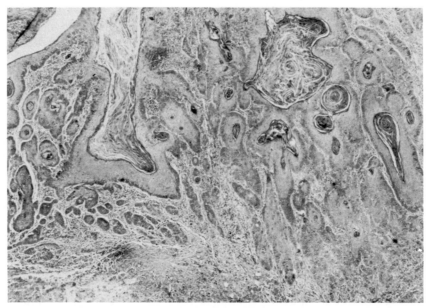

Figure 20:9. Squamous cell carcinoma. Irregular proliferation of keratinocytes with dermal invasion.

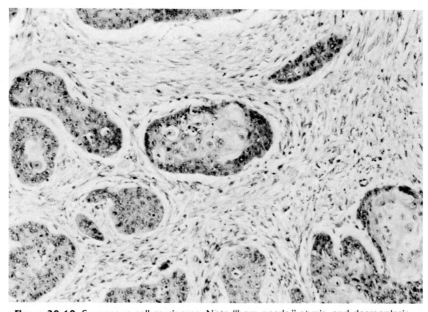

Figure 20:10. Squamous cell carcinoma. Note "horn pearls," atypia, and desmoplasia.

common melanotic feline skin neoplasm (Fig. 20:1*H*), and Siamese cats may be predisposed. Cocker spaniels and poodles appear to be the predisposed breeds among dogs.[145]

Usually, basal cell tumors are solitary, but they may occasionally be multiple.[65] In dogs, the most common sites of occurrence are the head and neck. There is no site predilection in cats. Basal cell tumors are usually firm, rounded, elevated, well circumscribed, and situated dermoepidermally, and they range from 0.5 to 10 cm in diameter (Fig. 20:11*A*). They frequently become ulcerated and alopecic and are occasionally cystic (Fig. 20:11*B*). Basal cell tumors are benign.

Histopathologically, basal cell tumors are characterized by a proliferation of basaloid cells (Figs. 20:12 and 20:13).[144] Frequent findings include uniform cell size, nuclear hyperchromasia, mitotic figures, and a lack of "intercellular bridges" (desmosomes). Several histologic patterns of basal cell tumors are described: solid, cystic, ribbon (garland), adenoid, basosquamous, and medusoid. It has been suggested that solid basal cell tumors may be more aggressive than the other histologic types,[46] but other investigators disagree.[125, 180] *Granular* basal cell tumors have been described as a distinct histopathologic entity in dogs.[181]

Clinical management of basal cell tumors may include surgical excision, cryotherapy, electrosurgery, or observation without treatment.[145, 199]

HAIR FOLLICLE TUMORS

Trichoepithelioma

Trichoepitheliomas are relatively common (in dogs) to rare (in cats) benign neoplasms that are thought to arise from keratinocytes in the hair follicle outer root sheath or the hair matrix, or both.[13, 37a, 51, 125, 144, 145, 147, 199] The cause of trichoepitheliomas in dogs and cats is unknown. In humans, a syndrome of multiple trichoepitheliomas is hereditary.[67]

Usually trichoepitheliomas occur in dogs and cats over 5 years of age. No sex predilection appears to exist in either species. In cats, there is no breed predilection, and the neoplasms may occur more commonly on the head. In dogs, there may be a predilection for the back, and cocker spaniels may be predisposed.

Although these neoplasms are usually solitary, they may occasionally be multiple. They are usually firm, rounded, elevated, well circumscribed, and dermoepidermal in position, ranging from 0.5 to 10 cm in diameter. Frequently, they become ulcerated and alopecic. Trichoepitheliomas are rarely invasive or metastatic (Fig. 20:11*C*).[180]

Histopathologically, trichoepitheliomas vary considerably, depending on the degree of differentiation and whether the tumor is primarily related to the follicular sheath of hair matrix.[120, 144] Frequent characteristics include horn cysts,

Figure 20:11. Firm rubbery nodule basal cell tumor that has ulcerated. *B*, BCT of the lower eyelid, a typical location. *C*, Multilobulated malignant trichoepithelioma over lateral neck and shoulder of a dog. (Courtesy W. H. Miller, Jr.) *D*, Dilated pore of Winer. Keratinaceous mass projecting from the surface pore. *E*, Multiple sebaceous hyperplasias on the face of a dog. (Courtesy W. H. Miller, Jr.) *F*, Sebaceous adenoma. Note multilobulated appearance and well-demarcated borders. *G*, Pigmented sebaceous epithelioma over the eye of a dog. *H*, Sebaceous adenocarcinoma that grew rapidly and is severely ulcerated.

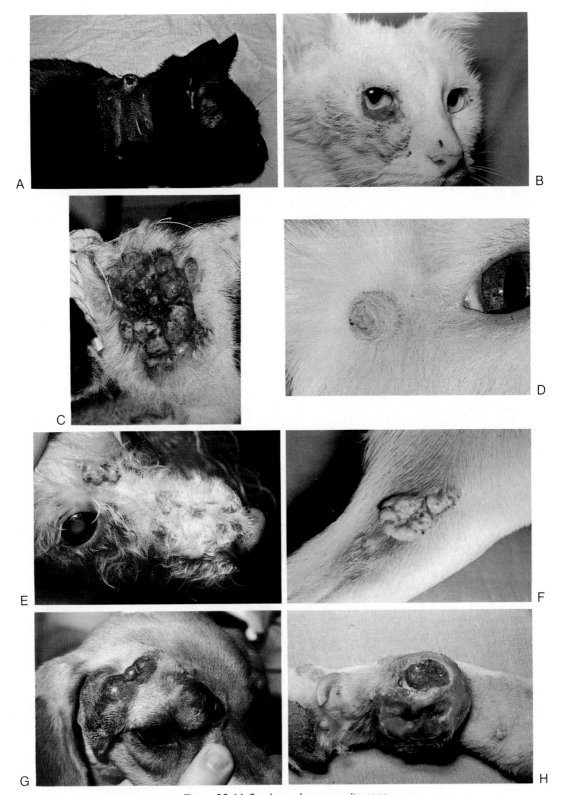

Figure 20:11 *See legend on opposite page*

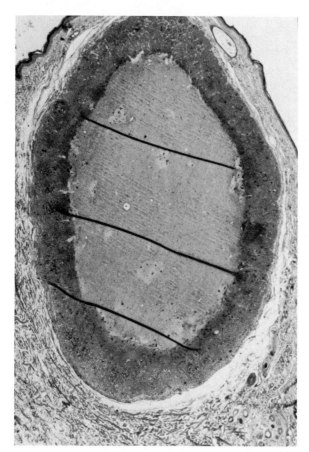

Figure 20:12. Pigmented cystic basal cell tumor from a cat.

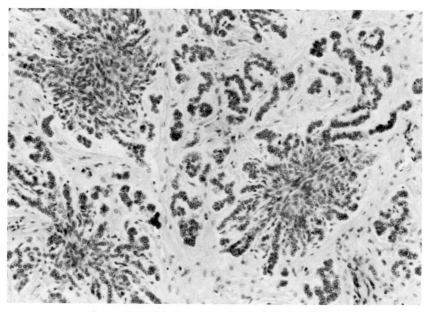

Figure 20:13. Medusoid basal cell tumor from a dog.

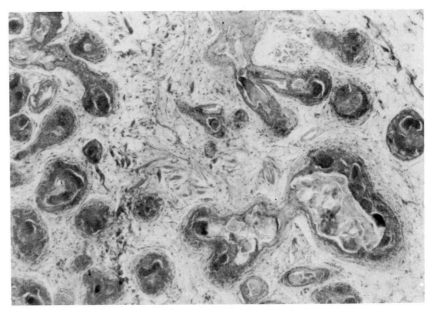

Figure 20:14. Trichoepithelioma. Disorganized proliferation of basaloid cells forming hair follicle–like structures and hairs.

lack of "intercellular bridges" (desmosomes), differentiation toward hair folli-cle–like structures, and formation of hairs (Fig. 20:14).

Clinical management of trichoepitheliomas may include surgical excision, cryotherapy, electrosurgery, or observation without treatment.[145, 199]

Tricholemmoma

Tricholemmomas are uncommon benign neoplasms of the dog that arise from keratinocytes of the outer root sheath of hair follicles.[57, 208] The cause of tricholemmomas is unknown. In humans, a syndrome of multiple tricholem-momas is hereditary.[67]

In dogs, tricholemmomas occur at 5 to 13 years of age. There appears to be no breed or sex predilection. These neoplasms occur most commonly on the head and neck and are usually firm, ovoid, and 1 to 7 cm in diameter.

Histopathologically, tricholemmomas are characterized by a nodular pro-liferation of keratinocytes, many of which are clear and PAS-positive, owing to their glycogen content (Fig. 20:15). The tumor lobules are surrounded by a distinct, often thickened basement membrane zone.

Clinical management of tricholemmomas may include surgical excision, cryotherapy, electrosurgery, or observation without treatment.

Trichofolliculoma
(Folliculoma, Hair Follicle Nevus)

Trichofolliculomas are rare benign neoplasms of dogs that are highly structured hamartomas of the pilosebaceous unit.[120, 180] The cause of trichofolliculomas is unknown.

Trichofolliculomas occur in dogs, with no apparent age, breed, sex, or site predilections. The lesions are solitary, dome-shaped, firm papules or nodules,

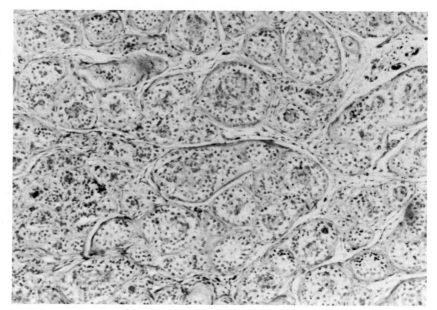

Figure 20:15. Tricholemmoma. Proliferation of predominantly clear, outer root sheathlike keratinocytes. Individual nodules are often surrounded by a distinct basement membrane zone.

often containing a central depression or pore that may exude sebaceous material, or contain a tuft of hairs.

Histopathologically, trichofolliculomas are characterized by a large dilated or cystic follicle with radiating follicles or follicle-like structures (Fig. 20:16).

Clinical management may include surgical excision or observation without treatment.

Dilated Pore of Winer

Dilated pore of Winer is a benign follicular tumor of cats.[176, 180] The cause of this lesion is unknown, although most evidence favors a developmental etiology based on the combining forces of obstruction and intrafollicular pressure leading to hair follicle hyperplasia.

Dilated pore is seen in older cats, especially males, with no apparent breed predilection. The lesions are solitary and occur on the face and neck (Fig. 20:11D). They are characterized by a well-demarcated, smooth, dermoepidermal cyst-like structure with a central, keratin-filled wide-mouthed pore.

Histopathologically, this disorder is characterized by a markedly dilated, keratinized, pilar infundibulum lined by an epithelium that is atrophic near the ostium, but increasingly hyperplastic toward the base of the lesion (Fig. 20:17). The epithelium at the base shows psoriasiform hyperplasia with rete ridges and irregular, thin projections into the surrounding dermis (Fig. 20:18).

Clinical management includes surgical excision or observation without treatment.

Warty Dyskeratoma

Warty dyskeratoma is a rare, benign, epithelial proliferation of dogs.[90a, 180] Although warty dyskeratoma is believed by many investigators to arise from

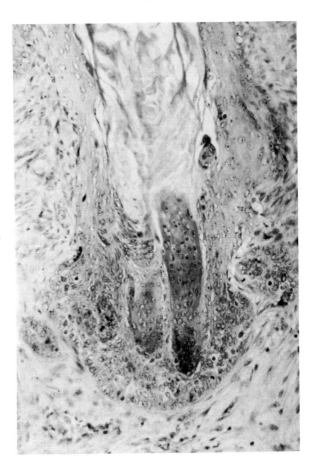

Figure 20:16. Trichofolliculoma. Large, dilated, keratin-filled follicle with peripheral proliferation of abortive hair follicle–like structures.

pilosebaceous structures, the fact that it occurs in the oral cavity of humans has challenged traditional interpretations.[120]

Warty dyskeratoma occurs in dogs, but too few cases have been recognized to infer age, breed, sex, or site predilections. The lesions are solitary, wartlike papules or nodules with a hyperkeratotic, umbilicated center.

Histopathologically, warty dyskeratoma is characterized by a cup-shaped invagination connected with the surface by a keratin-filled channel (Fig. 20:19). The large invagination contains numerous acantholytic, dyskeratotic cells (Fig. 20:20). The lower portion of the invagination is occupied by numerous villi (elongated dermal papillae lined with a single layer of basal cells) (Fig. 20:21). Typical corp ronds (dyskeratotic acanthocytes with a pyknotic nucleus surrounded by a clear halo) can usually be found.

Clinical management of warty dyskeratoma may include surgical excision or observation without treatment.

Pilomatrixoma

(Pilomatricoma, Benign Calcifying Epithelioma, Calcifying Epithelioma of Malherbe)

These uncommon benign neoplasms of the dog are thought to arise from the hair matrix.[144, 145, 199] Pilomatrixomas are extremely rare in cats.[37a, 125] The cause of pilomatrixomas is unknown.

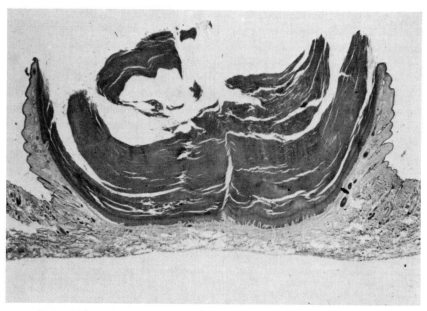

Figure 20:17. Dilated pore of Winer. Widely dilated, keratin-filled hair follicle.

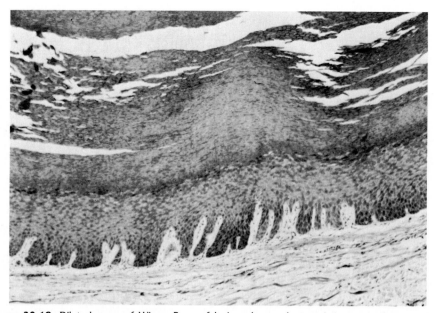

Figure 20:18. Dilated pore of Winer. Base of lesion shows characteristic psoriasiform epithelial hyperplasia.

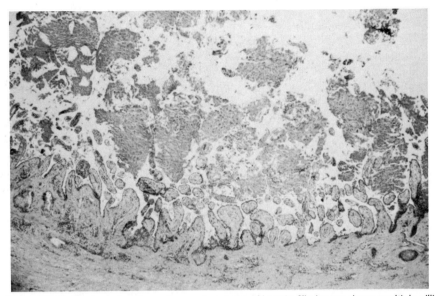

Figure 20:19. Warty dyskeratoma from a dog. Base of keratin-filled mass shows multiple villi.

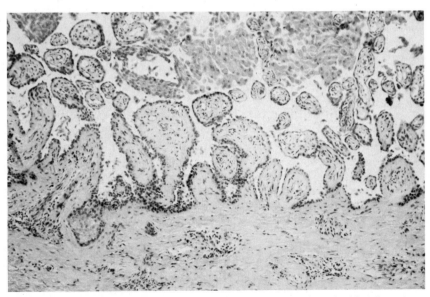

Figure 20:20. Warty dyskeratoma. Basal villi with single layer of attached keratinocytes.

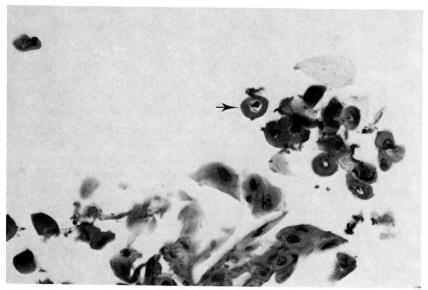

Figure 20:21. Warty dyskeratoma. Acantholytic cells and typical corps ronds (arrow).

Pilomatrixomas occur in dogs that are an average of 6 years of age. There is no apparent sex predilection. Kerry blue terriers and poodles appear to be predisposed.

Usually, pilomatrixomas are solitary. There may be site predilection of shoulders, back, flanks, and legs. Pilomatrixomas are usually firm, rounded, elevated, well circumscribed, and dermoepidermal in position, and they range from 2 to 10 cm in diameter (Fig. 20:22A,B). They frequently become ulcerated and alopecic, and are occasionally cystic. Pilomatrixomas are rarely invasive or metastatic.[100a, 136]

Histopathologically, pilomatrixomas are characterized by a variable proliferation of "basophilic cells" (which resemble hair matrix cells) and "shadow or ghost cells" (fully keratinized, faintly eosinophilic cells with a central, unstained nucleus) (Fig. 20:22C,D).[142, 161] "Shadow cells" are *not* pathognomonic, having been found in epidermoid cysts, inflamed hair follicles, and chronic hyperkeratotic dermatoses.[136] There is abrupt keratinization (no stratum granulosum), and the keratin is homogenous, relatively amorphous, and nonfibrillar (tricholemmal keratin). A frequent but not constant feature of pilomatrixomas is calcification within the areas of shadow cells.

Clinical management of pilomatrixomas may include surgical excision, cryotherapy, or observation without treatment.[145, 199]

SEBACEOUS GLAND TUMORS

Sebaceous gland tumors are common (in dogs) to rare (in cats) epithelial growths arising from sebaceous gland cells.[13, 37a, 125, 144, 145, 172, 199] Their cause is unknown.

These tumors occur in dogs and cats at an average of 9 to 10 years of age. No apparent sex predilection exists. There is no breed predilection in cats. In dogs, however, cocker spaniels, Kerry blue terriers, Boston terriers, poodles,

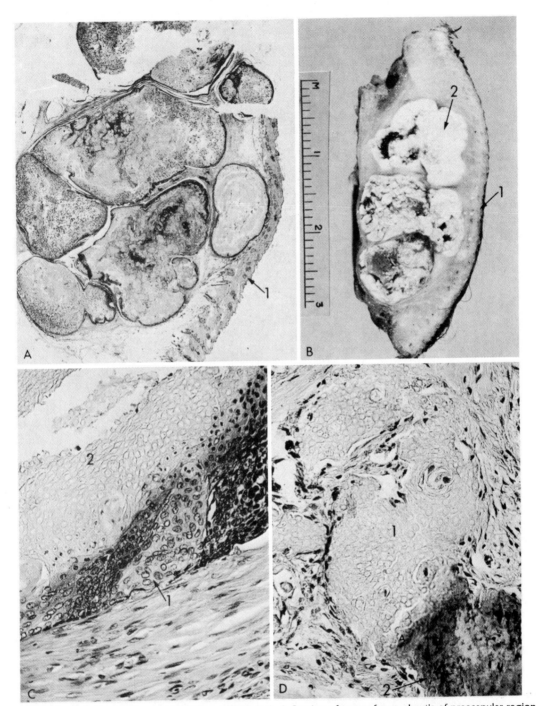

Figure 20:22. Pilomatrixoma (benign calcifying epithelioma). *A,* Section of tumor from subcutis of prescapular region of 3-year-old female French poodle. *B,* Gross appearance of same tumor. Epidermis (1), chalky granular and lobulated tumor (2). (Courtesy Armed Forces Institute of Pathology and M. G. Rhoades.) *C,* Section of similar tumor from 2-year-old Kerry blue terrier. Epithelial cells simulating hair matrix (1), cells in center of lesion stain poorly but maintain their outlines as "shadow" or "ghost" cells (2). *D,* Another section of tumor in *C.* "Ghost cells" in center of lesion (1), calcification present at (2). (Courtesy Armed Forces Institute of Pathology and G. A. Goode.) (From Smith, H. A., Jones, T. C., and Hunt, R. D.: Veterinary Pathology. 4th ed., Lea & Febiger, Philadelphia, 1972, p. 231, with permission.)

beagles, dachshunds, Norwegian elkhounds, and basset hounds are thought to be predisposed.

Sebaceous gland tumors may be single or multiple. They may occur anywhere in the skin, but the head is especially common. *Nodular sebaceous hyperplasia* is the most common type of sebaceous gland tumor in dogs and cats, and is usually firm, elevated, well circumscribed, dermoepidermal in position, alopecic, shiny, lobulated (cauliflower-like), pinkish to yellowish, and small (2 to 10 mm in diameter) (Fig. 20:11E). *Sebaceous adenomas* tend to be larger (up to 2 cm in diameter) and less lobulated (Fig. 20:13F). *Sebaceous epitheliomas* are similar to basal cell tumors in appearance (Fig. 20:11G). *Sebaceous adenocarcinomas* tend to be larger than 2 cm in diameter,[115] firm, poorly circumscribed, and ulcerated (Fig. 20:11H). Sebaceous gland tumors are usually benign in both dogs and cats. In dogs, sebaceous adenocarcinomas rarely metastasize.[145]

Histopathologically, sebaceous gland tumors are classified as *nodular sebaceous hyperplasia* (greatly enlarged sebaceous glands composed of numerous lobules grouped around centrally located sebaceous ducts) (Fig. 20:23); *sebaceous adenoma* (lobules of sebaceous cells of irregular shape and size, well demarcated from the surrounding tissue, and containing mostly mature sebaceous cells and fewer undifferentiated germinative cells); *sebaceous epithelioma* (similar to basal cell tumor but containing mostly undifferentiated germinative cells and fewer mature sebaceous cells) (Fig. 20:24); and *sebaceous adenocarcinoma* (pleomorphism, atypia) (Fig. 20:25).[95, 121, 142]

Clinical management of sebaceous gland tumors may include surgical excision, cryotherapy, electrosurgery, and observation without treatment.[145, 199] Recently, oral retinoids have been reported to be an effective treatment for sebaceous hyperplasia in humans.[33, 80]

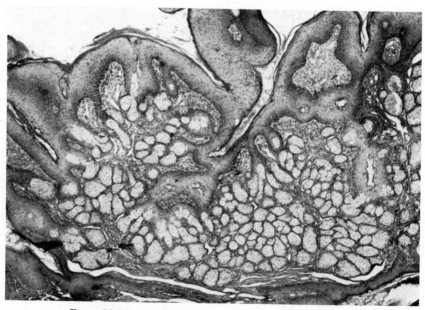

Figure 20:23. Nodular sebaceous gland hyperplasia in a dog.

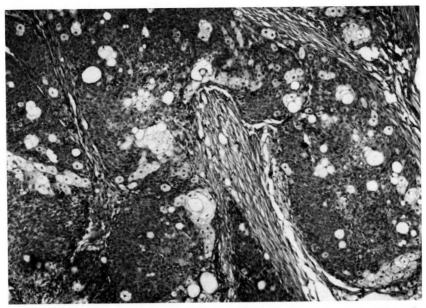

Figure 20:24. Sebaceous epithelioma in a dog. A neoplastic proliferation of basaloid cells with occasional sebaceous differentiation.

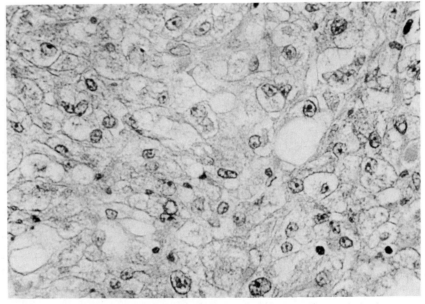

Figure 20:25. Sebaceous adenocarcinoma. Proliferation of pleomorphic, atypical sebaceous cells.

SWEAT GLAND TUMORS

Apocrine sweat gland tumors are uncommon growths in the dog and cat arising from apocrine sweat gland cells.[13, 37a, 46, 125, 144, 145, 172, 199] *Eccrine sweat gland tumors* are rare in the dog[145] and the cat.[37a] The cause of sweat gland tumors is unknown.

Sweat gland tumors usually occur in dogs and cats over 8 years old. Cats show no apparent breed or sex predilection. In dogs, it has been reported that cocker spaniels and males are predisposed.

Apocrine gland neoplasms are usually solitary and may have a predilection for the back and flanks. However, in dogs, *apocrine cysts* (cystic hyperplasia) are often multiple ("apocrine cystomatosis") and tend to occur more frequently on the head and neck (Fig. 20:26). They are elevated, rounded, fluctuant, well circumscribed, dermoepidermal in location, and often light blue to purplish in color (Fig. 20:27A). *Apocrine adenomas* are usually firm, elevated, well circumscribed, dermoepidermal in location, and 1 to 4 cm in diameter. *Apocrine adenocarcinomas* may be grossly indistinguishable from adenomas or may be firm, infiltrative (Fig. 20:27B), poorly circumscribed, with or without ulceration and surface infection, and mistaken for pyotraumatic dermatitis or pyoderma. Apocrine cysts and adenomas are benign, but apocrine adenocarcinomas frequently are highly invasive and metastatic.

The eccrine sweat gland tumors are *eccrine adenomas and adenocarcinomas.* These are solitary, firm, well-circumscribed to poorly circumscribed, often ulcerated masses arising from the eccrine sweat glands in the footpads (Fig. 20:27C). Too few cases have been recognized to comment on their biologic behavior.

Histopathologically, canine and feline apocrine sweat gland tumors have been classified into numerous types as follows: (1) apocrine cyst (cystic hyperplasia, apocrine hamartoma or nevus) (Figs. 20:28 and 20:29), (2) cystadenoma (Fig. 20:30), (3) papillary syringoadenoma (Figs. 20:31 and 20:32), (4) spiraden-

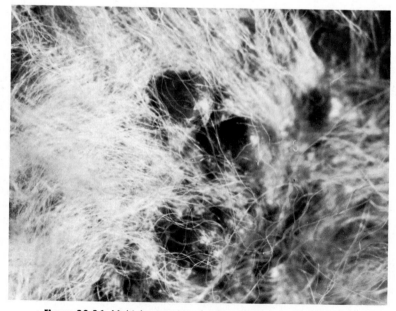

Figure 20:26. Multiple apocrine gland cysts on the neck of a dog.

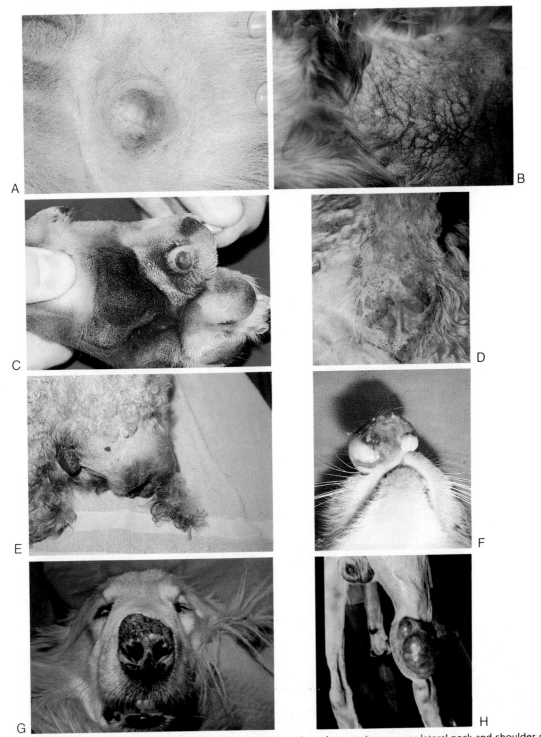

Figure 20:27. *A,* Apocrine cyst over the thorax of a dog. *B,* Apocrine adenocarcinoma over lateral neck and shoulder of a dog. *C,* Eccrine adenoma on the footpad of a dog. *D,* Perianal adenoma with ulceration in an aged wire-haired fox terrier. *E,* Perianal gland adenocarcinoma. *F,* Fibroma on the nose of a cat. *G,* Grossly deformed nose from fibrosarcoma. The patient also has nasal solar dermatitis. *H,* Schwannoma. This large mass recurred after two previous surgical excisions. (Courtesy G. E. Ross.)

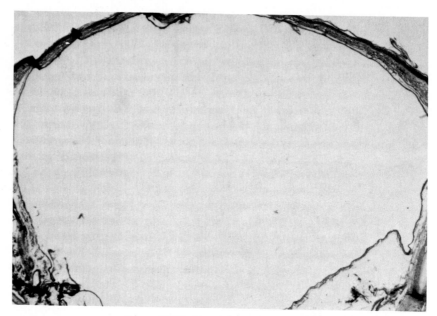

Figure 20:28. Apocrine cyst from a dog.

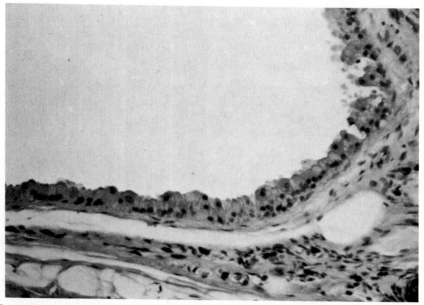

Figure 20:29. Apocrine cyst from a dog. Columnar glandular epithelium with apical budding.

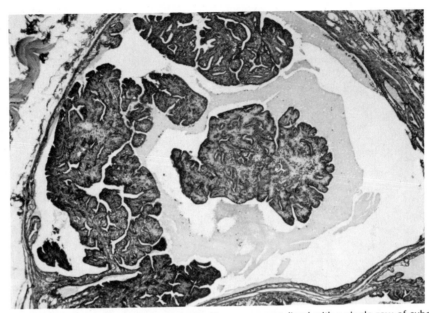

Figure 20:30. Feline papillary cystadenoma. Papillary processes, lined with a single row of cuboidal to columnar apocrine gland epithelial cells, projecting into a cyst cavity that also contains amorphous secretory material.

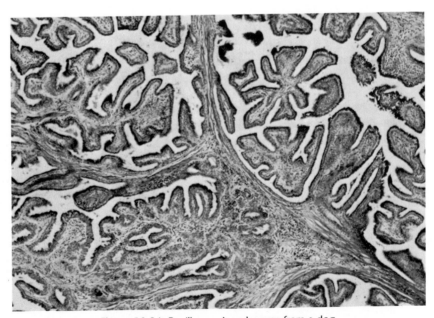

Figure 20:31. Papillary syringadenoma from a dog.

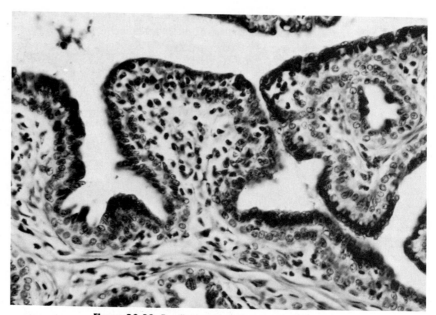

Figure 20:32. Papillary syringadenoma (higher power).

oma, (5) cylindroma, (6) hidradenoma papilliferum, (7) adenocarcinomas (papillary, tubular, solid, signet ring) (Fig. 20:33), (8) clear-cell hidradenocarcinoma, and (9) eccrine adenoma (Fig. 20:34).[96, 120, 144, 145, 199] The clinical significance of these various histologic types, except where benign or malignant, is not known. In humans, enzyme histochemistry and immunohistochemistry have been useful in distinguishing between neoplasms of apocrine or eccrine origin. Carcinoembryonic antigen, phosphorylase, and lactic dehydrogenase are found in eccrine tissue, while acid-phosphatase and β-glucuronidase are found in apocrine tissue.[127, 134]

Clinical management of sweat gland tumors may include surgical excision, cryosurgery, electrosurgery, or observation without treatment.[145, 199]

PERIANAL GLAND TUMOR

These tumors, which are common in the dog, arise most frequently from perianal glands (hepatoid or circumanal glands, modified sebaceous glands) and less commonly from apocrine anal glands (apocrine glands in skin of anal canal) or anal sac glands (apocrine glands of the anal sacs).[131, 135, 144, 145, 165a, 168, 199] The cause of perianal gland tumors is unknown. However, the "hepatoid" glands and their tumors are known to be modulated by sex hormones.

Perianal (hepatoid) gland tumors occur in dogs with an average age of 11 years. They are about nine times more frequent in males than in females. Perianal adenocarcinomas occur with equal frequency in males and females. Cocker spaniels, English bulldogs, Samoyeds, Afghans, dachshunds, and beagles are predisposed to the development of perianal gland tumors. Apocrine neoplasms of anal sac origin are most common in old female dogs and are often associated with pseudohyperparathyroidism.[135, 168] Perianal (hepatoid) gland neoplasms may be solitary or multiple. Most occur adjacent to the anus,

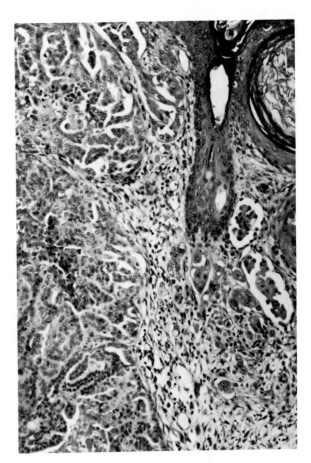

Figure 20:33. Canine apocrine gland carcinoma. A proliferation of atypical apocrine gland epithelial cells, in cords and glandular structures, with lymphatic invasion (right).

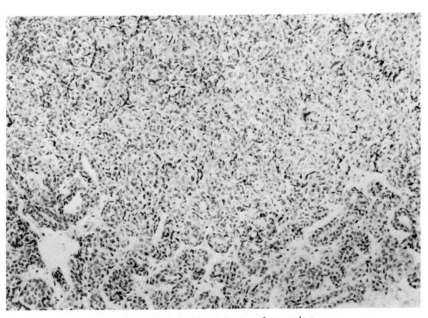

Figure 20:34. Eccrine adenoma from a dog.

but they may occur on the tail, perineum, prepuce, thigh, and dorsal lumbosacral area (see Fig. 20:27D). The smaller (less than 1 cm in diameter) neoplasms are spherical or ovoid and tend to become multinodular and ulcerated as they become larger (up to 10 cm in diameter). Perianal neoplasms are usually firm, dermoepidermal in location, and well-circumscribed to poorly circumscribed.

Nodular perianal gland hyperplasia may occur as multiple discrete nodules of varying size that are impossible to distinguish from perianal adenomas and apocrine anal gland tumors, or as a diffuse bulging ring around the anus (Fig. 20:35). Most perianal gland tumors are benign.

Perianal (hepatoid) adenocarcinomas (Fig. 20:27E) tend to grow more rapidly, attain a larger size, and ulcerate more extensively than adenomas. Metastasis may be widespread.

Apocrine tumors of anal sac origin are usually adenocarcinomas, often produce pseudohyperparathyroidism, and usually metastasize.

Histologically, perianal gland tumors are classified into two basic types: (1) perianal or hepatoid gland tumors (Fig. 20:36) (hyperplasia, adenoma, adenocarcinoma),[144] and (2) apocrine anal gland tumors.[131] Apocrine tumors of anal sac origin are a separate type.[135]

Clinical management of perianal gland tumors may include surgical excision, cryosurgery, electrosurgery, radiotherapy, castration, or the administration of estrogens.[144, 145, 199] Castration is usually the treatment of choice for perianal (hepatoid) gland hyperplasias and adenomas, with 95 per cent of the dogs responding well. Concurrent surgical excision is usually needed only with ulcerated or recurrent neoplasms in male dogs, but is usually mandatory for perianal gland neoplasms in females. Castration is not effective for adenocar-

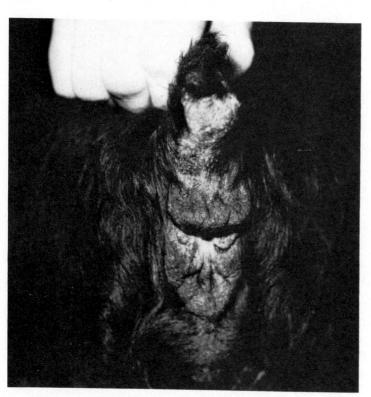

Figure 20:35. Diffuse perianal gland hyperplasia around the anus of a dog.

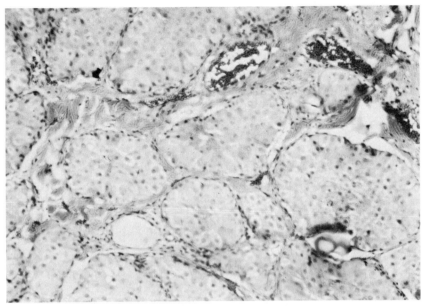

Figure 20:36. Perianal gland hyperplasia.

cinomas. Estrogen therapy is not usually recommended, since any tumor regressions induced are transient. Recurrence of perianal hyperplasia/adenoma after surgical resection and castration, or occurrence of these lesions in female dogs, suggests that these animals should be evaluated for hyperadrenocorticism (elevated androgen levels; see Chapter 10).[159a] For the much less common apocrine anal gland neoplasms, surgical excision is the therapy of choice, as there is no information to suggest that they are hormone dependent.

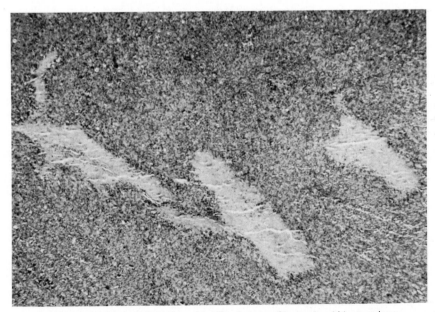

Figure 20:37. Epithelial sarcoma. Multifocal areas of necrosis within neoplasm.

EPITHELIOID SARCOMA

Epithelioid sarcoma is a malignant neoplasm that is probably epithelial in origin.[40, 217] The cause of this tumor is unknown.

Epithelioid sarcoma has been recognized in adult cats.[175] Lesions are solitary and occur on the upper extremities. They begin as firm, poorly circumscribed, dermal or subcutaneous nodules that may ulcerate as they enlarge. Metastasis may occur. In humans, epithelioid sarcomas have a recurrence rate of 77 per cent following surgery and metastasize (lymph nodes, lungs) in about 45 per cent of the cases.[40]

Histopathologically, epithelioid sarcomas are characterized by a nodular arrangement of plump spindle cells and large, round-to-polygonal epithelioid cells (Figs. 20:37 and 20:38).[40, 175] Mitoses are frequent, and necrosis is characteristically present, especially in the center of large nodules. In humans, immunocytochemical studies have shown that epithelioid sarcomas contain cytokeratin.[40, 217]

The therapy of choice is early, radical surgical excision.

Mesenchymal Neoplasms

FIBROMA
(Dermatofibroma, Nodular Subepidermal Fibrosis)

Fibromas are uncommon benign neoplasms of the dog and cat arising from dermal or subcutaneous fibroblasts.[37a, 144, 145, 172, 199] The cause of fibromas is unknown.

These neoplasms usually occur in older dogs and cats. There is no breed or sex predilection in cats. In dogs, however, fibromas are reported to occur

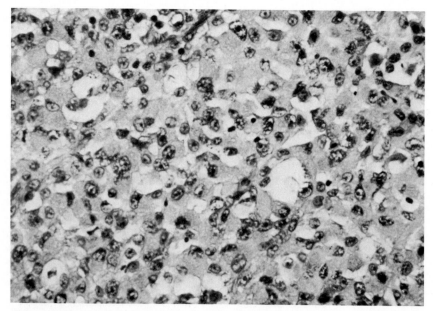

Figure 20:38. Epithelioid sarcoma. Proliferation of pleomorphic, atypical epithelioid cells.

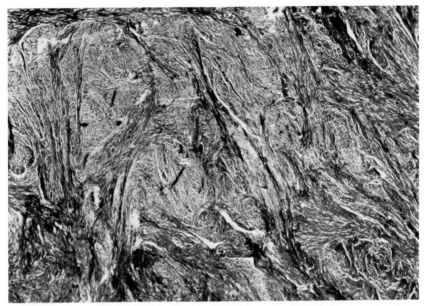

Figure 20:39. Canine fibroma. An interlacing proliferation of well-differentiated fibroblasts and collagen fibrils.

most commonly in boxers, Boston terriers, and fox terriers. Females are predisposed.

Usually these lesions are solitary (Fig. 20:27F) and may be more common on the limbs, flanks, and groin. They are usually well circumscribed, firm (fibroma durum) to soft (fibroma molle), dome shaped to pedunculated, and dermoepidermal to subcutaneous in location. In dogs, fibromas may be melanotic or "pin-feathered," or both. Fibromas are noninvasive and nonmetastatic.

Histologically, fibromas are characterized by whorls and interlacing bundles of fibroblasts and collagen fibers (Fig. 20:39).[144] The neoplastic cells are usually fusiform in shape, and mitoses are rare. Fibromas containing focal areas of mucinous or myxomatous degeneration are often called fibromyxomas.[18]

Clinical management of fibromas may include surgical excision, cryosurgery, electrosurgery, or observation without treatment.[145, 199]

FIBROVASCULAR PAPILLOMA
(Skin Tag, Acrochordon, Soft Fibroma)

Fibrovascular papillomas are common benign tumors of fibrovascular origin in dogs.[145, 180] The cause of these growths is unknown. No sex predilection is established, but large and giant breeds appear to be predisposed. The lesions may be solitary or multiple, filiform to pedunculated, smooth or hyperkeratotic, soft, and small (less than 1 cm in length) (Fig. 20:40). Fibrovascular papillomas occur most commonly on the proximal extremities and ventral thorax.

Histopathologically, fibrovascular papillomas are characterized by a fibrovascular core exhibiting papillomatosis and irregular hyperplasia of the overlying epidermis (Fig. 20:41).[145]

Clinical management of fibrovascular papillomas may include surgical excision, cryosurgery, electrosurgery, or observation without treatment.[145]

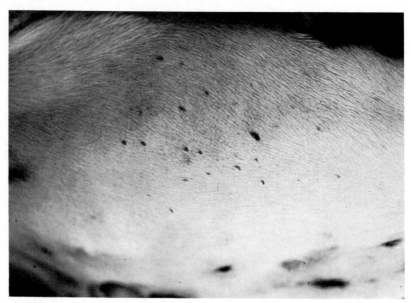

Figure 20:40. Multiple fibrovascular papillomas (acrochordons) on the sternum of a dog.

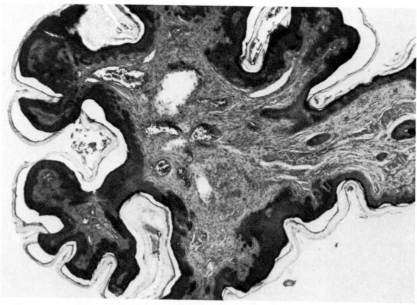

Figure 20:41. Canine fibrovascular papilloma. Papillomatous proliferation of epidermis and fibrovascular tissue.

FIBROSARCOMA
(Fibroblastic Spindle-Cell Sarcoma)

Fibrosarcomas are common malignant neoplasms of the dog and cat arising from dermal or subcutaneous fibroblasts.[37a, 144, 145, 172, 199] The cause of fibrosarcomas in older animals is unknown.

Some feline fibrosarcomas are virus induced.[84, 172, 199] Such fibrosarcomas, and cell-free extracts derived from them, contain C-type virus particles. Cell-free extracts produce multicentric fibrosarcomas when injected into kittens and puppies. Cats over 4 months old appear to be resistant to the oncogenic effects of this feline sarcoma virus (FeSV) and usually develop no neoplasms or develop benign neoplasms that spontaneously regress. The FeSV is a mutant of the feline leukemia virus (FeLV), and cats with FeSV–induced fibrosarcomas are FeLV–positive. FeSV is apparently *not* associated with the solitary fibrosarcomas in old cats.

Although fibrosarcomas usually occur in older dogs and cats, the FeSV–induced fibrosarcomas are seen in young cats. There are no apparent breed or sex predilections in cats. However, in dogs there may be a predilection for females, and cocker spaniels appear to be a predisposed breed.

Fibrosarcomas are usually solitary, except for the FeSV–induced multicentric form in young cats. There is a predilection for the limbs and trunk. Fibrosarcomas are usually irregular and nodular in shape, firm to fleshy, variable in size, poorly circumscribed, and dermoepidermal to subcutaneous in location (Fig. 20:27G). They are often ulcerated. Most fibrosarcomas demonstrate rapid, infiltrative growth, with metastasis occurring in less than 25 per cent of the cases.[144, 145, 172, 199] Immune-mediated thrombocytopenia has been reported in association with canine fibrosarcoma.[89]

Histopathologically, fibrosarcomas are characterized by interwoven bundles of immature fibroblasts and moderate numbers of collagen fibers.[144] The neoplastic cells are usually fusiform in shape, mitotic figures are common, and

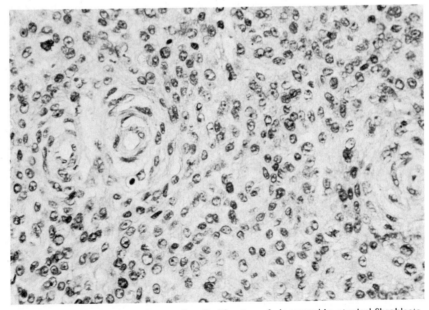

Figure 20:42. Fibrosarcoma from a dog. Proliferation of pleomorphic, atypical fibroblasts.

cellular atypia is pronounced (Fig. 20:42). Fibrosarcomas with focal areas of mucinous or myxomatous degeneration are often called *fibromyxosarcomas*.[18]

In a study of 44 cats with fibrosarcomas, it was found that the mitotic index and tumor site correlated with prognosis, whereas histologic appearance, tumor size, and duration of tumor growth did not.[22] Cats with fibrosarcomas of the head, back, or limbs and with a mitotic index of six or greater had the poorest prognosis. In a study of 84 dogs with fibrosarcomas, it was found that the site of tumor occurrence, tumor size, and delay between detection of the tumor and surgical excision had little influence on the prognosis for recurrence or metastasis.[23] Mitotic index of the neoplasms was shown to have a significant predictive value for recurrence, postsurgical survival time, and metastasis.

The clinical management of choice for fibrosarcomas is wide surgical excision.[145, 199] In dogs, local recurrence following surgical excision was reported in 30 per cent of the cases.[23] Radiotherapy, chemotherapy (doxorubicin, cyclophosphamide, methotrexate, vincristine), immunotherapy (mixed bacterial vaccine, levamisole), and cryosurgery have been of limited benefit.[25, 26, 145, 199]

MYXOMA AND MYXOSARCOMA

Myxomas and myxosarcomas are rare neoplasms of the dog and cat arising from dermal or subcutaneous fibroblasts,[13, 144, 145, 199] the cause of which is unknown. These neoplasms usually occur in older dogs and cats, with no breed or sex predilections. In dogs, they may occur more frequently on the limbs, back, or groin. They are usually solitary infiltrative growths that are soft, slimy, poorly circumscribed, and without definite shape. Myxomas are benign. Myxosarcomas are malignant but apparently do not commonly metastasize. Both neoplasms frequently recur following surgery, owing to their infiltrative growth patterns.

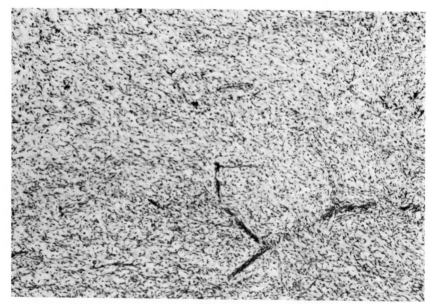

Figure 20:43. Feline myxosarcoma. An infiltrative proliferation of atypical fibroblasts (fusiform to stellate) with abundant ground substance production (mucinous degeneration).

Histopathologically, myxomas and myxosarcomas are characterized by stellate-to-fusiform cells distributed in a vacuolated, basophilic, mucinous stroma that may be partitioned by collagenous connective tissue septae (Fig. 20:43).[144]

In clinical management, the therapy of choice for myxomas and myxosarcomas is radical surgical excision.[145, 199]

UNDIFFERENTIATED SARCOMA
(Spindle-Cell Sarcoma)

Classification of some mesenchymal neoplasms may be difficult or impossible.[18, 25, 144, 145, 199] Such anaplastic sarcomas are usually called "undifferentiated sarcomas" or "spindle-cell sarcomas." Such sarcomas usually occur in older dogs and cats, with no breed or sex predilection. In cats, undifferentiated sarcoma may present as a pododermatitis restricted to the footpads of one or more feet.[172] Affected cats are usually lame, and the affected pads are usually soft, mushy, and painful, and they may be ulcerated.

Undifferentiated sarcomas are malignant and radical surgical excision is the therapy of choice.[145, 199]

NODULAR FASCIITIS
(Pseudosarcomatous Fasciitis)

Nodular fasciitis is a rare, benign, non-neoplastic growth of the dog and cat.[144] Nodular fasciitis is thought to represent a proliferative inflammatory process arising from the subcutaneous fascia and exhibiting a clinically aggressive behavior that suggests a locally invasive neoplasm.[120, 144]

There are no age, breed, or sex predilections for dogs and cats. Nodular fasciitis can occur anywhere on the body but may favor the head, face, and eyelids. The masses are usually solitary, firm, poorly circumscribed, 0.2 to 5 cm in diameter, and subcutaneous in location. In humans, nodular fasciitis is self-limited in duration, and thus, even if it is incompletely excised, it regresses. Cutaneous nodular fasciitis in dogs and cats is also benign, but spontaneous regression has not been reported. It is likely that the invasive, recurrent "nodular fasciitis" associated with the eye and eyelid[144] and the steroid-responsive "nodular fasciitis" in cats[172] actually represent fibrous histiocytoma.

Histopathologically, nodular fasciitis is characterized by a poorly circumscribed, infiltrative proliferation of pleomorphic fibroblasts growing haphazardly in a highly vascularized stroma with varying amounts of mucoid ground substance.[120, 144] Mitoses and giant cells are common, and a chronic inflammatory infiltrate is often present.

The clinical management of nodular fasciitis in dogs and cats has consisted of surgical excision.

LEIOMYOMA AND LEIOMYOSARCOMA

Leiomyomas and leiomyosarcomas are extremely rare neoplasms of dogs and cats arising from smooth muscle cells of arrector pili muscles or cutaneous blood vessels.[37a, 46, 51, 144, 145, 199] The cause of these neoplasms is unknown.

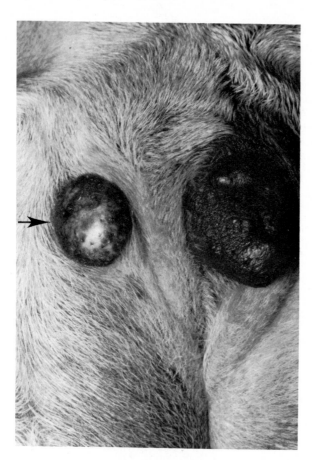

Figure 20:44. Leiomyoma (arrow) in the groin of a bitch.

They are usually solitary, firm, well circumscribed, dermoepidermal in location, and variable in size. There are no reported age, breed, or sex predilections. They may occur more frequently in the groin (Fig. 20:44).

Histopathologically, leiomyomas and leiomyosarcomas are characterized by interlacing bundles of smooth muscle fibers that tend to interact at right angles (Fig. 20:45).[120, 144] Cell nuclei are usually cigar shaped with rounded blunt ends. Masson's trichrome stain is often helpful in distinguishing between tumors of muscle, collagen, and neural origin.

In clinical management the therapy of choice is surgical excision.[145, 199]

TUMORS OF NEURAL ORIGIN

Schwannoma
(Neurofibroma, Neurilemmoma, Neurinoma, Perineural Fibroblastoma)

Schwannomas are rare neoplasms of the dog and cat arising from dermal or subcutaneous Schwann cells (nerve sheath).[37a, 104, 144, 145, 157, 172, 199] The cause of schwannomas is unknown.

There is much confusion over terminology concerning these neoplasms in the veterinary literature. In humans, there are two distinct clinical, histopathologic, and ultrastructural types of schwannomas,[120] *neurofibroma* and *neurilem-*

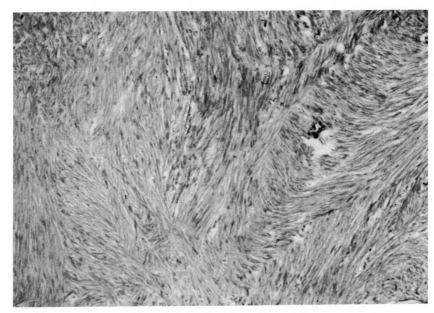

Figure 20:45. Leiomyoma from a dog.

moma. There is histopathologic and ultrastructural evidence that the same two types occur in dogs and cats. Unfortunately, most reports do not make this distinction and simply refer to them as "schwannomas" or "nerve sheath tumors"; consequently, meaningful clinicopathologic data on the two types do not exist.

Schwannomas usually occur in older dogs and cats, with no sex predilection. In cats, no breed predilection exists, but in dogs the fox terrier may be predisposed.

Schwannomas are usually solitary. They occur most commonly on the thoracic limb, head and neck in cats but may occur more commonly on the limbs in dogs (Fig. 20:27H). Schwannomas are usually firm, well-circumscribed to poorly circumscribed, variable in size, and dermoepidermal to subcutaneous in location. Rarely, schwannomas may be plexiform (multinodular). There may be obvious nerve involvement with or without neurologic deficit. Most schwannomas in dogs appear to be benign but recur frequently after surgery. In cats, most schwannomas are malignant.

Histopathologically, schwannomas are characterized by two patterns: (1) *neurofibroma*—faintly eosinophilic, thin, waxy fibers lying in loosely textured strands that extend in various directions, with spindle-shaped cells that may exhibit nuclear palisading, and (2) *neurilemmoma*—areas of spindle-shaped cells exhibiting nuclear palisading and twisting bands or rows (Antoni type A tissue), alternating with an edematous stroma containing relatively few haphazardly arranged cells (Antoni type B tissue) (Fig. 20:46).[144]

In the clinical management of schwannomas the therapy of choice is surgical excision.[145, 199] Radiotherapy, chemotherapy, immunotherapy, and cryosurgery appear to be of minimal benefit.[145, 199]

Neurothekeoma

Neurothekeomas are benign cutaneous neoplasms of Schwann cell origin.[70] The cause of these neoplasms is unknown.

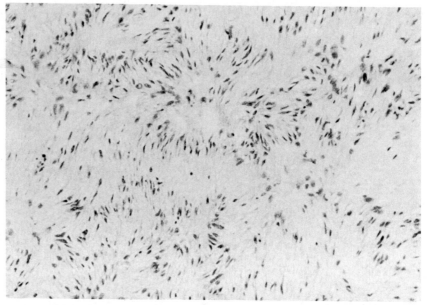

Figure 20:46. Schwannoma from a dog. Antoni A and B Type tissue.

Neurothekeomas occur in dogs,[180] but not enough cases have been seen to generate age, breed, or sex data. The lesions are solitary, firm, nodular, and subcutaneous to dermal in location. They occur on the legs.

Histopathologically, neurothekeomas are characterized by nests and cords of cells in a variably mucinous matrix (Fig. 20:47). Close relationship to small nerves may be seen.

Clinical management includes surgical excision or observation without treatment.

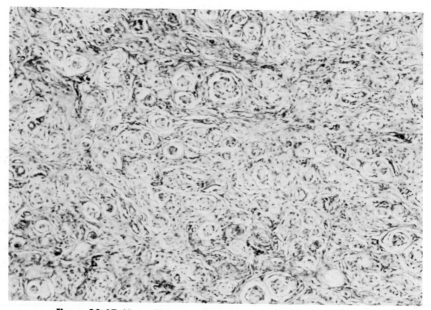

Figure 20:47. Neurothekeoma from a dog. Nests of neuroid tissue.

Granular Cell Tumor
(Granular Cell Myoblastoma, Granular Cell Schwannoma)

Granular cell tumors are rare neoplasms of the dog.[144, 145, 199, 206] Although the cell of origin is not established with certainty, current evidence suggests a neural source. In humans, granular cell tumors contain neuron-specific enolase and myelin basic protein.[153, 161] The cause of granular cell tumors is unknown.

Granular cell tumors have been reported in dogs from 2.5 to 13 years old, with no breed or sex predilection. Most of the neoplasms have occurred as solitary, firm, round, well-circumscribed masses within the tongue. Other dogs had a solitary subcutaneous neoplasm near the shoulder or on the lip, and one dog had multiple dermoepidermal and subcutaneous malignant neoplasms with visceral metastasis (Fig. 20:48). Most canine granular cell tumors have been benign.

Histopathologically, granular cell tumors are characterized by a circumscribed mass of ovoid-to-polyhedral cells with central or eccentric nuclei and pale cytoplasm containing numerous small, faintly eosinophilic granules.[120, 207] The tumor cells may be arranged diffusely or in "nests" and rows (Fig. 20:49). The cytoplasmic granules are periodic acid-Schiff (PAS) positive. The pseudo-carcinomatous hyperplasia that so frequently overlies granular cell tumors in humans is rarely seen in dogs.

In clinical management the therapy of choice for granular cell tumors is surgical excision.[145]

Amputation Neuroma

A specific neuropathy was identified in dogs that had aberrant healing after tail docking.[37b] Historically, affected dogs had inflicted self-trauma to the tail since puppyhood, beginning soon after tail docking. Physical examination revealed a chronic, painful, excoriated dermatosis at the tip of the tail.

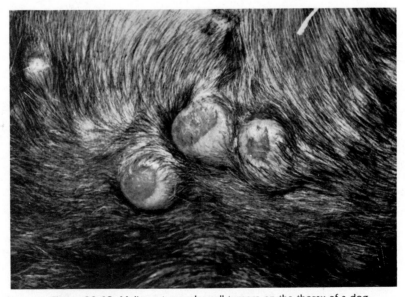

Figure 20:48. Malignant granular cell tumors on the thorax of a dog.

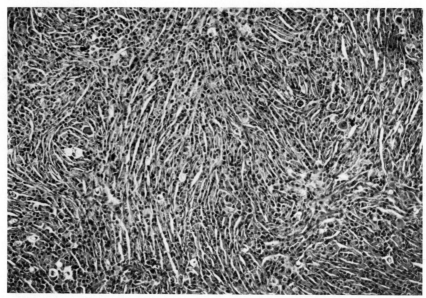

Figure 20:49. Malignant granular cell tumor in a dog. Cords and clusters of anaplastic cells with fine, eosinophilic cytoplasmic granules.

Histopathology revealed axonal sprouting with secondary remyelination in a bed of fibrous connective tissue. Surgical excision was curative.

LIPOMA

Lipomas are common (in dogs) to uncommon (in cats) benign neoplasms arising from subcutaneous lipocytes (adipocytes).[13, 37a, 125, 144, 145, 172, 199] The cause of lipomas is unknown.

Usually, these neoplasms occur in dogs and cats over 8 years old. There are no breed or sex predilections in cats. However, in dogs, lipomas are reported to occur more frequently in cocker spaniels, dachshunds, Weimaraners, Labrador retrievers, and small terriers, and in obese females.

Lipomas may be single or multiple and occur most often over the thorax, brisket, abdomen, and the proximal limbs (Fig. 20:50A). They are usually dome shaped or pedunculated, well circumscribed, soft to flabby, variable in size (1 to 30 cm in diameter), often multilobulated, and subcutaneous in location. Some lipomas are firm, owing to the presence of fibrous tissue or inflammation, or both. Some lipomas are painful and are invariably found to be *angiolipomas* histologically.[180]

Figure 20:50. A, Huge subcutaneous lipoma in an aged spaniel. Repeated trauma to the distended skin may cause secondary erythema and ulceration. Lipomas grow slowly. Surgical excision is usually easy because the tumor has a thin capsule and is relatively avascular. B, Bluish colored hemangioma on the pinna of a cat. C, Hemangiosarcoma on the face of a cat (Courtesy W. H. Miller, Jr.) D, Large hemangiopericytoma affecting the foreleg. Notice the smooth lobulated appearance of this firm mass. E, Canine lymphangioma. Erythematoses, cystic mass in groin. (Courtesy W. H. Miller, Jr.) F, Canine lymphangioma. Purpuric mass in groin. (Courtesy W. H. Miller, Jr.) G, Feline lymphangiosarcoma. Purpuric, nodular plaque on abdomen. H, Feline lymphangiosarcoma. Oozing, purpuric plaque.

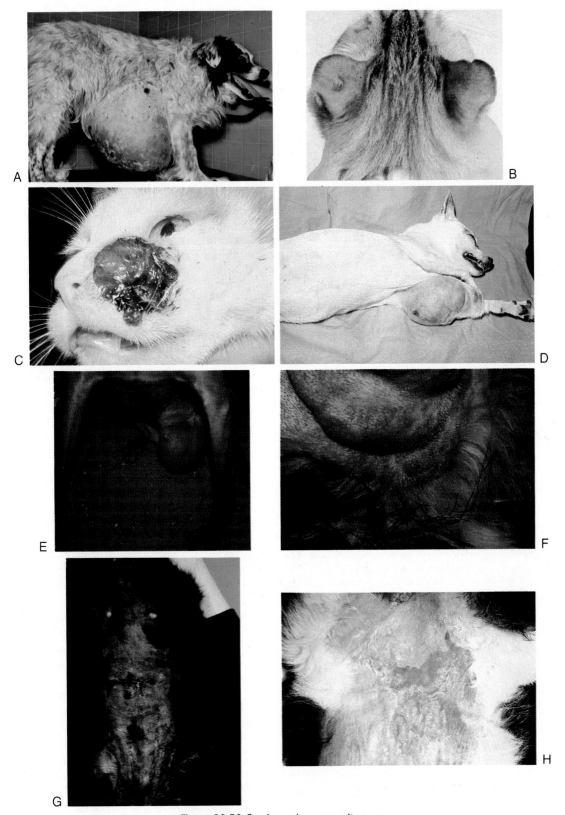

Figure 20:50 *See legend on opposite page*

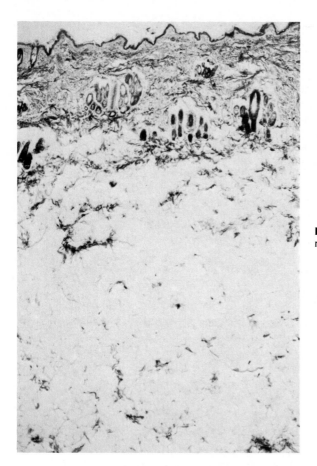

Figure 20:51. Lipoma from a cat. Proliferation of normal-appearing fat.

Infiltrative lipomas (lipomatosis) have been reported in dogs and cats.[37a, 63, 112] In dogs, these tumors occur in middle-aged animals with a predilection for females. Obesity does not appear to be a prerequisite. These tumors occur most frequently on the extremities and neck. The neoplasms are poorly circumscribed, soft masses in connective tissue and muscle that may cause dysfunction because of mechanical interference or pressure pain.

Histologically, lipomas are characterized by a well-circumscribed proliferation of normal-appearing lipocytes (Figs. 20:51 and 20:52).[144] Some neoplasms have a marked fibrous tissue component and are called *fibrolipomas*. Infiltrative lipomas are characterized by a poorly circumscribed proliferation of normal-appearing lipocytes that infiltrate surrounding tissues, especially muscle and collagen.[112] *Angiolipomas* are characterized by mature adipose tissue with a complex, branching blood vascular component (Fig. 20:53).[59, 180]

In clinical management the treatment of choice for all types of lipomas is surgical excision.[145, 199] In obese animals, a restricted diet for a few weeks prior to surgery often reduces the size of the neoplasms and improves the definition from surrounding tissues. Small, asymptomatic lipomas are often merely observed, unless they grow large. Lipomas that are large can usually be easily "peeled out," because they are well circumscribed and have a poor blood supply. Recently, the intratumoral injection of 10 per cent calcium chloride solution was found to cause complete remission in 4 of 18 canine lipomas treated, with a 50 per cent reduction in size of the other 14 treated tumors.[3]

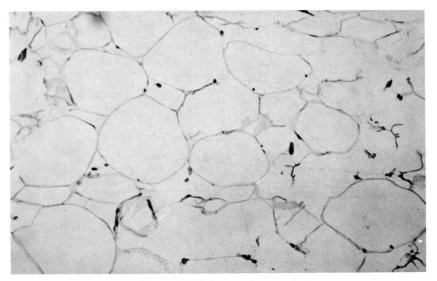

Figure 20:52. Lipoma from a cat.

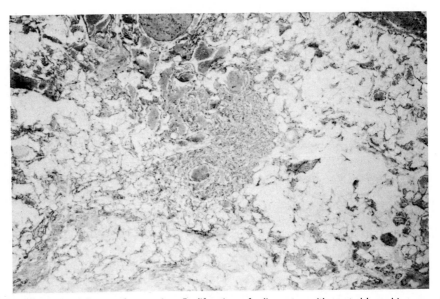

Figure 20:53. Angiolipoma from a dog. Proliferation of adipocytes with central branching vascular component.

LIPOSARCOMA

Liposarcomas are rare malignant neoplasms of the dog and cat arising from subcutaneous lipoblasts.[13, 37a, 59a, 144, 145, 172, 199] The cause of liposarcomas is unknown, although they can be induced in cats by injection of feline leukemia virus.[189, 190]

Liposarcomas occur in dogs and cats at an average of about 10 years of age. In cats, there are no breed or sex predilections. In dogs, liposarcomas may be more common in dachshunds and Brittany spaniels and in males.

Although they may be multiple, liposarcomas are usually solitary. In dogs, they occur most frequently on the ventral abdomen and thorax. Liposarcomas are usually poorly circumscribed, firm, variable in size (1 to 10 cm in diameter), and subcutaneous in location. Liposarcomas are malignant and infiltrative but rarely metastasize.

Histologically, liposarcomas are characterized by a cellular, infiltrative proliferation of atypical lipocytes with abundant, eosinophilic, finely vacuolated cytoplasm (Fig. 20:54).[144]

In clinical management, the therapy of choice for liposarcomas is wide surgical excision.[13, 151]

DIFFUSE LIPOMATOSIS

Lipomatosis is a benign proliferation of adipose tissue characterized by overgrowth of unencapsulated fat.[67, 120] Multiple symmetric lipomatosis is a rare condition in humans, currently thought to reflect a defect in lipid mobilization in which multiple areas of fat proliferation develop simultaneously on the neck, trunk, and proximal extremities.

Diffuse truncal lipomatosis was reported in a 5-year-old, spayed female dachshund that presented with a recent history of rapidly expanding pendulous

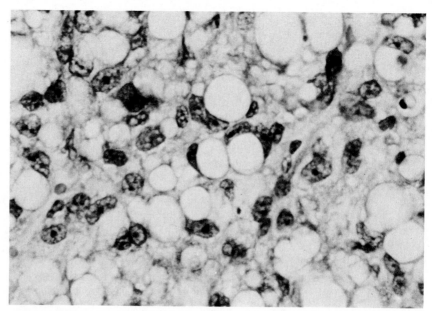

Figure 20:54. Liposarcoma from a cat. Proliferation of pleomorphic, atypical lipocytes.

skin folds on the neck, trunk, and rump.[71a] Skin biopsies revealed fat proliferation with occasional primitive mesenchymal cells and mucin deposits in the connective tissue septa. The dog was euthanized when the disease became so severe that she could not walk and had severe trauma to the skin.

TUMORS OF VASCULAR ORIGIN

Hemangioma
(Angioma)

Hemangiomas are uncommon (in dogs) to rare (in cats) benign neoplasms arising from the endothelial cells of blood vessels.[37a, 144, 145, 172, 199] The cause of hemangiomas is unknown. C-type virus particles have been found in cells from a subcutaneous hemangioma in a cat.

Hemangiomas occur in dogs and cats with an average age of 9 years. Cats show no breed or sex predilection. In dogs, there is no sex predilection, but boxers may be a breed at risk.

Hemangiomas are usually solitary (Fig. 20:50*B*) but may be multiple. In dogs and cats they usually occur in the limbs, flank, neck, and face. Hemangiomas are usually well circumscribed, firm to fluctuant, rounded, bluish to reddish black, 0.5 to 3 cm in diameter, and dermoepidermal to subcutaneous in location.

Histologically, hemangiomas are characterized by the proliferation of blood-filled vascular spaces lined by single layers of well-differentiated endothelial cells.[144] Hemangiomas are often subclassified as *cavernous or capillary*, depending on the size of the vascular spaces and the amount of intervening fibrous tissues (Figs. 20:55 and 20:56). Electron microscopy may be beneficial in determining the vascular origin of a neoplasm, as Weibel-Palade bodies are a specific cytoplasmic marker for endothelial cells.[38, 122] In addition, immunohistochemistry may be useful, as factor VIII–related antigen, UEA-1 lectin, and type IV collagen and laminin are found in vascular proliferations.[197]

Clinical management of hemangiomas may include surgical excision, cryosurgery, electrosurgery, or observation without treatment.[145, 199] Surgery of any vascular tumor can be difficult because of the rich blood supply. It is useful to first locate and ligate the main vessels.

Hemangiosarcoma
(Angiosarcoma, Malignant Hemangioendothelioma)

These are uncommon malignant neoplasms of dogs and cats arising from the endothelial cells of blood vessels.[29, 37a, 144, 145, 170, 199] The cause of hemangiosarcomas is unknown. In humans, they have been associated with exposure to thorium dioxide, arsenicals, and vinyl chloride.

Hemangiosarcomas occur in dogs and cats at an average of 10 years of age. In cats, there are no breed or sex predilections. In dogs, German shepherds, boxers, Bernese Mountain dogs, and males are most commonly affected.

Usually solitary (Fig. 20:50*C*), hemangiosarcomas occur most commonly on the trunk and extremities. They are usually rapidly growing, poorly circumscribed, soft and friable, 1 to 10 cm in diameter, and dermoepidermal to subcutaneous in location, and they often undergo necrosis, ulceration, and bleeding. They are highly invasive and malignant in dogs, with an average

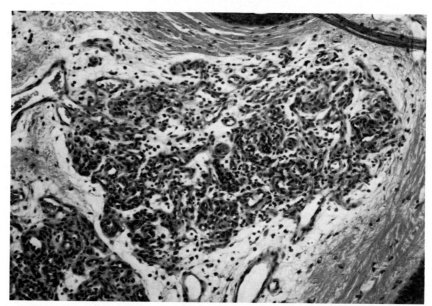

Figure 20:55. Canine capillary hemangioma. A benign proliferation of normal-appearing endothelial cells and blood vessels.

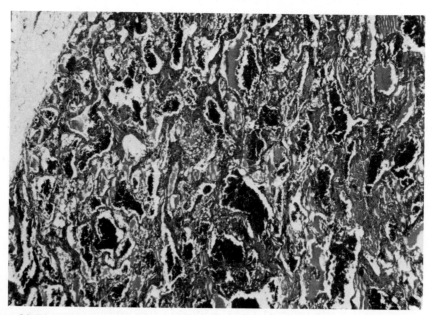

Figure 20:56. Canine cavernous hemangioma. A deep dermal proliferation of widely dilated, blood-filled vessels.

survival time of 4 months after diagnosis.[29] In cats, the tumors frequently recur following surgical excision but may not commonly metastasize.[37a, 170] Immune-mediated thrombocytopenia has been reported in association with canine hemangiosarcoma.[89]

Histopathologically, hemangiosarcomas are characterized by an invasive proliferation of atypical endothelial cells with areas of vascular space formation.[144]

In clinical management the therapy of choice for hemangiosarcomas is radical surgical excision.[145, 199] However, following *any* form of therapy, the prognosis for animals with hemangiosarcoma is poor, with local recurrence and metastasis being common.

Hemangiopericytoma
(Perithelioma, Dermatofibroma, Spindle-Cell Sarcoma)

Hemangiopericytomas are common benign neoplasms of the dog.[13, 78a, 144, 145, 165a] Rare cases of hemangiopericytoma in cats have been reported.[37a, 147] The cause of hemangiopericytomas is unknown.

Hemangiopericytomas occur in dogs with a mean of 10 years of age. Boxers, German shepherds, cocker spaniels, springer spaniels, fox terriers, and females are predisposed.

Hemangiopericytomas are usually solitary and occur most commonly on the limbs. They are usually firm, multinodular, well circumscribed, 2 to 25 cm in diameter, and dermoepidermal to subcutaneous in location (Fig. 20:50D). Hemangiopericytomas rarely metastasize.[78a]

Histopathologically, hemangiopericytomas are characterized by whorls ("fingerprint" pattern) of spindle-shaped to ovoid cells around blood vessels (Fig. 20:57).[78a, 144, 222a]

In clinical management the therapy of choice for hemangiopericytomas is surgical excision or amputation.[145, 199] Recurrent tumors have fewer whorls and

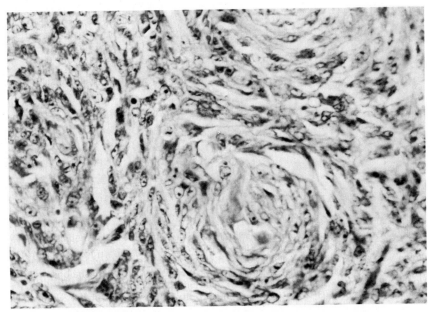

Figure 20:57. Canine hemangiopericytoma. Whorling of pericytes.

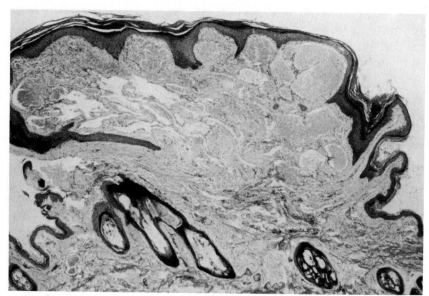

Figure 20:58. Canine angiokeratoma. Dilated, blood-filled vessels surrounded by hyperplastic epidermal collarettes.

look more like fibrosarcomas.[78a] Recent studies revealed that tumor cells are factor VIII negative (thus not endothelial in origin) and have a characteristic electron microscopic appearance of concentric arrangement of tumor cells around a central endothelium-lined capillary.[222a] About 30 per cent or more of these neoplasms recur 4 months to 4 years after surgical excision, and about 60 per cent were reported to recur after surgery and orthovoltage radiation therapy.[64a, 78a]

Angiokeratoma

Angiokeratomas are benign superficial cutaneous telangiectases with an associated epithelial proliferation.[34, 120, 180] The cause of angiokeratoma is unknown.

Angiokeratomas occur on the conjunctiva and skin of dogs. The lesions are usually discrete soft papules that may be heavily melanized. Their color varies from red to black.

Histopathologically, angiokeratomas are characterized by dilated and engorged superficial dermal blood vessels with a hyperplastic overlying epidermis (Fig. 20:58).

Clinical management of angiokeratomas includes surgical excision or observation without treatment.

Lymphangioma
(Angioma)

Lymphangiomas are very rare benign neoplasms of the dog and cat, arising from the endothelial cells of lymphatic vessels.[13, 37a, 187, 199] Their cause is unknown, and some authors consider them to be hamartomas.

Lymphangiomas have been reported in dogs from 11 months to 8 years old, with no apparent breed or sex predilection. The neoplasms were large,

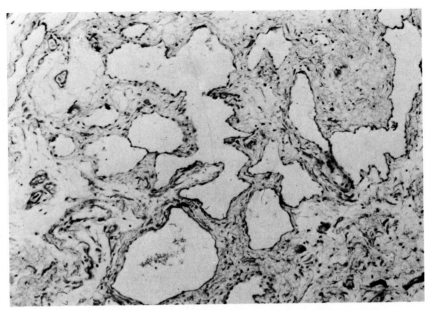

Figure 20:59. Canine lymphangioma. Proliferation of lymphatic vessels.

solitary, often red in color, fluctuant masses in the axillary and inguinal regions (Fig. 20:50E,F).

Histologically, lymphangiomas are characterized by a proliferation of variably sized cystic spaces, lined by a single layer of flattened endothelial cells, within the dermis or subcutis, or both (Fig. 20:59).[187]

In clinical management the therapy of choice for lymphangiomas is surgical excision.

Lymphangiosarcoma
(Angiosarcoma)

Lymphangiosarcoma is a rare malignant neoplasm arising from the endothelial cells of lymphatic vessels.[37a, 68, 107, 177, 209, 215] The cause of lymphangiosarcoma is unknown, although in humans the neoplasm often arises in areas of chronic lymphedema.

Lymphangiosarcoma has been reported in dogs from 7 months to 11 years of age. Lesions were characterized by poorly circumscribed, edematous to purpuric swellings in the skin. Lymphangiosarcoma has occurred in adult and aged cats, most commonly as a diffuse area of plaquelike thickenings of the ventral abdominal skin or draining-sinus to cyst-like lesions on the forelimb (Fig. 20:50G,H). Affected skin is erythematous to purplish and soft to spongy, and often oozes a serosanguineous discharge.

Histologically, lymphangiosarcoma is characterized by the proliferation of bizarre, atypical endothelial cells that tend to form variable-sized vascular spaces and surround collagen fibrils (Figs. 20:60 and 20:61).[209] The neoplastic vessels are characterized by tortuous shapes, a lack of pericytes, and little or no blood. A pleomorphic inflammatory infiltrate is usually present.

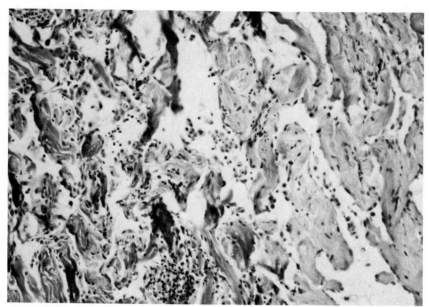

Figure 20:60. Feline lymphangiosarcoma. Atypical endothelial cells forming vessels and infiltrating between collagen bundles.

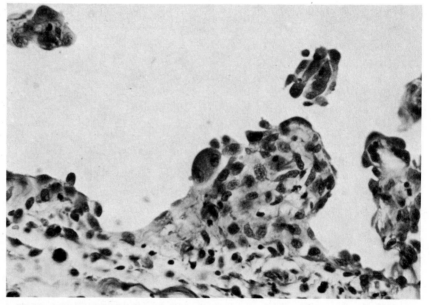

Figure 20:61. Feline lymphangiosarcoma. Pleomorphic and atypical endothelial cells lining vessels and budding off into vascular lumen.

MAST CELL TUMOR
(Mastocytoma, Mast Cell Sarcoma, Mastocytosis)

Mast cell tumors are common benign-to-malignant neoplasms of the dog and cat arising from mast cells.[12, 13, 37a, 124a, 125, 144, 145, 172, 175, 198, 199, 218] The cause of mast cell tumors is unknown. In dogs, mast cell tumors have been experimentally transmitted using tissues and cell-free extracts, which suggests a viral cause. However, ultrastructural examination of mast cell tumors has occasionally revealed viral particles.[124a] It has been theorized that boxers and Boston terriers possess oncogenes that are transmitted to offspring and combine with a genetically determined deficiency of immune surveillance to result in an increased incidence of mast cell tumors in these breeds. Rarely, canine mast cell tumor has been thought to arise within scars and chronic dermatoses.[124a, 154] In cats, transmission studies with various mast cell tumor extracts have failed to produce neoplasms in normal individuals. Multiple "histiocytic" mast cell tumors have been described in 6- to 8-week-old Siamese kittens, where multiple kittens of two litters (sired by the same tom) were affected.[90a]

Mast cell tumors may occur in dogs and cats of any age but occur in dogs with an average age of about 8.5 years. In dogs, there is no sex predilection, but boxers, Boston terriers, English bulldogs, bull terriers, fox terriers, Staffordshire terriers, Labrador retrievers, dachshunds, and Weimaraners are predisposed. In cats, mast cell tumors are more common in older males.

The clinical appearance of cutaneous mast cell tumors in dogs and cats is quite variable. Mast cell tumors are usually solitary, but may occasionally be multiple (Figs. 20:62A–H). Canine mast cell tumors occur most frequently on the trunk, perineum, and limbs, and they may be dome-shaped, nodular, or pedunculated; well to poorly circumscribed; firm to soft; dermoepidermal to subcutaneous in location; and 1 to 10 cm in diameter. They are frequently "pinfeathered," edematous, ulcerated, and may be melanotic (Figs. 20:63 and 20:64). Feline mast cell tumors occur most commonly on the head and neck and may present as (1) multiple raised, soft, round, poorly demarcated, edematous, pinkish, variable-sized (0.5 to 5 cm in diameter) masses that are fixed to the overlying skin; (2) multiple raised, firm, round, well-circumscribed, white-to-yellow, small (2 to 10 mm in diameter) papules and nodules that are fixed to the overlying skin; (3) single or multiple raised, firm, erythematous, well-circumscribed, variable-sized (1 to 7 cm in diameter) plaques that are frequently ulcerated and pruritic; and (4) solitary, firm-to-soft, well-circumscribed, variable-sized (0.5 to 3 cm in diameter) dermoepidermal nodules. Flushing (sudden, symmetric, diffuse reddening of large areas of skin) has been rarely seen in dogs with mast cell tumors.[141]

Urticaria pigmentosa is a proliferative mast cell disorder of humans.[67, 120] A syndrome with some clinicopathologic similarities to the human disorder has been seen in cats.[180] All cats have been young (less than 1 year of age) Himalayans with asymptomatic macular erythema and hyperpigmentation around the mouth, chin, neck, and eyes. The condition regressed spontaneously after several months. Skin biopsies revealed hyperplastic superficial perivascular dermatitis with numerous mast cells and epidermal hypermelanosis.

Noncutaneous symptomatology that may be seen in association with canine and feline mast cell tumors includes gastric and duodenal ulcers (thought to be histamine induced) and defective blood coagulation (thought to be heparin induced). In dogs, focal glomerulitis and defective antibody production have

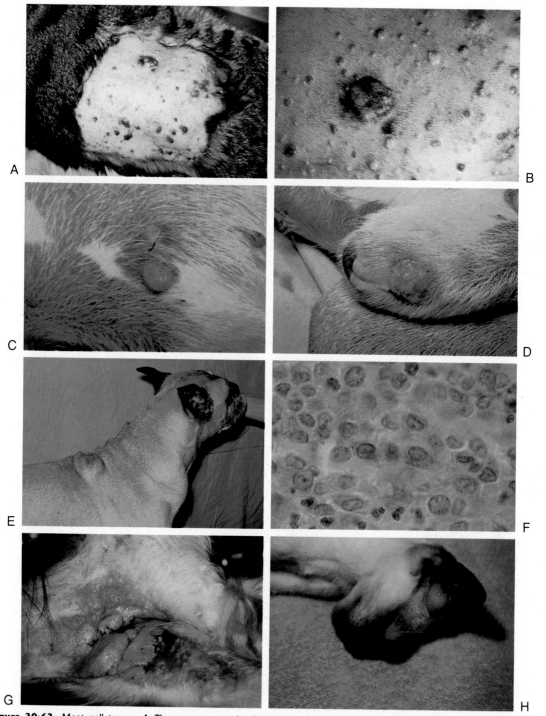

Figure 20:62. *Mast cell tumor. A,* The masses vary in size and many are ulcerated. Only a few metastatic foci were found at autopsy. *B,* Closer view of tumor masses on skin of patient in *A. Mastocytoma. C,* Initial mastocytoma lesion may be quiescent for many years. *D,* Mastocytoma on the sheath, a typical location. *E,* With generalized mastocytosis multiple lesions appear. They are fast-growing, firm, or edematous and spread rapidly. *F,* Histologic section of mastocytoma stained with toluidine blue. Note reddish purple staining cytoplasmic granules (high power, oil immersion). *G,* Malignant mastocytoma in inguinal region. *H,* Mast cell tumor of cat.

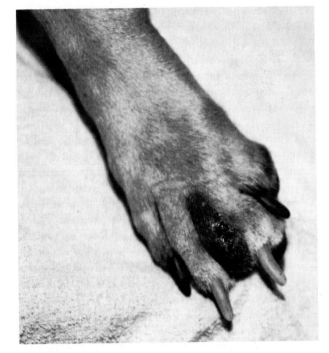

Figure 20:63. Canine mast cell tumor. Pigmented interdigital tumor in a boxer.

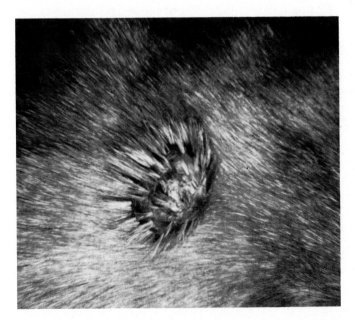

Figure 20:64. Canine mast cell tumor. Characteristic "pin-feathered" appearance.

been reported in association with mast cell tumors. Immune-mediated throm-bocytopenia has been reported in association with canine mast cell tumors.[89] Mast cell tumors in dogs should *always* be treated as potentially malignant neoplasms. In cats, the majority of cutaneous mast cell tumors are benign.[31, 218] In dogs, the frequency of malignancy is unclear, approaching about 30 per cent of all cases. Canine mast cell tumors arising from the perineum, prepuce, scrotum, and digits appear to be more commonly malignant.

This is one tumor in which stained impression smears of ulcerated sectioned tissue are useful in establishing a tentative immediate diagnosis. This procedure should not replace a complete histologic examination. Smears of cutaneous mast cell tumors in cats may reveal endocytosis of erythrocytes by the neoplastic mast cells.[126a]

Histologically, mast cell tumors are characterized by a diffuse-to-multino-dular proliferation of mast cells (Figs. 20:65–20:68).[144] Frequent findings in canine mast cell tumors include tissue eosinophilia, focal areas of collagen degeneration, and a wide variety of vascular lesions (hyalinization, fibrinoid degeneration, eosinophilic vasculitis) (Fig. 20:66). In cats, special caution is warranted to avoid confusing mast cell tumors with other round cell tumors and eosinophilic plaques. However, the striking tissue eosinophilia and collagen degeneration seen commonly in canine mast cell tumors is rare in cats.[31, 218] In addition, a "histiocytic" mast cell tumor has been described in cats (especially Siamese), wherein the diagnosis can be confirmed only by electron microscopic demonstration of mast cell granules.[218]

Clinical management of mast cell tumors may include surgical excision, cryosurgery, electrosurgery, chemotherapy, radiotherapy, immunotherapy, or some combination of these.[145, 198, 199] A histologic grading system (Table 20:7) and a clinical staging system (Table 20:8) have been developed for canine mast cell tumors.[198] The recommended therapeutic approach for each canine mast cell tumor case is based on an amalgamation of these systems (Table 20:9).

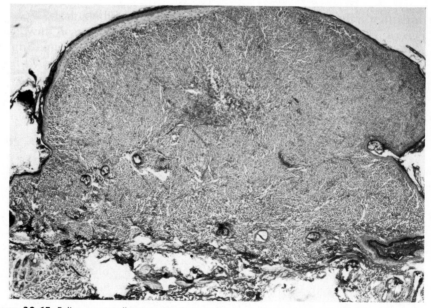

Figure 20:65. Feline mast cell tumor. Well-circumscribed, dome-shaped proliferation of mast cells.

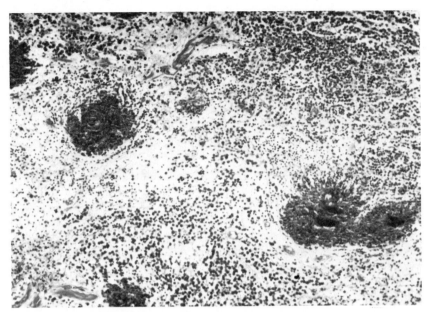

Figure 20:66. Canine mast cell tumor. Diffuse proliferation of mast cells with marked edema and focal areas of collagenolysis.

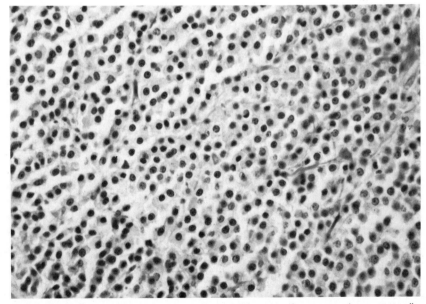

Figure 20:67. Feline mast cell tumor. Diffuse proliferation of monomorphous mast cells.

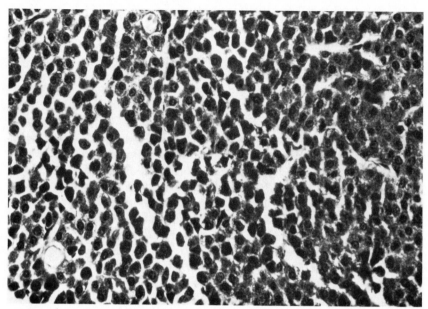

Figure 20:68. Feline mast cell tumor. Same lesion as in Figure 20:67 stained with AOG to highlight mast cell granules.

Early surgical excision is indicated in animals with a solitary neoplasm. Wide surgical margins, at least 3 cm between the palpable tumor and the incision, are recommended when possible. Approximately 50 per cent of canine mast cell tumors recur, even following a wide surgical excision.[20, 124a] In dogs with mast cell tumors, the survival time is related to the degree of histologic differentiation:[20, 151] Grade I mean survival time is 18 weeks after diagnosis; grade II is 28 weeks; and grade III is 51 weeks. A similar grading system was evaluated in feline mast cell tumors, and found *not* to correlate with biologic behavior.[31] The "histiocytic" mast cell tumor of cats, which is often characterized clinically by multiple cutaneous nodules in Siamese cats less than 4 years old, appears to frequently undergo spontaneous remission.[90a, 124a, 218]

Chemotherapy has been advocated for disseminated mast cell tumors. Oral prednisolone or prednisone (0.5 mg/kg SID) or intralesional triamcinolone (1 mg for every 1 cm of diameter of tumor) have been recommended (see Table 20:9). This treatment causes temporary regression of the tumors that may last

Table 20:7. HISTOLOGIC CLASSIFICATION OF MAST CELL TUMORS*

Grade	Microscopic Description
I. Anaplastic, immature, undifferentiated	Highly cellular, indistinct cytoplasmic boundaries; irregular size and shape of nuclei; often frequent mitotic figures; low number of cytoplasmic granules
II. Intermediate, differentiated	Cells are closely packed with indistinct cytoplasmic boundaries; nucleus-to-cytoplasm ratio lower than that of Grade I; mitotic figures infrequent; more granules than in Grade I tumors
III. Well differentiated, mature	Clearly defined cytoplasmic boundary with regular, spherical, or ovoid nucleus; mitotic figures rare; cytoplasmic granules large, deep staining, and plentiful

*From Tams, T. R., and Macy, D. W.: Canine mast cell tumors. Comp. Cont. Ed. *3*:873, 1981.

Table 20:8. CLINICAL STAGING SYSTEM FOR MAST CELL TUMORS*

Stage I: **One tumor confined to the dermis without regional lymph node involvement**
 a. Without systemic signs
 b. With systemic signs
Stage II: **One tumor confined to dermis, with regional lymph node involvement**
 a. Without systemic signs
 b. With systemic signs
Stage III: **Multiple dermal tumors; large infiltrating tumors with or without regional node involvement**
 a. Without systemic signs
 b. With systemic signs
Stage IV: **Any tumor with distant metastasis or recurrence with metastasis**

*From Tams, T. R., and Macy, D. W.: Canine mast cell tumors. Compend. Cont. Ed. *3*:873, 1981.

Table 20:9. SUGGESTED TREATMENT OF MAST CELL TUMORS BASED ON CLINICAL STAGES*

Stage	Treatment
I	Surgical excision only. (Surgery is defined as the excision of the tumor with a minimum margin of 3 cm between palpable tumor and incision line; such excision should include regional lymph node when possible.)
II	Surgical excision plus radiation. (Radiation therapy is defined as the administration of 4000 rad divided into 10 fractions to be administered every other day for 10 treatments.)
III	Intralesional steroids plus cimetidine. (Intralesional steroid is defined as the intralesional injection of 1 mg of triamcinolone for every centimeter diameter of tumor. This dosage is to be administered every 2 weeks.)
IV	Systemic steroids† plus cimetidine‡

*From Tams, T. R., and Macy, D. W.: Canine mast cell tumors. Compend. Cont. Ed. *3*:876, 1981.
†A dose of .5 mg/kg body weight of prednisolone to be administered every 2 weeks.
‡Cimetidine should be given daily at a dose of 4 mg/kg QID.

several months. Combination chemotherapy (glucocorticoids plus cyclophosphamide, vincristine, or vinblastine, for example) has been recommended by some, but no evidence suggests that this is superior to glucocorticoids alone in dogs and cats.[145, 199]

It has been recommended that cimetidine (Tagamet), 4 mg/kg orally QID, should be used in dogs with evidence of systemic or lymph node involvement, or if there is evidence of gastrointestinal hemorrhage. Cimetidine acts by competitively inhibiting the action of histamine on the H_2 receptors of gastric parietal cells, thus reducing gastric acid output and concentration.

In dogs, there is a frequent tendency for local hemorrhage during surgery and delayed wound healing at the site of tumor removal.[124a] Cryosurgery or hyperthermia may precipitate a shocklike reaction in dogs that have not been pretreated with antihistamines.[124a]

Recently, a dog with multicentric mast cell tumors was reported to respond well to immunomodulatory therapy with *Propionibacterium acnes* (Immuno-Regulin).[202a]

OSTEOMA AND OSTEOSARCOMA

Extraskeletal osteomas and osteosarcomas are very rare in cats and dogs. The cause of these tumors is not known.

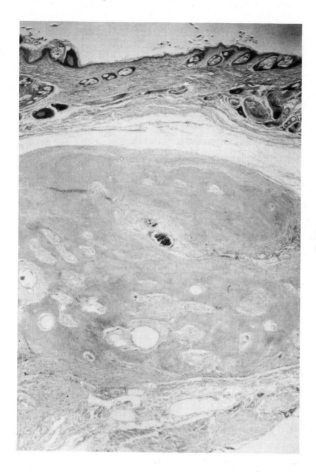

Figure 20:69. Feline osteoma cutis. Bone formation in subcutis.

Osteoma cutis was recognized in adult cats.[97, 180] The lesions were solitary, discrete, firm nodules involving proximal extremities. Histopathologically, numerous trabeculae consisting of both woven and lamellar bone, normal osteocytes within lacunae, and multinucleated osteoclasts are seen (Fig. 20:69). Surgical excision is curative. Because osteoma-like changes may be seen in certain non-neoplastic lesions (nevi) or as heterotypic ossification in response to repeated tissue injury (chronic inflammation, calcinosis cutis), true osteomas must satisfy the following criteria: (1) growth unattached to periosteum or periarticular structures, (2) spontaneous occurrence (*not* secondary to trauma or inflammation), and (3) *not* developmental in origin.

Extraskeletal osteosarcomas have been reported in the subcutaneous tissues (perianal, axillary, proximal limb) of aged dogs.[9] Metastatic lesions were present in most dogs. Histopathologically, a proliferation of malignant osteoblasts and variable amounts of osteoid is seen.

The treatment of choice for osteomas and osteosarcomas is surgical excision.

Lymphohistiocytic Neoplasms

HISTIOCYTOMA
(Button Tumor)

Histiocytomas are common benign neoplasms of the dog arising from histiocytes.[75, 144, 145, 199] They are very rare in the cat.[37a, 125, 172] Their cause is unknown, although evidence for an infectious etiology has been presented.

Characteristically, histiocytomas affect young dogs, with about 50 per cent of the cases occurring in dogs under 2 years old. However, old dogs may also be affected.[165a] Boxers, dachshunds, cocker spaniels, Great Danes, and Shetland sheepdogs are predisposed. There is no sex predilection.

Histiocytomas are usually solitary and occur most commonly on the head, pinnae, and limbs (Fig. 20:70A–C). They are usually small (less than 3 cm in diameter), firm, dome or button shaped, well circumscribed, dermoepidermal in location, and frequently ulcerated. Histiocytomas are fast-growing but benign. The rare reports of alleged generalized histiocytomas in older dogs were not confirmed ultrastructurally or cytochemically, and probably represent "histiocytic" lymphosarcoma.

Histopathologically, histiocytomas are characterized by uniform sheets of pleomorphic histiocytic cells infiltrating the dermis and subcutis and displacing the collagen fibers and adnexae (Figs. 20:71 and 20:72).[43, 144] A characteristic feature of this neoplasm is a high mitotic index. Lymphocytic infiltration and areas of necrosis develop in regressing neoplasms.

Clinical management of histiocytomas may include surgical excision, cryosurgery, electrosurgery, or observation without treatment.[145, 199] The majority of these neoplasms undergo spontaneous regression within 3 months.

MALIGNANT HISTIOCYTOSIS

Malignant histiocytosis is a rare, malignant neoplasm of histiocytic origin in dogs.[143, 165, 171, 214] The cause of the neoplasm is unknown.

Malignant histiocytosis has been recognized in several breeds of dogs with no sex predilection; typically, older animals are affected. This neoplasm has also been reported in closely related Bernese Mountain dogs, predominantly males.[143] Cutaneous lesions are rarely seen and are characterized by multiple, firm, dermal-to-subcutaneous nodules anywhere on the body. Lesions may or may not be alopecic or ulcerated. Typical clinical signs of malignant histiocytosis include lethargy, weight loss, lymphadenopathy, hepatosplenomegaly, and pancytopenia. The course is rapidly progressive and invariably fatal.

Histopathologically, malignant histiocytosis is characterized by nodular-to-diffuse, deep dermal and subcutaneous infiltration, with cytologically atypical histiocytes exhibiting cytophagocytosis and high mitotic index (Figs. 20:73 and 20:74).[143, 171, 214] Tumor cells are positive for lysozyme and α-1-antitrypsin.

Presently there is no effective treatment.

SYSTEMIC HISTIOCYTOSIS

Systemic histiocytosis is a histiocytic proliferative disorder of dogs.[142, 178] The cause of the condition is unknown.

Systemic histiocytosis was described in closely related Bernese Mountain dogs of 2 to 8 years of age, with males predominating.[142] The disorder has rarely been recognized in other breeds of dogs. Clinical signs include anorexia, weight loss, respiratory stertor, and multiple cutaneous papules, plaques, nodules, and ulcers over the entire body, especially the face (Fig. 20:70D,E). The course may be prolonged and fluctuating, with alternating episodes of exacerbation and remission, or rapidly progressive and fatal. Ultimately, most

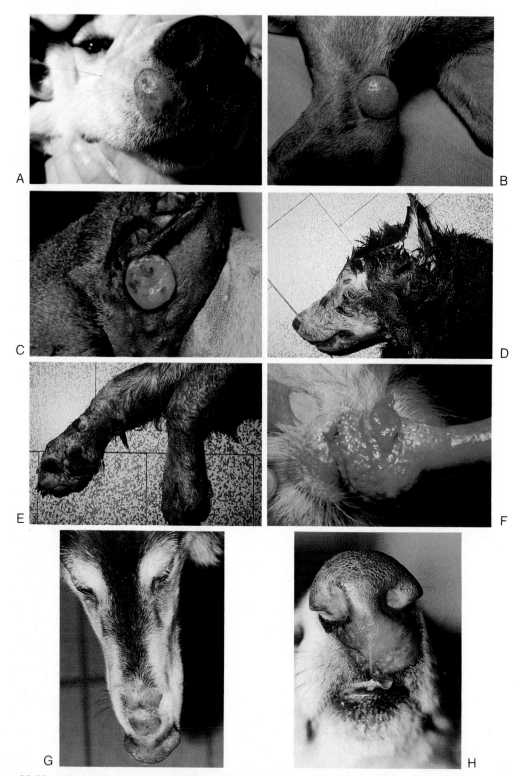

Figure 20:70. *A*, Typical location and appearance of histiocytoma. Note hairless surface with crusted exudate. *B*, Firm, circumscribed solitary nodule in the characteristic "button" shape. *C*, Large ulcerated histiocytoma at the base of the ear of a young Great Dane. *D*, Canine systemic histiocytosis. Alopecia, erythema, and ulceration of face. (Courtesy M. Suter.) *E*, Canine systemic histiocytosis. Same lesions on front legs. (Courtesy M. Suter.) *F*, Bright red nodule is a transmissible venereal tumor on the mucosa of the penis. Note multiple lymphoid follicles, a common finding on male dogs. *G*, Canine malignant fibrous histiocytoma. Nodules on bridge of nose. *H*, Canine malignant fibrous histiocytoma. Nodules on nose.

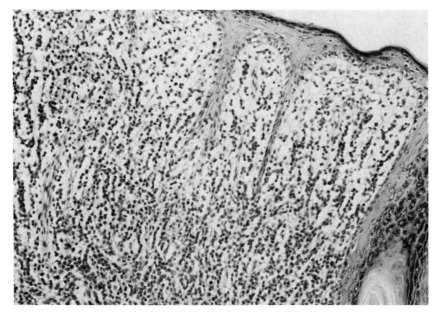

Figure 20:71. Canine histiocytoma.

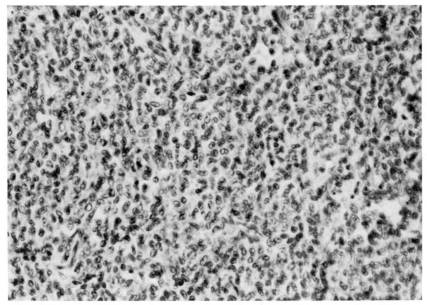

Figure 20:72. Canine histiocytoma. Proliferation of pleomorphic, hyperchromatic histiocytes.

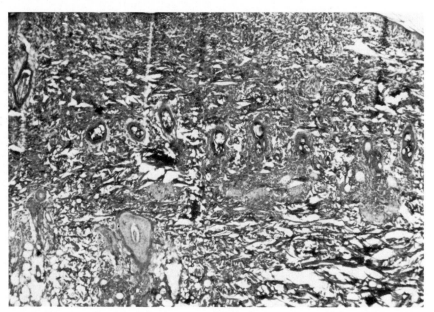

Figure 20:73. Canine malignant histiocytosis. Diffuse dermal and subcutaneous proliferation of atypical histiocytes.

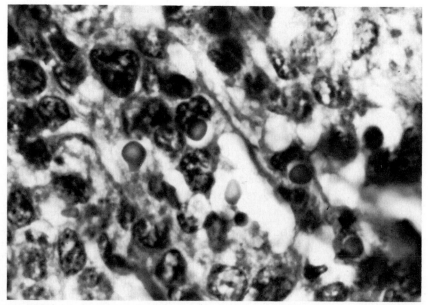

Figure 20:74. Canine malignant histiocytosis. Atypical histiocytes exhibiting erythrophagocytosis.

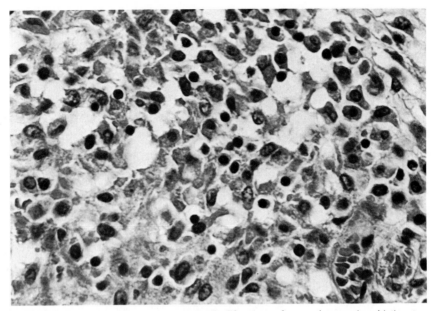

Figure 20:75. Canine systemic histiocytosis. Proliferation of normal-appearing histiocytes and occasional lymphocytes.

dogs were euthanized and showed histiocytic infiltration of multiple organ systems, especially lung, liver, spleen, bone marrow, and lymph nodes.

Histopathologically, systemic histiocytosis is characterized by superficial and deep perivascular, nodular, or diffuse dermal and subcutaneous infiltrations of cytologically normal histiocytes (Fig. 20:75).[142, 178] Electron microscopic examination revealed typical histiocytes with convoluted nuclei, filopodia, and abundant lysosomes. Enzyme histochemical studies revealed that the cells were positive for typical histiocyte markers: acid phosphate and nonspecific esterase.

Treatment with large doses of glucocorticoids and cytotoxic drugs has been generally ineffective. Preliminary reports indicate that treatment with bovine thymosin fraction 5 may be beneficial.[142]

CUTANEOUS HISTIOCYTOSIS

Cutaneous histiocytosis is a benign histiocytic proliferative disorder of dogs.[130] The cause of the disorder is unknown.

Cutaneous histiocytosis was reported in dogs, with no apparent age, breed, or sex predilections. Lesions were characterized as multiple, erythematous, dermal or subcutaneous plaques or nodules, 1 to 5 cm in diameter, anywhere on the body. Lesions often waxed and waned and appeared in new sites. Systemic involvement and lymphadenopathy were not reported.

Histopathologically, cutaneous histiocytosis is characterized by nodular-to-diffuse dermal or subcutaneous infiltrations of cytologically normal histiocytes.[130] Electron microscopy revealed typical histiocytes, and enzyme histochemical studies resulted in findings that the cells were positive for nonspecific esterase.

Treatment with large doses of glucocorticoids and cytotoxic drugs gave variable results.

TRANSMISSIBLE VENEREAL TUMOR

(Infectious Sarcoma, Contagious Venereal
Tumor, Venereal Granuloma, Canine Condyloma, Transmissible
Lymphosarcoma, Transmissible Reticulum Cell Tumor,
Histiocytoma, Sticker Tumor)

This tumor is an uncommon benign-to-malignant neoplasm of the dog.[144, 145, 199] The cell of origin is unknown. It is considered to be a naturally occurring allograft with transmission occurring by transplantation of viable neoplastic cells to a susceptible host. The tumor cells contain 59 chromosomes, as compared with the normal canine complement of 78. A viral origin has been investigated but not verified.[6] The neoplasm is usually transmitted by coitus but may be inoculated into multiple sites by licking, biting, and scratching. Transmission may be accomplished by subcutaneous, intravenous, and intra-peritoneal injections and by skin or mucosal scarification (incubation period about 3 weeks). Apparently, transmissible venereal tumor is more prevalent in temperate zones and in large cities.

Transmissible venereal tumor can grow for extended periods of time in an immunocompetent allogenic host. During progressive growth of the tumor, cell-mediated immune responses to tumor cells are impaired, and serum antibodies are present that when incubated with tumor cells can block complement-mediated lysis of tumor cells by serum antibodies from dogs with regressing transmissible venereal tumors.[149] Circulating immune complexes have been detected in dogs with transmissible venereal tumor, but the pathogenetic significance of this finding is unknown.[149]

Occurring in sexually active dogs (especially those young and unconfined), transmissible venereal tumor shows no apparent breed or sex predilection. Neoplasms occur commonly on the external genitalia (penis and vagina) and the skin (especially the face and limbs) (Figs. 20:70F and 20:76) and may be single or multiple, nodular, pedunculated, multilobular, or cauliflower-like, firm or friable, 1 to 20 cm in diameter, and dermoepidermal to subcutaneous in location, and they may frequently be ulcerated.

In experimental or laboratory dogs, these tumors frequently regress spontaneously. In one experimental dog colony, the neoplasm was transmitted through 40 generations, comprising 564 dogs.[106] Neoplasms developed in 68 per cent of the dogs and spontaneously regressed permanently in 87 per cent of these dogs within 180 days. However, there is no such evidence of general benignity in the naturally occurring disease.[5, 145, 207] The overall frequency of spontaneous regression in naturally occurring cases of transmissible venereal tumor is unknown, and many instances of metastasis and extragenital occurrence have been reported.

Histopathologically, transmissible venereal tumor is characterized by compact masses or sheets of uniform round-to-polyhedral neoplastic cells, often growing in rows in a delicate stroma (Fig. 20:77).[144] Mitoses are plentiful. Tumors undergoing spontaneous regression display necrosis, increasing numbers of infiltrating leukocytes (especially lymphocytes), and increasing numbers of collagen bundles.[90]

Because of (1) the inconclusive evidence regarding spontaneous regression in naturally occurring neoplasms, and (2) the numerous reports of metastasis, clinical management of transmissible venereal tumors is *always* indicated. Both radiotherapy and surgical excision have been reported to be successful, although

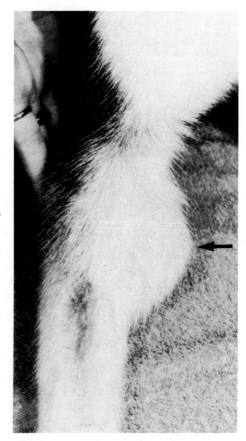

Figure 20:76. Transmissible venereal tumor near the elbow of a dog.

recurrence following surgery is not uncommon.[145, 199] Chemotherapy has also produced good results. Ninety-three per cent of dogs treated had complete regression of their neoplasms with no recurrence, after combination chemotherapy (vincristine 0.0125 to 0.025 mg/kg intravenously, weekly; cyclophosphamide 1 mg/kg orally, daily, or 50 mg/m^2 body surface area (BSA) orally, every other day; and methotrexate 0.3 to 0.5 mg/kg intravenously, weekly, or 2.5 mg/m^2 BSA orally, every other day).[28, 160] The average length of time to the point at which no disease was evident was 4 to 6 weeks. Two of the dogs that were cured had regional lymph node metastasis. Eighty-two per cent of dogs treated with single agent chemotherapy (vincristine 0.025 mg/kg intravenously once weekly) underwent a complete remission within an average of 4 weeks.[28, 160] Doxorubicin administered at a dosage of 0.5 mg/m^2 BSA intravenously once weekly for an average of 6 weeks is also reported to be effective.[160] Immunoadsorption of immune complexes with protein A was of no benefit.[44] Interestingly, when a modified-live parvovirus vaccine (feline panleukopenia virus) was inoculated into dogs at the same time transmissible venereal tumor transplantation was attempted, tumor growth did not occur.[222b]

FIBROUS HISTIOCYTOMA
(Dermatofibroma)

Fibrous histiocytomas are uncommon (in dogs) to rare (in cats).[145, 186] Their origin is controversial and may be an undifferentiated mesenchymal cell.[76] The

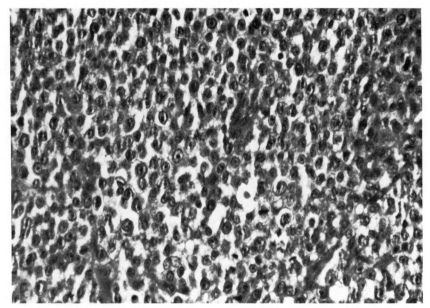

Figure 20:77. Canine transmissible venereal tumor. Sheets of neoplastic mononuclear cells containing vesicular nuclei.

cause of fibrous histiocytomas is unknown. Recently the neoplastic nature of at least the ocular form of this condition has been challenged.[151a] It was suggested that the ocular lesions are in fact granulomatous.

Fibrous histiocytomas occur most commonly in dogs 2 to 4 years of age, with no sex predilection. Collies appear to be predisposed.

Cutaneous fibrous histiocytomas are usually multiple and occur most commonly on the face (Fig. 20:78). They are usually firm, well circumscribed,

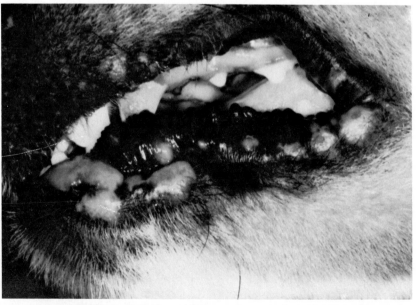

Figure 20:78. Multiple fibrous histiocytomas on the lower lip of a collie.

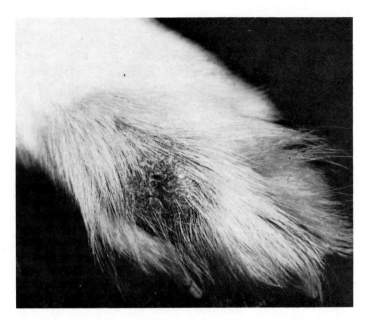

Figure 20:79. Fibrous histiocytoma on the paw of a collie.

0.5 to 7 cm in diameter, and dermoepidermal in location (Fig. 20:79). The overlying skin may be normal or alopecic. Histologically identical lesions occur in the cornea, with or without concurrent skin lesions (Fig. 20:80). These neoplasms appear to be benign.

Histologically, fibrous histiocytomas are characterized by a poorly circumscribed cellular infiltrate permeated by a swirling stroma.[145, 186] The majority of cells are fibroblasts and histiocytes (Fig. 20:81). Collagen formation is minimal. Lymphoid cells and plasma cells are commonly present, especially at the periphery of the masses. In humans, immunohistochemical studies of fibrous histiocytomas have shown that only about 33 per cent of the tumors are positive

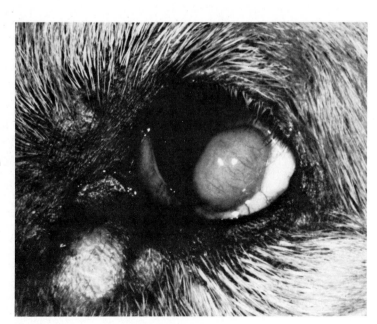

Figure 20:80. Fibrous histiocytoma on the sclera of a collie.

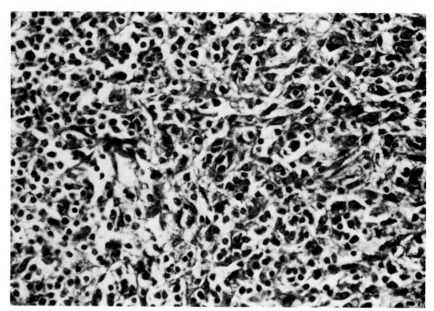

Figure 20:81. Canine fibrous histiocytoma. Proliferation of histiocytic and fibroblastic cells with intermingling lymphoid cells.

for traditional histiocytic markers (α-1-antitrypsin, α-1-antichymotrypsin, and lysozyme).[76]

Clinical management of fibrous histiocytomas may include surgical excision or glucocorticoids.[151a] Sublesional injections of 10 to 40 mg of methylprednisolone (Depo-Medrol) may be effective for single lesions. Multiple lesions are best treated with prednisolone or prednisone, 2 to 4 mg/kg orally SID until they have completely regressed (1 to 2 weeks). Recurrent lesions may require long-term alternate-day steroid therapy. Some cases are initially unresponsive to, or become refractory to, systemic glucocorticoids. Azathioprine, 2 mg/kg orally every 48 hours, is usually effective in these cases.[116, 151a, 180]

MALIGNANT FIBROUS HISTIOCYTOMA
(Extraskeletal Giant Cell Tumor,
Giant Cell Tumor of Soft Parts, Dermatofibrosarcoma)

Malignant fibrous histiocytomas are rare malignant neoplasms of the cat and dog.[3a, 117a, 145, 159, 172, 175] These neoplasms are believed to arise from undifferentiated mesenchymal cells.[163] The cause of malignant fibrous histiocytomas is unknown.

Malignant fibrous histiocytomas occur in older cats and dogs, with no apparent breed or sex predilection. They are usually solitary, firm, poorly circumscribed, variable in size and shape, and dermoepidermal and subcutaneous in location (Figs. 20:70G,H). There may be a predilection for limbs and the neck. These neoplasms are locally invasive (muscle, bone) but apparently slow to metastasize. In humans, these tumors occur most commonly on the extremities, demonstrate recurrence rates of 37.5 per cent and 0 per cent following surgical excision or amputation, respectively, and the 5-year survival rate is 36 per cent.[16]

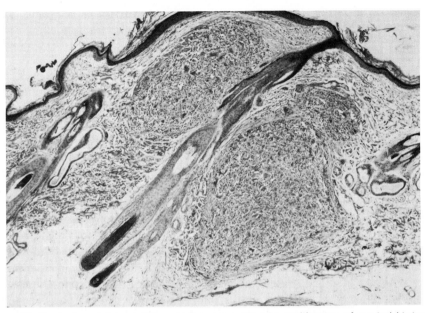

Figure 20:82. Canine malignant fibrous histiocytoma. Nodular proliferation of atypical histiocytes, fibroblasts, and histiocytic giant cells.

Histologically, malignant fibrous histiocytomas are characterized by an infiltrative mass composed of varying mixtures of pleomorphic histiocytes, fibroblasts, and multinucleated giant cells (Figs. 20:82 and 20:83).[145] Mitotic figures and a "storiform" (cartwheel) arrangement of fibroblasts and histiocytes are common features.

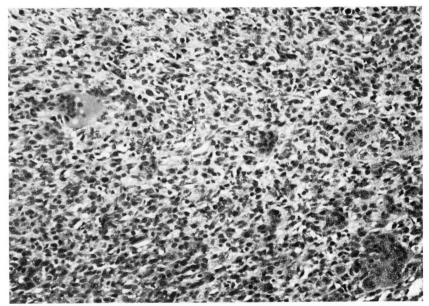

Figure 20:83. Canine malignant fibrous histiocytoma. Proliferation of atypical histiocytic and fibroblastic cells along with multinucleated giant cells.

In clinical management, the therapy of choice for malignant fibrous histiocytomas is radical surgical excision or amputation.

CUTANEOUS LYMPHOSARCOMA
(Malignant Lymphoma, Lymphoreticular Neoplasm, Lymphomatosis, Reticulum Cell Sarcoma)

Cutaneous lymphosarcoma is a rare malignant neoplasm of the dog and cat.[27, 35, 47, 132, 140, 145, 160, 172, 199] In cats, the cause of most types of lymphosarcoma is the feline leukemia virus (FeLV), although cats with cutaneous lymphosarcoma are usually FeLV–negative. In dogs, the cause of lymphosarcoma is unknown, although (1) lymphosarcoma can be transmitted to puppies by the injection of whole-cell preparations of malignant lymphocytes, (2) C-type viruses were found in neoplastic cells from dogs with lymphosarcoma, and (3) lymphosarcoma has been induced in neonatal puppies by injections of FeLV.

This neoplasm occurs in older dogs (although young dogs are also affected), with no sex predisposition but with a predilection for boxers, St. Bernards, basset hounds, cocker spaniels, beagles, German shepherds, golden retrievers, and Scottish terriers. In cats, no breed or sex predilections are apparent, and older animals are more commonly affected.

Cutaneous lymphosarcoma in dogs and cats is usually generalized or multifocal and has a variety of manifestations: nodules (dermoepidermal or subcutaneous), plaques, ulcers, erythroderma, and exfoliative dermatitis (Figs. 20:84A–H). The disorder may occur with or without other systemic involvement. Pruritus is common. Rarely, dogs and cats display solitary nodular skin lesions. The course may be acute or chronic, but it is ultimately fatal, except in those rare instances in which a solitary primary cutaneous lesion can be excised. Oral mucosal involvement may be seen in the form of erythematous nodules and plaques. Rarely, cutaneous lymphosarcoma in dogs and cats has been associated with monoclonal or biclonal gammopathies, serum hyperviscosity, and hypercalcemia.[47, 62, 98, 199]

Histologically, cutaneous lymphosarcoma can be divided into epitheliotropic and nonepitheliotropic types.[32] Epitheliotropic forms of cutaneous lymphosarcoma are usually of T-lymphocyte origin, while nonepitheliotropic forms are usually of B-lymphocyte origin. Nonepitheliotropic (B cell) lymphosarcomas are characterized by diffuse dermal and subcutaneous infiltration by malignant lymphocytes (lymphocytic, well-differentiated, or poorly differentiated; lymphoblastic; or histiocytic in cytologic form) (Figs. 20:85 and 20:86).[47, 79, 93, 94, 199]

Clinical management of cutaneous lymphosarcoma is usually unsuccessful.[47, 123, 145, 160] Traditional regimens of combined chemotherapy or chemoimmunotherapy may occasionally be useful for inducing short-term (average 8 months) remission. Cryosurgical treatment of some of the cutaneous lesions of lymphosarcoma in a dog resulted in regression of all lesions with a follow-up period of 1 year.[71] Rarely, surgical excision of a solitary cutaneous lymphosarcoma lesion results in long-term remission or, perhaps, cure.

Epitheliotropic Lymphosarcoma

Epitheliotropic lymphosarcoma is a rare cutaneous malignancy of dogs and cats.[2, 36, 145, 210] In humans, epitheliotropic lymphosarcomas are usually of T-lymphocyte origin.[32] In dogs, a T-cell origin is presumed, but not documented.[210]

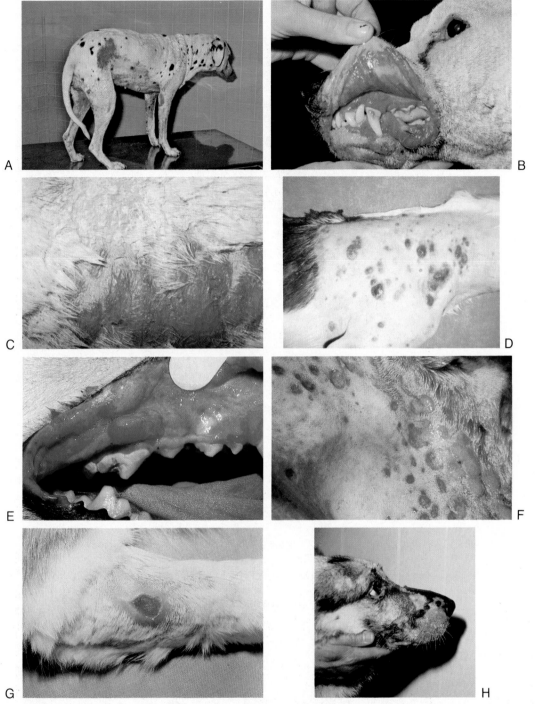

Figure 20:84. Cutaneous lymphosarcoma. *A,* Characteristic skin lesions can be seen as alopecic, red patches on this critically ill Dalmatian. *B,* Ecchymotic hemorrhages on the oral mucosa. Note the mucous eye discharge and anguished expression. *C,* Erythematous plaque with erosions is surrounded by thin, scaly skin. *D,* Cutaneous lymphosarcoma (reticulum cell sarcoma) of high malignancy. The lesions were numerous in most areas of the skin and affected some internal organs. *E,* Lymphosarcoma on the lips of a German shepherd. *F,* Multiple nodules and erythematous plaques on the abdomen of a cat with lymphosarcoma. (From Scott, D. W.: Feline dermatology 1900–1978: a monograph. J.A.A.H.A. *16:*331, 1980.) *G,* Solitary nodule lymphosarcoma. *H,* Erythroderma, ulcerated plaques, and diffuse cutaneous lymphosarcoma.

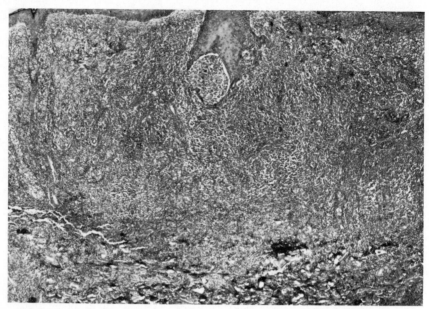

Figue 20:85. Feline lymphosarcoma. Diffuse dermal proliferation of neoplastic lymphoid cells, which spares the epidermis (B-cell pattern).

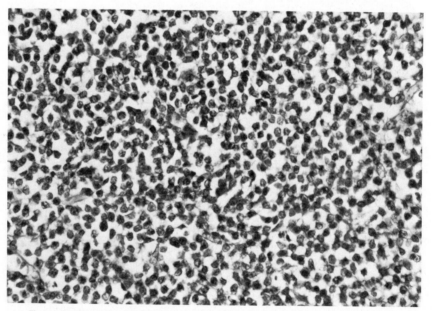

Figure 20:86. Feline lymphosarcoma. Proliferation of neoplastic lymphoid cells.

In cats, four cases of epitheliotropic lymphosarcoma were recognized and were shown to be of T-cell origin.[36, 141, 180]

In most instances, the cause of epitheliotropic lymphosarcomas is unknown. In human mycosis fungoides, the prototypical epitheliotropic (T-cell) lymphosarcoma, there is controversy about whether the disease begins as a reactive process, or as a neoplastic process.[200] In human adult T-cell leukemia-lymphosarcoma, the causative factor is believed to be the human T-cell lymphotropic virus type I (HTLV-I).[212] Epitheliotropic lymphosarcoma of dogs and cats is of unknown etiology, and all affected cats have been FeLV negative.

MYCOSIS FUNGOIDES

In humans, mycosis fungoides is defined clinically and immunologically as a neoplasm of helper T cells.[39, 200, 224] In dogs and cats, immunohistochemical studies documenting the precise cell of origin have not been reported. In cats, four cases of mycosis fungoides were shown to be of T-cell origin, on the basis of guinea pig erythrocyte rosetting of tumor cells and by marking with an anti-theta (T-cell) serum.[36, 141, 180]

In dogs and cats, mycosis fungoides usually affects older animals (5 to 16 years old, average of 11 years), with no apparent breed or sex predilections. Four clinical presentations are described: (1) generalized pruritic erythema and scaling (exfoliative erythroderma), usually misdiagnosed as allergy or seborrhea; (2) mucocutaneous ulceration and depigmentation, usually misdiagnosed as immune-mediated disease (pemphigus vulgaris, bullous pemphigoid, lupus erythematosus); (3) solitary or multiple cutaneous plaques or nodules; and (4) infiltrative and ulcerative oral mucosal disease, usually misdiagnosed as a non-neoplastic, chronic stomatitis (Figs. 20:87A,B,D).[210] Affected animals may or may not have peripheral lymphadenopathy or signs of systemic illness. In humans, mycosis fungoides may present as palmoplantar hyperkeratosis[188] or macular depigmentation.[53]

Histopathologically, mycosis fungoides is characterized by epitheliotropism, Pautrier's microabscesses (focal accumulations of pleomorphic, atypical lymphocytes within the epithelium) (Figs. 20:88 and 20:89), and the presence of "mycosis cells" (large, 20- to 30-μm lymphocytes with hyperchromatic, indented or folded nuclei) and "Sézary or Lutzner cells" (smaller, 8- to 20-μm lymphocytes that have markedly hyperconvoluted nuclei with numerous finger-like projections, producing a classic "cerebriform" appearance).[120, 174, 224] Often, a lichenoid band of pleomorphic lymphoid cells, with or without plasma cells, neutrophils, and eosinophils, is present in the superficial dermis and surrounding appendages. Epidermal mucinosis (acid mucopolysaccharides) and mild fibrosis of the immediate subepidermal superficial dermis may be seen.[146, 180] Electron microscopy reveals many tumor cells characterized by a high ratio of nucleus to cytoplasm, deep invaginations of the nuclear membrane (convoluted or cerebriform nucleus), a relatively wide rim of peripheral chromatin, a paucity of organelles, and peripheral cytoplasmic villi or projections (Fig. 20:90).[120, 191] Direct immunofluorescence testing may show the intercellular deposition of immunoglobulin in the epithelium, falsely suggesting a diagnosis of pemphigus.[191] Extensive immunocytochemical, nuclear contour indexing, DNA cytophotometric, and genotyping studies have been conducted on human epitheliotropic and nonepitheliotropic lymphosarcomas,[32, 99, 200, 203, 222] but such studies have not been reported for dogs and cats.

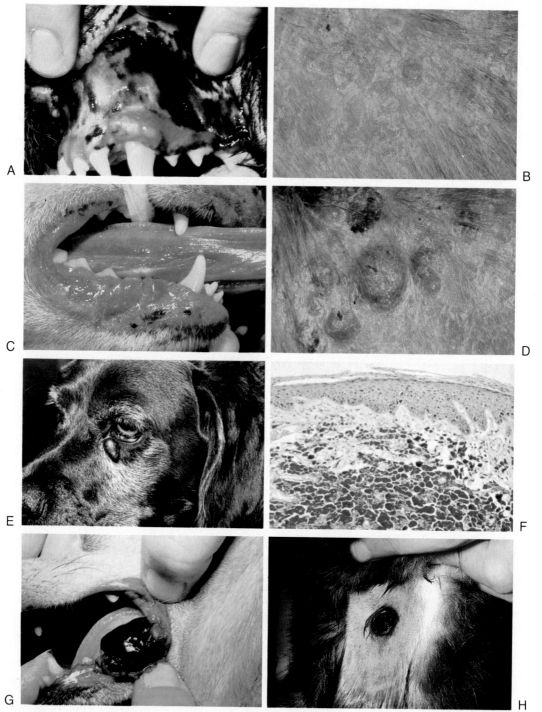

Figure 20:87. *Cutaneous lymphosarcoma.* *A,* Mycosis fungoides affecting gum of a dog (nodule and ulcers). *B,* Mycosis fungoides showing erythroderma, alopecia, scales, nodules, and plaques. *C,* Pagetoid reticulosis showing erythema, plaques, and ulcers of oral mucosa. *D,* Closer view of skin shown in *B* with nodules, ulcers, crusts, alopecia, and scales. *Melanoma. E,* Benign melanoma in cocker spaniel. *F,* Histologic section of *E* showing acanthotic epidermis with masses of heavily pigmented benign tumor cells in the dermis (low power). *G,* Malignant melanomas are commonly located in the oral region. *H,* Malignant melanoma on the neck of a cat.

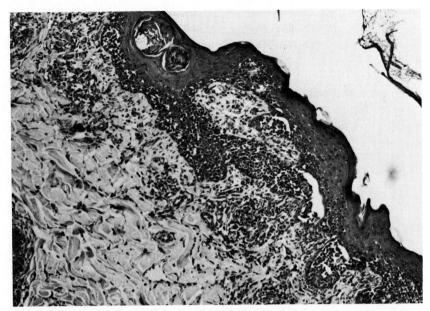

Figure 20:88. Canine mycosis fungoides. Infiltration of the lower portion of the epidermis with neoplastic lymphoid cells, and formation of several Pautrier microabscesses (T-cell pattern).

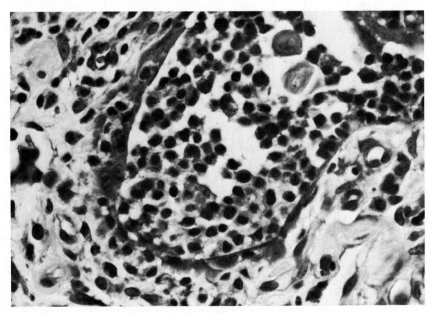

Figure 20:89. Canine mycosis fungoides. Pautrier microabscess containing pleomorphic and atypical lymphoid cells.

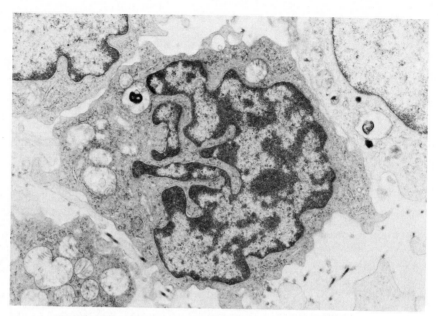

Figure 20:90. Feline mycosis fungoides. Typical Sezary or Lutzner cell.

The prognosis for canine and feline mycosis fungoides is grave.[2, 210] In a review of 49 canine cases, it was reported that the average duration of clinical signs prior to diagnosis was about 6 months, and average survival time after diagnosis was about 4 months, with or without treatment.[210] Exceptionally, dogs and cats with mycosis fungoides may live for over 2 years after a diagnosis is made. Death is due to septicemia, metastatic lymphosarcoma, or euthanasia.

Therapy for mycosis fungoides in dogs and cats has usually been of little or no benefit.[210] Chemotherapy with various combinations of prednisolone, chlorambucil, vincristine, cyclophosphamide, and methotrexate have occasionally produced some degree of clinical improvement for 1 to 5 months. The combination of oral prednisolone and intradermal injections of placental lysate was reported to be beneficial in one dog[14] but was ineffective in other dogs and one cat.[180]

The most commonly effective treatment for canine mycosis fungoides is the topical application of mechlorethamine (nitrogen mustard).[2, 140] Mechlorethamine hydrochloride, 10 mg, is dissolved in 50 ml of water and applied to the clipped surface (total body) two or three times weekly, until lesions have regressed. The solution is then applied as needed for maintenance (every 2 to 4 weeks). No signs of toxicity or drug hypersensitivity have been reported in dogs. Occasionally, dogs have developed demodicosis.[140] As mechlorethamine is a potent sensitizing agent in humans, gloves should be worn when applying the drug, and the dog should not be handled for the first few hours after application. In addition, exposure to the powder form or vapors from the drug can produce burning of the eyes and throat.[164] Although topical mechlorethamine appears to be very useful for managing the "dermatitic" and plaque stages of mycosis fungoides, no evidence suggests that it alters in any way the ultimately fatal course of eventual systemic involvement. In addition, mechlorethamine is a topical carcinogen and cocarcinogen and may be associated with the subsequent development of cutaneous epithelial malignancies (e.g., squamous cell carcinoma).[1, 225]

In humans, topical carmustine (BCNU) has been reported to be effective in mycosis fungoides, with fewer toxicities and hypersensitivity reactions than seen with topical mechlorethamine, and no development of secondary skin neoplasms.[225] Other therapies reported to be of benefit in humans with mycosis fungoides include oral retinoids,[42] interferon,[221] PUVA (oral 8-methoxypsoralen and subsequent exposure to UV-A),[224] cyclosporine,[88a] photophoresis,[88b] and electron beam therapy.[224] These modalities have not been evaluated in dogs and cats. An eicosapentaenoic acid–containing product (Dermcaps) has been used in a few dogs with mycosis fungoides.[180] Erythema was decreased, but no other benefit was seen. Recently, isotretinoin has produced encouraging responses in a few dogs (1 mg/kg BID orally) and cats (2 mg/kg SID orally) with epitheliotropic lymphoma.[239]

ALOPECIA MUCINOSA

In humans, alopecia mucinosa (follicular mucinosis) is characterized by well-demarcated areas of alopecia, fine scaling, and prominent hair follicle orifices, with or without slightly raised and mildly erythematous papules or plaques.[67, 120] There are three clinical patterns. The first, and most common, is seen in young adults; it is restricted to the head and neck, and it resolves in about 2 years. The second form is seen in a slightly older age group, lesions are more generalized, and resolution takes longer. The third form is seen in aged people, and plaques of mycosis fungoides eventually develop within the areas of alopecia. The pathomechanism of alopecia mucinosa is unknown.

Alopecia mucinosa was recognized in two adult cats with asymptomatic, well-demarcated alopecia and fine scaling on the head, ears, and neck (Fig. 20:91).[177] Biopsy specimens initially revealed mucinous degeneration of epidermis and hair follicle outer root sheath (Fig. 20:92). Several months later, both cats developed plaques in the areas of alopecia. Biopsy results at this time were typical of mycosis fungoides. Both cats were lost to follow-up.

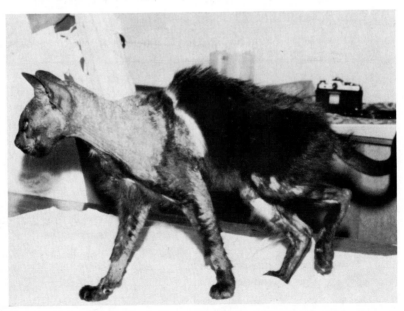

Figure 20:91. Feline alopecia mucinosa. Alopecia and scaling of head, neck, and front legs. (Courtesy V. Studdert.)

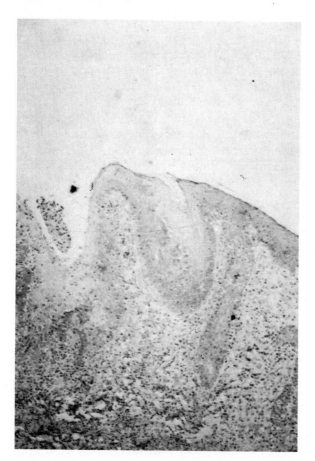

Figure 20:92. Feline alopecia mucinosa. Mucinous degeneration of hair follicle epithelium.

PAGETOID RETICULOSIS

In humans, pagetoid reticulosis is a controversial epitheliotropic lymphosarcoma.[54, 108, 128, 226] There is controversy about (1) the cell of origin (T lymphocyte versus histiocyte), (2) the relative benignity or malignancy of the disease, and (3) the relationship of pagetoid reticulosis to mycosis fungoides. Pagetoid reticulosis in humans is usually characterized by (1) a solitary, often erythematous and scaly plaque or tumor on the distal extremities, (2) extreme epitheliotropism (no subepidermal component) featuring relatively monomorphous cells (polymorphous in mycosis fungoides) with peripheral "halos," and (3) a relatively benign course wherein surgical excision or radiation therapy is curative.

A pagetoid reticulosis-like disease was described in dogs.[100, 210] However, many features of the canine disease are unlike the human disease: (1) Clinical signs were generalized and indistinguishable from mycosis fungoides (Fig. 20:87C), (2) internal metastasis was recorded, and (3) subepidermal involvement with neoplastic cells was seen late in the disease. Early histopathologic findings included extreme epitheliotropism, monomorphous and "haloed" neoplastic round cells (Fig. 20:93). It may be that so-called canine pagetoid reticulosis is simply a variant of mycosis fungoides with more precise epitheliotropism and cellular monomorphism.

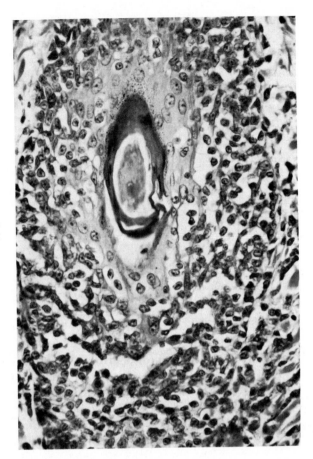

Figure 20:93. Canine pagetoid reticulosis. Proliferation of monomorphous lymphoid cells within the outer root sheath of a hair follicle.

SÉZARY SYNDROME

The Sézary syndrome is an epitheliotropic T-cell lymphosarcoma characterized by erythroderma (generalized erythema), pruritus, peripheral lymphadenopathy, and the presence of "Sézary" or "Lutzner" cells (see Mycosis Fungoides in this chapter) in the cutaneous infiltrate and in the peripheral blood.[67, 120, 200] Histopathologically, the skin biopsies are usually indistinguishable from mycosis fungoides. Most authors believe that the Sézary syndrome and mycosis fungoides are simply variants of the same T-cell lymphosarcoma.

A single case of Sézary-like syndrome has been reported in the dog.[202] The dog had generalized pruritus, multiple skin plaques and nodules, and lymphocytic leukemia. Skin biopsies revealed epitheliotropic lymphosarcoma. Sézary-like cells were found in the peripheral blood and the skin. In humans, the Sézary syndrome has been treated with many modalities, a current favorite being chlorambucil and prednisone, administered orally.[67, 219] The dog was treated with doxorubicin and prednisolone, failed to respond, and was euthanized. Necropsy examination revealed lymphosarcoma in many internal organs.

LEUKEMIA CUTIS

Leukemia cutis is generally regarded as a dissemination of aggressive systemic leukemia to the skin, and is seen in about 5 to 20 per cent of humans with leukemia.[67, 192] Cutaneous lesions seen with leukemia may be *specific* (leukemic infiltrates presenting as macules, papules, plaques, nodules, purpura, ulcers) or *nonspecific* (infectious dermatoses, erythema multiforme, urticaria, exfoliative dermatitis, pruritus). In dogs, leukemia cutis (patchy alopecia, erythema, and papules of the trunk) was reported in an English bulldog with chronic lymphocytic leukemia.[48] Nonspecific skin lesions of leukemia (recurrent pyoderma) were reported in 9 per cent of a series of dogs with chronic lymphocytic leukemia.[118]

Histopathologically, specific leukemia cutis is characterized by a perivascular, lichenoid, or diffuse monomorphous infiltration of leukemia cells.[192] The leukemia cells often infiltrate between collagen bundles. Extensive involvement and disruption of blood vessels and appendages may be seen.

Treatment includes various combinations of chemotherapeutic agents, the prognosis being poor.[67, 192] The English bulldog with chronic lymphocytic leukemia and specific leukemia cutis responded favorably to prednisone, vincristine, and chlorambucil.[48]

PSEUDOLYMPHOMA

Pseudolymphomas have been defined as disorders in which a histologic picture suggesting malignant lymphoma stands in sharp contrast to benign biologic behavior.[32, 67] Cutaneous pseudolymphomas have been subclassified into simulators of B-cell and T-cell lymphomas.[32] In humans, pseudolymphomas have been associated with reactions to sunlight, drugs, arthropods, viruses, and contact allergens, as well as with idiopathy. Other authors prefer to reserve the term "pseudolymphoma" for benign, non-neoplastic but hyperplastic lymphoproliferative processes that mimic malignant lymphoma, but which do not show adequate criteria for diagnosis of a specific disease and have a strong tendency for spontaneous regression.[39] Thus, according to this definition (1) pseudolymphomas are of unknown etiology and do not include specific disease entities of known cause, and (2) pseudolymphomatous disorders of known cause are referred to as "pseudopseudolymphomas"!

Pseudolymphomas usually present as plaques or nodules, usually solitary, often erythematous, and occasionally ulcerated. Age, breed, sex, and site predilections are not clear in small animals. Pseudolymphomas have been recognized in dogs in association with arthropod (especially tick) bites and topical or systemic medicaments.[180]

Histopathologically, the distinction between malignant lymphoma and pseudolymphoma of the skin is one of the most difficult problems in dermatopathology. (Fig. 20:94)[32, 39, 120] Major points of differentiation are presented in Table 20:10.

Treatment of pseudolymphoma is best directed at the underlying cause. Surgical excision of solitary lesions is usually curative.

CUTANEOUS PLASMACYTOMA

Multiple myeloma with skin involvement and primary cutaneous plasmacytomas are rare.[67, 145] Multiple myeloma with cutaneous plasmacytomas was reported in an 8-month-old boxer and an aged cat.[37a, 211] The dog had over 180 firm, circumscribed masses covering the neck, trunk, and limbs, 0.5 to 7 cm in

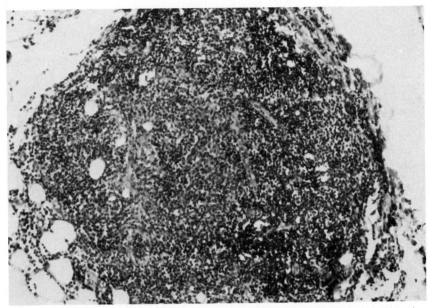

Figure 20:94. Canine pseudolymphoma. Nodular subcutaneous proliferation of normal lymphocytes and plasma cells.

diameter, and dermoepidermal to subcutaneous in location. Occasionally, solitary cutaneous plasmacytomas have been the initial clinical sign of multiple myeloma, and may precede the detection of myeloma by several months.[119, 204] Solitary cutaneous plasmacytomas (rounded, soft, erythematous, 0.5 to 5 cm diameter, subepidermal) have been recognized in adult to aged dogs (pinna, trunk) that were free of multiple myeloma for as long as 3 years after excision.[180] Oral extramedullary plasmacytomas have also been described in dogs.[143a] Histologically, plasmacytomas are characterized by dermal and subcutaneous infiltrations of normal-appearing to pleomorphic, atypical plasma cells (Figs. 20:95 and 20:96). Definitive diagnosis may require electron microscopy or immunofluorescent/immunohistochemical techniques, which confirm a monoclonal proliferation of immunoglobulin-producing cells.[143a]

Table 20:10. HISTOLOGIC CRITERIA FOR THE DIFFERENTIATION OF MALIGNANT LYMPHOMA FROM PSEUDOLYMPHOMA

Malignant Lymphoma	Pseudolymphoma
Cellular infiltrate greater in deep dermis ("bottom heavy")	Cellular infiltrate greater in superficial dermis ("top heavy")
Monomorphous cellular infiltrate	Polymorphous (mixed-cell) cellular infiltrate
Medium or large lymphocytes usually predominate	Small lymphocytes usually predominate
Germinal centers rare	Germinal centers common
Polychrome (tingible body) macrophages, rare	Polychrome (tingible body) macrophages, common
Necrosis en masse may be present	No necrosis en masse
Epithelial and vascular structures often involved	Epithelial and vascular structures spared
Cytologic atypia common	Cytologic atypia rare
Monoclonal immmunocytologic pattern	Polyclonal immunocytologic pattern

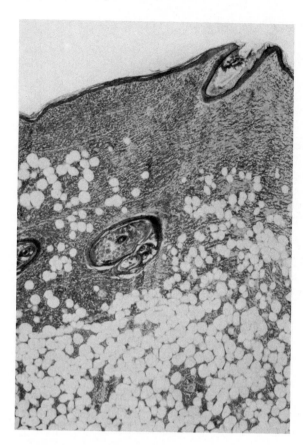

Figure 20:95. Canine plasmacytoma. Diffuse infiltration of dermis.

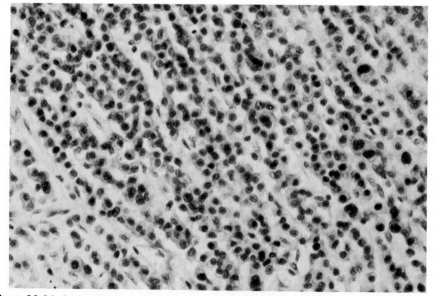

Figure 20:96. Canine plasmacytoma. Cordlike proliferation of pleomorphic, atypical plasma cells.

PRIMARY CUTANEOUS NEUROENDOCRINE TUMOR
(Merkel Cell Tumor, "Atypical Histiocytoma")

Primary cutaneous neuroendocrine tumors are uncommon neoplasms of humans[184] and dogs.[73, 138] The cause of these tumors is unknown. The cell of origin may be the Merkel cell, which, like this neoplasm, shows dual epithelial and neural differentiation.[61, 92]

In humans, primary cutaneous neuroendocrine tumors occur in the dermis and subcutis of the head, neck, and limbs of elderly people. One large study recorded 30 per cent local recurrence following surgery, regional lymph node metastasis in 65 per cent of the patients, and distant metastasis in 40 per cent.[184]

In dogs, primary cutaneous neuroendocrine tumors have been reported to be malignant and metastatic,[73] or benign with rare recurrence following surgery.[138] Most dogs are over 8 years of age, and most have solitary lesions, especially on the lips, ears, or digits.[73a, 146a] Neuroendocrine tumors may also occur in the oral cavity of dogs.[216a]

Histopathologically, primary cutaneous neuroendocrine tumors are characterized by sheets, solid nests, or anastomosing trabeculae of uniformly round tumor cells with abundant amphophilic cytoplasm, hyperchromatic and vesicular nuclei, and frequent mitoses.[73, 146a, 184] Giant and multinucleated tumor cells may be seen. Electron microscopic examination reveals characteristic cytoplasmic dense-core membrane-bound granules, and a perinuclear whorl of intermediate filaments.[83, 184] The characteristic cytoplasmic neurosecretory granules are lost in formalin-fixed tissues.[83] Immunohistochemical studies have shown that the primary cutaneous neuroendocrine tumors of humans contain cytokeratin, neurofilament, neuron-specific enolase, and common epithelial antigen.[61, 92, 117, 185]

Clinical management of these tumors is best accomplished with early radical surgical excision.[184] The vast majority of dogs appear to be cured following surgery.[73a, 146a]

Melanocytic Neoplasms

MELANOMA
(Melanocytic Nevus, Melanocytoma, Melanosarcoma)*

Melanomas are relatively common (in dogs) to rare (in cats) benign or malignant neoplasms arising from melanocytes and melanoblasts.[12, 37a, 125, 144, 145, 165a, 172, 199] The cause of melanomas is unknown. In cats, malignant melanomas have been produced with injections of feline fibrosarcoma virus.[199] In humans, there is a correlation between exposure to ultraviolet light and the development of malignant melanoma.[67] Canine melanomas can be transplanted to neonatal dogs (after treatment with antilymphocyte serum) and to nude mice.[220a]

Melanomas occur in dogs and cats with an average age of 9 years. In cats, there is no apparent breed or sex predilection. In dogs, Scottish terriers, Boston terriers, Airedales, cocker spaniels, springer spaniels, boxers, Irish setters, Irish

---

*The veterinary classification of melanomas differs markedly from the terminology used for these tumors in human beings.

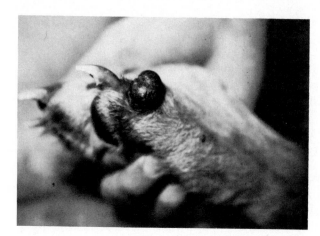

Figure 20:97. Malignant melanoma on the digit of a dog.

terriers, chow chows, Chihuahuas, Doberman pinschers, and males appear to be predisposed.

Melanomas are usually solitary. In dogs, they occur most commonly in the face, trunk, feet, and scrotum. In cats, the head and pinnae may be more commonly involved.

Benign melanomas vary in appearance from brown to black macules and plaques to firm, dome-shaped nodules 0.5 to 2 cm in diameter (Fig. 20:87E, p. 922). *Malignant melanomas* are usually rapidly growing, larger than 2 cm in diameter, and frequently ulcerated. In cats, most cutaneous melanomas are malignant (Fig. 20:87H).[95, 172] In dogs, over 90 per cent of the oral and mucocutaneous melanomas are malignant (Fig. 20:87G). Canine cutaneous melanomas may be malignant in up to 25 to 50 per cent of the cases, especially if they arise from the digits or scrotum (Fig. 20:97).[45, 75, 144, 145]

Histopathologically, cutaneous melanomas are divided into the categories shown in the following outline (Fig. 20:87F):[45, 75, 144, 145]

I. Benign Melanomas
    A. Benign melanoma with junctional activity (nevus pigmentosus or melanocytic nevus, junctional and compound types)
    B. Benign dermal melanoma (blue nevus)
        1. Cellular type
        2. Fibrous type
II. Malignant Melanomas
    A. Epithelioid type
    B. Spindle-cell type
    C. Epithelioid and spindle-cell type
    D. Dendritic and whorled type

Melanomas are particularly frustrating because no reliable correlation can be made between biologic behavior (prognosis) and the microscopic appearance of the neoplasm (mitotic index, size of nucleoli, degree of pigmentation, and so on).[21, 69, 75, 87, 145] In dogs, cutaneous *clear cell* melanomas have been described,[58] which require electron microscopic examination for confirmation of the diagnosis. In addition, *pilar neurocristic melanomas*—wherein the melanocytes proliferate exclusively perifollicularly—have recently been recognized in dogs.[6c]

In clinical management, the therapy of choice for *any* melanoma is radical surgical excision.[145, 199] In one large study of surgically treated cutaneous melanomas in dogs, animals with histologically malignant melanomas had a median survival time of 12 months and a death rate of 54 per cent within 2 years if their neoplasm was small, and a median survival time of 4 months and a death rate of 100 per cent within 2 years if their neoplasm was large.[69] In the same study, 6 per cent of the dogs with surgically treated cutaneous melanomas that were histologically benign were euthanized within 2 years because of recurrence or metastasis, or both. The mean survival time of dogs with surgically treated oral melanomas was 3 months.[87] In another large study,[21] 10 per cent of the dogs with histologically benign cutaneous melanomas died of the disease.

Secondary Skin Neoplasms

Secondary skin neoplasms result from the metastasis of primary neoplasms in other organs to the skin. In humans, the frequency of metastases to the skin varies from 1 to 4.5 per cent.[67, 120] The neoplasms most frequently associated with cutaneous metastases in humans originate in the breast, stomach, lung, uterus, kidney, ovary, colon, and urinary bladder. Skin metastases usually portend an extremely poor prognosis, and the patient often dies within 3 to 6 months. Areas of the skin that are predisposed to metastases are the scalp (breast, lung, genitourinary carcinomas), thorax (breast cancer), and abdominal wall (gastrointestinal carcinomas).

Secondary skin neoplasms are apparently rare in dogs and cats. Circumscribed, solid, subcutaneous nodules were recognized on the heads of cats with metastatic mammary adenocarcinoma and gastric carcinoma.[145] Multiple purpuric papules, plaques, and nodules of the neck have been seen in dogs with metastatic pharyngeal carcinomas (Fig. 20:98A).[141] Nodular to ulcerative to edematous ("pseudocellulitis," "inflammatory carcinoma") lesions have been recognized in the inguinal skin of dogs and cats with metastatic mammary adenocarcinoma (Fig. 20:98B)[196, 216] and colonic adenocarcinoma (Fig. 20:99).[145] Nodules in the umbilical skin have been recognized in dogs and cats with metastatic pancreatic ductal adenocarcinoma, jejunal adenocarcinoma, and teratoma.[52] Ulcerative, destructive lesions on the digits (multiple digits, multiple paws) have been seen in aged cats with asymptomatic bronchiogenic carcinomas (Figs. 20:98C,D and 20:100).[37a, 98a, 141, 158] Exfoliative erythroderma has been seen in cats with thymomas.[37]

Non-Neoplastic Tumors

CUTANEOUS CYSTS

Cutaneous cysts are common (in dogs) to uncommon (in cats) benign nonneoplastic lesions characterized by an epithelial wall with secretory or keratinous contents.[66, 145] Cutaneous keratinous cysts are subdivided into four types based on histopathologic findings.

Epidermoid cysts (epidermal inclusion cysts, epidermal cysts, "sebaceous" cysts, wens) are thought to be acquired lesions arising from displaced (traumatic?) fragments of epithelium or occluded pilosebaceous follicles.[66, 145] They may be single or multiple, and there appear to be no age, sex, or breed predilections. The lesions are round, smooth and well-circumscribed, firm to

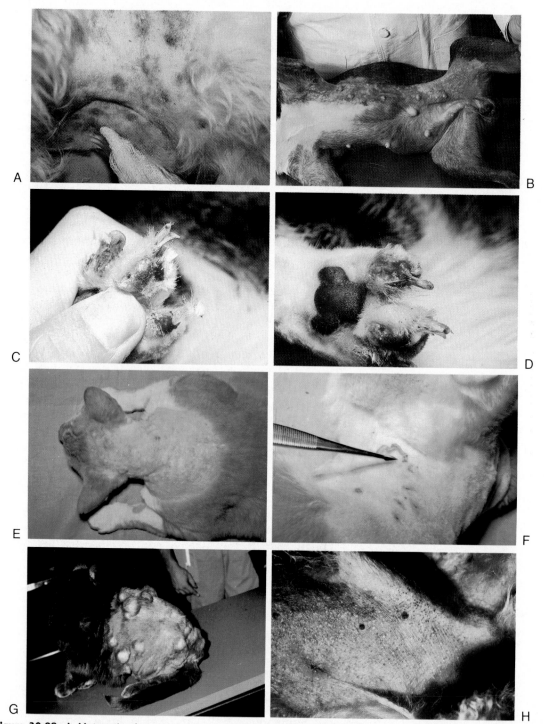

Figure 20:98. *A,* Metastatic pharyngeal carcinoma. Purpuric plaques on neck of a dog. (Courtesy W. H. Miller, Jr.) *B,* Metastatic mammary adenocarcinoma. *C,* Metastatic bronchiogenic carcinoma. Ulcerative digital lesions in a cat. (Courtesy W. H. Miller, Jr.) *D,* Same cat as in *C.* (Courtesy W. H. Miller, Jr.) *E,* Multiple epidermal cysts on neck of a cat (the area has been clipped). *F,* When incised, the cyst matrix can be expressed as a grayish white cheesy material resembling toothpaste. *G,* Multiple epidermal cysts in a cat. *H,* Multiple follicular cysts in the groin of a dog.

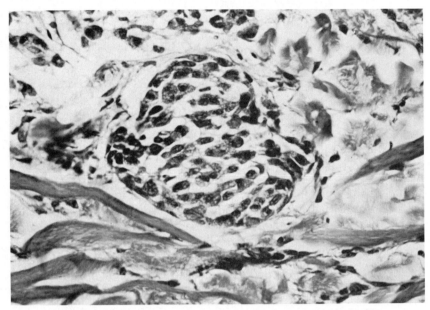

Figure 20:99. Colonic adenocarcinoma. Lymphatic metastasis in skin.

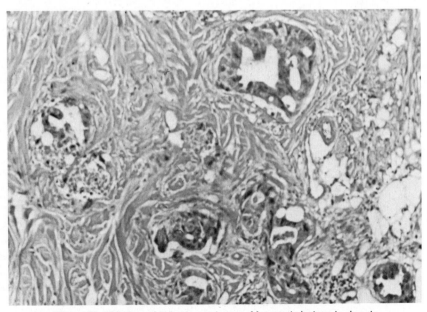

Figure 20:100. Bronchiogenic carcinoma. Metastatic lesions in dermis.

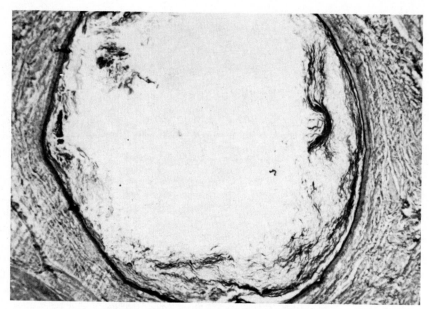

Figure 20:101. Epidermal cyst (low power).

fluctuant, 5 mm to 5 cm in diameter, often bluish, and dermoepidermal to subcutaneous in location (Fig. 20:98E–G). They may open and discharge a grayish to whitish brown, cheesy material. Epidermoid cysts tend to occur most commonly on the head, neck, trunk, and proximal limbs. Histopathologically, they are characterized by an epithelial lining that undergoes maturation and keratinization typical of epidermis but that contains no adnexal structures (Fig. 20:101).

Dermoid cysts are usually congenital and/or hereditary lesions, which may be single or multiple. Boxers, Kerry blue terriers, and Rhodesian ridgebacks are predisposed.[66, 129, 145] There is no sex predilection, and the lesions are recognized in young animals. The dermoid cyst (dermoid sinus, pilonidal sinus) of Rhodesian ridgebacks and their crosses is thought to be inherited as a simple recessive trait and occurs as single or multiple sinuses along the dorsal midline of the neck and sacrum (see p. 675). Rarely, dermoid cyst-sinus is seen in other breeds of dogs.[182] Histopathologically, dermoid cysts are characterized by a stratified epithelial lining that contains adnexae (hair follicles, sebaceous and apocrine glands) and a keratinous material.

Follicular cysts (milia) are reported to be common in animals[66, 145] and develop by retention of follicular or glandular products, owing to congenital or acquired loss or obliteration of follicular orifices. There are no age, breed, sex, or site predilections. Follicular cysts are usually small (2 to 5 mm in diameter) and white to yellow in color, and they may grossly resemble pustules or calcinosis cutis. (Fig. 20:98H). Histopathologically, they are characterized by a greatly enlarged, dilated, keratin-filled hair follicle with sebaceous or apocrine sweat glands or atrophic secondary hair follicles entering the base of the cyst (Fig. 20:102).

Trichilemmal or pilar cysts are seen in dogs.[46, 180] No age, breed, sex, or site predilections are apparent. Grossly, the lesions resemble epidermoid and dermoid cysts. Histopathologically, trichilemmal cysts are greatly enlarged and

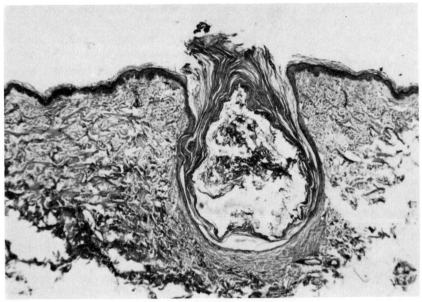

Figure 20:102. Follicular cyst or milium.

dilated hair follicles with a proliferative wall exhibiting trichilemmal keratinization, and homogeneous keratin filling the cyst cavity (Fig. 20:103 and 20:104). Squamous eddies are frequently present. A so-called *hybrid cyst* (combined epidermoid and trichilemmal cyst components) in humans has been described.[30]

All types of cysts may be complicated by rupture and resulting foreign body granuloma reaction and secondary bacterial infection. Such cysts often appear inflamed and infected grossly, and they may be painful or pruritic, or both.

In clinical management the therapy for most cutaneous cysts is surgical excision or observation without treatment. Dermoid cysts of Rhodesian ridgebacks and their crosses should always be surgically excised (see p. 675). Cysts should *never* be squeezed hard or manually evacuated, as such procedures greatly increase the chance of expressing cyst contents into the dermis or subcutis and inciting foreign body reaction and infection.

NEVI
(Hamartomas)

A nevus is a circumscribed developmental defect of the skin.[173] Nevi may arise from any skin component or combination thereof. They may or may not be congenital and are uncommonly reported in dogs and cats.

The mechanism of nevus formation is not understood. A failure in the normal orderly embryonic inductive process has been theorized. In addition, the distribution of certain epidermal and vascular nevi has prompted speculation that a relationship to dermatomes or peripheral nerves exists. Finally, some nevi have a hereditary occurrence.

Collagenous nevi have been recognized in many breeds of dogs as solitary or multiple cutaneous lesions, especially on the head, neck, and proximal

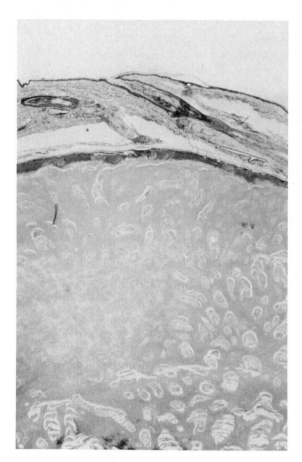

Figure 20:103. Tricholemmal cyst from a dog. Large cyst lined with basaloid cells and filled with homogenous tricholemmal keratin.

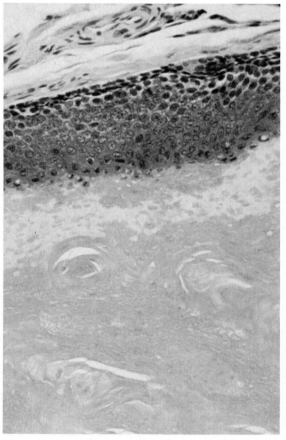

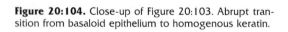

Figure 20:104. Close-up of Figure 20:103. Abrupt transition from basaloid epithelium to homogenous keratin.

extremities (Fig. 20:105*A,B*).[101, 173] In German shepherds, a syndrome of multiple, often symmetric collagenous nevi ("nodular dermatofibrosis") on the limbs, head, neck, and ventral trunk, associated with bilateral multifocal renal cystad-enocarcinomas and multiple uterine leiomyomas has been reported.[113, 121, 173] In these German shepherds, the syndrome appears to be autosomal dominant in inheritance and is characterized by the sudden onset of skin lesions at 3 to 5 years of age, which precede signs referable to renal disease by 3 to 5 years. Most collagenous nevi are firm, well circumscribed, and 0.5 to 5 cm in diameter. Some of the lesions are alopecic, variably hyperpigmented, and have pitted surfaces ("cobblestone" or "orange peel" appearance) (Fig. 20:105*C,D*). Lesions on the feet may cause pain and lameness. Histopathologically, the lesions are characterized by nodular areas of collagenous hyperplasia (Figs. 20:106 and 107).

Organoid nevi were reported in dogs and cats, with no age, breed, or sex predilection.[145] The lesions are single or multiple, firm to mushy, 3 mm to 3 cm in diameter, and dome shaped to pedunculated (Fig. 20:108). They occur primarily on the face, head, and proximal extremities. Histopathologically, they are characterized by hyperplasia of hair follicles, sebaceous glands, and, rarely, apocrine sweat glands (Fig. 20:109).

Vascular nevi ("varicose tumors of the scrotum") were reported in the scrotum of dogs.[144, 145] They are most common in dogs past middle age and in breeds with pigmented skin, such as Scottish terriers, Airedales, Kerry blue terriers, and Labrador retrievers. The lesions are characterized by single or multiple, slowly enlarging and hyperpigmenting plaques on the scrotum. Periodic hemorrhage from the lesions may be seen. Vascular nevi are occasionally seen at other cutaneous sites.[166, 180] Histopathologically, the scrotal lesions are characterized by cavernous dilatation (telangiectasia) of blood vessels and epidermal melanosis.

A *sebaceous gland nevus* was recognized in a 1-year-old male poodle.[173] The lesion had been present on the cranial right thigh since birth and had been slowly enlarging. It was linear, multinodular, alopecic, smooth, shiny, greasy, and orange-yellow (Fig. 20:105*E*). Histopathologically, it was characterized by sebaceous gland hyperplasia and overlying papillated epidermal hyperplasia (Fig. 20:110, p. 944).

Epidermal nevi have been recognized in dogs. In a 2-month-old male miniature schnauzer, the lesions developed as wavy, linear bands of closely set, hyperpigmented, hyperkeratotic papules and plaques over the trunk.[173] Other dogs have had single linear, hyperpigmented, hyperkeratotic lesions of the trunk or proximal extremities.[180] Histologically, orthokeratotic hyperkeratosis, papillated epidermal hyperplasia, and papillomatosis are seen (Fig. 20:111). In some instances, granular degeneration of the epidermis is present.

Melanocytic nevi are seen in the dog and cat. The lesions may be single or multiple and occur most commonly on the trunk.[37a, 45, 110, 145, 180] They vary from brown to black, and from macular (junctional nevi) to papular or pedunculated (compound and intradermal nevi) (Fig. 20:105*F,G*). There are no recorded instances of malignant transformation. Histopathologically, melanocytic nevi are characterized by intraepidermal and/or dermal nests (theques) of benign, hyperplastic melanocytes ("nevus cells").

The schnauzer comedo syndrome bears a striking clinical and histopathologic resemblance to *nevus comedonicus* in humans (see p. 733).

In clinical management, the therapy of choice for nevi, when necessary and feasible, is surgical excision or cryosurgery.

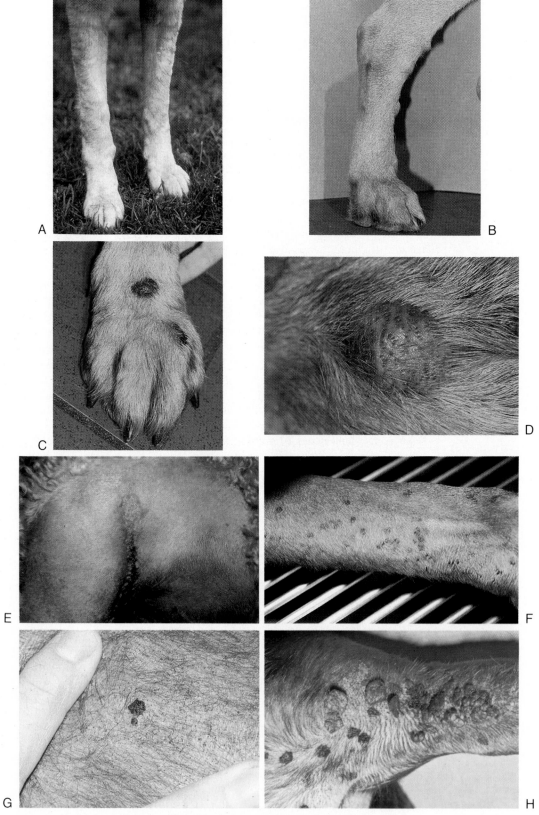

Figure 20:105 *See legend on opposite page*

Keratoses are firm, elevated, circumscribed areas of excessive keratin production.[145] In humans, keratoses are common and of numerous types. Keratoses are uncommonly reported in dogs and cats.

Seborrheic keratoses have been recognized in dogs.[74, 145] The cause of seborrheic keratoses is unknown, and they have nothing to do with seborrhea. They may be single or multiple and have no apparent age, breed, sex, or site predilections. The lesions are elevated plaques and nodules with a hyperkeratotic, often greasy surface (Fig. 20:105H). They are frequently hyperpigmented. Histologically, seborrheic keratoses are characterized by hyperkeratosis, hyperplasia (basaloid and squamoid), and papillomatosis (Fig. 20:112).

Actinic (solar) keratoses have been recognized in dogs and cats.[64, 85, 145, 175] They are caused by excessive exposure to ultraviolet light. Actinic keratoses may be single or multiple, appear in lightly haired and lightly pigmented skin, and vary in appearance from ill-defined areas of erythema, hyperkeratosis, and crusting to indurated, crusted, hyperkeratotic plaques (Figs. 20:113A and 20:114). Histopathologically, they are characterized by atypia and dysplasia of the epidermis, hyperkeratosis (especially parakeratotic) and occasionally by solar elastosis of the underlying dermis (Fig. 20:115). Actinic keratoses are premalignant lesions capable of becoming invasive squamous cell carcinomas.

Lichenoid keratoses have been recognized in dogs.[6b, 174, 180] Generally, solitary asymptomatic lesions are seen on the pinnae of adult dogs. Lesions are well circumscribed, erythematous, and scaly-to-markedly hyperkeratotic plaques or papillomas. Histologically, an irregular-to-papillated epidermal hyperplasia with overlying hyperkeratosis and an underlying subepidermal lichenoid band of inflammation are seen.

Cutaneous horns have been recognized in dogs and cats. The cause of cutaneous horns may be unknown, or they may originate from papillomas, basal cell tumors, squamous cell carcinomas, keratinous cysts, keratoacanthomas, or other keratoses. Cutaneous horns may be single or multiple and have no apparent age, sex, or site predilections. They are firm, hornlike projections of up to 5 cm in length (Fig. 20:113B,C). Multiple cutaneous horns have been seen on the footpads of cats with feline leukemia virus (FeLV) infection.[175] Generally, multiple horns are seen on multiple footpads (Fig. 20:113D). Occasionally lesions are seen on the face. Histopathologically, cutaneous horns are characterized by extensive, compact, laminated hyperkeratosis (Figs. 20:116 and 20:117). The base of a cutaneous horn must always be inspected for the possible underlying cause. FeLV–associated cutaneous horns in cats have been characterized by dyskeratosis and multinucleated epidermal giant cells.

In clinical management, the therapy of choice for most keratoses is surgical excision. Actinic keratoses are always premalignant lesions, and cutaneous

Figure 20:105. *A,* Collagenous nevi. Multiple papules on the front legs of a German shepherd. (Courtesy J. Yager.) *B,* Collagenous nevi. Papules and nodules on rear leg. *C,* Collagenous nevus. Alopecic, pigmented nodule on paw. *D,* Collagenous nevus. Alopecic, pitted ("orange peel") nodule. *E,* Sebaceous nevus in the flank of a dog (the area has been clipped). *F,* Multiple melanocytic nevi on the leg of a dog. (Courtesy W. H. Miller, Jr.) *G,* Melanocytic nevus on the back of a dog. *H,* Seborrheic keratoses on the medial surface of the foreleg in a French bulldog. They are multiple, slightly raised, verrucous nodules. Since they vary in color from brown to black, they must be differentiated histopathologically from melanomas. Individual susceptible dogs can have numerous seborrheic keratoses. Histologically, they are raised above the level of the surrounding epidermis through the formation of layers of keratin that originate from pilosebaceous follicles and the epidermis itself. They usually are innocuous but, if necessary, can be removed by a shave biopsy and electric desiccation.

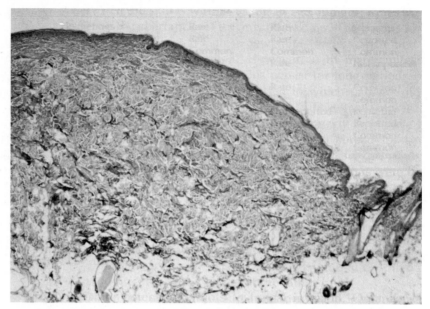

Figure 20:106. Collagenous nevus. Exophylic, nodular hyperplasia of collagen.

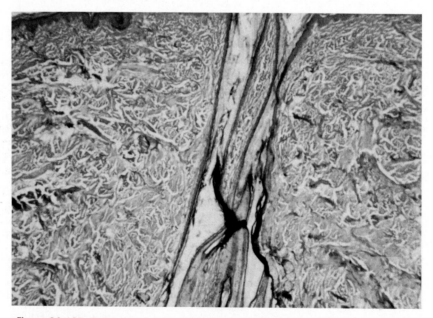

Figure 20:107. Collagenous nevus. Collagenous hyperplasia surrounding a hair follicle.

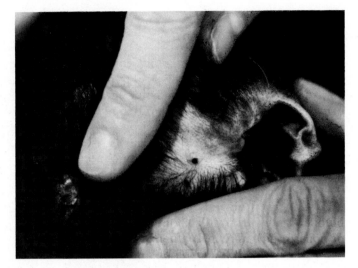

Figure 20:108. Organoid nevus in a cat. Pigmented, hairy, papillomatous lesion in the temporal area. (From Scott, D. W.: Feline dermatology 1900–1978: a monograph. J.A.A.H.A., *16*:331, 1980.)

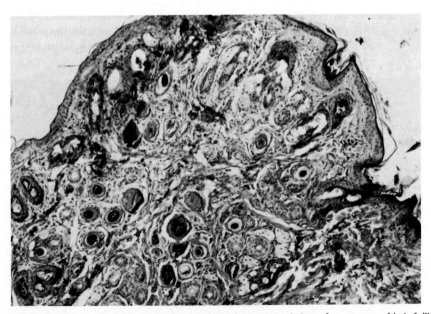

Figure 20:109. Feline organoid nevus. Dome-shaped mass consisting of an excess of hair follicles and sebaceous glands. (From Scott, D. W.: Feline dermatology 1900–1978: a monograph. J.A.A.H.A., *16*:331, 1980.)

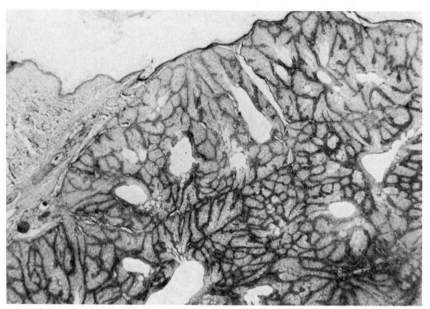

Figure 20:110. Canine sebaceous gland nevus. Nodular sebaceous gland hyperplasia.

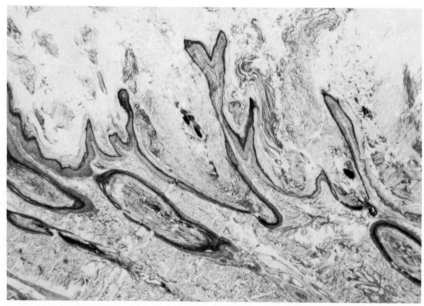

Figure 20:111. Canine epidermal nevus. Orthokeratotic hyperkeratosis, papillated epidermal hyperplasia, and papillomatosis.

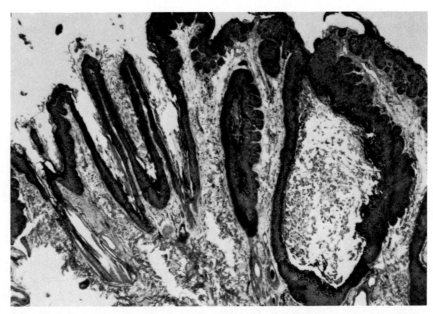

Figure 20:112. Canine seborrheic keratosis. Papillomatosis and basosquamous proliferation.

horns may have a neoplastic process at their bases. In humans, topical 5-fluorouracil has been extensively and successfully used for the treatment of actinic keratoses.[67] The usefulness of this modality in dogs and cats is unknown. There is presently no satisfactory treatment for the multiple FeLV–associated cutaneous horns of cats.

KELOIDS

Keloids are benign, post-traumatic proliferations of fibrous tissue in humans.[67] The cause of keloids in humans is unknown. Undetailed and unsubstantiated reports of keloids occurring in dogs have appeared in the literature.[18, 145]

XANTHOMAS

Xanthomas are benign granulomatous lesions usually associated with abnormal concentrations or composition of plasma lipids.[67] Multiple cutaneous xanthomas were reported in a dog with diabetes mellitus and hypertriglyceridemia.[41] The lesions were yellow and erythematous, having the gross appearance of pustules, and they involved predominantly the ventrum, head, and ears. The lesions regressed as the diabetes mellitus and hypertriglyceridemia were controlled. Xanthomas have also been seen in cats with naturally occurring or megestrol acetate-induced diabetes mellitus.[102, 115, 175] Lesions consisted of multiple whitish to erythematous papules and plaques, ulcers, and subcutaneous nodules over the head and bony prominences (Fig. 20:113E).

Xanthomatosis has also been reported in cats with a presumed hereditary hyperlipoproteinemia (hypercholesterolemia, hypertriglyceridemia, and decreased lipoprotein lipase activity).[103]

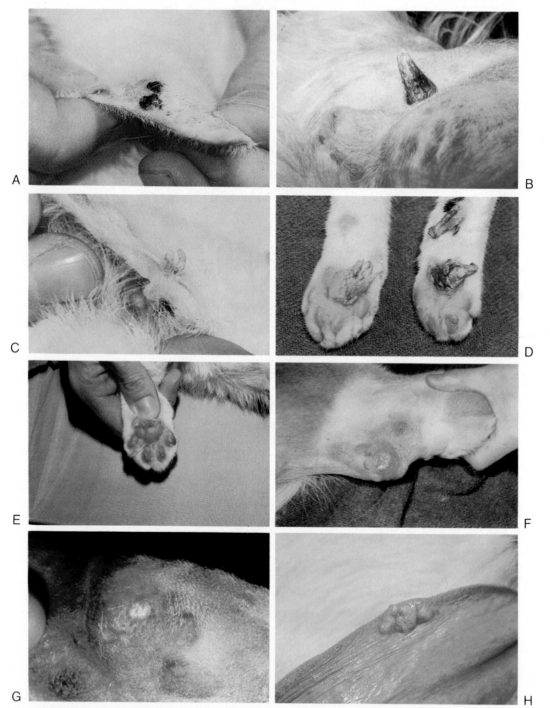

Figure 20:113. *A,* Feline actinic keratosis. Two crusted plaques in a field of solar dermatitis. *B,* Anteriorly to the vulva, a cutaneous horn is seen, which grew from a reddened and slightly thickened base. *C,* Two cutaneous horns on the pinna of a cat. *D,* Multiple cutaneous horns on the footpads of an FeLV-infected cat. *E,* Xanthomas on the footpads of a cat with diabetes mellitus caused by megestrol acetate. (Courtesy K. Kwochka.) *F,* Calcinosis circumscripta on the elbow of a dog. *G,* Closer view of the lesion in *F.* Note the white area of calcific discharge. *H,* Calcinosis circumscripta on the tongue of a dog.

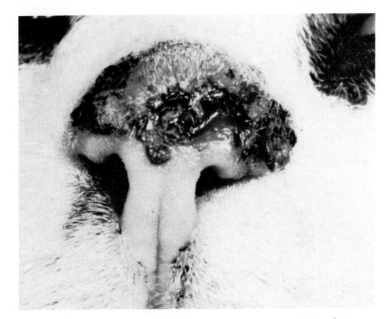

Figure 20:114. Feline actinic keratosis. Erythema, scaling, and crusting on the nose.

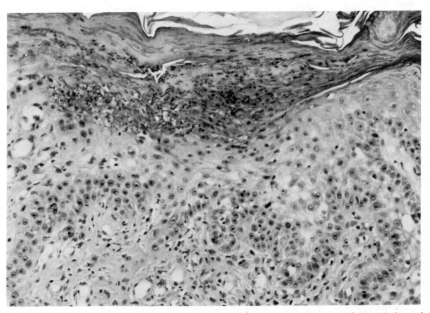

Figure 20:115. Feline actinic keratosis. Epidermal dysplasia with overlying parakeratotic hyperkeratosis.

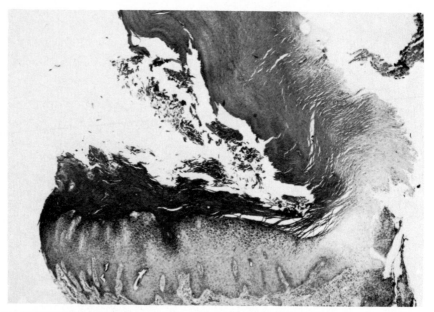

Figure 20:116. Feline cutaneous horn. Hornlike projection of dense, parakeratotic keratin arising from hyperplastic, hypergranulotic, hyperkeratotic footpad epithelium.

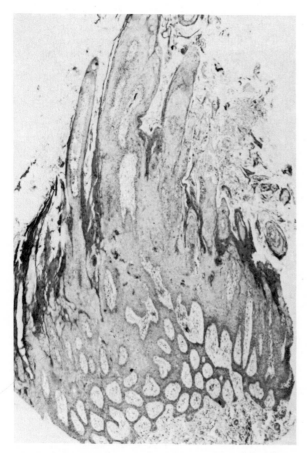

Figure 20:117. Feline cutaneous horn. Hornlike projection from footpad of FeLV-infected cat.

Histopathologically, xanthomas are characterized by an infiltration of "foamy" macrophages (xanthoma cells) with or without concurrent granulomatous inflammation and fibroplasia (Fig. 20:118).

Diabetes mellitus–associated xanthomas regress as the diabetes is controlled.

CALCINOSIS CUTIS

Calcinosis cutis is an uncommon disorder of the dog.[145, 179] Calcification of the skin may occur in a wide variety of unrelated disorders (Table 20:11). The complex biologic process whereby inorganic ions are deposited as a solid phase in soft tissues is not understood. It is probable that abnormal skin calcifications are usually associated with collagen and elastin.

Widespread calcinosis cutis has frequently been reported in dogs in association with naturally occurring or iatrogenic hyperglucocorticoidism (see p. 597). Cutaneous lesions consist of papules, plaques, and nodules that are firm, often gritty, frequently ulcerated and secondarily infected, and yellowish white to pinkish yellow. These lesions may occur anywhere but are especially common along the dorsum and in the axillae and groin. Histologically, calcium salts are deposited along collagen and elastin fibers in the dermis and basement membrane zones and are frequently surrounded by a foreign body granuloma reaction. This form of calcinosis cutis in dogs is thought to be *dystrophic* in nature, since blood calcium and phosphorus levels are invariably normal. Correcting the hyperglucocorticoidism causes this type of calcinosis cutis to regress within 2 to 6 months. A syndrome of calcinosis cutis grossly and histologically identical to glucocorticoid-associated calcinosis cutis has rarely been seen in healthy dogs less than 1 year old.[180] Lesions spontaneously regress within 1 year. Recently, calcinosis cutis was reported in dogs secondary to percutaneous penetration of calcium chloride (contact with a commercial hy-

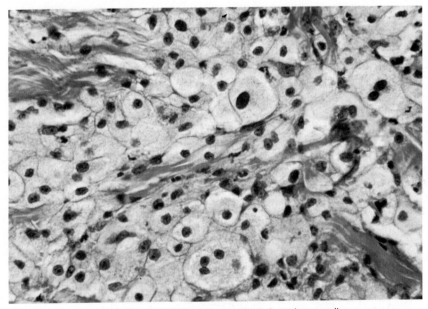

Figure 20:118. Feline xanthoma. Typical xanthoma cells.

Table 20:11. CAUSES OF CALCINOSIS CUTIS IN DOGS

Dystrophic calcification (deposition of calcium salts in injured, degenerating, or dead tissue)

Localized areas (calcinosis circumscripta)
    Inflammatory lesions (tuberculosis, foreign body granuloma, demodicosis, staphylococcal
       pododermatitis)
    Degenerative lesions (epidermoid cysts)
    Neoplastic lesions (pilomatrixoma, others)

Widespread areas (calcinosis universalis)
    Hyperglucocorticoidism (naturally occurring or iatrogenic)
    Diabetes mellitus
    Percutaneous penetration of calcium

Idiopathic calcification (deposition of calcium salts with no appreciable tissue damage or demonstrable metabolic defect)

Localized areas (idiopathic calcinosis circumscripta of large breed dogs)
Widespread areas (idiopathic calcinosis universalis of young dogs)

Metastatic calcification deposition of calcium salts associated with abnormal metabolism of calcium and phosphorus with demonstrable serum level changes)

Chronic renal disease

groscopic landscaping product).[170a] Spontaneous recovery followed avoidance of further contact with the substance.

Localized areas of calcinosis cutis (*calcinosis circumscripta*) are seen most commonly in younger dogs (less than 2 years of age) of either sex.[179] About 80 per cent of all reported cases have been in large breeds of dogs, and over 50 per cent of the cases have been in German shepherds. Lesions are usually dome shaped, fluctuant or firm, and 1 to 10 cm in diameter (Fig. 20:113*F*). Initially, the overlying skin may be freely movable and covered with hair. As the lesions progress, however, ulceration frequently occurs, as does the discharge of a chalky white, pasty-to-gritty material (Fig. 20:113*G*). Lesions may be single or multiple and are occasionally bilaterally symmetric. They are most frequently seen over or near pressure points and bony prominences: tarsometatarsal (24 per cent of reported cases), phalangeal (19 per cent), elbow (17 per cent), and neck, near the fourth to sixth cervical vertebrae (10 per cent). They may also occur in the tongue (Fig. 20:113*H*). Boxers and Boston terriers appear to be predisposed to lesions at the base of the pinna and on the cheek, respectively. Calcinosis circumscripta is extremely rare in cats.[6a]

Histologically, this localized type of calcinosis cutis is characterized by multifocal areas of granular amorphous material surrounded by a zone of granulomatous inflammation and separated by fibrous trabeculae (Fig. 20:119). Cartilaginous and osseous metaplasia, as well as transepidermal elimination of minerals, may be seen in some lesions. A cross section of a gross specimen is seen in Fig. 20:120.[130] The amorphous masses are usually strongly periodic acid-Schiff (PAS) positive and Alcian-blue positive. The cause of this localized type of calcinosis cutis is idiopathic. No evidence to support traumatic, myxomatous degenerative, or apocrine sweat gland origin of this lesion has been found. The therapy of choice is surgical excision.

Metastatic calcinosis cutis is occasionally seen in the dog.[145, 179] All reported cases have occurred in association with chronic renal disease. Cutaneous lesions

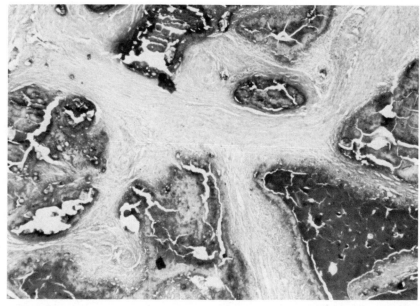

Figure 20:119. Canine calcinosis circumscripta. Multinodular areas of mineralization separated by fibrous trabeculae.

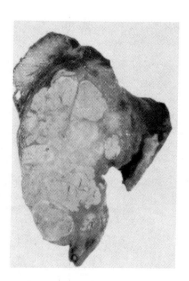

Figure 20:120. Cross section of multilocular mass of tissue, calcinosis circum-scripta, dog. (From Jubb, K. V. F., and Kennedy, D. C.: Pathology of Domestic Animals, vol. 2. Academic Press, Inc., New York, 1963.)

have been localized to the footpads. Affected pads are enlarged, painful, firm, and often ulcerated and discharging a chalky white, pasty-to-gritty material. Histopathologic findings are as described above for calcinosis circumscripta. No therapy is beneficial.

CUTANEOUS MUCINOSIS

Cutaneous mucinoses are a heterogeneous group of skin disorders characterized by the excessive accumulation or deposition of mucin (acid mucopolysaccharide) in the dermis and/or epithelial structures.[55, 67] The mucinosis may be primary or secondary, or focal to diffuse. In dogs, cutaneous mucinosis may be seen with hypothyroidism, lupus erythematosus, dermatomyositis, mycosis fungoides, and as a normal finding in the Chinese Shar Pei. In cats, cutaneous mucinosis may be seen with alopecia mucinosa and mycosis fungoides.

Focal cutaneous mucinosis has been reported in dogs.[55] Three dogs (two Doberman pinschers; all three females, 3.5 to 6 years old) had solitary, asymptomatic, firm and rubbery-to-soft nodules (1 to 3 cm in diameter) on the head or leg. The primary histopathologic finding was an accumulation of excessive mucin (Alcian-blue positive or colloidal-iron positive) within the dermis or subcutis, which disrupted and separated collagen fibers (Fig. 20:121). In addition, a mild-to-extensive proliferation of fibroblasts and a mild lymphohistiocytic infiltrate were seen. Surgical excision was apparently curative.

In the same paper, focal cutaneous mucinosis was reported in three Chinese Shar Pei. The clinicopathologic information about these three dogs is difficult to interpret, but it is likely that the alleged "mucinosis" is simply normal for this breed. "Mucinosis" is present to one degree or another in all skin biopsies from Chinese Shar Pei, regardless of the dermatosis!

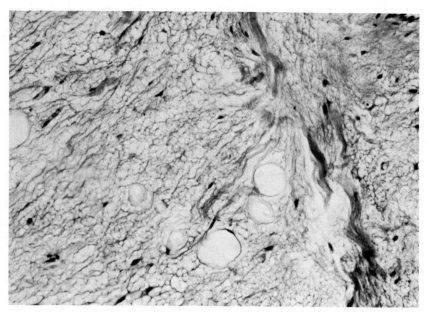

Figure 20:121. Canine focal cutaneous mucinosis. Dermal mucinous degeneration.

References

1. Abel, E. A., et al.: Cutaneous malignancies and metastatic squamous cell carcinoma following topical therapies for mycosis fungoides. J. Am. Acad. Dermatol. *14*:1029, 1986.

2. Ackerman, L.: Cutaneous T cell–like lymphoma in the dog. Compend. Cont. Ed. *6*:37, 1984.

3. Albers, G. W., and Theilen, G. H.: Calcium chloride for treatment of subcutaneous lipomas in dogs. J.A.V.M.A. *186*:492, 1985.

3a. Allen, S. W., and Duncan, J. R.: Malignant fibrous histiocytoma in a cat. J.A.V.M.A. *192*:90, 1988.

4. Allen, S. W., and Prasse, K. W.: Cytologic diagnosis of neoplasia and perioperative implementation. Compend. Cont. Ed. *8*:872, 1986.

5. Amber, E. I., and Henderson, R. A.: Canine transmissible venereal tumor: Evaluation of surgical excision of primary and metastatic lesions in Zaria-Nigeria. J.A.A.H.A. *18*:350, 1982.

6. Amber, E. I., et al.: Viral-like particles associated with naturally occurring transmissible venereal tumor in two dogs: Preliminary report. A.J.V.R. *46*:2613, 1985.

6a. Anderson, W. I., and Scott, D. W.: Calcinosis circumscripta in a domestic short-haired cat. Cornell Vet. *77*:348, 1987.

6b. Anderson, W. I., et al.: Lichenoid keratosis on the pinna of the ear in four dogs. (Submitted for publication, 1988.)

6c. Anderson, W. I., et al.: Pilar neurocristic melanoma in four dogs. (Submitted for publication, 1988.)

7. Androphy, E. J., et al.: Response of warts in epidermodysplasia verruciformis to treatment with systemic and intralesional alpha interferon. J. Am. Acad. Dermatol. *11*:197, 1984.

8. Austin, V. H.: The skin. *In* Catcott, E. J., ed.: *Feline Medicine and Surgery.* 2nd ed. American Veterinary Publications, Inc., Santa Barbara, 1975, pp. 461–484.

9. Bardet, J. F., et al.: Extraskeletal osteosarcomas: Literature review and a case presentation. J.A.A.H.A. *19*:601, 1983.

10. Barr, R. J.: Cutaneous cytology. J. Am. Acad. Dermatol. *10*:163, 1984.

11. Barton, C. L.: Cytologic diagnosis of cutaneous neoplasia: An algorithmic approach. Comp. Cont. Ed. *9*:20, 1987.

12. Bastianello, S. S.: A survey of neoplasia in domestic species over a 40-year period from 1935 to 1974 in the Republic of South Africa. V. Tumours occurring in the cat. Onderstepoort J. Vet. Res. *50*:105, 1983.

13. Bastianello, S. S.: A survey of neoplasia in domestic species over a 40-year period from 1935 to 1974 in the Republic of South Africa. VI. Tumours occurring in dogs. Onderstepoort J. Vet. Res. *50*:199, 1983.

14. Bender, W. M.: Nontraditional treatment of mycosis fungoides in a dog. J.A.V.M.A. *185*:900, 1984.

15. Benoldi, D., and Alinovi, A.: Multiple persistent keratoacanthomas: Treatment with oral etretinate. J. Am. Acad. Dermatol. *10*:1035, 1984.

16. Bertoni, F., et al.: Malignant fibrous histiocytoma of soft tissue. An analysis of 78 cases located and deeply seated in the extremities. Cancer *56*:356, 1985.

17. Bevier, D. E., and Goldschmidt, M. H.: Skin tumors in the dog, part I. Epithelial tumors and tumor-like lesions. Compend. Cont. Ed. *3*:389, 1981.

18. Bevier, D. E., and Goldschmidt, M. H.: Skin tumors in the dog, part II. Tumors of the soft (mesenchymal) tissues. Compend. Cont. Ed. *3*:506, 1981.

19. Bostock, D. E.: Prognosis in cats bearing squamous cell carcinoma. J. Small Anim. Pract. *13*:119, 1972.

20. Bostock, D. E.: The prognosis following surgical removal of mastocytomas in dogs. J. Small Anim. Pract. *14*:27, 1973.

21. Bostock, D. E.: Prognosis after surgical excision of canine melanomas. Vet. Pathol. *16*:32, 1979.

22. Bostock, D. E., and Dye, M. T.: Prognosis after surgical excision of fibrosarcomas in cats. J.A.V.M.A. *175*:727, 1979.

23. Bostock, D. E., and Dye, M. T.: Prognosis after surgical excision of canine fibrous connective tissue sarcomas. Vet. Pathol. *17*:581, 1980.

23a. Bregman, C. L., et al.: Cutaneous neoplasms in dogs associated with canine oral papillomavirus vaccine. Vet. Pathol. *24*:477, 1987.

24. Brodey, R. S.: Canine and feline neoplasia. Adv. Vet. Sci. *14*:309, 1970.

25. Brown, N. O., et al.: Soft tissue sarcomas in the cat. J.A.V.M.A. *173*:744, 1978.

26. Brown, N. O., et al.: Combined modality therapy in the treatment of solid tumors in cats. J.A.A.H.A. *16*:719, 1980.

27. Brown, N. O., et al.: Cutaneous lymphosarcoma in the dog: A disease with variable clinical and histologic manifestations. J.A.A.H.A. *16*:565, 1980.

28. Brown, N. O., et al.: Transmissible venereal tumor in the dog. Calif. Vet. *35*:6, 1981.

29. Brown, N. O., et al.: Canine hemangiosarcoma: Retrospective analysis of 104 cases. J.A.V.M.A. *186*:56, 1985.

30. Brownstein, M. H.: Hybrid cyst: A combined epidermoid and trichilemmal cyst. J. Am. Acad. Dermatol. *9*:872, 1983.

31. Buerger, R. G., and Scott, D. W.: Cutaneous mast cell neoplasia in the cat: 14 cases (1975–1985). J.A.V.M.A. *190*:1440, 1987.

32. Burg, G., and Braun-Falco, O.: *Cutaneous Lymphomas, Pseudolymphomas, and Related Disorders.* Springer-Verlag, New York, 1983.

33. Burton, C. S., and Sawchuk, W. S.: Premature sebaceous gland hyperplasia: Successful treatment with isotretinoin. J. Am. Acad. Dermatol. *12*:182, 1985.

34. Buyukmihci, N., and Stannard, A. A.: Canine conjunctival angiokeratomas. J.A.V.M.A. *178*:1279, 1981.

35. Caciolo, P. L., et al.: Cutaneous lymphosarcoma in the cat: A report of nine cases. J.A.A.H.A. *20*:491, 1984.

36. Caciolo, P. L., et al.: A case of mycosis fungoides in a cat and literature review. J.A.A.H.A. *20*:505, 1984.

36a. Campbell, K. L., et al.: Cutaneous inverted papillomas in dogs. Vet. Pathol. *25*:67, 1988.

37. Carpenter, J. L., and Holzworth, J.: Thymoma in 11 cats. J.A.V.M.A. *181*:248, 1982.

37a. Carpenter, J. L., et al.: Tumors and tumor-like lesions. *In* Holzworth, J. (ed.): Diseases of the Cat, Vol. 1. W. B. Saunders Co., Philadelphia, 1987, p. 406.

37b. Carr, S. H., and Gross, T. L.: Caudal neuropathy subsequent to tail docking. Ann. Meet. Am. Acad. Vet. Dermatol., Am. Coll. Vet. Dermatol., 1988.

38. Carstens, P. H. B.: The Weibel-Palade body in

the diagnosis of endothelial tumors. Ultrastruct. Pathol. 2:315, 1981.

39. Cerio, R., and MacDonald, D. M.: Benign cutaneous lymphoid infiltrates. J. Cut. Pathol. 12:442, 1985.

40. Chase, D. R., and Enzinger, F. M.: Epithelioid sarcoma. Diagnosis, prognostic indicators, and treatment. Am. J. Surg. Pathol. 9:241, 1985.

41. Chastain, C. B., and Graham, C. L.: Xanthomatosis secondary to diabetes mellitus in a dog. J.A.V.M.A. 172:1209, 1978.

41a. Chastain, C. B., and Turk, M. A. M.: Benign cutaneous mastocytomas in litters of Siamese kittens. Ann. Meet. Am. Acad. Vet. Dermatol., Am. Coll. Vet. Dermatol., 1987.

42. Claudy, A. L., et al.: Treatment of cutaneous lymphoma with etretinate. Br. J. Dermatol. 109:49, 1983.

43. Cockerell, G. L., and Slauson, D. O.: Patterns of lymphoid infiltrate in the canine cutaneous histiocytoma. J. Comp. Pathol. 89:193, 1979.

44. Cohen, D., et al.: Treatment of canine transmissible venereal tumor by intravenous administration of protein A. J. Biol. Resp. Modif. 3:271, 1984.

45. Conroy, J. D.: Melanocytic tumors of domestic animals. Arch. Dermatol. 96:372, 1967.

46. Conroy, J. D.: Canine skin tumors. J.A.A.H.A. 19:91, 1983.

47. Couto, C. G.: Canine lymphomas: Something old, something new. Compend. Cont. Ed. 7:291, 1985.

48. Couto, C. G., and Sousa, C.: Chronic lymphocytic leukemia with cutaneous involvement in a dog. J.A.A.H.A. 22:374, 1986.

49. Craig, J. A., et al.: A practical guide to clinical oncology—4: Chemotherapy and immunotherapy. Vet. Med. 82:226, 1986.

50. Cristofolini, M., et al.: The role of etretinate (Tegison; Tigason) in the management of keratoacanthoma. J. Am. Acad. Dermatol. 12:633, 1985.

51. Crow, S. E., et al.: Skin tumors in dogs and cats. Dermatol. Rep. 3:1, 1984.

52. Crowe, D. T., and Todoroff, R. J.: Umbilical masses and discolorations as signs of intra-abdominal disease. J.A.A.H.A. 18:295, 1982.

53. Dabski, K., et al.: Unusual clinical presentation of epidermotropic cutaneous lymphoma. Small hypopigmented macules. Int. J. Dermatol. 24:108, 1985.

54. Deneau, D. G., et al.: Woringer-Kolopp disease (pagetoid reticulosis). Four cases with histopathologic, ultrastructural, and immunohistologic observations. Arch. Dermatol. 120:1045, 1984.

55. Dillberger, J. E., and Altman, N. H.: Focal mucinosis in dogs: Seven cases and review of cutaneous mucinoses of man and animals. Vet. Pathol. 23:132, 1986.

56. Diters, R. W., and Walsh, K. M.: Feline basal cell tumors: A review of 124 cases. Vet. Pathol. 21:51, 1984.

57. Diters, R. W., and Goldschmidt, M. H.: Hair follicle tumors resembling tricholemmomas in six dogs. Vet. Pathol. 20:123, 1983.

58. Diters, R. W., and Walsh, K. M.: Cutaneous clear cell melanomas: A report of three cases. Vet. Pathol. 21:355, 1984.

59. Dixon, A. Y., et al.: Angiolipomas: An ultrastructural and clinicopathological study. Human Pathol. 12:739, 1981.

59a. Doster, A. R., et al.: Canine liposarcoma. Vet. Pathol. 23:84, 1986.

60. Draelos, Z. K., and Levine, N.: Hyperthermic treatment of cutaneous malignancies. J. Am. Acad. Dermatol. 9:623, 1983.

61. Dreno, B., et al.: A study of intermediate filaments (cytokeratin, vimentin, neurofilament) in

two cases of Merkel cell tumor. J. Cut. Pathol. 12:37, 1985.

62. Dust, A., et al.: Cutaneous lymphosarcoma with IgG monoclonal gammopathy, serum hyperviscosity, and hypercalcemia in a cat. Can. Vet. J. 23:235, 1982.

63. Esplin, D. G.: Infiltrating lipoma in a cat. Feline Pract. 14:24, 1984.

64. Evans, A. G., et al.: A trial of 13-cis-retinoic acid for treatment of squamous cell carcinoma and preneoplastic lesions of the head in cats. A.J.V.R. 46:2553, 1985.

64a. Evans, S. M.: Canine hemangiosarcoma: a retrospective analysis of response to surgery and orthovoltage radiation. Vet. Radiol. 28:13, 1987.

65. Fehrer, S. L., and Lin, S. H.: Multicentric basal cell tumors in a cat. J.A.V.M.A. 189:1469, 1986.

66. Fezer, G., and Weiss, E.: Die zystischen Bildungen in der Haut der Haustiere. Arch. Exper. Vet. Med. 23:60, 1969.

67. Fitzpatrick, T. B., et al.: Dermatology in General Medicine III. McGraw-Hill Book Company, New York, 1987.

68. Franklin, R. T., et al.: Lymphangiosarcoma in a dog. J.A.V.M.A. 184:474, 1984.

69. Frese, K.: Verlaufsuntersuchungen beim Melanomen der Haut und der Mundschleimhaut des Hundes. Vet. Pathol. 15:461, 1978.

70. Gallagher, R. L., and Helwig, E. B.: Neurothekeoma: A benign cutaneous tumor of neural origin. Am. J. Clin. Pathol. 74:759, 1980.

71. Giannone, J. A.: Cryotherapy of cutaneous lymphosarcoma in a German shepherd. Mod. Vet. Pract. 65:725, 1984.

71a. Gilbert, P. A., and Griffin, C. E.: Diffuse trunkal lipomatosis in a dog. Ann. Meet. Am. Acad. Vet. Dermatol., Am. Coll. Vet. Dermatol., 1988.

72. Gleiser, C. A., et al.: Malignant fibrous histiocytoma in dogs and cats. Vet. Pathol. 16:199, 1979.

73. Glick, A. D., et al.: Neuroendocrine carcinoma of the skin in a dog. Vet. Pathol. 20:761, 1983.

73a. Goldschmidt, M. H.: Small animal dermatopathology: "What's old, what's new, what's borrowed, what's useful." Semin. Vet. Med. Surg. 2:162, 1987.

74. Goldschmidt, M. H., and Kunkle, G.: Inverted follicular keratosis in a dog. Vet. Pathol. 16:374, 1979.

75. Goldschmidt, M. H., and Bevier, D. E.: Skin tumors in the dog, part III. Lymphohistiocytic and melanocytic tumors. Compend. Cont. Ed. 3:588, 1981.

76. Gonzalez, S. B.: Benign fibrous histiocytoma of the skin. An immunohistochemical analysis of 30 cases. Pathol. Res. Pract. 180:486, 1985.

77. Gourley, I. M., et al.: Burn scar malignancy in a dog. J.A.V.M.A. 180:1095, 1982.

78. Grain, E., and Walder, E. J.: Hypercalcemia associated with squamous cell carcinoma in a dog. J.A.V.M.A. 181:165, 1982.

78a. Graves, G. M., et al.: Canine hemangiopericytoma: 23 cases (1967–1984). J.A.V.M.A. 192:99, 1988.

79. Gray, K. N., et al.: Histologic classification as an indication of therapeutic response in malignant lymphoma of dogs. J.A.V.M.A. 184:814, 1984.

80. Grekin, R. C., and Ellis, C. N.: Isotretinoin for the treatment of sebaceous hyperplasia. Cutis 34:90, 1984.

81. Grier, R. L., et al.: Hyperthermic treatment of superficial tumors in cats and dogs. J.A.V.M.A. 177:227, 1980.

82. Grier, R. L., et al.: Pilot study in the treatment with thioproline of 24 small animals with tumors. A.J.V.R. 45:2162, 1984.

83. Haneke, E.: Electron microscopy of Merkel cell

carcinoma from formalin-fixed tissue. J. Am. Acad. Dermatol. *12*:487, 1985.

84. Harasen, G. L. G.: Multicentric fibrosarcoma in a cat and a review of the literature. Can. Vet. J. *24*:207, 1984.

85. Hargis, A. M., and Thomassen, R. W.: Solar keratosis (solar dermatosis, senile keratosis) and solar keratosis with squamous cell carcinoma. Am. J. Pathol. *94*:193, 1979.

86. Harris, M.: Spindle cell squamous carcinoma: Ultrastructural observations. Histopathol. *6*:197, 1982.

87. Harvey, H. J., et al.: Prognostic criteria for dogs with oral melanoma. J.A.V.M.A. *178*:580, 1981.

88. Headington, J. T.: Tumors of the hair follicle. A review. Am. J. Pathol. *85*:480, 1976.

88a. Heald, P. W., and Edelson, R. L.: New therapies for cutaneous T-cell lymphoma. Arch. Dermatol. *123*:189, 1987.

88b. Heald, P. W., and Edelson, R. L.: Photopheresis for T cell mediated diseases. *In* Callen, J. P., et al. (eds.): Advances in Dermatology III. Year Book Medical Publishers, Chicago, 1988, p. 25.

89. Helfand, S. C., et al.: Immune-mediated thrombocytopenia associated with solid tumors in dogs. J.A.A.H.A. *21*:787, 1985.

90. Hill, D. L., et al.: Canine transmissible venereal sarcoma: Tumor cell and infiltrating leukocyte ultrastructure at different growth stages. Vet. Pathol. *21*:39, 1984.

90a. Hill, J. R.: Warty dyskeratoma in two dogs. Ann. Meet. Am. Acad. Vet. Dermatol., Am. Coll. Vet. Dermatol., 1987.

91. Hinsel, C. A., et al.: Cisplatin chemotherapy for metastatic squamous cell carcinoma in two dogs. J.A.V.M.A. *189*:1575, 1986.

92. Hofler, H., et al.: The intermediate filament cystoskeleton of cutaneous neuroendocrine carcinoma (Merkel cell tumor). Virchows Arch. Pathol. Anat. *406*:339, 1985.

93. Holmberg, C. A., et al.: Canine malignant lymphomas: Comparison of morphologic and immunologic parameters. J. Natl. Cancer Inst. *56*:125, 1976.

94. Holmberg, C. A., et al.: Feline malignant lymphomas: Comparison of morphologic and immunologic characteristics. A.J.V.R. *37*:1455, 1976.

95. Howard-Martin, M. O., and Qualls, C. W.: Metastatic melanoma in a cat. Feline Pract. *16*:6, 1986.

96. Jabara, A. G., and Finnie, J. W.: Four cases of clear-cell hidradenocarcinomas in the dog. J. Comp. Pathol. *88*:525, 1978.

97. Jabara, A. G., and Paton, J. S.: Extraskeletal osteoma in a cat. Aust. Vet. J. *61*:405, 1984.

98. Jacobs, R. M., et al.: Biclonal gammopathy in a dog with myeloma and cutaneous lymphoma. Vet. Pathol. *23*:211, 1986.

98a. Jensen, H. E., and Arnbjerg, J.: Bone metastasis of undifferentiated pulmonary adenocarcinoma in a cat. Nord. Vet. Med. *38*:288, 1986.

99. Jimbo, K., and Takami, T.: Cutaneous T-cell lymphoma and related disorders. Int. J. Dermatol. *25*:485, 1986.

100. Johnson, J. A., and Patterson, J. M.: Canine epidermotropic lymphoproliferative disease resembling pagetoid reticulosis in man. Vet. Pathol. *18*:487, 1981.

100a. Johnson, R. P., et al.: Malignant pilomatrixoma in an Old English Sheepdog. Can. Vet. J. *24*:392, 1983.

101. Jones, B. R., et al.: Cutaneous collagen nodules in a dog. J. Small Anim. Pract. *26*:445, 1985.

102. Jones, B. R., et al.: Cutaneous xanthomata associated with diabetes mellitus in a cat. J. Small Anim. Pract. *26*:33, 1985.

103. Jones, B. R., et al.: Inherited hyperchylomicronemia in the cat. Feline Pract. *16*:7, 1986.

104. Jones, S. A., and Strafuss, A. C.: Scanning electron microscopy of nerve sheath neoplasms. A.J.V.R. *39*:1069, 1978.

105. Kabay, M. J., and Jones, B. R.: Local current field radiofrequency treatment of superficial skin tumours in cats. N. Z. Vet. J. *31*:173, 1983.

105a. Kaplan, R. P.: Cancer complicating chronic ulcerative and scarifying mucocutaneous disorders. *In* Callen, J. P., et al. (eds.): Advances in Dermatology II. Year Book Medical Publishers, Chicago, 1987, p. 19.

106. Kavison, A. G., and Mann, F. C.: The transmissible venereal tumor of dogs. Observations on 40 generations of experimental transfers. Ann. N.Y. Acad. Sci. *54*:1197, 1952.

107. Kelly, W. R., et al.: Canine angiosarcoma (lymphangiosarcoma): A case report. Vet. Pathol. *18*:224, 1981.

108. Kendall, F. A., and MacDonald, D. M.: Pagetoid reticulosis. Histiocytic marker studies. Arch. Dermatol. *120*:76, 1984.

109. Knowles, D. P., and Hargis, A. M.: Solar elastosis associated with neoplasia in two dalmatians. Vet. Pathol. *23*:512, 1986.

110. Kraft, I., and Frese, K.: Histological studies on canine pigmented moles. J. Comp. Pathol. *86*:143, 1976.

111. Kraft, I., and Frese, K.: Lentigo-ähnliche Proliferation des Zitzenepithels beim Hund. Zbl. Veterinaermed. *A23*:234, 1976.

112. Kramek, B. A., et al.: Infiltrative lipoma in three dogs. J.A.V.M.A. *186*:81, 1985.

113. Krieger-Huber, S., and Faussner, M.: Nierenkarzinom und nodulare Dermatofibrose mit erblicher Disposition—Eine "neue" Erkrankung beim Deutschen Schaferhund. Kleintier Praxis *30*:235, 1985.

114. Kripke, M. L.: Immunology and photocarcinogenesis. J. Am. Acad. Dermatol. *14*:149, 1986.

114a. Kwochka, K. W.: Retinoids in dermatology. *In* Kirk, R. W. (ed.): Current Veterinary Therapy X. W. B. Saunders Company, Philadelphia (in press).

115. Kwochka, K. W., and Short, B. G.: Cutaneous xanthomatosis and diabetes mellitus following long-term therapy with megestrol acetate in cat. Compend. Cont. Ed. *6*:185, 1984.

116. Latimer, C. A., et al.: Azathioprine in the management of fibrous histiocytoma in two dogs. J.A.A.H.A. *19*:155, 1983.

117. Layfield, L., et al.: Neuroendocrine carcinoma of the skin: An immunohistochemical study of tumor markers and neuroendocrine products. J. Cut. Pathol. *13*:268, 1986.

117a. Legrand, J. J., et al.: Histiocytome fibreux malin chez un chat. Étude d'un cas clinique et comparison avec les donnees de la litterature. Prat. Med. Chirurg. Anim. Comp. *22*:401, 1987.

118. Leifer, C. E., and Matus, R. E.: Chronic lymphocytic leukemia in the dog: 22 cases (1974–1984). J.A.V.M.A. *189*:214, 1986.

119. Lester, S. J., and Mesfin, G. M.: A solitary plasmacytoma in a dog with progression to a disseminated myeloma. Can. Vet. J. *21*:284, 1980.

120. Lever, W. F., and Schaumburg-Lever, G.: *Histopathology of the Skin VI.* J. B. Lippincott Company, Philadelphia, 1983.

121. Lium, B., and Moe, L.: Hereditary and multifocal renal cystadenocarcinomas and nodular dermatofibrosis in the German shepherd dog: Macroscopic and histopathologic changes. Vet. Pathol. *22*:447, 1985.

122. Llombart-Bosch, A., et al.: Ultrastructure of vascular neoplasms. Pathol. Res. Pract. *174*:1, 1982.

123. MacEwen, E. G., et al.: Levamisole as adjuvant to chemotherapy for canine lymphosarcoma. J. Biol. Resp. Modif. *4*:427, 1985.

124. MacEwen, E. G.: Anti-tumor evaluation of benzaldehyde in the dog and cat. A.J.V.R. 47:451, 1986.

124a. Macy, D. W.: Canine and feline mast cell tumors: biologic behavior, diagnosis, and therapy. Semin. Vet. Med. Surg. 1:72, 1986.

125. Macy, D. W., and Reynolds, H. A.: The incidence, characteristics, and clinical management of skin tumors of cats. J.A.A.H.A. 17:1026, 1981.

126. Madewell, B. R., et al.: Multiple subungual squamous cell carcinomas in five dogs. J.A.V.M.A. 180:731, 1982.

126a. Madewell, B. R., et al.: Endocytosis of erythrocytes in vivo and particulate substances in vitro by feline neoplastic mast cells. Can. J. Vet. Res. 51:517, 1987.

127. Maiorana, A., et al.: Immunohistochemical markers of sweat gland tumors. J. Cutan. Pathol. 13:187, 1986.

128. Mandojana, R. M., and Helwig, E. B.: Localized epidermotropic reticulosis (Woringer-Kolopp disease). J. Am. Acad. Dermatol. 8:813, 1983.

129. Mann, G. E., and Stratton, J.: Dermoid sinus in the Rhodesian ridgeback. J. Small Anim. Pract. 7:631, 1966.

130. Mays, M. B. C., and Bergeron, J. A.: Cutaneous histiocytosis in dogs. J.A.V.M.A. 188:377, 1986.

131. McGavin, M. D., and Fisburn, F.: Perianal adenoma of apocrine origin in a dog. J.A.V.M.A. 166:388, 1975.

132. McKeever, P. J., et al.: Canine cutaneous lymphoma. J.A.V.M.A. 18:531, 1982.

133. McNutt, M. A., et al.: Coexpression of intermediate filaments in human epithelial neoplasms. Ultrastruct. Pathol. 9:31, 1985.

134. Mehregan, A. H.: The origin of the adnexal tumors of the skin: A viewpoint. J. Cutan. Pathol. 12:459, 1985.

135. Meuten, D. J., et al.: Hypercalcemia in dogs with adenocarcinoma derived from apocrine glands of the anal sac. Biochemical and histomorphometric investigations. Lab. Invest. 48:428, 1983.

136. Meyer, D. J., and Franks, P.: Clinical cytology part 1: Management of tissue specimens. Mod. Vet. Pract. 67:255, 1986.

137. Meyer, D. J., and Franks, P.: Clinical cytology part 2: Cytologic characteristics of tumors. Mod. Vet. Pract. 67:440, 1986.

138. Mickoloff, B. J., et al.: Canine regressing atypical histiocytoma: A neuroendocrine tumor. Arch. Dermatol. 120:1613, 1984.

139. Miettinen, M., et al.: Antibodies to intermediate filament proteins in the diagnosis and classification of human tumors. Ultrastruct. Pathol. 7:83, 1984.

140. Miller, W. H.: Canine cutaneous lymphomas. In Kirk, R. W., (ed.): Current Veterinary Therapy VII. W. B. Saunders Company, Philadelphia, 1980, pp. 493–495.

141. Miller, W. H.: Unpublished observations.

142. Moore, P. F.: Systemic histiocytosis of Bernese Mountain dogs. Vet. Pathol. 21:554, 1984.

143. Moore, P. F., and Rosin, A.: Malignant histiocytosis of Bernese Mountain dogs. Vet. Pathol. 23:1, 1986.

143a. Morton, L. D., et al.: Oral extramedullary plasmacytomas in two dogs. Vet. Pathol. 23:637, 1986.

144. Moulton, J. E.: Tumors in Domestic Animals. 2nd ed. University of California Press, Berkeley, 1978.

145. Muller, G. H., et al.: Small Animal Dermatology. 3rd ed. W. B. Saunders Company, Philadelphia, 1983.

146. Nickoloff, B. J.: Epidermal mucinosis in mycosis fungoides. J. Am. Acad. Dermatol. 15:83, 1986.

146a. Nickoloff, B. J. et al.: Canine neuroendocrine carcinoma: a tumor resembling histiocytoma. Am. J. Dermatopathol. 7:579, 1985.

147. Nielsen, S. W.: Classification of tumors in dogs and cats. J.A.A.H.A. 19:13, 1983.

148. O'Rourke, M.: Multiple digital squamous-cell carcinomas in 2 dogs. Mod. Vet. Pract. 66:644, 1985.

149. Palker, T. J., and Yang, T. J.: Detection of immune complexes in sera of dogs with canine transmissible venereal sarcoma (CTVS) by a conglutinin-binding assay. J. Comp. Pathol. 95:247, 1985.

150. Parker, C. M., and Hanke, C. W.: Large keratoacanthomas in difficult locations treated with intralesional 5-fluorouracil. J. Am. Acad. Dermatol. 14:770, 1986.

151. Patnaik, A. K., et al.: Canine cutaneous mast cell tumor: Morphologic grading and survival time in 83 dogs. Vet. Pathol. 21:469, 1984.

151a. Paulsen, M. E., et al.: Nodular granulomatous episclerokeratitis in dogs: 19 cases (1973–1985). J.A.V.M.A. 190:1581, 1987.

152. Peirce, A. R. J., et al.: Immunotherapy using mycobacterial cell-wall immunostimulants. Mod. Vet. Pract. 67:813, 1986.

153. Penneys, N. S., et al.: Granular cell tumors of the skin contain myelin basic protein. Arch. Pathol. Lab. Med. 107:302, 1983.

154. Peterson, S. L.: Scar-associated canine mast cell tumor. Canine Pract. 12:23, 1985.

155. Podkonjak, K. R.: Veterinary cryotherapy—1. Vet. Med. Small Anim. Clin. 77:51, 1982.

156. Podkonjak, K. R.: Veterinary cryotherapy—2. Vet. Med. Small Anim. Clin. 77:183, 1972.

157. Pollak, M., et al.: Metastatic squamous cell carcinoma in multiple digits of a cat: Case report. J.A.A.H.A. 20:835, 1984.

158. Pool, R. R., et al.: Primary lung carcinoma with skeletal metastasis in the cat. Feline Pract. 4:36, 1974.

159. Renlund, R. C., and Prhzker, K. P. H.: Malignant fibrous histiocytoma involving the digit in a cat. Vet. Pathol. 21:442, 1984.

159a. Richardson, R. C.: Tumors of the skin and subcutis. Proc. Ann. Kal Kan Symp. Treat. Small Anim. Dis. 10:113, 1986.

160. Richardson, R. C., et al.: Common skin tumors of the dog: A clinical approach to diagnosis and treatment. Compend. Cont. Ed. 6:1080, 1984.

161. Rode, J., et al.: Immunohistochemical staining of granular cell tumors for neurone specific enolase: Evidence in support of a neural origin. Diagn. Histopathol. 5:205, 1982.

162. Roholl, P. J. M., et al.: Application of markers in the diagnosis of soft tissue tumours. Histopathol. 9:1019, 1985.

163. Roholl, P. J. M., et al.: Characterization of tumour cells in malignant fibrous histiocytomas and other soft tissue tumours in comparison with malignant histiocytes. I. Immunohistochemical study on paraffin sections. J. Pathol. 147:87, 1985.

164. Rosenthal, R. C., and Kingston, R. E.: Nitrogen mustard: Human exposure and toxicity in a veterinary hospital. J.A.A.H.A. 20:821, 1984.

165. Rosin, A., et al.: Malignant histiocytosis in Bernese Mountain dogs. J.A.V.M.A. 188:1041, 1986.

165a. Rothwell, T. L. W., et al.: Skin neoplasms of dogs in Sydney, Aust. Vet. J. 64:161, 1987.

166. Roudebush, P., and MacDonald, J. M.: Mucocutaneous angiomatous hamartoma in a dog. J.A.A.H.A. 20:168, 1984.

167. Roundtable discussion: Veterinary immunotherapy: Today's treatments, tomorrow's possibilities. Vet. Med. 82:1131, 1986.

168. Rubin, S., and Shivaprasad, H. L.: Hypercalcemia associated with an anal sac adenocarcinoma in a castrated male dog. Compend. Cont. Ed. 7:348, 1985.

169. Rudd, R. G., et al.: A practical guide to clinical oncology—2: Surgical treatments. Vet. Med. 81:29, 1985.

169a. Sandusky, G. E., et al.: Diagnostic immunohistochemistry of canine round cell tumors. Vet. Pathol. 24:495, 1987.

170. Scavelli, T. D., et al.: Hemangiosarcoma in the cat: Retrospective evaluation of 31 surgical cases. J.A.V.M.A. 187:817, 1985.

170a. Schick, M. P., et al.: Calcinosis cutis secondary to percutaneous penetration of calcium chloride in dogs. J.A.V.M.A. 191:207, 1987.

171. Scott, D. W., et al.: Lymphoreticular neoplasia in a dog resembling malignant histiocytosis (histiocytic medullary reticulosis) in man. Cornell Vet. 69:176, 1979.

172. Scott, D. W.: Feline dermatology 1900–1978: A monograph. J.A.A.H.A. 16:331, 1980.

173. Scott, D. W., et al.: Nevi in the dog. J.A.A.H.A. 20:505, 1984.

174. Scott, D. W.: Lichenoid reactions in the skin of dogs: Clinicopathologic correlations. J.A.A.H.A. 20:305, 1984.

175. Scott, D. W.: Feline dermatology 1979–1982: Introspective retrospections. J.A.A.H.A. 20:537, 1984.

176. Scott, D. W., and Flanders, J. A.: Dilated pore of Winer in a cat. Feline Pract. 14:33, 1984.

177. Scott, D. W.: Feline dermatology 1983–1985: "The secret sits." J.A.A.H.A. 23:255, 1987.

178. Scott, D. W., et al.: Systemic histiocytosis in two dogs (submitted for publication).

179. Scott, D. W., and Buerger, R. G.: Idiopathic calcinosis circumscripta in the dog: A retrospective analysis of 130 cases. J.A.A.H.A. (in press).

180. Scott, D. W.: Unpublished observations.

181. Seiler, R. J.: Granular basal cell tumors in the skin of three dogs: A distinct histopathologic entity. Vet. Pathol. 18:23, 1981.

182. Selcer, E. A., et al.: Dermoid sinus in a Shih Tzu and a boxer. J.A.A.H.A. 20:634, 1984.

183. Shumer, S. M., and O'Keefe, E. J.: Bleomycin in the treatment of recalcitrant warts. J. Am. Acad. Dermatol. 9:91, 1983.

184. Sibley, R. K., et al.: Primary neuroendocrine (Merkel cell?) carcinoma of the skin. I. A clinicopathologic and ultrastructural study of 43 cases. Am. J. Surg. Pathol. 9:95, 1985.

185. Sibley, R. K., et al.: Primary neuroendocrine (Merkel cell?) carcinoma of the skin. II. An immunocytochemical study of 21 cases. Am. J. Surg. Pathol. 9:109, 1985.

186. Smith, J. S., et al.: Infiltrative corneal lesions resembling fibrous histiocytoma: Clinical and pathologic findings in 6 dogs and 1 cat. J.A.V.M.A. 169:722, 1976.

187. Stambaugh, J. E., et al.: Lymphangioma in 4 dogs. J.A.V.M.A. 173:759, 1978.

188. Stasko, T., et al.: Hyperkeratotic mycosis fungoides restricted to the palms. J. Am. Acad. Dermatol. 7:792, 1982.

189. Stephens, L. C., et al.: Virus-associated liposarcoma and malignant lymphoma in a kitten. J.A.V.M.A. 183:123, 1983.

190. Stephens, L. C., et al.: Attempted transmission of a feline virus–associated liposarcoma to newborn kittens. Vet. Pathol. 21:614, 1984.

191. Stoeckli, R., et al.: Canine epidermotropic lymphoma associated with the intercellular deposition of immunoglobulin on direct immunofluorescence testing. Companion. Anim. Pract. 1:36, 1988.

192. Su, W. P. D., et al.: Clinicopathologic correlations in leukemia cutis. J. Am. Acad. Dermatol. 11:121, 1984.

193. Sundberg, J. P., et al.: Immunoperoxidase localization of papillomaviruses in hyperplastic and neoplastic epithelial lesions of animals. Am. J. Vet. Res. 45:1441, 1984.

194. Sundberg, J. P., et al.: Cloning and characterization of a canine oral papillomavirus. Am. J. Vet. Res. 47:1142, 1986.

195. Susaneck, S. J.: Feline skin tumors. Compend. Cont. Ed. 5:251, 1983.

196. Susaneck, S. J., et al.: Inflammatory mammary carcinoma in the dog. J.A.A.H.A. 19:971, 1983.

197. Suzuki, Y., et al.: The value of blood group-specific lectin and endothelial associated antibodies in the diagnosis of vascular proliferations. J. Cutan. Pathol. 13:408, 1986.

198. Tams, T. R., and Macy, D. W.: Canine mast cell tumors. Compend. Cont. Ed. 3:869, 1981.

199. Theilen, G. H., and Madewell, B. R.: Veterinary Cancer Medicine. 2nd ed. Lea & Febiger, Philadelphia, 1987.

200. Thiers, B. H.: Controversies in mycosis fungoides. J. Am. Acad. Dermatol. 7:1, 1982.

201. Thoma, R. E., et al.: Phototherapy: A promising cancer therapy. Vet. Med. (S.A.C.) 78:1693, 1983.

202. Thrall, M. A., et al.: Cutaneous lymphosarcoma and leukemia in a dog resembling Sézary syndrome in man. Vet. Pathol. 21:182, 1984.

202a. Tinsley, P. E., and Taylor, D. O.: Immunotherapy for multicentric malignant mastocytoma in a dog. Mod. Vet. Pract. 68:225, 1987.

203. Tosca, A. D., et al.: Mycosis fungoides. Evaluation of immunohistochemical criteria for the early diagnosis of the disease and differentiation between stages. J. Am. Acad. Dermatol. 15:237, 1986.

204. Trigo, F. J., and Hargis, A. M.: Canine cutaneous plasmacytoma with regional lymph node metastasis. Vet. Med. (S.A.C.) 78:1749, 1983.

205. Tseng-tong, K.: Clear cell carcinoma of the skin. Am. J. Surg. Pathol. 4:573, 1980.

206. Turk, M. A. M., et al.: Canine granular cell tumour (myoblastoma): A report of four cases and review of the literature. J. Small Anim. Pract. 24:637, 1983.

207. Van Rensburg, I. B. J., and Petrick, S. W. T.: Extragenital malignant transmissible venereal tumour in a bitch. J. S. Afr. Vet. Assoc. 51:199, 1980.

207a. Wagner, R. F., and Krontiris, T. G.: Oncogenes and human malignancy. In Callen, J. P., et al. (eds.): Advances in Dermatology III. Year Book Medical Publishers, Chicago, 1988, p. 277.

208. Walsh, K. M., and Corapi, W. V.: Tricholemmomas in three dogs. J. Comp. Pathol. 96:115, 1986.

209. Walton, D. K., et al.: Cutaneous lymphangiosarcoma in a cat. Feline Pract. 13:21, 1983.

210. Walton, D. K.: Canine epidermotropic lymphoma (mycosis fungoides and pagetoid reticulosis). In Kirk, R. W., (ed.): Current Veterinary Therapy IX. W. B. Saunders Company, Philadelphia, 1986, p. 609.

211. Walton, G. S., and Gopinath, C.: Multiple myeloma in a dog with some unusual features. J. Small Anim. Pract. 13:703, 1972.

212. Wantzin, G. L., et al.: Occurrence of human T cell lymphotropic virus (type I) antibodies. J. Am. Acad. Dermatol. 15:598, 1986.

213. Weller, R. E., et al.: Histologic classification as a prognostic criterion for canine lymphosarcomas. A.J.V.R. 41:1310, 1980.

214. Wellman, M. L., et al.: Malignant histiocytosis in four dogs. J.A.V.M.A. 187:919, 1985.

215. White, J. V., and Dunstan, R. W.: Clinical and

histopathologic evaluation of canine dermal angiosarcoma: A case report. J.A.A.H.A. *20*:607, 1984.

216. White, S. D., et al.: Cutaneous matastases of a mammary adenocarcinoma resembling eosinophilic plaques in a cat. Feline Pract. *15*:27, 1985.

216a. Whiteley, L. O., and Leininger, J. R.: Neuroendocrine (Merkel) cell tumors of the canine oral cavity. Vet. Pathol. *24*:570, 1987.

217. Wick, M. R., and Manivel, J. C.: Epithelioid sarcoma and isolated necrobiotic granuloma: A comparative immunocytochemical study. J. Cutan. Pathol. *13*:253, 1986.

218. Wilcock, B. P., et al.: The morphology and behavior of feline cutaneous mastocytomas. Vet. Pathol. *23*:320, 1986.

219. Winkelman, R. K., et al.: The treatment of Sézary syndrome. J. Am. Acad. Dermatol. *10*:1000, 1984.

220. Withrow, S. J.: Symposium on cryosurgery. Vet. Clin. North Am. *10*:753, 1980.

220a. Wolfe, L. G., et al.: Biologic characterization of canine melanoma cell lines. Am. J. Vet. Res. *48*:1642, 1987.

221. Wolff, J. M., et al.: Intralesional interferon in the treatment of early mycosis fungoides. J. Am. Acad. Dermatol. *13*:604, 1985.

222. Wood, G. S., et al.: Leu-8 and Leu-9 antigen phenotypes: Immunologic criteria for the distinction of mycosis fungoides from cutaneous inflammation. J. Am. Acad. Dermatol. *14*:1006, 1986.

222a. Xu, F. N.: Ultrastructure of canine hemangiopericytoma. Vet. Pathol. *23*:643, 1986.

222b. Yang, T. J.: Parvovirus-induced regression of canine transmissible venereal sarcoma. Am. J. Vet. Res. *48*:799, 1987.

223. Yuspa, S. H.: Cutaneous chemical carcinogenesis. J. Am. Acad. Dermatol. *15*:1031, 1986.

224. Zackheim, H. S.: Cutaneous T-cell lymphomas. A review of the recent literature. Arch. Dermatol. *117*:295, 1981.

225. Zackheim, H. S., et al.: Topical carmustine (BCNU) for mycosis fungoides and related disorders. J. Am. Acad. Dermatol. *9*:363, 1983.

226. Zackheim, H. S.: Is "localized epidermotropic reticulosis" (Woringer-Kolopp disease) benign? J. Am. Acad. Dermatol. *11*:276, 1984.

21

Chronology of Veterinary Dermatology (1900–1988)

An overview of the history of veterinary dermatology, Historical Highlights—Ancient and Modern, can be found in chapter 90, pages 711 to 735, of the second edition of this book (1976). This material was updated for the third edition of this book (1983). Since the historical material is unchanged, it will not be repeated in the fourth edition. Instead, the chronology is given here and updated to 1988.

1900 Joseph Bayer and Eugene Fröhner of Vienna, Austria, persuaded Hugo Schindelka to write a book on skin diseases of domestic animals.

1903 Publication of the first book on veterinary dermatology *Hautkrankheiten bei Haustieren* (Skin Diseases of Domestic Animals) by Hugo Schindelka at Vienna.

1908 Publication of the second and final edition of Schindelka's book *Hautkrankheiten bei Haustieren.*

1910 Publication of the first book on comparative dermatology *Die Vergleichende Pathologie der Haut* (The Comparative Pathology of the Skin) by Julius Heller at Berlin, Germany.

1926 Publication of *Animal Dermatology* by Leblois in France.

1930 Publication of the book *Course in Skin Diseases of Domestic Animals* by N. N. Bogdanov at Moscow.

1931 Publication of *Die Klinik der Wichtigsten Tierdermatosen* (The Clinic of the Most Important Animal Dermatoses) by Julius Heller at Berlin, Germany.

1931 Publication of *Veterinari Dermatologie* by Frantisek Kral (Frank Kral) at Brno, Czechoslovakia.

1948 Frank Kral emigrated to the United States and joined the faculty of the School of Veterinary Medicine, University of Pennsylvania in Philadelphia. He formed the Veterinary Dermatology Clinic, which was the first teaching unit of animal skin diseases in the United States.

1953 Publication of *Veterinary Dermatology* by Frank Kral and Benjamin J. Novak, first veterinary dermatologic book in English: a complete revision, expansion and translation of Kral's 1931 book (325 pages).

1958 Formation of the Dermatology Subcommittee of the Committee on General Medicine of the American Animal Hospital Association on April 23, 1958. R. W. Worley and G. H. Muller, Cochairmen: first organization of veterinary dermatology.

1958   E. M. Farber appoints G. H. Muller to the clinical faculty of Stanford University's Dermatology Department and establishes the first center of comparative dermatology in America.

1959   R. M. Schwartzman obtains the first Ph.D. degree in Veterinary Dermatology and shortly thereafter joins F. Kral's veterinary dermatology section at the University of Pennsylvania.

1959   Formation of the Dermatology Committee of the American Animal Hospital Association on February 5, 1959. G. H. Muller, Chairman. Committee functioned for 7 years.

1959   Publication of the *Compendium of Veterinary Dermatology* by Frank Kral. Hand-out for Kral's cross-country symposia in 1959 (69 pages).

1962   Publication of *A Comparative Study of Skin Diseases of Dog and Man* by Robert M. Schwartzman and Milton Orkin: the first book in English on comparative dermatology (365 pages).

1963   Transatlantic Conference on Canine and Feline Dermatology at Chicago and London on April 26, 1963. Knowles, Muller, and Schwartzman for the United States; Singleton, Joshua, and Wilkinson for England.

1964   Publication of section on Dermatologic Diseases (edited by G. H. Muller) in R. W. Kirk's *Current Veterinary Therapy,* revised four times from 1966 to 1974, and two times from 1977 to 1980 (edited by R. E. W. Halliwell).

1964   Publication of chapter on "Feline diseases of the skin" by J. D. Conroy in *Feline Medicine.*

1964   The American Academy of Veterinary Dermatology was organized at Philadelphia by Conroy, Kral (President), Muller, and Schwartzman.

1964   Symposium on Comparative Physiology and Pathology of the Skin at London, England, in April, 1964. A. J. Rook and G. S. Walton, Chairmen. Proceedings were published in 1965.

1964   Publication of *Veterinary and Comparative Dermatology* by F. Kral and R. M. Schwartzman: a revision and expansion of Kral and Novak's *Veterinary Dermatology* (444 pages).

1964   First Symposium on Comparative Dermatology sponsored by the American Academy of Dermatology at Chicago on December 8, 1964. Milton Orkin was chairman of this and the next three symposia.

1965   Second Symposium on Comparative Dermatology, December 7, 1965, at Chicago.

1965   Publication of *Comparative Physiology and Pathology* by A. J. Rook and G. S. Walton.

1966   Third Symposium on Comparative Dermatology, December 5, 1966, at Miami, Florida.

1966   Symposium on Skin Diseases Common to Man and Animals at Palm Springs, California, on November 2, 1966. Orkin and Muller, Cochairmen.

1967   Fourth Symposium on Comparative Dermatology, December 4, 1967, at Chicago.

1967   Publication of *Atlas of Canine and Feline Dermatoses* by R. M. Schwartzman and Frank Kral.

1968   Publication of the atlas *Canine Skin Lesions* by G. H. Muller.

1968   J. D. Conroy receives a Ph.D. degree and thereby launches the first career devoted exclusively to veterinary dermatohistopathology in America.

1969   Publication of *Small Animal Dermatology* by G. H. Muller and R. W. Kirk (485 pages): the first complete textbook devoted exclusively to skin diseases of dogs and cats. Used as textbook by many schools of veterinary medicine. Translated into Japanese and French and reprinted in Taiwan.

1970   Formation of an organizing committee of the American College of Veterinary Dermatologists consisting of Blakemore, Conroy, Muller (Chairman), Schwartzman, Kirk, and Kral.

1973   The formation of the *Task Force on Comparative Dermatology* as part of the *National Program for Dermatology* of the *American Academy of Dermatology.*

1974   Publication of the atlas *Feline Skin Lesions* by G. H. Muller.

1974   Publication of a stereoscopic atlas of *Clinical Dermatology of Small Animals* by G. G. Doering and H. E. Jensen (211 pages).

1974   Dermatology Specialty Group of the American College of Veterinary Internal Medicine (ACVIM) receives approval of the Advisory Board of Veterinary Specialties of the American Veterinary Medical Association (AVMA) on April 5, 1974.

1974   The first meeting of the Dermatology Specialty Group of the ACVIM was held on April 20, 1974, at San Francisco.

1974   The Dermatology Specialty Group was officially recognized by receiving probationary approval of the ACVIM and Council of Education of the AVMA on July 20, 1974, at Denver, Colorado.

1976   Formation of the British Veterinary Dermatology Study Group on February 20, 1976. Honorary Secretary Brian G. Bagnal; committee members Michael R. Geary, Raymond Hopes, David H. Lloyd, and Keith L. Thoday.

1976   Publication of the *Veterinary Dermatology Newsletter* (Vol. 1, No. 1) in May 1976 by the British Veterinary Dermatology Study Group.

1976   Publication of the second edition of *Small Animal Dermatology* by G. H. Muller and R. W. Kirk. Translated into Italian (809 pages).

1979   Publication of *The Skin and Internal Disease* (edited by G. H. Muller), the Veterinary Clinics of North America, 1979, W. B. Saunders Company (152 pages).

1980   Publication of *Feline Dermatology 1900–1978: A Monograph* by D. W. Scott (128 pages).

1980   Frank Kral deceased September 7, 1980.

1981   Membership list of the diplomates of the Veterinary Dermatology Specialty Group of the ACVIM: R. K. Anderson, V. H. Austin, B. B. Baker, J. C. Blakemore, P. T. Breen, D. K. Chester, J. D. Conroy, G. G. Doering, C. E. Griffin, R. E. W. Halliwell, P. J. Ihrke, R. W. Kirk, G. A. Kunkle, J. M. MacDonald, T. O. Manning, W. H. Miller, G. H. Muller, G. H. Nesbitt, L. M. Reedy, R. M. Schwartzman, D. W. Scott, E. Small, and A. A. Stannard.

1981   Formation of a French veterinary dermatologic organization: Groupe D'Étude en Dermatologie des Animaux de Compagnie (GEDAC). President Pierre Fourrier, Secretary Didier Carlotti.

1981   Publication of *Canine Dermatoses* by J. M. Keep (Australia).

1981   Publication of *Feline Dermatoses* by J. M. Keep (Australia).

1982   On March 9, 1982, the American Board of Veterinary Specialties of the AVMA granted probationary approval to the American College of Veterinary Dermatology as a certifying body in Veterinary Dermatology. This group replaces the Dermatology Specialty Group of the ACVIM.

The organizing committee of the American College of Veterinary Dermatology consists of Doctors J. C. Blakemore, J. D. Conroy, R. E. W. Halliwell, G. H. Muller, and E. Small.

1982   The American College of Veterinary Dermatology was approved by the Council of Education of the AVMA on April 23, 1982, and approved by the House of Delegates of the AVMA on July 20, 1982. The charter members of the group are the diplomates of the ACVIM (Dermatology) listed under 1981. There were 24 diplomates at the end of 1982.

1982   Formation of a German veterinary dermatology organization called the "Freundeskreis Hautkrankheiten Interessierter Tierärtzte." The organizing members are H. Koch (President), B. Beardi, G. Feslev, H. Gehrig, G. Kasa, F. Kasa, G. H. Muller, and C. Terling. The first meeting was held on October 12, 1982, at Birkenfeld, West Germany. The name of this organization was later changed to: Arbeitskreis Veterinär Dermatologie.

1983   Publication of the third edition of *Small Animal Dermatology* by G. H. Muller, R. W. Kirk, and D. W. Scott (889 pages). Translated into Portuguese and Japanese.

1983   Publication of *Canine and Feline Dermatology: A Systematic Approach* by G. H. Nesbitt (244 pages).

1984   Formation of the European Society of Veterinary Dermatology (ESVD) on September 18, 1984. President Hans Koch (Germany), Vice President Ton Willemse (Holland), Secretary David Lloyd (England), Treasurer Didier Carlotti (France), Membership Secretary Pierre Fourrier (France), Meeting Secretary Claudia Von Tscharner (Switzerland). Honorary Members Richard Halliwell, Peter Ihrke, Robert Kirk, George Muller, and Danny Scott (USA).

1984   Formation of an Australian veterinary dermatology organization began; started informally that year under the auspices of the Australian College of Veterinary Scientists. It granted full fellowship by examination in veterinary dermatology to Kenneth V. Mason on August 28, 1984. Two other veterinarians, George Wilkinson and Susan Shaw, are qualified in internal medicine and practicing veterinary dermatology within university organizations. It is hoped that dermatology will soon be accepted as a full specialty under the umbrella of the Australian College of Veterinary Scientists.

1984   Publication of *Equine Dermatoses* by R. Pascoe (Australia).

1985   Publication of the *Color Atlas of Small Animal Dermatology* by G. T. Wilkinson (272 pages), Australia.

1986   Publication of *Skin Diseases in the Dog and Cat* by D. I. Grant (187 pages), England.

1986   Formation of the Canadian Academy of Veterinary Dermatology. President Lowell Ackerman, Secretary B. P. Pukay.

1987   Publication of *Contemporary Issues in Small Animal Practice: Dermatology* Volume 8, New York (332 pages) (edited by G. H. Nesbitt).

1987   In addition to the diplomates listed in 1981, new diplomates of the American College of Veterinary Dermatology who have passed the board examination recently are L. Ackerman, D. E. Bevier, R. G. Buerger, P. L. Caciolo, D. J. DeBoer, A. G. Evans, V. A. Fadok, C. S. Foil, K. A. Helton-Rhodes, K. W. Kwochka, L. Medleau, P. J. McKeever, W. S. Rosenkrantz, E. J. Rosser, V. J. Scheidt, K. J. Shanley, C. Sousa, D. Walton Angarano, and S. D. White.

1987   Formation, on October 23, of the Italian Veterinary Dermatology Group as part of the Italian Small Animal Veterinary Association (SCIVAC). President, Alessandra Fondati.

1988   Publication of *Large Animal Dermatology* by D. W. Scott (487 pages).

1989   Publication of the fourth edition of *Small Animal Dermatology* by G. H. Muller, R. W. Kirk, and D. W. Scott (1007 pages). Translated into German.

References

Bogdanov, N. N.: Course in Skin Diseases of Domestic Animals. Government Publishing House, Moscow, 1930.

Heller, J.: Die Vergleichende Pathologie der Haut. August Hirschwald, Berlin, 1910.

Heller, J.: Die Klinik der Wichtigsten Tierdermatosen. *In* Jadassohn: Handbuch der Haut und Geschlechtskrankheiten. Julius Springer, Berlin, 1930.

Kirk, R. W.: Current Veterinary Therapy V. W. B. Saunders Company, Philadelphia, 1974.

Kral, F., and Novak, B. J.: Veterinary Dermatology. J. B. Lippincott Company, Philadelphia, 1953.

Kral, F., and Schwartzman, R. M.: Veterinary and Comparative Dermatology. J. B. Lippincott Company, Philadelphia, 1964.

Leblois, C.: Documents pour servir à l'édification d'une dermatologie animale (chien et chat). Vigot Frères Editeurs, Paris, 1926.

Muller, G. H., and Kirk, R. W.: Small Animal Dermatology. 1st ed. W. B. Saunders Company, Philadelphia, 1969.

Orkin, M.: Symposium of skin diseases common to man and animals. J.A.M.A. *197*, 1966.

Rook, A. J., and Walton, G. S.: Comparative Physiology and Pathology of the Skin. F. A. Davis Company, Philadelphia, 1965.

Schindelka, H.: Hautkrankheiten bei Haustieren. Wilhelm Braumüller, Vienna, 1902.

Schneidemühl, G.: Lehrbuch der Vergleichenden Pathologie und Therapie des Menchen und der Haustiere. Wilhelm Engelmann, Leipzig, 1898.

Schwartzman, R. M.: Atlas of Canine and Feline Dermatoses. Lea & Febiger, Philadelphia, 1968.

Schwartzman, R. M., and Orkin, M.: A Comparative Study of Skin Diseases of Dog and Man. Charles C. Thomas, Springfield, Illinois, 1962.

Scott, D. W.: Feline dermatology 1900–1978: a monograph. J.A.A.H.A. *16*:331, 1980.

Glossary

Abrasion—Superficial removal of epidermis resulting in oozing and crusting.

Abscess—Localized collection of pus in a cavity formed by disintegration of tissue.

Acantholysis—Loss of cohesion between keratinocytes.

Acanthosis—A diffuse hypertrophy of the prickle cell layer of the epidermis.

Acanthosis nigricans—A cutaneous reaction pattern with multiple causes. It is characterized by axillary hyperpigmentation and lichenification.

Acariasis—An infestation caused by any mite.

Acarus—A mite.

Acne—A dermatosis characterized by a primary lesion called a comedo or blackhead. These are often inflamed or infected.

Acral—Pertaining to distal parts of the body, especially the extremities.

Actinic—Refers to the injurious effect of ultraviolet light.

Actinodermatitis—An inflammatory condition of the skin caused by visible or ultraviolet light.

Actinomycotic mycetoma—A lesion caused by bacteria of the order Actinomycetales.

Adenoma—Benign neoplasia of a gland.

Adnexa—Pertaining to the skin, it means structures that are bound to it, i.e., hair, claws, and eccrine, sebaceous, and apocrine glands. Extruded hair shafts and claws are more accurately called appendages.

Aleuriospore—A terminal or lateral spore attached by a wide base to the conidiophore; it is released by fracture of the cell wall below the spore.

Aleurioconidium (pl. aleurioconidia)—A thick-walled terminal conidium formed from the blown-out ends of a conidiogenous cell, as in *Microsporum* sp.

Allergen—A substance that is capable of inducing an allergic state.

Allergy—The specific immunologic process that serves to preserve the biologic identity of animal organisms; often used interchangeably with "hypersensitivity."

Alopecia—Loss of hair.

Amyloid—A mucopolysaccharide related to chondroitin sulfuric acid that may make up the ground substance of some tissue.

Anagen—The phase of the hair cycle during which synthesis of hair takes place.

Anaphylactic—Possessing anaphylaxis.

Anaphylaxis—An unusual or exaggerated reaction of the organism to foreign protein or other substances.

Anaplasia—A loss of differentiation of cells and their orientation to one another and to their axial framework and blood vessels. A characteristic of tumor tissue.

965

Annelide—A conidiogenous cell producing conidia that develop from a proliferation through the scars left by the previous conidia, as in *Scopulariopsis* sp.

Annelloconidium (pl. *annelloconidia*)—A conidium that develops from an annelide, as in *Scopulariopsis* sp.

Annular—Shaped like a ring.

Anonychia—Congenital absence of a nail or claw.

Anthropophilic—Having a preference for man. Used dermatologically, pertaining to anthropophilic fungi whose primary host is man.

Antibody—A modified type of serum globulin synthesized by lymphoid tissue in response to antigenic stimulus, each differing haptenic structure of one antigen molecule being capable of inciting a distinct response.

Antigen—A substance or complex of high molecular weight, usually protein or protein-polysaccharide complex in nature, which, when foreign to the blood stream of an animal or gaining access to the tissues of such an animal, stimulates the formation of a specific antibody and reacts specifically in vivo or in vitro with its homologous antibody.

Antitoxin—An antibody that neutralizes an antigen that is a toxin.

Aplasia—A condition of failure or lack of full development or growth.

Apocrine—Denoting that type of glandular secretion in which the secretory products become concentrated at the free end of the secreting cell and are thrown off together with the portion of the cell where they have accumulated, as in the mammary gland.

Appendages—Claw plates and hair shafts that hang from the skin. "Adnexa" is a better word for skin glands, claw matrix, and the pilosebaceous apparatus.

Arciform—Shaped in curves (refers to the shape of lesions).

Arthroconidium (pl. *arthroconidia*)—conidium that results from fragmentation of a hypha at the septum, as in *Geotrichum* sp.

Arthrospore—A spore formed by septation of hyphae with subsequent separation of cells.

Ascomycota—A division of fungi that produce asci.

Ascospore—A spore that results from karyogamy and meiosis and is formed within an ascus.

Ascus (pl. *asci*)—A sac-shaped cell in the Ascomycota that after karyogamy and meiosis produces ascospores.

Atopy—A clinical hypersensitivity state that is subject to hereditary influences. Canine atopy is characterized by scratching, paw licking, face rubbing, and, rarely, sneezing.

Atrophy—A defect or failure of nutrition manifested as a wasting away or diminution in the size of a cell, tissue, organ, or part.

Autoimmunization—The production in an organism of reactivity to its own tissues, with appearance of certain clinical and laboratory manifestations as a result of the altered immunologic response.

Bacterial pseudomycetoma—Preferred term for botryomycosis, a bacterial granuloma.

Basidiomycota—A division of fungi that produce basidia.

Basidiospore—A spore that results from karyogamy and meiosis and is formed on a basidium.

Basidium (pl. *basidia*)—A club-shaped cell in the Basidiomycota that after karyogamy and meiosis supports the basidiospores.

Benign—Mild or not serious; not malignant.

Biopsy—The examination of a specimen from live tissue, usually with a microscope.

Blastoconidium (pl. blastoconidia)—An asexual unit produced by budding, as in *Cladosporium* or *Candida* sp.

Blister—A thin-walled structure containing air or fluid; dermatologically, vesicles and bullae.

Botryomycosis—A bacterial granuloma (especially staphylococcal).

Budding—Asexual reproduction producing blastoconidia, as in *Cladosporium* or *Candida* sp.

Bulla—A large vesicle or blister.

Calcinosis—A pathologic condition in which calcium in abnormal amounts has been abnormally deposited. The condition of calcium deposits occurring in the skin is called "calcinosis cutis"; those occurring in localized small nodules in the subcutaneous tissue or muscle are called "calcinosis circumscripta."

Callus—Hypertrophy of the horny layer (stratum corneum) in localized areas, especially over pressure points.

Capsule—A hyaline gelatinous sheath that surrounds a cell, as seen in *Cryptococcus* sp.

Carbuncle—A lesion consisting of multiple cutaneous abscesses that are connected by sinuses.

Carcinoma—A malignant new growth made up of epithelial cells tending to infiltrate the surrounding tissues and give rise to metastases.

Catagen—That phase of the hair cycle in which there is a transition from growth (anagen) to cessation of growth and inception of an end stage (telogen).

Cerumen—The waxlike secretion of the specialized apocrine glands of the ear canal.

Chalazion—A small tumor of the eyelid formed by a chronic inflammation of the meibomian gland.

Chlamydospore—A thick-walled, intercalary or terminal vegetative cell that by thickening of the wall has become modified into a resting spore; as in *Candida albicans*.

Chromo body—A sclerotic body consisting of dematiaceous, muriform, thick-walled cells in chromoblastomycosis.

Chromoblastomycosis—A mycotic infection of cutaneous and subcutaneous tissues characterized by sclerotic bodies. There are no valid reports of chromoblastomycosis in animals.

Chromomycosis—A fungal infection that is characterized by dematiaceous fungal elements in tissue. This term includes both phaeohyphomycosis and chromoblastomycosis.

Civatte's body—Necrotic epidermal basal cell; also called a "colloid," "hyaline," or "apoptotic" body.

Clavate—Club-shaped.

Clear cell—A kind of cell found regularly in the basal cell layer of the epidermis (melanocyte, Langhans' cell, and others).

Cleft—A slitlike space within the epidermis.

Cleistothecium—A closed fruit body containing asci.

Collagen—The normal fibrillar substance of the connective tissue of the dermis.

Columella (pl. *columellae*)—The sterile domelike inflated area at the tip of a sporangiophore, as in *Absidia* sp.

Comedo (pl. *comedones*)—A plug of keratin and dried sebum in an excretory duct (or hair follicle) of the skin.

Confluent—Becoming merged or running together; not discrete.

Conidiogenous cell—A cell that produces conidia.

Conidiophore—A specialized hypha upon which conidia develop.

Conidium (pl. *conidia*)—An asexual reproductive structure that gives rise to genetically identical organisms.

Contact dermatitis—Inflammation of skin resulting from external application of a primary irritant (primary irritant contact dermatitis) or of an ordinarily harmless substance toward which a state of sensitization has been established (allergic contact dermatitis).

Cornification—The process of callosity or becoming horny; hyperkeratosis.

Crust—A dried exudate on the surface of a lesion.

Cutaneous—Pertaining to skin.

Cutaneous asthenia—A loss of strength in the skin and subcutaneous tissues. The Ehlers-Danlos syndrome.

Cutis—The entire skin; frequently, the dermis.

Cyst—A sac, bladder, or fluid-filled, circumscribed, walled process that is not inflamed.

Dalmatian bronzing syndrome—Old term for a cutaneous reaction now recognized as a generalized folliculitis and hypersensitivity dermatitis.

Dandruff—A word used by laymen to indicate excessive scaliness of the scalp or of hairy skin.

Degeneration—Deterioration; change of a tissue from a higher to a lower or less active functional form.

Dematiaceous—Darkly pigmented, usually black to brown, as in *Alternaria* sp.

Demodex—A genus of mites. *Demodex canis* causes demodicosis in dogs.

Demodicosis—A skin disease associated with infestation by demodectic mites.

Depigmentation—The act or result of removing pigment (in skin usually implies melanin).

Dermal—Pertaining to the skin.

Dermatitis (pl. *dermatitides*)—Inflammation of the skin. Never a synonym for all skin disease.

Dermatoglyphics—Surface characteristics of the skin with respect to its folds, furrows, ridges, and wrinkles.

Dermatology—The study of everything that relates to the skin in health and disease.

Dermatomycosis (pl. *dermatomycoses*)—A fungal infection of the skin or its appendages. The term includes dermatophytosis as well as deep fungal infections.

Dermatophyte—A fungus parasitic upon the skin, hair, or claws. The term embraces imperfect fungi of the genera *Microsporum, Epidermophyton,* or *Trichophyton*.

Dermatophytosis (pl. *dermatophytoses*)—A fungal infection of the skin caused by *Microsporum, Trichophyton,* or *Epidermophyton*. Of the three genera, *Microsporum* and *Trichophyton* are the most common in animals.

Dermatosis—A pathologic condition of the skin.

Dermis—The corium or layer of skin between the epidermis and the subcutaneous tissue.

Desensitization—The process of reducing sensitivity. An immunologic transformation to a new state of insensitivity.

Diffuse—Not definitely limited or localized; widely distributed.

Dimorphic—Having two morphologic forms, such as *Histoplasma capsulatum*, which has a yeast and mycelium form.

Discrete—Made up of separate parts or characterized by lesions that do not become blended.

Disseminated—Disposed in separate patches.

Distichiasis—A double row of eyelashes.

Dopa—Dihydroxyphenylalanine.

Dry pyoderma—Old term for skin reaction, seen with zinc-responsive dermatoses.

Dyskeratosis—Abnormal, premature, or imperfect keratinization of the keratinocytes.

Ecchymosis—Dermal hemorrhage greater than 1 cm in diameter.

Eccrine—Secreting outward (as sweat). Exocrine.

Echinulate—Delicately spiny, as the macroconidia or *Microsporum* sp.

Ectoderm—The "external skin," the outermost of the three primary layers of the developing embryo.

Ectothrix—A fungal infection of hair characterized by arthroconidia on the external surface of the hair shaft with hyphae penetrating and invading the hair shaft. Ectothrix invasion of hair may be observed with *Microsporum canis* and *Trichophyton mentagrophytes* infection.

Ectropion—Turning out of the eyelids.

Eczema—An inflammatory, superficial skin disease that in an early stage is erythematous, papulovesicular, oozing, and crusting and that later becomes red-purple, scaly, lichenified, and possibly pigmented. Through misuse, its meaning has become vague and indefinite.

Edema—Swelling caused by abnormal amounts of fluid in tissues.

Elastic fibers—Stretchable fibers consisting of elastin fibrils held together by a cementing substance, and entwined among collagen bundles of the dermis.

Elastin—The normal material of elastic fibers.

Emollient—Softening, or a softening agent.

Emulsion—A preparation of one liquid distributed in small globules throughout the body of a second liquid; "a milklike product."

Endocrine—Secreting within, or dispersing into, the circulation; applied to the organs that secrete into blood or lymph a substance, especially hormones, that has a specific effect on another organ.

Endoderm—The "inner skin," the innermost of the three primary layers of the developing embryo.

Endospore—See Sporangiospore.

Endothelium—Layer of epithelial cells lining the cavities of heart, blood, and lymph vessels and the serous body cavities.

Endothrix—A fungal infection of hair characterized by fungal invasion within the hair shaft. The hair cuticle is not broken.

Entity—A specific, distinct condition.

Entropion—Turning in of the eyelids.

Eosinophilic—Taking the color of eosin (pink).

Epidermal atrophy—A lack of full development of the epidermis.

Epidermal collarette—A peeling edge of epithelium surrounding an erosion or ulcer.

Epidermal papilla—See Tylotrich pad.

Epidermis—The outer layer of the skin just above the dermis.

Epidermolysis—Separation of the epidermis and dermis with the formation of clefts and vesicles or bullae.

Epilate—To remove hair.

Epilation—Removal of hair.

Epithelioma—Neoplasia of the epithelium.

Epulis—A growth (fibroma or sarcoma) of the gingiva or underlying bone.

Erosion—A superficial breakdown or shallow ulceration of the skin that involves only the epidermis and heals without scarring.

Eruption—A rapidly developing lesion of the skin due to disease and marked by redness, prominence, or both.

Erythema—A redness of the skin produced by congestion of the capillaries.

Erythematous—Possessing a redness of the skin.

Eschar—A necrotic scab or crust usually caused by a burn.

Eukaryote—An organism whose cells have a true nucleus bounded by a nuclear membrane.

Excoriation—Erosions and ulcers caused by scratching, biting, or other physical damage.

Exfoliation—The shedding of leaflike scales or layers.

Exocrine—Separating (or secreting) to the outside.

Exocytosis—The migration of inflammatory cells or erythrocytes or both through the intercellular spaces of epidermis.

Exudation—The escape of fluid, cells, and cellular debris from blood vessels and their deposition in or on the tissues. Usually the result of inflammation.

Feline endocrine alopecia—Old term for a cutaneous reaction pattern now known as feline symmetric alopecia and caused by hypersensitivity, psychogenic, or idiopathic factors.

Feline eosinophilic granuloma complex—Old term for a cutaneous reaction pattern caused by feline flea bite hypersensitivity, food allergy, or atopy.

Feline miliary dermatitis—Old term for a cutaneous reaction pattern caused by multiple factors, but especially feline flea bite hypersensitivity, food allergy, and atopy.

Festoons—Dermal papillae, devoid of attached epidermal cells, that project into a vesicle.

Fibril—A single fine thread structure (in the dermis).

Fibroblast—The parenchymal cells of the dermis that produce the collagen bundles.

Fibroma—A hard papule, nodule, or tumor that histologically shows fibroblasts and their product (collagen bundles) in a dense formation.

Fibroplasia—The formation and development of fibrous tissue in increased amounts.

Fissure—A splitting or discontinuity of a surface, especially one that persists.

Fistula—A deep, sinuous ulcer, often leading to an internal hollow organ.

Flexuose—Winding or wavy.

Foam cell—A histiocyte that has imbibed various materials and has thus come to appear bubbled.

Follicle—A tiny, saclike structure. In dermatology it particularly refers to the housing of the hair apparatus.

Follicular plug—An accumulation of excess keratin in an inactive hair follicle.

Folliculitis—Inflammation of a follicle or follicles.

Fungal—Caused by or relating to a fungus. Synonymous with the adjective "fungous."

Fungicidal—An agent or procedure that kills fungi.

Fungistatic—An agent or process that arrests the growth of fungi.

Fungi Imperfecti (Deuteromycota)—Fungi whose asexual state is known but whose sexual state is unknown.

Fungus (pl. fungi)—The kingdom of eukaryotic achlorophyllous organisms that may have unicellular and/or multicellular forms. The kingdom of the fungi contains five divisions: Chytridiomycota, Zygomycota, Basidiomycota, Ascomycota, and Fungi Imperfecti or Deuteromycota.

Furunculosis—Rupture of hair follicles due to severe inflammation.

Fusiform—Spindle-shaped; narrowing toward the ends.

Geniculate—Bent like a knee.

Geophilic—Pertaining to organisms that normally inhabit the soil, such as *Microsporum gypseum*.

Germ tube—Initial formation of a hypha.

Glabrous—Smooth, referring to hairless skin.

Gland—An aggregation of cells specialized to secrete or excrete materials not related to their ordinary metabolic needs.

Glands of Krause and Wolfring—Accessory lacrimal glands located on the inner surface of the eyelids.

Glands of Manz—Glandular depressions at the margin of the eyelid.

Glands of Moll—Apocrine glands of the cilia.

Glands of Zeis—Sebaceous glands of the cilia.

Glomus—A body shaped like a ball of wool or yarn.

Granuloma—A circumscribed tissue reaction wherein the histiocyte or macrophage is a predominant cell type.

Grenz zone—Marginal zone of relatively normal dermis that separates the epidermis from an underlying pathologic process.

Group—An assemblage of lesions having certain things in common, such as location or form.

Guttate—Characterized by lesions that are drop-shaped.

Gynecomastia—Enlargement of the male mammary gland.

Haarscheiben—See Tylotrich pad.

Hair—A single thread of keratin.

Hapten—A substance that becomes antigenic when it complexes with proteins.

Hemangioma—A massing, overdevelopment, or tumefaction of blood vessels.

Herpetiform—Marked by a cluster of vesicles, or having the form of herpes.

Histiocyte—A dermal cell of monocyte origin.

Hives—A condition characterized by wheals.

Holocrine—Entirely secretory. Applied to the sebaceous gland whose product is a complete shedding of cellular substance.

Hordeolum—An acutely painful, pyogenic infection of a sebaceous gland of the eyelid; a sty. External hordeolum involves a gland of Zeis; internal hordeolum involves a meibomian gland.

Horn—Hard keratin.

Hyaline—Colorless, transparent, glassy.

Hydropic degeneration—Intracellular edema and disintegration of epidermal basal cells.

Hypergranulosis—An increased thickness of the granular layer in the epidermis.

Hyperhidrosis—Increased sweating.

Hyperkeratosis—An increased thickness (cornification) of the horny layer of the skin.

Hyperpigmentation—Excessive coloration of the skin caused by increased deposition of pigment (especially melanin).

Hyperplasia—Excessive growth (of cells).

Hypersensitivity—A specific immunologic response that is injurious.

Hypertrophy—Overdevelopment.

Hypha (pl. *hyphae*)—A vegetative filament of a fungus.

Hypopigmentation—Less than normal pigmentation.

Hyposensitization—Desensitization; the procedure of decreasing or eliminating sensitivity to offending substances.

Hypotrichosis—Presence of less than the normal amount of hair.

Ichthyosis—Any of several congenital skin disorders characterized by dryness, roughness, and scaliness owing to hyperkeratosis. A result of excess production or excess retention of keratin, or a molecular defect in keratin.

Imperfect state (or stage)—The portion of a fungal life cycle characterized by asexual reproduction.

Impetigo—A superficial pyogenic infection with pustules and friable, adherent crusts.

Indurated—Hardened.

Infectious—Caused by microbial agents; may imply communicability.

Infestation—The state of harboring metazoal parasites on or in the body.

Infiltrate—To penetrate into tissue; used especially of invasion by cells that are not normal to the location. Also, material deposited by infiltration.

Inflammation—A condition of tissues reacting to injury. There are pain, heat, redness, swelling, and sometimes loss of function.

Intertrigo—Dermatitis caused by chafing of the skin between two adjacent areas, as between toes or flanks.

Intradermal—Within the dermis.

Intraepidermal—Within the epidermis.

Inunction—The action and result of rubbing or smearing oil or salve into the skin.

Ischemia—Deficiency of blood in a part resulting from severe interference with circulation.

Itching—An unpleasant cutaneous sensation that provokes the desire to scratch or rub the skin.

Karyogamy—Cell conjugation with union of nuclei.

Keratin—Any of various sulfur-containing fibrous proteins that form the chemical basis of horny epidermal tissue.

Keratohyaline granules—Specks seen within the cells of the granular layer that appear glassy (hyaline) and of the character of horn (kerato-) in conventional histologic staining. They may be precursor substances of finished keratin.

Keratolysis—Dissolving or peeling of keratin from the epidermis.

Keratolytic—Causing keratolysis.

Keratosis—A condition of excessive development of horny tissue.

Kerion—A nodular, boggy, circumscribed fungal and bacterial infection of the skin and hair follicles.

Lacuna—A slitlike space within the epidermis.

Lanugo—The fine down or woolly hair.

Lentigo—A lentil-shaped, pigmented spot like a freckle.

Lesion—Any pathologic or traumatic deviation from normal tissue.

Leukocytoclasis—Karyorrhexis of neutrophils, resulting in "nuclear dust."

Leukocytosis—An increased number of white blood cells.

Leukoderma—Acquired lack of pigment in skin; also called acromoderma.

Leukonychia—Whitish discoloration of nail or claw.

Leukoplakia—Flat, white patches of hyperkeratinization on mucous membranes.

Leukotrichia—Acquired lack of pigment in hair; also called achromotrichia.

Lichenification—A thickening and hardening of the skin characterized by an exaggeration of the superficial skin markings and usually accompanied by hyperpigmentation.

Lichenoid—*Grossly*, refers to flat-topped papules; *microscopically*, refers to a dense band of mononuclear cells that obscure the dermoepidermal junction.

Lotion—A liquid preparation that is applied to the skin as a paint rather than as a wash.

Lupus—A chronic local skin condition attended more or less with hypertrophy, absorption, and ulceration. It is rarely used alone, but with a modifier, e.g., lupus erythematosus.

Maceration—The softening and disintegration of tissue by wetting.

Macroconidium (pl. *macroconidia*)—The larger of two different sizes of conidia produced by a single fungus, as in *Fusarium*.

Macule—A perceptible circumscribed change in color on, in, or of the skin that is not visibly raised above or depressed below the surrounding general level of the skin. Macules larger than 1 cm in diameter are referred to as patches.

Malassezia pachydermatitis—Preferred term for *Pityrosporum canis*.

Mange—A skin disease of animals caused by a mite. Sarcoptic mange (*Sarcoptes scabiei*) and demodectic mange (*Demodex canis*) are now called canine scabies and demodicosis.

Mast cell—A large cell containing metachromatically staining cytoplasmic granules that contain heparin and histamine.

Mastocytosis—A condition in which mast cells are abnormally abundant.

Matrix—The source from which development takes place, a parental stem.

Max Joseph spaces—Subepidermal clefts resulting from severe hydropic degeneration of epidermal basal cells.

Medlar body—See Chromo body.

Meibomian gland—A modified sebaceous gland of the eyelid that is not associated with cilia or hairs.

Melanin—Colored protein complexes formed in many organisms by specialized cells. In shades of tan or black, the material results from polymerization of tyrosine and desoxyphenylalanine under the influence of tyrosinase.

Melanocyte—A mature cell that produces melanin.

Melanoderma—Increased dermal melanin.

Melanoma—A neoplasm consisting of melanocytes.

Melanophage—A cell that engulfs melanin.

Melanotrichia—Increased pigment in hair.

Merocrine—"Separating"; applied to apocrine glands whose product consists of some part of their cellular material that separates and is shed.

Mesoderm—The "middle skin," the embryonal layer (between ectoderm and endoderm) that gives rise to connective tissue, muscle, blood, bone, and other components.

Metaplasia—A condition in which there has been a change in cellular development.

Metastasis—The transfer of disease from one organ to another not directly connected with it.

Microconidium (pl. *microconidia*)—The smaller of two different sizes of conidia produced by a single fungus, as in *Fusarium* sp.

Microsporum—A genus of fungi.

Miliary—Resembling a millet seed.

Mould—A filamentous fungus.

Mucinous degeneration—Increased amounts of mucin within connective tissue.

Multiple—Occurring in various parts of the body at once.

Munro's microabscess—Small, dessicated accumulation of neutrophils within or below the horny layer of the epidermis.

Muriform—Having horizontal and vertical crosswalls, as in *Alternaria* sp.

Mycelium—A mass or mat of hyphae.

Mycetoma (maduromycetoma, maduromycosis)—A localized mycotic or actinomycotic infection that involves cutaneous and subcutaneous tissue, fascia, and bone. A mycetoma is characterized by swelling, draining sinuses, and granules.

Mycology—The study of fungi.

Mycosis (pl. *mycoses*)—Any disease of animals caused by a fungus.

Myiasis—Deposition of ova by flies in open wounds and development of larvae therein.

Myxedema—*Grossly,* the nonpitting cutaneous edema seen with hypothyroidism; *microscopically,* the diffuse, noninflammatory deposition of excessive mucin in the dermis.

Necrolysis—Separation or exfoliation of tissue due to necrosis.

Necrosis—Death of cells or tissues in a living organism.

Nevus—A circumscribed developmental defect of the skin.

Nictitans gland—Gland of the third eyelid (formerly called "Harderian gland").

Nigricans—Blackening.

Nikolsky's sign—The ability to dislodge or excessively wrinkle normal-appearing epidermis with sliding digital pressure.

Nodule—A small node or circumscribed solid elevation that usually extends into the deeper layers of the skin.

Nummular—Like a little coin or round disk.

Onychauxis—Overgrowth or thickening of nail or claw.

Onychia—Ulceration of matrix of a claw.

Onychogryphosis—Deformed overgrowth of nails or claws.

Onycholysis—Separation of nail from nail bed.

Onychomadesis—Complete shedding of the nails or claws.

Onychomalacia—Softening of a claw.

Onychomycosis—A fungal infection of a claw.

Onychorrhexis—A breakage or brittleness of a claw.

Onychoschisis—Fissuring of nails or claws.

Onychosis—Disease or deformity of nails or claws.

Oozing—A continuing process of exudation of fluid.

Pachyonychia—Hypertrophy of nail bed, causing thickening and elevation of nail plate.

Panniculitis—Inflammation of cutaneous adipose tissue.

Papillomatosis—The projection of dermal papillae above the surface of the skin.

Papule—A small, solid elevation of the skin up to 1 cm in diameter. Larger, solid, elevated lesions are called nodules or tumors. Larger, flat-topped elevations are called plaques.

Parakeratosis—A condition of abnormal cornification. Clinically there is excess scaling; histologically the keratinized cells of the horny layer still possess nuclei.

Paronychia—Inflammation or ulceration involving the tissue fold around the claw.

Patch—A flat, circumscribed change in color of the skin that is larger than 1 cm in diameter (therefore, a larger macule).

Pautrier's microabscess—Small accumulation of abnormal lymphoid cells within the epidermis, especially in the basal layer.

Pectinate hyphae—Hyphae that resembles a comb.

Pediculosis—Infestation with lice.

Pemphigus—A serious vesicular disease characterized histologically by acantholysis and thought to be of autoimmune origin.

Penicillus (pl. penicilli)—A brushlike structure seen in *Penicillium*, including conidia, phialides, and metula if present.

Perfect state (or stage)—The portion of a fungal life cycle characterized by sexual reproduction.

Petechia—A dermal hemorrhage less than 1 cm in diameter.

Phaeohyphomycosis—A subcutaneous and systemic infection characterized by dark-walled, septate mycelial or yeast elements in the host tissue. There are no chromo or medlar bodies, however.

Phialide—An open-ended cell from which phialioconidia are produced. The cell does not increase in length, since the conidia are produced from an open growing point. Phialides are seen in *Aspergillus* and *Penicillium* spp.

Phialoconidium (pl. phialoconidia)—A conidium that develops from a phialide, as in *Penicillium* sp.

Photodermatitis—An inflammatory condition of the skin caused by the influence of light.

Pigmentary incontinence—Melanin granules in the superficial dermis and in dermal macrophages, usually secondary to hydropic degeneration of epidermal basal cells.

Pili—Plural of *pilus*, hair.

Pilosebaceous—Referring to hair and sebaceous gland as an organized apparatus.

Pityriasis—Conditions of the skin characterized by branny scaling.

Plaque—A flat-topped, solid skin elevation larger than 1 cm in diameter.

Pleomorphic—Having more than one form.

Poliosis—Premature grayness of hair.

Polycyclic—Consisting of several circular lesions.

Polymorphous—Referring to the simultaneous presence of several different types of primary and secondary lesions, as opposed to *monomorphous*, in which all lesions of the dermatosis are the same.

Poroconidium (pl. poroconidia)—A conidium produced through a pore in the wall of the conidiogenous cell or hypha, as in *Alternaria* sp.

Prickle cell—An epidermal cell of the malpighian layer. *Prickles* are the desmosomes visible in this layer of the epidermis.

Prokaryote—An organism, e.g., bacterium, that does not have a true nucleus.

Pruritus—Intense and persistent itching.

Pseudoallescheria boydii—Preferred term for *Allescheria boydii* or *Petriellidium boydii*.

Pseudoepitheliomatous hyperplasia—Increased formation of epithelium that is not malignantly neoplastic. It is seen in long-enduring dermatitides, granulomas, and ulcerations.

Pseudohypha (pl. *pseudohyphae)*—A chain of blastoconidia that have remained attached to each other.

Pseudomycetoma—Subcutaneous infection caused by a dermatophyte.

Purpura—Gross or microscopic hemorrhage into the skin.

Pustule—A small, circumscribed elevation of the skin filled with pus.

Pyoderma—A skin disease characterized by purulence.

Pyogenic—Producing pus or purulence.

Pyriform—Pear-shaped.

Racquet hyphae—A hypha with racquet-shaped or club-shaped cells, the clubbed end of one cell being attached to the small end of an adjacent cell.

Reticulum fibers—Fine, thready, young collagen fibers.

Rhizoid—A rootlike structure, as in *Rhizopus* sp.

Ringworm—Ring-shaped patches of cutaneous disease caused by dermatophytes. A synonym for fungous infection that is becoming outmoded as a medical term.

Rodent ulcer—Basal cell epithelioma; also, a synonym for eosinophilic granuloma (especially in cats).

Rugose—Full of wrinkles.

Russell's body—Globular plasma cell inclusions. Mucoprotein in nature, containing surface gamma globulin, and probably resulting from condensation of internal cellular secretions.

Saprophyte—Any plant organism that obtains its nourishment from dead organic matter.

Sarcoma—Malignancy that develops from tissues of mesodermal origin.

Sarcoptes—A genus of mites.

Scab—A hard concretion on superficial wounds. It is composed of clotted blood and tissue debris. Scab is a lay term for which *crust* is medically more acceptable.

Scabies—Infestation with *Sarcoptes scabiei* or *Notoedres cati.*

Scale—An accumulation of fragments of the horny layer.

Scar—A hard plaque of dense fibrous tissue that has replaced damaged dermis. It is often covered by atrophic epidermis.

Sclerosis—Hardening.

Sclerotic bodies—Large dark-walled cells 4 to 12 μm in diameter observed in chromoblastomycosis.

Scurf—Obsolete word for scales and crusts.

Sebaceous—Adjective from "sebum"; pertaining to sebaceous gland or its product.

Seborrhea—An increase in scaling of the skin with or without increase in sebum production.

Seborrheic dermatitis—An inflammatory type of seborrhea.

Sebum—The waxy, oily product of the sebaceous gland.

Septate—Having cross walls.

Septum (pl. *septa*)—A cross wall produced in a hypha, spore, or conidium.

Serpiginous—Creeping; referring to lesions that slowly enlarge in the shape of a crawling snake.

Sessile—Having no stem.

Shampoo—Massaging and washing the hair with soap and water. Also, a preparation used for washing hair.

Slough—Separation of a membrane or necrotic debris en masse.

Solar—Pertaining to the sun.

Spiral hyphae—Hyphae ending in flat or helical coils, as in *Trichophyton*.

Spongiosis—Intercellular edema within the epidermis having a spongy appearance.

Sporangium (pl. *sporangia*)—A saclike structure in which the entire contents are cleaved into asexual spores.

Sporangiophore—A specialized hypha upon which a sporangium develops.

Spore—A sexual reproductive structure.

Squame—A scale or scalelike substance.

Squamous—Full of scales.

Stolon—A hypha that arches away from the substrate, then touches it again some distance away.

Stratum—A layer, especially of the epidermis.

Stria (pl. *striae*)—A rather shallow linear depression; a furrow or channel.

Subcorneal—Just under the stratum corneum.

Subcutis—Tissue directly beneath the skin.

Suspension—A pharmaceutic preparation in which ingredients are dispersed as visible particles and which is consequently turbid.

Sympoduloconidium (pl. *sympoduloconidia*)—A conidium produced from a main axis extending by growth of a succession of apices, each of which develops behind and to one side of the previous apex, as in *Sporothrix* sp.

Tattoo—Permanent coloration of the skin with pigments driven into the skin by puncture. It usually refers to a planned procedure, but the term also describes accidental introduction of pigments.

Telogen—The resting or final phase of a hair cycle. That long period before a hair is shed or falls.

Thallus—A vegetative body of undifferentiated cells.

Tinea—Superficial fungous infection of human skin.

Trachyonychia—Roughness of surface of nail plate.

Tricho—A prefix denoting hair.

Trichophyton—A genus of fungi.

Trombicula—A genus of mites.

Tumor—A swelling or enlargement of varying size that may involve any structure of the skin. Usually, but not always, neoplastic.

Tylotrich pad—A half-millimeter, round, dermoepidermal disc in close proximity to hairs and recognized as a nerve end organ that is a slow-adapting touch receptor.

Ulcer—A break in continuity of the epidermis with loss of substance and exposure of underlying tissue. It is slow to heal or tends not to heal at all.

Urticaria—A condition of the skin characterized by wheals.

Vacuolization—The process of development of small empty spaces in cells or tissues.

Vasculitis—Inflammation of blood vessels.

Vellus—Fine hair that succeeds the lanugo hair.

Verruca—A warty growth, often caused by a virus.

Verrucose—Having small rounded processes or "warts."

Vesicle—A blister, or small sharply circumscribed elevation of the skin filled with clear fluid. Lesions larger than 1 cm in diameter are called *bullae.*

Vibrissae—Long coarse hairs growing about the nose or muzzle. "Whiskers."

Villi—Dermal papillae, covered by one to two layers of epidermal cells, that project into a vesicle.

Vitiligo—A characteristic leukoderma of humans.

Wart—A small callous growth. May be caused by a virus.

Weeping—A superficial inflammatory process in which there is considerable exudation of clear serum from rupture of vesicles or discontinuity of the epidermis.

Wheal—A sharply circumscribed raised lesion caused by dermal edema. Many wheals produce a condition known as urticaria or hives.

Wood's light—Electromagnetic energy with a wavelength of about 3650 Å; an apparatus equipped with a nickel oxide filter that produces ultraviolet light of that quality.

Xanthoma—A papule, nodule, or plaque of a yellow color in the skin usually due to deposits of lipids.

Xerosis—A condition of abnormal dryness of the skin.

X-rays—Electromagnetic energy of wavelengths between 0.5 and 2 Å; roentgen rays.

Yeast—A unicellular budding fungus, such as *Cryptococcus* sp.

Zoonosis—A disease of animals that may be communicated to humans.

Zoophilic—Pertaining to organisms that have become adapted to animals, such as *Microsporum canis.*

Zoospore—A motile sporangiospore having a flagellum.

Zygomycosis—A mycotic infection of humans or animals caused by members of the Zygomycota. Preferred term for phycomycosis.

Zygospore—A spore that results from fusion of gametes of the Zygomycota.

Index

Note: Page numbers in *italics* refer to illustrations; page numbers followed by t refer to tables.

979